QUICK LOOK DRUGBOOK

NOTICE

This data is intended to serve the user as a handy reference and not as a complete drug information resource. It does not include information on every therapeutic agent available. The publication covers over 1850 commonly used drugs and is specifically designed to present important aspects of drug data in a more concise format than is typically found in medical literature or product material supplied by manufacturers.

The nature of drug information is that it is constantly evolving because of ongoing research and clinical experience and is often subject to interpretation. While great care has been taken to ensure the accuracy of the information and recommendations presented, the reader is advised that the authors, editors, reviewers, contributors, and publishers cannot be responsible for the continued currency of the information or for any errors, omissions, or the application of this information, or for any consequences arising therefrom. Therefore, the author(s) and/or the publisher shall have no liability to any person or entity with regard to claims, loss, or damage caused, or alleged to be caused, directly or indirectly, by the use of information contained herein. Because of the dynamic nature of drug information, readers are advised that decisions regarding drug therapy must be based on the independent judgment of the clinician, changing information about a drug (eg, as reflected in the literature and manufacturer's most current product information), and changing medical practices. Therefore, this data is designed to be used in conjunction with other necessary information and is not designed to be solely relied upon by any user. The user of this data hereby and forever releases the authors and publishers of this data from any and all liability of any kind that might arise out of the use of this data. The editors are not responsible for any inaccuracy of quotation or for any false or misleading implication that may arise due to the text or formulas as used or due to the quotation of revisions no longer official.

Certain of the authors, editors, and contributors have written this book in their private capacities. No official support or endorsement by any federal or state agency or pharmaceutical company is intended or inferred.

The publishers have made every effort to trace any third party copyright holders, if any, for borrowed material. If they have inadvertently overlooked any, they will be pleased to make the necessary arrangements at the first opportunity.

Book revisions are available at our website at http://www.lexi.com/home/revisions/.

This manual was produced using Lexi-Comp's Information Management System™ (LIMS) — a complete publishing service of Lexi-Comp, Inc.

Lexicomp®

1100 Terex Road • Hudson, Ohio • 44236
(330) 650-6506

Wolters Kluwer
Health

TABLE OF CONTENTS

Visit thePoint http://thepoint.lww.com/QL2013 for exclusive access to:

- Apothecary/Metric Conversions
- Pounds/Kilograms Conversion
- Temperature Conversion
- Pharmaceutical Manufacturers and Distributors
- Multivitamin Products

Refer to the inside front cover of this book for your online access code.

EDITORIAL ADVISORY PANEL

Julie A. Dopheide, PharmD, BCPP
Associate Professor of Clinical Pharmacy, Psychiatry and the Behavioral Sciences
Schools of Pharmacy and Medicine
University of Southern California

Teri Dunsworth, PharmD, FCCP, BCPS
Pharmacotherapy Specialist
Lexi-Comp, Inc

Eve Echt, MD
Medical Staff
Department of Radiology
Akron General Medical Center

Michael S. Edwards, PharmD, MBA, BCOP
Chief, Oncology Pharmacy
and *Director, Oncology Pharmacy Residency Program*
Walter Reed Army Medical Center

Vicki L. Ellingrod, PharmD, BCPP
Head, Clinical Pharmacogenomics Laboratory
and *Associate Professor*
Department of Psychiatry
Colleges of Pharmacy and Medicine
University of Michigan

Kelley K. Engle, BSPharm
Medical Science Pharmacist
Lexi-Comp, Inc

Christopher Ensor, PharmD, BCPS (AQ-CV)
Clinical Specialist
Cardiothoracic Transplantation
and Mechanical Circulatory Support
The Johns Hopkins Hospital

Erin Fabian, PharmD, RPh
Pharmacotherapy Specialist
Lexi-Comp, Inc

Elizabeth A. Farrington, PharmD, FCCP, FCCM, FPPAG, BCPS
Pharmacist III - Pediatrics
New Hanover Regional Medical Center

Margaret A. Fitzgerald, MS, APRN, BC, NP-C, FAANP
President
Fitzgerald Health Education Associates, Inc.
Family Nurse Practitioner
Greater Lawrence Family Health Center

Lawrence A. Frazee, PharmD, BCPS
Pharmacotherapy Specialist in Internal Medicine
Akron General Medical Center

Matthew A. Fuller, PharmD, BCPS, BCPP, FASHP
Clinical Pharmacy Specialist, Psychiatry
Cleveland Department of Veterans Affairs Medical Center
Associate Clinical Professor of Psychiatry and *Clinical Instructor of Psychology*
Case Western Reserve University
Adjunct Associate Professor of Clinical Pharmacy
University of Toledo

Jason C. Gallagher, PharmD, BCPS
Clinical Pharmacy Specialist, Infectious Diseases
and *Clinical Associate Professor*
Temple University Hospital

Jennifer L. Gardner, PharmD
Neonatal Clinical Pharmacy Specialist
Texas Children's Hospital

Meredith D. Girard, MD, FACP
Medical Staff
Department of Internal Medicine
Summa Health Systems
Assistant Professor Internal Medicine
Northeast Ohio Medical University (NEOMED)

Morton P. Goldman, RPh, PharmD, BCPS, FCCP
Senior Editor
Lexi-Comp, Inc

Julie A. Golembiewski, PharmD
Clinical Associate Professor and *Clinical Pharmacist, Anesthesia/Pain*
Colleges of Pharmacy and Medicine
University of Illinois

Jeffrey P. Gonzales, PharmD, BCPS
Critical Care Clinical Pharmacy Specialist
University of Maryland Medical Center

Roland Grad, MDCM, MSc, CCFP, FCFP
Associate Professor
Department of Family Medicine
McGill University

Larry D. Gray, PhD, ABMM
Director, Clinical Microbiology
TriHealth Laboratories
Bethesda and Good Samaritan Hospitals

Tracy Hagemann, PharmD
Associate Professor
College of Pharmacy
The University of Oklahoma

JoEllen L. Hanigosky, PharmD
Clinical Coordinator
Department of Hematology/Oncology/Bone Marrow Transplant
Children's Hospital of Akron

Martin D. Higbee, PharmD
Associate Professor
Department of Pharmacy Practice and Science
The University of Arizona

Jane Hurlburt Hodding, PharmD
Executive Director, Inpatient Pharmacy Services and Clinical Nutrition Services
Long Beach Memorial Medical Center and Miller Children's Hospital

Mark T. Holdsworth, PharmD, BCOP
Associate Professor of Pharmacy & Pediatrics
and *Pharmacy Practice Area Head*
College of Pharmacy
The University of New Mexico

Edward Horn, PharmD, BCPS
Clinical Specialist, Transplant Surgery
Allegheny General Hospital

Barrie McCombs, MD, FCFP
Medical Information Service Coordinator
The Alberta Rural Physician Action Plan

Christopher McPherson, PharmD
Clinical Pharmacist
Neonatal Intensive Care Unit
St. Louis Children's Hospital

Timothy F. Meiller, DDS, PhD
Professor
Oncology and Diagnostic Sciences
Baltimore College of Dental Surgery
Professor of Oncology
Marlene and Stewart Greenebaum Cancer Center
University of Maryland Medical System

Geralyn M. Meny, MD
Medical Director
American Red Cross, Penn-Jersey Region

Charla E. Miller, RPh, PharmD
Neonatal Clinical Pharmacy Specialist
Wolfson Children's Hospital

Julie Miller, PharmD
Pharmacy Clinical Specialist, Cardiology
Columbus Children's Hospital

Katherine Mills, PharmD
Pharmacotherapy Contributor
Lexi-Comp, Inc

Leah Millstein, MD
Assistant Professor
Division of General Internal Medicine
University of Maryland School of Medicine

Stephanie S. Minich, PharmD, BCOP
Pharmacotherapy Specialist
Lexi-Comp, Inc

Kim Moeller, RN, MSN, OCN, ACNS-BC
Advanced Practice Nurse
Summit Oncology Associates

Kevin M. Mulieri, BS, PharmD
Pediatric Hematology/Oncology Clinical Specialist
Penn State Milton S. Hershey Medical Center
Instructor of Pharmacology
Penn State College of Medicine

Elizabeth A. Neuner, PharmD, BCPS
Infectious Diseases Clinical Specialist
The Cleveland Clinic Foundation

Tom Palma, MS, RPh
Medical Science Pharmacist
Lexi-Comp, Inc

Susie H. Park, PharmD, BCPP
Assistant Professor of Clinical Pharmacy
University of Southern Califormia

Nicole Passerrello, PharmD, BCPS
Pharmacotherapy Specialist
Lexi-Comp, Inc

Alpa Patel, PharmD
Antimicrobial Clinical Pharmacist
University of Louisville Hospital

Gayle Pearson, BSPharm, MSA
Drug Information Pharmacist
Peter Lougheed Centre
Alberta Health Services

James A. Ponto, MS, RPh, BCNP
Chief Nuclear Pharmacist
Department of Radiology
University of Iowa, Hospitals and Clinics
Professor of Clinical Pharmacy
Department of Pharmacy Practice and Science
University of Iowa College of Pharmacy

Amy L. Potts, PharmD, BCPS
Assistant Director
Department of Pharmacy
PGY1 & PGY2 Residency Program Director
Monroe Carell Jr. Children's Hospital at Vanderbilt

James Reissig, PharmD
Assistant Director, Clinical Services
Akron General Medical Center

A.J. (Fred) Remillard, PharmD
Assistant Dean, Research and Graduate Affairs
College of Pharmacy and Nutrition
University of Saskatchewan

Curtis M. Rimmermann, MD, MBA, FACC
Gus P. Karos Chair
Clinical Cardiovascular Medicine
The Cleveland Clinic Foundation

P. David Rogers, PharmD, PhD, FCCP
Director, Clinical and Translational Therapeutics
University of Tennessee College of Pharmacy

James L. Rutkowski, DMD, PhD
Editor-in-Chief
Journal of Oral Implantology

Amy Rybarczyk, PharmD, BCPS
Pharmacotherapy Specialist, Internal Medicine
Akron General Medical Center

Jennifer K. Sekeres, PharmD, BCPS
Infectious Diseases Clinical Specialist
The Cleveland Clinic Foundation

Todd P. Semla, MS, PharmD, BCPS, FCCP, AGSF
Clinical Pharmacy Specialist
Department of Veterans Affairs
Pharmacy Benefits Management Services
Associate Professor, Clinical
Department of Medicine and
Psychiatry and Behavioral Health
Feinberg School of Medicine
Northwestern University

Pamela J. Sims, PharmD, PhD
Professor
Department of Pharmaceutical, Social, and
Administrative Sciences
McWhorter School of Pharmacy
Samford University

PREFACE

Working with clinical pharmacists, hospital pharmacy and therapeutics committees, and hospital drug information centers, the editors of this handbook have directly assisted in the development and production of hospital-specific formulary documentation for several hundred major U.S. and International medical institutions. The resultant documentation provides relevant detail concerning use of medications within the hospital and other clinical settings. Current information on medications has been extracted from pertinent sources, reviewed, coalesced, and cross-referenced by the editors to create this *Quick Look Drug Book*.

Designed to meet the unique needs of medical transcription, this handbook gives the user quick access to data on over 1850 medications with cross-referencing to 7457 U.S. and Canadian brand or trade names. Selection of the included medications was based on the analysis of those medications offered in a wide range of hospital formularies. The concise standardized format for data used in this handbook was developed to ensure a consistent presentation of information for all medications.

All generic drug names and synonyms appear in lower case, whereas brand or trade names appear in upper/lower case with the proper trademark information. These three items appear as individual entries in the alphabetical listing of drugs and, thus, there is no requirement for an alphabetical index of drugs names.

Chemotherapy regimens along with an index are provided in the section directly following the alphabetical listing of drugs. The mailing and web site addresses for pharmaceutical manufacturers and drug distributors can be accessed online using the code located on the inside front cover of this book.

The Indication/Therapeutic Category Index is an expedient mechanism for locating the medication of choice along with its classification. This index will help the user, with knowledge of the disease state, to identify medications which are most commonly used in treatment. All disease states are cross-referenced to a varying number of medications with the most frequently used medication(s) noted.

USE OF THE HANDBOOK

The *Quick Look Drug Book* is organized into a drug information section, an appendix, and an indication/ therapeutic category index.

The drug information section of the handbook, wherein all drugs are listed alphabetically, details information pertinent to each drug. Extensive cross-referencing is provided by brand name and synonyms.

Drug information is presented in a consistent format and for quick reference will provide the following:

Generic Name	U.S. Adopted Name (USAN) or International Nonproprietary Name (INN) If a drug product is only available in Canada, a ***(Canada only)*** will be attached to that product and will appear with every occurrence of that drug throughout the book
Pronunciation Guide	Subjective aid for pronouncing drug names
Medication Safety Issues	In an effort to promote the safe use of medications, this field is intended to highlight possible sources of medication errors such as sound-alike/look-alike drugs or highly concentrated formulations which require vigilance on the part of healthcare professionals. In addition, medications which have been associated with severe consequences in the event of a medication error are also identified in this field.
Synonyms	Includes names or accepted abbreviations of the generic drug; may include common brand names no longer available; this field is used to create cross-references to monographs
Tall-Man	"Tall-Man" lettering revisions recommended by the FDA
U.S. Brand Names	Trade names (manufacturer-specific) found in the United States. The symbol [DSC] appears after trade names that have been recently discontinued.
Canadian Brand Names	Trade names found in Canada
Therapeutic Category	Lexicomp's own system of logical medication classification
Controlled Substance	Contains controlled substance schedule information as assigned by the United States Drug Enforcement Administration (DEA) or Canadian Controlled Substance Act (CDSA). CDSA information is only provided for drugs available in Canada and not available in the U.S.
Use	Information pertaining to appropriate FDA-approved indications of the drug.
General Dosage Range	The range of dosing typically used during therapy in children and adults based upon route of administration. The information included is useful for confirming the dose is within the range but should not be used for prescribing purposes. Medications with a variety of indication-specific doses that cannot be encompassed by a range will not have a dose.
Product Availability	Provides availability information on products that have been approved by the FDA, but not yet available for use. Estimates for when a product may be available are included, when this information is known. May also provide any unique or critical drug availability issues.
Dosage Forms	Information with regard to form, strength, and availability of the drug in the United States.
Dosage Forms - Canada	Information with regard to form, strength, and availability of products that are uniquely available in Canada, but currently not available in the United States.

Appendix

The appendix offers a compilation of tables, guidelines, and conversion information that can often be helpful when considering patient care.

Indication/Therapeutic Category Index

This index provides a listing of accepted drugs for various disease states thus focusing attention on selection of medications most frequently prescribed in relation to a clinical diagnosis. Diseases may have other nonofficial drugs for their treatment and this indication/therapeutic category index should not be used by itself to determine the appropriateness of a particular therapy. The listed indications may encompass varying degrees of severity and, since certain medications may not be appropriate for a given degree of severity, it should not be assumed that the agents listed for specific indications are interchangeable. Also included as a valuable reference is each medication's therapeutic category.

FDA NAME DIFFERENTIATION PROJECT: THE USE OF TALL-MAN LETTERS

Confusion between similar drug names is an important cause of medication errors. For years, The Institute For Safe Medication Practices (ISMP), has urged generic manufacturers to use a combination of large and small letters as well as bolding (ie, chlorpro**MAZINE** and chlorpro**PAMIDE**) to help distinguish drugs with look-alike names, especially when they share similar strengths. Recently the FDA's Division of Generic Drugs began to issue recommendation letters to manufacturers suggesting this novel way to label their products to help reduce this drug name confusion. Although this project has had marginal success, the method has successfully eliminated problems with products such as diphenhydr**AMINE** and dimenhy**DRINATE**. Hospitals should also follow suit by making similar changes in their own labels, preprinted order forms, computer screens and printouts, and drug storage location labels.

Lexi-Comp, Inc. Medical Publishing will use "Tall-Man" letters for the drugs suggested by the FDA or recommended by ISMP.

The following is a list of generic and brand name product names and recommended revisions.

Drug Product	Recommended Revision
acetazolamide	aceta**ZOLAMIDE**
alprazolam	**ALPRAZ**olam
amiloride	a**MIL**oride
amlodipine	am**LODIP**ine
aripiprazole	**ARIP**iprazole
atomoxetine	ato**MOX**etine
atorvastatin	atorva**STAT**in
Avinza	**AVIN**za
azacitidine	aza**CITID**ine
azathioprine	aza**THIO**prine
bupropion	bu**PROP**ion
buspirone	bus**PIR**one
carbamazepine	car**BAM**azepine
carboplatin	**CARBO**platin
cefazolin	ce**FAZ**olin
cefotetan	cefo**TE**tan
cefoxitin	cef**OX**itin
ceftazidime	cef**TAZ**idime
ceftriaxone	cef**TRIAX**one
Celebrex	Cele**BREX**
Celexa	Cele**XA**
chlordiazepoxide	chlordiaze**POXIDE**
chlorpromazine	chlorpro**MAZINE**
chlorpropamide	chlorpro**PAMIDE**
cisplatin	**CIS**platin
clomiphene	clomi**PHENE**
clomipramine	clomi**PRAMINE**
clonazepam	clonaze**PAM**
clonidine	clo**NID**ine
clozapine	clo**ZAP**ine
cycloserine	cyclo**SERINE**
cyclosporine	cyclo**SPORINE**
dactinomycin	**DACTIN**omycin
daptomycin	**DAPTO**mycin
daunorubicin	**DAUNO**rubicin
dimenhydrinate	dimenhy**DRINATE**
diphenhydramine	diphenhydr**AMINE**
dobutamine	**DOBUT**amine
docetaxel	**DOCE**taxel
dopamine	**DOP**amine

Drug Product	Recommended Revision
doxorubicin	**DOXO**rubicin
duloxetine	**DUL**oxetine
ephedrine	e**PHED**rine
epinephrine	**EPINEPH**rine
epirubicin	**EPI**rubicin
eribulin	eri**BUL**in
fentanyl	fenta**NYL**
flavoxate	flavox**ATE**
fluoxetine	**FLU**oxetine
fluphenazine	flu**PHENAZ**ine
fluvoxamine	fluvoxa**MINE**
glipizide	glipi**ZIDE**
glyburide	gly**BURIDE**
guaifenesin	guai**FEN**esin
guanfacine	guan**FACINE**
Humalog	Huma**LOG**
Humulin	Humu**LIN**
hydralazine	hydr**ALAZINE**
hydrocodone	**HYDRO**codone
hydromorphone	**HYDRO**morphone
hydroxyzine	hydr**OXY**zine
idarubicin	**IDA**rubicin
infliximab	in**FLIX**imab
Invanz	**INV**anz
isotretinoin	**ISO**tretinoin
Klonopin	Klono**PIN**
Lamictal	La**MIC**tal
Lamisil	Lam**ISIL**
lamivudine	lami**VUD**ine
lamotrigine	lamo**TRI**gine
levetiracetam	Lev**ETIRA**cetam
levocarnitine	lev**OCARN**itine
lorazepam	**LOR**azepam
medroxyprogesterone	medroxy**PROGESTER**one
metformin	met**FORMIN**
methylprednisolone	methyl**PREDNIS**olone
methyltestosterone	methyl**TESTOSTER**one
metronidazole	metro**NIDAZOLE**
mitomycin	mito**MY**cin
mitoxantrone	Mito**XAN**trone
Nexavar	Nex**AVAR**
Nexium	Nex**IUM**
nicardipine	ni**CAR**dipine
nifedipine	**NIFE**dipine
nimodipine	ni**MOD**ipine
Novolin	Novo**LIN**
Novolog	Novo**LOG**
olanzapine	**OLANZ**apine
oxcarbazepine	**OX**carbazepine
oxycodone	oxy**CODONE**
Oxycontin	Oxy**CONTIN**
paclitaxel	**PACL**itaxel
paroxetine	**PAR**oxetine
pemetrexed	**PEME**trexed
penicillamine	penicill**AMINE**
pentobarbital	**PENT**obarbital
phenobarbital	**PHEN**obarbital

Drug Product	Recommended Revision
pralatrexate	**PRALA**trexate
prednisolone	predniso**LONE**
prednisone	predni**SONE**
Prilosec	Pri**LOSEC**
Prozac	**PRO**zac
quetiapine	**QUE**tiapine
quinidine	qui**NID**ine
quinine	qui**NINE**
rabeprazole	**RABE**prazole
Risperdal	Risper**DAL**
risperidone	risperi**DONE**
rituximab	ri**TUX**imab
romidepsin	romi**DEP**sin
romiplostim	romi**PLOS**tim
ropinirole	r**OPINIR**ole
Sandimmune	sand**IMMUNE**
Sandostatin	Sando**STATIN**
Seroquel	**SERO**quel
Sinequan	**SINE**quan
sitagliptin	sita**GLIP**tin
Solu-Cortef	Solu-**CORTEF**
Solu-Medrol	Solu-**MEDROL**
sorafenib	**SORA**fenib
sufentanil	**SUF**entanil
sulfadiazine	sulf**ADIAZINE**
sulfasalazine	sulfa**SALA**zine
sumatriptan	**SUMA**triptan
sunitinib	**SUNI**tinib
Tegretol	**TEG**retol
tiagabine	tia**GAB**ine
tizanidine	ti**ZAN**idine
tolazamide	**TOLAZ**amide
tolbutamide	**TOLBUT**amide
tramadol	tra**MAD**ol
trazodone	tra**ZOD**one
Trental	**TREN**tal
valacyclovir	val**ACY**clovir
valganciclovir	val**GAN**ciclovir
vinblastine	vin**BLAS**tine
vincristine	vin**CRIS**tine
zolmitriptan	**ZOLM**itriptan
Zyprexa	Zy**PREXA**
Zyrtec	Zyr**TEC**

"FDA and ISMP Lists of Look-Alike Drug Names with Recommended Tall Man Letter." Available at http://www.ismp.org/tools/tallmanletters.pdf. Last accessed January 6, 2011.

"Name Differentiation Project." Available at http://www.fda.gov/Drugs/DrugSafety/MedicationErrors/ucm164587.htm. Last accessed January 6, 2011.

U.S. Pharmacopeia, "USP Quality Review: Use Caution-Avoid Confusion," March 2001, No. 76. Available at http://www.usp.org

PREVENTING PRESCRIBING ERRORS

Prescribing errors account for the majority of reported medication errors and have prompted healthcare professionals to focus on the development of steps to make the prescribing process safer. Prescription legibility has been attributed to a portion of these errors and legislation has been enacted in several states to address prescription legibility. However, eliminating handwritten prescriptions and ordering medications through the use of technology (eg, computerized prescriber order entry [CPOE]) has been the primary recommendation. Whether a prescription is electronic, typed, or hand-printed, additional safe practices should be considered for implementation to maximize the safety of the prescribing process. Listed below are suggestions for safer prescribing:

- Ensure correct patient by using at least 2 patient identifiers on the prescription (eg, full name, birth date, or address). Review prescription with the patient or patient's caregiver.
- If pediatric patient, document patient's birth date or age and most recent weight. If geriatric patient, document patient's birth date or age.
- Prevent drug name confusion:
  - Use TALLman lettering (eg, buPROPion, busPIRone, predniSONE, prednisoLONE). For more information see http://www.fda.gov/Drugs/DrugSafety/MedicationErrors/ucm164587.htm.
  - Avoid abbreviated drug names (eg, MSO_4, $MgSO_4$, MS, HCT, 6MP, MTX), as they may be misinterpreted and cause error.
  - Avoid investigational names for drugs with FDA approval (eg, FK-506, CBDCA).
  - Avoid chemical names such as 6-mercaptopurine or 6-thioguanine, as sixfold overdoses have been given when these were not recognized as chemical names. The proper names of these drugs are mercaptopurine or thioguanine.
  - Use care when prescribing drugs that look or sound similar (eg, look-alike, sound-alike drugs). Common examples include: Celebrex® vs Celexa®, hydroxyzine vs hydralazine, Zyprexa® vs Zyrtec®.
- Avoid dangerous, error-prone abbreviations (eg, regardless of letter-case: U, IU, QD, QOD, µg, cc, @). Do not use apothecary system or symbols. Additionally, text messaging abbreviations (eg, "2Day") should never be used.
  - For more information see http://www.ismp.org/Tools/errorproneabbreviations.pdf
- Always use a leading zero for numbers less than 1 (0.5 mg is correct and .5 mg is **incorrect**) and never use a trailing zero for whole numbers (2 mg is correct and 2.0 mg is **incorrect**).
- Always use a space between a number and its units as it is easier to read. There should be no periods after the abbreviations mg or mL (10 mg is correct and 10mg is **incorrect**).
- For doses that are greater than 1,000 dosing units, use properly placed commas to prevent 10-fold errors (100,000 units is correct and 100000 units is **incorrect**).
- Do not prescribe drug dosage by the type of container in which the drug is available (eg, do not prescribe "1 amp", "2 vials", etc).
- Do not write vague or ambiguous orders which have the potential for misinterpretation by other healthcare providers. Examples of vague orders to avoid: "Resume pre-op medications," "give drug per protocol," or "continue home medications."
- Review each prescription with patient (or patient's caregiver) including the medication name, indication, and directions for use.
- Take extra precautions when prescribing *high alert drugs* (drugs that can cause significant patient harm when prescribed in error). Common examples of these drugs include: Anticoagulants, chemotherapy, insulins, opiates, and sedatives.
  - For more information see http://www.ismp.org/Tools/highalertmedications.pdf

To Err Is Human: Building a Safer Health System, Kohn LT, Corrigan JM, and Donaldson MS, eds, Washington, D.C.: National Academy Press, 2000.

A Complete Outpatient Prescription[1]

A complete outpatient prescription can prevent the prescriber, the pharmacist, and/or the patient from making a mistake and can eliminate the need for further clarification. The complete outpatient prescription should contain:

- Patient's full name
- Medication indication
- Allergies
- Prescriber name and telephone or pager number
- For pediatric patients: Their birth date or age and current weight
- For geriatric patients: Their birth date or age
- Drug name, dosage form and strength
- For pediatric patients: Intended daily weight-based dose so that calculations can be checked by the pharmacist (ie, mg/kg/day or units/kg/day)
- Number or amount to be dispensed
- Complete instructions for the patient or caregiver, including the purpose of the medication, directions for use (including dose), dosing frequency, route of administration, duration of therapy, and number of refills.
- Dose should be expressed in convenient units of measure.
- When there are recognized contraindications for a prescribed drug, the prescriber should indicate knowledge of this fact to the pharmacist (ie, when prescribing a potassium salt for a patient receiving an ACE inhibitor, the prescriber should write "K serum leveling being monitored").

Upon dispensing of the final product, the pharmacist should ensure that the patient or caregiver can effectively demonstrate the appropriate administration technique. An appropriate measuring device should be provided or recommended. Household teaspoons and tablespoons should not be used to measure liquid medications due to their variability and inaccuracies in measurement; oral medication syringes are recommended.

For additional information see http://www.ppag.org/attachments/files/111/Guidelines_Peds.pdf

[1]Levine SR, Cohen MR, Blanchard NR, et al, "Guidelines for Preventing Medication Errors in Pediatrics," *J Pediatr Pharmacol Ther*, 2001, 6:426-42.

ALPHABETICAL LISTING OF DRUGS

A-25 [OTC] *see* vitamin A *on page 949*
A200® Lice [OTC] *see* permethrin *on page 709*
A-200® Lice Treatment Kit [OTC] *see* pyrethrins and piperonyl butoxide *on page 776*
A-200® Maximum Strength [OTC] *see* pyrethrins and piperonyl butoxide *on page 776*
A+D® Original [OTC] *see* vitamin A and vitamin D (topical) *on page 949*

abacavir (a BAK a veer)

Synonyms abacavir sulfate; ABC
U.S. Brand Names Ziagen®
Canadian Brand Names Ziagen®
Therapeutic Category Antiretroviral Agent, Nucleoside Reverse Transcriptase Inhibitor (NRTI)
Use Treatment of HIV infections in combination with other antiretroviral agents
General Dosage Range Dosage adjustment recommended in patients with hepatic impairment
Oral:
Infants and Children ≥3 months to <16 years: 8 mg/kg twice daily (maximum: 300 mg twice daily)
Adolescents ≥16 years and Adults: 600 mg/day in 1-2 divided doses (maximum: 600 mg/day)
Dosage Forms
Solution, oral:
Ziagen®: 20 mg/mL (240 mL)
Tablet, oral: 300 mg
Ziagen®: 300 mg

abacavir and lamivudine (a BAK a veer & la MI vyoo deen)

Synonyms abacavir sulfate and lamivudine; lamivudine and abacavir
U.S. Brand Names Epzicom®
Canadian Brand Names Kivexa™
Therapeutic Category Antiretroviral Agent, Nucleoside Reverse Transcriptase Inhibitor (NRTI)
Use Treatment of HIV infections in combination with other antiretroviral agents
General Dosage Range Oral: *Adults:* One tablet (abacavir 600 mg and lamivudine 300 mg) once daily
Dosage Forms
Tablet:
Epzicom®: Abacavir 600 mg and lamivudine 300 mg

abacavir, lamivudine, and zidovudine
(a BAK a veer, la MI vyoo deen, & zye DOE vyoo deen)

Synonyms 3TC, abacavir, and zidovudine; azidothymidine, abacavir, and lamivudine; AZT, abacavir, and lamivudine; compound S, abacavir, and lamivudine; lamivudine, abacavir, and zidovudine; ZDV, abacavir, and lamivudine; zidovudine, abacavir, and lamivudine
U.S. Brand Names Trizivir®
Canadian Brand Names Trizivir®
Therapeutic Category Antiretroviral Agent, Nucleoside Reverse Transcriptase Inhibitor (NRTI)
Use Treatment of HIV infection (either alone or in combination with other antiretroviral agents) in patients whose regimen would otherwise contain the components of Trizivir®
General Dosage Range Oral: *Adolescents ≥40 kg and Adults:* 1 tablet twice daily
Dosage Forms
Tablet, oral:
Trizivir®: Abacavir 300 mg, lamivudine 150 mg, and zidovudine 300 mg

abacavir sulfate *see* abacavir *on page 16*
abacavir sulfate and lamivudine *see* abacavir and lamivudine *on page 16*

abatacept (ab a TA sept)

Medication Safety Issues
Sound-alike/look-alike issues:
Orencia® may be confused with Oracea®
Synonyms BMS-188667; CTLA-4Ig
U.S. Brand Names Orencia®
Canadian Brand Names Orencia®

Therapeutic Category Antirheumatic, Disease Modifying

Use

Treatment of moderately- to severely-active adult rheumatoid arthritis (RA); may be used as monotherapy or in combination with other DMARDs

Treatment of moderately- to severely-active juvenile idiopathic arthritis (JIA); may be used as monotherapy or in combination with methotrexate

Note: Abatacept should **not** be used in combination with anakinra or TNF-blocking agents

General Dosage Range

I.V.: Repeat dose at 2 weeks and 4 weeks, then every 4 weeks thereafter

Children ≥6 years and <75 kg: 10 mg/kg/dose

Children ≥6 years and 75-100 kg: 750 mg/dose

Children ≥6 years and >100 kg: 1000 mg/dose

Adults <60 kg: 500 mg/dose

Adults 60-100 kg: 750 mg/dose

Adults >100 kg: 1000 mg/dose

SubQ: *Adults:* 125 mg/dose once weekly

Dosage Forms

Injection, powder for reconstitution [preservative free]:

Orencia®: 250 mg

Injection, solution [preservative free]:

Orencia®: 125 mg/mL (1 mL)

abbott-43818 *see* leuprolide *on page 527*

ABC *see* abacavir *on page 16*

ABCD *see* amphotericin B cholesteryl sulfate complex *on page 71*

abciximab (ab SIK si mab)

Medication Safety Issues

High alert medication:

The Institute for Safe Medication Practices (ISMP) includes this medication among its list of drugs which have a heightened risk of causing significant patient harm when used in error.

Synonyms 7E3; C7E3

U.S. Brand Names Reopro®

Canadian Brand Names ReoPro®

Therapeutic Category Platelet Aggregation Inhibitor

Use Prevention of cardiac ischemic complications in patients undergoing percutaneous coronary intervention (PCI); prevention of cardiac ischemic complications in patients with unstable angina (UA)/ non-ST-elevation myocardial infarction (NSTEMI) unresponsive to conventional therapy when PCI is scheduled within 24 hours

Note: Intended for use with aspirin and heparin, at a minimum.

General Dosage Range **I.V.:** *Adults:* Bolus: 0.25 mg/kg; Infusion: 0.125 mcg/kg/minute (maximum: 10 mcg/minute)

Dosage Forms

Injection, solution [preservative free]:

Reopro®: 2 mg/mL (5 mL)

Abelcet® *see* amphotericin B lipid complex *on page 72*

Abenol® (Can) *see* acetaminophen *on page 20*

ABI-007 *see* paclitaxel (protein bound) *on page 684*

Abilify® *see* aripiprazole *on page 90*

Abilify Discmelt® *see* aripiprazole *on page 90*

abiraterone *see* abiraterone acetate *on page 17*

abiraterone acetate (a bir A ter one AS e tate)

Synonyms abiraterone; CB7630

U.S. Brand Names Zytiga™

Canadian Brand Names Zytiga™

Therapeutic Category Antiandrogen

Use Treatment of metastatic, castration-resistant prostate cancer (in combination with prednisone) in patients previously treated with docetaxel

General Dosage Range Dosage adjustment recommended in patients with hepatic impairment or who develop toxicity.

Oral: *Adults:* 1000 mg once daily

Dosage Forms

Tablet, oral:

Zytiga™: 250 mg

Ablavar® *see* gadofosveset *on page 415*

ABLC *see* amphotericin B lipid complex *on page 72*

abobotulinumtoxinA (aye bo BOT yoo lin num TOKS in aye)

Medication Safety Issues

Other safety concerns:

Botulinum products are not interchangeable; potency differences may exist between the products.

Synonyms botulinum toxin type A

U.S. Brand Names Dysport™

Therapeutic Category Neuromuscular Blocker Agent, Toxin

Use Treatment of cervical dystonia in both toxin-naive and previously treated patients; temporary improvement in the appearance of moderate-severe glabellar lines associated with procerus and corrugator muscle activity

General Dosage Range I.M.:

Adults: Cervical dystonia: Initial: 500 units/treatment; subsequent doses: 250-1000 units

Adults <65 years: Reduction of glabellar lines: 10 units (0.05 mL or 0.08 mL) into each site (total dose: 50 units)

Dosage Forms

Injection, powder for reconstitution:

Dysport™: 500 units

Abraxane® *see* paclitaxel (protein bound) *on page 684*

Abraxane® for Injectable Suspension (Can) *see* paclitaxel (protein bound) *on page 684*

Abreva® [OTC] *see* docosanol *on page 304*

absorbable cotton *see* cellulose, oxidized regenerated *on page 188*

absorbable gelatin sponge *see* gelatin (absorbable) *on page 421*

absorica *see* isotretinoin *on page 505*

Abstral® *see* fentanyl *on page 377*

Abstral™ (Can) *see* fentanyl *on page 377*

ABT-335 *see* fenofibric acid *on page 376*

ABX-EGF *see* panitumumab *on page 688*

AC 2993 *see* exenatide *on page 369*

ACAM2000® *see* smallpox vaccine *on page 839*

acamprosate (a kam PROE sate)

Synonyms acamprosate calcium; calcium acetylhomotaurinate

U.S. Brand Names Campral®

Canadian Brand Names Campral®

Therapeutic Category GABA Agonist/Glutamate Antagonist

Use Maintenance of alcohol abstinence

General Dosage Range Dosage adjustment recommended in patients with renal impairment.

Oral: *Adults:* 666 mg 3 times/day (maximum: 1998 mg/day)

Dosage Forms

Tablet, delayed release, enteric coated, oral:

Campral®: 333 mg

acamprosate calcium *see* acamprosate *on page 18*

Acanya® *see* clindamycin and benzoyl peroxide *on page 219*

acarbose (AY car bose)

Medication Safety Issues

Sound-alike/look-alike issues:

Precose® may be confused with PreCare®

High alert medication:

The Institute for Safe Medication Practices (ISMP) includes this medication among its list of drug classes which have a heightened risk of causing significant patient harm when used in error.

International issues:

Precose® [U.S., Malaysia] may be confused with Precosa brand name for *Saccharomyces boulardii* [Finland, Sweden]

U.S. Brand Names Precose®

Canadian Brand Names Glucobay™

Therapeutic Category Antidiabetic Agent, Oral

Use Adjunct to diet and exercise to lower blood glucose in patients with type 2 diabetes mellitus (noninsulin-dependent, NIDDM)

General Dosage Range Dosage adjustment recommended in patients on concomitant therapy

Oral: *Adults:* Initial: 25 mg 1-3 times/day; Maintenance: 75-300 mg/day in 3 divided doses (maximum: ≤60 kg: 150 mg/day; >60 kg: 300 mg/day)

Dosage Forms

Tablet, oral: 25 mg, 50 mg, 100 mg

Precose®: 25 mg, 50 mg, 100 mg

A-Caro-25 [OTC] *see* beta-carotene *on page 128*
Accel-Amlodipine (Can) *see* amlodipine *on page 65*
Accel-Pioglitazone (Can) *see* pioglitazone *on page 725*
Accolate® *see* zafirlukast *on page 958*
AccuNeb® *see* albuterol *on page 41*
Accupril® *see* quinapril *on page 781*
Accuretic® *see* quinapril and hydrochlorothiazide *on page 782*
Accutane *see* isotretinoin *on page 505*
Accutane® (Can) *see* isotretinoin *on page 505*
ACE *see* captopril *on page 171*

acebutolol (a se BYOO toe lole)

Medication Safety Issues

Sound-alike/look-alike issues:

Sectral® may be confused with Seconal®, Septra®

Synonyms acebutolol hydrochloride

U.S. Brand Names Sectral®

Canadian Brand Names Apo-Acebutolol®; Ava-Acebutolol; Mylan-Acebutolol; Mylan-Acebutolol (Type S); Nu-Acebutolol; Rhotral; Sandoz-Acebutolol; Sectral®; Teva-Acebutolol

Therapeutic Category Antiarrhythmic Agent, Class II; Beta-Adrenergic Blocker

Use Treatment of hypertension; management of ventricular arrhythmias

General Dosage Range Dosage adjustment recommended in patients with renal impairment

Oral:

Adults: 200-1200 mg/day in 2 divided doses (maximum: 1200 mg/day)

Elderly: 200-800 mg/day in 2 divided doses (maximum: 800 mg/day)

Dosage Forms

Capsule, oral: 200 mg, 400 mg

Sectral®: 200 mg, 400 mg

acebutolol hydrochloride *see* acebutolol *on page 19*
Aceon® *see* perindopril erbumine *on page 709*
Acephen™ [OTC] *see* acetaminophen *on page 20*
Acerola [OTC] *see* ascorbic acid *on page 94*
Acetadote® *see* acetylcysteine *on page 32*

acetaminophen (a seet a MIN oh fen)

Medication Safety Issues

Sound-alike/look-alike issues:

Acephen® may be confused with AcipHex®
FeverALL® may be confused with Fiberall®
Triaminic™ Children's Fever Reducer Pain Reliever may be confused with Triaminic® cough and cold products
Tylenol® may be confused with atenolol, timolol, Tylenol® PM, Tylox®

Other safety concerns:

Duplicate therapy issues: This product contains acetaminophen, which may be a component of combination products. Do not exceed the maximum recommended daily dose of acetaminophen.

Infant concentration change: The new infant acetaminophen concentration (160 mg/5 mL) is available. All children's liquid acetaminophen products will now be the same 160 mg/5 mL concentration. However, the former infant acetaminophen concentration (80 mg/0.8 mL) may still be available in some pharmacies until supplies run out. Check concentrations closely prior to administering or dispensing (November 2011).

Injection: Reports of 10-fold overdose errors using the parenteral product have occurred in the U.S. and Europe; calculation of doses in "mg" and subsequent administration of the dose in "mL" using the commercially available concentration of 10 mg/mL contributed to these errors. Expressing doses as mg **and** mL, as well as pharmacy preparation of doses, may decrease error potential (Dart, 2012; ISMP, 2012).

International issues:

Depon [Greece] may be confused with Depen brand name for penicillamine [U.S.]; Depin brand name for nifedipine [India]; Dipen brand name for diltiazem [Greece]
Duorol [Spain] may be confused with Diuril brand name for chlorothiazide [U.S., Canada]
Paralen [Czech Republic] may be confused with Aralen brand name for chloroquine [U.S., Mexico]

Synonyms APAP (abbreviation is not recommended); n-acetyl-p-aminophenol; paracetamol

U.S. Brand Names Acephen™ [OTC]; APAP 500 [OTC]; Aspirin Free Anacin® Extra Strength [OTC]; Cetafen® Extra [OTC]; Cetafen® [OTC]; Excedrin® Tension Headache [OTC]; Feverall® [OTC]; Infantaire [OTC]; Little Fevers™ [OTC]; Mapap® Arthritis Pain [OTC]; Mapap® Children's [OTC]; Mapap® Extra Strength [OTC]; Mapap® Infant's [OTC]; Mapap® Junior Rapid Tabs [OTC]; Mapap® [OTC]; Non-Aspirin Pain Reliever [OTC]; Nortemp Children's [OTC]; Ofirmev™; Pain & Fever Children's [OTC]; Pain Eze [OTC]; Q-Pap Children's [OTC]; Q-Pap Extra Strength [OTC]; Q-Pap Infant's [OTC]; Q-Pap [OTC]; RapiMed® Children's [OTC]; RapiMed® Junior [OTC]; Silapap Children's [OTC]; Silapap Infant's [OTC]; Triaminic™ Children's Fever Reducer Pain Reliever [OTC]; Tylenol® 8 Hour [OTC]; Tylenol® Arthritis Pain Extended Relief [OTC]; Tylenol® Children's Meltaways [OTC]; Tylenol® Children's [OTC]; Tylenol® Extra Strength [OTC]; Tylenol® Infant's Concentrated [OTC]; Tylenol® Jr. Meltaways [OTC]; Tylenol® [OTC]; Valorin Extra [OTC]; Valorin [OTC]

Canadian Brand Names Abenol®; Apo-Acetaminophen®; Atasol®; Novo-Gesic; Pediatrix; Tempra®; Tylenol®

Therapeutic Category Analgesic, Nonnarcotic; Antipyretic

Use Treatment of mild-to-moderate pain and fever (analgesic/antipyretic)

I.V.: Additional indication: Management of moderate-to-severe pain when combined with opioid analgesia

General Dosage Range Dosage adjustment recommended in patients with renal impairment

Oral, rectal:

Children 0-3 months: 10-15 mg/kg/dose **or** 40 mg/dose every 4-6 hours as needed (maximum: 2.6 g daily)

Children 4-11 months: 10-15 mg/kg/dose **or** 80 mg/dose every 4-6 hours as needed (maximum: 2.6 g daily)

Children 1-2 years: 10-15 mg/kg/dose **or** 120 mg/dose every 4-6 hours as needed (maximum: 2.6 g daily)

Children 2-3 years: 10-15 mg/kg/dose **or** 160 mg/dose every 4-6 hours as needed (maximum: 2.6 g daily)

Children 4-5 years: 10-15 mg/kg/dose **or** 240 mg/dose every 4-6 hours as needed (maximum: 2.6 g daily)

Children 6-8 years: 10-15 mg/kg/dose **or** 320 mg/dose every 4-6 hours as needed (maximum: 2.6 g daily)

Children 9-10 years: 10-15 mg/kg/dose **or** 400 mg/dose every 4-6 hours as needed (maximum: 2.6 g daily)

Children 11 years: 10-15 mg/kg/dose **or** 480 mg/dose every 4-6 hours as needed (maximum: 2.6 g daily)

Children ≥12 years, Adolescents, and Adults: Regular release: 325-650 mg every 4-6 hours as needed **or** 1000 mg 3-4 times daily as needed (maximum: 4 g daily); Extended release: 1300 mg every 8 hours (maximum: 3.9 g daily)

I.V.:

Children 2-12 years: 15 mg/kg every 6 hours **or** 12.5 mg/kg every 4 hours; maximum single dose: 15 mg/kg/dose; maximum daily dose: 75 mg/kg/day (≤3.75 g daily)

Adolescents and Adults <50 kg: 15 mg/kg every 6 hours **or** 12.5 mg/kg every 4 hours; maximum daily dose: 75 mg/kg/day (≤3.75 g daily)

Adolescents and Adults ≥50 kg: 650 mg every 4 hours **or** 1000 mg every 6 hours; maximum daily dose: 4 g daily

Dosage Forms

Caplet, oral: 500 mg
- Cetafen® Extra [OTC]: 500 mg
- Mapap® Extra Strength [OTC]: 500 mg
- Pain Eze [OTC]: 650 mg
- Tylenol® [OTC]: 325 mg
- Tylenol® Extra Strength [OTC]: 500 mg

Caplet, extended release, oral:
- Mapap® Arthritis Pain [OTC]: 650 mg
- Tylenol® 8 Hour [OTC]: 650 mg
- Tylenol® Arthritis Pain Extended Relief [OTC]: 650 mg

Capsule, oral:
- Mapap® Extra Strength [OTC]: 500 mg

Captab, oral: 500 mg

Elixir, oral:
- Mapap® Children's [OTC]: 160 mg/5 mL (118 mL, 480 mL)

Gelcap, oral: 500 mg
- Mapap® [OTC]: 500 mg

Gelcap, rapid release, oral: 500 mg
- Tylenol® Extra Strength [OTC]: 500 mg

Geltab, oral: 500 mg
- Excedrin® Tension Headache [OTC]: 500 mg

Injection, solution [preservative free]:
- Ofirmev™: 10 mg/mL (100 mL)

Liquid, oral: 160 mg/5 mL (120 mL, 473 mL); 500 mg/5 mL (240 mL)
- APAP 500 [OTC]: 500 mg/5 mL (237 mL)
- Q-Pap Children's [OTC]: 160 mg/5 mL (118 mL, 473 mL)
- Silapap Children's [OTC]: 160 mg/5 mL (118 mL, 237 mL, 473 mL)
- Tylenol® Extra Strength [OTC]: 500 mg/15 mL (240 mL)

Solution, oral: 160 mg/5 mL (5 mL, 10 mL, 20 mL, 118 mL, 473 mL); 80 mg/0.8 mL (15 mL)
- Infantaire [OTC]: 80 mg/0.8 mL (15 mL, 30 mL)
- Little Fevers™ [OTC]: 80 mg/mL (30 mL)
- Mapap® [OTC]: 80 mg/0.8 mL (15 mL)
- Pain & Fever Children's [OTC]: 160 mg/5 mL (118 mL, 473 mL)
- Q-Pap Infant's [OTC]: 80 mg/0.8 mL (15 mL)
- Silapap Infant's [OTC]: 80 mg/0.8 mL (15 mL, 30 mL)

Suppository, rectal: 120 mg (12s, 50s, 100s); 325 mg (12s); 650 mg (12s, 50s, 100s)
- Acephen™ [OTC]: 120 mg (12s, 50s, 100s); 325 mg (6s, 12s, 50s, 100s); 650 mg (12s, 50s, 100s)
- Feverall® [OTC]: 80 mg (6s, 50s); 120 mg (6s, 50s); 325 mg (6s, 50s); 650 mg (50s)

Suspension, oral: 160 mg/5 mL (5 mL, 10 mL, 10.15 mL, 20 mL, 20.3 mL); 80 mg/0.8 mL (0.8 mL, 2 mL)
- Mapap® Children's [OTC]: 160 mg/5 mL (118 mL)
- Mapap® Infant's [OTC]: 80 mg/0.8 mL (15 mL, 30 mL)
- Nortemp Children's [OTC]: 160 mg/5 mL (118 mL)
- Pain & Fever Children's [OTC]: 160 mg/5 mL (60 mL)
- Q-Pap Children's [OTC]: 160 mg/5 mL (118 mL)
- Tylenol® Children's [OTC]: 160 mg/5 mL (60 mL, 120 mL)
- Tylenol® Infant's Concentrated [OTC]: 80 mg/0.8 mL (15 mL, 30 mL)

Syrup, oral:
- Triaminic™ Children's Fever Reducer Pain Reliever [OTC]: 160 mg/5 mL (118 mL)

Tablet, oral: 325 mg, 500 mg
Aspirin Free Anacin® Extra Strength [OTC]: 500 mg
Cetafen® [OTC]: 325 mg
Mapap® [OTC]: 325 mg
Non-Aspirin Pain Reliever [OTC]: 325 mg
Q-Pap [OTC]: 325 mg
Q-Pap Extra Strength [OTC]: 500 mg
Tylenol® [OTC]: 325 mg
Tylenol® Extra Strength [OTC]: 500 mg
Valorin [OTC]: 325 mg
Valorin Extra [OTC]: 500 mg
Tablet, chewable, oral: 80 mg
Mapap® Children's [OTC]: 80 mg
Tablet, orally disintegrating, oral: 80 mg, 160 mg
Mapap® Children's [OTC]: 80 mg
Mapap® Junior Rapid Tabs [OTC]: 160 mg
RapiMed® Children's [OTC]: 80 mg
RapiMed® Junior [OTC]: 160 mg
Tylenol® Children's Meltaways [OTC]: 80 mg
Tylenol® Jr. Meltaways [OTC]: 160 mg

acetaminophen and butalbital *see* butalbital and acetaminophen *on page* 154

acetaminophen and chlorpheniramine *see* chlorpheniramine and acetaminophen *on page* 199

acetaminophen and codeine (a seet a MIN oh fen & KOE deen)

Medication Safety Issues

Sound-alike/look-alike issues:
Tylenol® may be confused with atenolol, timolol, Tylox®

High alert medication:
The Institute for Safe Medication Practices (ISMP) includes this medication among its list of drug classes which have a heightened risk of causing significant patient harm when used in error.

Other safety concerns:
Duplicate therapy issues: This product contains acetaminophen, which may be a component of other combination products. Do not exceed the maximum recommended daily dose of acetaminophen.
T3 is an error-prone abbreviation (mistaken as liothyronine)

International issues:
Codex: Brand name for acetaminophen/codeine [Brazil], but also the brand name for *saccharomyces boulardii* [Italy]
Codex [Brazil] may be confused with Cedax brand name for ceftibuten [U.S. and multiple international markets]

Synonyms codeine and acetaminophen; Tylenol #2; Tylenol #3; Tylenol Codeine

U.S. Brand Names Capital® and Codeine; Tylenol® with Codeine No. 3; Tylenol® with Codeine No. 4

Canadian Brand Names ratio-Emtec; ratio-Lenoltec; Triatec-30; Triatec-8; Triatec-8 Strong; Tylenol Elixir with Codeine; Tylenol No. 1; Tylenol No. 1 Forte; Tylenol No. 2 with Codeine; Tylenol No. 3 with Codeine; Tylenol No. 4 with Codeine

Therapeutic Category Analgesic, Narcotic

Controlled Substance C-III; C-V

Use Relief of mild-to-moderate pain

General Dosage Range Dosage adjustment recommended in patients with renal impairment

Oral:
Acetaminophen:
Children ≤12 years: 10-15 mg/kg/dose every 4-6 hours as needed (maximum: 2.6 g/day)
Children >12 years and Adults: 325-650 mg every 4-6 hours as needed (maximum: 4 g/day)
Codeine:
Children: 0.5-1 mg/kg/dose every 4-6 hours (maximum: 60 mg/dose)
Adults: 15-60 mg/dose every 4-6 hours (maximum: 360 mg/day)

Dosage Forms
Solution, oral [C-V]: Acetaminophen 120 mg and codeine 12 mg per 5 mL
Suspension, oral [C-V]: Acetaminophen 120 mg and codeine 12 mg per 5 mL
Capital® and Codeine [C-V]: Acetaminophen 120 mg and codeine 12 mg per 5 mL

Tablet, oral [C-III]: Acetaminophen 300 mg and codeine 15 mg; acetaminophen 300 mg and codeine 30 mg; acetaminophen 300 mg and codeine 60 mg

Tylenol® with Codeine No. 3: Acetaminophen 300 mg and codeine 30 mg

Tylenol® with Codeine No. 4: Acetaminophen 300 mg and codeine 60 mg

Dosage Forms - Canada Note: In countries outside of the U.S., some formulations of Tylenol® with Codeine include caffeine.

Caplet:

ratio-Lenoltec No. 1, Tylenol No. 1: Acetaminophen 300 mg, codeine 8 mg, and caffeine 15 mg

Tylenol No. 1 Forte: Acetaminophen 500 mg, codeine 8 mg, and caffeine 15 mg

Solution, oral:

Tylenol Elixir with Codeine: Acetaminophen 160 mg and codeine 8 mg per 5 mL

Tablet:

ratio-Emtec, Triatec-30: Acetaminophen 300 mg and codeine 30 mg

ratio-Lenoltec No. 1: Acetaminophen 300 mg, codeine 8 mg, and caffeine 15 mg

ratio-Lenoltec No. 2, Tylenol No. 2 with Codeine: Acetaminophen 300 mg, codeine 15 mg, and caffeine 15 mg

ratio-Lenoltec No. 3, Tylenol No. 3 with Codeine: Acetaminophen 300 mg, codeine 30 mg, and caffeine 15 mg

ratio-Lenoltec No. 4, Tylenol No. 4 with Codeine: Acetaminophen 300 mg and codeine 60 mg

Triatec-8: Acetaminophen 325 mg, codeine 8 mg, and caffeine 30 mg

Triatec-8 Strong: Acetaminophen 500 mg, codeine 8 mg, and caffeine 30 mg

acetaminophen and diphenhydramine (a seet a MIN oh fen & dye fen HYE dra meen)

Medication Safety Issues

Sound-alike/look-alike issues:

Excedrin® may be confused with Dexedrine®

Percogesic® may be confused with paregoric, Percodan®

Tylenol® may be confused with atenolol, timolol, Tylox®

Tylenol® PM may be confused with Tylenol®

Other safety concerns:

Duplicate therapy issues: This product contains acetaminophen, which may be a component of other combination products. Do not exceed the maximum recommended daily dose of acetaminophen.

Synonyms diphenhydramine and acetaminophen

U.S. Brand Names Excedrin PM® [OTC]; Goody's PM® [OTC]; Legatrin PM® [OTC]; Mapap PM [OTC]; Percogesic® Extra Strength [OTC]; TopCare® Pain Relief PM [OTC]; Tylenol® PM [OTC]; Tylenol® Severe Allergy [OTC]

Therapeutic Category Analgesic, Nonnarcotic

Use Aid in the relief of insomnia accompanied by minor pain

General Dosage Range Oral: *Children ≥12 years and Adults:* 50 mg of diphenhydramine HCl (76 mg diphenhydramine citrate) at bedtime

Dosage Forms

Caplet, oral:

Excedrin PM® [OTC]: Acetaminophen 500 mg and diphenhydramine 38 mg

Legatrin PM® [OTC]: Acetaminophen 500 mg and diphenhydramine 50 mg

Mapap PM [OTC], TopCare® Pain Relif PM [OTC], Tylenol® PM [OTC]: Acetaminophen 500 mg and diphenhydramine 25 mg

Percogesic® Extra Strength [OTC]: Acetaminophen 500 mg and diphenhydramine 12.5 mg

Tylenol® Severe Allergy [OTC]: Acetaminophen 500 mg and diphenhydramine 12.5 mg

Captab, oral: Acetaminophen 500 mg and diphenhydramine 25 mg

Gelcap, rapid release, oral:

Tylenol® PM [OTC]: Acetaminophen 500 mg and diphenhydramine 25 mg

Geltab, oral: Acetaminophen 500 mg and diphenhydramine 25 mg

Excedrin® PM [OTC]: Acetaminophen 500 mg and diphenhydramine 38 mg

Tylenol® PM [OTC]: Acetaminophen 500 mg and diphenhydramine 25 mg

Liquid, oral:

Tylenol® PM [OTC]: Acetaminophen 500 mg and diphenhydramine 25 mg per 15 mL

Powder for solution, oral:

Goody's PM® [OTC]: Acetaminophen 500 mg and diphenhydramine 38 mg

Tablet, oral: Acetaminophen 500 mg and diphenhydramine 25 mg

Excedrin® PM [OTC]: Acetaminophen 500 mg and diphenhydramine 38 mg

acetaminophen and hydrocodone *see* hydrocodone and acetaminophen *on page 454*

acetaminophen and oxycodone *see* oxycodone and acetaminophen *on page 679*

acetaminophen and pamabrom (a seet a MIN oh fen & PAM a brom)

Medication Safety Issues

Other safety concerns:

Duplicate therapy issues: This product contains acetaminophen, which may be a component of other combination products. Do not exceed the maximum recommended daily dose of acetaminophen.

Synonyms pamabrom and acetaminophen

U.S. Brand Names Cramp Tabs [OTC]; Midol® Teen Formula [OTC]; Tylenol® Women's Menstrual Relief [OTC]

Therapeutic Category Analgesic, Miscellaneous; Diuretic, Combination

Use Temporary relief of symptoms associated with premenstrual and menstrual symptoms (eg, cramps, bloating, water-weight gain, headache, backache, muscle aches)

General Dosage Range Oral: *Children ≥12 years and Adults:* Acetaminophen 650-1000 mg and pamabrom 50 mg every 4-6 hours as needed (maximum: 8 caplets/tablets/24 hours)

Dosage Forms

Caplet:

Midol® Teen Formula: Acetaminophen 500 mg and pamabrom 25 mg

Tylenol® Women's Menstrual Relief: Acetaminophen 500 mg and pamabrom 25 mg

Tablet:

Cramp Tabs: Acetaminophen 325 mg and pamabrom 25 mg

acetaminophen and pentazocine *see* pentazocine and acetaminophen *on page 705*

acetaminophen and phenylephrine (a seet a MIN oh fen & fen il EF rin)

Medication Safety Issues

Other safety concerns:

Duplicate therapy issues: This product contains acetaminophen, which may be a component of combination products. Do not exceed the maximum recommended daily dose of acetaminophen.

Synonyms phenylephrine hydrochloride and acetaminophen

U.S. Brand Names Cetafen Cold® [OTC]; Contac® Cold + Flu Maximum Strength Non-Drowsy [OTC]; Excedrin® Sinus Headache [OTC]; Mapap® Sinus PE [OTC]; Robitussin® Peak Cold Nasal Relief [OTC]; Sinus Pain & Pressure [OTC]; Sudafed PE® Pressure + Pain [OTC]; Tylenol® Sinus Congestion & Pain Daytime [OTC]; Vicks® DayQuil® Sinex® Daytime Sinus [OTC]

Therapeutic Category Analgesic, Miscellaneous; Decongestant

Use Temporary relief of sinus/nasal congestion and pressure, headache, and minor aches and pains

General Dosage Range Oral: *Children ≥12 years and Adults:* Acetaminophen 325 mg and phenylephrine 5 mg/caplet: Take 2 caplets every 4 hours as needed (maximum: 12 caplets/24 hours; maximum acetaminophen: 4 g/day)

Dosage Forms

Caplet, oral:

Contac® Cold + Flu Maximum Strength Non Drowsy [OTC]: Acetaminophen 500 mg and phenylephrine 5 mg

Excedrin® Sinus Headache [OTC], Mapap® Sinus PE [OTC], Sudafed PE® Pressure + Pain [OTC]: Acetaminophen 325 mg and phenylephrine 5 mg

Tylenol® Sinus Congestion & Pain Daytime [OTC]: Acetaminophen 325 mg and phenylephrine 5 mg [Cool Burst® flavor]

Capsule, liquid filled, oral:

Vicks® DayQuil® Sinex® Daytime Sinus [OTC]: Acetaminophen 325 mg and phenylephrine 5 mg

Gelcap, rapid release, oral:

Tylenol® Sinus Congestion & Pain Daytime [OTC]: Acetaminophen 325 mg and phenylephrine 5 mg

Tablet, oral:

Cetafen Cold® [OTC], Sinus Pain & Pressure [OTC]: Acetaminophen 500 mg and phenylephrine 5 mg

Robitussin® Peak Cold Nasal Relief [OTC]: Acetaminophen 325 mg and phenylephrine 5 mg

acetaminophen and phenyltoloxamine (a seet a MIN oh fen & fen il to LOKS a meen)

Medication Safety Issues

Sound-alike/look-alike issues:

Percogesic® may be confused with paregoric, Percodan®

Other safety concerns:

Duplicate therapy issues: This product contains acetaminophen, which may be a component of other combination products. Do not exceed the maximum recommended daily dose of acetaminophen.

Synonyms phenyltoloxamine citrate and acetaminophen

U.S. Brand Names RhinoFlex™ [DSC]; RhinoFlex™-650 [DSC]; Zgesic

Therapeutic Category Analgesic, Nonnarcotic

Use Relief of mild-to-moderate pain

General Dosage Range Oral: Based on acetaminophen component:

Children <12 years: 10-15 mg/kg/dose every 4-6 hours as needed (maximum: 2.6 g/day)

Children ≥12 years and Adults: 325-650 mg every 4-6 hours as needed (maximum: 4 g/day)

Dosage Forms

Tablet: Acetaminophen 325 mg and phenyltoloxamine 30 mg

Tablet, prolonged release, oral:

Zgesic: Acetaminophen 600 mg and phenyltoloxamine 66 mg

acetaminophen and pseudoephedrine (a seet a MIN oh fen & soo doe e FED rin)

Medication Safety Issues

Sound-alike/look-alike issues:

Ornex® may be confused with Orexin®, Orinase®

Other safety concerns:

Duplicate therapy issues: This product contains acetaminophen, which may be a component of other combination products. Do not exceed the maximum recommended daily dose of acetaminophen.

Synonyms pseudoephedrine and acetaminophen; pseudoephedrine hydrochloride and acetaminophen

U.S. Brand Names Ornex® Maximum Strength [OTC]; Ornex® [OTC]

Canadian Brand Names Contac® Cold and Sore Throat, Non Drowsy, Extra Strength; Dristan® N.D.; Dristan® N.D., Extra Strength; Sinutab® Non Drowsy; Sudafed® Head Cold and Sinus Extra Strength; Tylenol® Decongestant; Tylenol® Sinus

Therapeutic Category Decongestant/Analgesic

Use Temporary relief of nasal congestion, and minor aches and pains associated with colds, flu, sinusitis, or allergies

General Dosage Range Oral:

Children 6-11 years: Acetaminophen 325 mg/pseudoephedrine 30 mg every 4-6 hours (maximum: 120 mg/day pseudoephedrine)

Children ≥12 years and Adults: Acetaminophen 625-1000 mg/pseudoephedrine 60 mg every 4-6 hours (maximum: 240 mg/day pseudoephedrine)

Dosage Forms

Caplet:

Ornex® [OTC]: Acetaminophen 325 mg and pseudoephedrine 30 mg

Ornex® Maximum Strength [OTC]: Acetaminophen 500 mg and pseudoephedrine 30 mg

acetaminophen and tramadol (a seet a MIN oh fen & TRA ma dole)

Medication Safety Issues

Sound-alike/look-alike issues:

Ultracet® may be confused with Ultane®, Ultram®

Other safety concerns:

Duplicate therapy issues: This product contains acetaminophen, which may be a component of other combination products. Do not exceed the maximum recommended daily dose of acetaminophen.

Synonyms tramadol hydrochloride and acetaminophen

U.S. Brand Names Ultracet®

Canadian Brand Names Apo-Tramadol/Acet®; Tramacet

Therapeutic Category Analgesic, Miscellaneous; Analgesic, Nonnarcotic

Use Short-term (≤5 days) management of acute pain

General Dosage Range Dosage adjustment recommended in patients with renal impairment

Oral: *Adults:* Two tablets every 4-6 hours as needed (maximum: 8 tablets/day)

Dosage Forms

Tablet: Acetaminophen 325 mg and tramadol 37.5 mg

Ultracet®: Acetaminophen 325 mg and tramadol 37.5 mg

acetaminophen, aspirin, and caffeine (a seet a MIN oh fen, AS pir in, & KAF een)

Medication Safety Issues

Sound-alike/look-alike issues:

Excedrin® may be confused with Dexedrine®

Other safety concerns:

Duplicate therapy issues: This product contains acetaminophen, which may be a component of other combination products. Do not exceed the maximum recommended daily dose of acetaminophen.

Synonyms aspirin, acetaminophen, and caffeine; aspirin, caffeine, and acetaminophen; caffeine, acetaminophen, and aspirin; caffeine, aspirin, and acetaminophen

U.S. Brand Names Anacin® Advanced Headache Formula [OTC]; Excedrin® Extra Strength [OTC]; Excedrin® Migraine [OTC]; Fem-Prin® [OTC]; Goody's® Extra Strength Headache Powder [OTC]; Goody's® Extra Strength Pain Relief [OTC]; Pain-Off [OTC]; Vanquish® Extra Strength Pain Reliever [OTC]

Therapeutic Category Analgesic, Nonnarcotic

Use Relief of mild-to-moderate pain; mild-to-moderate pain associated with migraine headache

General Dosage Range Oral: *Children >12 years and Adults:* 1-2 doses every 4-6 hours as needed (maximum: 4 g/day [based on acetaminophen and aspirin component])

Dosage Forms

Caplet: Acetaminophen 250 mg, aspirin 250 mg, and caffeine 65 mg; acetaminophen 194 mg, aspirin 227 mg, and caffeine 33 mg

Excedrin® Extra Strength [OTC], Excedrin® Migraine [OTC]: Acetaminophen 250 mg, aspirin 250 mg, and caffeine 65 mg

Vanquish® Extra Strength Pain Reliever [OTC]: Acetaminophen 194 mg, aspirin 227 mg, and caffeine 33 mg

Geltab: Acetaminophen 250 mg, aspirin 250 mg, and caffeine 65 mg

Excedrin® Extra Strength [OTC], Excedrin® Migraine [OTC]: Acetaminophen 250 mg, aspirin 250 mg, and caffeine 65 mg

Powder: Acetaminophen 260 mg, aspirin 520 mg, and caffeine 32.5 mg

Goody's® Extra Strength Headache Powder [OTC]: Acetaminophen 260 mg, aspirin 520 mg, and caffeine 32.5 mg

Tablet:

Anacin® Advanced Headache Formula [OTC], Excedrin® Extra Strength [OTC], Excedrin® Migraine [OTC], Pain-Off [OTC]: Acetaminophen 250 mg, aspirin 250 mg, and caffeine 65 mg

Fem-Prin® [OTC]: Acetaminophen 194.4 mg, aspirin 226.8 mg, and caffeine 32.4 mg

Goody's® Extra Strength Pain Relief [OTC]: Acetaminophen 130 mg, aspirin 260 mg, and caffeine 16.25 mg

acetaminophen, butalbital, and caffeine *see* butalbital, acetaminophen, and caffeine *on page 153*

acetaminophen, caffeine, and dihydrocodeine
(a seet a MIN oh fen, KAF een, & dye hye droe KOE deen)

Medication Safety Issues

Sound-alike/look-alike issues:

Panlor® may be confused with Pamelor™

High alert medication:

The Institute for Safe Medication Practices (ISMP) includes this medication among its list of drug classes which have a heightened risk of causing significant patient harm when used in error.

Other safety concerns:

Duplicate therapy issues: This product contains acetaminophen, which may be a component of other combination products. Do not exceed the maximum recommended daily dose of acetaminophen.

Synonyms caffeine, dihydrocodeine, and acetaminophen; dihydrocodeine bitartrate, acetaminophen, and caffeine

U.S. Brand Names Trezix™

Therapeutic Category Analgesic Combination (Opioid)

Controlled Substance C-III

Use Relief of moderate- to moderately-severe pain

General Dosage Range Oral: *Adults:* 1 tablet or 2 capsules every 4 hours as needed (maximum: 5 tablets/day or 10 capsules/day)

Dosage Forms

Capsule:

Trezix™: Acetaminophen 356.4 mg, caffeine 30 mg, and dihydrocodeine 16 mg

Tablet: Acetaminophen 712.8 mg, caffeine 60 mg, and dihydrocodeine bitartrate 32 mg

acetaminophen, caffeine, codeine, and butalbital *see* butalbital, acetaminophen, caffeine, and codeine *on page 153*

acetaminophen, chlorpheniramine, phenylephrine, and phenyltoloxamine (a seet a MIN oh fen, klor fen IR a meen, fen il EF rin, & fen il tole LOKS a meen)

Synonyms chlorpheniramine maleate, acetaminophen, phenylephrine hydrochloride, and phenyltoloxamine citrate; phenylephrine, chlorpheniramine, acetaminophen, and phenyltoloxamine; phenyltoloxamine, chlorpheniramine, phenylephrine, and acetaminophen

U.S. Brand Names norel® SR

Therapeutic Category Alkylamine Derivative; Alpha/Beta Agonist; Analgesic, Miscellaneous; Decongestant; Ethanolamine Derivative; Histamine H_1 Antagonist; Histamine H_1 Antagonist, First Generation

Use Temporary relief of cold, allergy, or sinus symptoms caused from inhalation of airborne irritants

General Dosage Range Oral: *Children >12 years and Adults:* One tablet every 12 hours

Dosage Forms

Tablet, extended release, oral:

norel® SR: Acetaminophen 325 mg, chlorpheniramine maleate 8 mg, phenylephrine hydrochloride 40 mg, and phenyltoloxamine citrate 50 mg [scored]

acetaminophen, codeine, and doxylamine *(Canada only)*

(a seet a MIN oh fen, KOE deen, & dox IL a meen)

Medication Safety Issues

High alert medication:

The Institute for Safe Medication Practices (ISMP) includes this medication among its list of drug classes which have a heightened risk of causing significant patient harm when used in error.

Other safety concerns:

Duplicate therapy issues: This product contains acetaminophen, which may be a component of other combination products. Do not exceed the maximum recommended daily dose of acetaminophen.

Synonyms codeine, doxylamine, and acetaminophen; doxylamine succinate, codeine phosphate, and acetaminophen

Canadian Brand Names Mersyndol® With Codeine

Therapeutic Category Analgesic, Opioid; Antihistamine

Controlled Substance CDSA-1

Use Relief of headache, cold symptoms, neuralgia, and muscular aches/pain

General Dosage Range Oral: *Children >12 years and Adults:* 1-2 tablets every 4 hours as needed (maximum: 12 tablets/day)

Product Availability Not available in U.S.

Dosage Forms - Canada

Tablet, oral:

Mersyndol® With Codeine: Acetaminophen 325 mg, codeine 8 mg, and doxylamine 5 mg

acetaminophen, dextromethorphan, and doxylamine

(a seet a MIN oh fen, deks troe meth OR fan, & dox IL a meen)

Medication Safety Issues

Other safety concerns:

Duplicate therapy issues: This product contains acetaminophen, which may be a component of other combination products. Do not exceed the maximum recommended daily dose of acetaminophen.

Synonyms dextromethorphan hydrobromide, acetaminophen, and doxylamine succinate; doxylamine, acetaminophen, and dextromethorphan

U.S. Brand Names All-Nite Multi-Symptom Cold/Flu Relief [OTC]; Night Time Multi-Symptom Cold/Flu Relief [OTC]; Tylenol® Cold & Cough Nighttime [OTC]; Tylenol® Cough & Sore Throat Nighttime [OTC]; Vicks® Nature Fusion™ Cold & Flu Nighttime Relief [OTC]; Vicks® NyQuil® Cold & Flu Multi-Symptom [OTC] [DSC]; Vicks® NyQuil® Cold & Flu Nighttime Relief [OTC]

Therapeutic Category Analgesic, Miscellaneous; Antitussive; Histamine H_1 Antagonist; Histamine H_1 Antagonist, First Generation

Use Temporary relief of common cold and flu symptoms (eg, minor aches and pain, fever, cough, runny nose, sneezing, sore throat)

General Dosage Range Oral: *Children ≥12 years and Adults:* Two capsules **or** 30 mL every 6 hours (maximum: 8 capsules **or** 120 mL/24 hours [Vicks® NyQuil® Cold & Flu, Vicks® Nature Fusion™ Cold & Flu, All-Nite] **or** 240 mL/24 hours [Tylenol® Cold and Cough])

Dosage Forms

Capsule, liquid filled, oral: Acetaminophen 325 mg, dextromethorphan hydrobromide 15 mg, and doxylamine succinate 6.25 mg

Night Time Multi-Symptom Cold/Flu Relief [OTC], Vicks® NyQuil® Cold & Flu Nighttime Relief [OTC]: Acetaminophen 325 mg, dextromethorphan 15 mg, and doxylamine 6.25 mg

Liquid, oral:

All-Nite Multi-Symptom Cold/Flu Relief [OTC], Tylenol® Cold & Cough Nighttime [OTC], Tylenol® Cough & Sore Throat Nighttime [OTC]: Acetaminophen 500 mg, dextromethorphan 15 mg, and doxylamine 6.25 mg per 15 mL

Vicks® Nature Fusion™ Cold & Flu Nighttime Relief [OTC]: Acetaminophen 650 mg, dextromethorphan 30 mg, and doxylamine 7.5 mg per 30 mL

Vicks® NyQuil® Cold & Flu Nighttime Relief [OTC]: Acetaminophen 650 mg, dextromethorphan 30 mg, and doxylamine 12.5 mg per 30 mL

acetaminophen, dextromethorphan, and phenylephrine

(a seet a MIN oh fen, deks troe meth OR fan, & fen il EF rin)

Medication Safety Issues

Other safety concerns:

Duplicate therapy issues: This product contains acetaminophen, which may be a component of other combination products. Do not exceed the maximum recommended daily dose of acetaminophen.

Synonyms dextromethorphan hydrobromide, acetaminophen, and phenylephrine hydrochloride; phenylephrine, acetaminophen, and dextromethorphan; phenylephrine, dextromethorphan, and acetaminophen

U.S. Brand Names Alka-Seltzer Plus® Day Cold [OTC]; Comtrex® Maximum Strength, Non-Drowsy Cold & Cough [OTC]; Mapap® Multi-Symptom Cold [OTC]; Theraflu Warming Relief® Daytime Multi-Symptom Cold [OTC]; Theraflu Warming Relief® Daytime Severe Cold & Cough [OTC]; Theraflu® Daytime Severe Cold & Cough [OTC]; Tylenol® Cold Head Congestion Daytime [OTC]; Tylenol® Cold Multi-Symptom Daytime [OTC]; Vicks® DayQuil® Cold & Flu Multi-Symptom [OTC]; Vicks® Nature Fusion™ Cold & Flu Multi-Symptom Relief [OTC]

Therapeutic Category Analgesic, Miscellaneous; Antitussive; Decongestant

Use Temporary relief of common cold and flu symptoms (eg, pain, fever, cough, congestion)

General Dosage Range Oral: *Children ≥6 years and Adults:* Dosage varies greatly depending on product

Dosage Forms

Caplet, oral:

Comtrex® Maximum Strength, Non-Drowsy Cold & Cough [OTC], Mapap® Multi-Symptom Cold [OTC], Theraflu Warming Relief® Daytime Multi-Symptom Cold [OTC], Tylenol® Cold Head Congestion Daytime [OTC], Tylenol® Cold Multi-Symptom Daytime [OTC], Vicks® Nature Fusion™ Cold & Flu Multi-Symptom Relief [OTC]: Acetaminophen 325 mg, dextromethorphan 10 mg, and phenylephrine 5 mg

Capsule, liquid filled, oral:

Alka-Seltzer Plus® Day Cold [OTC]: Acetaminophen 325 mg, dextromethorphan 10 mg, and phenylephrine 5 mg

Vicks® DayQuil® Cold & Flu Multi-Symptom [OTC], Tylenol® Cold Multi-Symptom Daytime [OTC]: Acetaminophen 325 mg, dextromethorphan 10 mg, and phenylephrine 5 mg

Gelcap, rapid release, oral:

Tylenol® Cold Multi-Symptom Daytime [OTC]: Acetaminophen 325 mg, dextromethorphan 10 mg, and phenylephrine 5 mg

Liquid, oral:

Tylenol® Cold Multi-Symptom Daytime [OTC], Vicks® DayQuil® Cold & Flu Multi-Symptom [OTC]: Acetaminophen 325 mg, dextromethorphan 10 mg, and phenylephrine 5 mg per 15 mL

Powder for solution, oral:

Theraflu® Daytime Severe Cold & Cough [OTC]: Acetaminophen 650 mg, dextromethorphan 20 mg, and phenylephrine 10 mg per packet

Syrup, oral:

Theraflu Warming Relief® Daytime Severe Cold & Cough [OTC]: Acetaminophen 325 mg, dextromethorphan 10 mg, and phenylephrine 5 mg per 15 mL

acetaminophen, dichloralphenazone, and isometheptene *see* acetaminophen, isometheptene, and dichloralphenazone *on page 30*

acetaminophen, diphenhydramine, and phenylephrine

(a seet a MIN oh fen, dye fen HYE dra meen, & fen il EF rin)

Medication Safety Issues

Other safety concerns:

Duplicate therapy issues: This product contains acetaminophen, which may be a component of combination products. Do not exceed the maximum recommended daily dose of acetaminophen.

Synonyms acetaminophen, phenylephrine, and diphenhydramine; diphenhydramine, phenylephrine hydrochloride, and acetaminophen; phenylephrine hydrochloride, acetaminophen, and diphenhydramine

U.S. Brand Names Benadryl® Allergy and Cold [OTC]; Benadryl® Allergy and Sinus Headache [OTC]; Benadry® Maximum Strength Severe Allergy and Sinus Headache [OTC]; Cold Control PE [OTC]; One Tab™ Allergy & Sinus [OTC]; One Tab™ Cold & Flu [OTC]; Robitussin® Peak Cold Nighttime Multi-Symptom Cold [OTC]; Sudafed PE® Nighttime Cold [OTC]; Sudafed PE® Severe Cold [OTC]; Theraflu® Nighttime Severe Cold & Cough [OTC]; Theraflu® Sugar-Free Nighttime Severe Cold & Cough [OTC]; Theraflu® Warming Relief™ Flu & Sore Throat [OTC]; Theraflu® Warming Relief™ Nighttime Severe Cold & Cough [OTC]; Tylenol® Allergy Multi-Symptom Nighttime [OTC]; Tylenol® Children's Plus Cold and Allergy [OTC]

Therapeutic Category Analgesic, Miscellaneous; Decongestant; Histamine H_1 Antagonist

Use Temporary relief of symptoms of hay fever and the common cold, including sinus/nasal congestion and pain/pressure, headache, sneezing, runny nose, itchy/watery eyes, sore throat, fever, cough, and minor aches and pains

General Dosage Range Oral:

Caplet:

Children 6-11 years: One caplet every 4 hours as needed (maximum: 5 doses/caplets)

Children ≥12 years and Adults: Two caplets every 4 hours as needed (maximum: 12 caplets/24 hours)

Liquid: *Children 6-11 years and 48-95 lbs:* 10 mL every 4 hours as needed (maximum: 5 doses/24 hours)

Powder for solution: *Children ≥12 years and Adults:* One packet every 4 hours as needed (maximum: 6 doses/24 hours)

Syrup: *Children ≥12 years and Adults:* 30 mL every 4 hours as needed (maximum: 6 doses/24 hours)

Dosage Forms

Caplet, oral:

Benadryl® Allergy and Cold [OTC], Benadryl® Allergy and Sinus Headache [OTC], Sudafed PE® Severe Cold [OTC]: Acetaminophen 325 mg, diphenhydramine 12.5 mg, and phenylephrine 5 mg

Benadry® Maximum Strength Severe Allergy and Sinus Headache [OTC], Sudafed PE® Nighttime Cold [OTC], Tylenol® Allergy Multi-Symptom Nighttime [OTC]: Acetaminophen 325 mg, diphenhydramine 25 mg, and phenylephrine 5 mg

Cold Control PE [OTC]: Acetaminophen 650 mg, diphenhydramine 25 mg, and phenylephrine 10 mg

One Tab™ Allergy & Sinus, One Tab™ Cold and Flu: Acetaminophen 650 mg, diphenhydramine 25 mg, and phenylephrine 10 mg

Liquid, oral:

Robitussin® Peak Cold Nighttime Multi-Symptom Cold: Acetaminophen 160 mg, diphenhydramine 6.25 mg, and phenylephrine 2.5 mg per 5 mL

Tylenol® Children's Plus Cold and Allergy [OTC]: Acetaminophen 160 mg, diphenhydramine 12.5 mg, and phenylephrine 2.5 mg per 5 mL

Powder for solution, oral:

Theraflu® Nighttime Severe Cold & Cough [OTC], Theraflu® Sugar-Free Nighttime Severe Cold & Cough [OTC]: Acetaminophen 650 mg, diphenhydramine 25 mg, and phenylephrine 10 mg per packet (6s)

Syrup, oral:

Theraflu® Warming Relief™ Flu & Sore Throat [OTC], Theraflu® Warming Relief™ Nighttime Severe Cold & Cough [OTC]: Acetaminophen 325 mg, diphenhydramine 12.5 mg, and phenylephrine 5 mg per 15 mL (245.5 mL)

acetaminophen, isometheptene, and dichloralphenazone

(a seet a MIN oh fen, eye soe me THEP teen, & dye KLOR al FEN a zone)

Medication Safety Issues

Sound-alike/look-alike issues:

Midrin® may be confused with midodrine, Mydfrin®

Other safety concerns:

Duplicate therapy issues: This product contains acetaminophen, which may be a component of other combination products. Do not exceed the maximum recommended daily dose of acetaminophen.

Synonyms acetaminophen, dichloralphenazone, and isometheptene; dichloralphenazone, acetaminophen, and isometheptene; dichloralphenazone, isometheptene, and acetaminophen; isometheptene, acetaminophen, and dichloralphenazone; isometheptene, dichloralphenazone, and acetaminophen; Midrin

Therapeutic Category Analgesic, Nonnarcotic

Controlled Substance C-IV

Use Relief of migraine and tension headache

General Dosage Range Oral: *Adults:* 2 capsules initially, then 1 capsule every hour until relief; alternatively, 1-2 capsules every 4 hours (maximum: 5 capsules/12 hours or 8 capsules/day)

Dosage Forms

Capsule, oral: Acetaminophen 325 mg, isometheptene mucate 65 mg, and dichloralphenazone 100 mg

acetaminophen, phenylephrine, and diphenhydramine *see* acetaminophen, diphenhydramine, and phenylephrine *on page 29*

Acetasol® HC *see* acetic acid, propylene glycol diacetate, and hydrocortisone *on page 31*

Acetazolam (Can) *see* acetazolamide *on page 30*

acetazolamide (a set a ZOLE a mide)

Medication Safety Issues

International issues:

Diamox [Canada and multiple international markets] may be confused with Diabinese brand name for chlorpropamide [Multiple international markets]; Dobutrex brand name for dobutamine [Multiple international markets]; Trimox brand name for amoxicillin [Brazil]; Zimox brand name for amoxicillin [Italy] and carbidopa/levodopa [Greece]

Tall-Man aceta**ZOLAMIDE**

U.S. Brand Names Diamox® Sequels®

Canadian Brand Names Acetazolam; Diamox®

Therapeutic Category Anticonvulsant; Carbonic Anhydrase Inhibitor

Use Treatment of glaucoma (chronic simple open-angle, secondary glaucoma, preoperatively in acute angle-closure); drug-induced edema or edema due to congestive heart failure (adjunctive therapy; I.V. and immediate release dosage forms); centrencephalic epilepsies (I.V. and immediate release dosage forms); prevention or amelioration of symptoms associated with acute mountain sickness (immediate and extended release dosage forms)

General Dosage Range Dosage adjustment recommended in patients with renal impairment

I.V.: *Adults:* 250-1000 mg/day

Oral:

Immediate release:

Children: 8-30 mg/kg/day divided in 1-4 doses (maximum: 30 mg/kg/day or 1 g/day)

Adults: 250-1000 mg/day **or** 8-30 mg/kg/day in 1-4 divided doses (maximum: 30 mg/kg/day or 1 g/day) **or** 125-250 mg every 4 hours

Elderly: Initial: 250-500 mg/day

Extended release:

Adults: 500-1000 mg/day

Dosage Forms

Capsule, extended release, oral: 500 mg

Capsule, sustained release, oral:

Diamox® Sequels®: 500 mg

Injection, powder for reconstitution: 500 mg

Tablet, oral: 125 mg, 250 mg

acetic acid (a SEE tik AS id)

Medication Safety Issues

Sound-alike/look-alike issues:

Acetic acid for irrigation may be confused with glacial acetic acid

VoSol® may be confused with Vexol®,VoSol® HC

Synonyms ethanoic acid

U.S. Brand Names VoSoL®

Therapeutic Category Antibacterial, Otic; Antibacterial, Topical

Use Irrigation of the bladder; periodic irrigation of indwelling catheters; treatment of superficial bacterial infections of the external auditory canal

General Dosage Range

Irrigation:

Adults: Continuous: 0.25% at a rate approximate to urine flow; usually 500-1500 mL/day; Periodic: 50 mL of 0.25%

Otic:

Children ≥3 years: Instill 3-5 drops 3-4 times/day

Adults: Instill 5 drops 3-4 times/day

Dosage Forms

Solution, for irrigation: 0.25% (1000 mL)

Solution, for irrigation [preservative free]: 0.25% (250 mL, 500 mL, 1000 mL)

Solution, otic: 2% (15 mL, 60 mL)

VoSoL®: 2% (15 mL)

acetic acid, hydrocortisone, and propylene glycol diacetate *see* acetic acid, propylene glycol diacetate, and hydrocortisone *on page* 31

acetic acid, propylene glycol diacetate, and hydrocortisone

(a SEE tik AS id, PRO pa leen GLY kole dye AS e tate, & hye droe KOR ti sone)

Medication Safety Issues

Sound-alike/look-alike issues:

VoSol® may be confused with Vexol®

Synonyms acetic acid, hydrocortisone, and propylene glycol diacetate; hydrocortisone, acetic acid, and propylene glycol diacetate; propylene glycol diacetate, acetic acid, and hydrocortisone

U.S. Brand Names Acetasol® HC; VoSol® HC

Therapeutic Category Antibiotic/Corticosteroid, Otic

Use Treatment of superficial infections of the external auditory canal caused by organisms susceptible to the action of the antimicrobial, complicated by swelling

General Dosage Range Otic: *Children ≥3 years and Adults:* Instill 3-5 drops in ear(s) every 4-6 hours

Dosage Forms

Solution, otic [drops]: Acetic acid 2%, propylene glycol diacetate 3%, and hydrocortisone 1% (10 mL)

Acetasol® HC, VoSol® HC: Acetic acid 2%, propylene glycol diacetate 3%, and hydrocortisone 1% (10 mL)

acetohydroxamic acid (a SEE toe hye droks am ik AS id)

Medication Safety Issues

Sound-alike/look-alike issues:

Lithostat® may be confused with Lithobid®

Synonyms AHA

U.S. Brand Names Lithostat®

Canadian Brand Names Lithostat®

Therapeutic Category Urinary Tract Product

Use Adjunctive therapy in chronic urea-splitting urinary infection

General Dosage Range Oral:

Children: Initial: 10 mg/kg/day

Adults: 250 mg 3-4 times/day (maximum: 10-15 mg/kg/day)

Dosage Forms

Tablet, oral:

Lithostat®: 250 mg

Acetoxyl® (Can) *see* benzoyl peroxide *on page 124*
acetoxymethylprogesterone *see* medroxyprogesterone *on page 567*

acetylcholine (a se teel KOE leen)

Medication Safety Issues

Sound-alike/look-alike issues:

Acetylcholine may be confused with acetylcysteine

Synonyms acetylcholine chloride

U.S. Brand Names Miochol®-E

Canadian Brand Names Miochol®-E

Therapeutic Category Cholinergic Agent

Use Produces complete miosis in cataract surgery, keratoplasty, iridectomy, and other anterior segment surgery where rapid miosis is required

General Dosage Range Intraocular: *Adults:* Instill 0.5-2 mL of 1% injection (5-20 mg)

Dosage Forms

Powder for solution, intraocular:

Miochol®-E: 20 mg (2 mL)

acetylcholine chloride *see* acetylcholine *on page 32*

acetylcysteine (a se teel SIS teen)

Medication Safety Issues

Sound-alike/look-alike issues:

Acetylcysteine may be confused with acetylcholine
Mucomyst® may be confused with Mucinex®

Synonyms *N* acetylcysteine; *N*-acetyl-L-cysteine; *N*-acetylcysteine; acetylcysteine sodium; mercapturic acid; Mucomyst; NAC

U.S. Brand Names Acetadote®

Canadian Brand Names Acetylcysteine Injection; Acetylcysteine Solution; Mucomyst®; Parvolex®

Therapeutic Category Mucolytic Agent

Use Antidote for acute acetaminophen poisoning; repeated supratherapeutic ingestion (RSTI) of acetaminophen; adjunctive mucolytic therapy in patients with abnormal or viscid mucous secretions in acute and chronic bronchopulmonary diseases; pulmonary complications of surgery and cystic fibrosis; diagnostic bronchial studies

General Dosage Range

Inhalation:

Nebulization:

Infants: 1-2 mL of 20% solution or 2-4 mL 10% solution 3-4 times/day

Children and Adults: 1-10 mL of 20% solution or 2-20 mL of 10% solution every 2-6 hours

Direct instillation: *Adults:* 1-4 mL of 10% or 1-2 mL of 20% solution every 1-4 hours

I.V.: Acetadote®:

Children and Adults: 21-hour regimen: Consists of 3 doses; total dose delivered: 300 mg/kg

Loading dose: 150 mg/kg (maximum: 15 g) infused over 60 minutes

Second dose: 50 mg/kg (maximum: 5 g) infused over 4 hours

Third dose: 100 mg/kg (maximum: 10 g) infused over 16 hours

Oral:

Children and Adults: Acetaminophen poisoning: 72-hour regimen: Consists of 18 doses; total dose delivered: 1330 mg/kg

Loading dose: 140 mg/kg

Maintenance dose: 70 mg/kg every 4 hours

Dosage Forms

Injection, solution [preservative free]:

Acetadote®: 20% [200 mg/mL] (30 mL)

Solution, for inhalation/oral: 10% [100 mg/mL] (10 mL, 30 mL); 20% [200 mg/mL] (10 mL, 30 mL)

Solution, for inhalation/oral [preservative free]: 10% [100 mg/mL] (4 mL, 10 mL); 20% [200 mg/mL] (4 mL, 10 mL, 30 mL)

Acetylcysteine Injection (Can) *see* acetylcysteine *on page 32*
acetylcysteine, methylcobalamin, and methylfolate *see* methylfolate, methylcobalamin, and acetylcysteine *on page 590*

acetylcysteine, methylfolate, and methylcobalamin *see* methylfolate, methylcobalamin, and acetylcysteine *on page 590*
acetylcysteine sodium *see* acetylcysteine *on page 32*
Acetylcysteine Solution (Can) *see* acetylcysteine *on page 32*
acetylsalicylic acid *see* aspirin *on page 96*
achromycin *see* tetracycline *on page 884*
aciclovir *see* acyclovir (systemic) *on page 34*
aciclovir *see* acyclovir (topical) *on page 35*
Acid Control (Can) *see* famotidine *on page 372*
Acid Gone [OTC] *see* aluminum hydroxide and magnesium carbonate *on page 55*
Acid Gone Extra Strength [OTC] *see* aluminum hydroxide and magnesium carbonate *on page 55*
Acid Reducer (Can) *see* ranitidine *on page 788*
acidulated phosphate fluoride *see* fluoride *on page 393*
Acilac (Can) *see* lactulose *on page 519*
AcipHex® *see* rabeprazole *on page 784*

acitretin (a si TRE tin)

Medication Safety Issues

Sound-alike/look-alike issues:

Soriatane® may be confused with Loxitane®, sertraline, Sonata®

U.S. Brand Names Soriatane®

Canadian Brand Names Soriatane®

Therapeutic Category Retinoid-like Compound

Use Treatment of severe psoriasis

General Dosage Range Oral: *Adults:* 25-50 mg/day as a single dose

Dosage Forms

Capsule, oral:

Soriatane®: 10 mg, 17.5 mg, 25 mg

Aclaro® *see* hydroquinone *on page 461*
Aclaro PD® *see* hydroquinone *on page 461*
Aclasta® (Can) *see* zoledronic acid *on page 965*

aclidinium (a kli DIN ee um)

Synonyms aclidinium bromide; Tudorza® Pressair®

Therapeutic Category Anticholinergic Agent

Use Maintenance treatment of bronchospasm associated with chronic obstructive pulmonary disease (COPD), including chronic bronchitis and emphysema

Product Availability Tudorza® Pressair®: FDA approved July 2012; availability anticipated in the fourth quarter of 2012

aclidinium bromide *see* aclidinium *on page 33*
Aclovate® *see* alclometasone *on page 43*
Acne Clear Maximum Strength [OTC] *see* benzoyl peroxide *on page 124*

acrivastine and pseudoephedrine (AK ri vas teen & soo doe e FED rin)

Synonyms pseudoephedrine hydrochloride and acrivastine

U.S. Brand Names Semprex®-D

Therapeutic Category Antihistamine/Decongestant Combination

Use Relief of symptoms associated with seasonal allergic rhinitis

General Dosage Range Oral: *Children ≥12 years and Adults:* One capsule every 4-6 hours (maximum: 4 doses/24 hours)

Dosage Forms

Capsule:

Semprex®-D: Acrivastine 8 mg and pseudoephedrine 60 mg

Act® [OTC] *see* fluoride *on page 393*
ACT-D *see* dactinomycin *on page 251*

Actemra® *see* tocilizumab *on page 902*
ACTH *see* corticotropin *on page 237*
Acthar *see* corticotropin *on page 237*
ActHIB® *see Haemophilus* B conjugate vaccine *on page 439*
Acthrel® *see* corticorelin *on page 237*
Actidose®-Aqua [OTC] *see* charcoal, activated *on page 193*
Actidose® with Sorbitol [OTC] *see* charcoal, activated *on page 193*
Actifed® (Can) *see* triprolidine and pseudoephedrine *on page 922*
Actigall® *see* ursodiol *on page 932*
Actimmune® *see* interferon gamma-1b *on page 492*
actinomycin *see* dactinomycin *on page 251*
actinomycin D *see* dactinomycin *on page 251*
actinomycin CI *see* dactinomycin *on page 251*
Actiq® *see* fentanyl *on page 377*
Activase® *see* alteplase *on page 53*
Activase® rt-PA (Can) *see* alteplase *on page 53*
activated carbon *see* charcoal, activated *on page 193*
activated charcoal *see* charcoal, activated *on page 193*
activated dimethicone *see* simethicone *on page 834*
activated ergosterol *see* ergocalciferol *on page 339*
activated factor XIII *see* factor XIII concentrate (human) *on page 372*
activated methylpolysiloxane *see* simethicone *on page 834*
activated protein C, human, recombinant *see* drotrecogin alfa (activated) *on page 318*
Activella® *see* estradiol and norethindrone *on page 349*
Act® Kids [OTC] *see* fluoride *on page 393*
Actonel® *see* risedronate *on page 803*
Actonel® DR (Can) *see* risedronate *on page 803*
Actoplus Met® *see* pioglitazone and metformin *on page 725*
Actoplus Met® XR *see* pioglitazone and metformin *on page 725*
Actos® *see* pioglitazone *on page 725*
Act® Restoring™ [OTC] *see* fluoride *on page 393*
Act® Total Care™ [OTC] *see* fluoride *on page 393*
Acular® *see* ketorolac (ophthalmic) *on page 513*
Acular LS® *see* ketorolac (ophthalmic) *on page 513*
Acuvail® *see* ketorolac (ophthalmic) *on page 513*
ACV *see* acyclovir (systemic) *on page 34*
ACV *see* acyclovir (topical) *on page 35*
acycloguanosine *see* acyclovir (systemic) *on page 34*
acycloguanosine *see* acyclovir (topical) *on page 35*

acyclovir (systemic) (ay SYE kloe veer)

Medication Safety Issues

Sound-alike/look-alike issues:

Acyclovir may be confused with ganciclovir, Retrovir®, valacyclovir

Zovirax® may be confused with Doribax®, Valtrex®, Zithromax®, Zostrix®, Zyloprim®, Zyvox®

Synonyms aciclovir; ACV; acycloguanosine

U.S. Brand Names Zovirax®

Canadian Brand Names Apo-Acyclovir®; Mylan-Acyclovir; Nu-Acyclovir; ratio-Acyclovir; Teva-Acyclovir; Zovirax®

Therapeutic Category Antiviral Agent

Use Treatment of genital herpes simplex virus (HSV) and HSV encephalitis

General Dosage Range Dosage adjustment recommended in patients with renal impairment

I.V.:

Children <12 years: 10-20 mg/kg/dose every 8 hours (maximum: 60 mg/kg/day)

Children ≥12 years and Adults: 5-10 mg/kg/dose **or** 500 mg/m^2/dose every 8 hours (maximum: 45 mg/kg/day)

Oral:

Children ≥2 years and ≤40 kg: 20 mg/kg/dose 4 times/day (maximum: 800 mg/dose)

Children ≥2 years and >40 kg: 800 mg/dose 4 times/day

Adults: 200-800 mg/dose 3-5 times/day

Dosage Forms

Capsule, oral: 200 mg

Zovirax®: 200 mg

Injection, powder for reconstitution: 500 mg, 1000 mg

Injection, solution [preservative free]: 50 mg/mL (10 mL, 20 mL)

Suspension, oral: 200 mg/5 mL (473 mL)

Zovirax®: 200 mg/5 mL (473 mL)

Tablet, oral: 400 mg, 800 mg

Zovirax®: 400 mg, 800 mg

acyclovir (topical) (ay SYE kloe veer)

Medication Safety Issues

Sound-alike/look-alike issues:

Acyclovir may be confused with ganciclovir, Retrovir®, valacyclovir

Zovirax® may be confused with Doribax®, Valtrex®, Zithromax®, Zostrix®, Zyloprim®, Zyvox®

International issues:

Opthavir [Mexico] may be confused with Optivar brand name for azelastine [U.S.]

Synonyms aciclovir; ACV; acycloguanosine

U.S. Brand Names Zovirax®

Canadian Brand Names Zovirax®

Therapeutic Category Antiviral Agent, Topical

Use Treatment of herpes labialis (cold sores), mucocutaneous HSV in immunocompromised patients

General Dosage Range Topical:

Children ≥12 years: Cream: Apply 5 times/day

Adults: Cream: Apply 5 times/day; Ointment: 1/2" ribbon for a 4" square surface area 6 times/day

Dosage Forms

Cream, topical:

Zovirax®: 5% (2 g, 5 g)

Ointment, topical:

Zovirax®: 5% (15 g, 30 g)

acyclovir and hydrocortisone (ay SYE kloe veer & hye droe KOR ti sone)

Synonyms hydrocortisone and acyclovir; ME-609; Xerclear

U.S. Brand Names Xerese™

Therapeutic Category Antiviral Agent, Topical; Corticosteroid, Topical

Use Treatment of recurrent herpes labialis (cold sores)

General Dosage Range Topical: *Children ≥12 years and Adults:* Apply 5 times/day

Dosage Forms

Cream, topical:

Xerese®: Acyclovir 5% and hydrocortisone 1% (5 g)

ACZ885 *see* canakinumab *on page* 168

Aczone® *see* dapsone (topical) *on page* 254

Aczone™ (Can) *see* dapsone (topical) *on page* 254

AD32 *see* valrubicin *on page* 935

Adacel® *see* diphtheria and tetanus toxoids, and acellular pertussis vaccine *on page* 298

Adacel®-Polio (Can) *see* diphtheria and tetanus toxoids, acellular pertussis, and poliovirus vaccine *on page* 296

Adagen® *see* pegademase (bovine) *on page* 695

Adalat® XL® (Can) *see* nifedipine *on page* 641

Adalat® CC *see* nifedipine *on page 641*

adalimumab (a da LIM yoo mab)

Medication Safety Issues

Sound-alike/look-alike issues:

Humira® may be confused with Humulin®, Humalog®

Humira® Pen may be confused with HumaPen® Memoir®

Synonyms antitumor necrosis factor alpha (human); D2E7; human antitumor necrosis factor alpha

U.S. Brand Names Humira®; Humira® Pen

Canadian Brand Names Humira®

Therapeutic Category Antirheumatic, Disease Modifying; Monoclonal Antibody

Use

Treatment of active rheumatoid arthritis (moderate-to-severe) and active psoriatic arthritis; may be used alone or in combination with disease-modifying antirheumatic drugs (DMARDs); treatment of ankylosing spondylitis

Treatment of moderately- to severely-active Crohn disease in patients with inadequate response to conventional treatment, or patients who have lost response to or are intolerant of infliximab

Treatment of moderate-to-severe plaque psoriasis

Treatment of moderately- to severely-active juvenile idiopathic arthritis

General Dosage Range SubQ:

Children ≥4 years: 15 kg to <30 kg: 20 mg every other week; ≥30 kg: 40 mg every other week

Adults: Initial: 80-160 mg; Maintenance: 40 mg every other week (maximum: 40 mg every week)

Dosage Forms

Injection, solution [preservative free]:

Humira®: 20 mg/0.4 mL (0.4 mL); 40 mg/0.8 mL (0.8 mL)

Humira® Pen: 40 mg/0.8 mL (0.8 mL)

adamantanamine hydrochloride *see* amantadine *on page 58*

adapalene (a DAP a leen)

U.S. Brand Names Differin®

Canadian Brand Names Differin®; Differin® XP

Therapeutic Category Acne Products

Use Treatment of acne vulgaris

General Dosage Range Topical: *Children >12 years and Adults:* Apply once daily at bedtime

Dosage Forms

Cream, topical: 0.1% (45 g)

Differin®: 0.1% (45 g)

Gel, topical: 0.1% (45 g)

Differin®: 0.1% (45 g); 0.3% (45 g)

Lotion, topical:

Differin®: 0.1% (59 mL)

adapalene and benzoyl peroxide (a DAP a leen & BEN zoe il peer OKS ide)

Synonyms benzoyl peroxide and adapalene

U.S. Brand Names Epiduo®

Canadian Brand Names Tactuo™

Therapeutic Category Acne Products; Topical Skin Product; Topical Skin Product, Acne

Use Topical treatment of acne vulgaris

General Dosage Range Topical: *Children ≥12 years and Adults:* Apply once daily

Dosage Forms

Gel, topical:

Epiduo®: Adapalene 0.1% and benzoyl peroxide 2.5% (45 g)

Adcetris™ *see* brentuximab vedotin *on page 140*

Adcirca® *see* tadalafil *on page 866*

ADD 234037 *see* lacosamide *on page 517*

Addaprin [OTC] *see* ibuprofen *on page 468*

Adderall® *see* dextroamphetamine and amphetamine *on page 271*

Adderall XR® *see* dextroamphetamine and amphetamine *on page 271*

adefovir (a DEF o veer)

Synonyms adefovir dipivoxil; bis-POM PMEA

U.S. Brand Names Hepsera®

Canadian Brand Names Hepsera™

Therapeutic Category Antiretroviral Agent, Nonnucleoside Reverse Transcriptase Inhibitor (NNRTI)

Use Treatment of chronic hepatitis B with evidence of active viral replication (based on persistent elevation of ALT/AST or histologic evidence), including patients with lamivudine-resistant hepatitis B

General Dosage Range Dosage adjustment recommended in patients with renal impairment

Oral: *Children ≥12 years and Adults:* 10 mg once daily

Dosage Forms

Tablet, oral:

Hepsera®: 10 mg

adefovir dipivoxil *see* adefovir *on page 37*

ADEKs® [OTC] *see* vitamins (multiple/pediatric) *on page 952*

Adenocard® (Can) *see* adenosine *on page 37*

Adenocard® IV *see* adenosine *on page 37*

Adenoscan® *see* adenosine *on page 37*

adenosine (a DEN oh seen)

Medication Safety Issues

High alert medication:

The Institute for Safe Medication Practices (ISMP) includes this medication among its list of drugs which have a heightened risk of causing significant patient harm when used in error.

Synonyms 9-beta-d-ribofuranosyladenine

U.S. Brand Names Adenocard® IV; Adenoscan®

Canadian Brand Names Adenocard®; Adenosine Injection, USP; PMS-Adenosine

Therapeutic Category Antiarrhythmic Agent, Class IV; Diagnostic Agent

Use

Adenocard®: Treatment of paroxysmal supraventricular tachycardia (PSVT) including that associated with accessory bypass tracts (Wolff-Parkinson-White syndrome); when clinically advisable, appropriate vagal maneuvers should be attempted prior to adenosine administration; **not effective for conversion of atrial fibrillation, atrial flutter, or ventricular tachycardia**

Adenoscan®: Pharmacologic stress agent used in myocardial perfusion thallium-201 scintigraphy

General Dosage Range I.V.:

Children <50 kg: Initial: 0.05-0.1 mg/kg/dose (maximum initial dose: 6 mg); repeat: 0.05-0.3 mg/kg/dose (maximum: 0.3 mg/kg/dose or 12 mg/dose)

Children ≥50 kg and Adults: Initial: 6 mg; if not effective, 12 mg may be given; may repeat 12 mg if needed (maximum: 12 mg/dose)

Dosage Forms

Injection, solution [preservative free]: 3 mg/mL (2 mL, 4 mL)

Adenocard® IV: 3 mg/mL (2 mL, 4 mL)

Adenoscan®: 3 mg/mL (20 mL, 30 mL)

Adenosine Injection, USP (Can) *see* adenosine *on page 37*

adenovirus type 4 and type 7 vaccine *see* adenovirus (types 4, 7) vaccine *on page 37*

adenovirus (types 4, 7) vaccine (ad e noh VYE rus typs for SEV en vak SEEN)

Synonyms adenovirus type 4 and type 7 vaccine; adenovirus vaccine; adenovirus vaccine (types 4 and 7); type 4 and type 7 adenovirus vaccine

Therapeutic Category Vaccine, Live (Viral)

Use Prevention of acute febrile respiratory disease caused by adenovirus types 4 and 7 (approved for use in military populations)

General Dosage Range Oral: *Adolescents ≥17 years and Adults ≤50 years:* One tablet each of type 4 and type 7 as a single vaccine dose

Dosage Forms

Tablet, enteric coated, oral [combination package]:

Adenovirus type 4 ≥4.5 log_{10} $TCID_{50}$ [contains albumin (human); 100 white tablets]

Adenovirus type 7 ≥4.5 log_{10} $TCID_{50}$ [contains albumin (human); 100 white tablets]

adenovirus vaccine *see* adenovirus (types 4, 7) vaccine *on page 37*
adenovirus vaccine (types 4 and 7) *see* adenovirus (types 4, 7) vaccine *on page 37*
ADH *see* vasopressin *on page 940*
Adipex-P® *see* phentermine *on page 714*
A&D Jr. [OTC] *see* vitamin A and vitamin D (systemic) *on page 949*
ADL-2698 *see* alvimopan *on page 57*
Adoxa® *see* doxycycline *on page 314*
Adrenalin® *see* epinephrine (nasal) *on page 335*
Adrenalin® *see* epinephrine (systemic, oral inhalation) *on page 334*
adrenaline *see* epinephrine (nasal) *on page 335*
adrenaline *see* epinephrine (systemic, oral inhalation) *on page 334*
adrenocorticotropic hormone *see* corticotropin *on page 237*
ADR (error-prone abbreviation) *see* doxorubicin *on page 313*
AdreView™ *see* iobenguane I 123 *on page 493*
Adria *see* doxorubicin *on page 313*
Adriamycin® *see* doxorubicin *on page 313*
Adrucil® *see* fluorouracil (systemic) *on page 395*
adsorbent charcoal *see* charcoal, activated *on page 193*
Advagraf® (Can) *see* tacrolimus (systemic) *on page 865*
Advair® (Can) *see* fluticasone and salmeterol *on page 401*
Advair Diskus® *see* fluticasone and salmeterol *on page 401*
Advair® HFA *see* fluticasone and salmeterol *on page 401*
Advanced Eye Relief™ Dry Eye Environmental [OTC] *see* artificial tears *on page 93*
Advanced Eye Relief™ Dry Eye Rejuvenation [OTC] *see* artificial tears *on page 93*
Advate *see* antihemophilic factor (recombinant) *on page 78*
Advicor® *see* niacin and lovastatin *on page 639*
Advil® [OTC] *see* ibuprofen *on page 468*
Advil® (Can) *see* ibuprofen *on page 468*
Advil® Allergy Sinus *see* ibuprofen, pseudoephedrine, and chlorpheniramine *on page 470*
Advil® Children's [OTC] *see* ibuprofen *on page 468*
Advil® Cold and Sinus Nighttime (Can) *see* ibuprofen, pseudoephedrine, and chlorpheniramine *on page 470*
Advil® Cold and Sinus Plus (Can) *see* ibuprofen, pseudoephedrine, and chlorpheniramine *on page 470*
Advil® Cold & Sinus [OTC] *see* pseudoephedrine and ibuprofen *on page 773*
Advil® Cold & Sinus (Can) *see* pseudoephedrine and ibuprofen *on page 773*
Advil® Cold & Sinus Daytime (Can) *see* pseudoephedrine and ibuprofen *on page 773*
Advil® Infants' [OTC] *see* ibuprofen *on page 468*
Advil® Migraine [OTC] *see* ibuprofen *on page 468*
Advil® Multi-Symptom Cold *see* ibuprofen, pseudoephedrine, and chlorpheniramine *on page 470*
Aerius® (Can) *see* desloratadine *on page 263*
Aerius® Kids (Can) *see* desloratadine *on page 263*
Afeditab® CR *see* nifedipine *on page 641*
Afinitor® *see* everolimus *on page 367*
Afinitor® Disperz *see* everolimus *on page 367*

aflibercept (ophthalmic) (a FLIB er sept)

Medication Safety Issues

Sound-alike/look-alike issues:

Aflibercept may be confused with Ziv-aflibercept

Synonyms AVE 0005; AVE 005; AVE-0005; VEGF trap; VEGF trap-eye
U.S. Brand Names Eylea™
Therapeutic Category Ophthalmic Agent; Vascular Endothelial Growth Factor (VEGF) Inhibitor
Use Treatment of neovascular (wet) age-related macular degeneration (AMD)
General Dosage Range Intravitreal: *Adults:* 2 mg (0.05 mL) every 4-8 weeks
Dosage Forms
Injection, solution, intravitreal [preservative free]:
Eylea™: 40 mg/mL (0.05 mL)

aflibercept I.V. *see* ziv-aflibercept (systemic) *on page 964*
Afluria® *see* influenza virus vaccine (inactivated) *on page 482*
A-Free Prenatal [OTC] *see* vitamins (multiple/prenatal) *on page 952*
Afrin® Extra Moisturizing [OTC] *see* oxymetazoline (nasal) *on page 681*
Afrin® Original [OTC] *see* oxymetazoline (nasal) *on page 681*
Afrin® Severe Congestion [OTC] *see* oxymetazoline (nasal) *on page 681*
Afrin® Sinus [OTC] *see* oxymetazoline (nasal) *on page 681*
AG-013736 *see* axitinib *on page 105*

agalsidase alfa *(Canada only)* (aye GAL si days AL fa)

Medication Safety Issues
Sound-alike/look-alike issues:
Agalsidase alfa may be confused with agalsidase beta, alglucerase, alglucosidase alfa
Synonyms agalsidase alpha; alpha-galactosidase-A (gene-activated)
Canadian Brand Names Replagal®
Therapeutic Category Enzyme
Use Replacement therapy for Fabry disease
General Dosage Range I.V.: *Children and Adults:* 0.2 mg/kg every 2 weeks
Product Availability Not available in U.S.
Dosage Forms - Canada
Injection, solution [preservative free]:
Replagal™: 1 mg/1 mL (3.5 mL)

agalsidase alpha *see* agalsidase alfa *(Canada only) on page 39*

agalsidase beta (aye GAL si days BAY ta)

Medication Safety Issues
Sound-alike/look-alike issues:
Agalsidase beta may be confused with agalsidase alfa, alglucerase, alglucosidase alfa
Synonyms alpha-galactosidase-A (recombinant); r-h α-GAL
U.S. Brand Names Fabrazyme®
Canadian Brand Names Fabrazyme®
Therapeutic Category Enzyme
Use Replacement therapy for Fabry disease
General Dosage Range I.V.: *Children ≥8 years and Adults:* 1 mg/kg every 2 weeks
Dosage Forms
Injection, powder for reconstitution:
Fabrazyme®: 5 mg, 35 mg

Aggrastat® *see* tirofiban *on page 900*
Aggrenox® *see* aspirin and dipyridamole *on page 98*
AGN 1135 *see* rasagiline *on page 789*
$AgNO_3$ *see* silver nitrate *on page 833*
Agriflu™ (Can) *see* influenza virus vaccine (inactivated) *on page 482*
Agrylin® *see* anagrelide *on page 74*
AHA *see* acetohydroxamic acid *on page 31*
AHF (human) *see* antihemophilic factor (human) *on page 78*
AHF (human) *see* antihemophilic factor/von Willebrand factor complex (human) *on page 78*

albendazole (al BEN da zole)

Medication Safety Issues

Sound-alike/look-alike issues:

Albenza® may be confused with Aplenzin™, Relenza®

International issues:

Albenza [U.S.] may be confused with Avanza brand name for mirtazapine [Australia]

U.S. Brand Names Albenza®

Therapeutic Category Anthelmintic

Use Treatment of parenchymal neurocysticercosis caused by *Taenia solium* and cystic hydatid disease of the liver, lung, and peritoneum caused by *Echinococcus granulosus*

General Dosage Range Oral:

Children and Adults <60 kg: 15 mg/kg/day in 2 divided doses (maximum: 800 mg/day)

Children and Adults ≥60 kg: 800 mg/day in 2 divided doses (maximum: 800 mg/day)

Dosage Forms

Tablet, oral:

Albenza®: 200 mg

albumin (al BYOO min)

Medication Safety Issues

Sound-alike/look-alike issues:

Albutein® may be confused with albuterol

Buminate® may be confused with bumetanide

Synonyms albumin (human); normal human serum albumin; normal serum albumin (human); salt-poor albumin; SPA

U.S. Brand Names Albuked™ 25; Albuked™ 5; Albuminar®-25; Albuminar®-5; AlbuRx® 25; AlbuRx® 5; Albutein®; Buminate; Flexbumin 25%; Human Albumin Grifols® 25%; Kedbumin™; Plasbumin®-25; Plasbumin®-5

Canadian Brand Names Alburex® 25; Alburex® 5; Albutein 25%; Albutein 5%; Buminate-25%; Buminate-5%; Plasbumin®-25; Plasbumin®-5

Therapeutic Category Blood Product Derivative

Use Plasma volume expansion and maintenance of cardiac output in the treatment of certain types of shock or impending shock; may be useful for burn patients, ARDS, and cardiopulmonary bypass; other uses considered by some investigators (but not proven) are retroperitoneal surgery, peritonitis, and ascites; unless the condition responsible for hypoproteinemia can be corrected, albumin can provide only symptomatic relief or supportive treatment

Note: Nutritional supplementation is not an appropriate indication.

General Dosage Range I.V.:

Children: 0.5-1 g/kg/dose (10-20 mL/kg/dose) as needed

Adults: 0.5-1 g/kg/dose as needed **or** 25 g/dose may repeat in 15-30 minutes if response inadequate (maximum: 250 g/48 hours)

Dosage Forms

Injection, solution [preservative free]: 5% [50 mg/mL] (250 mL, 500 mL); 20% [200 mg/mL] (50 mL, 100 mL); 25% [250 mg/mL] (50 mL, 100 mL)

Albuked™ 5: 5% [50 mg/mL] (250 mL)

Albuked™ 25: 25% [250 mg/mL] (50 mL)

Albuminar®-5: 5% [50 mg/mL] (250 mL, 500 mL)

Albuminar®-25: 25% [250 mg/mL] (50 mL, 100 mL)

AlbuRx® 5: 5% [50 mg/mL] (250 mL, 500 mL)

AlbuRx® 25: 25% [250 mg/mL] (50 mL, 100 mL)

Albutein®: 5% [50 mg/mL] (250 mL, 500 mL); 25% [250 mg/mL] (50 mL, 100 mL)

Buminate: 5% [50 mg/mL] (250 mL, 500 mL); 25% [250 mg/mL] (20 mL)

Flexbumin 25%: 25% [250 mg/mL] (50 mL, 100 mL)

Human Albumin Grifols® 25%: 25% [250 mg/mL] (50 mL, 100 mL)

Kedbumin™: 25% [250 mg/mL] (50 mL)

Plasbumin®-5: 5% [50 mg/mL] (50 mL, 250 mL)

Plasbumin®-25: 25% [250 mg/mL] (20 mL, 50 mL, 100 mL)

^{131}I-albumin *see* iodinated I 131 albumin *on page* 493

Albuminar®-5 *see* albumin *on page* 41

Albuminar®-25 *see* albumin *on page* 41

albumin-bound paclitaxel *see* paclitaxel (protein bound) *on page* 684

albumin (human) *see* albumin *on page* 41

albumin-stabilized nanoparticle paclitaxel *see* paclitaxel (protein bound) *on page* 684

Alburex® 5 (Can) *see* albumin *on page* 41

Alburex® 25 (Can) *see* albumin *on page* 41

AlbuRx® 5 *see* albumin *on page* 41

AlbuRx® 25 *see* albumin *on page* 41

Albutein® *see* albumin *on page* 41

Albutein 5% (Can) *see* albumin *on page* 41

Albutein 25% (Can) *see* albumin *on page* 41

albuterol (al BYOO ter ole)

Medication Safety Issues

Sound-alike/look-alike issues:

Albuterol may be confused with Albutein®, atenolol

Proventil® may be confused with Bentyl®, PriLOSEC®, Prinivil®
Salbutamol may be confused with salmeterol
Ventolin® may be confused with phentolamine, Benylin®, Vantin

Synonyms albuterol sulfate; salbutamol; salbutamol sulphate

U.S. Brand Names AccuNeb®; ProAir® HFA; Proventil® HFA; Ventolin® HFA; VoSpire ER®

Canadian Brand Names Airomir; Apo-Salvent®; Apo-Salvent® AEM; Apo-Salvent® CFC Free; Apo-Salvent® Sterules; Dom-Salbutamol; Mylan-Salbutamol Respirator Solution; Mylan-Salbutamol Sterinebs P.F.; Novo-Salbutamol HFA; Nu-Salbutamol; PHL-Salbutamol; PMS-Salbutamol; ratio-Ipra-Sal; ratio-Salbutamol; Sandoz-Salbutamol; Teva-Salbutamol; Ventolin®; Ventolin® Diskus; Ventolin® HFA; Ventolin® I.V. Infusion; Ventolin® Nebules P.F.

Therapeutic Category Adrenergic Agonist Agent

Use Treatment or prevention of bronchospasm in patients with reversible obstructive airway disease; prevention of exercise-induced bronchospasm

General Dosage Range

Inhalation via metered-dose inhaler (90 mcg/puff): *Children and Adults:* 2 puffs every 4-6 hours **or** 4-8 puffs every 1-4 hours [acute symptoms] **or** 1-2 puffs prior to exercise

Nebulization:

Children <12 years: 0.15-0.3 mg/kg (maximum: 10 mg) every 1-4 hours **or** 0.63-1.25 mg 3-4 times/day **or** 0.5 mg/kg/hour by continuous nebulization

Children ≥12 years: 2.5-10 mg every 1-4 hours **or** 10-15 mg/hour by continuous nebulization

Adults: 2.5-10 mg every 1-4 hours **or** 10-15 mg/hour by continuous nebulization

Oral:

Regular release:

Children 2-6 years: 0.1-0.2 mg/kg/dose 3 times/day (maximum: 12 mg/day)

Children 6-12 years: 2 mg/dose 3-4 times/day (maximum: 24 mg/day)

Children >12 years and Adults: 2-4 mg/dose 3-4 times/day (maximum: 32 mg/day)

Extended release:

Children 6-12 years: 4 mg every 12 hours (maximum: 24 mg/day)

Children >12 years and Adults: 8 mg every 12 hours (maximum: 32 mg/day)

Dosage Forms

Aerosol, for oral inhalation:

ProAir® HFA: 90 mcg/inhalation (8.5 g)

Proventil® HFA: 90 mcg/inhalation (6.7 g)

Ventolin® HFA: 90 mcg/inhalation (8 g, 18 g)

Solution, for nebulization: 0.083% [2.5 mg/3 mL] (25s, 30s, 60s); 0.5% [100 mg/20 mL] (1s)

Solution, for nebulization [preservative free]: 0.021% [0.63 mg/3 mL] (25s); 0.042% [1.25 mg/3 mL] (25s, 30s); 0.083% [2.5 mg/3 mL] (10s, 24s, 25s, 30s, 60s); 0.5% [2.5 mg/0.5 mL] (10s, 30s)

AccuNeb®: 0.021% [0.63 mg/3 mL] (25s); 0.042% [1.25 mg/3 mL] (25s)

Syrup, oral: 2 mg/5 mL (473 mL, 480 mL)

Tablet, oral: 2 mg, 4 mg

Tablet, extended release, oral: 4 mg, 8 mg

VoSpire ER®: 4 mg, 8 mg

Dosage Forms - Canada

Injection, solution:

Ventolin® I.V.: 1 mg/1mL (5 mL)

albuterol and ipratropium *see* ipratropium and albuterol *on page* 499

albuterol sulfate *see* albuterol *on page* 41

alcaftadine (al KAF ta deen)

U.S. Brand Names Lastacaft™

Therapeutic Category Histamine H_1 Antagonist; Mast Cell Stabilizer

Use Prevention of itching associated with allergic conjunctivitis

General Dosage Range Ophthalmic: *Children ≥2 years and Adults:* Instill 1 drop into each eye once daily

Dosage Forms

Solution, ophthalmic:

Lastacaft™: 0.25% (3 mL)

Alcaine® *see* proparacaine *on page* 766

Alcalak [OTC] *see* calcium carbonate *on page* 161

alclometasone (al kloe MET a sone)

Medication Safety Issues

Sound-alike/look-alike issues:

Aclovate® may be confused with Accolate®

International issues:

Cloderm: Brand name for alclometasone [Indonesia], but also brand name for clobetasol [China, India, Malaysia, Singapore, Thailand]; clocortolone [U.S., Canada]; clotrimazole [Germany]

Synonyms alclometasone dipropionate

U.S. Brand Names Aclovate®

Therapeutic Category Corticosteroid, Topical

Use Treatment of inflammation of corticosteroid-responsive dermatosis (low-to-medium potency topical corticosteroid)

General Dosage Range Topical: *Children ≥1 year and Adults:* Apply a thin film to the affected area 2-3 times/day

Dosage Forms

Cream, topical: 0.05% (15 g, 45 g, 60 g)

Aclovate®: 0.05% (15 g, 60 g)

Ointment, topical: 0.05% (15 g, 45 g, 60 g)

Aclovate®: 0.05% (15 g, 60 g)

alclometasone dipropionate *see* alclometasone *on page 43*

alcohol, absolute *see* alcohol (ethyl) *on page 43*

alcohol, dehydrated *see* alcohol (ethyl) *on page 43*

alcohol (ethyl) (AL koe hol, ETH il)

Medication Safety Issues

Sound-alike/look-alike issues:

Ethanol may be confused with Ethyol®, Ethamolin®

Synonyms alcohol, absolute; alcohol, dehydrated; ethanol; ethyl alcohol; EtOH

U.S. Brand Names Epi-Clenz™ [OTC]; Gel-Stat™ [OTC]; GelRite™ [OTC]; Isagel® [OTC]; Lavacol® [OTC]; Prevacare® [OTC]; Protection Plus® [OTC]; Purell® 2 in 1 [OTC]; Purell® Lasting Care [OTC]; Purell® Moisture Therapy [OTC]; Purell® with Aloe [OTC]; Purell® [OTC]

Canadian Brand Names Biobase-G™; Biobase™

Therapeutic Category Intravenous Nutritional Therapy; Pharmaceutical Aid

Use Topical antiinfective; pharmaceutical aid; therapeutic neurolysis (nerve or ganglion block); replenishment of carbohydrate calories

General Dosage Range

I.V.:

Infusion: *Adults:* Dosage varies depending on indication

Intraneural: *Adults:* Dosage varies depending on indication

Topical: *Children and Adults:* Apply 1-3 times/day as needed

Dosage Forms

Aerosol, foam, topical:

Epi-Clenz™ [OTC]: 70% (240 mL)

Gel, topical: 62% (1.5 mL, 118 mL, 354 mL, 473 mL)

Epi-Clenz™ [OTC]: 70% (45 mL, 120 mL, 480 mL)

Gel-Stat™ [OTC]: 62% (120 mL, 480 mL)

GelRite™ [OTC]: 67% (120 mL, 480 mL, 800 mL)

Isagel® [OTC]: 60% (59 mL, 118 mL, 621 mL, 800 mL)

Prevacare® [OTC]: 60% (120 mL, 240 mL, 960 mL, 1200 mL, 1500 mL)

Purell® [OTC]: 62% (15 mL, 30 mL, 59 mL, 60 mL, 120 mL, 236 mL, 240 mL, 250 mL, 360 mL, 500 mL, 800 mL, 1000 mL, 2000 mL)

Purell® Lasting Care [OTC]: 62% (120 mL, 240 mL, 1000 mL)

Purell® Moisture Therapy [OTC]: 62% (75 mL)

Purell® with Aloe [OTC]: 62% (15 mL, 59 mL, 60 mL, 120 mL, 236 mL, 354 mL, 800 mL, 1000 mL, 2000 mL)

Injection, solution [preservative free]: ≥ 98% (1 mL, 5 mL)

Liquid, topical: 70% (480 mL, 3840 mL)

Lavacol® [OTC]: 70% (473 mL)

Lotion, topical:
Purell® 2 in 1 [OTC]: 62% (60 mL, 360 mL, 1000 mL)
Pad, topical:
Isagel® [OTC]: 60% (50s, 300s)
Purell® [OTC]: 62% (24s, 35s, 175s)
Solution, topical:
Protection Plus® [OTC]: 62% (800 mL)

Alcortin® A *see* iodoquinol and hydrocortisone *on page 495*

Aldactazide® *see* hydrochlorothiazide and spironolactone *on page 453*

Aldactazide 25® (Can) *see* hydrochlorothiazide and spironolactone *on page 453*

Aldactazide 50® (Can) *see* hydrochlorothiazide and spironolactone *on page 453*

Aldactone® *see* spironolactone *on page 852*

Aldara® *see* imiquimod *on page 476*

aldesleukin (al des LOO kin)

Medication Safety Issues

Sound-alike/look-alike issues:
Aldesleukin may be confused with oprelvekin
Proleukin® may be confused with oprelvekin

High alert medication:
The Institute for Safe Medication Practices (ISMP) includes this medication among its list of drug classes which have a heightened risk of causing significant patient harm when used in error.

Synonyms IL-2; interleukin 2; interleukin-2; lymphocyte mitogenic factor; recombinant human interleukin-2; T-cell growth factor; TCGF; thymocyte stimulating factor

U.S. Brand Names Proleukin®

Canadian Brand Names Proleukin®

Therapeutic Category Biological Response Modulator

Use Treatment of metastatic renal cell cancer, metastatic melanoma

General Dosage Range Dosage adjustment recommended in patients who develop toxicities
I.V.: *Adults:* 600,000 units/kg every 8 hours (maximum: 14 doses); may repeat after 9 days for a total of 28 doses/course

Dosage Forms
Injection, powder for reconstitution:
Proleukin®: 22 x 10^6 units

Aldex® AN *see* doxylamine *on page 315*

Aldex® CT *see* diphenhydramine and phenylephrine *on page 294*

Aldomet *see* methyldopa *on page 588*

Aldoril *see* methyldopa and hydrochlorothiazide *on page 588*

Aldroxicon I [OTC] *see* aluminum hydroxide, magnesium hydroxide, and simethicone *on page 56*

Aldroxicon II [OTC] *see* aluminum hydroxide, magnesium hydroxide, and simethicone *on page 56*

Aldurazyme® *see* laronidase *on page 524*

alefacept (a LE fa sept)

Synonyms B 9273; BG 9273; human LFA-3/IgG(1) fusion protein; LFA-3/IgG(1) fusion protein, human

U.S. Brand Names Amevive® [DSC]

Canadian Brand Names Amevive®

Therapeutic Category Monoclonal Antibody

Use Treatment of moderate-to-severe chronic plaque psoriasis in adults who are candidates for systemic therapy or phototherapy

General Dosage Range I.M.: *Adults:* 15 mg once weekly

Dosage Forms
Injection, powder for reconstitution:
Amevive®: 15 mg

alemtuzumab (ay lem TU zoo mab)

Medication Safety Issues

High alert medication:

This medication is in a class the Institute for Safe Medication Practices (ISMP) includes among its list of drug classes which have a heightened risk of causing significant patient harm when used in error.

Synonyms anti-CD52 monoclonal antibody; campath-1H; humanized IgG1 anti-CD52 monoclonal antibody; MoAb CD52; monoclonal antibody campath-1H; monoclonal antibody CD52

U.S. Brand Names Campath® [DSC]

Canadian Brand Names MabCampath®

Therapeutic Category Antineoplastic Agent, Monoclonal Antibody

Use Campath®: Treatment (as a single agent) of B-cell chronic lymphocytic leukemia (B-CLL)

General Dosage Range Dosage adjustment recommended in patients who develop toxicities

I.V. (infusion): *Adults:* Initial: 3 mg/day, then 10 mg/day; Maintenance: 30 mg/day 3 times/week on alternate days; Maximum dose: 30 mg/day; 90 mg/week (cumulative)

alendronate (a LEN droe nate)

Medication Safety Issues

Sound-alike/look-alike issues:

Alendronate may be confused with risedronate

Fosamax® may be confused with Flomax®, Fosamax Plus D®, fosinopril, Zithromax®

International issues:

Fosamax [U.S., Canada, and multiple international markets] may be confused with Fisamox brand name for amoxicillin [Australia]

Synonyms alendronate sodium; alendronic acid monosodium salt trihydrate; MK-217

U.S. Brand Names Binosto™; Fosamax®

Canadian Brand Names Alendronate-FC; Apo-Alendronate®; CO Alendronate; Dom-Alendronate; Fosamax®; JAMP-Alendronate; Mylan-Alendronate; PHL-Alendronate; PMS-Alendronate; PMS-Alendronate-FC; Q-Alendronate; ratio-Alendronate; Riva-Alendronate; Sandoz-Alendronate; Teva-Alendronate

Therapeutic Category Bisphosphonate Derivative

Use Treatment and prevention of osteoporosis in postmenopausal females; treatment of osteoporosis in males; Paget disease of the bone in patients who are symptomatic, at risk for future complications, or with alkaline phosphatase ≥2 times the upper limit of normal; treatment of glucocorticoid-induced osteoporosis in males and females with low bone mineral density who are receiving a daily dosage ≥7.5 mg of prednisone (or equivalent)

General Dosage Range Oral: *Adults:* 5-10 mg/day **or** 35-70 mg once weekly (maximum: 70 mg/week) **or** 40 mg once daily [Paget disease]

Dosage Forms

Tablet, oral: 5 mg, 10 mg, 35 mg, 40 mg, 70 mg

Fosamax®: 70 mg

Tablet for solution, oral:

Binosto™: 70 mg

alendronate and cholecalciferol (a LEN droe nate & kole e kal SI fer ole)

Medication Safety Issues

Sound-alike/look-alike issues:

Fosamax Plus D® may be confused with Fosamax®

Synonyms alendronate sodium and cholecalciferol; cholecalciferol and alendronate; vitamin D_3 and alendronate

U.S. Brand Names Fosamax Plus D®

Canadian Brand Names Fosavance

Therapeutic Category Bisphosphonate Derivative; Vitamin D Analog

Use Treatment of osteoporosis in postmenopausal females; increase bone mass in males with osteoporosis

General Dosage Range Oral: *Adults:* One tablet (alendronate 70 mg/cholecalciferol 2800-5600 units) once weekly

Dosage Forms

Tablet:

Fosamax Plus D® 70/2800: Alendronate 70 mg and cholecalciferol 2800 units

Fosamax Plus D® 70/5600: Alendronate 70 mg and cholecalciferol 5600 units

Alendronate-FC (Can) *see* alendronate *on page* 45

alendronate sodium *see* alendronate *on page* 45

alendronate sodium and cholecalciferol *see* alendronate and cholecalciferol *on page* 45

alendronic acid monosodium salt trihydrate *see* alendronate *on page* 45

Aler-Cap [OTC] *see* diphenhydramine (systemic) *on page* 292

Aler-Dryl [OTC] *see* diphenhydramine (systemic) *on page* 292

Aler-Tab [OTC] *see* diphenhydramine (systemic) *on page* 292

Alertec® (Can) *see* modafinil *on page* 609

Alesse® (Can) *see* ethinyl estradiol and levonorgestrel *on page* 357

Aleve® [OTC] *see* naproxen *on page* 628

Aleve®-D Sinus & Cold [OTC] *see* naproxen and pseudoephedrine *on page* 629

Aleve®-D Sinus & Headache [OTC] *see* naproxen and pseudoephedrine *on page* 629

1alfacalcidol *see* alfacalcidol *(Canada only) on page* 46

alfacalcidol *(Canada only)* (Al fa CAL ce dol)

Medication Safety Issues

Sound-alike/look-alike issues:

Alfacalcidol may be confused with calcitriol, cholecalciferol, ergocalciferol, paricalcitol

Synonyms 1-α-hydroxycholecalciferol; 1-α-hydroxyvitamin D_3; 1alfacalcidol; $_1$alfa-hydroxyvitamin D3

Canadian Brand Names One-Alpha®

Therapeutic Category Vitamin D Analog

Use Management of hypocalcemia, secondary hyperparathyroidism, and osteodystrophy in patients with chronic renal failure

General Dosage Range Individualize dosage:

Oral: *Adults:* 0.25-3 mcg/day

I.V.: *Adults:* 1-12 mcg/week (with dialysis)

Product Availability Not available in the U.S.

Dosage Forms - Canada

Capsule, softgel, oral:

One-Alpha®: 0.25 mcg, 1 mcg [contains sesame oil]

Injection, solution:

One-Alpha®: 2 mcg/mL

Solution, oral [drops]:

One-Alpha®: 2 mcg/mL

$_1$alfa-hydroxyvitamin D3 *see* alfacalcidol *(Canada only) on page* 46

Alfenta® *see* alfentanil *on page* 46

alfentanil (al FEN ta nil)

Medication Safety Issues

Sound-alike/look-alike issues:

Alfentanil may be confused with Anafranil®, fentanyl, remifentanil, sufentanil

Alfenta® may be confused with Sufenta®

High alert medication:

The Institute for Safe Medication Practices (ISMP) includes this medication among its list of drug classes which have a heightened risk of causing significant patient harm when used in error.

Synonyms alfentanil hydrochloride

U.S. Brand Names Alfenta®

Canadian Brand Names Alfentanil Injection, USP; Alfenta®

Therapeutic Category Analgesic, Narcotic; General Anesthetic

Controlled Substance C-II

Use Analgesic adjunct for the induction and maintenance of general anesthesia; analgesic component for monitored anesthesia care (MAC)

General Dosage Range I.V.:
Anesthetic induction: *Children ≥12 years and Adults:* Initial: 130-245 mcg/kg; Maintenance: 0.5-1.5 mcg/kg/minute
Continuous infusion: *Children ≥12 years and Adults:* Initial: 50-75 mcg/kg; Maintenance: 0.5-3 mcg/kg/minute
Incremental injection: *Children ≥12 years and Adults:*
≤30 minutes anesthesia: Initial: 8-20 mcg/kg; Maintenance: 3-5 mcg/kg **or** 0.5-1 mcg/kg/minute (maximum: 40 mcg/kg total dose)
≥30 minutes anesthesia: Initial: 20-50 mcg/kg; Maintenance: 5-15 mcg/kg (maximum: 75 mcg/kg total dose)

Dosage Forms
Injection, solution [preservative free]: 500 mcg/mL (2 mL, 5 mL, 10 mL, 20 mL)
Alfenta®: 500 mcg/mL (2 mL, 5 mL)

alfentanil hydrochloride *see* alfentanil *on page 46*

Alfentanil Injection, USP (Can) *see* alfentanil *on page 46*

Alferon® N *see* interferon alfa-n3 *on page 491*

alfuzosin (al FYOO zoe sin)

Synonyms alfuzosin hydrochloride
U.S. Brand Names Uroxatral®
Canadian Brand Names Apo-Alfuzosin®; Sandoz-Alfuzosin; Teva-Alfuzosin PR; Xatral
Therapeutic Category Alpha-Adrenergic Blocking Agent
Use Treatment of the functional symptoms of benign prostatic hyperplasia (BPH)
General Dosage Range Oral: *Adults:* 10 mg once daily
Dosage Forms
Tablet, extended release, oral: 10 mg
Uroxatral®: 10 mg

alfuzosin hydrochloride *see* alfuzosin *on page 47*

alglucosidase *see* alglucosidase alfa *on page 47*

alglucosidase alfa (al gloo KOSE i dase AL fa)

Medication Safety Issues
Sound-alike/look-alike issues:
Alglucosidase alfa may be confused with agalsidase alfa, agalsidase beta, alglucerase
Synonyms alglucosidase; GAA; rhGAA
U.S. Brand Names Lumizyme®; Myozyme®
Canadian Brand Names Myozyme®
Therapeutic Category Enzyme
Use
Lumizyme™: Replacement therapy for late-onset (noninfantile) Pompe disease without evidence of cardiac hypertrophy in patients 8 years and older
Myozyme®: Replacement therapy for infantile-onset Pompe disease
General Dosage Range I.V.:
Myozyme®: *Children 1 month to 3.5 years:* 20 mg/kg every 2 weeks
Lumizyme™: *Children ≥8 years and Adults:* 20 mg/kg every 2 weeks
Dosage Forms
Injection, powder for reconstitution:
Lumizyme®: 50 mg
Myozyme®: 50 mg

Aliclen™ *see* salicylic acid *on page 816*

Alimta® *see* pemetrexed *on page 700*

Alinia® *see* nitazoxanide *on page 643*

aliskiren (a lis KYE ren)

Medication Safety Issues
Sound-alike/look-alike issues:
Tekturna® may be confused with Valturna®

Synonyms aliskiren hemifumarate; SPP100

U.S. Brand Names Tekturna®

Canadian Brand Names Rasilez®

Therapeutic Category Renin Inhibitor

Use Treatment of hypertension, alone or in combination with other antihypertensive agents

General Dosage Range Oral: *Adults:* 150-300 mg once daily (maximum: 300 mg/day)

Dosage Forms

Tablet, oral:

Tekturna®: 150 mg, 300 mg

aliskiren, amlodipine, and hydrochlorothiazide

(a lis KYE ren, am LOE di peen, & hye droe klor oh THYE a zide)

Medication Safety Issues

Sound-alike/look-alike issues:

Amturnide™ may be confused with AMILoride

Synonyms aliskiren, hydrochlorothiazide, and amlodipine; amlodipine besylate, aliskiren hemifumarate, and hydrochlorothiazide; amlodipine, aliskiren, and hydrochlorothiazide; amlodipine, hydrochlorothiazide, and aliskiren; hydrochlorothiazide, aliskiren, and amlodipine; hydrochlorothiazide, amlodipine, and aliskiren

U.S. Brand Names Amturnide™

Therapeutic Category Calcium Channel Blocker; Calcium Channel Blocker, Dihydropyridine; Diuretic, Thiazide; Renin Inhibitor

Use Treatment of hypertension (not for initial therapy)

General Dosage Range Oral: *Adults:* Aliskiren 150-300 mg and Amlodipine 5-10 mg and Hydrochlorothiazide 12.5-25 mg once daily (maximum recommended daily dose: Aliskiren 300 mg; amlodipine 10 mg; hydrochlorothiazide 25 mg)

Dosage Forms

Tablet, oral:

Amturnide™: Aliskiren 150 mg, amlodipine 5 mg, and hydrochlorothiazide 12.5 mg; Aliskiren 300 mg, amlodipine 5 mg, and hydrochlorothiazide 12.5 mg; Aliskiren 300 mg, amlodipine 5 mg, and hydrochlorothiazide 25 mg; Aliskiren 300 mg, amlodipine 10 mg, and hydrochlorothiazide 12.5 mg; Aliskiren 300 mg, amlodipine 10 mg, and hydrochlorothiazide 25 mg

aliskiren and amlodipine (a lis KYE ren & am LOE di peen)

Synonyms aliskiren hemifumarate and amlodipine besylate; amlodipine and aliskiren

U.S. Brand Names Tekamlo™

Therapeutic Category Calcium Channel Blocker; Calcium Channel Blocker, Dihydropyridine; Renin Inhibitor

Use Treatment of hypertension, alone or in combination with other antihypertensive agents, including use as initial therapy in patients likely to need multiple antihypertensives for adequate control

General Dosage Range Oral: *Adults:* Aliskiren 150-300 mg and amlodipine 5-10 mg once daily (maximum: 300 mg/day [aliskiren]; 10 mg/day [amlodipine])

Dosage Forms

Tablet, oral:

Tekamlo™: 150/5: Aliskiren 150 mg and amlodipine 5 mg, 300/5: Aliskiren 300 mg and amlodipine 5 mg, 150/10: Aliskiren 150 mg and amlodipine 10 mg, 300/10: Aliskiren 300 mg and amlodipine 10 mg

aliskiren and hydrochlorothiazide (a lis KYE ren & hye droe klor oh THYE a zide)

Synonyms aliskiren hemifumarate and hydrochlorothiazide; hydrochlorothiazide and aliskiren

U.S. Brand Names Tekturna HCT®

Canadian Brand Names Rasilez HCT®

Therapeutic Category Antihypertensive Agent, Combination; Diuretic, Thiazide; Renin Inhibitor

Use Treatment of hypertension, including use as initial therapy in patients likely to need multiple antihypertensives for adequate control

General Dosage Range Oral: *Adults:* Aliskiren 150-300 mg and hydrochlorothiazide 12.5-25 mg once daily (maximum: 300 mg/day [aliskiren]; 25 mg/day [hydrochlorothiazide])

Dosage Forms

Tablet:

Tekturna HCT®: 150/12.5: Aliskiren 150 mg and hydrochlorothiazide 12.5 mg; 150/25: Aliskiren 150 mg and hydrochlorothiazide 25 mg; 300/12.5: Aliskiren 300 mg and hydrochlorothiazide 12.5 mg; 300/25: Aliskiren 300 mg and hydrochlorothiazide 25 mg

aliskiren and valsartan (a lis KYE ren & val SAR tan)

Medication Safety Issues

Sound-alike/look-alike issues:

Valturna® may be confused with Tekturna®, valsartan

Synonyms aliskiren hemifumarate and valsartan; valsartan and aliskiren

U.S. Brand Names Valturna® [DSC]

Therapeutic Category Angiotensin II Receptor Blocker; Renin Inhibitor

Use Treatment of hypertension, including use as initial therapy in patients likely to need multiple antihypertensives for adequate control

General Dosage Range Oral: *Adults:* Aliskiren 150-300 mg and valsartan 160-320 mg once daily (maximum: 300 mg/day [aliskiren]; 320 mg/day [valsartan])

aliskiren hemifumarate *see* aliskiren *on page 47*

aliskiren hemifumarate and amlodipine besylate *see* aliskiren and amlodipine *on page 48*

aliskiren hemifumarate and hydrochlorothiazide *see* aliskiren and hydrochlorothiazide *on page 48*

aliskiren hemifumarate and valsartan *see* aliskiren and valsartan *on page 49*

aliskiren, hydrochlorothiazide, and amlodipine *see* aliskiren, amlodipine, and hydrochlorothiazide *on page 48*

alitretinoin (a li TRET i noyn)

Medication Safety Issues

Sound-alike/look-alike issues:

Panretin® may be confused with pancreatin

High alert medication:

The Institute for Safe Medication Practices (ISMP) includes this medication among its list of drugs which have a heightened risk of causing significant patient harm when used in error.

U.S. Brand Names Panretin®

Therapeutic Category Antineoplastic Agent; Retinoic Acid Derivative

Use Orphan drug: Topical treatment of cutaneous lesions in AIDS-related Kaposi sarcoma

General Dosage Range Topical: *Adults:* Apply twice daily

Dosage Forms

Gel, topical:

Panretin®: 0.1% (60 g)

Alka-Mints® [OTC] *see* calcium carbonate *on page 161*

Alka-Seltzer Plus® Day Cold [OTC] *see* acetaminophen, dextromethorphan, and phenylephrine *on page 28*

Alkeran® *see* melphalan *on page 570*

All Day Allergy [OTC] *see* cetirizine *on page 190*

All Day Relief [OTC] *see* naproxen *on page 628*

Allegra® *see* fexofenadine *on page 381*

Allegra-D® (Can) *see* fexofenadine and pseudoephedrine *on page 382*

Allegra-D® 12 Hour *see* fexofenadine and pseudoephedrine *on page 382*

Allegra-D® 24 Hour *see* fexofenadine and pseudoephedrine *on page 382*

Allegra® Allergy 12 Hour [OTC] *see* fexofenadine *on page 381*

Allegra® Allergy 24 Hour [OTC] *see* fexofenadine *on page 381*

Allegra® Children's Allergy [OTC] *see* fexofenadine *on page 381*

Allegra® Children's Allergy ODT [OTC] *see* fexofenadine *on page 381*

Aller-chlor® [OTC] *see* chlorpheniramine *on page 199*

Allerdryl® (Can) *see* diphenhydramine (systemic) *on page 292*

Allerest *see* chlorpheniramine and pseudoephedrine *on page 200*

Allergy Relief [OTC] *see* chlorpheniramine *on page* 199
AllerMax® [OTC] *see* diphenhydramine (systemic) *on page* 292
Allernix (Can) *see* diphenhydramine (systemic) *on page* 292
Aller-Relief [OTC] (Can) *see* cetirizine *on page* 190
Allfen [OTC] *see* guaifenesin *on page* 433
Allfen CD *see* guaifenesin and codeine *on page* 434
Allfen CDX *see* guaifenesin and codeine *on page* 434
Alli® [OTC] *see* orlistat *on page* 671
All-Nite Multi-Symptom Cold/Flu Relief [OTC] *see* acetaminophen, dextromethorphan, and doxylamine *on page* 27
Alloprin® (Can) *see* allopurinol *on page* 50

allopurinol (al oh PURE i nole)

Medication Safety Issues
Sound-alike/look-alike issues:
Allopurinol may be confused with Apresoline
Zyloprim® may be confused with ZORprin®, Zovirax®

Synonyms allopurinol sodium

U.S. Brand Names Aloprim®; Zyloprim®

Canadian Brand Names Alloprin®; Novo-Purol; Zyloprim®

Therapeutic Category Xanthine Oxidase Inhibitor

Use
Oral: Management of primary or secondary gout (acute attack, tophi, joint destruction, uric acid lithiasis, and/or nephropathy); management of hyperuricemia associated with cancer treatment for leukemia, lymphoma, or solid tumor malignancies; management of recurrent calcium oxalate calculi (with uric acid excretion >800 mg/day in men and >750 mg/day in women)
I.V.: Management of hyperuricemia associated with cancer treatment for leukemia, lymphoma, or solid tumor malignancies

General Dosage Range Dosage adjustment recommended in patients with renal impairment
I.V.:
Children: Initial: 200 mg/m^2/day as a single infusion or in equally divided doses at 6-, 8-, or 12-hour intervals
Adults: 200-400 mg/m^2/day as a single infusion or in equally divided doses at 6-, 8-, or 12-hour intervals (maximum: 600 mg/day)
Oral:
Children <6 years: 150 mg/day
Children 6-10 years: 10 mg/kg/day
Children >10 years and Adults: 100-800 mg/day in 1-3 divided doses (maximum: 800 mg/day)

Dosage Forms
Injection, powder for reconstitution: 500 mg (base)
Aloprim®: 500 mg (base)
Tablet, oral: 100 mg, 300 mg
Zyloprim®: 100 mg, 300 mg

allopurinol sodium *see* allopurinol *on page* 50
all-*trans* retinoic acid *see* tretinoin (systemic) *on page* 913
all-*trans* vitamin A acid *see* tretinoin (systemic) *on page* 913
Almacone® [OTC] *see* aluminum hydroxide, magnesium hydroxide, and simethicone *on page* 56
Almacone® Double Strength [OTC] *see* aluminum hydroxide, magnesium hydroxide, and simethicone *on page* 56

almotriptan (al moh TRIP tan)

Medication Safety Issues
Sound-alike/look-alike issues:
Axert® may be confused with Antivert®

Synonyms almotriptan malate

U.S. Brand Names Axert®

Canadian Brand Names Axert®

Therapeutic Category Serotonin 5-HT$_{1D}$ Receptor Agonist

Use Acute treatment of migraine with or without aura in adults (with a history of migraine) and adolescents (with a history of migraine lasting ≥4 hours when left untreated)

General Dosage Range Dosage adjustment recommended in patients with hepatic or renal impairment and/or on concomitant therapy

Oral: *Children ≥12 years and Adults:* 6.25-12.5 mg in a single dose; may repeat after 2 hours (maximum daily dose: 25 mg)

Dosage Forms

Tablet, oral:

Axert®: 6.25 mg, 12.5 mg

almotriptan malate *see* almotriptan *on page* 50
Alocril® *see* nedocromil *on page* 631
Alodox™ *see* doxycycline *on page* 314
Aloe Vesta® Antifungal [OTC] *see* miconazole (topical) *on page* 599
Alomide® *see* lodoxamide *on page* 546
Alophen® [OTC] *see* bisacodyl *on page* 134
Aloprim® *see* allopurinol *on page* 50
Alora® *see* estradiol (systemic) *on page* 347

alosetron (a LOE se tron)

Medication Safety Issues

Sound-alike/look-alike issues:

Lotronex® may be confused with Lovenox®, Protonix®

U.S. Brand Names Lotronex®

Therapeutic Category 5-HT$_3$ Receptor Antagonist

Use Treatment of women with severe diarrhea-predominant irritable bowel syndrome (IBS) who have failed to respond to conventional therapy

General Dosage Range Oral: *Adults:* Initial: 0.5 mg twice daily; may increase to 1 mg twice daily if needed (maximum: 2 mg/day)

Dosage Forms

Tablet, oral:

Lotronex®: 0.5 mg, 1 mg

Aloxi® *see* palonosetron *on page* 686
alpha$_1$-antiprotease *see* alpha$_1$-proteinase inhibitor *on page* 51
alpha$_1$-antitrypsin *see* alpha$_1$-proteinase inhibitor *on page* 51
A$_1$-PI *see* alpha$_1$-proteinase inhibitor *on page* 51
alpha$_1$-PI *see* alpha$_1$-proteinase inhibitor *on page* 51
alpha$_1$-proteinase inhibitor, human *see* alpha$_1$-proteinase inhibitor *on page* 51

alpha$_1$-proteinase inhibitor (al fa won PRO tee in ase in HI bi tor)

Synonyms A$_1$-PI; alpha$_1$-antiprotease; alpha$_1$-antitrypsin; alpha$_1$-PI; alpha$_1$-proteinase inhibitor, human; α_1-PI

U.S. Brand Names Aralast NP; Glassia™; Prolastin®-C; Zemaira®

Canadian Brand Names Prolastin®-C

Therapeutic Category Antitrypsin Deficiency Agent

Use Replacement therapy in congenital alpha$_1$-proteinase inhibitor (alpha$_1$-antitrypsin, A$_1$-PI) deficiency with clinical emphysema

General Dosage Range I.V.: *Adults:* 60 mg/kg once weekly

Dosage Forms

Injection, powder for reconstitution [preservative free]:

Aralast NP: ~500 mg, ~1000 mg
Prolastin®-C: ~1000 mg
Zemaira®: ~1000 mg

Injection, solution [preservative free]:

Glassia™: ~1000 mg (50 mL)

alpha-galactosidase (AL fa ga lak TOE si days)

Medication Safety Issues

Sound-alike/look-alike issues:

beano® may be confused with B&O (belladonna and opium)

Synonyms *Aspergillus niger*

U.S. Brand Names beano® Meltaways [OTC]; beano® [OTC]

Therapeutic Category Enzyme

Use Prevention of flatulence and bloating attributed to a variety of grains, cereals, nuts, and vegetables

General Dosage Range Oral: *Children ≥12 years and Adults:*

Tablet, chewable (beano®): Usual dose: 2-3 tablets/meal

Tablet, orally disintegrating (beano® Meltaways): One tablet per meal

Dosage Forms

Tablet, chewable, oral:

beano® [OTC]: 150 Galactosidase units

Tablet, orally disintegrating, oral:

beano® Meltaways [OTC]: 300 Galactosidase units

alpha-galactosidase-A (gene-activated) *see* agalsidase alfa *(Canada only) on page 39*
alpha-galactosidase-A (recombinant) *see* agalsidase beta *on page 39*
1α-hydroxyergocalciferol *see* doxercalciferol *on page 313*
Alphagan® (Can) *see* brimonidine *on page 141*
Alphagan® P *see* brimonidine *on page 141*
Alphanate® *see* antihemophilic factor/von Willebrand factor complex (human) *on page 78*
AlphaNine® SD *see* factor IX *on page 371*
Alphaquin HP® *see* hydroquinone *on page 461*
Alph-E [OTC] *see* vitamin E *on page 950*
Alph-E-Mixed [OTC] *see* vitamin E *on page 950*

alprazolam (al PRAY zoe lam)

Medication Safety Issues

Sound-alike/look-alike issues:

ALPRAZolam may be confused with alprostadil, LORazepam, triazolam

Xanax® may be confused with Fanapt®, Lanoxin®, Tenex®, Tylox®, Xopenex®, Zantac®, ZyrTEC®

BEERS Criteria medication:

This drug may be potentially inappropriate for use in geriatric patients (Quality of evidence - high; Strength of recommendation - strong).

Tall-Man **ALPRAZ**olam

U.S. Brand Names Alprazolam Intensol™; Niravam™; Xanax XR®; Xanax®

Canadian Brand Names Apo-Alpraz®; Apo-Alpraz® TS; Mylan-Alprazolam; NTP-Alprazolam; Nu-Alpraz; Teva-Alprazolam; Xanax TS™; Xanax®

Therapeutic Category Benzodiazepine

Controlled Substance C-IV

Use Treatment of anxiety disorder (GAD); short-term relief of symptoms of anxiety; panic disorder, with or without agoraphobia; anxiety associated with depression

General Dosage Range Dosage adjustment recommended in patients with hepatic impairment

Oral:

Immediate release:

Adults: Initial: 0.25-0.5 mg 3 times/day; titrate as needed and tolerated (maximum: 10 mg/day)

Elderly: Initial: 0.25 mg 2-3 times/day; titrate gradually if needed and tolerated

Extended release:

Adults: Initial: 0.5-1 mg once daily; Maintenance: 3-6 mg/day (maximum: 6 mg/day)

Elderly: Initial: 0.5 mg/day; titrate gradually if needed and tolerated

Dosage Forms

Solution, oral:

Alprazolam Intensol™: 1 mg/mL (30 mL)

Tablet, oral: 0.25 mg, 0.5 mg, 1 mg, 2 mg

Xanax®: 0.25 mg, 0.5 mg, 1 mg, 2 mg

Tablet, extended release, oral: 0.5 mg, 1 mg, 2 mg, 3 mg
Xanax XR®: 0.5 mg, 1 mg, 2 mg, 3 mg
Tablet, orally disintegrating, oral: 0.25 mg, 0.5 mg, 1 mg, 2 mg
Niravam™: 0.25 mg, 0.5 mg, 1 mg, 2 mg

Alprazolam Intensol™ *see* alprazolam *on page* 52

alprostadil (al PROS ta dill)

Medication Safety Issues

Sound-alike/look-alike issues:
Alprostadil may be confused with alPRAZolam

Synonyms PGE_1; prostaglandin E_1

U.S. Brand Names Caverject Impulse®; Caverject®; Edex®; Muse®; Prostin VR Pediatric®

Canadian Brand Names Alprostadil Injection USP; Caverject®; Muse® Pellet; Prostin® VR

Therapeutic Category Prostaglandin

Use

Prostin VR Pediatric®: Temporary maintenance of patency of ductus arteriosus in neonates with ductal-dependent congenital heart disease until surgery can be performed. These defects include cyanotic (eg, pulmonary atresia, pulmonary stenosis, tricuspid atresia, Fallot tetralogy, transposition of the great vessels) and acyanotic (eg, interruption of aortic arch, coarctation of aorta, hypoplastic left ventricle) heart disease.

Caverject®: Treatment of erectile dysfunction of vasculogenic, psychogenic, or neurogenic etiology; adjunct in the diagnosis of erectile dysfunction

Edex®, Muse®: Treatment of erectile dysfunction of vasculogenic, psychogenic, or neurogenic etiology

General Dosage Range

I.V.: *Neonates:* Initial: 0.05-0.1 mcg/kg/minute; Maintenance: 0.01-0.4 mcg/kg/minute

Intracavernous: *Adults:* Initial: 1.25-2.5 mcg; Maintenance: Increase to effective dose no more than 3 times/week with at least 24 hours between doses (maximum: 40 mcg/dose [Edex®]; 60 mcg/dose [Caverject®])

Intraurethral: *Adults:* Initial: 125-250 mcg; Maintenance: As needed (maximum: 2 doses/day)

Dosage Forms

Injection, powder for reconstitution:
Caverject Impulse®: 10 mcg, 20 mcg
Caverject®: 20 mcg, 40 mcg
Edex®: 10 mcg, 20 mcg, 40 mcg
Injection, solution: 500 mcg/mL (1 mL)
Prostin VR Pediatric®: 500 mcg/mL (1 mL)
Pellet, urethral:
Muse®: 125 mcg (1s, 6s); 250 mcg (1s, 6s); 500 mcg (1s, 6s); 1000 mcg (1s, 6s)

Alprostadil Injection USP (Can) *see* alprostadil *on page* 53
Alrex® *see* loteprednol *on page* 552
Alsuma™ *see* sumatriptan *on page* 863
Altabax™ *see* retapamulin *on page* 795
Altacaine *see* tetracaine (ophthalmic) *on page* 883
Altace® *see* ramipril *on page* 786
Altace® HCT (Can) *see* ramipril and hydrochlorothiazide *(Canada only) on page* 787
Altace® Plus Felodipine (Can) *see* ramipril and felodipine *(Canada only) on page* 786
Altachlore [OTC] *see* sodium chloride *on page* 840
Altafrin *see* phenylephrine (ophthalmic) *on page* 716
Altamist [OTC] *see* sodium chloride *on page* 840
Altaryl [OTC] *see* diphenhydramine (systemic) *on page* 292
Altavera™ *see* ethinyl estradiol and levonorgestrel *on page* 357

alteplase (AL te plase)

Medication Safety Issues

Sound-alike/look-alike issues:
Activase® may be confused with Cathflo® Activase®, TNKase®
Alteplase may be confused with Altace®

"tPA" abbreviation should not be used when writing orders for this medication; has been misread as TNKase (tenecteplase)

High alert medication:

The Institute for Safe Medication Practices (ISMP) includes this medication (I.V.) among its list of drugs which have a heightened risk of causing significant patient harm when used in error.

Synonyms alteplase, recombinant; alteplase, tissue plasminogen activator, recombinant; tPA

U.S. Brand Names Activase®; Cathflo® Activase®

Canadian Brand Names Activase® rt-PA; Cathflo® Activase®

Therapeutic Category Thrombolytic Agent

Use Management of ST-elevation myocardial infarction (STEMI) for the lysis of thrombi in coronary arteries; management of acute ischemic stroke (AIS); management of acute pulmonary embolism (PE)

Recommended criteria for treatment:

STEMI: Chest pain ≥20 minutes duration, onset of chest pain within 12 hours of treatment (or within prior 12-24 hours in patients with continuing ischemic symptoms), and ST-segment elevation >0.1 mV in at least two contiguous precordial leads or two adjacent limb leads on ECG or new or presumably new left bundle branch block (LBBB)

AIS: Onset of stroke symptoms within 3 hours of treatment

Acute pulmonary embolism: Age ≤75 years: Documented massive PE (defined as acute PE with sustained hypotension [SBP <90 mm Hg for ≤15 minutes or requiring inotropic support], persistent profound bradycardia [HR <40 bpm with signs or symptoms of shock], or pulselessness); alteplase may be considered for submassive PE with clinical evidence of adverse prognosis (eg, new hemodynamic instability, worsening respiratory insufficiency, severe RV dysfunction, or major myocardial necrosis) and low risk of bleeding complications. **Note:** Not recommended for patients with low-risk PE (eg, normotensive, no RV dysfunction, normal biomarkers) or submassive acute PE with minor RV dysfunction, minor myocardial necrosis, and no clinical worsening (Jaff, 2011).

Cathflo® Activase®: Restoration of central venous catheter function

General Dosage Range

Intracatheter:

Children <30 kg: 110% of the internal lumen volume of the catheter; retain in catheter for 0.5-2 hours; may repeat once (maximum: 2 mg/2 mL/dose)

Children ≥30 kg and Adults: 2 mg (2 mL) retain in catheter for 0.5-2 hours; may repeat once

I.V. infusion: *Adults:* Dosage varies greatly depending on indication

Dosage Forms

Injection, powder for reconstitution:

Activase®: 50 mg, 100 mg

Cathflo® Activase®: 2 mg

alteplase, recombinant *see* alteplase *on page* 53

alteplase, tissue plasminogen activator, recombinant *see* alteplase *on page* 53

ALternaGel® [OTC] *see* aluminum hydroxide *on page* 55

Alti-Doxazosin (Can) *see* doxazosin *on page* 311

Alti-Flurbiprofen (Can) *see* flurbiprofen (systemic) *on page* 399

Alti-Fluvoxamine (Can) *see* fluvoxamine *on page* 403

Alti-Ipratropium (Can) *see* ipratropium (nasal) *on page* 499

Alti-MPA (Can) *see* medroxyprogesterone *on page* 567

Alti-Nadolol (Can) *see* nadolol *on page* 623

Alti-Sulfasalazine (Can) *see* sulfasalazine *on page* 861

Altoprev® *see* lovastatin *on page* 553

altretamine (al TRET a meen)

Medication Safety Issues

High alert medication:

This medication is in a class the Institute for Safe Medication Practices (ISMP) includes among its list of drug classes which have a heightened risk of causing significant patient harm when used in error.

International issues:

Hexalen: Brand name altretamine [U.S., Canada, and Thailand], but also brand name for hexetidine [Greece]

Synonyms hexamethylmelamine; HMM; HXM

U.S. Brand Names Hexalen®

Canadian Brand Names Hexalen®

Therapeutic Category Antineoplastic Agent

Use Palliative treatment of persistent or recurrent ovarian cancer

General Dosage Range Dosage adjustment recommended in patients who develop toxicities

Oral: *Adults:* 260 mg/m^2/day in 4 divided doses for 14 or 21 days of a 28-day cycle

Dosage Forms

Capsule, oral:

Hexalen®: 50 mg

aluminum chloride hexahydrate (a LOO mi num KLOR ide heks a HYE drate)

Medication Safety Issues

Sound-alike/look-alike issues:

Drysol™ may be confused with Drisdol®

U.S. Brand Names Certain Dri® [OTC]; Drysol™; Hypercare™; Xerac™ AC

Therapeutic Category Topical Skin Product

Use Astringent in the management of hyperhidrosis

General Dosage Range Topical: *Adults:* Apply once daily

Dosage Forms

Solution, topical:

Certain Dri® [OTC]: 12% (36 mL)
Drysol™: 20% (35 mL, 37.5 mL, 60 mL)
Hypercare™: 20% (35 mL, 37.5 mL, 60 mL)
Xerac™ AC: 6.25% (35 mL, 60 mL)

aluminum hydroxide (a LOO mi num hye DROKS ide)

U.S. Brand Names ALternaGel® [OTC]; Dermagran® [OTC]

Canadian Brand Names Amphojel®; Basaljel®

Therapeutic Category Antacid

Use Treatment of hyperacidity; hyperphosphatemia; temporary protection of minor cuts, scrapes, and burns

General Dosage Range

Oral:

Children: 50-150 mg/kg/day in divided doses every 4-6 hours
Adults: 300-1200 mg 3-4 times/day

Topical: *Children and Adults:* Apply to affected area as needed; reapply at least every 12 hours

Dosage Forms

Ointment, topical:

Dermagran® [OTC]: 0.275% (113 g)

Suspension, oral: 320 mg/5 mL (30 mL, 355 mL, 360 mL, 473 mL, 480 mL)

ALternaGel® [OTC]: 600 mg/5 mL (360 mL)

aluminum hydroxide and magnesium carbonate

(a LOO mi num hye DROKS ide & mag NEE zhum KAR bun nate)

Medication Safety Issues

International issues:

Remegel [Netherlands] may be confused with Renagel brand name for sevelamer [U.S., Canada, and multiple international markets]

Remegel: Brand name for aluminum hydroxide and magnesium carbonate [Netherlands], but also the brand name for calcium carbonate [Great Britain, Hungary, and Ireland]

Synonyms magnesium carbonate and aluminum hydroxide

U.S. Brand Names Acid Gone Extra Strength [OTC]; Acid Gone [OTC]; Gaviscon® Extra Strength [OTC]; Gaviscon® Liquid [OTC]

Therapeutic Category Antacid

Use Temporary relief of symptoms associated with gastric acidity

General Dosage Range Oral: *Adults:* 15-30 mL **or** 2-4 tablets 4 times/day

Dosage Forms

Liquid: Aluminum hydroxide 31.7 mg and magnesium carbonate 119.3 mg per 5 mL; aluminum hydroxide 84.6 mg and magnesium carbonate 79.1 mg per 5 mL

Acid Gone [OTC], Gaviscon® [OTC]: Aluminum hydroxide 31.7 mg and magnesium carbonate 119.3 mg per 5 mL

Gaviscon® Extra Strength [OTC]: Aluminum hydroxide 84.6 mg and magnesium carbonate 79.1 mg per 5 mL

Tablet, chewable: Aluminum hydroxide 160 mg and magnesium carbonate 105 mg

Acid Gone Extra Strength [OTC], Gaviscon® Extra Strength [OTC]: Aluminum hydroxide 160 mg and magnesium carbonate 105 mg

aluminum hydroxide and magnesium hydroxide

(a LOO mi num hye DROKS ide & mag NEE zhum hye DROK side)

Synonyms magnesium hydroxide and aluminum hydroxide

U.S. Brand Names Alamag [OTC]; Mag-Al Ultimate [OTC]; Mag-Al [OTC]

Canadian Brand Names Diovol®; Diovol® Ex; Gelusil® Extra Strength; Mylanta™

Therapeutic Category Antacid

Use Antacid for symptoms related to hyperacidity associated with heartburn, hiatal hernia, upset stomach, peptic ulcer, peptic esophagitis, or gastritis

General Dosage Range Oral: *Children ≥12 years and Adults:* 10-20 mL 4 times/day (maximum: magnesium hydroxide 4500 mg/day; aluminum hydroxide 4500 mg/day) **or** 1-2 tablets as needed (maximum: 16 tablets)

Dosage Forms

Liquid, oral:

Mag-Al [OTC]: Aluminum hydroxide 200 mg and magnesium hydroxide 200 mg per 5 mL

Suspension, oral:

Mag-Al Ultimate [OTC]: Aluminum hydroxide 500 mg and magnesium hydroxide 500 mg per 5 mL

Tablet, chewable:

Alamag [OTC]: Aluminum hydroxide 300 mg and magnesium hydroxide 150 mg

aluminum hydroxide and magnesium trisilicate

(a LOO mi num hye DROKS ide & mag NEE zhum trye SIL i kate)

Synonyms magnesium trisilicate and aluminum hydroxide

U.S. Brand Names Gaviscon® Tablet [OTC]

Therapeutic Category Antacid

Use Temporary relief of hyperacidity

General Dosage Range Oral: *Adults:* 2-4 tablets 4 times/day

Dosage Forms

Tablet, chewable: Aluminum hydroxide 80 mg and magnesium trisilicate 20 mg

Gaviscon® [OTC]: Aluminum hydroxide 80 mg and magnesium trisilicate 20 mg

aluminum hydroxide, magnesium hydroxide, and simethicone

(a LOO mi num hye DROKS ide, mag NEE zhum hye DROKS ide, & sye METH i kone)

Medication Safety Issues

Sound-alike/look-alike issues:

Maalox® may be confused with Maox®, Monodox®

Mylanta® may be confused with Mynatal®

Other safety concerns:

Liquid Maalox® products contain a different formulation than Maalox® Total Relief® which contains bismuth subsalicylate.

Synonyms magnesium hydroxide, aluminum hydroxide, and simethicone; simethicone, aluminum hydroxide, and magnesium hydroxide

U.S. Brand Names Alamag Plus [OTC]; Aldroxicon I [OTC]; Aldroxicon II [OTC]; Almacone® Double Strength [OTC]; Almacone® [OTC]; Gelusil® [OTC]; Maalox® Advanced Maximum Strength [OTC]; Maalox® Advanced Regular Strength [OTC]; Mi-Acid Maximum Strength [OTC] [DSC]; Mi-Acid [OTC]; Mintox Plus [OTC]; Mylanta® Classic Maximum Strength Liquid [OTC]; Mylanta® Classic Regular Strength Liquid [OTC]; Rulox [OTC]

Canadian Brand Names Diovol Plus®; Gelusil®; Mylanta® Double Strength; Mylanta® Extra Strength; Mylanta® Regular Strength

Therapeutic Category Antacid; Antiflatulent

Use Temporary relief of hyperacidity associated with gas; may also be used for indications associated with other antacids

General Dosage Range Oral: *Adults:* 10-20 mL or 2-4 tablets 4-6 times/day

Dosage Forms

Liquid: Aluminum hydroxide 200 mg, magnesium hydroxide 200 mg, and simethicone 20 mg per 5 mL; aluminum hydroxide 400 mg, magnesium hydroxide 400 mg, and simethicone 40 mg per 5 mL

Aldroxicon I [OTC], Almacone® [OTC], Maalox® Advanced Regular Strength [OTC], Mi-Acid [OTC], Mylanta® Classic Regular Strength [OTC]: Aluminum hydroxide 200 mg, magnesium hydroxide 200 mg, and simethicone 20 mg per 5 mL

Aldroxicon II [OTC], Almacone® Double Strength [OTC], Maalox® Advanced Maximum Strength [OTC], Mi-Acid Maximum Strength [OTC], Mylanta® Classic Maximum Strength [OTC]: Aluminum hydroxide 400 mg, magnesium hydroxide 400 mg, and simethicone 40 mg per 5 mL

Suspension: Aluminum hydroxide 225 mg, magnesium hydroxide 200 mg, and simethicone 25 mg per 5 mL

Rulox [OTC]: Aluminum hydroxide 200 mg, magnesium hydroxide 200 mg, and simethicone 25 mg per 5 mL

Tablet, chewable: Aluminum hydroxide 200 mg, magnesium hydroxide 200 mg, and simethicone 25 mg

Alamag Plus [OTC], Gelusil® [OTC], Mintox Plus [OTC]: Aluminum hydroxide 200 mg, magnesium hydroxide 200 mg, and simethicone 25 mg

Almacone® [OTC]: Aluminum hydroxide 200 mg, magnesium hydroxide 200 mg, and simethicone 20 mg

aluminum sucrose sulfate, basic *see* sucralfate *on page* 856

aluminum sulfate and calcium acetate (a LOO mi num SUL fate & KAL see um AS e tate)

Synonyms calcium acetate and aluminum sulfate

U.S. Brand Names Domeboro® [OTC]; Gordon Boro-Packs [OTC]; Pedi-Boro® [OTC]

Therapeutic Category Topical Skin Product

Use Astringent wet dressing for relief of inflammatory conditions of the skin; reduce weeping that may occur in dermatitis

General Dosage Range Topical: *Adults:* Soak affected area or wet dressing in the solution 2-4 times/day

Dosage Forms

Powder, for solution, topical: Aluminum sulfate 1191 mg and calcium acetate 839 mg per packet (12s)

Domeboro®: Aluminum sulfate tetradecahydrate 1347 mg and calcium acetate monohydrate 952 mg per packet (12s, 100s)

Gordon Boro-Packs: Aluminum sulfate 49% and calcium acetate 51% per packet (100s)

Pedi-Boro®: Aluminum sulfate tetradecahydrate 1191 mg and calcium acetate monohydrate 839 mg per packet (12s, 100s)

Alupent *see* metaproterenol *on page* 579
Aluvea™ *see* urea *on page* 930
Alvesco® *see* ciclesonide (oral inhalation) *on page* 207

alvimopan (al VI moe pan)

Medication Safety Issues

Sound-alike/look-alike issues:

Alvimopan may be confused with almotriptan

Synonyms ADL-2698; LY246736

U.S. Brand Names Entereg®

Therapeutic Category Gastrointestinal Agent, Miscellaneous; Opioid Antagonist, Peripherally-Acting

Use Accelerate the time to upper and lower GI recovery following partial large or small bowel resection surgery with primary anastomosis

General Dosage Range Oral: *Adults:* Initial: 12 mg prior to surgery; Maintenance: 12 mg twice daily (maximum: 15 doses)

Dosage Forms

Capsule, oral:

Entereg®: 12 mg

Alyacen 1/35 *see* ethinyl estradiol and norethindrone *on page* 359
Alyacen 7/7/7 *see* ethinyl estradiol and norethindrone *on page* 359

amantadine (a MAN ta deen)

Medication Safety Issues

Sound-alike/look-alike issues:

Amantadine may be confused with ranitidine, rimantadine

Symmetrel may be confused with Synthroid®

Synonyms adamantanamine hydrochloride; amantadine hydrochloride; Symmetrel

Canadian Brand Names Dom-Amantadine; Mylan-Amantadine; PHL-Amantadine; PMS-Amantadine

Therapeutic Category Anti-Parkinson Agent (Dopamine Agonist); Antiviral Agent

Use Prophylaxis and treatment of influenza A viral infection (per manufacturer labeling; also refer to current ACIP guidelines for recommendations during current flu season); treatment of parkinsonism; treatment of drug-induced extrapyramidal symptoms

General Dosage Range Dosage adjustment recommended in patients with renal impairment

Oral:

Children 1-9 years: 4.4-8.8 mg/kg/day in 2 divided doses (maximum: 150 mg/day)

Children ≥10 years and <40 kg: 5 mg/kg/day in 2 divided doses

Children ≥10 years and ≥40 kg: 100 mg twice daily (maximum: 200 mg/day)

Adults: 200-400 mg/day in 2 divided doses (maximum: 400 mg/day)

Elderly: 100-400 mg/day in 2 divided doses (maximum: 400 mg/day)

Dosage Forms

Capsule, oral: 100 mg

Capsule, softgel, oral: 100 mg

Solution, oral: 50 mg/5 mL (473 mL)

Syrup, oral: 50 mg/5 mL (10 mL, 473 mL, 480 mL)

Tablet, oral: 100 mg

amantadine hydrochloride *see* amantadine *on page 58*

Amaryl® *see* glimepiride *on page 426*

Amatine® (Can) *see* midodrine *on page 601*

ambenonium (am be NOE nee um)

Synonyms ambenonium chloride

U.S. Brand Names Mytelase® [DSC]

Therapeutic Category Cholinergic Agent

Use Treatment of myasthenia gravis

General Dosage Range Oral: *Adults:* Usual dose: 5-25 mg 3-4 times/day; some patients may require as much as 50-75 mg/dose

ambenonium chloride *see* ambenonium *on page 58*

Ambi 10PEH/400GFN [OTC] *see* guaifenesin and phenylephrine *on page 435*

Ambien® *see* zolpidem *on page 966*

Ambien CR® *see* zolpidem *on page 966*

Ambifed DM *see* guaifenesin, pseudoephedrine, and dextromethorphan *on page 437*

Ambifed-G [OTC] *see* guaifenesin and pseudoephedrine *on page 436*

Ambifed-G DM *see* guaifenesin, pseudoephedrine, and dextromethorphan *on page 437*

AmBisome® *see* amphotericin B liposomal *on page 72*

ambrisentan (am bri SEN tan)

Synonyms BSF208075

U.S. Brand Names Letairis®

Canadian Brand Names Volibris®

Therapeutic Category Endothelin Antagonist

Use Treatment of pulmonary artery hypertension (PAH) World Health Organization (WHO) Group I to improve exercise ability and decrease the rate of clinical deterioration

General Dosage Range Dosage adjustment recommended in patients on concomitant therapy.

Oral: *Adults:* Initial: 5 mg once daily (maximum: 10 mg/day)

Dosage Forms

Tablet, oral:

Letairis®: 5 mg, 10 mg

amcinonide (am SIN oh nide)

Canadian Brand Names Amcort®; Cyclocort®; ratio-Amcinonide; Taro-Amcinonide

Therapeutic Category Corticosteroid, Topical

Use Relief of the inflammatory and pruritic manifestations of corticosteroid-responsive dermatoses (high potency corticosteroid)

General Dosage Range Topical: *Adults:* Apply in a thin film 2-3 times/day

Dosage Forms

Cream, topical: 0.1% (15 g, 30 g, 60 g)
Lotion, topical: 0.1% (60 mL)
Ointment, topical: 0.1% (15 g, 30 g, 60 g)

Amcort® (Can) *see* amcinonide *on page* 59
AMD3100 *see* plerixafor *on page* 729
Amerge® *see* naratriptan *on page* 629
Americaine® Hemorrhoidal [OTC] *see* benzocaine *on page* 121
A-Methapred® *see* methylprednisolone *on page* 591
Amethia™ *see* ethinyl estradiol and levonorgestrel *on page* 357
Amethia™ Lo *see* ethinyl estradiol and levonorgestrel *on page* 357
amethocaine hydrochloride *see* tetracaine (ophthalmic) *on page* 883
amethocaine hydrochloride *see* tetracaine (systemic) *on page* 883
amethocaine hydrochloride *see* tetracaine (topical) *on page* 884
amethopterin *see* methotrexate *on page* 584
Amethyst™ *see* ethinyl estradiol and levonorgestrel *on page* 357
Ametop™ (Can) *see* tetracaine (topical) *on page* 884
Amevive® [DSC] *see* alefacept *on page* 44
Amevive® (Can) *see* alefacept *on page* 44
amfepramone *see* diethylpropion *on page* 283
AMG 073 *see* cinacalcet *on page* 209
AMG-162 *see* denosumab *on page* 261
AMG 531 *see* romiplostim *on page* 810
Amicar® *see* aminocaproic acid *on page* 61
Amidate® *see* etomidate *on page* 365

amifostine (am i FOS teen)

Medication Safety Issues

Sound-alike/look-alike issues:
Ethyol® may be confused with ethanol

Synonyms ethiofos; gammaphos; WR-2721; YM-08310

U.S. Brand Names Ethyol®

Canadian Brand Names Ethyol®

Therapeutic Category Antidote

Use Reduce the incidence of moderate-to-severe xerostomia in patients undergoing postoperative radiation treatment for head and neck cancer, where the radiation port includes a substantial portion of the parotid glands; reduce the cumulative renal toxicity associated with repeated administration of cisplatin

General Dosage Range I.V.: *Adults:* 910 mg/m^2 once daily 30 minutes prior to cytotoxic therapy **or** 200 mg/m^2/day 15-30 minutes prior to radiation therapy

Dosage Forms

Injection, powder for reconstitution: 500 mg
Ethyol®: 500 mg

Amigesic® (Can) *see* salsalate *on page* 820
Ami-Hydro (Can) *see* amiloride and hydrochlorothiazide *on page* 60

amikacin (am i KAY sin)

Medication Safety Issues

Sound-alike/look-alike issues:

Amikacin may be confused with Amicar®, anakinra

Amikin® may be confused with Amicar®, Kineret®

Synonyms amikacin sulfate

Canadian Brand Names Amikacin Sulfate Injection, USP; Amikin®

Therapeutic Category Aminoglycoside (Antibiotic)

Use Treatment of serious infections (bone infections, respiratory tract infections, endocarditis, and septicemia) due to organisms resistant to gentamicin and tobramycin, including *Pseudomonas*, *Proteus*, *Serratia*, and other gram-negative bacilli; documented infection of mycobacterial organisms susceptible to amikacin

General Dosage Range Dosage adjustment recommended in patients with renal impairment

I.M.: *Infants, Children, and Adults:* 5-7.5 mg/kg/dose every 8 hours (maximum: 20 mg/kg/day)

I.V.:

Infants and Children: 5-7.5 mg/kg/dose every 8 hours (maximum: 20 mg/kg/day)

Adults: 5-7.5 mg/kg/dose every 8 hours **or** 15-20 mg/kg as a single daily dose (maximum: 20 mg/kg/day)

Dosage Forms

Injection, solution: 250 mg/mL (2 mL, 4 mL)

amikacin sulfate *see* amikacin *on page 60*

Amikacin Sulfate Injection, USP (Can) *see* amikacin *on page 60*

Amikin® (Can) *see* amikacin *on page 60*

amiloride (a MIL oh ride)

Medication Safety Issues

Sound-alike/look-alike issues:

AMILoride may be confused with amiodarone, amLODIPine, inamrinone

Synonyms amiloride hydrochloride

Tall-Man a**MIL**oride

Canadian Brand Names Apo-Amiloride®; Midamor

Therapeutic Category Diuretic, Potassium Sparing

Use Counteracts potassium loss induced by other diuretics in the treatment of hypertension or edematous conditions including CHF, hepatic cirrhosis, and hypoaldosteronism; usually used in conjunction with more potent diuretics such as thiazides or loop diuretics

General Dosage Range Dosage adjustment recommended in patients with renal impairment

Oral:

Adults: 5-10 mg/day in 1-2 divided doses (maximum: 20 mg/day)

Elderly: Initial: 5 mg once daily or every other day

Dosage Forms

Tablet, oral: 5 mg

amiloride and hydrochlorothiazide (a MIL oh ride & hye droe klor oh THYE a zide)

Synonyms hydrochlorothiazide and amiloride

Canadian Brand Names Ami-Hydro; Apo-Amilzide®; Gen-Amilazide; Moduret; Novamilor; Nu-Amilzide

Therapeutic Category Diuretic, Combination

Use Potassium-sparing diuretic; antihypertensive

General Dosage Range Dosage adjustment recommended in patients with renal impairment

Oral:

Adults: 1-2 tablets (amiloride 5 mg/HCTZ 50 mg per tablet) once daily (maximum: 2 tablets/day)

Elderly: Initial: 1/2 to 1 tablet/day (maximum: 2 tablets/day)

Dosage Forms

Tablet: 5/50: Amiloride 5 mg and hydrochlorothiazide 50 mg

amiloride hydrochloride *see* amiloride *on page 60*

2-amino-6-mercaptopurine *see* thioguanine *on page 890*

2-amino-6-methoxypurine arabinoside *see* nelarabine *on page 632*

2-amino-6-trifluoromethoxy-benzothiazole *see* riluzole *on page* 801

amino acid injection (a MEE noe AS id in JEK shun)

Medication Safety Issues

Sound-alike/look-alike issues:

TrophAmine® may be confused with tromethamine

U.S. Brand Names Aminosyn®; Aminosyn® II; Aminosyn®-HBC; Aminosyn®-PF; Aminosyn®-RF; BranchAmin® [DSC]; Clinisol®; FreAmine® HBC; FreAmine® III; HepatAmine®; Hepatasol®; NephrAmine®; PremaSol™; Prosol; Travasol®; TrophAmine®

Canadian Brand Names Aminosyn; Aminosyn-PF; Aminosyn-RF; Aminosyn® II; Primene®

Therapeutic Category Intravenous Nutritional Therapy

Use As part of parenteral nutrition to prevent nitrogen loss or treat negative nitrogen balance when alimentary tract cannot be used (eg, GI absorption is impaired, bowel rest is needed). Specialty amino acid formulas may be considered only in certain instances.

General Dosage Range Dosage adjustment recommended in patients with hepatic or renal impairment

I.V.:

Children: 1-3.85 g/kg/day

Adults: 0.8-2 g/kg/day

Dosage Forms

Injection, solution:

Aminosyn®: 8.5% (500 mL); 10% (500 mL, 1000 mL)
Aminosyn® II: 8.5% (500 mL); 10% (500 mL, 1000 mL, 2000 mL); 15% (2000 mL)
Aminosyn®-HBC: 7% (500 mL)
Aminosyn®-PF: 7% (500 mL); 10% (1000 mL)
Aminosyn®-RF: 5.2% (500 mL)
Clinisol®: 15% (500 mL, 2000 mL)
FreAmine® HBC: 6.9% (750 mL)
FreAmine® III: 3% (1000 mL); 8.5% (500 mL); 10% (500 mL, 1000 mL)
HepatAmine®: 8% (500 mL)
Hepatasol®: 8% (500 mL)
NephrAmine®: 5.4% (250 mL)
PremaSol™: 6% (500 mL); 10% (500 mL, 1000 mL, 2000 mL)
Prosol: 20% (2000 mL)
Travasol®: 10% (500 mL, 1000 mL, 2000 mL)
TrophAmine®: 6% (500 mL); 10% (500 mL)

aminobenzylpenicillin *see* ampicillin *on page* 73

aminocaproic acid (a mee noe ka PROE ik AS id)

Medication Safety Issues

Sound-alike/look-alike issues:

Amicar® may be confused with amikacin, Amikin®

International issues:

Amicar [U.S.] may be confused with Omacor brand name for Omega-3-Acid Ethyl Esters [multiple international markets]

Synonyms EACA; epsilon aminocaproic acid

U.S. Brand Names Amicar®

Therapeutic Category Hemostatic Agent

Use To enhance hemostasis when fibrinolysis contributes to bleeding (causes may include cardiac surgery, hematologic disorders, neoplastic disorders, abruptio placentae, hepatic cirrhosis, and urinary fibrinolysis)

General Dosage Range

I.V.: *Adults:* Dosage varies greatly depending on indication

Oral: *Adults:* Initial: Loading dose: 4-5 g for first hour; Maintenance: 1 g/hour (or 1.25 g/hour using oral solution) for 8 hours or until bleeding controlled (maximum: 30 g/day)

Dosage Forms

Injection, solution: 250 mg/mL (20 mL)

Solution, oral: 1.25 g/5 mL (237 mL, 473 mL)

Syrup, oral:
Amicar®: 1.25 g/5 mL (473 mL)
Tablet, oral: 500 mg
Amicar®: 500 mg, 1000 mg

aminolevulinic acid (a MEE noh lev yoo lin ik AS id)

Medication Safety Issues
Sound-alike/look-alike issues:
Aminolevulinic acid may be confused with methyl aminolevulinate
Synonyms 5-ALA; 5-aminolevulinic acid; ALA; amino levulinic acid; aminolevulinic acid hydrochloride
U.S. Brand Names Levulan® Kerastick®
Canadian Brand Names Levulan® Kerastick®
Therapeutic Category Photosensitizing Agent, Topical; Porphyrin Agent, Topical
Use Treatment of minimally to moderately thick actinic keratoses (grade 1 or 2) of the face or scalp; to be used in conjunction with blue light illumination
General Dosage Range Topical: *Adults:* Apply to actinic keratoses once; may repeat after 8 weeks
Dosage Forms
Powder for solution, topical:
Levulan® Kerastick®: 20% (6s)

amino levulinic acid *see* aminolevulinic acid *on page* 62
5-aminolevulinic acid *see* aminolevulinic acid *on page* 62
aminolevulinic acid hydrochloride *see* aminolevulinic acid *on page* 62

aminophylline (am in OFF i lin)

Medication Safety Issues
Sound-alike/look-alike issues:
Aminophylline may be confused with amitriptyline, ampicillin
Synonyms theophylline ethylenediamine
Canadian Brand Names Aminophylline Injection; JAA-Aminophylline
Therapeutic Category Theophylline Derivative
Use Treatment of symptoms and reversible airway obstruction due to asthma or other chronic lung diseases (eg, emphysema, chronic bronchitis)

Note: The National Heart, Lung, and Blood Institute Guidelines (2007) do not recommend aminophylline I.V. for the treatment of asthma exacerbations.
General Dosage Range
I.V.:
Infants to Adults: Loading dose: 5.7 mg/kg
Children 6 weeks to 1 year: Maintenance: Equivalent theophylline dose: mg/kg/hour = (0.008)(age in weeks) + 0.21
Children 1-9 years: Maintenance: 1.01 mg/kg/hour
Children 9-12 years: Maintenance: 0.89 mg/kg/hour
Adolescents 12-16 years (smokers): Maintenance: 0.89 mg/kg/hour
Adolescents 12-16 years (nonsmokers): Maintenance: 0.63 mg/kg/hour
Adolescents >16 years and Adults ≤60 years (nonsmokers): Maintenance: 0.51 mg/kg/hour (maximum: 900 mg/day)
Adults >60 years (nonsmokers): Maintenance: 0.38 mg/kg/hour (maximum: 400 mg/day)
Oral:
Children 1-15 years and <45 kg (without risk factors for impaired clearance): Initial: 15.2-17.7 mg/kg/day divided every 4-6 hours for 3 days (maximum: 380 mg), then increase to 20.3 mg/kg/day divided every 4-6 hours for 3 days (maximum: 400 mg/day); Maintenance: 25.3 mg/kg/day divided every 4-6 hours (maximum: 760 mg/day)
Children ≥45 kg and Adults: Initial: 380 mg/day divided every 6-8 hours for 3 days, then 507 mg/day divided every 6-8 hours for 3 days; Maintenance: 760 mg/day divided every 6-8 hours
Dosage Forms
Injection, solution: 25 mg/mL (10 mL, 20 mL)
Injection, solution [preservative free]: 25 mg/mL (10 mL, 20 mL)

Dosage Forms - Canada

Injection, solution [preservative free]: 25 mg/mL (10 mL); 50 mg/mL (10 mL)

Tablet, oral: 100 mg

Aminophylline Injection (Can) *see* aminophylline *on page 62*

4-aminopyridine *see* dalfampridine *on page 251*

aminosalicylate sodium *see* aminosalicylic acid *on page 63*

aminosalicylic acid (a mee noe sal i SIL ik AS id)

Synonyms 4-aminosalicylic acid; aminosalicylate sodium; para-aminosalicylate sodium; PAS; sodium PAS

U.S. Brand Names Paser®

Therapeutic Category Nonsteroidal Antiinflammatory Drug (NSAID)

Use Adjunctive treatment of tuberculosis used in combination with other antitubercular agents

General Dosage Range Dosage adjustment recommended in patients with renal impairment

Oral:

Children: 200-300 mg/kg/day in 2-4 divided doses

Adults: 8-12 g/day in 2-3 divided doses

Dosage Forms

Granules, delayed release, oral:

Paser®: 4 g/packet (30s)

4-aminosalicylic acid *see* aminosalicylic acid *on page 63*

5-aminosalicylic acid *see* mesalamine *on page 577*

Aminosyn® *see* amino acid injection *on page 61*

Aminosyn (Can) *see* amino acid injection *on page 61*

Aminosyn® II *see* amino acid injection *on page 61*

Aminosyn®-HBC *see* amino acid injection *on page 61*

Aminosyn®-PF *see* amino acid injection *on page 61*

Aminosyn-PF (Can) *see* amino acid injection *on page 61*

Aminosyn®-RF *see* amino acid injection *on page 61*

Aminosyn-RF (Can) *see* amino acid injection *on page 61*

Aminoxin® [OTC] *see* pyridoxine *on page 777*

amiodarone (a MEE oh da rone)

Medication Safety Issues

Sound-alike/look-alike issues:

Amiodarone may be confused with aMILoride, inamrinone

Cordarone® may be confused with Cardura®, Cordran®

High alert medication:

The Institute for Safe Medication Practices (ISMP) includes this medication among its list of drugs which have a heightened risk of causing significant patient harm when used in error.

BEERS Criteria medication:

This drug may be potentially inappropriate for use in geriatric patients (Quality of evidence - high; Strength of recommendation - strong).

Synonyms amiodarone hydrochloride

U.S. Brand Names Cordarone®; Nexterone®; Pacerone®

Canadian Brand Names Amiodarone Hydrochloride Injection; Apo-Amiodarone®; Ava-Amiodarone; Cordarone®; Dom-Amiodarone; Mylan-Amiodarone; PHL-Amiodarone; PMS-Amiodarone; PRO-Amiodarone; ratio-Amiodarone; Riva-Amiodarone; Sandoz-Amiodarone; Teva-Amiodarone

Therapeutic Category Antiarrhythmic Agent, Class III

Use Management of life-threatening recurrent ventricular fibrillation (VF) or hemodynamically-unstable ventricular tachycardia (VT) refractory to other antiarrhythmic agents or in patients intolerant of other agents used for these conditions

General Dosage Range

I.O.: *Children (PALS dosing):* 5 mg/kg (maximum: 300 mg/day); may repeat up to maximum dose of 15 mg/kg/day

I.V.:

Children (PALS dosing): 5 mg/kg (maximum: 300 mg/day); may repeat up to maximum dose of 15 mg/kg/day

Adults: Initial: 150-300 mg bolus **or** 5-7 mg/kg; Maintenance: 1200-1800 mg/day continuous infusion until 10 g total **or** 1 mg/minute infusion for 6 hours, then 0.5 mg/minute infusion for 18 hours (maximum: 2.1 g/day)

Oral: *Adults:* Initial: 600-1600 mg/day until 10 g total; Maintenance: 100-400 mg/day

Dosage Forms

Infusion, premixed iso-osmotic dextrose solution:

Nexterone®: 150 mg (100 mL); 360 mg (200 mL)

Injection, solution: 50 mg/mL (3 mL, 9 mL, 18 mL)

Tablet, oral: 200 mg, 400 mg

Cordarone®: 200 mg

Pacerone®: 100 mg, 200 mg, 400 mg

amiodarone hydrochloride *see* amiodarone *on page 63*

Amiodarone Hydrochloride Injection (Can) *see* amiodarone *on page 63*

Amitiza® *see* lubiprostone *on page 554*

amitriptyline (a mee TRIP ti leen)

Medication Safety Issues

Sound-alike/look-alike issues:

Amitriptyline may be confused with aminophylline, imipramine, nortriptyline

Elavil® may be confused with Aldoril®, Eldepryl®, enalapril, Equanil®, Plavix®

BEERS Criteria medication:

This drug may be potentially inappropriate for use in geriatric patients (Quality of evidence - high [moderate for SIADH]; Strength of recommendation - strong).

Synonyms amitriptyline hydrochloride; Elavil

Canadian Brand Names Bio-Amitriptyline; Dom-Amitriptyline; Elavil; Levate®; Novo-Triptyn; PMS-Amitriptyline

Therapeutic Category Antidepressant, Tricyclic (Tertiary Amine)

Use Relief of symptoms of depression

General Dosage Range Oral:

Adolescents: Initial: 25-50 mg/day; Maintenance: 25-100 mg/day (maximum: 100 mg/day)

Adults: 50-300 mg/day as a single dose at bedtime or in divided doses (maximum: 300 mg/day)

Elderly: Initial: 10-25 mg at bedtime; Maintenance: 25-150 mg/day (maximum: 150 mg/day)

Dosage Forms

Tablet, oral: 10 mg, 25 mg, 50 mg, 75 mg, 100 mg, 150 mg

amitriptyline and chlordiazepoxide (a mee TRIP ti leen & klor dye az e POKS ide)

Medication Safety Issues

BEERS Criteria medication:

This drug may be potentially inappropriate for use in geriatric patients (Quality of evidence - high [moderate for SIADH]; Strength of recommendation - strong).

Synonyms chlordiazepoxide and amitriptyline hydrochloride; Limbitrol

Therapeutic Category Antidepressant, Tricyclic (Tertiary Amine)

Controlled Substance C-IV

Use Treatment of moderate-to-severe anxiety and/or agitation and depression

General Dosage Range Oral: *Adults:* 2-6 tablets (amitriptyline 12.5-25 mg/chlordiazepoxide 5-10 mg per tablet)/day (maximum: 6 tablets/day)

Dosage Forms

Tablet: 12.5/5: Amitriptyline 12.5 mg and chlordiazepoxide 5 mg; 25/10: Amitriptyline 25 mg and chlordiazepoxide 10 mg

amitriptyline and perphenazine (a mee TRIP ti leen & per FEN a zeen)

Medication Safety Issues

BEERS Criteria medication:

This drug may be potentially inappropriate for use in geriatric patients (Quality of evidence - high [moderate for SIADH]; Strength of recommendation - strong).

Synonyms perphenazine and amitriptyline hydrochloride

Canadian Brand Names PMS-Levazine

Therapeutic Category Antidepressant/Phenothiazine

Use Treatment of patients with moderate-to-severe anxiety and/or agitation and depression; schizophrenia with depressive symptoms

General Dosage Range Oral: *Adults:* Initial: Amitriptyline 25 mg/perphenazine 2-4 mg 3-4 times/day **or** amitriptyline 50 mg/perphenazine 4-8 mg 2-3 times/day; Maintenance: Amitriptyline 25 mg/perphenazine 2-4 mg 2-4 times/day **or** amitriptyline 50 mg/perphenazine 4 mg 2 times/day; maximum daily dose: amitriptyline 200 mg/perphenazine 16 mg

Dosage Forms

Tablet: 2-10: Amitriptyline 10 mg and perphenazine 2 mg; 2-25: Amitriptyline 25 mg and perphenazine 2 mg; 4-10: Amitriptyline 10 mg and perphenazine 4 mg; 4-25: Amitriptyline 25 mg and perphenazine 4 mg; 4-50: Amitriptyline 50 mg and perphenazine 4 mg

amitriptyline hydrochloride *see* amitriptyline *on page 64*

AMJ 9701 *see* palifermin *on page 684*

AmLactin® [OTC] *see* lactic acid and ammonium hydroxide *on page 517*

amlexanox (am LEKS an oks)

U.S. Brand Names Aphthasol®

Therapeutic Category Antiinflammatory Agent, Locally Applied

Use Treatment of aphthous ulcers (ie, canker sores)

General Dosage Range Topical: *Adults:* ~1/4 inch (0.5 cm) directly on ulcers 4 times/day

Dosage Forms

Paste, oral:

Aphthasol®: 5% (3 g)

amlodipine (am LOE di peen)

Medication Safety Issues

Sound-alike/look-alike issues:

AmLODIPine may be confused with aMILoride

Norvasc® may be confused with Navane®, Norvir®, Vascor®

International issues:

Norvasc [U.S., Canada, and multiple international markets] may be confused with Vascor brand name for imidapril [Philippines] and simvastatin [Malaysia, Singapore, and Thailand]

Synonyms amlodipine besylate

Tall-Man am**LODIP**ine

U.S. Brand Names Norvasc®

Canadian Brand Names Accel-Amlodipine; Amlodipine-Odan; Apo-Amlodipine®; CO Amlodipine; Dom-Amlodipine; GD-Amlodipine; JAMP-Amlodipine; Manda-Amlodipine; Mint-Amlodipine; Mylan-Amlodipine; Norvasc®; PHL-Amlodipine; PMS-Amlodipine; Q-Amlodipine; RAN™-Amlodipine; ratio-Amlodipine; Riva-Amlodipine; Sandoz Amlodipine; Septa-Amlodipine; Teva-Amlodipine; ZYM-Amlodipine

Therapeutic Category Calcium Channel Blocker

Use Treatment of hypertension; treatment of symptomatic chronic stable angina, vasospastic (Prinzmetal) angina (confirmed or suspected); prevention of hospitalization due to angina with documented CAD (limited to patients without heart failure or ejection fraction <40%)

General Dosage Range Dosage adjustment recommended in patients with hepatic impairment

Oral:

Children 6-17 years: 2.5-5 mg once daily

Adults: Initial: 5 mg once daily; Maintenance: 2.5-10 mg once daily (maximum: 10 mg/day)

Elderly: 2.5-5 mg once daily

Dosage Forms

Tablet, oral: 2.5 mg, 5 mg, 10 mg

Norvasc®: 2.5 mg, 5 mg, 10 mg

amlodipine, aliskiren, and hydrochlorothiazide *see* aliskiren, amlodipine, and hydrochlorothiazide *on page 48*

amlodipine and aliskiren *see* aliskiren and amlodipine *on page 48*

amlodipine and atorvastatin (am LOW di peen & a TORE va sta tin)

Synonyms atorvastatin and amlodipine; atorvastatin calcium and amlodipine besylate

U.S. Brand Names Caduet®

Canadian Brand Names Caduet®

Therapeutic Category Antilipemic Agent, HMG-CoA Reductase Inhibitor; Calcium Channel Blocker

Use For use when treatment with both amlodipine and atorvastatin is appropriate:

Amlodipine: Treatment of hypertension; treatment of chronic stable angina, vasospastic (Prinzmetal) angina (confirmed or suspected); prevention of hospitalization or to decrease coronary revascularization procedure due to angina with documented CAD (limited to patients without heart failure or ejection fraction <40%)

Atorvastatin: Treatment of dyslipidemias or primary prevention of cardiovascular disease (atherosclerotic) as detailed here:

Primary prevention of cardiovascular disease (high-risk for CVD): To reduce the risk of MI or stroke in patients without evidence of coronary heart disease who have multiple CVD risk factors or type 2 diabetes; also reduces the risk for angina or revascularization procedures in patients with multiple CVD risk factors without evidence of coronary heart disease

Secondary prevention of cardiovascular disease: To reduce the risk of MI, stroke, revascularization procedures, angina, and hospitalization for heart failure

Treatment of dyslipidemias: To reduce elevations in total cholesterol, LDL-C, apolipoprotein B, and triglycerides in patients with elevations of one or more components, and/or to increase low HDL-C as present in heterozygous familial/nonfamilial hypercholesterolemia and mixed dyslipidemia (Fredrickson type IIa and IIb hyperlipidemias); treatment of primary dysbetalipoproteinemia (Fredrickson type III), elevated serum TG levels (Fredrickson type IV), and homozygous familial hypercholesterolemia

Treatment of heterozygous familial hypercholesterolemia (HeFH) in adolescent patients (10-17 years of age, females >1 year postmenarche) having LDL-C ≥190 mg/dL or LDL-C ≥160 mg/dL with positive family history of premature cardiovascular disease (CVD) or with two or more CVD risk factors.

General Dosage Range Dosage adjustment recommended in patients on concomitant therapy

Oral:

Children 10-17 years (females >1 year postmenarche): 2.5-5 mg (amlodipine) and 10-20 mg (atorvastatin) once daily (maximum: amlodipine 5 mg/day; atorvastatin 20 mg/day)

Adults: 2.5-10 mg (amlodipine) and 10-80 mg (atorvastatin) once daily (maximum: amlodipine 10 mg/day; atorvastatin 80 mg/day)

Dosage Forms

Tablet, oral: Amlodipine 2.5 mg and atorvastatin 10 mg; Amlodipine 2.5 mg and atorvastatin 20 mg; Amlodipine 2.5 mg and atorvastatin 40 mg; Amlodipine 5 mg and atorvastatin 10 mg; Amlodipine 5 mg and atorvastatin 20 mg; Amlodipine 5 mg and atorvastatin 40 mg; Amlodipine 5 mg and atorvastatin 80 mg; Amlodipine 10 mg and atorvastatin 10 mg; Amlodipine 10 mg and atorvastatin 20 mg; Amlodipine 10 mg and atorvastatin 40 mg; Amlodipine 10 mg and atorvastatin 80 mg

Caduet®:

2.5/10: Amlodipine 2.5 mg and atorvastatin 10 mg; 2.5/20: Amlodipine 2.5 mg and atorvastatin 20 mg; 2.5/40: Amlodipine 2.5 mg and atorvastatin 40 mg

5/10: Amlodipine 5 mg and atorvastatin 10 mg; 5/20: Amlodipine 5 mg and atorvastatin 20 mg; 5/40: Amlodipine 5 mg and atorvastatin 40 mg; 5/80: Amlodipine 5 mg and atorvastatin 80 mg

10/10: Amlodipine 10 mg and atorvastatin 10 mg; 10/20: Amlodipine 10 mg and atorvastatin 20 mg; 10/40: Amlodipine 10 mg and atorvastatin 40 mg; 10/80: Amlodipine 10 mg and atorvastatin 80 mg

amlodipine and benazepril (am LOE di peen & ben AY ze pril)

Synonyms benazepril hydrochloride and amlodipine besylate

U.S. Brand Names Lotrel®

Therapeutic Category Antihypertensive Agent, Combination

Use Treatment of hypertension

General Dosage Range Dosage adjustment recommended in patients with hepatic impairment

Oral:

Adults: 2.5-10 mg (amlodipine) and 10-40 mg (benazepril) once daily (maximum: amlodipine 10 mg/day; benazepril 80 mg/day)

Elderly: Initial: 2.5 mg/day (based on amlodipine component)

Dosage Forms

Capsule, oral: 2.5/10: Amlodipine 2.5 mg and benazepril 10 mg; 5/10: Amlodipine 5 mg and benazepril 10 mg; 5/20: Amlodipine 5 mg and benazepril 20 mg; 5/40: Amlodipine 5 mg and benazepril hydrochloride 40 mg; 10/20: Amlodipine 10 mg and benazepril 20 mg; 10/40: Amlodipine 10 mg and benazepril hydrochloride 40 mg

Lotrel®: 2.5/10: Amlodipine 2.5 and benazepril 10 mg; 5/10: Amlodipine 5 mg and benazepril 10 mg; 5/20: Amlodipine 5 mg and benazepril 20 mg; 5/40: Amlodipine 5 mg and benazepril 40 mg; 10/20: Amlodipine 10 mg and benazepril 20 mg; 10/40: Amlodipine 10 mg and benazepril 40 mg

amlodipine and olmesartan (am LOE di peen & olme SAR tan)

Synonyms amlodipine besylate and olmesartan medoxomil; olmesartan and amlodipine

U.S. Brand Names Azor™

Therapeutic Category Angiotensin II Receptor Blocker Combination; Antihypertensive Agent, Combination; Calcium Channel Blocker

Use Treatment of hypertension, including initial treatment in patients who will require multiple antihypertensives for adequate control

General Dosage Range Oral: *Adults:* Amlodipine 5-10 mg and olmesartan 20-40 mg once daily (maximum: 10 mg/day [amlodipine]; 40 mg/day [olmesartan])

Dosage Forms

Tablet:

Azor™: 5/20: Amlodipine 5 mg and olmesartan medoxomil 20 mg; 5/40: Amlodipine 5 mg and olmesartan medoxomil 40 mg; 10/20: Amlodipine 10 mg and olmesartan medoxomil 20 mg; 10/40: Amlodipine 10 mg and olmesartan medoxomil 40 mg

amlodipine and telmisartan *see* telmisartan and amlodipine *on page* 874

amlodipine and valsartan (am LOE di peen & val SAR tan)

Synonyms amlodipine besylate and valsartan; valsartan and amlodipine

U.S. Brand Names Exforge®

Therapeutic Category Angiotensin II Receptor Blocker Combination; Antihypertensive Agent, Combination; Calcium Channel Blocker

Use Treatment of hypertension

General Dosage Range Oral: *Adults:* Amlodipine 5-10 mg and valsartan 160-320 mg once daily (maximum: 10 mg/day [amlodipine]; 320 mg/day [valsartan])

Dosage Forms

Tablet:

Exforge®: 5/160: Amlodipine 5 mg and valsartan 160 mg; 5/320 mg: Amlodipine 5 mg and valsartan 320 mg; 10/160: Amlodipine 10 mg and valsartan 160 mg; 10/320: Amlodipine 10 mg and valsartan 320 mg

amlodipine besylate *see* amlodipine *on page* 65

amlodipine besylate, aliskiren hemifumarate, and hydrochlorothiazide *see* aliskiren, amlodipine, and hydrochlorothiazide *on page* 48

amlodipine besylate and olmesartan medoxomil *see* amlodipine and olmesartan *on page* 67

amlodipine besylate and telmisartan *see* telmisartan and amlodipine *on page* 874

amlodipine besylate and valsartan *see* amlodipine and valsartan *on page* 67

amlodipine besylate, olmesartan medoxomil, and hydrochlorothiazide *see* olmesartan, amlodipine, and hydrochlorothiazide *on page* 662

amlodipine besylate, valsartan, and hydrochlorothiazide *see* amlodipine, valsartan, and hydrochlorothiazide *on page* 68

amlodipine, hydrochlorothiazide, and aliskiren *see* aliskiren, amlodipine, and hydrochlorothiazide *on page* 48

amlodipine, hydrochlorothiazide, and olmesartan *see* olmesartan, amlodipine, and hydrochlorothiazide *on page* 662

amlodipine, hydrochlorothiazide, and valsartan *see* amlodipine, valsartan, and hydrochlorothiazide *on page* 68

Amlodipine-Odan (Can) *see* amlodipine *on page* 65

amlodipine, valsartan, and hydrochlorothiazide

(am LOE di peen, val SAR tan, & hye droe klor oh THYE a zide)

Synonyms amlodipine besylate, valsartan, and hydrochlorothiazide; amlodipine, hydrochlorothiazide, and valsartan; hydrochlorothiazide, amlodipine, and valsartan; valsartan, hydrochlorothiazide, and amlodipine

U.S. Brand Names Exforge HCT®

Therapeutic Category Angiotensin II Receptor Blocker; Calcium Channel Blocker; Diuretic, Thiazide

Use Treatment of hypertension (not for initial therapy)

General Dosage Range Oral: *Adults:* Amlodipine 5-10 mg and valsartan 160-320 mg and hydrochlorothiazide 12.5-25 mg once daily (maximum: 10 mg/day [amlodipine]; 25 mg/day [hydrochlorothiazide]; 320 mg/day [valsartan])

Dosage Forms

Tablet, oral:

Exforge HCT®: Amlodipine 5 mg, valsartan 160 mg, and hydrochlorothiazide 12.5 mg; Amlodipine 5 mg, valsartan 160 mg, and hydrochlorothiazide 25 mg; Amlodipine 10 mg, valsartan 160 mg, and hydrochlorothiazide 12.5 mg; Amlodipine 10 mg, valsartan 160 mg, and hydrochlorothiazide 25 mg; Amlodipine 10 mg, valsartan 320 mg, and hydrochlorothiazide 25 mg

Ammens® Original Medicated [OTC] *see* zinc oxide *on page 963*

Ammens® Shower Fresh [OTC] *see* zinc oxide *on page 963*

ammonapse *see* sodium phenylbutyrate *on page 845*

ammonia spirit (aromatic) (a MOE nee ah SPEAR it, air oh MAT ik)

Synonyms smelling salts

Therapeutic Category Respiratory Stimulant

Use Prevention or treatment of fainting

General Dosage Range Inhalation: *Children >12 years and Adults:* Slowly inhale the vapors of one crushed ampul or opened bottle of solution until fainting resolves

Dosage Forms

Solution, for inhalation: 1.7% to 2.1% (0.33 mL, 60 mL)

ammonium chloride (a MOE nee um KLOR ide)

Therapeutic Category Electrolyte Supplement, Oral

Use Treatment of hypochloremic states or metabolic alkalosis

General Dosage Range Metabolic alkalosis: The following equations represent different methods of correction utilizing either the serum HCO_3^-, the serum chloride, or the base excess

Dosing of mEq NH_4Cl via the chloride-deficit method (hypochloremia):

Dose of mEq NH_4Cl = [0.2 L/kg x body weight (kg)] x [103 - observed serum chloride]; administer 50% of dose over 12 hours, then re-evaluate

Note: 0.2 L/kg is the estimated chloride volume of distribution and 103 is the average normal serum chloride concentration (mEq/L)

Dosing of mEq NH_4Cl via the bicarbonate-excess method (refractory hypochloremic metabolic alkalosis):

Dose of NH_4Cl = [0.5 L/kg x body weight (kg)] x (observed serum HCO_3^- - 24); administer 50% of dose over 12 hours, then re-evaluate

Note: 0.5 L/kg is the estimated bicarbonate volume of distribution and 24 is the average normal serum bicarbonate concentration (mEq/L)

These equations will yield different requirements of ammonium chloride

Dosage Forms

Injection, solution: Ammonium 5 mEq/mL and chloride 5 mEq/mL (20 mL)

ammonium hydroxide and lactic acid *see* lactic acid and ammonium hydroxide *on page 517*

ammonium lactate *see* lactic acid and ammonium hydroxide *on page 517*

Ammonul® *see* sodium phenylacetate and sodium benzoate *on page 844*

AMN107 *see* nilotinib *on page 642*

Amnesteem® *see* isotretinoin *on page 505*

amobarbital (am oh BAR bi tal)

Medication Safety Issues

BEERS Criteria medication:

This drug may be potentially inappropriate for use in geriatric patients (Quality of evidence - high; Strength of recommendation - strong).

Synonyms amobarbital sodium; amylobarbitone

U.S. Brand Names Amytal®

Canadian Brand Names Amytal®

Therapeutic Category Barbiturate

Controlled Substance C-II

Use Hypnotic in short-term treatment of insomnia; reduce anxiety and provide sedation preoperatively

General Dosage Range Dosage adjustment recommended in patients with hepatic or renal impairment

I.M., I.V.:

Children 6-12 years: Sedative: 65-500 mg/dose

Adults:

Hypnotic: 65-200 mg at bedtime (maximum single dose: 1000 mg)

Sedative: 30-50 mg 2-3 times/day (maximum single dose: 1000 mg)

Dosage Forms

Injection, powder for reconstitution:

Amytal®: 0.5 g

amobarbital sodium *see* amobarbital *on page* 69

Amoclan *see* amoxicillin and clavulanate *on page* 70

amoxapine (a MOKS a peen)

Medication Safety Issues

Sound-alike/look-alike issues:

Amoxapine may be confused with amoxicillin, Amoxil

Asendin may be confused with aspirin

BEERS Criteria medication:

This drug may be potentially inappropriate for use in geriatric patients (Quality of evidence - moderate; Strength of recommendation - strong).

Synonyms Asendin [DSC]

Therapeutic Category Antidepressant, Tricyclic (Secondary Amine)

Use Treatment of depression (including endogenous, neurotic, psychotic, and reactive depression); treatment of depression accompanied by anxiety or agitation

General Dosage Range Oral:

Adults: 50 mg 2-3 times/day; usual effective dose: 200-300 mg/day; maximum: 600 mg/day (inpatient); 400 mg/day (outpatient)

Elderly: 25 mg 2-3 times/day; usual effective dose: 100-150 mg/day; maximum: 300 mg/day

Dosage Forms

Tablet, oral: 25 mg, 50 mg, 100 mg, 150 mg

amoxicillin (a moks i SIL in)

Medication Safety Issues

Sound-alike/look-alike issues:

Amoxicillin may be confused with amoxapine, Augmentin®

Amoxil may be confused with amoxapine

International issues:

Fisamox [Australia] may be confused with Fosamax brand name for alendronate [U.S., Canada, and multiple international markets] and Vigamox brand name for moxifloxacin [U.S., Canada, and multiple international markets]

Limoxin [Mexico] may be confused with Lanoxin brand name for digoxin [U.S., Canada, and multiple international markets]; Lincocin brand name for lincomycin [U.S., Canada, and multiple international markets]

Zimox: Brand name for amoxicillin [Italy], but also the brand name for carbidopa/levodopa [Greece]

Zimox [Italy] may be confused with Diamox which is the brand name for acetazolamide [Canada and multiple international markets]

Synonyms *p*-hydroxyampicillin; amoxicillin trihydrate; Amoxil; amoxycillin

U.S. Brand Names Moxatag™

Canadian Brand Names Apo-Amoxi®; Mylan-Amoxicillin; Novamoxin®; NTP-Amoxicillin; Nu-Amoxi; PHL-Amoxicillin; PMS-Amoxicillin; Pro-Amox-250; Pro-Amox-500

Therapeutic Category Penicillin

Use Treatment of otitis media, sinusitis, and infections caused by susceptible organisms involving the upper and lower respiratory tract, skin, and urinary tract; prophylaxis of infective endocarditis in patients undergoing surgical or dental procedures; as part of a multidrug regimen for *H. pylori* eradication; periodontitis

General Dosage Range Dosage adjustment recommended in patients with renal impairment

Oral:

Immediate release:

Infants ≤3 months: 20-30 mg/kg/day divided every 12 hours

Children >3 months and <40 kg: 20-100 mg/kg/day divided every 8-12 hours

Adults: 250-500 mg every 8 hours **or** 500-875 mg twice daily (maximum: 875 mg/dose)

Extended release: *Children ≥12 years and Adults:* 775 mg once daily

Dosage Forms

Capsule, oral: 250 mg, 500 mg

Powder for suspension, oral: 125 mg/5 mL (80 mL, 100 mL, 150 mL); 200 mg/5 mL (50 mL, 75 mL, 100 mL); 250 mg/5 mL (80 mL, 100 mL, 150 mL); 400 mg/5 mL (50 mL, 75 mL, 100 mL)

Tablet, oral: 500 mg, 875 mg

Tablet, chewable, oral: 125 mg, 200 mg, 250 mg, 400 mg

Tablet, extended release, oral:

Moxatag™: 775 mg

amoxicillin and clavulanate (a moks i SIL in & klav yoo LAN ate)

Medication Safety Issues

Sound-alike/look-alike issues:

Augmentin® may be confused with amoxicillin, Azulfidine®

Synonyms amoxicillin and clavulanate potassium; amoxicillin and clavulanic acid; clavulanic acid and amoxicillin

U.S. Brand Names Amoclan; Augmentin XR®; Augmentin®

Canadian Brand Names Amoxi-Clav; Apo-Amoxi-Clav®; Clavulin®; Novo-Clavamoxin; ratio-Aclavulanate

Therapeutic Category Penicillin

Use Treatment of otitis media, sinusitis, and infections caused by susceptible organisms involving the lower respiratory tract, skin and skin structure, and urinary tract; spectrum same as amoxicillin with additional coverage of beta-lactamase producing *B. catarrhalis*, *H. influenzae*, *N. gonorrhoeae*, and *S. aureus* (not MRSA). The expanded coverage of this combination makes it a useful alternative when amoxicillin resistance is present and patients cannot tolerate alternative treatments.

General Dosage Range Dosage adjustment recommended in patients with renal impairment

Oral:

Immediate release:

Infants <3 months: 30 mg/kg/day divided every 12 hours

Children ≥3 months and <40 kg: 25-90 mg/kg/day divided every 12 hours **or** 20-40 mg/kg/day divided every 8 hours

Children >40 kg and Adults: 250-500 mg every 8 hours **or** 875 mg every 12 hours

Extended release: *Children ≥16 years and Adults:* 2000 mg every 12 hours (maximum: 2000 mg/dose)

Dosage Forms

Powder for suspension, oral: 200: Amoxicillin 200 mg and clavulanate potassium 28.5 mg per 5 mL; 250: Amoxicillin 250 mg and clavulanate potassium 62.5 mg per 5 mL; 400: Amoxicillin 400 mg and clavulanate potassium 57 mg per 5 mL; 600: Amoxicillin 600 mg and clavulanate potassium 42.9 mg per 5 mL

Amoclan:

200: Amoxicillin 200 mg and clavulanate potassium 28.5 mg per 5 mL

400: Amoxicillin 400 mg and clavulanate potassium 57 mg per 5 mL

600: Amoxicillin 600 mg and clavulanate potassium 42.9 mg per 5 mL

Augmentin®:

125: Amoxicillin 125 mg and clavulanate potassium 31.25 mg per 5 mL

250: Amoxicillin 250 mg and clavulanate potassium 62.5 mg per 5 mL

Tablet, oral: 250: Amoxicillin 250 mg and clavulanate potassium 125 mg; 500: Amoxicillin 500 mg and clavulanate potassium 125 mg; 875: Amoxicillin 875 mg and clavulanate potassium 125 mg

Augmentin®:

500: Amoxicillin 500 mg and clavulanate potassium 125 mg

875: Amoxicillin 875 mg and clavulanate potassium 125 mg

Tablet, chewable, oral: 200: Amoxicillin 200 mg and clavulanate potassium 28.5 mg; 400: Amoxicillin 400 mg and clavulanate potassium 57 mg

Tablet, extended release, oral: Amoxicillin 1000 mg and clavulanate acid 62.5 mg

Augmentin XR®: 1000: Amoxicillin 1000 mg and clavulanate acid 62.5 mg

amoxicillin and clavulanate potassium *see* amoxicillin and clavulanate *on page 70*

amoxicillin and clavulanic acid *see* amoxicillin and clavulanate *on page 70*

amoxicillin, clarithromycin, and lansoprazole *see* lansoprazole, amoxicillin, and clarithromycin *on page 523*

amoxicillin, clarithromycin, and omeprazole *see* omeprazole, clarithromycin, and amoxicillin *on page 666*

amoxicillin trihydrate *see* amoxicillin *on page 69*

Amoxi-Clav (Can) *see* amoxicillin and clavulanate *on page 70*

Amoxil *see* amoxicillin *on page 69*

amoxycillin *see* amoxicillin *on page 69*

Amphadase™ *see* hyaluronidase *on page 451*

amphetamine and dextroamphetamine *see* dextroamphetamine and amphetamine *on page 271*

Amphojel® (Can) *see* aluminum hydroxide *on page 55*

Amphotec® *see* amphotericin B cholesteryl sulfate complex *on page 71*

amphotericin B cholesteryl sulfate complex

(am foe TER i sin bee kole LES te ril SUL fate KOM plecks)

Medication Safety Issues

High alert medication:

The Institute for Safe Medication Practices (ISMP) includes this medication among its list of drugs which have a heightened risk of causing significant patient harm when used in error.

Other safety concerns:

Lipid-based amphotericin formulations (Amphotec®) may be confused with conventional formulations (Amphocin®, Fungizone®)

Large overdoses have occurred when conventional formulations were dispensed inadvertently for lipid-based products. Single daily doses of conventional amphotericin formulation never exceed 1.5 mg/kg.

Synonyms ABCD; amphotericin B colloidal dispersion

U.S. Brand Names Amphotec®

Canadian Brand Names Amphotec®

Therapeutic Category Antifungal Agent

Use Treatment of invasive aspergillosis in patients who have failed amphotericin B deoxycholate treatment, or who have renal impairment or experience unacceptable toxicity which precludes treatment with amphotericin B deoxycholate in effective doses.

General Dosage Range I.V.: *Children and Adults:* 3-4 mg/kg/day

Dosage Forms

Injection, powder for reconstitution:

Amphotec®: 50 mg, 100 mg

amphotericin B colloidal dispersion *see* amphotericin B cholesteryl sulfate complex *on page 71*

amphotericin B (conventional) (am foe TER i sin bee con VEN sha nal)

Medication Safety Issues

High alert medication:

The Institute for Safe Medication Practices (ISMP) includes this medication (intrathecal administration) among its list of drugs which have a heightened risk of causing significant patient harm when used in error.

Other safety concerns:

Conventional amphotericin formulations (Amphocin®, Fungizone®) may be confused with lipid-based formulations (AmBisome®, Abelcet®, Amphotec®).

Large overdoses have occurred when conventional formulations were dispensed inadvertently for lipid-based products. Single daily doses of conventional amphotericin formulation never exceed 1.5 mg/kg.

Synonyms amphotericin B deoxycholate; amphotericin B desoxycholate; conventional amphotericin B

Canadian Brand Names Fungizone®

Therapeutic Category Antifungal Agent

Use Treatment of severe systemic and central nervous system infections caused by susceptible fungi such as *Candida* species, *Histoplasma capsulatum*, *Cryptococcus neoformans*, *Aspergillus* species, *Blastomyces dermatitidis*, *Torulopsis glabrata*, and *Coccidioides immitis*; fungal peritonitis; irrigant for bladder fungal infections; used in fungal infection in patients with bone marrow transplantation, amebic meningoencephalitis, ocular aspergillosis (intraocular injection), candidal cystitis (bladder irrigation), chemoprophylaxis (low-dose I.V.), immunocompromised patients at risk of aspergillosis (intranasal/nebulized), refractory meningitis (intrathecal), coccidioidal arthritis (intraarticular/I.M.).

Low-dose amphotericin B has been administered after bone marrow transplantation to reduce the risk of invasive fungal disease.

General Dosage Range Dosage adjustment recommended in patients who develop toxicities

I.V.:

Infants and Children: Test dose: 0.1 mg/kg/dose (maximum: 1 mg); Maintenance: 0.25-1 mg/kg/day given once daily; 1-1.5 mg/kg every other day may be given once therapy is established (maximum: 1.5-4 g cumulative dose)

Adults: Test dose: 1 mg infused; Maintenance: 0.3-1.5 mg/kg/day given once daily; 1-1.5 mg/kg every other day may be given once therapy is established (maximum: 1.5 mg/kg/day)

Dosage Forms

Injection, powder for reconstitution: 50 mg

amphotericin B deoxycholate *see* amphotericin B (conventional) *on page 71*

amphotericin B desoxycholate *see* amphotericin B (conventional) *on page 71*

amphotericin B lipid complex (am foe TER i sin bee LIP id KOM pleks)

Medication Safety Issues

High alert medication:

The Institute for Safe Medication Practices (ISMP) includes this medication among its list of drugs which have a heightened risk of causing significant patient harm when used in error.

Other safety concerns:

Lipid-based amphotericin formulations (Abelcet®) may be confused with conventional formulations (Fungizone®) or with other lipid-based amphotericin formulations (amphotericin B liposomal [AmBisome®]; amphotericin B cholesteryl sulfate complex [Amphotec®])

Large overdoses have occurred when conventional formulations were dispensed inadvertently for lipid-based products. Single daily doses of conventional amphotericin formulation never exceed 1.5 mg/kg.

Synonyms ABLC

U.S. Brand Names Abelcet®

Canadian Brand Names Abelcet®

Therapeutic Category Antifungal Agent

Use Treatment of invasive fungal infection in patients who are refractory to or intolerant of conventional amphotericin B (amphotericin B deoxycholate) therapy

General Dosage Range I.V.: *Children and Adults:* 5 mg/kg once daily

Dosage Forms

Injection, suspension [preservative free]:

Abelcet®: 5 mg/mL (20 mL)

amphotericin B liposomal (am foe TER i sin bee lye po SO mal)

Medication Safety Issues

High alert medication:

The Institute for Safe Medication Practices (ISMP) includes this medication among its list of drugs which have a heightened risk of causing significant patient harm when used in error.

Other safety concerns:

Lipid-based amphotericin formulations (AmBisome®) may be confused with conventional formulations (Amphocin®, Fungizone®) or with other lipid-based amphotericin formulations (Abelcet®, Amphotec®)

Large overdoses have occurred when conventional formulations were dispensed inadvertently for lipid-based products. Single daily doses of conventional amphotericin formulation never exceed 1.5 mg/kg.

Synonyms L-AmB

U.S. Brand Names AmBisome®

Canadian Brand Names AmBisome®

Therapeutic Category Antifungal Agent, Systemic

Use Empirical therapy for presumed fungal infection in febrile, neutropenic patients; treatment of patients with *Aspergillus* species, *Candida* species, and/or *Cryptococcus* species infections refractory to amphotericin B desoxycholate (conventional amphotericin), or in patients where renal impairment or unacceptable toxicity precludes the use of amphotericin B desoxycholate; treatment of cryptococcal meningitis in HIV-infected patients; treatment of visceral leishmaniasis

General Dosage Range **I.V.:** *Children and Adults:* 3-6 mg/kg/day as a single daily dose (maximum: 6 mg/kg/day)

Dosage Forms

Injection, powder for reconstitution:

AmBisome®: 50 mg

ampicillin (am pi SIL in)

Medication Safety Issues

Sound-alike/look-alike issues:

Ampicillin may be confused with aminophylline

Synonyms aminobenzylpenicillin; ampicillin sodium; ampicillin trihydrate

Canadian Brand Names Ampicillin for Injection; Apo-Ampi®; Novo-Ampicillin; Nu-Ampi

Therapeutic Category Penicillin

Use Treatment of susceptible bacterial infections (nonbeta-lactamase-producing organisms); treatment or prophylaxis of infective endocarditis; susceptible bacterial infections caused by streptococci, pneumococci, nonpenicillinase-producing staphylococci, *Listeria*, meningococci; some strains of *H. influenzae*, *Salmonella*, *Shigella*, *E. coli*, *Enterobacter*, and *Klebsiella*

General Dosage Range Dosage adjustment recommended in patients with renal impairment

I.M., I.V.:

Infants and Children: 100-400 mg/kg/day divided every 6 hours (maximum: 12 g/day)

Adults: 1-2 g every 4-6 hours or 50-250 mg/kg/day in divided doses (maximum: 12 g/day)

Oral:

Infants and Children: 50-100 mg/kg/day divided every 6 hours (maximum: 2-4 g/day)

Adults: 250-500 mg every 6 hours

Dosage Forms

Capsule, oral: 250 mg, 500 mg

Injection, powder for reconstitution: 125 mg, 250 mg, 500 mg, 1 g, 2 g, 10 g

Powder for suspension, oral: 125 mg/5 mL (100 mL, 200 mL); 250 mg/5 mL (100 mL, 200 mL)

ampicillin and sulbactam (am pi SIL in & SUL bak tam)

Synonyms sulbactam and ampicillin

U.S. Brand Names Unasyn®

Canadian Brand Names Unasyn®

Therapeutic Category Penicillin

Use Treatment of susceptible bacterial infections involved with skin and skin structure, intraabdominal infections, gynecological infections; spectrum is that of ampicillin plus organisms producing beta-lactamases such as *S. aureus*, *H. influenzae*, *E. coli*, *Klebsiella*, *Acinetobacter*, *Enterobacter*, and anaerobes

General Dosage Range Dosage adjustment recommended in patients with renal impairment

I.M.: *Adults:* 1-2 g (1.5-3 g Unasyn®) ampicillin every 6 hours (maximum: 8 g ampicillin/day)

I.V.:

Children ≥1 year: 100-400 mg ampicillin/kg/day divided every 6 hours (maximum: 8 g ampicillin/day)

Adults: 1-2 g (1.5-3 g Unasyn®) ampicillin every 6 hours (maximum: 8 g ampicillin/day)

Dosage Forms

Injection, powder for reconstitution: 1.5 g [ampicillin 1 g and sulbactam 0.5 g]; 3 g [ampicillin 2 g and sulbactam 1 g]; 15 g [ampicillin 10 g and sulbactam 5 g]

Unasyn®: 1.5 g [ampicillin 1 g and sulbactam 0.5 g]; 3 g [ampicillin 2 g and sulbactam 1 g]; 15 g [ampicillin 10 g and sulbactam 5 g]; 15 g [ampicillin 10 g and sulbactam 5 g

Ampicillin for Injection (Can) *see* ampicillin *on page 73*

ampicillin sodium *see* ampicillin *on page 73*

ampicillin trihydrate *see* ampicillin *on page* *73*

AMPT *see* metyrosine *on page* *598*

Ampyra™ *see* dalfampridine *on page* *251*

AMR101 *see* icosapent ethyl *on page* *472*

Amrix® *see* cyclobenzaprine *on page* *243*

Amturnide™ *see* aliskiren, amlodipine, and hydrochlorothiazide *on page* *48*

Amvisc® *see* hyaluronate and derivatives *on page* *450*

Amvisc® Plus *see* hyaluronate and derivatives *on page* *450*

amylase, lipase, and protease *see* pancrelipase *on page* *687*

amyl nitrite (AM il NYE trite)

Synonyms isoamyl nitrite

Therapeutic Category Vasodilator

Use Coronary vasodilator in angina pectoris

Note: Given the widespread use of newer nitrate compounds, the use of amyl nitrite for patients experiencing angina pectoris has fallen out of favor.

General Dosage Range **Inhalation:** *Adults:* 2-6 nasal inhalations from 1 crushed ampul; may repeat in 3-5 minutes

Dosage Forms

Liquid, for inhalation: USP: 85% to 103% (0.3 mL)

amyl nitrite, sodium nitrite, and sodium thiosulfate *see* sodium nitrite, sodium thiosulfate, and amyl nitrite *on page* *844*

amylobarbitone *see* amobarbital *on page* *69*

Amytal® *see* amobarbital *on page* *69*

Amyvid™ *see* florbetapir F18 *on page* *387*

AN100226 *see* natalizumab *on page* *630*

Anacin® Advanced Headache Formula [OTC] *see* acetaminophen, aspirin, and caffeine *on page* *26*

Anadrol®-50 *see* oxymetholone *on page* *682*

Anafranil® *see* clomipramine *on page* *223*

anagrelide (an AG gre lide)

Medication Safety Issues

Sound-alike/look-alike issues:

Anagrelide may be confused with anastrozole

Synonyms anagrelide hydrochloride; BL4162A

U.S. Brand Names Agrylin®

Canadian Brand Names Agrylin®; Dom-Anagrelide; Mylan-Anagrelide; PMS-Anagrelide; Sandoz-Anagrelide

Therapeutic Category Platelet Reducing Agent

Use Treatment of thrombocythemia associated with myeloproliferative disorders (eg, chronic myelogenous leukemia, essential thrombocythemia, polycythemia vera, myeloid metaplasia with myelofibrosis, or other myeloproliferative disorder) to reduce the risk of thrombosis and reduce associated symptoms (including thrombo-hemorrhagic events)

General Dosage Range Dosage adjustment recommended in patients with hepatic impairment

Oral:

Children: Initial: 0.5 mg/day; Maintenance: 0.5 mg 1-4 times/day (maximum: 10 mg/day; 2.5 mg/dose)

Adults: Initial: 0.5 mg 4 times/day **or** 1 mg twice daily (maximum: 10 mg/day; 2.5 mg/dose)

Dosage Forms

Capsule, oral: 0.5 mg, 1 mg

Agrylin®: 0.5 mg

anagrelide hydrochloride *see* anagrelide *on page* *74*

anakinra (an a KIN ra)

Medication Safety Issues

Sound-alike/look-alike issues:

Anakinra may be confused with amikacin, Ampyra™

Kineret® may be confused with Amikin®

Synonyms IL-1Ra; interleukin-1 receptor antagonist

U.S. Brand Names Kineret®

Canadian Brand Names Kineret®

Therapeutic Category Antirheumatic, Disease Modifying

Use Treatment of moderately- to severely-active rheumatoid arthritis in adult patients who have failed one or more disease-modifying antirheumatic drugs (DMARDs); may be used alone or in combination with DMARDs (other than tumor necrosis factor-blocking agents)

General Dosage Range Dosage adjustment recommended in patients with renal impairment

SubQ: *Adults:* 100 mg once daily

Dosage Forms

Injection, solution [preservative free]:

Kineret®: 100 mg/0.67 mL (0.67 mL)

Ana-Kit® *see* epinephrine and chlorpheniramine *on page* *335*
Analpram E™ *see* pramoxine and hydrocortisone *on page* *751*
Analpram HC® *see* pramoxine and hydrocortisone *on page* *751*
AnaMantle HC® Cream *see* lidocaine and hydrocortisone *on page* *538*
AnaMantle HC® Forte *see* lidocaine and hydrocortisone *on page* *538*
AnaMantle HC® Gel *see* lidocaine and hydrocortisone *on page* *538*
Anandron® (Can) *see* nilutamide *on page* *642*
Anaplex® DM *see* brompheniramine, pseudoephedrine, and dextromethorphan *on page* *144*
Anaprox® *see* naproxen *on page* *628*
Anaprox® DS *see* naproxen *on page* *628*
Anascorp® *see Centruroides* immune $F(ab')_2$ (equine) *on page* *189*
Anaspaz® *see* hyoscyamine *on page* *465*

anastrozole (an AS troe zole)

Medication Safety Issues

Sound-alike/look-alike issues:

Anastrozole may be confused with anagrelide, letrozole

Arimidex® may be confused with Aromasin®

Synonyms ICI-D1033; ZD1033

U.S. Brand Names Arimidex®

Canadian Brand Names Arimidex®

Therapeutic Category Antineoplastic Agent

Use First-line treatment of locally-advanced or metastatic breast cancer (hormone receptor-positive or unknown) in postmenopausal women; treatment of advanced breast cancer in postmenopausal women with disease progression following tamoxifen therapy; adjuvant treatment of early hormone receptor-positive breast cancer in postmenopausal women

General Dosage Range Oral: *Adults:* 1 mg once daily

Dosage Forms

Tablet, oral: 1 mg

Arimidex®: 1 mg

A-Natural [OTC] *see* vitamin A *on page* *949*
A-Natural-25 [OTC] *see* vitamin A *on page* *949*
Anbesol® [OTC] *see* benzocaine *on page* *121*
Anbesol® Baby [OTC] *see* benzocaine *on page* *121*
Anbesol® Baby (Can) *see* benzocaine *on page* *121*
Anbesol® Cold Sore Therapy [OTC] *see* benzocaine *on page* *121*
Anbesol® Jr. [OTC] *see* benzocaine *on page* *121*
Anbesol® Maximum Strength [OTC] *see* benzocaine *on page* *121*

ancef *see* cefazolin *on page* 181
anchoic acid *see* azelaic acid *on page* 107
Ancobon® *see* flucytosine *on page* 389
Andriol® (Can) *see* testosterone *on page* 881
Androcur® (Can) *see* cyproterone *(Canada only) on page* 246
Androcur® Depot (Can) *see* cyproterone *(Canada only) on page* 246
Androderm® *see* testosterone *on page* 881
AndroGel® *see* testosterone *on page* 881
Android® *see* methyltestosterone *on page* 593
Andropository (Can) *see* testosterone *on page* 881
Androvite® [OTC] *see* vitamins (multiple/oral) *on page* 951
Androxy™ *see* fluoxymesterone *on page* 397
AneCream™ [OTC] *see* lidocaine (topical) *on page* 535
Anectine® *see* succinylcholine *on page* 855
Anestafoam™ [OTC] *see* lidocaine (topical) *on page* 535
aneurine hydrochloride *see* thiamine *on page* 890
Anexate® (Can) *see* flumazenil *on page* 390
Angeliq® *see* drospirenone and estradiol *on page* 317
Angiomax® *see* bivalirudin *on page* 137
anhydrous glucose *see* dextrose *on page* 275

anidulafungin (ay nid yoo la FUN jin)

Synonyms LY303366
U.S. Brand Names Eraxis™
Canadian Brand Names Eraxis™
Therapeutic Category Antifungal Agent, Parenteral; Echinocandin
Use Treatment of candidemia and other forms of *Candida* infections (including those of intraabdominal, peritoneal, and esophageal locus)
General Dosage Range I.V.: *Adults:* Loading dose: 100-200 mg as a single dose; Maintenance: 50-100 mg daily
Dosage Forms
Injection, powder for reconstitution:
Eraxis™: 50 mg, 100 mg

Anolor 300 *see* butalbital, acetaminophen, and caffeine *on page* 153
Ansaid® (Can) *see* flurbiprofen (systemic) *on page* 399
ansamycin *see* rifabutin *on page* 799
Antabuse® *see* disulfiram *on page* 302
antagon *see* ganirelix *on page* 419
Antara® *see* fenofibrate *on page* 375
Anthraforte® (Can) *see* anthralin *on page* 76

anthralin (AN thra lin)

Synonyms dithranol
U.S. Brand Names Dritho-Creme®; Dritho-Scalp®; Zithranol®-RR
Canadian Brand Names Anthraforte®; Anthranol®; Anthrascalp®; Micanol®
Therapeutic Category Keratolytic Agent
Use Treatment of psoriasis (quiescent or chronic psoriasis)
General Dosage Range Topical: *Adults:* Generally, apply once a day or as directed
Dosage Forms
Cream, topical:
Dritho-Creme®: 1% (50 g)
Dritho-Scalp®: 0.5% (50 g)
Zithranol®-RR: 1.2% (45 g)

Anthranol® (Can) *see* anthralin *on page* 76
Anthrascalp® (Can) *see* anthralin *on page* 76

anthrax vaccine, adsorbed (AN thraks vak SEEN ad SORBED)

Synonyms AVA

U.S. Brand Names BioThrax®

Therapeutic Category Vaccine

Use Immunization against *Bacillus anthracis* in persons at high risk for exposure.

The Advisory Committee on Immunization Practices (ACIP) recommends routine vaccination (pre-exposure vaccination) for the following (CDC, 2010):

- Persons who work directly with the organism in the laboratory
- Persons who handle animals or animal products only when
  - potentially infected in research settings;
  - in areas of high incidence of enzootic anthrax; or
  - where standards and restrictions are not sufficient to prevent exposure
- Military personnel deployed to areas with high risk of exposure as recommended by the Department of Defense (DoD)
- Persons engaged in environmental investigations or remediation efforts

Routine immunization for the general population is not recommended. Routine vaccination may be offered to emergency and other responders (police and fire departments, the National Guard, etc) on a voluntary basis under the direction of a comprehensive occupational health and safety program.

The ACIP recommends postexposure prophylaxis after inhalation exposure to aerosolized *Bacillus anthracis* spores for the following (in the absence of completing a pre-exposure, routine vaccination schedule):

- The general public, including pregnant and breast-feeding women
- Medical professionals
- Children ages 0-18 years as determined on an event-by-event basis
- Persons engaged in handling certain animals or animal products
- Persons who work directly with the organism in the laboratory (postexposure vaccination dependant upon pre-event vaccination status)
- Military personnel as recommended by the DoD
- Persons engaged in environmental investigations or remediation efforts (postexposure vaccination dependent upon pre-event vaccination status)
- Emergency and other responders (police and fire departments, the National Guard, etc)
- Persons working in postal facilities

General Dosage Range

I.M.: *Adults ≤65 years:* 0.5 mL

SubQ: *Adults:* 0.5 mL

Dosage Forms

Injection, suspension:

BioThrax®: *Bacillus anthracis* proteins (5 mL)

anti-4 alpha integrin *see* natalizumab *on page 630*

anti-D immunoglobulin *see* Rh_o(D) immune globulin *on page 797*

131 I anti-B1 antibody *see* tositumomab and iodine I 131 tositumomab *on page 907*

131 I-anti-B1 monoclonal antibody *see* tositumomab and iodine I 131 tositumomab *on page 907*

antibody-drug conjugate SGN-35 *see* brentuximab vedotin *on page 140*

anti-CD20 monoclonal antibody *see* rituximab *on page 805*

anti-CD20-murine monoclonal antibody I-131 *see* tositumomab and iodine I 131 tositumomab *on page 907*

anti-CD30 ADC SGN-35 *see* brentuximab vedotin *on page 140*

anti-CD30 antibody-drug conjugate SGN-35 *see* brentuximab vedotin *on page 140*

anti-CD52 monoclonal antibody *see* alemtuzumab *on page 45*

anti-c-erB-2 *see* trastuzumab *on page 911*

Anti-Diarrheal [OTC] *see* loperamide *on page 547*

antidigoxin fab fragments, ovine *see* digoxin immune Fab *on page 286*

antidiuretic hormone *see* vasopressin *on page 940*

anti-ERB-2 *see* trastuzumab *on page 911*

Anti-Fungal™ [OTC] *see* clotrimazole (topical) *on page 227*

antihemophilic factor (human) (an tee hee moe FIL ik FAK tor HYU man)

Medication Safety Issues

Sound-alike/look-alike issues:

Factor VIII may be confused with Factor XIII

Other safety concerns:

Confusion may occur due to the omitting of "Factor VIII" from some product labeling. Review product contents carefully prior to dispensing any antihemophilic factor.

Synonyms AHF (human); factor VIII (human)

U.S. Brand Names Hemofil M; Koāte®-DVI; Monoclate-P®

Canadian Brand Names Hemofil M

Therapeutic Category Blood Product Derivative

Use Prevention and treatment of hemorrhagic episodes in patients with hemophilia A (classic hemophilia); perioperative management of hemophilia A; can be of significant therapeutic value in patients with acquired factor VIII inhibitors not exceeding 10 Bethesda units/mL

General Dosage Range I.V.: *Children and Adults:* Dosage varies greatly depending on indication

Dosage Forms

Injection, powder for reconstitution:

Hemofil M: ~250 units, ~500 units, ~1000 units, ~1700 units
Koāte®-DVI: ~250 units, ~500 units, ~1000 units
Monoclate-P®: ~250 units, ~500 units, ~1000 units, ~1500 units

antihemophilic factor (recombinant) (an tee hee moe FIL ik FAK tor ree KOM be nant)

Medication Safety Issues

Sound-alike/look-alike issues:

Factor VIII may be confused with Factor XIII

Other safety concerns:

Confusion may occur due to the omitting of "Factor VIII" from some product labeling. Review product contents carefully prior to dispensing any antihemophilic factor.

Synonyms AHF (recombinant); factor VIII (recombinant); rAHF

U.S. Brand Names Advate; Helixate® FS; Kogenate® FS; Recombinate; Xyntha®; Xyntha® Solofuse™

Canadian Brand Names Advate; Helixate® FS; Kogenate® FS; Xyntha®

Therapeutic Category Blood Product Derivative

Use Prevention and treatment of hemorrhagic episodes in patients with hemophilia A (classic hemophilia or congenital factor VIII deficiency); perioperative management of hemophilia A; routine prophylaxis in patients with hemophilia A to prevent bleeding episodes (Advate, Helixate® FS, Kogenate® FS)

Note: Helixate® FS and Kogenate® FS are also approved in children with hemophilia A with no pre-existing joint damage to reduce risk of joint damage. In addition, Recombinate can be of therapeutic value in patients with acquired factor VIII inhibitors ≤10 Bethesda units/mL.

General Dosage Range I.V.: *Children and Adults:* Dosage varies greatly depending on indication

Dosage Forms

Injection, powder for reconstitution [preservative free]:

Advate: 250 units, 500 units, 1000 units, 1500 units, 2000 units, 3000 units, 4000 units
Helixate® FS: 250 units, 500 units, 1000 units, 2000 units, 3000 units
Kogenate® FS: 250 units, 500 units, 1000 units, 2000 units, 3000 units
Recombinate: 250 units, 500 units, 1000 units, 1500 units, 2000 units
Xyntha®: 250 units, 500 units, 1000 units, 2000 units
Xyntha® Solofuse™: 1000 units, 2000 units, 3000 units

antihemophilic factor/von Willebrand factor complex (human)

(an tee hee moe FIL ik FAK tor von WILL le brand FAK tor KOM plex HYU man)

Medication Safety Issues

Sound-alike/look-alike issues:

Factor VIII may be confused with Factor XIII

Synonyms AHF (human); factor VIII (human); factor VIII concentrate; FVIII/vWF; von willebrand factor/factor VIII complex; VWF/FVIII concentrate; VWF:RCo; vWF:RCof

U.S. Brand Names Alphanate®; Humate-P®; Wilate®

Canadian Brand Names Humate-P®

Therapeutic Category Antihemophilic Agent; Blood Product Derivative

Use

Factor VIII deficiency: Alphanate®, Humate-P®: Prevention and treatment of hemorrhagic episodes in patients with hemophilia A (classical hemophilia) or acquired factor VIII deficiency (Alphanate® only); **Note:** Wilate® is not approved for use in patients with hemophilia A or acquired factor VIII deficiency

von Willebrand disease (VWD):

Alphanate®: Prophylaxis with surgical and/or invasive procedures in patients with VWD when desmopressin is either ineffective or contraindicated; **Note:** Not indicated for patients with severe VWD undergoing major surgery

Humate-P®: Treatment of spontaneous or trauma-induced bleeding, as well as prevention of excessive bleeding during and after surgery in patients with severe VWD, including mild or moderate disease where use of desmopressin is known or suspected to be inadequate; **Note:** Not indicated for the prophylaxis of spontaneous bleeding episodes

Wilate®: Treatment of spontaneous and trauma-induced bleeding in patients with severe VWD, including mild or moderate disease where use of desmopressin is known or suspected to be inadequate or contraindicated; **Note:** Not indicated for prophylaxis of spontaneous bleeding or prevention of excessive bleeding during and after surgery)

General Dosage Range I.V.: *Children and Adults:* Dosage varies greatly depending on indication

Dosage Forms

Injection, powder for reconstitution [human derived]:

Alphanate®:

250 units [Factor VIII and VWF:RCo ratio varies by lot]
500 units [Factor VIII and VWF:RCo ratio varies by lot]
1000 units [Factor VIII and VWF:RCo ratio varies by lot]
1500 units [Factor VIII and VWF:RCo ratio varies by lot]

Humate-P®:

FVIII 250 units and VWF:RCo 600 units
FVIII 500 units and VWF:RCo 1200 units
FVIII 1000 units and VWF:RCo 2400 units

Wilate®:

FVIII 500 units and VWF:RCo 500 units
FVIII 1000 units and VWF:RCo 1000 units

Anti-Hist [OTC] *see* diphenhydramine (systemic) *on page 292*

antiinhibitor coagulant complex (an TEE in HI bi tor coe AG yoo lant KOM pleks)

Synonyms AICC; aPCC; coagulant complex inhibitor

U.S. Brand Names Feiba NF; Feiba VH [DSC]

Canadian Brand Names Feiba NF

Therapeutic Category Hemophilic Agent

Use Hemophilia A & B patients with inhibitors who are to undergo surgery or those who are bleeding

General Dosage Range I.V.: *Children and Adults:* 50-100 units/kg every 6-12 hours (maximum: 200 units/kg/day)

Dosage Forms

Injection, powder for reconstitution:

Feiba NF: ~500 units, ~1000 units, ~2500 units

Antiphlogistine Rub A-535 No Odour (Can) *see* trolamine *on page 923*

antipyrine and benzocaine (an tee PYE reen & BEN zoe kane)

Synonyms benzocaine and antipyrine

U.S. Brand Names Aurodex®

Canadian Brand Names Auralgan®

Therapeutic Category Otic Agent, Analgesic; Otic Agent, Ceruminolytic

Use Temporary relief of pain and reduction of swelling associated with acute congestive and serous otitis media; facilitates ear wax removal

General Dosage Range Otic: *Children and Adults:* Instill drops 3 times/day (ear wax removal) or fill ear canal every 1-2 hours (otitis media)

Dosage Forms

Solution, otic [drops]: Antipyrine 5.4% and benzocaine 1.4% (10 mL, 15 mL)

Aurodex™: Antipyrine 5.4% and benzocaine 1.4% (10 mL)

antithrombin III (an tee THROM bin)

Synonyms antithrombin alfa; AT; AT-III; hpAT; rhAT; rhATIII

U.S. Brand Names Atryn®; Thrombate III®

Canadian Brand Names Thrombate III®

Therapeutic Category Blood Product Derivative

Use Prophylaxis (ATryn®, Thrombate III®) of thromboembolic events in patients with hereditary antithrombin (AT or AT-III) deficiency undergoing surgical or obstetrical procedures (eg, childbirth); treatment (Thrombate III®) of thromboembolism in patients with hereditary AT deficiency

General Dosage Range I.V.: *Adults:* Dosage varies greatly depending on indication

Dosage Forms

Injection, powder for reconstitution [preservative free]:

Atryn®: ~1750 units

Thrombate III®: ~500 units

antithrombin alfa *see* antithrombin III *on page* 80

antithymocyte globulin (equine) (an te THY moe site GLOB yu lin, E kwine)

Medication Safety Issues

Sound-alike/look-alike issues:

Antithymocyte globulin equine (Atgam®) may be confused with antithymocyte globulin rabbit (Thymoglobulin®)

Atgam® may be confused with Ativan®

Synonyms antithymocyte immunoglobulin; ATG; horse antihuman thymocyte gamma globulin; lymphocyte immune globulin

U.S. Brand Names Atgam®

Canadian Brand Names Atgam®

Therapeutic Category Immunosuppressant Agent

Use Prevention and treatment of acute renal allograft rejection; treatment of moderate-to-severe aplastic anemia in patients not considered suitable candidates for bone marrow transplantation

General Dosage Range I.V.:

Children: Initial: 5-25 mg/kg/day administered daily for 8-14 days; may be followed by administration every other day (maximum: 21 doses in 28 days)

Adults: Initial: 10-20 mg/kg/day administered daily; may be followed by administration every other day (maximum: 21 doses in 28 days)

Dosage Forms

Injection, solution:

Atgam®: 50 mg/mL (5 mL)

antithymocyte globulin (rabbit) (an te THY moe site GLOB yu lin RAB bit)

Medication Safety Issues

Sound-alike/look-alike issues:

Antithymocyte globulin rabbit (Thymoglobulin®) may be confused with antithymocyte globulin equine (Atgam®)

Synonyms antithymocyte immunoglobulin; rATG

U.S. Brand Names Thymoglobulin®

Therapeutic Category Immunosuppressant Agent

Use Treatment of acute rejection of renal transplant; used in conjunction with concomitant immunosuppression

General Dosage Range I.V.: *Children and Adults:* 1.5 mg/kg/day as a single daily dose

Dosage Forms

Injection, powder for reconstitution:

Thymoglobulin®: 25 mg

antithymocyte immunoglobulin *see* antithymocyte globulin (equine) *on page* 80

antithymocyte immunoglobulin *see* antithymocyte globulin (rabbit) *on page* 80

antitumor necrosis factor alpha (human) *see* adalimumab *on page* 36

anti-VEGF monoclonal antibody *see* bevacizumab *on page* 132

anti-VEGF rhuMAb *see* bevacizumab *on page* 132

antivenin (*Centruroides*) immune F(ab')$_2$ (equine) *see Centruroides* immune F(ab')$_2$ (equine) *on page 189*

antivenin (crotalidae) polyvalent, FAB (ovine) *see* crotalidae polyvalent immune FAB (ovine) *on page 241*

antivenin *(Latrodectus mactans)* (an tee VEN in lak tro DUK tus MAK tans)

Synonyms *Latrodectus mactans* antivenin; *Latrodectus mactans* antivenom; *Latrodectus* antivenin; *Latrodectus* antivenom; black widow spider species antivenin; black widow spider species antivenom

Therapeutic Category Antivenin

Use Treatment of patients with moderate-to-severe symptoms (eg, cramping, intractable pain, hypertension) due to *Latrodectus mactans* (black widow spider) envenomation

General Dosage Range

I.M.: *Children ≥12 years and Adults:* 1-2 vials (2.5-5 mL)

I.V.: *Children and Adults:* 1-2 vials (2.5-5 mL)

Dosage Forms

Injection, powder for reconstitution: 6000 Antivenin units

antivenin *(Micrurus fulvius)* (an tee VEN in mye KRU rus FUL vee us)

Synonyms *Micrurus fulvius* antivenin; *Micrurus fulvius* antivenom; coral snake antivenin; coral snake antivenom; NACSA; North American coral snake antivenin; North American coral snake antivenom

Therapeutic Category Antivenin

Use Treatment of envenomation by an Eastern coral snake (*Micrurus fulvius*) or Texas coral snake (*Micrurus tener*)

General Dosage Range I.V.: *Children and Adults:* 3-5 vials; some patients may need more than 10 vials

antivenin scorpion *see Centruroides* immune F(ab')$_2$ (equine) *on page 189*

antivenom (*Centruroides*) immune F(ab')$_2$ (equine) *see Centruroides* immune F(ab')$_2$ (equine) *on page 189*

antivenom (crotalidae) polyvalent, FAB (ovine) *see* crotalidae polyvalent immune FAB (ovine) *on page 241*

antivenom scorpion *see Centruroides* immune F(ab')$_2$ (equine) *on page 189*

Antivert® *see* meclizine *on page 566*

Antizol® *see* fomepizole *on page 405*

Anucort-HC™ *see* hydrocortisone (topical) *on page 457*

Anu-Med [OTC] *see* phenylephrine (topical) *on page 717*

Anu-med HC *see* hydrocortisone (topical) *on page 457*

Anusol-HC® *see* hydrocortisone (topical) *on page 457*

Anuzinc (Can) *see* zinc sulfate *on page 963*

Anzemet® *see* dolasetron *on page 306*

4-AP *see* dalfampridine *on page 251*

APAP 500 [OTC] *see* acetaminophen *on page 20*

APAP (abbreviation is not recommended) *see* acetaminophen *on page 20*

APC8015 *see* sipuleucel-T *on page 836*

aPCC *see* antiinhibitor coagulant complex *on page 79*

ApexiCon™ *see* diflorasone *on page 284*

ApexiCon® E *see* diflorasone *on page 284*

Aphthasol® *see* amlexanox *on page 65*

Apidra® *see* insulin glulisine *on page 487*

Apidra® SoloStar® *see* insulin glulisine *on page 487*

apixaban *(Canada only)* (a PIX a ban)

Medication Safety Issues

High alert medication:

This medication is in a class the Institute for Safe Medication Practices (ISMP) includes among its list of drug classes which have a heightened risk of causing significant patient harm when used in error.

Canadian Brand Names Eliquis™

Therapeutic Category Factor Xa Inhibitor

Use Postoperative prophylaxis of venous thromboembolism (VTE) following elective knee or hip replacement surgery

General Dosage Range Oral: *Adults:* 2.5 mg twice daily

Product Availability Not available in the U.S.

Dosage Forms - Canada

Tablet, oral:

Eliquis™: 2.5 mg

apomorphine (a poe MOR feen)

Synonyms apomorphine hydrochloride; apomorphine hydrochloride hemihydrate
U.S. Brand Names Apokyn®
Therapeutic Category Anti-Parkinson Agent (Dopamine Agonist)

Use Treatment of hypomobility, "off" episodes with Parkinson disease

General Dosage Range Dosage adjustment recommended in patients with renal impairment

SubQ: *Adults:* Initial test dose: 2 mg; Starting dose: 2-3 mg/dose at time of "off" episode; Maintenance dose: 2-6 mg/dose at time of "off" episode (maximum: 20 mg/day; 6 mg/dose; 5 doses/day)

Dosage Forms

Injection, solution:

Apokyn®: 10 mg/mL (3 mL)

apomorphine hydrochloride *see* apomorphine *on page* 85
apomorphine hydrochloride hemihydrate *see* apomorphine *on page* 85
Apo-Mycophenolate (Can) *see* mycophenolate *on page* 619
Apo-Nabumetone® (Can) *see* nabumetone *on page* 623
Apo-Nadol® (Can) *see* nadolol *on page* 623
Apo-Napro-Na® (Can) *see* naproxen *on page* 628
Apo-Napro-Na DS® (Can) *see* naproxen *on page* 628
Apo-Naproxen® (Can) *see* naproxen *on page* 628
Apo-Naproxen EC® (Can) *see* naproxen *on page* 628
Apo-Naproxen SR® (Can) *see* naproxen *on page* 628
Apo-Nifed PA® (Can) *see* nifedipine *on page* 641
Apo-Nitrazepam® (Can) *see* nitrazepam *(Canada only) on page* 644
Apo-Nitrofurantoin® (Can) *see* nitrofurantoin *on page* 644
Apo-Nizatidine® (Can) *see* nizatidine *on page* 647
Apo-Norflox® (Can) *see* norfloxacin *on page* 649
Apo-Nortriptyline® (Can) *see* nortriptyline *on page* 650
Apo-Oflox® (Can) *see* ofloxacin (systemic) *on page* 659
Apo-Olanzapine® (Can) *see* olanzapine *on page* 660
Apo-Olanzapine ODT® (Can) *see* olanzapine *on page* 660
Apo-Omeprazole® (Can) *see* omeprazole *on page* 665
Apo-Ondansetron® (Can) *see* ondansetron *on page* 667
Apo-Orciprenaline® (Can) *see* metaproterenol *on page* 579
Apo-Oxaprozin® (Can) *see* oxaprozin *on page* 675
Apo-Oxazepam® (Can) *see* oxazepam *on page* 676
Apo-Oxcarbazepine® (Can) *see* oxcarbazepine *on page* 676
Apo-Oxybutynin® (Can) *see* oxybutynin *on page* 677
Apo-Paclitaxel® (Can) *see* paclitaxel *on page* 683
Apo-Pantoprazole® (Can) *see* pantoprazole *on page* 689
Apo-Paroxetine® (Can) *see* paroxetine *on page* 693
Apo-Pentoxifylline SR® (Can) *see* pentoxifylline *on page* 707
Apo-Pen VK® (Can) *see* penicillin V potassium *on page* 704
Apo-Perindopril® (Can) *see* perindopril erbumine *on page* 709
Apo-Perphenazine® (Can) *see* perphenazine *on page* 710
Apo-Pimozide® (Can) *see* pimozide *on page* 723
Apo-Pindol® (Can) *see* pindolol *on page* 724
Apo-Pioglitazone® (Can) *see* pioglitazone *on page* 725
Apo-Piroxicam® (Can) *see* piroxicam *on page* 727
Apo-Pramipexole® (Can) *see* pramipexole *on page* 749
Apo-Pravastatin® (Can) *see* pravastatin *on page* 752
Apo-Prazo® (Can) *see* prazosin *on page* 753
Apo-Prednisone® (Can) *see* prednisone *on page* 755
Apo-Primidone® (Can) *see* primidone *on page* 758
Apo-Procainamide® (Can) *see* procainamide *on page* 759
Apo-Prochlorperazine® (Can) *see* prochlorperazine *on page* 760
Apo-Propafenone® (Can) *see* propafenone *on page* 765
Apo-Propranolol® (Can) *see* propranolol *on page* 767
Apo-Quetiapine® (Can) *see* quetiapine *on page* 781

apraclonidine (a pra KLOE ni deen)

Medication Safety Issues

Sound-alike/look-alike issues:

Iopidine® may be confused with indapamide, iodine, Lodine®

Synonyms aplonidine; apraclonidine hydrochloride; p-aminoclonidine

U.S. Brand Names Iopidine®

Canadian Brand Names Iopidine®

Therapeutic Category $Alpha_2$ Agonist, Ophthalmic

Use Prevention and treatment of postsurgical intraocular pressure (IOP) elevation; short-term, adjunctive therapy in patients who require additional reduction of IOP

General Dosage Range **Ophthalmic:** *Adults:* 0.5%: Instill 1-2 drops in the affected eye(s) 3 times/day; 1%: Instill 1 drop in operative eye 1 hour prior to and upon completion of surgery

Dosage Forms

Solution, ophthalmic: 0.5% (5 mL, 10 mL)

Iopidine®: 0.5% (5 mL, 10 mL); 1% (0.1 mL)

apraclonidine hydrochloride *see* apraclonidine *on page 88*

aprepitant (ap RE pi tant)

Medication Safety Issues

Sound-alike/look-alike issues:

Aprepitant may be confused with fosaprepitant

Emend® (aprepitant) oral capsule formulation may be confused with Emend® for injection (fosaprepitant)

Synonyms L 754030; MK 869

U.S. Brand Names Emend®

Canadian Brand Names Emend®

Therapeutic Category Antiemetic

Use Prevention of acute and delayed nausea and vomiting associated with moderately- and highly-emetogenic chemotherapy (in combination with other antiemetics); prevention of postoperative nausea and vomiting (PONV)

General Dosage Range **Oral:** *Adults:* 125 mg on day 1, followed by 80 mg on days 2 and 3 **or** 40 mg within 3 hours prior to induction with anesthesia

Dosage Forms

Capsule, oral:

Emend®: 40 mg, 80 mg, 125 mg

Combination package, oral:

Emend®: Capsule: 80 mg (2s) and Capsule: 125 mg (1s)

aprepitant injection *see* fosaprepitant *on page 408*

Apresoline [DSC] *see* hydralazine *on page 451*

Apresoline® (Can) *see* hydralazine *on page 451*

Apri® *see* ethinyl estradiol and desogestrel *on page 356*

Apriso™ *see* mesalamine *on page 577*

Aprodine [OTC] *see* triprolidine and pseudoephedrine *on page 922*

aprotinin (a proe TYE nin)

Canadian Brand Names Trasylol®

Therapeutic Category Hemostatic Agent

Use Prevention of perioperative blood loss in patients who are at increased risk for blood loss and blood transfusions in association with cardiopulmonary bypass in coronary artery bypass graft (CABG) surgery

Note: Aprotinin has been withdrawn from the worldwide market due to evidence demonstrating an increased risk of renal dysfunction, myocardial infarction, and mortality in patients undergoing cardiac surgery (Canada has lifted this suspension); use limited to investigational use in the U.S. only according to a special treatment protocol allowing for treatment in select patients at increased risk of blood loss and transfusion during CABG surgery when alternative therapies are unacceptable.

General Dosage Range I.V.: *Adults:* Test dose: 1 mL (1.4 mg) 10 minutes prior to loading dose; Loading dose: 1-2 million KIU (140-280 mg; 100-200 mL); Pump prime volume: 1-2 million KIU (140-280 mg, 100-200 mL); Infusion: 250,000-500,000 KIU/hour (35-70 mg/hour; 25-50 mL/hour)

Dosage Forms

Injection, solution:

Trasylol®: 1.4 mg/mL [10,000 KIU/mL] (100 mL, 200 mL)

Aptivus® *see* tipranavir *on page* 899
Aqua-Ban® Maximum Strength [OTC] *see* pamabrom *on page* 686
Aqua Care® [OTC] *see* urea *on page* 930
Aquacort® (Can) *see* hydrocortisone (topical) *on page* 457
AquADEKs™ [OTC] *see* vitamins (multiple/pediatric) *on page* 952
Aqua Gem-E™ [OTC] *see* vitamin E *on page* 950
AquaLase® *see* balanced salt solution *on page* 113
AquaMEPHYTON® (Can) *see* phytonadione *on page* 722
Aquanil HC® [OTC] *see* hydrocortisone (topical) *on page* 457
Aquaphilic® with Carbamide [OTC] *see* urea *on page* 930
Aquasol A® *see* vitamin A *on page* 949
Aquasol E® [OTC] *see* vitamin E *on page* 950
aquavan *see* fospropofol *on page* 410
aqueous procaine penicillin G *see* penicillin G procaine *on page* 703
Aquoral™ *see* saliva substitute *on page* 819
ara-C *see* cytarabine (conventional) *on page* 248
arabinosylcytosine *see* cytarabine (conventional) *on page* 248
Aralast NP *see* alpha$_1$-proteinase inhibitor *on page* 51
Aralen® *see* chloroquine *on page* 198
Aranelle® *see* ethinyl estradiol and norethindrone *on page* 359
Aranesp® *see* darbepoetin alfa *on page* 254
Aranesp® SingleJect® *see* darbepoetin alfa *on page* 254
Arava® *see* leflunomide *on page* 525
Arbinoxa™ *see* carbinoxamine *on page* 175
Arcalyst® *see* rilonacept *on page* 801
Arcapta™ Neohaler™ *see* indacaterol *on page* 479
Aredia® *see* pamidronate *on page* 686
Arestin Microspheres (Can) *see* minocycline *on page* 604

arformoterol (ar for MOE ter ol)

Synonyms (R,R)-formoterol L-tartrate; arformoterol tartrate

U.S. Brand Names Brovana®

Therapeutic Category Beta$_2$-Adrenergic Agonist, Long-Acting

Use Long-term maintenance treatment of bronchoconstriction in chronic obstructive pulmonary disease (COPD), including chronic bronchitis and emphysema

General Dosage Range Nebulization: *Adults:* 5 mcg twice daily (maximum: 30 mcg/day)

Dosage Forms

Solution, for nebulization:

Brovana®: 15 mcg/2 mL (30s, 60s)

arformoterol tartrate *see* arformoterol *on page* 89

argatroban (ar GA troh ban)

Medication Safety Issues

Sound-alike/look-alike issues:

Argatroban may be confused with Aggrastat®, Orgaran®

High alert medication:

The Institute for Safe Medication Practices (ISMP) includes this medication among its list of drugs which have a heightened risk of causing significant patient harm when used in error.

Therapeutic Category Anticoagulant, Thrombin Inhibitor

Use Prophylaxis or treatment of thrombosis in patients with heparin-induced thrombocytopenia (HIT); adjunct to percutaneous coronary intervention (PCI) in patients who have or are at risk of thrombosis associated with HIT

General Dosage Range Dosage adjustment recommended in patients with hepatic impairment

I.V.:

Children: Initial dose: 0.75 mcg/kg/minute; dosage may be adjusted in increments of 0.1-0.25 mcg/kg/minute

Adults: Bolus dose: 150-350 mcg/kg during procedure; Infusion: Initial: 2 mcg/kg/minute **or** 25 mcg/kg/minute during procedure; Maintenance: 0.5-10 mcg/kg/minute (maximum: 10 mcg/kg/minute) **or** 25-40 mcg/kg/minute during procedure

Adults (critically-ill): Initial: 0.2 mcg/kg/minute; Maintenance: 0.5-1.3 mcg/kg/minute

Dosage Forms

Infusion, premixed in NS: 125 mg (125 mL)

Infusion, premixed in water for injection: 50 mg (50 mL)

Injection, solution: 100 mg/mL (2.5 mL)

arginine (AR ji neen)

Medication Safety Issues

Administration issues:

The Food and Drug Administration (FDA) has identified several cases of fatal arginine overdose in children and has recommended that healthcare professionals always recheck dosing calculations prior to administration of arginine. Doses used in children should not exceed usual adult doses.

Synonyms arginine HCl; arginine hydrochloride; L-arginine; L-arginine hydrochloride

U.S. Brand Names R-Gene® 10

Therapeutic Category Diagnostic Agent

Use Pituitary function test (growth hormone)

General Dosage Range I.V.:

Children: 0.5 g/kg/dose as a single dose

Adults: 30 g (300 mL) as a single dose

Dosage Forms

Injection, solution:

R-Gene® 10: 10% [100 mg/mL] (300 mL)

arginine HCl *see* arginine *on page* 90

arginine hydrochloride *see* arginine *on page* 90

8-arginine vasopressin *see* vasopressin *on page* 940

Aricept® *see* donepezil *on page* 309

Aricept® ODT *see* donepezil *on page* 309

Aricept® RDT (Can) *see* donepezil *on page* 309

Aridol™ *see* mannitol *on page* 561

Arimidex® *see* anastrozole *on page* 75

aripiprazole (ay ri PIP ray zole)

Medication Safety Issues

Sound-alike/look-alike issues:

Abilify® may be confused with Ambien®

ARIPiprazole may be confused with proton pump inhibitors (dexlansoprazole, esomeprazole, lansoprazole, omeprazole, pantoprazole, RABEprazole)

BEERS Criteria medication:

This drug may be potentially inappropriate for use in geriatric patients (Quality of evidence - moderate; Strength of recommendation - strong).

Synonyms BMS 337039; OPC-14597

Tall-Man **ARIP**iprazole

U.S. Brand Names Abilify Discmelt®; Abilify®

Canadian Brand Names Abilify®

Therapeutic Category Antipsychotic Agent, Quinolone

Use

Oral: Acute and maintenance treatment of schizophrenia; acute (manic and mixed episodes) and maintenance treatment of bipolar I disorder as monotherapy or as an adjunct to lithium or valproic acid; adjunctive treatment of major depressive disorder; treatment of irritability associated with autistic disorder

Injection: Agitation associated with schizophrenia or bipolar I disorder

General Dosage Range Dosage adjustment recommended in patients on concomitant therapy or CYP2D6 metabolizer status

Oral:

Children 6-9 years: 5-15 mg once daily (maximum: 15 mg/day)

Children ≥10 years: 5-30 mg once daily (maximum: 30 mg/day)

Adults: 10-30 mg once daily (maximum: 30 mg/day)

I.M.: *Adults:* 5.25-30 mg/day (maximum: 30 mg/day)

Dosage Forms

Injection, solution:

Abilify®: 7.5 mg/mL (1.3 mL)

Solution, oral:

Abilify®: 1 mg/mL (150 mL)

Tablet, oral:

Abilify®: 2 mg, 5 mg, 10 mg, 15 mg, 20 mg, 30 mg

Tablet, orally disintegrating, oral:

Abilify Discmelt®: 10 mg, 15 mg

Aristospan® *see* triamcinolone (systemic) *on page 914*

Arixtra® *see* fondaparinux *on page 406*

armodafinil (ar moe DAF i nil)

Synonyms R-modafinil

U.S. Brand Names Nuvigil®

Therapeutic Category Stimulant

Controlled Substance C-IV

Use Improve wakefulness in patients with excessive daytime sleepiness associated with narcolepsy and shift work sleep disorder (SWSD); adjunctive therapy for obstructive sleep apnea/hypopnea syndrome (OSAHS)

General Dosage Range Dosage adjustment recommended in patients with hepatic impairment

Oral: *Adults:* 150-250 mg once daily

Dosage Forms

Tablet, oral:

Nuvigil®: 50 mg, 150 mg, 250 mg

Armour® Thyroid *see* thyroid, desiccated *on page 893*

Aromasin® *see* exemestane *on page 368*

Arranon® *see* nelarabine *on page 632*

arsenic trioxide (AR se nik tri OKS id)

Medication Safety Issues

High alert medication:

This medication is in a class the Institute for Safe Medication Practices (ISMP) includes among its list of drugs which have a heightened risk of causing significant patient harm when used in error.

Synonyms As_2O_3

U.S. Brand Names Trisenox®

Therapeutic Category Antineoplastic Agent, Miscellaneous

Use Remission induction and consolidation in patients with relapsed or refractory acute promyelocytic leukemia (APL) characterized by t(15;17) translocation or PML/RAR-alpha gene expression

General Dosage Range Dosage adjustment recommended for renal impairment.

I.V.: *Children ≥4 years and Adults:* Induction: 0.15 mg/kg/day (maximum: 60 doses); Consolidation: 0.15 mg/kg/day (maximum: 25 doses over a period of up to 5 weeks)

Dosage Forms

Injection, solution [preservative free]:

Trisenox®: 1 mg/mL (10 mL)

Artane *see* trihexyphenidyl *on page* 919

artemether and benflumetol *see* artemether and lumefantrine *on page* 92

artemether and lumefantrine (ar TEM e ther & loo me FAN treen)

Synonyms artemether and benflumetol; benflumetol and artemether; lumefantrine and artemether

U.S. Brand Names Coartem®

Therapeutic Category Antimalarial Agent

Use Treatment of acute, uncomplicated malaria infections due to *Plasmodium falciparum*, including geographical regions where chloroquine resistance has been reported

General Dosage Range Oral:

Children 2 months to ≤16 years:

5 to <15 kg: Artemether 20 mg/lumefantrine 120 mg twice daily (maximum: 6 tablets per treatment course)

15 to <25 kg: Artemether 40 mg/lumefantrine 240 mg twice daily (maximum: 12 tablets per treatment course)

25 to <35 kg: Artemether 60 mg/lumefantrine 360 mg twice daily (maximum: 18 tablets per treatment course)

≥35 kg: Artemether 80 mg/lumefantrine 480 mg twice daily (maximum: 24 tablets per treatment course)

Children >16 years and Adults:

25 to <35 kg: Artemether 60 mg/lumefantrine 360 mg twice daily (maximum: 18 tablets per treatment course)

≥35 kg: Artemether 80 mg/lumefantrine 480 mg twice daily (maximum: 24 tablets per treatment course)

Dosage Forms

Tablet:

Coartem®: Artemether 20 mg and lumefantrine 120 mg

artemisinin derivative *see* artesunate *on page* 92

artesunate (ar TES oo nate)

Synonyms artemisinin derivative; artesunic acid; dihydroartemisinin hemisuccinate sodium; dihydroqinghaosu hemisuccinate sodium; Nuartez™; P01BE03; qinghao derivative; qinghaosu derivative; sodium artesunate

Therapeutic Category Antimalarial Agent; Artemisinin Derivative

General Dosage Range

I.V.: *Children and Adults:* 2.4 mg/kg/dose initially, followed by 2.4 mg/kg/dose at 12 hours, 24 hours, and 48 hours after the initial dose for a total of 4 doses

artesunic acid *see* artesunate *on page* 92

Arthrotec® *see* diclofenac and misoprostol *on page* 281

Articadent™ *see* articaine and epinephrine *on page* 92

articaine and epinephrine (AR ti kane & ep i NEF rin)

Synonyms epinephrine and articaine hydrochloride

U.S. Brand Names Articadent™; Orabloc™; Septocaine® with epinephrine 1:100,000; Septocaine® with epinephrine 1:200,000; Zorcaine™

Canadian Brand Names Astracaine® with epinephrine 1:200,000; Astracaine® with epinephrine forte 1:100,000; Posicaine N; Posicaine SP; Septanest® N; Septanest® SP; Ultracaine® DS; Ultracaine® DS Forte; Zorcaine™

Therapeutic Category Local Anesthetic

Use Local, infiltrative, or conductive anesthesia during simple and complex dental procedures

General Dosage Range Local injection:

Children 4-16 years: Maximum: 7 mg/kg (0.175 mL/kg)

Complex procedures: 0.37-7.48 mg/kg (0.7-3.9 mL)

Simple procedures: 0.76-5.65 mg/kg (0.9-5.1 mL)

Adults: Maximum: 7 mg/kg (0.175 mL/kg)

Infiltration: 0.5-2.5 mL of 4% solution; Total dose: 20-100 mg

Nerve block: 0.5-3.4 mL of 4% solution; Total dose: 20-136 mg

Oral surgery: 1-5.1 mL of 4% solution; Total dose: 40-204 mg

Elderly 65-75 years:
Complex procedures: 1.05-4.27 mg/kg (1.3-6.8 mL)
Simple procedures: 0.43-4.76 mg/kg (0.9-11.9 mL)
Elderly ≥75 years:
Complex procedures: 1.12-2.17 mg/kg (1.3-5.1 mL)
Simple procedures: 0.78-4.76 mg/kg (1.3-11.9 mL)

Dosage Forms

Injection, solution [for dental use]:
Articadent™: Articaine hydrochloride 4% [40 mg/mL] and epinephrine 1:100,000 (1.7 mL)
Articadent™: Articaine hydrochloride 4% [40 mg/mL] and epinephrine 1:200,000 (1.7 mL)
Orabloc™: Articaine hydrochloride 4% [40 mg/mL] and epinephrine 1:100,000 (1.8 mL)
Orabloc™: Articaine hydrochloride 4% [40 mg/mL] and epinephrine 1:200,000 (1.8 mL)
Septocaine® with epinephrine 1:100,000: Articaine 4% [40 mg/mL] and epinephrine 1:100,000 (1.7 mL)
Septocaine® with epinephrine 1:200,000: Articaine 4% [40 mg/mL] and epinephrine 1:200,000 (1.7 mL)
Zorcaine™: Articaine 4% [40 mg/mL] and epinephrine 1:100,000 (1.7 mL)

Dosage Forms - Canada

Injection, solution [for dental use]:
Astracaine® with epinephrine 1:200,000: Articaine 4% and epinephrine 1:200,000 (1.8 mL)
Astracaine® Forte with epinephrine forte 1:100,000: Articaine 4% and epinephrine 1:100,000 (1.8 mL)
Septanest® N: Articaine 4% and epinephrine 1:200,000 (1.7 mL)
Septanest® SP: Articaine 4% and epinephrine 1:100,000 (1.7 mL)
Ultracaine® DS: Articaine 4% and epinephrine 1:200,000 (1.7 mL)
Ultracaine® DS Forte: Articaine 4% and epinephrine 1:100,000 (1.7 mL)

artificial saliva *see* saliva substitute *on page 819*

artificial tears (ar ti FISH il tears)

Medication Safety Issues

Sound-alike/look-alike issues:
Isopto® Tears may be confused with Isoptin®

Synonyms hydroxyethylcellulose; polyvinyl alcohol

U.S. Brand Names Advanced Eye Relief™ Dry Eye Environmental [OTC]; Advanced Eye Relief™ Dry Eye Rejuvenation [OTC]; Bion® Tears [OTC]; HypoTears [OTC]; Murine Tears® [OTC]; Soothe® Hydration [OTC]; Soothe® [OTC]; Systane® Ultra [OTC]; Systane® [OTC]; Tears Again® [OTC]; Tears Naturale® Forte [OTC]; Tears Naturale® Free [OTC]; Tears Naturale® II [OTC]; Viva-Drops® [OTC]

Canadian Brand Names Teardrops®

Therapeutic Category Ophthalmic Agent, Miscellaneous

Use Ophthalmic lubricant; for temporary relief of burning and eye irritation due to dry eyes

General Dosage Range Ophthalmic: *Children and Adults:* 1-2 drops into eye(s) as needed

Dosage Forms

Solution, ophthalmic:
Advanced Eye Relief™ Dry Eye Environmental [OTC]: Glycerin 1% (15 mL)
Advanced Eye Relief™ Dry Eye Rejuvenation [OTC]: Glycerin 0.3% and propylene glycol 1.0% (30 mL)
HypoTears [OTC]: Polyvinyl alcohol 1% and polyethylene glycol 400 1% (30 mL)
Murine Tears® [OTC]: Polyvinyl alcohol 0.5% and povidone 0.6% (15 mL)
Soothe® Hydration [OTC]: Povidone 1.25% (15 mL)
Systane® Ultra [OTC]: Polyethylene glycol 400 0.4% and propylene glycol 0.3% (5 mL, 10 mL)
Systane® [OTC]: Polyethylene glycol 400 0.4% and propylene glycol 0.3% (5 mL, 15 mL, 30 mL)
Tears Again® [OTC]: Polyvinyl alcohol 1.4% (30 mL)
Tears Naturale® II [OTC]: Dextran 70 0.1% and hydroxypropyl methylcellulose 2910 0.3% (30 mL)
Tears Naturale® Forte [OTC]: Dextran 70 1%, glycerin 0.2%, and hydroxypropyl methylcellulose 2910 0.3% (30 mL)

Solution, ophthalmic [preservative free]:
Bion® Tears [OTC]: Dextran 70 0.1% and hydroxypropyl methylcellulose 2910 0.3% per 0.4 mL (28s)
Soothe® [OTC]: Glycerin 0.6% and propylene glycol 0.6% per 0.6 mL (28s)
Systane® Ultra [OTC]: Polyethylene glycol 400 0.4% and propylene glycol 0.3% per 0.4 mL (24s)
Tears Naturale® Free [OTC]: Dextran 70 0.1% and hydroxypropyl methylcellulose 2910 0.3% per 0.5 mL (36s, 60s)
Viva-Drops® [OTC]: Polysorbate 80 1% (0.5 mL, 10 mL)

Artiss *see* fibrin sealant *on page 383*

Arzerra™ *see* ofatumumab *on page 659*

As_2O_3 *see* arsenic trioxide *on page 91*
ASA *see* aspirin *on page 96*
5-ASA *see* mesalamine *on page 577*
ASA and diphenhydramine *see* aspirin and diphenhydramine *on page 97*
Asacol® *see* mesalamine *on page 577*
Asacol® 800 (Can) *see* mesalamine *on page 577*
Asacol® HD *see* mesalamine *on page 577*
Asaphen (Can) *see* aspirin *on page 96*
Asaphen E.C. (Can) *see* aspirin *on page 96*
Asclera™ *see* polidocanol *on page 736*
Asco-Caps-500 [OTC] *see* ascorbic acid *on page 94*
Asco-Caps-1000 [OTC] *see* ascorbic acid *on page 94*
Ascocid® [OTC] *see* ascorbic acid *on page 94*
Ascocid®-500 [OTC] *see* ascorbic acid *on page 94*
Ascomp® with Codeine *see* butalbital, aspirin, caffeine, and codeine *on page 155*
Ascor L 500® [DSC] *see* ascorbic acid *on page 94*
Ascor L NC® [DSC] *see* ascorbic acid *on page 94*

ascorbic acid (a SKOR bik AS id)

Medication Safety Issues

International issues:

Rubex [Ireland] may be confused with Brivex brand name for brivudine [Switzerland]
Rubex: Brand name for ascorbic acid [Ireland], but also the brand name for doxorubicin [Brazil]

Synonyms vitamin C

U.S. Brand Names Acerola [OTC]; Asco-Caps-1000 [OTC]; Asco-Caps-500 [OTC]; Asco-Tabs-1000 [OTC]; Ascocid® [OTC]; Ascocid®-500 [OTC]; Ascor L 500® [DSC]; Ascor L NC® [DSC]; C-Gel [OTC]; C-Gram [OTC]; C-Time [OTC]; Cemill 1000 [OTC]; Cemill 500 [OTC]; Chew-C [OTC]; Dull-C® [OTC]; Mild-C® [OTC]; One Gram C [OTC]; Time-C® [OTC]; Vicks® Vitamin C [OTC]; Vita-C® [OTC]

Canadian Brand Names Proflavanol C™; Revitalose C-1000®

Therapeutic Category Vitamin, Water Soluble

Use Prevention and treatment of scurvy; acidify the urine

General Dosage Range

I.M., SubQ:

Children: 100-300 mg/day in divided doses
Adults: 100-250 mg 1-2 times/day

I.V., Oral:

Children: 100-300 mg/day in divided doses (maximum: 500 mg every 6-8 hours)
Adults: 100-250 mg 1-2 times/day (maximum: 4-12 g/day in 3-4 divided doses)

Dosage Forms

Caplet, oral: 1000 mg
Caplet, timed release, oral: 500 mg, 1000 mg
Capsule, oral:
Mild-C® [OTC]: 500 mg
Capsule, softgel, oral:
C-Gel [OTC]: 1000 mg
Capsule, sustained release, oral:
C-Time [OTC]: 500 mg
Capsule, timed release, oral: 500 mg
Asco-Caps-500 [OTC]: 500 mg
Asco-Caps-1000 [OTC]: 1000 mg
Time-C® [OTC]: 500 mg
Crystals for solution, oral: (170 g, 1000 g)
Mild-C® [OTC]: (170 g, 1000 g)
Vita-C® [OTC]: (113 g, 454 g)
Injection, solution: 500 mg/mL (50 mL)
Injection, solution [preservative free]: 500 mg/mL (50 mL)
Liquid, oral: 500 mg/5 mL (118 mL, 120 mL, 473 mL)

Lozenge, oral:
Vicks® Vitamin C [OTC]: 25 mg (20s)
Powder for solution, oral:
Ascocid® [OTC]: (227 g, 454 g)
Dull-C® [OTC]: (113 g, 454 g)
Tablet, oral: 100 mg, 250 mg, 500 mg, 1000 mg
Asco-Tabs-1000 [OTC]: 1000 mg
Ascocid®-500 [OTC]: 500 mg
C-Gram [OTC]: 1000 mg
One Gram C [OTC]: 1000 mg
Tablet, chewable, oral: 250 mg, 500 mg
Acerola [OTC]: 500 mg
Chew-C [OTC]: 500 mg
Mild-C® [OTC]: 250 mg
Tablet, timed release, oral: 500 mg, 1000 mg
Cemill 500 [OTC]: 500 mg
Cemill 1000 [OTC]: 1000 mg
Mild-C® [OTC]: 1000 mg

Asco-Tabs-1000 [OTC] *see* ascorbic acid *on page 94*
Ascriptin® Maximum Strength [OTC] *see* aspirin *on page 96*
Ascriptin® Regular Strength [OTC] *see* aspirin *on page 96*

asenapine (a SEN a peen)

Medication Safety Issues
BEERS Criteria medication:
This drug may be potentially inappropriate for use in geriatric patients (Quality of evidence - moderate; Strength of recommendation - strong).

U.S. Brand Names Saphris®
Canadian Brand Names Saphris®
Therapeutic Category Antimanic Agent; Antipsychotic Agent, Atypical
Use Acute and maintenance treatment of schizophrenia; treatment of acute mania or mixed episodes associated with bipolar I disorder (as monotherapy or in combination with lithium or valproate)
General Dosage Range Oral: *Adults:* 5-10 mg twice daily
Dosage Forms
Tablet, sublingual:
Saphris®: 5 mg, 10 mg

Asendin [DSC] *see* amoxapine *on page 69*
Asmanex® Twisthaler® *see* mometasone (oral inhalation) *on page 610*
asparaginase *see* asparaginase (*E. coli*) *on page 95*

asparaginase (*E. coli*) (a SPEAR a ji nase e ko lye)

Medication Safety Issues
Sound-alike/look-alike issues:
Asparaginase (*E. coli*) may be confused with asparaginase (*Erwinia*), pegaspargase
Elspar® may be confused with Elaprase®, Erwinaze™, Oncaspar®
High alert medication:
This medication is in a class the Institute for Safe Medication Practices (ISMP) includes among its list of drug classes which have a heightened risk of causing significant patient harm when used in error.

Synonyms *E. coli* asparaginase; asparaginase; L-asparaginase (*E. coli*)
U.S. Brand Names Elspar®
Canadian Brand Names Kidrolase®
Therapeutic Category Antineoplastic Agent
Use Treatment (in combination with other chemotherapy) of acute lymphoblastic leukemia (ALL)
General Dosage Range
I.M.: *Children and Adults:* 6000 units/m^2/dose 3 times/week **or** 6000 units/m^2 every ~3 days
I.V.: *Children and Adults:* Dosage varies greatly depending on indication
Intradermal: *Children and Adults:* Test dose: 0.1-0.2 mL of a 20-250 units/mL concentration

Dosage Forms
Injection, powder for reconstitution:
Elspar®: 10,000 units

asparaginase (*Erwinia*) (a SPEAR a ji nase er WIN i ah)

Medication Safety Issues
Sound-alike/look-alike issues:
Asparaginase *(Erwinia)* may be confused with asparaginase *(E. coli)*, pegaspargase
Erwinaze™ may be confused with Elaprase®, Elspar®, Oncaspar®
High alert medication:
This medication is in a class the Institute for Safe Medication Practices (ISMP) includes among its list of drug classes which have a heightened risk of causing significant patient harm when used in error.

Synonyms *Erwinia chrysanthemi*; asparaginase *Erwinia chrysanthemi*; L-asparaginase (*Erwinia*)

U.S. Brand Names Erwinaze™

Canadian Brand Names Erwinase®

Therapeutic Category Antineoplastic Agent, Miscellaneous; Enzyme

Use Treatment (in combination with other chemotherapy) of acute lymphoblastic leukemia (ALL) in patients with hypersensitivity to *E. coli*-derived asparaginase

General Dosage Range I.M.: *Children and Adults:* 25,000 units/m^2 3 times/week (Mon, Wed, Fri) for 6 doses for each planned pegaspargase dose **or** 25,000 units/m^2 for each planned asparaginase (*E. coli*) dose

Dosage Forms
Injection, powder for reconstitution:
Erwinaze™: 10,000 units

asparaginase *Erwinia chrysanthemi* *see* asparaginase (*Erwinia*) *on page 96*
aspart insulin *see* insulin aspart *on page 485*
Aspercin [OTC] *see* aspirin *on page 96*
Aspercreme® [OTC] *see* trolamine *on page 923*
Aspergillus niger *see* alpha-galactosidase *on page 52*
Aspergum® [OTC] *see* aspirin *on page 96*

aspirin (AS pir in)

Medication Safety Issues
Sound-alike/look-alike issues:
Aspirin may be confused with Afrin®
Ascriptin® may be confused with Aricept®
Ecotrin® may be confused with Edecrin®, Epogen®
Halfprin® may be confused with Haltran®
ZORprin® may be confused with Zyloprim®
International issues:
Cartia [multiple international markets] may be confused with Cartia XT brand name for diltiazem [U.S.]
BEERS Criteria medication:
This drug may be potentially inappropriate for use in geriatric patients (Quality of evidence - moderate; Strength of recommendation - strong).

Synonyms acetylsalicylic acid; ASA; baby aspirin

U.S. Brand Names Ascriptin® Maximum Strength [OTC]; Ascriptin® Regular Strength [OTC]; Aspercin [OTC]; Aspergum® [OTC]; Aspir-low [OTC]; Aspirtab [OTC]; Bayer® Aspirin Extra Strength [OTC]; Bayer® Aspirin Regimen Adult Low Strength [OTC]; Bayer® Aspirin Regimen Children's [OTC]; Bayer® Aspirin Regimen Regular Strength [OTC]; Bayer® Genuine Aspirin [OTC]; Bayer® Plus Extra Strength [OTC]; Bayer® Women's Low Dose Aspirin [OTC]; Buffasal [OTC]; Bufferin® Extra Strength [OTC]; Bufferin® [OTC]; Buffinol [OTC]; Ecotrin® Arthritis Strength [OTC]; Ecotrin® Low Strength [OTC]; Ecotrin® [OTC]; Halfprin® [OTC]; St Joseph® Adult Aspirin [OTC]; Tri-Buffered Aspirin [OTC]

Canadian Brand Names Asaphen; Asaphen E.C.; Entrophen®; Novasen; Praxis ASA EC 81 Mg Daily Dose

Therapeutic Category Analgesic, Nonnarcotic; Antiplatelet Agent; Antipyretic; Nonsteroidal Antiinflammatory Drug (NSAID)

Use Treatment of mild-to-moderate pain, inflammation, and fever; prevention and treatment of acute coronary syndromes (ST-elevation MI, non-ST-elevation MI, unstable angina), acute ischemic stroke, and transient ischemic episodes; management of rheumatoid arthritis, rheumatic fever, osteoarthritis; adjunctive therapy in revascularization procedures (coronary artery bypass graft [CABG], percutaneous transluminal coronary angioplasty [PTCA], carotid endarterectomy), stent implantation

General Dosage Range

Oral:

Children: 10-15 mg/kg/dose every 4-6 hours (maximum: 4 g/day) **or** 60-100 mg/kg/day divided every 4-8 hours **or** 1-20 mg/kg/day as a single dose

Adults: 325-650 mg every 4-6 hours (maximum: 4 g/day) **or** 2.4-5.4 g/day in divided doses **or** 40-325 mg/day as a single dose

Rectal:

Children: 10-15 mg/kg/dose every 4-6 hours (maximum: 4 g/day)

Adults: 300-600 mg every 4-6 hours (maximum: 4 g/day)

Dosage Forms

Caplet, oral: 500 mg

Ascriptin® Maximum Strength [OTC]: 500 mg
Bayer® Aspirin Extra Strength [OTC]: 500 mg
Bayer® Genuine Aspirin [OTC]: 325 mg
Bayer® Plus Extra Strength [OTC]: 500 mg
Bayer® Women's Low Dose Aspirin [OTC]: 81 mg

Caplet, enteric coated, oral:

Bayer® Aspirin Regimen Regular Strength [OTC]: 325 mg

Gum, chewing, oral:

Aspergum® [OTC]: 227 mg (12s)

Suppository, rectal: 300 mg (12s); 600 mg (12s)

Tablet, oral: 325 mg

Ascriptin® Regular Strength [OTC]: 325 mg
Aspercin [OTC]: 325 mg
Aspirtab [OTC]: 325 mg
Bayer® Genuine Aspirin [OTC]: 325 mg
Buffasal [OTC]: 325 mg
Bufferin® [OTC]: 325 mg
Bufferin® Extra Strength [OTC]: 500 mg
Buffinol [OTC]: 324 mg
Tri-Buffered Aspirin [OTC]: 325 mg

Tablet, chewable, oral: 81 mg

Bayer® Aspirin Regimen Children's [OTC]: 81 mg
St Joseph® Adult Aspirin [OTC]: 81 mg

Tablet, enteric coated, oral: 81 mg, 325 mg, 650 mg

Aspir-low [OTC]: 81 mg
Bayer® Aspirin Regimen Adult Low Strength [OTC]: 81 mg
Ecotrin® [OTC]: 325 mg
Ecotrin® Arthritis Strength [OTC]: 500 mg
Ecotrin® Low Strength [OTC]: 81 mg
Halfprin® [OTC]: 81 mg, 162 mg
St Joseph® Adult Aspirin [OTC]: 81 mg

aspirin, acetaminophen, and caffeine *see* acetaminophen, aspirin, and caffeine *on page* 26

aspirin and carisoprodol *see* carisoprodol and aspirin *on page* 178

aspirin and diphenhydramine (AS pir in & dye fen HYE dra meen)

Synonyms ASA and diphenhydramine; aspirin and diphenhydramine citrate; diphenhydramine and ASA; diphenhydramine and aspirin; diphenhydramine citrate and aspirin

U.S. Brand Names Bayer® PM [OTC]

Therapeutic Category Analgesic, Miscellaneous

Use Aid in the relief of insomnia accompanied by minor pain or headache

General Dosage Range Oral: *Children ≥12 years and Adults:* Two caplets (1000 mg aspirin/77 mg diphenhydramine citrate) at bedtime

Dosage Forms

Caplet, oral:

Bayer® PM [OTC]: Aspirin 500 mg and diphenhydramine 38.3 mg

aspirin and diphenhydramine citrate *see* aspirin and diphenhydramine *on page* *97*

aspirin and dipyridamole (AS pir in & dye peer ID a mole)

Medication Safety Issues

Sound-alike/look-alike issues:

Aggrenox® may be confused with Aggrastat®

Synonyms aspirin and extended-release dipyridamole; dipyridamole and aspirin

U.S. Brand Names Aggrenox®

Canadian Brand Names Aggrenox®

Therapeutic Category Antiplatelet Agent

Use Reduction in the risk of stroke in patients who have had transient ischemia of the brain or ischemic stroke due to thrombosis

General Dosage Range Oral: *Adults:* 1 capsule (200 mg dipyridamole, 25 mg aspirin) twice daily

Dosage Forms

Capsule:

Aggrenox®: Aspirin 25 mg [immediate release] and dipyridamole 200 mg [extended release]

aspirin and extended-release dipyridamole *see* aspirin and dipyridamole *on page* *98*

aspirin and oxycodone *see* oxycodone and aspirin *on page* *680*

aspirin, caffeine, and acetaminophen *see* acetaminophen, aspirin, and caffeine *on page* *26*

aspirin, caffeine, and butalbital *see* butalbital, aspirin, and caffeine *on page* *154*

aspirin, caffeine, and orphenadrine *see* orphenadrine, aspirin, and caffeine *on page* *672*

aspirin, caffeine, codeine, and butalbital *see* butalbital, aspirin, caffeine, and codeine *on page* *155*

aspirin, carisoprodol, and codeine *see* carisoprodol, aspirin, and codeine *on page* *178*

Aspirin Free Anacin® Extra Strength [OTC] *see* acetaminophen *on page* *20*

aspirin, orphenadrine, and caffeine *see* orphenadrine, aspirin, and caffeine *on page* *672*

Aspir-low [OTC] *see* aspirin *on page* *96*

Aspirtab [OTC] *see* aspirin *on page* *96*

Astelin® *see* azelastine (nasal) *on page* *107*

Astepro® *see* azelastine (nasal) *on page* *107*

Asthmanefrin™ [OTC] *see* epinephrine (systemic, oral inhalation) *on page* *334*

Astracaine® with epinephrine 1:200,000 (Can) *see* articaine and epinephrine *on page* *92*

Astracaine® with epinephrine forte 1:100,000 (Can) *see* articaine and epinephrine *on page* *92*

Astramorph®/PF *see* morphine (systemic) *on page* *612*

AstrinGyn® *see* ferric subsulfate *on page* *379*

AT *see* antithrombin III *on page* *80*

AT-III *see* antithrombin III *on page* *80*

Atacand® *see* candesartan *on page* *168*

Atacand HCT® *see* candesartan and hydrochlorothiazide *on page* *168*

Atacand® Plus (Can) *see* candesartan and hydrochlorothiazide *on page* *168*

Atarax® (Can) *see* hydroxyzine *on page* *464*

Atasol® (Can) *see* acetaminophen *on page* *20*

atazanavir (at a za NA veer)

Synonyms atazanavir sulfate; ATV; BMS-232632

U.S. Brand Names Reyataz®

Canadian Brand Names Reyataz®

Therapeutic Category Antiretroviral Agent, Protease Inhibitor

Use Treatment of HIV-1 infections in combination with at least two other antiretroviral agents

General Dosage Range Dosage adjustment recommended in patients with hepatic or renal impairment or on concomitant therapy

Oral:

Children 6 to <18 years:

15 to <20 kg: Atazanavir 150 mg once daily

20 to <40 kg: Atazanavir 200 mg once daily

≥40 kg: Atazanavir 300 mg once daily

Children ≥13 years (≥40 kg) and Adults: 400 mg once daily (antiretroviral-naive) **or** atazanavir 300 mg once daily

Dosage Forms

Capsule, oral:

Reyataz®: 100 mg, 150 mg, 200 mg, 300 mg

atazanavir sulfate *see* atazanavir *on page 98*

Atelvia™ *see* risedronate *on page 803*

atenolol (a TEN oh lole)

Medication Safety Issues

Sound-alike/look-alike issues:

Atenolol may be confused with albuterol, Altenol®, timolol, Tylenol®

Tenormin® may be confused with Imuran®, Norpramin®, thiamine, Trovan®

U.S. Brand Names Tenormin®

Canadian Brand Names Apo-Atenol®; Ava-Atenolol; CO Atenolol; Dom-Atenolol; JAMP-Atenolol; Mint-Atenolol; Mylan-Atenolol; Nu-Atenol; PMS-Atenolol; RAN™-Atenolol; ratio-Atenolol; Riva-Atenolol; Sandoz-Atenolol; Septa-Atenolol; Tenormin®; Teva-Atenolol

Therapeutic Category Beta-Adrenergic Blocker

Use Treatment of hypertension, alone or in combination with other agents; management of angina pectoris; secondary prevention postmyocardial infarction

General Dosage Range Dosage adjustment recommended in patients with renal impairment

Oral:

Children: 0.5-1 mg/kg/dose given daily; range of 0.5-1.5 mg/kg/day (maximum dose: 2 mg/kg/day up to 100 mg/day)

Adults: 25-100 mg/day as a single daily dose (maximum dose: 100 mg/day)

Dosage Forms

Tablet, oral: 25 mg, 50 mg, 100 mg

Tenormin®: 25 mg, 50 mg, 100 mg

atenolol and chlorthalidone (a TEN oh lole & klor THAL i done)

Synonyms chlorthalidone and atenolol

U.S. Brand Names Tenoretic®

Canadian Brand Names Apo-Atenidone®; Novo-Atenolthalidone; Tenoretic®; Teva-Atenolol Chlorthalidone

Therapeutic Category Antihypertensive Agent, Combination

Use Treatment of hypertension with a cardioselective beta-blocker and a diuretic

General Dosage Range Dosage adjustment recommended in patients with renal impairment.

Oral: *Adults:* Initial: Atenolol 50 mg and chlorthalidone 25 mg once daily; Maintenance: Atenolol 50-100 mg and chlorthalidone 25 mg once daily (maximum dose: Atenolol 100 mg/day; chlorthalidone 25 mg/day)

Dosage Forms

Tablet, oral: Atenolol 50 mg and chlorthalidone 25 mg; atenolol 100 mg and chlorthalidone 25 mg

Tenoretic®: Atenolol 50 mg and chlorthalidone 25 mg; atenolol 100 mg and chlorthalidone 25 mg

ATG *see* antithymocyte globulin (equine) *on page 80*

Atgam® *see* antithymocyte globulin (equine) *on page 80*

Ativan® *see* lorazepam *on page 550*

atlizumab *see* tocilizumab *on page 902*

ATNAA *see* atropine and pralidoxime *on page 103*

atomoxetine (AT oh mox e teen)

Medication Safety Issues

Sound-alike/look-alike issues:

AtoMOXetine may be confused with atorvaSTATin

Synonyms atomoxetine hydrochloride; LY139603; methylphenoxy-benzene propanamine; tomoxetine

Tall-Man ato**MOX**etine

U.S. Brand Names Strattera®

Canadian Brand Names Apo-Atomoxetine®; Mylan-Atomoxetine; PMS-Atomoxetine; Sandoz-Atomoxetine; Strattera®; Teva-Atomoxetine

Therapeutic Category Norepinephrine Reuptake Inhibitor, Selective

Use Treatment of attention-deficit/hyperactivity disorder (ADHD)

General Dosage Range Dosage adjustment recommended in patients with hepatic impairment or on concomitant therapy.

Oral:

Children ≥6 years and ≤70 kg: Initial: 0.5 mg/kg/day in 1-2 divided doses; Maintenance: 0.5-1.4 mg/kg/day in 1-2 divided doses (maximum: 1.4 mg/kg/day **or** 100 mg/day, whichever is less)

Children ≥6 years and >70 kg and Adults: Initial: 40 mg/day in 1-2 divided doses; Maintenance: 40-100 mg/day in 1-2 divided doses (maximum: 100 mg/day)

Dosage Forms

Capsule, oral:

Strattera®: 10 mg, 18 mg, 25 mg, 40 mg, 60 mg, 80 mg, 100 mg

atomoxetine hydrochloride *see* atomoxetine *on page 99*

Atopiclair® *see* emollients *on page 328*

atorvastatin (a TORE va sta tin)

Medication Safety Issues

Sound-alike/look-alike issues:

AtorvaSTATin may be confused with atoMOXetine, lovastatin, nystatin, pitavastatin, pravastatin, rosuvastatin, simvastatin

Lipitor® may be confused with labetalol, Levatol®, lisinopril, Loniten®, Lopid®, Mevacor®, Zocor®, ZyrTEC®

Synonyms atorvastatin calcium

Tall-Man atorva**STAT**in

U.S. Brand Names Lipitor®

Canadian Brand Names Apo-Atorvastatin®; Ava-Atorvastatin; CO Atorvastatin; Dom-Atorvastatin; GD-Atorvastatin; Lipitor®; Mylan-Atorvastatin; Novo-Atorvastatin; PMS-Atorvastatin; RAN™-Atorvastatin; ratio-Atorvastatin; Sandoz-Atorvastatin

Therapeutic Category HMG-CoA Reductase Inhibitor

Use Treatment of dyslipidemias or primary prevention of cardiovascular disease (atherosclerotic) as detailed below:

Primary prevention of cardiovascular disease (high-risk for CVD): To reduce the risk of MI or stroke in patients without evidence of heart disease who have multiple CVD risk factors or type 2 diabetes. Treatment reduces the risk for angina or revascularization procedures in patients with multiple risk factors.

Secondary prevention of cardiovascular disease: To reduce the risk of nonfatal MI, nonfatal stroke, revascularization procedures, hospitalization for heart failure, and angina in patients with evidence of coronary heart disease.

Treatment of dyslipidemias: To reduce elevations in total cholesterol (C), LDL-C, apolipoprotein B, and triglycerides in patients with elevations of one or more components, and/or to increase low HDL-C as present in Fredrickson type IIa, IIb, III, and IV hyperlipidemias, heterozygous familial and nonfamilial hypercholesterolemia, and homozygous familial hypercholesterolemia

Treatment of heterozygous familial hypercholesterolemia (HeFH) in adolescent patients (10-17 years of age, females >1 year postmenarche) having LDL-C ≥190 mg/dL or LDL-C ≥160 mg/dL with positive family history of premature cardiovascular disease (CVD) or with two or more CVD risk factors.

General Dosage Range

Dosage adjustment recommended in patients on concomitant therapy

Oral:

Children 10-17 years (females >1 year postmenarche): 10-20 mg/day (maximum: 20 mg/day)

Adults: Maintenance: 10-80 mg once daily (maximum: 80 mg/day)

Dosage Forms

Tablet, oral: 10 mg, 20 mg, 40 mg, 80 mg

Lipitor®: 10 mg, 20 mg, 40 mg, 80 mg

atorvastatin and amlodipine *see* amlodipine and atorvastatin *on page* 66
atorvastatin calcium *see* atorvastatin *on page* 100
atorvastatin calcium and amlodipine besylate *see* amlodipine and atorvastatin *on page* 66

atovaquone (a TOE va kwone)

U.S. Brand Names Mepron®
Canadian Brand Names Mepron®
Therapeutic Category Antiprotozoal
Use Acute oral treatment of mild-to-moderate *Pneumocystis jirovecii* pneumonia (PCP) in patients who are intolerant to co-trimoxazole; prophylaxis of PCP in patients who are intolerant to co-trimoxazole
General Dosage Range Oral: *Children 13-16 years and Adults:* 1500 mg/day in 1-2 divided doses
Dosage Forms
Suspension, oral:
Mepron®: 750 mg/5 mL (5 mL, 210 mL)

atovaquone and proguanil (a TOE va kwone & pro GWA nil)

Synonyms atovaquone and proguanil hydrochloride; proguanil and atovaquone; proguanil hydrochloride and atovaquone
U.S. Brand Names Malarone®
Canadian Brand Names Malarone®; Malarone® Pediatric
Therapeutic Category Antimalarial Agent
Use Prevention or treatment of acute, uncomplicated *P. falciparum* malaria
General Dosage Range Oral:
Children 5-8 kg: Treatment: 125 mg/50 mg as a single daily dose
Children 9-10 kg: Treatment: 187.5 mg/75 mg as a single daily dose
Children 11-20 kg: Prophylaxis: 62.5 mg/25 mg; Treatment: 250 mg/100 mg as a single daily dose
Children 21-30 kg: Prophylaxis: 125 mg/50 mg; Treatment: 500 mg/200 mg as a single daily dose
Children 31-40 kg: Prophylaxis: 187.5 mg/75 mg; Treatment: 750 mg/300 mg as a single daily dose
Children >40 kg and Adults: Prophylaxis: 250 mg/100 mg; Treatment: 1 g/400 mg as a single daily dose
Dosage Forms
Tablet: Atovaquone 250 mg and proguanil hydrochloride 100 mg
Malarone®: Atovaquone 250 mg and proguanil 100 mg
Tablet [pediatric]:
Malarone®: Atovaquone 62.5 mg and proguanil 25 mg

atovaquone and proguanil hydrochloride *see* atovaquone and proguanil *on page* 101
ATRA *see* tretinoin (systemic) *on page* 913

atracurium (a tra KYOO ree um)

Medication Safety Issues
High alert medication:
The Institute for Safe Medication Practices (ISMP) includes this medication among its list of drugs which have a heightened risk of causing significant patient harm when used in error.
Other safety concerns:
United States Pharmacopeia (USP) 2006: The Interdisciplinary Safe Medication Use Expert Committee of the USP has recommended the following:
- Hospitals, clinics, and other practice sites should institute special safeguards in the storage, labeling, and use of these agents and should include these safeguards in staff orientation and competency training.
- Healthcare professionals should be on **high alert** (especially vigilant) whenever a neuromuscular-blocking agent (NMBA) is stocked, ordered, prepared, or administered.

Synonyms atracurium besylate
Canadian Brand Names Atracurium Besylate Injection
Therapeutic Category Skeletal Muscle Relaxant
Use Adjunct to general anesthesia to facilitate endotracheal intubation and to relax skeletal muscles during surgery; to facilitate mechanical ventilation in ICU patients; does not relieve pain or produce sedation
General Dosage Range I.V.:
Children 1 month to 2 years: Initial: 0.3-0.4 mg/kg; Maintenance: Doses as needed to maintain neuromuscular blockade; Infusion: 10-20 mcg/kg/minute

Children >2 years and Adults: Initial: 0.4-0.5 mg/kg; Maintenance: 0.08-1 mg/kg at 15- to 25-minute intervals; Infusion: 5-13 mcg/kg/minute

Dosage Forms

Injection, solution: 10 mg/mL (10 mL)

Injection, solution [preservative free]: 10 mg/mL (5 mL)

atracurium besylate *see* atracurium *on page* 101

Atracurium Besylate Injection (Can) *see* atracurium *on page* 101

Atralin™ *see* tretinoin (topical) *on page* 914

Atrapro™ Antipruritic *see* emollients *on page* 328

Atrapro™ Dermal *see* sodium hypochlorite solution *on page* 842

Atriance™ (Can) *see* nelarabine *on page* 632

Atripla® *see* efavirenz, emtricitabine, and tenofovir *on page* 324

AtroPen® *see* atropine *on page* 102

atropine (A troe peen)

Medication Safety Issues

BEERS Criteria medication:

This drug may be potentially inappropriate for use in geriatric patients (Quality of evidence - varies based on comorbidity; Strength of recommendation - varies based on comorbidity)

Synonyms atropine sulfate

U.S. Brand Names AtroPen®; Atropine Care™; Isopto® Atropine

Canadian Brand Names Dioptic's Atropine Solution; Isopto® Atropine

Therapeutic Category Anticholinergic Agent

Use

Injection: Preoperative medication to inhibit salivation and secretions; treatment of symptomatic sinus bradycardia, AV block (nodal level); antidote for anticholinesterase poisoning (carbamate insecticides, nerve agents, organophosphate insecticides); adjuvant use with anticholinesterases (eg, edrophonium, neostigmine) to decrease their side effects during reversal of neuromuscular blockade

Note: Use is no longer recommended in the management of asystole or pulseless electrical activity (PEA) (ACLS, 2010).

Ophthalmic: Produce mydriasis and cycloplegia for examination of the retina and optic disc and accurate measurement of refractive errors; produce papillary dilation in inflammatory conditions (eg, uveitis)

General Dosage Range

I.M.; SubQ:

Children ≤5 kg: 0.02 mg/kg/dose every 4-6 hours as needed

Children >5 kg: 0.01-0.02 mg/kg/dose every 4-6 hours as needed (maximum: 0.4 mg/dose; minimum: 0.1 mg/dose)

Adults: 0.4-0.6 mg every 4-6 hours as needed

AtroPen® (I.M.):

Children <6.8 kg: 0.25 mg/dose (maximum: 3 doses)

Children 6.8-18 kg: 0.5 mg/dose (maximum: 3 doses)

Children 18-41 kg: 1 mg/dose (maximum: 3 doses)

Children >41 kg and Adults: 2 mg/dose (maximum: 3 doses)

I.V.: *Children and Adults:* Dosage varies greatly depending on indication

Ophthalmic: *Adults:* Ointment: Apply a small amount in the conjunctival sac up to 3 times/day; Solution (1%): Instill 1-2 drops up to 4 times/day

Dosage Forms

Injection, solution: 0.05 mg/mL (5 mL); 0.1 mg/mL (5 mL, 10 mL); 0.4 mg/mL (1 mL, 20 mL)

AtroPen®: 0.25 mg/0.3 mL (0.3 mL); 0.5 mg/0.7 mL (0.7 mL); 1 mg/0.7 mL (0.7 mL); 2 mg/0.7 mL (0.7 mL)

Injection, solution [preservative free]: 0.4 mg/mL (1 mL); 1 mg/mL (1 mL)

Ointment, ophthalmic: 1% (3.5 g)

Solution, ophthalmic: 1% (2 mL, 5 mL, 15 mL)

Atropine Care™: 1% (2 mL, 5 mL, 15 mL)

Isopto® Atropine: 1% (5 mL, 15 mL)

atropine and difenoxin *see* difenoxin and atropine *on page* 284

atropine and diphenoxylate *see* diphenoxylate and atropine *on page* 295

atropine and pralidoxime (A troe peen & pra li DOKS eem)

Synonyms atropine and pralidoxime chloride; Mark 1™; NAAK; nerve agent antidote kit; pralidoxime and atropine

U.S. Brand Names ATNAA; Duodote™

Therapeutic Category Anticholinergic Agent; Antidote

Use

ATNAA: Treatment of poisoning in patients who have been exposed to organophosphate nerve agents (eg, tabun, sarin, soman) that have acetylcholinesterase-inhibiting activity for self- or buddy-administration by military personnel

Duodote™: Treatment of poisoning by organophosphate nerve agents (eg, tabun, sarin, soman) or organophosphate insecticides for use by trained emergency medical services personnel

General Dosage Range I.M.: *Adults:* 1-3 injections (maximum: 3 injections)

Dosage Forms

Injection, solution:

ATNAA, Duodote™: Atropine 2.1 mg/0.7 mL and pralidoxime chloride 600 mg/2 mL [contains benzyl alcohol; prefilled autoinjector]

atropine and pralidoxime chloride *see* atropine and pralidoxime *on page* 103

Atropine Care™ *see* atropine *on page* 102

atropine, hyoscyamine, phenobarbital, and scopolamine *see* hyoscyamine, atropine, scopolamine, and phenobarbital *on page* 467

atropine sulfate *see* atropine *on page* 102

atropine sulfate and edrophonium chloride *see* edrophonium and atropine *on page* 324

Atrovent® *see* ipratropium (nasal) *on page* 499

Atrovent® HFA *see* ipratropium (oral inhalation) *on page* 499

Atryn® *see* antithrombin III *on page* 80

ATV *see* atazanavir *on page* 98

Augmentin® *see* amoxicillin and clavulanate *on page* 70

Augmentin XR® *see* amoxicillin and clavulanate *on page* 70

Auralgan® (Can) *see* antipyrine and benzocaine *on page* 79

auranofin (au RANE oh fin)

Medication Safety Issues

Sound-alike/look-alike issues:

Ridaura® may be confused with Cardura®

U.S. Brand Names Ridaura®

Canadian Brand Names Ridaura®

Therapeutic Category Gold Compound

Use Management of active stage classic or definite rheumatoid arthritis in patients who do not respond to or tolerate other agents

General Dosage Range Dosage adjustment recommended in patients with renal impairment

Oral: *Adults:* Initial: 6 mg/day; Maintenance: 6-9 mg/day (maximum: 9 mg/day)

Dosage Forms

Capsule, oral:

Ridaura®: 3 mg

Auraphene B® [OTC] *see* carbamide peroxide *on page* 173

Auro® [OTC] *see* carbamide peroxide *on page* 173

Auro-Cefprozil (Can) *see* cefprozil *on page* 185

Auro-Cefuroxime (Can) *see* cefuroxime *on page* 187

Auro-Ciprofloxacin (Can) *see* ciprofloxacin (systemic) *on page* 210

Auro-Citalopram (Can) *see* citalopram *on page* 213

Auro-Cyclobenzaprine (Can) *see* cyclobenzaprine *on page* 243

Aurodex® *see* antipyrine and benzocaine *on page* 79

Auro-Mirtazapine (Can) *see* mirtazapine *on page* 606

Auro-Nevirapine (Can) *see* nevirapine *on page* 637

Auro-Terbinafine (Can) *see* terbinafine (systemic) *on page* 878

Aurstat® *see* emollients *on page 328*
AVA *see* anthrax vaccine, adsorbed *on page 77*
Ava-Acebutolol (Can) *see* acebutolol *on page 19*
Ava-Amiodarone (Can) *see* amiodarone *on page 63*
Ava-Atenolol (Can) *see* atenolol *on page 99*
Ava-Atorvastatin (Can) *see* atorvastatin *on page 100*
Ava-Azithromycin (Can) *see* azithromycin (systemic) *on page 108*
Ava-Baclofen (Can) *see* baclofen *on page 112*
Ava-Bicalutamide (Can) *see* bicalutamide *on page 133*
Ava-Bisoprolol (Can) *see* bisoprolol *on page 136*
Ava-Bupropion SR (Can) *see* bupropion *on page 150*
Ava-Carvedilol (Can) *see* carvedilol *on page 179*
Ava-Cefprozil (Can) *see* cefprozil *on page 185*
Ava-Citalopram (Can) *see* citalopram *on page 213*
Ava-Clarithromycin (Can) *see* clarithromycin *on page 215*
Ava-Clindamycin (Can) *see* clindamycin (systemic) *on page 218*
Ava-Cyclobenzaprine (Can) *see* cyclobenzaprine *on page 243*
Ava-Diclofenac (Can) *see* diclofenac (systemic) *on page 279*
Ava-Diclofenac SR (Can) *see* diclofenac (systemic) *on page 279*
Ava-Diltiazem (Can) *see* diltiazem *on page 288*
Ava-Famciclovir (Can) *see* famciclovir *on page 372*
Ava-Fluoxetine (Can) *see* fluoxetine *on page 396*
Avagard™ [OTC] *see* chlorhexidine gluconate *on page 196*
Avage® *see* tazarotene *on page 869*
AVA-Gliclazide (Can) *see* gliclazide *(Canada only) on page 425*
avakine *see* infliximab *on page 481*
Ava-Levetiracetam (Can) *see* levetiracetam *on page 528*
Avalide® *see* irbesartan and hydrochlorothiazide *on page 501*
Ava-Metformin (Can) *see* metformin *on page 579*
Ava-Metoprolol (Can) *see* metoprolol *on page 595*
Ava-Metoprolol (Type L) (Can) *see* metoprolol *on page 595*
Ava-Mirtazapine (Can) *see* mirtazapine *on page 606*
Avamys® (Can) *see* fluticasone (nasal) *on page 400*

avanafil (a VAN a fil)

Medication Safety Issues

Sound-alike/look-alike issues:

Avanafil may be confused with sildenafil, tadalafil, vardenafil

Synonyms Stendra™

Therapeutic Category Phosphodiesterase-5 Enzyme Inhibitor

Use Treatment of erectile dysfunction (ED)

General Dosage Range Dosage adjustment recommended in patients on concomitant therapy.

Oral: *Adults:* Initial: 100 mg 30 minutes prior to sexual activity; to be given as one single dose and not given more than once daily; dosing range: 50-200 mg once daily

Product Availability Stendra™: FDA approved April 2012; availability currently undetermined.

Avandamet® *see* rosiglitazone and metformin *on page 812*
Avandaryl® *see* rosiglitazone and glimepiride *on page 811*
Avandia® *see* rosiglitazone *on page 811*
Ava-Nortriptyline (Can) *see* nortriptyline *on page 650*
Ava-Olanzapine (Can) *see* olanzapine *on page 660*
Ava-Pantoprazole (Can) *see* pantoprazole *on page 689*
Ava-Pioglitazone (Can) *see* pioglitazone *on page 725*
Ava-Pramipexole (Can) *see* pramipexole *on page 749*
Avapro® *see* irbesartan *on page 500*

axitinib (ax I ti nib)

Medication Safety Issues

Sound-alike/look-alike issues:

Axitinib may be confused with gefitinib, imatinib, pazopanib, SORAfenib, SUNItinib, vandetanib, vemurafenib

High alert medication:

This medication is in a class the Institute for Safe Medication Practices (ISMP) includes among its list of drug classes which have a heightened risk of causing significant patient harm when used in error.

Synonyms AG-013736

U.S. Brand Names Inlyta®

Therapeutic Category Antineoplastic Agent, Tyrosine Kinase Inhibitor; Vascular Endothelial Growth Factor (VEGF) Inhibitor

Use Treatment of advanced renal cell cancer (RCC) after failure of one prior systemic treatment

General Dosage Range Dosage adjustment recommended in patients with hepatic impairment, on concomitant therapy, or who develop toxicities.

Oral: *Adults:* 5 mg every 12 hours; maximum: 10 mg every 12 hours

Dosage Forms

Tablet, oral:

Inlyta®: 1 mg, 5 mg

AY-25650 *see* triptorelin *on page 922*
Aygestin® *see* norethindrone *on page 648*
Ayr® Allergy & Sinus [OTC] *see* sodium chloride *on page 840*
Ayr® Baby Saline [OTC] *see* sodium chloride *on page 840*
Ayr® Saline [OTC] *see* sodium chloride *on page 840*
Ayr® Saline Nasal Gel [OTC] *see* sodium chloride *on page 840*
Ayr® Saline No-Drip [OTC] *see* sodium chloride *on page 840*
5-Aza-2'-deoxycytidine *see* decitabine *on page 258*

azacitidine (ay za SYE ti deen)

Medication Safety Issues

Sound-alike/look-alike issues:
AzaCITIDine may be confused with azaTHIOprine

High alert medication:
This medication is in a class the Institute for Safe Medication Practices (ISMP) includes among its list of drug classes which have a heightened risk of causing significant patient harm when used in error.

Synonyms 5-azacytidine; 5-AZC; AZA-CR; azacytidine; ladakamycin

Tall-Man aza**CITID**ine

U.S. Brand Names Vidaza®

Canadian Brand Names Vidaza®

Therapeutic Category Antineoplastic Agent, Antimetabolite (Pyrimidine)

Use Treatment of myelodysplastic syndrome (MDS)

General Dosage Range Dosage adjustment recommended in patients who develop toxicities
I.V., SubQ: *Adults:* 75-100 mg/m^2/day for 7 days/28-day treatment cycle

Dosage Forms

Injection, powder for suspension:
Vidaza®: 100 mg

AZA-CR *see* azacitidine *on page 106*
Azactam® *see* aztreonam *on page 110*
azacytidine *see* azacitidine *on page 106*
5-azacytidine *see* azacitidine *on page 106*
5-Aza-dCyd *see* decitabine *on page 258*
azaepothilone B *see* ixabepilone *on page 508*
Azarga™ (Can) *see* brinzolamide and timolol *(Canada only) on page 142*
Azasan® *see* azathioprine *on page 106*
AzaSite® *see* azithromycin (ophthalmic) *on page 109*

azathioprine (ay za THYE oh preen)

Medication Safety Issues

Sound-alike/look-alike issues:
AzaTHIOprine may be confused with azaCITIDine, azidothymidine, azithromycin, Azulfidine®
Imuran® may be confused with Elmiron®, Enduron, Imdur®, Inderal®, Tenormin®

Other safety concerns:
Azathioprine is metabolized to mercaptopurine; concurrent use of these commercially-available products has resulted in profound myelosuppression.

Synonyms azathioprine sodium

Tall-Man aza**THIO**prine

U.S. Brand Names Azasan®; Imuran®

Canadian Brand Names Apo-Azathioprine®; Imuran®; Mylan-Azathioprine; Teva-Azathioprine

Therapeutic Category Immunosuppressant Agent

Use Adjunctive therapy in prevention of rejection of kidney transplants; management of active rheumatoid arthritis (RA)

General Dosage Range Dosage adjustment recommended in patients with renal impairment, on concomitant therapy, or who develop toxicities
I.V.: *Adults:* Transplant immunosuppression: Initial: 3-5 mg/kg/day as a single daily dose; Maintenance: 1-3 mg/kg/day as a single daily dose

Oral: *Adults:*

Transplant immunosuppression: Initial: 3-5 mg/kg/day in 1-2 divided doses; Maintenance: 1-3 mg/kg/day in 1-2 divided doses

Rheumatoid arthritis: Initial: 1 mg/kg/day (50-100 mg) in 1-2 divided doses; Maintenance: 0.5-2.5 mg/kg/day in 1-2 divided doses

Dosage Forms

Injection, powder for reconstitution: 100 mg

Tablet, oral: 50 mg

Azasan®: 75 mg, 100 mg

Imuran®: 50 mg

azathioprine sodium *see* azathioprine *on page 106*

5-AZC *see* azacitidine *on page 106*

AZD6140 *see* ticagrelor *on page 895*

AZD6474 *see* vandetanib *on page 937*

azelaic acid (a zeh LAY ik AS id)

Synonyms anchoic acid; lepargylic acid

U.S. Brand Names Azelex®; Finacea®; Finacea® Plus™

Canadian Brand Names Finacea®

Therapeutic Category Topical Skin Product

Use

Azelex®: Treatment of mild-to-moderate inflammatory acne vulgaris

Finacea®: Treatment of inflammatory papules and pustules of mild-to-moderate rosacea

General Dosage Range

Topical: *Children ≥12 years and Adults:* Apply to the affected area(s) twice daily.

Dosage Forms

Cream, topical:

Azelex®: 20% (30 g, 50 g)

Gel, topical:

Finacea®: 15% (50 g)

Finacea® Plus™: 15% (50 g)

azelastine (nasal) (a ZEL as teen)

Medication Safety Issues

Sound-alike/look-alike issues:

Astelin® may be confused with Astepro®

Synonyms azelastine hydrochloride

U.S. Brand Names Astelin®; Astepro®

Canadian Brand Names Astelin®

Therapeutic Category Histamine H_1 Antagonist; Histamine H_1 Antagonist, Second Generation

Use Treatment of the symptoms of seasonal allergic rhinitis such as rhinorrhea, sneezing, and nasal pruritus; treatment of the symptoms of vasomotor rhinitis

General Dosage Range Intranasal:

Children 5-11 years: 1 spray in each nostril twice daily

Children ≥12 years and Adults: 1-2 sprays in each nostril twice daily

Dosage Forms

Solution, intranasal: 0.1% [137 mcg/spray] (30 mL)

Astelin®: 0.1% [137 mcg/spray] (30 mL)

Astepro®: 0.15% [205.5 mcg/spray] (30 mL)

azelastine (ophthalmic) (a ZEL as teen)

Medication Safety Issues

Sound-alike/look-alike issues:

Optivar® may be confused with Optiray®, Optive™

International issues:

Optivar [U.S.] may be confused with Opthavir brand name for acyclovir [Mexico]

Synonyms azelastine hydrochloride

U.S. Brand Names Optivar®

Therapeutic Category Histamine H_1 Antagonist; Histamine H_1 Antagonist, Second Generation

Use Treatment of itching of the eye associated with seasonal allergic conjunctivitis

General Dosage Range Ophthalmic: *Children ≥3 years and Adults:* Instill 1 drop into affected eye(s) twice daily

Dosage Forms

Solution, ophthalmic: 0.05% (6 mL)

Optivar®: 0.05% (6 mL)

azelastine and fluticasone (a ZEL as teen & floo TIK a sone)

Synonyms Dymista™; fluticasone proprionate and azelastine hydrochloride

U.S. Brand Names Dymista™

Therapeutic Category Corticosteroid, Nasal; Histamine H_1 Antagonist, Second Generation

Use Symptomatic relief of seasonal allergic rhinitis

General Dosage Range Intranasal: *Children ≥12 years and Adults:* 1 spray (137 mcg azelastine/50 mcg fluticasone) per nostril twice daily

Dosage Forms

Suspension, intranasal [spray]:

Dymista™: Azelastine hydrochloride 0.1% [137 mcg/spray] and fluticasone propionate 0.037% [50 mcg/spray] (23 g)

azelastine hydrochloride *see* azelastine (nasal) *on page 107*
azelastine hydrochloride *see* azelastine (ophthalmic) *on page 107*
Azelex® *see* azelaic acid *on page 107*
azidothymidine *see* zidovudine *on page 961*
azidothymidine, abacavir, and lamivudine *see* abacavir, lamivudine, and zidovudine *on page 16*
Azilect® *see* rasagiline *on page 789*

azilsartan (ay zil SAR tan)

Synonyms azilsartan medoxomil; AZL-M

U.S. Brand Names edarbi™

Therapeutic Category Angiotensin II Receptor Blocker

Use Treatment of hypertension; may be used alone or in combination with other antihypertensives

General Dosage Range Oral: *Adults:* 40-80 mg once daily

Dosage Forms

Tablet, oral:

edarbi™: 40 mg, 80 mg

azilsartan and chlorthalidone (ay zil SAR tan & klor THAL i done)

Synonyms azilsartan medoxomil and chlorthalidone; chlorthalidone and azilsartan

U.S. Brand Names edarbyclor™

Therapeutic Category Angiotensin II Receptor Blocker; Diuretic, Thiazide

Use Treatment of hypertension

General Dosage Range Oral: *Adults:* 40 mg (azilsartan) and 12.5-25 mg (chlorthalidone) once daily; (maximum: azilsartan 40 mg/day; chlorthalidone 25 mg/day)

Dosage Forms

Tablet, oral:

edarbyclor™: 40/12.5: Azilsartan medoxomil 40 mg and chlorthalidone 12.5 mg

edarbyclor™: 40/25: Azilsartan medoxomil 40 mg and chlorthalidone 25 mg

azilsartan medoxomil *see* azilsartan *on page 108*
azilsartan medoxomil and chlorthalidone *see* azilsartan and chlorthalidone *on page 108*

azithromycin (systemic) (az ith roe MYE sin)

Medication Safety Issues

Sound-alike/look-alike issues:

Azithromycin may be confused with azathioprine, erythromycin

Zithromax® may be confused with Fosamax®, Zinacef®, Zovirax®

Synonyms azithromycin dihydrate; azithromycin hydrogencitrate; azithromycin monohydrate; Z-Pak

U.S. Brand Names Zithromax®; Zithromax® TRI-PAK™; Zithromax® Z-PAK®; Zmax®

Canadian Brand Names Apo-Azithromycin®; Ava-Azithromycin; Azithromycin for Injection; CO Azithromycin; Dom-Azithromycin; GD-Azithromycin; Mylan-Azithromycin; Novo-Azithromycin; PHL-Azithromycin; PMS-Azithromycin; PRO-Azithromycin; ratio-Azithromycin; Riva-Azithromycin; Sandoz-Azithromycin; Zithromax®; Zmax SR™

Therapeutic Category Antibiotic, Macrolide

Use Oral, I.V.: Treatment of acute otitis media due to *H. influenzae*, *M. catarrhalis*, or *S. pneumoniae*; pharyngitis/tonsillitis due to *S. pyogenes*; treatment of mild-to-moderate upper and lower respiratory tract infections, infections of the skin and skin structure, community-acquired pneumonia, pelvic inflammatory disease (PID), sexually-transmitted diseases (urethra/cervix/rectum), and genital ulcer disease (chancroid) due to susceptible strains of *Chlamydophila pneumoniae, C. trachomatis, M. catarrhalis, H. influenzae, S. aureus, S. pneumoniae, Mycoplasma genitalium, Mycoplasma pneumoniae*, and *C. psittaci*; acute bacterial exacerbations of chronic obstructive pulmonary disease (COPD) due to *H. influenzae, M. catarrhalis,* or *S. pneumoniae*; acute bacterial sinusitis; prevention, alone or in combination with rifabutin, of MAC in patients with advanced HIV infection; treatment, in combination with ethambutol, of disseminated MAC in patients with advanced HIV infection

General Dosage Range

I.V.: *Adults:* 500 mg as a single daily dose

Oral:

Immediate release:

Children ≥6 months to 2 years: 5-10 mg/kg as a single daily dose (maximum: 500 mg/dose) **or** 30 mg/kg as a single dose (maximum: 1500 mg/dose)

Children ≥2 years: 5-12 mg/kg as single daily dose (maximum: 500 mg/dose) **or** 30 mg/kg as a single dose (maximum: 1500 mg/dose)

Adults: 250-500 mg as a single daily dose **or** 1-2 g as a single dose

Extended release (suspension):

Children ≥6 months and <34 kg: 60 mg/kg as a single dose

Children ≥6 months and ≥34 kg and Adults: 2 g as a single dose

Dosage Forms

Injection, powder for reconstitution: 500 mg

Zithromax®: 500 mg

Microspheres for suspension, extended release, oral:

Zmax®: 2 g/bottle (60 mL)

Powder for suspension, oral: 100 mg/5 mL (15 mL); 200 mg/5 mL (15 mL, 22.5 mL, 30 mL); 1 g/packet (3s, 10s)

Zithromax®: 100 mg/5 mL (15 mL); 200 mg/5 mL (15 mL, 22.5 mL, 30 mL); 1 g/packet (3s, 10s)

Tablet, oral: 250 mg, 500 mg, 600 mg

Zithromax®: 250 mg, 500 mg, 600 mg

Zithromax® TRI-PAK™: 500 mg

Zithromax® Z-PAK®: 250 mg

azithromycin (ophthalmic) (az ith roe MYE sin)

Medication Safety Issues

Sound-alike/look-alike issues:

Azithromycin may be confused with azathioprine, erythromycin

U.S. Brand Names AzaSite®

Therapeutic Category Antibiotic, Macrolide; Antibiotic, Ophthalmic

Use Treatment of bacterial conjunctivitis caused by susceptible microorganisms

General Dosage Range Ophthalmic: *Children ≥1 year and Adults:* Days 1 and 2: 1 drop into affected eye(s) twice daily; Days 3-7: 1 drop into affected eye(s) once daily

Dosage Forms

Solution, ophthalmic:

AzaSite®: 1% (2.5 mL)

azithromycin dihydrate *see* azithromycin (systemic) *on page 108*

Azithromycin for Injection (Can) *see* azithromycin (systemic) *on page 108*

azithromycin hydrogencitrate *see* azithromycin (systemic) *on page 108*

azithromycin monohydrate *see* azithromycin (systemic) *on page 108*

AZL-M *see* azilsartan *on page 108*

Azo-Gesic™ [OTC] *see* phenazopyridine *on page 711*

Azopt® *see* brinzolamide *on page* 142
Azor™ *see* amlodipine and olmesartan *on page* 67
AZO Standard® [OTC] [DSC] *see* phenazopyridine *on page* 711
AZO Standard® Maximum Strength [OTC] [DSC] *see* phenazopyridine *on page* 711
AZO Urinary Pain Relief™ [OTC] *see* phenazopyridine *on page* 711
AZO Urinary Pain Relief™ Maximum Strength [OTC] *see* phenazopyridine *on page* 711
AZT™ (Can) *see* zidovudine *on page* 961
AZT + 3TC (error-prone abbreviation) *see* lamivudine and zidovudine *on page* 520
AZT, abacavir, and lamivudine *see* abacavir, lamivudine, and zidovudine *on page* 16
AZT (error-prone abbreviation) *see* zidovudine *on page* 961
azthreonam *see* aztreonam *on page* 110

aztreonam (AZ tree oh nam)

Medication Safety Issues

Sound-alike/look-alike issues:

Aztreonam may be confused with azidothymidine

Synonyms azthreonam

U.S. Brand Names Azactam®; Cayston®

Canadian Brand Names Cayston®

Therapeutic Category Antibiotic, Miscellaneous

Use

Injection: Treatment of patients with urinary tract infections, lower respiratory tract infections, septicemia, skin/skin structure infections, intraabdominal infections, and gynecological infections caused by susceptible gram-negative bacilli

Inhalation: Improve respiratory symptoms in cystic fibrosis (CF) patients with *Pseudomonas aeruginosa*

General Dosage Range Dosage adjustment recommended in patients with renal impairment

I.M.:

Children >1 month: 30-50 mg/kg/dose every 6-8 hours (maximum: 8 g/day)
Adults: 500 mg to 1 g every 8-12 hours

I.V.:

Children >1 month: 30-50 mg/kg/dose every 6-8 hours (maximum: 8 g/day)
Adults: 1-2 g every 6-12 hours (maximum: 8 g/day)

Oral inhalation: *Children ≥7 years and Adults:* 75 mg 3 times/day

Dosage Forms

Infusion, premixed iso-osmotic solution:
Azactam®: 1 g (50 mL); 2 g (50 mL)

Injection, powder for reconstitution: 1 g, 2 g
Azactam®: 1 g, 2 g

Powder for reconstitution, for oral inhalation [preservative free]:
Cayston®: 75 mg

Azulfidine® *see* sulfasalazine *on page* 861
Azulfidine EN-tabs® *see* sulfasalazine *on page* 861
Azurette™ *see* ethinyl estradiol and desogestrel *on page* 356
B6 *see* pyridoxine *on page* 777
B1939 *see* eribulin *on page* 341
B2036-PEG *see* pegvisomant *on page* 700
B 9273 *see* alefacept *on page* 44
baby aspirin *see* aspirin *on page* 96
BabyBIG® *see* botulism immune globulin (intravenous-human) *on page* 140
Bacid® [OTC] *see* Lactobacillus *on page* 518
Bacid® (Can) *see* Lactobacillus *on page* 518
Baciguent® [OTC] *see* bacitracin *on page* 111
Baciguent® (Can) *see* bacitracin *on page* 111
BACiiM™ *see* bacitracin *on page* 111
Baciject® (Can) *see* bacitracin *on page* 111
bacillus Calmette-Guérin (BCG) live *see* BCG *on page* 116

bacitracin (bas i TRAY sin)

Medication Safety Issues

Sound-alike/look-alike issues:

Bacitracin may be confused with Bactrim™, Bactroban®

U.S. Brand Names Baciguent® [OTC]; BACiiM™

Canadian Brand Names Baciguent®; Baciject®

Therapeutic Category Antibiotic, Miscellaneous; Antibiotic, Ophthalmic; Antibiotic, Topical

Use Treatment of susceptible bacterial infections mainly (has activity against gram-positive bacilli); due to toxicity risks, systemic and irrigant uses of bacitracin should be limited to situations where less toxic alternatives would not be effective

General Dosage Range

I.M.:

Infants ≤2.5 kg: 900 units/kg/day in 2-3 divided doses

Infants >2.5 kg: 1000 units/kg/day in 2-3 divided doses

Ophthalmic: *Children and Adults:* Instill 1/4" to 1/2" ribbon every 3-4 hours (acute infections) or 2-3 times/day (mild-to-moderate infections)

Oral: *Adults:* 25,000 units 4 times/day

Topical: *Children and Adults:* Apply 1-3 times/day

Dosage Forms

Injection, powder for reconstitution: 50,000 units

BACiiM™: 50,000 units

Ointment, ophthalmic: 500 units/g (3.5 g)

Ointment, topical: 500 units/g (0.9 g, 15 g, 30 g, 120 g, 454 g)

Baciguent® [OTC]: 500 units/g (30 g)

bacitracin and polymyxin B (bas i TRAY sin & pol i MIKS in bee)

Medication Safety Issues

Sound-alike/look-alike issues:

Betadine® may be confused with Betagan®, betaine

Synonyms polymyxin B and bacitracin

U.S. Brand Names AK-Poly-Bac™; Polycin™; Polysporin® [OTC]

Canadian Brand Names LID-Pack®; Optimyxin®

Therapeutic Category Antibiotic, Ophthalmic; Antibiotic, Topical

Use Treatment of superficial infections caused by susceptible organisms

General Dosage Range

Ophthalmic: *Children and Adults:* Instill 1/2" ribbon in the affected eye(s) every 3-4 hours (acute infections) **or** 2-3 times/day (mild-to-moderate infections)

Topical: *Children and Adults:* Apply to affected area 1-4 times/day

Dosage Forms

Ointment, ophthalmic: Bacitracin 500 units and polymyxin B 10,000 units per g (3.5 g)

AK-Poly-Bac™: Bacitracin 500 units and polymyxin B 10,000 units per g (3.5 g)

Polycin™: Bacitracin 500 units and polymyxin B 10,000 units per g (3.5 g)

Ointment, topical: Bacitracin 500 units and polymyxin B 10,000 units per g in white petrolatum (15 g, 30 g)

Polysporin®: Bacitracin 500 units and polymyxin B 10,000 units per g (0.9 g, 15 g, 30 g)

Powder, topical:

Polysporin®: Bacitracin 500 units and polymyxin B 10,000 units per g (10 g)

bacitracin, neomycin, and polymyxin B
(bas i TRAY sin, nee oh MYE sin, & pol i MIKS in bee)

Synonyms neomycin, bacitracin, and polymyxin B; polymyxin B, bacitracin, and neomycin; triple antibiotic

U.S. Brand Names Neo-Polycin™; Neosporin® Neo To Go® [OTC]; Neosporin® Topical [OTC]

Therapeutic Category Antibiotic, Ophthalmic; Antibiotic, Topical

Use Helps prevent infection in minor cuts, scrapes, and burns; short-term treatment of superficial external ocular infections caused by susceptible organisms

General Dosage Range

Ophthalmic: *Children and Adults:* Instill 1/2" every 3-4 hours

Topical: *Children and Adults:* Apply 1-3 times/day

Dosage Forms

Ointment, ophthalmic: Bacitracin 400 units, neomycin 3.5 mg, and polymyxin B 10,000 units per g (3.5 g)

Neo-Polycin™: Bacitracin 400 units, neomycin 3.5 mg, and polymyxin B 10,000 units per g (3.5 g)

Ointment, topical: Bacitracin 400 units, neomycin 3.5 mg, and polymyxin B 5000 units per g (0.9 g, 15 g, 30 g, 454 g)

Neosporin® [OTC]: Bacitracin 400 units, neomycin 3.5 mg, and polymyxin B 5000 units per g (15 g, 30 g)

Neosporin® Neo To Go® [OTC]: Bacitracin 400 units, neomycin 3.5 mg, and polymyxin B 5000 units per g (0.9 g)

bacitracin, neomycin, polymyxin B, and hydrocortisone

(bas i TRAY sin, nee oh MYE sin, pol i MIKS in bee, & hye droe KOR ti sone)

Synonyms hydrocortisone, bacitracin, neomycin, and polymyxin B; neomycin, bacitracin, polymyxin B, and hydrocortisone; polymyxin B, bacitracin, neomycin, and hydrocortisone

U.S. Brand Names Cortisporin® Ointment; Neo-Polycin™ HC

Canadian Brand Names Cortisporin® Topical Ointment

Therapeutic Category Antibiotic/Corticosteroid, Ophthalmic; Antibiotic/Corticosteroid, Topical

Use Prevention and treatment of susceptible inflammatory conditions where bacterial infection (or risk of infection) is present

General Dosage Range

Ophthalmic: *Children and Adults:* Instill 1/2 inch every 3-4 hours

Topical: *Children and Adults:* Apply sparingly 2-4 times/day

Dosage Forms

Ointment, ophthalmic: Bacitracin 400 units, neomycin sulfate 3.5 mg, polymyxin B 10,000 units, and hydrocortisone 10 mg per g (3.5 g)

Neo-Polycin™ HC: Bacitracin 400 units, neomycin 3.5 mg, polymyxin B 10,000 units, and hydrocortisone 10 mg per g (3.5 g)

Ointment, topical:

Cortisporin®: Bacitracin 400 units, neomycin 3.5 mg, polymyxin B 5000 units, and hydrocortisone 10 mg per g (15 g)

bacitracin, neomycin, polymyxin B, and pramoxine

(bas i TRAY sin, nee oh MYE sin, pol i MIKS in bee, & pra MOKS een)

Synonyms neomycin, bacitracin, polymyxin B, and pramoxine; polymyxin B, neomycin, bacitracin, and pramoxine; pramoxine, neomycin, bacitracin, and polymyxin B

U.S. Brand Names Neosporin® + Pain Relief Ointment [OTC]; Tri Biozene [OTC]

Therapeutic Category Antibiotic, Topical

Use Prevention and treatment of susceptible superficial topical infections and provide temporary relief of pain or discomfort

General Dosage Range Topical: *Children ≥2 years and Adults:* Apply 1-3 times/day to infected areas

Dosage Forms

Ointment, topical: Bacitracin 500 units, neomycin 3.5 mg, polymyxin B 10,000 units, and pramoxine 10 mg (15 g, 30 g)

Neosporin® + Pain Relief Ointment [OTC]: Bacitracin 500 units, neomycin 3.5 mg, polymyxin B 10,000 units, and pramoxine 10 mg (15 g, 30 g)

Tri Biozene [OTC]: Bacitracin 500 units, neomycin 3.5 mg, polymyxin B 10,000 units, and pramoxine 10 mg (15 g)

baclofen (BAK loe fen)

Medication Safety Issues

Sound-alike/look-alike issues:

Baclofen may be confused with Bactroban®

Lioresal® may be confused with lisinopril, Lotensin®

High alert medication:

The Institute for Safe Medication Practices (ISMP) includes this medication (intrathecal administration) among its list of drugs which have a heightened risk of causing significant patient harm when used in error.

U.S. Brand Names Gablofen®; Lioresal®

Canadian Brand Names Apo-Baclofen®; Ava-Baclofen; Dom-Baclofen; Lioresal®; Lioresal® D.S.; Lioresal® Intrathecal; Med-Baclofen; Mylan-Baclofen; Novo-Baclofen; Nu-Baclo; PHL-Baclofen; PMS-Baclofen; ratio-Baclofen; Riva-Baclofen

Therapeutic Category Skeletal Muscle Relaxant

Use Treatment of reversible spasticity associated with multiple sclerosis or spinal cord lesions

Orphan drug: Intrathecal: Treatment of intractable spasticity caused by spinal cord injury, multiple sclerosis, and other spinal disease (spinal ischemia or tumor, transverse myelitis, cervical spondylosis, degenerative myelopathy)

General Dosage Range

Intrathecal:

Children: Test dose: 25-100 mcg; Initial infusion: Infuse at a 24-hourly rate dosed at twice the test dose

Adults: Test dose: 50-100 mcg; Initial infusion: Infuse at a 24-hourly rate dosed at twice the test dose

Oral:

Adults: Initial: 5 mg 3 times/day; Maintenance: Up to 80 mg/day in 2-3 divided doses

Elderly: Initial: 5 mg 2-3 times/day, increasing gradually as needed

Dosage Forms

Injection, solution, intrathecal [preservative free]:

Gablofen®: 50 mcg/mL (1 mL); 500 mcg/mL (20 mL); 1000 mcg/mL (20 mL); 2000 mcg/mL (20 mL)

Lioresal®: 50 mcg/mL (1 mL); 500 mcg/mL (20 mL); 2000 mcg/mL (5 mL, 20 mL)

Tablet, oral: 10 mg, 20 mg

Bactoshield® CHG [OTC] *see* chlorhexidine gluconate *on page 196*

Bactrim™ *see* sulfamethoxazole and trimethoprim *on page 860*

Bactrim™ DS *see* sulfamethoxazole and trimethoprim *on page 860*

Bactroban® *see* mupirocin *on page 618*

Bactroban Cream® *see* mupirocin *on page 618*

Bactroban Nasal® *see* mupirocin *on page 618*

baking soda *see* sodium bicarbonate *on page 840*

BAL *see* dimercaprol *on page 290*

balanced salt solution (BAL anced salt soe LOO shun)

U.S. Brand Names AquaLase®; BSS Plus®; BSS®

Canadian Brand Names BSS Plus®; BSS®; Eye-Stream®

Therapeutic Category Ophthalmic Agent, Miscellaneous

Use

Irrigation solution for ophthalmic surgery:

AquaLase®, BSS®: Intraocular or extraocular irrigating solution

BSS Plus®: Intraocular irrigating solution

Irrigation solution for eyes, ears, nose, or throat

General Dosage Range Irrigation: *Children and Adults:* Based on standard for each surgical procedure

Dosage Forms

Solution, ophthalmic [irrigation; preservative free]: Sodium chloride 0.64%, potassium chloride 0.075%, calcium chloride 0.048%, magnesium chloride 0.03%, sodium acetate 0.39%, sodium citrate 0.17% (18 mL, 500 mL)

AquaLase®: Sodium chloride 0.64%, potassium chloride 0.075%, calcium chloride 0.048%, magnesium chloride 0.03%, sodium acetate 0.39%, sodium citrate 0.17% (90 mL)

BSS®: Sodium chloride 0.64%, potassium chloride 0.075%, calcium chloride 0.048%, magnesium chloride 0.03%, sodium acetate 0.39%, sodium citrate 0.17% (15 mL, 30 mL, 250 mL, 500 mL)

BSS Plus®: Sodium chloride 0.71%, potassium chloride 0.038%, calcium chloride 0.015%, magnesium chloride 0.02%, sodium phosphate 0.042%, sodium bicarbonate 0.21%, dextrose 0.092%, glutathione 0.018% (250 mL, 500 mL)

BAL in Oil® *see* dimercaprol *on page 290*

Balmex® [OTC] *see* zinc oxide *on page 963*

Balminil Decongestant (Can) *see* pseudoephedrine *on page 771*

Balminil DM D (Can) *see* pseudoephedrine and dextromethorphan *on page 772*

Balminil DM + Decongestant + Expectorant (Can) *see* guaifenesin, pseudoephedrine, and dextromethorphan *on page 437*

Balminil DM E (Can) *see* guaifenesin and dextromethorphan *on page 434*

Balminil Expectorant (Can) *see* guaifenesin *on page 433*
Balnetar® [OTC] *see* coal tar *on page 228*

balsalazide (bal SAL a zide)

Medication Safety Issues
Sound-alike/look-alike issues:
Colazal® may be confused with Clozaril®
Synonyms balsalazide disodium; Giazo™
U.S. Brand Names Colazal®
Therapeutic Category 5-Aminosalicylic Acid Derivative; Antiinflammatory Agent
Use Treatment of mildly- to moderately-active ulcerative colitis
Giazo™: Only approved in males ≥18 years; effectiveness in females was not demonstrated
General Dosage Range Oral:
Capsule:
Children ≥5 years: 750 mg **or** 2.25 g 3 times daily
Adults: 2.25 g 3 times daily
Tablet: *Adults: Males:* 3.3 g twice daily
Product Availability
Giazo™: FDA approved February 2012; availability expected third quarter 2012.
Giazo™ is a twice-daily balsalazide formulation approved for the treatment of mildly- to moderately-active ulcerative colitis in adult male patients.
Dosage Forms
Capsule, oral: 750 mg
Colazal®: 750 mg

balsalazide disodium *see* balsalazide *on page 114*
balsam Peru, castor oil, and trypsin *see* trypsin, balsam Peru, and castor oil *on page 925*
Balziva™ *see* ethinyl estradiol and norethindrone *on page 359*
Band-Aid® Hurt Free™ Antiseptic Wash [OTC] *see* lidocaine (topical) *on page 535*
Banophen™ [OTC] *see* diphenhydramine (systemic) *on page 292*
Banophen™ Anti-Itch [OTC] *see* diphenhydramine (topical) *on page 293*
Banzel® *see* rufinamide *on page 814*
Banzel™ (Can) *see* rufinamide *on page 814*
Baraclude® *see* entecavir *on page 333*
Baridium [OTC] *see* phenazopyridine *on page 711*

barium (BA ree um)

Synonyms barium sulfate
U.S. Brand Names Digibar™ 190; E-Z Cat® Dry; E-Z-Cat®; E-Z-Disk™; E-Z-Dose™ with Liquid Polibar Plus®; E-Z-HD™; E-Z-Paque®; E-Z-Paste®; Entero Vu™; Entero VU™ 24%; Entero-H™; Esopho-Cat®; Liquid Entero Vu™; Liquid Polibar Plus®; Liquid Polibar®; Maxibar™; Polibar® ACB; Readi-Cat®; Readi-Cat® 2; Sensatrast™; Tagitol™ V; Ultra-R®; Varibar® Honey; Varibar® Nectar; Varibar® Pudding; Varibar® Thin Honey; Varibar® Thin Liquid; VoLumen®
Therapeutic Category Radiopaque Agents
Use Diagnostic aid for computed tomography or x-ray examinations of the GI tract
Dosage Forms
Cream, oral:
E-Z-Paste®: 60% w/w (454 g)
Esopho-Cat®: 3% w/w (30 g)
Paste, oral:
Varibar® Pudding: 40% w/v (230 mL)
Powder for suspension, oral:
Digibar™ 190: 190% w/v after reconstitution (232 g)
E-Z Cat® Dry: 2% w/w after reconstitution (23 g)
E-Z-HD™: 98% w/w before reconstitution (340 g)
E-Z-Paque®: 96% w/w before reconstitution (176 g, 1200 g)
Entero Vu™: 13% w/v after reconstitution (100 g)
Ultra-R®: 95% w/w before reconstitution (170 g)
Varibar® Thin Liquid: 40% w/v after reconstitution (148 g)

Powder for suspension, oral/rectal:
Sensatrast™: 100% before reconstitution (120 g)
Powder for suspension, rectal:
Polibar® ACB: 96% w/w before reconstitution (397 g, 454 g)
Suspension, oral:
E-Z-Cat®: 4.9% w/v (255 mL)
Entero VU™ 24%: 24% w/v (600 mL)
Entero-H™: 80% w/v (1900 mL)
Liquid Entero Vu™: 13% w/v (600 mL)
Maxibar™: 210% w/v (120 mL)
Readi-Cat® 2: 2.1% w/v (250 mL, 450 mL)
Tagitol™ V: 40% w/v (20 mL)
Varibar® Honey: 40% w/v (250 mL)
Varibar® Nectar: 40% w/v (240 mL)
Varibar® Thin Honey: 40% w/v (250 mL)
VoLumen®: 0.1% w/v (450 mL)
Suspension, oral/rectal:
Liquid Polibar Plus®: 105% w/v (1900 mL)
Liquid Polibar®: 100% w/v (1900 mL)
Readi-Cat®: 1.3% w/v (450 mL, 900 mL, 1900 mL)
Readi-Cat® 2: 2.1% w/v (450 mL, 900 mL, 1900 mL)
Suspension, rectal:
E-Z-Dose™ with Liquid Polibar Plus®: 105% w/v (650 mL)
Tablet, oral:
E-Z-Disk™: 648 mg

barium sulfate *see* barium *on page* *114*
Basaljel® (Can) *see* aluminum hydroxide *on page* *55*
base ointment *see* zinc oxide *on page* *963*

basiliximab (ba si LIK si mab)

U.S. Brand Names Simulect®

Canadian Brand Names Simulect®

Therapeutic Category Immunosuppressant Agent

Use Prophylaxis of acute organ rejection in renal transplantation (in combination with cyclosporine and corticosteroids)

General Dosage Range I.V.:
Children <35 kg: 10 mg within 2 hours prior to transplant surgery, followed by a second 10 mg dose 4 days after transplantation
Children ≥35 kg and Adults: 20 mg within 2 hours prior to transplant surgery, followed by a second 20 mg dose 4 days after transplantation

Dosage Forms
Injection, powder for reconstitution:
Simulect®: 10 mg, 20 mg

BAY 43-9006 *see* sorafenib *on page* *850*
BAY 59-7939 *see* rivaroxaban *on page* *806*
Baycadron™ *see* dexamethasone (systemic) *on page* *266*
Bayer® Aspirin Extra Strength [OTC] *see* aspirin *on page* *96*
Bayer® Aspirin Regimen Adult Low Strength [OTC] *see* aspirin *on page* *96*
Bayer® Aspirin Regimen Children's [OTC] *see* aspirin *on page* *96*
Bayer® Aspirin Regimen Regular Strength [OTC] *see* aspirin *on page* *96*
Bayer® Genuine Aspirin [OTC] *see* aspirin *on page* *96*
Bayer® Plus Extra Strength [OTC] *see* aspirin *on page* *96*
Bayer® PM [OTC] *see* aspirin and diphenhydramine *on page* *97*
Bayer® Women's Low Dose Aspirin [OTC] *see* aspirin *on page* *96*
Baza® Antifungal [OTC] *see* miconazole (topical) *on page* *599*
Baza® Clear [OTC] *see* vitamin A and vitamin D (topical) *on page* *949*
B-Caro-T™ [OTC] *see* beta-carotene *on page* *128*

BCG (bee see jee)

Medication Safety Issues

Sound-alike/look-alike issues:

BCG (intravesical) may be confused with BCG for immunization

High alert medication:

The Institute for Safe Medication Practices (ISMP) includes this medication among its list of drugs which have a heightened risk of causing significant patient harm when used in error.

Synonyms bacillus Calmette-Guérin (BCG) live; BCG vaccine U.S.P. *(percutaneous use product)*; BCG, live

U.S. Brand Names BCG Vaccine; TheraCys®; TICE® BCG

Canadian Brand Names BCG Vaccine; ImmuCyst®; Oncotice™

Therapeutic Category Biological Response Modulator

Use

BCG intravesical: Treatment and prophylaxis of carcinoma *in situ* of the bladder; prophylaxis of primary or recurrent superficial or minimally invasive papillary tumors following transurethral resection

BCG vaccine: Immunization against *Mycobacterium tuberculosis* in persons not previously infected and who are at high risk for exposure

BCG vaccine is not routinely administered for the prevention of *M. tuberculosis* in the United States. The Advisory Committee on Immunization Practices (ACIP) recommends vaccination be considered for the following:

- Children with a negative tuberculin skin test who are continually exposed to (and cannot be separated from) adults who are untreated or ineffectively treated for TB disease when the child cannot be given long-term treatment for infection **or** if the adult has TB caused by strains resistant to isoniazid and rifampin.
- Healthcare workers with a high percentage of patients with *M. tuberculosis* strains resistant to both isoniazid and rifampin, if there is ongoing transmission of the resistant strains and subsequent infection is likely, or if comprehensive infection-control precautions have not been successful. In addition, healthcare workers should be counseled on the risks and benefits of vaccination and treatment of latent TB infection

General Dosage Range

Percutaneous:

Children <1 month: 0.2-0.3 mL (half-strength dilution)

Children >1 month and Adults: 0.2-0.3 mL (full-strength dilution)

Intravesicular: *Adults:*

TheraCys®: 1 dose instilled into bladder (retain for 2 hours) once weekly for 6 weeks followed by 1 treatment at 3, 6, 12, 18, and 24 months after initial treatment

TICE® BCG: 1 dose instilled into bladder (retain for 2 hours) once weekly for 6 weeks (may repeat cycle 1 time), followed by approximately once monthly for at least 6-12 months

Dosage Forms

Injection, powder for reconstitution, intravesical:

TICE® BCG: 50 mg

Injection, powder for reconstitution, intravesical [preservative free]:

TheraCys®: 81 mg

Injection, powder for reconstitution, percutaneous:

BCG Vaccine: 50 mg

BCG, live *see* BCG *on page 116*

BCG Vaccine *see* BCG *on page 116*

BCG vaccine U.S.P. *(percutaneous use product)* *see* BCG *on page 116*

BCNU *see* carmustine *on page 178*

B complex combinations *see* vitamin B complex combinations *on page 950*

BD™ Glucose [OTC] *see* dextrose *on page 275*

beano® [OTC] *see* alpha-galactosidase *on page 52*

beano® Meltaways [OTC] *see* alpha-galactosidase *on page 52*

Bebulin® VH *see* factor IX complex (human) *on page 371*

becaplermin (be KAP ler min)

Medication Safety Issues

Sound-alike/look-alike issues:

Regranex® may be confused with Granulex®, Repronex®

Synonyms recombinant human platelet-derived growth factor B; rPDGF-BB

U.S. Brand Names Regranex®

Therapeutic Category Topical Skin Product

Use Adjunctive treatment of diabetic neuropathic ulcers occurring on the lower limbs and feet that extend into subcutaneous tissue (or beyond) and have adequate blood supply

General Dosage Range Topical: *Adults:* Apply once daily; to determine the length of gel to apply to the ulcer, measure the greatest length of the ulcer by the greatest width of the ulcer. Tube size and unit of measure will determine the formula used in the calculation. Recalculate amount of gel needed every 1-2 weeks, depending on the rate of change in ulcer area.

Centimeters: 15 g tube: [ulcer length (cm) x width (cm)] divided by 4 = length of gel (cm); 2 g tube: [ulcer length (cm) x width (cm)] divided by 2 = length of gel (cm)

Inches: 15 g tube: [length (in) x width (in)] x 0.6 = length of gel (in); 2 g tube: [length (in) x width (in)] x 1.3 = length of gel (in)

Dosage Forms

Gel, topical:

Regranex®: 0.01% (15 g)

beclomethasone (oral inhalation) (be kloe METH a sone)

Synonyms Vanceril

U.S. Brand Names QVAR®

Canadian Brand Names QVAR®

Therapeutic Category Corticosteroid, Inhalant (Oral)

Use Oral inhalation: Maintenance and prophylactic treatment of asthma; includes those who require corticosteroids and those who may benefit from a dose reduction/elimination of systemically-administered corticosteroids. Not for relief of acute bronchospasm.

General Dosage Range Inhalation:

Children 5-11 years: Initial: 40 mcg twice daily; Maintenance: 80-160 mcg/day in 2 divided doses

Children ≥12 years and Adults: Initial: 40-160 mcg twice daily; Maintenance: 80-640 mcg/day in 2 divided doses

Dosage Forms

Aerosol, for oral inhalation:

QVAR®: 40 mcg/inhalation (8.7 g); 80 mcg/inhalation (8.7 g)

Dosage Forms - Canada

Aerosol, for oral inhalation:

QVAR™: 50 mcg/inhalation (6.5 g, 12.4 g); 100 mcg/inhalation (6.5 g, 12.4 g)

beclomethasone (nasal) (be kloe METH a sone)

Synonyms beclomethasone dipropionate

U.S. Brand Names Beconase AQ®; Qnasl™

Canadian Brand Names Apo-Beclomethasone®; Mylan-Beclo AQ; Nu-Beclomethasone; Rivanase AQ

Therapeutic Category Corticosteroid, Nasal

Use

Beconase AQ®: Symptomatic treatment of seasonal or perennial allergic rhinitis; nonallergic (vasomotor) rhinitis; prevent recurrence of nasal polyps following surgery

Qnasl™: Symptomatic treatment of seasonal or perennial allergic rhinitis

General Dosage Range Intranasal:

Children ≥6 years and Adults (Beconase AQ®): 1-2 inhalations each nostril twice daily (maximum: 336 mcg/day)

Children ≥12 years and Adults (Qnasl™): Two inhalations each nostril once daily (maximum: 320 mcg/day)

Dosage Forms

Aerosol, spray, intranasal:

Qnasl™: 80 mcg/inhalation (8.7 g)

Suspension, intranasal:

Beconase AQ®: 42 mcg/inhalation (25 g)

beclomethasone dipropionate *see* beclomethasone (nasal) *on page* 117

Beconase AQ® *see* beclomethasone (nasal) *on page* 117

behenyl alcohol *see* docosanol *on page* 304

belatacept (bel AT a sept)

Synonyms BMS-224818; LEA29Y

U.S. Brand Names Nulojix®

Therapeutic Category Selective T-Cell Costimulation Blocker

Use Prophylaxis of organ rejection concomitantly with basiliximab, mycophenolate, and corticosteroids in Epstein-Barr virus (EBV) seropositive kidney transplant recipients

General Dosage Range I.V.: *Adults:* Initial phase: 10 mg/kg/dose; maintenance phase: 5 mg/kg/dose

Dosage Forms

Injection, powder for reconstitution:

Nulojix®: 250 mg

belimumab (be LIM yoo mab)

U.S. Brand Names Benlysta®

Canadian Brand Names Benlysta®

Therapeutic Category Monoclonal Antibody

Use Treatment of autoantibody-positive (antinuclear antibody [ANA] and/or antidouble-stranded DNA [anti-ds-DNA]) active systemic lupus erythematosus (SLE) in addition to standard therapy

General Dosage Range I.V.: *Adults:* 10 mg/kg every 2 weeks for 3 doses; Maintenance: 10 mg/kg every 4 weeks

Dosage Forms

Injection, powder for reconstitution:

Benlysta®: 120 mg, 400 mg

belladonna alkaloids with phenobarbital *see* hyoscyamine, atropine, scopolamine, and phenobarbital *on page* 467

belladonna and opium (bel a DON a & OH pee um)

Medication Safety Issues

Sound-alike/look-alike issues:

B&O may be confused with beano®

High alert medication:

The Institute for Safe Medication Practices (ISMP) includes this medication among its list of drug classes which have a heightened risk of causing significant patient harm when used in error.

BEERS Criteria medication:

This drug may be potentially inappropriate for use in geriatric patients (Quality of evidence - moderate; Strength of recommendation - strong).

Synonyms B&O; opium and belladonna

Therapeutic Category Analgesic, Narcotic

Controlled Substance C-II

Use Relief of moderate-to-severe pain associated with ureteral spasms not responsive to nonopioid analgesics and to space intervals between injections of opiates

General Dosage Range Rectal: *Children >12 years and Adults:* 1 suppository 1-2 times/day (maximum: 4 doses/day)

Dosage Forms

Suppository: Belladonna extract 16.2 mg and opium 30 mg; belladonna extract 16.2 mg and opium 60 mg

Belviq® *see* lorcaserin *on page* 551

Benadryl® (Can) *see* diphenhydramine (systemic) *on page* 292

Benadryl-D® Allergy & Sinus [OTC] *see* diphenhydramine and phenylephrine *on page* 294

Benadryl-D® Children's Allergy & Sinus [OTC] *see* diphenhydramine and phenylephrine *on page* 294
Benadryl® Allergy [OTC] *see* diphenhydramine (systemic) *on page* 292
Benadryl® Allergy and Cold [OTC] *see* acetaminophen, diphenhydramine, and phenylephrine *on page* 29
Benadryl® Allergy and Sinus Headache [OTC] *see* acetaminophen, diphenhydramine, and phenylephrine *on page* 29
Benadryl® Allergy Quick Dissolve [OTC] *see* diphenhydramine (systemic) *on page* 292
Benadryl® Children's Allergy [OTC] *see* diphenhydramine (systemic) *on page* 292
Benadryl® Children's Allergy FastMelt® [OTC] *see* diphenhydramine (systemic) *on page* 292
Benadryl® Children's Allergy Perfect Measure™ [OTC] *see* diphenhydramine (systemic) *on page* 292
Benadryl® Children's Dye Free Allergy [OTC] *see* diphenhydramine (systemic) *on page* 292
Benadryl® Cream (Can) *see* diphenhydramine (topical) *on page* 293
Benadryl® Dye-Free Allergy [OTC] *see* diphenhydramine (systemic) *on page* 292
Benadryl® Extra Strength Itch Stopping [OTC] *see* diphenhydramine (topical) *on page* 293
Benadryl® Itch Relief Extra Strength [OTC] *see* diphenhydramine (topical) *on page* 293
Benadryl® Itch Relief Stick (Can) *see* diphenhydramine (topical) *on page* 293
Benadryl® Itch Stopping [OTC] *see* diphenhydramine (topical) *on page* 293
Benadryl® Itch Stopping Extra Strength [OTC] *see* diphenhydramine (topical) *on page* 293
Benadryl® Spray (Can) *see* diphenhydramine (topical) *on page* 293
Benadry® Maximum Strength Severe Allergy and Sinus Headache [OTC] *see* acetaminophen, diphenhydramine, and phenylephrine *on page* 29

benazepril (ben AY ze pril)

Medication Safety Issues

Sound-alike/look-alike issues:

Benazepril may be confused with Benadryl®
Lotensin® may be confused with Lioresal®, lovastatin

Synonyms benazepril hydrochloride

U.S. Brand Names Lotensin®

Canadian Brand Names Lotensin®

Therapeutic Category Angiotensin-Converting Enzyme (ACE) Inhibitor

Use Treatment of hypertension, either alone or in combination with other antihypertensive agents

General Dosage Range Dosage adjustment recommended in patients with renal impairment

Oral:

Children ≥6 years: Initial: 0.2 mg/kg/day (up to 10 mg/day); Maintenance: 0.1-0.6 mg/kg/day (maximum: 40 mg/day)
Adults: Initial: 5-10 mg/day; Maintenance: 20-80 mg/day in 1-2 divided doses

Dosage Forms

Tablet, oral: 5 mg, 10 mg, 20 mg, 40 mg
Lotensin®: 10 mg, 20 mg, 40 mg

benazepril and hydrochlorothiazide (ben AY ze pril & hye droe klor oh THYE a zide)

Synonyms benazepril hydrochloride and hydrochlorothiazide; hydrochlorothiazide and benazepril

U.S. Brand Names Lotensin HCT®

Therapeutic Category Antihypertensive Agent, Combination

Use Treatment of hypertension

General Dosage Range Oral: *Adults:* Benazepril 5-20 mg and hydrochlorothiazide 6.25-25 mg daily

Dosage Forms

Tablet:

Generics:
5/6.25: Benazepril 5 mg and hydrochlorothiazide 6.25 mg
10/12.5: Benazepril 10 mg and hydrochlorothiazide 12.5 mg
20/12.5: Benazepril 20 mg and hydrochlorothiazide 12.5 mg
20/25: Benazepril 20 mg and hydrochlorothiazide 25 mg

Brands:
Lotensin HCT® 10/12.5: Benazepril 10 mg and hydrochlorothiazide 12.5 mg
Lotensin HCT® 20/12.5: Benazepril 20 mg and hydrochlorothiazide 12.5 mg
Lotensin HCT® 20/25: Benazepril 20 mg and hydrochlorothiazide 25 mg

benazepril hydrochloride *see* benazepril *on page* *119*
benazepril hydrochloride and amlodipine besylate *see* amlodipine and benazepril *on page* *66*
benazepril hydrochloride and hydrochlorothiazide *see* benazepril and hydrochlorothiazide *on page* *119*

bendamustine (ben da MUS teen)

Medication Safety Issues
Sound-alike/look-alike issues:
Bendamustine may be confused with brentuximab, carmustine, lomustine
High alert medication:
This medication is in a class the Institute for Safe Medication Practices (ISMP) includes among its list of drug classes which have a heightened risk of causing significant patient harm when used in error.

Synonyms bendamustine hydrochloride; cytostasan; SDX-105
U.S. Brand Names Treanda®
Canadian Brand Names Treanda®
Therapeutic Category Antineoplastic Agent, Alkylating Agent
Use Treatment of chronic lymphocytic leukemia (CLL); treatment of progressed indolent B-cell non-Hodgkin lymphoma (NHL)
General Dosage Range Dosage adjustment recommended in patients who develop toxicities
I.V.: *Adults:* 100 mg/m^2 on days 1 and 2 of a 28-day treatment cycle **or** 120 mg/m^2 on days 1 and 2 of a 21-day treatment cycle
Dosage Forms
Injection, powder for reconstitution:
Treanda®: 25 mg, 100 mg

bendamustine hydrochloride *see* bendamustine *on page* *120*
bendroflumethiazide and nadolol *see* nadolol and bendroflumethiazide *on page* *624*
Benefiber® [OTC] *see* wheat dextrin *on page* *955*
Benefiber® Plus Calcium [OTC] *see* wheat dextrin *on page* *955*
BeneFix® *see* factor IX *on page* *371*
Benemid [DSC] *see* probenecid *on page* *758*
benflumetol and artemether *see* artemether and lumefantrine *on page* *92*
BenGay® [OTC] *see* methyl salicylate and menthol *on page* *592*
Benicar® *see* olmesartan *on page* *662*
Benicar HCT® *see* olmesartan and hydrochlorothiazide *on page* *663*
Benlysta® *see* belimumab *on page* *118*
Benoxyl® (Can) *see* benzoyl peroxide *on page* *124*

benserazide and levodopa *(Canada only)* (ben SER a zide & lee voe DOE pa)

Synonyms levodopa and benserazide
Canadian Brand Names Prolopa®
Therapeutic Category Anti-Parkinson Agent (Dopamine Agonist)
Use Treatment of Parkinson disease (except drug-induced parkinsonism)
General Dosage Range **Oral:** *Adults:* Initial: Levodopa 100 mg/benserazide 25 mg 1-2 times/day; Maintenance: Levodopa 400-800 mg/benserazide 100-200 mg daily in 4-6 divided doses (maximum during first year of treatment: Levodopa/benserazide 1200/300 mg/day)
Product Availability Not available in U.S.
Dosage Forms - Canada
Capsule:
Prolopa®: 50-12.5: Levodopa 50 mg and benserazide 12.5 mg; 100-25: Levodopa 100 mg and benserazide 25 mg; 200-50: Levodopa 200 mg and benserazide 50 mg

bentoquatam (BEN toe kwa tam)

Synonyms quaternium-18 bentonite

U.S. Brand Names Ivy Block® [OTC]

Therapeutic Category Protectant, Topical

Use Skin protectant for the prevention of allergic contact dermatitis to poison oak, ivy, and sumac

General Dosage Range Topical: *Children >6 years and Adults:* Apply to skin 15 minutes prior to potential exposure to poison ivy, poison oak, or poison sumac, and reapply every 4 hours

Dosage Forms

Lotion, topical:

Ivy Block® [OTC]: 5% (120 mL)

Bentyl® *see* dicyclomine *on page* 282
Bentylol® (Can) *see* dicyclomine *on page* 282
Benuryl™ (Can) *see* probenecid *on page* 758
Benylin® 3.3 mg-D-E (Can) *see* guaifenesin, pseudoephedrine, and codeine *on page* 437
Benylin® D for Infants (Can) *see* pseudoephedrine *on page* 771
Benylin® DM-D (Can) *see* pseudoephedrine and dextromethorphan *on page* 772
Benylin® DM-D-E (Can) *see* guaifenesin, pseudoephedrine, and dextromethorphan *on page* 437
Benylin® DM-E (Can) *see* guaifenesin and dextromethorphan *on page* 434
Benylin® E Extra Strength (Can) *see* guaifenesin *on page* 433
Benzac AC® (Can) *see* benzoyl peroxide *on page* 124
BenzaClin® *see* clindamycin and benzoyl peroxide *on page* 219
Benzac W® Gel (Can) *see* benzoyl peroxide *on page* 124
Benzac W® Wash (Can) *see* benzoyl peroxide *on page* 124
Benzamycin® *see* erythromycin and benzoyl peroxide *on page* 344
Benzamycin® Pak *see* erythromycin and benzoyl peroxide *on page* 344
benzathine benzylpenicillin *see* penicillin G benzathine *on page* 702
benzathine penicillin G *see* penicillin G benzathine *on page* 702
Benzedrex® [OTC] *see* propylhexedrine *on page* 768
BenzEFoam™ *see* benzoyl peroxide *on page* 124
BenzEFoam Ultra™ *see* benzoyl peroxide *on page* 124
benzene hexachloride *see* lindane *on page* 541
benzhexol hydrochloride *see* trihexyphenidyl *on page* 919
Benziq™ *see* benzoyl peroxide *on page* 124
benzmethyzin *see* procarbazine *on page* 760

benzocaine (BEN zoe kane)

Medication Safety Issues

Sound-alike/look-alike issues:

Orabase® may be confused with Orinase

Synonyms ethyl aminobenzoate

U.S. Brand Names Americaine® Hemorrhoidal [OTC]; Anbesol® Baby [OTC]; Anbesol® Cold Sore Therapy [OTC]; Anbesol® Jr. [OTC]; Anbesol® Maximum Strength [OTC]; Anbesol® [OTC]; Benzodent® [OTC]; Bi-Zets [OTC]; Boil-Ease® Pain Relieving [OTC]; Cepacol® Fizzlers™ [OTC]; Cepacol® Sore Throat & Coating [OTC]; Cepacol® Sore Throat Pain Relief [OTC] [DSC]; Cepacol® Sore Throat Plus Coating Relief [OTC]; Cepacol® Sore Throat [OTC]; Cepacol® Ultra Sore Throat [OTC]; Chiggerex® Plus [OTC]; ChiggerTox® [OTC]; Dent's Extra Strength Toothache Gum [OTC]; Dentapaine [OTC]; Dermoplast® Antibacterial [OTC]; Dermoplast® Pain Relieving [OTC]; Detane® [OTC]; Foille® [OTC]; HDA® Toothache [OTC]; HurriCaine ONE™; Hurricaine® [OTC]; Ivy-Rid® [OTC]; Kank-A® Soft Brush [OTC]; Lanacane® Maximum Strength [OTC]; Lanacane® [OTC]; Little Teethers® [OTC]; Medicone® Hemorrhoidal [OTC]; Mycinettes® [OTC]; Orabase® with Benzocaine [OTC]; Orajel® Baby Daytime and Nighttime [OTC]; Orajel® Baby Teething Nighttime [OTC]; Orajel® Baby Teething [OTC]; Orajel® Cold Sore [OTC]; Orajel® Denture Plus [OTC]; Orajel® Maximum Strength [OTC]; Orajel® Medicated Mouth Sore [OTC]; Orajel® Medicated Toothache [OTC]; Orajel® Mouth Sore [OTC]; Orajel® Multi-Action Cold Sore [OTC]; Orajel® PM Maximum Strength [OTC]; Orajel® Ultra Mouth Sore [OTC]; Orajel® [OTC]; Outgro® [OTC]; Red Cross™ Canker Sore [OTC]; Rid-A-Pain Dental [OTC]; Sepasoothe® [OTC]; Skeeter Stik® [OTC]; Sore Throat Relief [OTC]; Sting-Kill® [OTC]; Tanac® [OTC]; Thorets [OTC]; Trocaine® [OTC]; Zilactin® Tooth & Gum Pain [OTC]; Zilactin®-B [OTC]

Canadian Brand Names Anbesol® Baby; Zilactin Baby®; Zilactin-B®

Therapeutic Category Local Anesthetic

Use Temporary relief of pain associated with pruritic dermatosis, pruritus, minor burns, acute congestive, bee stings, and insect bites; mouth and gum irritations (toothache, minor sore throat pain, canker sores, dentures, orthodontia, teething, mucositis, stomatitis); sunburn; hemorrhoids; anesthetic lubricant for passage of catheters and endoscopic tubes

General Dosage Range

Oral: *Children ≥5 years and Adults:* 1 lozenge (10-15 mg) every 2 hours as needed

Rectal: *Children ≥12 years and Adults:* Apply externally to affected area up to 6 times/day

Topical: *Children ≥2 years and Adults:* Apply to affected area 3-4 times/day as needed

Topical (oral): *Children ≥4 months and Adults:* Apply thin layer to affected area up to 4 times/day

Topical (oral) spray: Children ≥6 years and Adults: Apply 1 spray to affected area up to 4 times/day

Dosage Forms

Aerosol, spray, oral:
Hurricaine® [OTC]: 20% (60 mL)

Aerosol, spray, topical:
Dermoplast® Antibacterial [OTC]: 20% (82.5 mL)
Dermoplast® Pain Relieving [OTC]: 20% (60 mL, 82.5 mL)
Ivy-Rid® [OTC]: 2% (85 g)
Lanacane® Maximum Strength [OTC]: 20% (120 mL)

Combination package, oral:
Orajel® Baby Daytime and Nighttime [OTC]: gel, oral (Daytime Regular formula): benzocaine 7.5% (5.3 g) [1 tube] and gel, oral (Nighttime formula): benzocaine 10% (5.3 g) [1 tube]

Cream, oral:
Benzodent® [OTC]: 20% (7.5 g, 30 g)
Orajel® PM Maximum Strength [OTC]: 20% (5.3 g, 7 g)

Cream, topical:
Lanacane® [OTC]: 6% (28 g, 60 g)
Lanacane® Maximum Strength [OTC]: 20% (28 g)

Gel, oral: 20% (15 g)
Anbesol® [OTC]: 10% (7.1 g)
Anbesol® Baby [OTC]: 7.5% (7.1 g)
Anbesol® Jr. [OTC]: 10% (7.1 g)
Anbesol® Maximum Strength [OTC]: 20% (7.1 g, 10 g)
Dentapaine [OTC]: 20% (11 g)
HDA® Toothache [OTC]: 6.5% (15 mL)
Hurricaine® [OTC]: 20% (30 g); 20% (5.25 g, 30 g)
Kank-A® Soft Brush [OTC]: 20% (2 g)
Little Teethers® [OTC]: 7.5% (9.4 g)
Orabase® with Benzocaine [OTC]: 20% (7 g)
Orajel® [OTC]: 10% (5.3 g, 7 g, 9.4 g)
Orajel® Baby Teething [OTC]: 7.5% (11.9 g); 7.5% (9.4 g)
Orajel® Baby Teething Nighttime [OTC]: 10% (5.3 g)
Orajel® Denture Plus [OTC]: 15% (9 g)
Orajel® Maximum Strength [OTC]: 20% (5.4 g, 7 g, 9.4 g, 11.9 g)
Orajel® Mouth Sore [OTC]: 20% (5.3 g, 9.4 g, 11.9 g)
Orajel® Multi-Action Cold Sore [OTC]: 20% (9.4 g)
Orajel® Ultra Mouth Sore [OTC]: 15% (9.4 g)
Zilactin®-B [OTC]: 10% (7.5 g)

Gel, topical:
Detane® [OTC]: 7.5% (15 g)

Liquid, oral: 20% (15 mL)
Anbesol® [OTC]: 10% (9.3 mL)
Anbesol® Maximum Strength [OTC]: 20% (9.3 mL)
Cepacol® Ultra Sore Throat [OTC]: 5% (22.2 mL)
HurriCaine ONE™: 20% (0.5 mL)
Hurricaine® [OTC]: 20% (30 mL)
Orajel® Baby Teething [OTC]: 7.5% (13.3 mL)
Orajel® Maximum Strength [OTC]: 20% (13.5 mL)
Rid-A-Pain Dental [OTC]: 6.3% (30 mL)
Tanac® [OTC]: 10% (13 mL)

Liquid, topical:
ChiggerTox® [OTC]: 2% (30 mL)
Outgro® [OTC]: 20% (9.3 mL)
Skeeter Stik® [OTC]: 5% (14 mL)
Lozenge, oral:
Bi-Zets [OTC]: 15 mg (10s)
Cepacol® Sore Throat [OTC]: 15 mg (16s)
Cepacol® Sore Throat & Coating [OTC]: 15 mg (16s)
Cepacol® Sore Throat Plus Coating Relief [OTC]: 15 mg (18s)
Mycinettes® [OTC]: 15 mg (12s)
Sepasoothe® [OTC]: 10 mg (6s, 24s, 100s, 250s, 500s)
Sore Throat Relief [OTC]: 10 mg (100s, 250s, 500s)
Thorets [OTC]: 18 mg (300s)
Trocaine® [OTC]: 10 mg (50s, 300s)
Ointment, oral:
Anbesol® Cold Sore Therapy [OTC]: 20% (7.1 g)
Red Cross™ Canker Sore [OTC]: 20% (7.5 g)
Ointment, rectal:
Americaine® Hemorrhoidal [OTC]: 20% (30 g)
Medicone® Hemorrhoidal [OTC]: 20% (28.4 g)
Ointment, topical:
Boil-Ease® Pain Relieving [OTC]: 20% (30 g)
Chiggerex® Plus [OTC]: 6% (50 g)
Foille® [OTC]: 5% (3.5 g, 14 g, 28 g)
Pad, topical:
Sting-Kill® [OTC]: 20% (8s)
Paste, oral:
Orabase® with Benzocaine [OTC]: 20% (6 g)
Swab, oral:
Hurricaine® [OTC]: 20% (8s, 72s)
Orajel® Baby Teething [OTC]: 7.5% (12s)
Orajel® Cold Sore [OTC]: 20% (12s)
Orajel® Medicated Mouth Sore [OTC]: 20% (8s, 12s)
Orajel® Medicated Toothache [OTC]: 20% (8s, 12s)
Zilactin® Tooth & Gum Pain [OTC]: 20% (8s)
Swab, topical:
Boil-Ease® Pain Relieving [OTC]: 20% (12s)
Sting-Kill® [OTC]: 20% (5s)
Tablet, orally dissolving, oral:
Cepacol® Fizzlers™ [OTC]: 6 mg (12s)
Wax, oral:
Dent's Extra Strength Toothache Gum [OTC]: 20% (1 g)

benzocaine and antipyrine *see* antipyrine and benzocaine *on page 79*

benzocaine, butamben, and tetracaine (BEN zoe kane, byoo TAM ben, & TET ra kane)

Synonyms benzocaine, butamben, and tetracaine hydrochloride; benzocaine, butyl aminobenzoate, and tetracaine; butamben, tetracaine, and benzocaine; tetracaine, benzocaine, and butamben

U.S. Brand Names Cetacaine®; Exactacain®

Therapeutic Category Local Anesthetic

Use Topical anesthetic to control pain in surgical or endoscopic procedures; anesthetic for accessible mucous membranes except for the eyes

General Dosage Range Topical: *Adults:*
Cetacaine®: Aerosol: Apply for ≤1 second (maximum: 2 seconds); Gel: Apply ~1/2" (13 mm) x 3/16" (5 mm) (maximum: 1" [26 cm] x 3/16" [5 mm]); Liquid: Apply 6-7 drops (0.2 mL) (maximum: 12 drops)
Exactacain™: 3 metered sprays (maximum: 6 metered sprays)

Dosage Forms
Aerosol, spray, topical [kit]:
Cetacaine®: Benzocaine 14%, butamben 2%, and tetracaine 2% (56 g)
Aerosol, spray, topical:
Cetacaine®: Benzocaine 14%, butamben 2%, and tetracaine 2% (56 g)
Exactacain®: Benzocaine 14%, butamben 2%, and tetracaine 2% (60 g)

Gel, topical:
Cetacaine®: Benzocaine 14%, butamben 2%, and tetracaine 2% (32 g)
Liquid, topical, kit:
Cetacaine®: Benzocaine 14%, butamben 2%, and tetracaine 2% (14 g)
Liquid, topical:
Cetacaine®: Benzocaine 14%, butamben 2%, and tetracaine 2% (14 g, 30 g)

benzocaine, butamben, and tetracaine hydrochloride *see* benzocaine, butamben, and tetracaine *on page 123*

benzocaine, butyl aminobenzoate, and tetracaine *see* benzocaine, butamben, and tetracaine *on page 123*

Benzodent® [OTC] *see* benzocaine *on page 121*

benzoic acid, hyoscyamine, methenamine, methylene blue, and phenyl salicylate *see* methenamine, phenyl salicylate, methylene blue, benzoic acid, and hyoscyamine *on page 583*

benzoic acid, methenamine, methylene blue, phenyl salicylate, and hyoscyamine *see* methenamine, phenyl salicylate, methylene blue, benzoic acid, and hyoscyamine *on page 583*

benzoin (BEN zoin)

Synonyms gum benjamin

U.S. Brand Names Benz-Protect Swabs™ [OTC]; Sprayzoin™ [OTC]

Therapeutic Category Pharmaceutical Aid; Protectant, Topical

Use Protective application for irritations of the skin; sometimes used in boiling water as steam inhalants for its expectorant and soothing action

General Dosage Range Topical: *Children and Adults:* Apply 1-2 times/day

Dosage Forms

Tincture, topical: Benzoin Compound USP: Benzoin 10% (30 mL, 59 mL, 60 mL, 120 mL, 473 mL); Benzoin NFXI (59 mL)
Benz-Protect Swabs™: Benzoin Compound USP: Benzoin 10% (3 mL)
Tincture, topical [spray]:
Sprayzoin™: Benzoin Compound USP: Benzoin 10% (120 mL)

benzonatate (ben ZOE na tate)

Synonyms tessalon perles

U.S. Brand Names Tessalon®; Zonatuss™

Therapeutic Category Antitussive

Use Symptomatic relief of nonproductive cough

General Dosage Range Oral: *Children >10 years and Adults:* 100-200 mg 3 times/day as needed (maximum: 600 mg/day)

Dosage Forms

Capsule, oral:
Zonatuss™: 150 mg
Capsule, softgel, oral: 100 mg, 200 mg
Tessalon®: 100 mg, 200 mg

benzoyl peroxide (BEN zoe il peer OKS ide)

Medication Safety Issues

Sound-alike/look-alike issues:
Benzoyl peroxide may be confused with benzyl alcohol
Benoxyl® may be confused with Brevoxyl®, Peroxyl®
Benzac® may be confused with Benza®
Brevoxyl® may be confused with Benoxyl®
Fostex® may be confused with pHisoHex®

U.S. Brand Names Acne Clear Maximum Strength [OTC]; BenzEFoam Ultra™; BenzEFoam™; Benziq™; BP Cleanser [OTC]; BP Cleansing Lotion [OTC]; BP Wash [OTC]; BPO; Clean & Clear® advantage® 3-in-1 [OTC]; Clean & Clear® continuous control® [OTC]; Clean & Clear® persa-gel® 10 [OTC]; Clearskin [OTC]; Desquam-X® 10 [OTC]; Desquam-X® 5 [OTC]; Inova®; Neutrogena® On The Spot® Acne Treatment [OTC]; OXY® Clinical Clearing Treatment [OTC]; OXY® Maximum Face Wash [OTC]; OXY® Maximum Spot Treatment [OTC]; Pacnex®; Pacnex® HP; Pacnex® LP; Pacnex® MX; PanOxyl® Bar [OTC]; PanOxyl® [OTC]; PanOxyl®-4 [OTC]; PanOxyl®-8 [OTC]; PR™ Wash; SE BPO; TL BPO MX; Zapzyt® [OTC]

Canadian Brand Names Acetoxyl®; Benoxyl®; Benzac AC®; Benzac W® Gel; Benzac W® Wash; Desquam-X®; Oxyderm™; PanOxyl®; Solugel®

Therapeutic Category Acne Products

Use Treatment of mild-to-moderate acne vulgaris and acne rosacea

General Dosage Range Topical: *Children ≥12 years, Adolescents, and Adults:*

Cleanser: Wash once or twice daily

Topical formulations: Apply sparingly once daily; gradually increase to 2-3 times/day if needed

Dosage Forms

Aerosol, foam, topical:
- BenzEFoam Ultra™: 9.8% (100 g)
- BenzEFoam™: 5.3% (60 g, 100 g)

Bar, topical:
- PanOxyl® Bar [OTC]: 10% (113 g)

Cloth, topical:
- BPO: 3% (60s); 6% (60s); 9% (60s)

Cream, topical:
- Clean & Clear® continuous control® [OTC]: 10% (141 g)
- Clearskin [OTC]: 10% (28 g)
- Neutrogena® On The Spot® Acne Treatment [OTC]: 2.5% (21 g)
- OXY® Maximum Spot Treatment [OTC]: 10% (18.4 g)

Gel, topical: 2.5% (60 g); 5% (42.5 g, 60 g, 90 g, 150 g, 240 g); 10% (42.5 g, 60 g, 90 g, 150 g, 240 g)
- Acne Clear Maximum Strength [OTC]: 10% (42.5 g)
- Benziq™: 5.25% (50 g)
- BPO: 4% (42.5 g); 8% (42.5 g)
- Clean & Clear® persa-gel® 10 [OTC]: 10% (28 g)
- Zapzyt® [OTC]: 10% (28 g)

Liquid, topical: 5% (148 g, 237 g); 10% (148 g, 237 g)
- Benziq™: 5.25% (175 g)
- BP Cleanser [OTC]: 4.25% (480 g)
- BP Wash [OTC]: 5.25% (175 g)
- Desquam-X® 5 [OTC]: 5% (140 g)
- Desquam-X® 10 [OTC]: 10% (140 g)
- OXY® Maximum Face Wash [OTC]: 10% (177 mL)
- Pacnex®: 7% (480 mL)
- Pacnex® MX: 4.25% (480 g)
- PanOxyl®-4 [OTC]: 4% (170 g)
- PanOxyl®-8 [OTC]: 8% (170 g)
- PanOxyl® [OTC]: 10% (156 g)
- SE BPO: 7% (180 g)
- TL BPO MX: 4.25% (480 g)

Lotion, topical: 5% (30 mL); 10% (30 mL); 6% (170 g, 355 g)
- BP Cleansing Lotion [OTC]: 4% (297 g)
- Clean & Clear® advantage® 3-in-1 [OTC]: 5% (141 g)
- OXY® Clinical Clearing Treatment [OTC]: 5% (35.4 g)
- PR™ Wash: 7% (473 mL)

Pad, topical:
- Inova®: 4% (30s); 8% (30s)
- Pacnex® HP: 7% (60s)
- Pacnex® LP: 4.25% (60s)

benzoyl peroxide and adapalene *see* adapalene and benzoyl peroxide *on page 36*
benzoyl peroxide and clindamycin *see* clindamycin and benzoyl peroxide *on page 219*
benzoyl peroxide and erythromycin *see* erythromycin and benzoyl peroxide *on page 344*

benzoyl peroxide and hydrocortisone (BEN zoe il peer OKS ide & hye droe KOR ti sone)

Synonyms hydrocortisone and benzoyl peroxide

U.S. Brand Names Vanoxide-HC®

Canadian Brand Names Vanoxide-HC®

Therapeutic Category Acne Products

Use Treatment of acne vulgaris and oily skin

General Dosage Range Topical: *Adolescents ≥12 years and Adults:* Apply thin film 1-3 times/day

Dosage Forms

Lotion, topical:

Vanoxide-HC®: Benzoyl peroxide 5% and hydrocortisone 0.5% (25 mL)

Lotion, topical [kit]:

Vanoxide-HC®: Benzoyl peroxide 5% and hydrocortisone 0.5% (25 g) packaged with cleanser

benzphetamine (benz FET a meen)

Synonyms benzphetamine hydrochloride

U.S. Brand Names Didrex®

Therapeutic Category Anorexiant

Controlled Substance C-III

Use Short-term (few weeks) adjunct to caloric restriction in exogenous obesity

Pharmacotherapy for weight loss is recommended only for obese patients with a body mass index ≥30 kg/m^2, or ≥27 kg/m^2 in the presence of other risk factors such as hypertension, diabetes, and/or dyslipidemia or a high waist circumference; therapy should be used in conjunction with a comprehensive weight management program.

General Dosage Range Oral: *Children ≥12 years and Adults:* Initial: 25-50 mg once daily; Maintenance: 25-50 mg 1-3 times/day (maximum: 150 mg/day)

Dosage Forms

Tablet, oral: 50 mg

Didrex®: 50 mg

benzphetamine hydrochloride *see* benzphetamine *on page 126*

Benz-Protect Swabs™ [OTC] *see* benzoin *on page 124*

benztropine (BENZ troe peen)

Medication Safety Issues

Sound-alike/look-alike issues:

Benztropine may be confused with bromocriptine

BEERS Criteria medication:

This drug may be potentially inappropriate for use in geriatric patients (Parkinson's disease: Quality of evidence - moderate; Strength of recommendation - strong).

Synonyms benztropine mesylate

U.S. Brand Names Cogentin®

Canadian Brand Names Apo-Benztropine®; Benztropine Omega; PMS-Benztropine

Therapeutic Category Anti-Parkinson Agent; Anticholinergic Agent

Use Adjunctive treatment of Parkinson disease; treatment of drug-induced extrapyramidal symptoms (except tardive dyskinesia)

General Dosage Range I.M., I.V., Oral: *Adults:* Range: 0.5-8 mg/day

Dosage Forms

Injection, solution: 1 mg/mL

Cogentin®: 1 mg/mL

Tablet, oral: 0.5 mg, 1 mg, 2 mg

benztropine mesylate *see* benztropine *on page 126*

Benztropine Omega (Can) *see* benztropine *on page 126*

benzydamine *(Canada only)* (ben ZID a meen)

Synonyms benzydamine hydrochloride

Canadian Brand Names Apo-Benzydamine®; Dom-Benzydamine; Novo-Benzydamine; PMS-Benzydamine; Tantum®

Therapeutic Category Analgesic, Topical

Use Symptomatic treatment of pain associated with acute pharyngitis; treatment of pain associated with radiation-induced oropharyngeal mucositis

General Dosage Range Oral rinse: *Adults:* Gargle with 15 mL every 1½-3 hours until symptoms resolve **or** 3-4 times/day

Product Availability Not available in U.S.

Dosage Forms - Canada

Oral rinse: 0.15% (100 mL, 250 mL)

benzydamine hydrochloride *see* benzydamine *(Canada only) on page 126*

benzyl alcohol (BEN zill AL koe hol)

Medication Safety Issues

Sound-alike/look-alike issues:

Benzyl alcohol may be confused with benzoyl peroxide

U.S. Brand Names Ulesfia®; Zilactin®-L [OTC]

Therapeutic Category Antiparasitic Agent, Topical; Pediculocide

Use

Liquid (Zilactin®-L): Temporary relief of pain from cold sores/fever blisters

Lotion (Ulesfia™): Treatment of head lice infestation

General Dosage Range Topical:

Liquid: *Children ≥2 years and Adults:* Apply to affected area up to 4 times/day

Lotion: *Children ≥6 months and Adults:* 4-48 ounces per application based upon hair length; repeat in 7 days

Dosage Forms

Liquid, topical:

Zilactin®-L [OTC]: 10% (5.9 mL)

Lotion, topical:

Ulesfia®: 5% (227 g)

benzylpenicillin benzathine *see* penicillin G benzathine *on page 702*

benzylpenicillin potassium *see* penicillin G (parenteral/aqueous) *on page 703*

benzylpenicillin sodium *see* penicillin G (parenteral/aqueous) *on page 703*

benzylpenicilloyl polylysine (BEN zil pen i SIL oyl pol i LIE seen)

Synonyms benzylpenicilloyl-polylysine; penicilloyl-polylysine; PPL

U.S. Brand Names Pre-Pen®

Therapeutic Category Diagnostic Agent

Use Adjunct in assessing the risk of administering penicillin (penicillin G or benzylpenicillin) in patients suspected of clinical penicillin hypersensitivity

General Dosage Range

Intradermal: *Children and Adults:* Inject a volume of skin test solution sufficient to raise a small intradermal bleb ~3 mm in diameter, in duplicate

Puncture test (first step): *Children and Adults:* Apply a small drop of solution to make a single shallow puncture of the epidermis

Dosage Forms

Injection, solution:

Pre-Pen®: 6 x 10^{-5} M (0.25 mL)

benzylpenicilloyl-polylysine *see* benzylpenicilloyl polylysine *on page 127*

bepotastine (be poe TAS teen)

Synonyms bepotastine besilate

U.S. Brand Names Bepreve®

Therapeutic Category Histamine H_1 Antagonist; Histamine H_1 Antagonist, Second Generation; Mast Cell Stabilizer

Use Treatment of itching associated with allergic conjunctivitis

General Dosage Range Ophthalmic: *Children ≥2 years and Adults:* Instill 1 drop into the affected eye(s) twice daily

Dosage Forms

Solution, ophthalmic:

Bepreve®: 1.5% (5 mL, 10 mL)

bepotastine besilate *see* bepotastine *on page 127*

Bepreve® *see* bepotastine *on page 127*

beractant (ber AKT ant)

Medication Safety Issues

Sound-alike/look-alike issues:

Survanta® may be confused with Sufenta®

Synonyms bovine lung surfactant; natural lung surfactant

U.S. Brand Names Survanta®

Canadian Brand Names Survanta®

Therapeutic Category Lung Surfactant

Use Prevention and treatment of respiratory distress syndrome (RDS) in premature infants

Prophylactic therapy: Body weight <1250 g in infants at risk for developing, or with evidence of, surfactant deficiency (administer within 15 minutes of birth)

Rescue therapy: Treatment of infants with RDS confirmed by x-ray and requiring mechanical ventilation (administer as soon as possible - within 8 hours of age)

General Dosage Range Endotracheal: *Premature infants:* Administer 4 mL/kg (100 mg phospholipids/kg); may repeat if needed, no more frequently than every 6 hours to a maximum of 4 doses/48 hours

Dosage Forms

Suspension, intratracheal [preservative free]:

Survanta®: Phospholipids 25 mg/mL (4 mL, 8 mL)

Berinert® *see* C1 inhibitor (human) *on page 156*

besifloxacin (be si FLOX a sin)

Synonyms besifloxacin hydrochloride; BOL-303224-A; SS734

U.S. Brand Names Besivance™

Therapeutic Category Antibiotic, Ophthalmic; Antibiotic, Quinolone

Use Treatment of bacterial conjunctivitis

General Dosage Range Ophthalmic: *Children ≥1 year and Adults:* 1 drop into affected eye(s) 3 times/day (4-12 hours apart)

Dosage Forms

Suspension, ophthalmic:

Besivance™: 0.6% (5 mL)

besifloxacin hydrochloride *see* besifloxacin *on page 128*

Besivance™ *see* besifloxacin *on page 128*

β,β-dimethylcysteine *see* penicillamine *on page 701*

Betacaine® (Can) *see* lidocaine (topical) *on page 535*

beta-carotene (BAY ta KARE oh teen)

U.S. Brand Names A-Caro-25 [OTC]; B-Caro-T™ [OTC]; Lumitene™ [OTC]

Therapeutic Category Vitamin, Fat Soluble

Use Prophylaxis against photosensitivity reactions in erythropoietic protoporphyria (EPP)

General Dosage Range Oral:

Children <14 years: 30-150 mg/day

Adults: 30-300 mg/day

Dosage Forms

Capsule, oral:

Lumitene™ [OTC]: 50,000 units

Capsule, softgel, oral: 25,000 units

A-Caro-25 [OTC]: 25,000 units

B-Caro-T™ [OTC]: 25,000 units

Tablet, oral: 10,000 units

Betaderm (Can) *see* betamethasone *on page 129*

Betadine® *see* povidone-iodine (ophthalmic) *on page 747*

Betadine® [OTC] *see* povidone-iodine (topical) *on page 747*

Betadine® (Can) *see* povidone-iodine (topical) *on page 747*

Betadine® Swab Aids [OTC] *see* povidone-iodine (topical) *on page 747*

9-beta-d-ribofuranosyladenine *see* adenosine *on page 37*

Betagan® *see* levobunolol *on page 529*
Beta-HC® [OTC] *see* hydrocortisone (topical) *on page 457*

betahistine *(Canada only)* (bay ta HISS teen)

Synonyms betahistine dihydrochloride
Canadian Brand Names CO Betahistine; Novo-Betahistine; Serc®
Therapeutic Category Antihistamine
Use Treatment of Ménière disease (to decrease episodes of vertigo)
General Dosage Range Oral: *Adults:* 8-16 mg 3 times/day or 24 mg twice daily
Product Availability Not available in U.S.
Dosage Forms - Canada
Tablet, oral:
Novo-Betahistine: 8 mg, 16 mg, 24 mg
Serc®: 16 mg, 24 mg

betahistine dihydrochloride *see* betahistine *(Canada only) on page 129*

betaine (BAY ta een)

Medication Safety Issues
Sound-alike/look-alike issues:
Betaine may be confused with Betadine®
Cystadane® may be confused with cysteamine, cysteine
Synonyms betaine anhydrous
U.S. Brand Names Cystadane®
Canadian Brand Names Cystadane®
Therapeutic Category Homocystinuria Agent
Use Treatment of homocystinuria (eg, deficiencies or defects in cystathionine beta-synthase [CBS], 5,10-methylene tetrahydrofolate reductase [MTHFR], and cobalamin cofactor metabolism [CBL])
General Dosage Range Oral:
Children <3 years: Initial: 100 mg/kg/day, then increase weekly by 50 mg/kg increments, as needed
Children ≥3 years and Adults: 3 g twice daily (maximum: 20 g/day)
Dosage Forms
Powder for solution, oral:
Cystadane®: 1 g/scoop (180 g)

betaine anhydrous *see* betaine *on page 129*
Betaject™ (Can) *see* betamethasone *on page 129*
Betaloc® (Can) *see* metoprolol *on page 595*
BetaMed™ [OTC] *see* pyrithione zinc *on page 779*

betamethasone (bay ta METH a sone)

Medication Safety Issues
Sound-alike/look-alike issues:
Luxiq® may be confused with Lasix®
International issues:
Beta-Val [U.S.] may be confused with Betanol brand name for metipranolol [Monaco]
Synonyms betamethasone dipropionate; betamethasone dipropionate, augmented; betamethasone sodium phosphate; betamethasone valerate; flubenisolone
U.S. Brand Names Celestone®; Celestone® Soluspan®; Diprolene®; Diprolene® AF; Luxiq®
Canadian Brand Names Betaderm; Betaject™; Betnesol®; Betnovate®; Celestone® Soluspan®; Diprolene®; Diprolene® Glycol; Diprosone®; Ectosone; Prevex® B; ratio-Ectosone; Ratio-Topilene; ratio-Topilene; Ratio-Topisone; ratio-Topisone; Rivasone; Rolene; Rosone; Taro-Sone; Valisone® Scalp Lotion
Therapeutic Category Adrenal Corticosteroid; Corticosteroid, Topical
Use Inflammatory dermatoses such as seborrheic or atopic dermatitis, neurodermatitis, anogenital pruritus, psoriasis, inflammatory phase of xerosis
General Dosage Range
I.M.:
Children ≤12 years: 0.0175-0.125 mg base/kg/day **or** 0.5-7.5 mg base/m^2/day divided every 6-12 hours
Children ≥13 years and Adults: 0.6-9 mg/day divided every 12-24 hours

Intrabursal, intraarticular, intradermal: *Adults:* 0.25-2 mL
Intralesional: *Adults:* Very large joints: 1-2 mL; Large joints: 1 mL; Medium joints: 0.5-1 mL; Small joints: 0.25-0.5 mL
Oral:
Children ≤12 years: 0.0175-0.25 mg/kg/day **or** 0.5-7.5 mg/m^2/day divided every 6-8 hours
Children ≥13 years and Adults: 0.6-7.2 mg/day in 2-4 divided doses
Topical: *Children ≥13 years and Adults:* Apply once or twice daily (maximum: 45-50 g/week; 50 mL/week)

Dosage Forms
Aerosol, foam, topical:
Luxiq®: 0.12% (50 g, 100 g)
Cream, topical: 0.05% (15 g, 45 g, 50 g); 0.1% (15 g, 45 g)
Diprolene® AF: 0.05% (15 g, 50 g)
Gel, topical: 0.05% (15 g, 50 g)
Injection, suspension: Betamethasone sodium phosphate 3 mg and betamethasone acetate 3 mg per 1 mL (5 mL)
Celestone® Soluspan®: Betamethasone sodium phosphate 3 mg and betamethasone acetate 3 mg per 1 mL (5 mL)
Lotion, topical: 0.05% (30 mL, 60 mL); 0.1% (60 mL)
Diprolene®: 0.05% (30 mL, 60 mL)
Ointment, topical: 0.05% (15 g, 45 g, 50 g); 0.1% (15 g, 45 g)
Diprolene®: 0.05% (15 g, 50 g)
Solution, oral:
Celestone®: 0.6 mg/5 mL (118 mL)

betamethasone and clotrimazole (bay ta METH a sone & kloe TRIM a zole)

Medication Safety Issues
Sound-alike/look-alike issues:
Clotrimazole may be confused with co-trimoxazole
Lotrisone® may be confused with Lotrimin®

Synonyms clotrimazole and betamethasone
U.S. Brand Names Lotrisone®
Canadian Brand Names Lotriderm®
Therapeutic Category Antifungal/Corticosteroid
Use Topical treatment of various dermal fungal infections (including tinea pedis, cruris, and corpora in patients ≥17 years of age)
General Dosage Range Topical: *Adults:* Apply to affected area twice daily (maximum: 45 g cream/week; 45 mL lotion/week)

Dosage Forms
Cream: Betamethasone 0.05% and clotrimazole 1% (15 g, 45 g)
Lotrisone®: Betamethasone 0.05% and clotrimazole 1% (15 g, 45 g)
Lotion: Betamethasone 0.05% and clotrimazole 1% (30 mL)
Lotrisone®: Betamethasone 0.05% and clotrimazole 1% (30 mL)

betamethasone dipropionate *see* betamethasone *on page* 129
betamethasone dipropionate and calcipotriene hydrate *see* calcipotriene and betamethasone *on page* 159
betamethasone dipropionate, augmented *see* betamethasone *on page* 129
betamethasone sodium phosphate *see* betamethasone *on page* 129
betamethasone valerate *see* betamethasone *on page* 129
Betapace® *see* sotalol *on page* 851
Betapace AF® *see* sotalol *on page* 851
Beta Sal® [OTC] *see* salicylic acid *on page* 816
Betasept® [OTC] *see* chlorhexidine gluconate *on page* 196
Betaseron® *see* interferon beta-1b *on page* 492
Betatar Gel® [OTC] *see* coal tar *on page* 228
Betaxin® (Can) *see* thiamine *on page* 890

betaxolol (systemic) (be TAKS oh lol)

Medication Safety Issues

Sound-alike/look-alike issues:

Betaxolol may be confused with bethanechol, labetalol

Synonyms betaxolol hydrochloride

U.S. Brand Names Kerlone®

Therapeutic Category Beta-Blocker, Beta-1 Selective

Use Management of hypertension

General Dosage Range Dosage adjustment recommended in patients with renal impairment

Oral:

Adults: 5-20 mg/day

Elderly: Initial dose: 5 mg/day

Dosage Forms

Tablet, oral: 10 mg, 20 mg

Kerlone®: 10 mg, 20 mg

betaxolol (ophthalmic) (be TAKS oh lol)

Medication Safety Issues

Sound-alike/look-alike issues:

Betoptic® S may be confused with Betagan®, Timoptic®

Synonyms betaxolol hydrochloride

U.S. Brand Names Betoptic S®

Canadian Brand Names Betoptic® S; Sandoz-Betaxolol

Therapeutic Category Ophthalmic Agent, Antiglaucoma

Use Treatment of chronic open-angle glaucoma or ocular hypertension

General Dosage Range Ophthalmic:

Children: Suspension: Instill 1 drop twice daily

Adults:

Solution: Instill 1-2 drops twice daily

Suspension: Instill 1 drop twice daily

Dosage Forms

Solution, ophthalmic: 0.5% (5 mL, 10 mL, 15 mL)

Suspension, ophthalmic:

Betoptic S®: 0.25% (10 mL, 15 mL)

betaxolol hydrochloride *see* betaxolol (ophthalmic) *on page 131*

betaxolol hydrochloride *see* betaxolol (systemic) *on page 131*

bethanechol (be THAN e kole)

Medication Safety Issues

Sound-alike/look-alike issues:

Bethanechol may be confused with betaxolol

Synonyms bethanechol chloride

U.S. Brand Names Urecholine®

Canadian Brand Names Duvoid®; PHL-Bethanechol; PMS-Bethanechol

Therapeutic Category Cholinergic Agent

Use Treatment of acute postoperative and postpartum nonobstructive (functional) urinary retention; treatment of neurogenic atony of the urinary bladder with retention

General Dosage Range Oral: *Adults:* 10-100 mg 2-4 times/day

Dosage Forms

Tablet, oral: 5 mg, 10 mg, 25 mg, 50 mg

Urecholine®: 5 mg, 10 mg, 25 mg, 50 mg

Dosage Forms - Canada

Tablet:

Duvoid®: 10 mg, 25 mg, 50 mg

bethanechol chloride *see* bethanechol *on page 131*

Betimol® *see* timolol (ophthalmic) *on page 897*

Betnesol® (Can) *see* betamethasone *on page 129*
Betnovate® (Can) *see* betamethasone *on page 129*
Betoptic S® *see* betaxolol (ophthalmic) *on page 131*
Betoptic® S (Can) *see* betaxolol (ophthalmic) *on page 131*

bevacizumab (be vuh SIZ uh mab)

Medication Safety Issues

Sound-alike/look-alike issues:
Avastin® may be confused with Astelin®
Bevacizumab may be confused with brentuximab, cetuximab, riTUXimab

High alert medication:
This medication is in a class the Institute for Safe Medication Practices (ISMP) includes among its list of drug classes which have a heightened risk of causing significant patient harm when used in error.

International issues:
Avastin [U.S., Canada, and multiple international markets] may be confused with Avaxim, a brand name for hepatitis A vaccine [Canada and multiple international markets]

Synonyms anti-VEGF monoclonal antibody; anti-VEGF rhuMAb; rhuMAb-VEGF

U.S. Brand Names Avastin®

Canadian Brand Names Avastin®

Therapeutic Category Antineoplastic Agent, Monoclonal Antibody; Vaccine, Recombinant

Use Treatment of metastatic colorectal cancer; treatment of unresectable, locally advanced, recurrent or metastatic nonsquamous, nonsmall cell lung cancer; treatment of progressive glioblastoma; treatment of metastatic renal cell cancer (not an approved use in Canada)

Note: For the treatment of glioblastoma, effectiveness is based on improvement in objective response rate.

General Dosage Range I.V.: *Adults:* 5 or 10 mg/kg every 2 weeks **or** 15 mg/kg every 3 weeks

Dosage Forms

Injection, solution [preservative free]:
Avastin®: 25 mg/mL (4 mL, 16 mL)

bexarotene (systemic) (beks AIR oh teen)

Medication Safety Issues

High alert medication:
The Institute for Safe Medication Practices (ISMP) includes this medication among its list of drugs which have a heightened risk of causing significant patient harm when used in error.

U.S. Brand Names Targretin®

Therapeutic Category Antineoplastic Agent, Miscellaneous

Use Treatment of cutaneous manifestations of cutaneous T-cell lymphoma in patients who are refractory to at least one prior systemic therapy

General Dosage Range Oral: *Adults:* 300-400 mg/m^2 once daily

Dosage Forms

Capsule, oral:
Targretin®: 75 mg

bexarotene (topical) (beks AIR oh teen)

Medication Safety Issues

High alert medication:
The Institute for Safe Medication Practices (ISMP) includes this medication among its list of drugs which have a heightened risk of causing significant patient harm when used in error.

U.S. Brand Names Targretin®

Therapeutic Category Antineoplastic Agent, Miscellaneous

Use Treatment of cutaneous lesions in patients with refractory cutaneous T-cell lymphoma (stage 1A and 1B) or who have not tolerated other therapies

General Dosage Range Topical: *Adults:* Initial: Apply once every other day for first week; Maintenance: Apply 1-4 times/day

Dosage Forms

Gel, topical:
Targretin®: 1% (60 g)

Bexxar® *see* tositumomab and iodine I 131 tositumomab *on page 907*
Beyaz™ *see* ethinyl estradiol, drospirenone, and levomefolate *on page 363*

bezafibrate *(Canada only)* (be za FYE brate)

Canadian Brand Names Bezalip® SR
Therapeutic Category Antihyperlipidemic Agent, Miscellaneous
Use Adjunct to diet and other therapeutic measures for treatment of type IIa and IIb mixed hyperlipidemia, to regulate lipid and apoprotein levels (reduce serum TG, LDL-cholesterol, and apolipoprotein B, increase HDL-cholesterol and apolipoprotein A); treatment of adult patients with high to very high triglyceride levels (Fredrickson classification type IV and V hyperlipidemias) who are at high risk of sequelae and complications from their dyslipidemia
General Dosage Range
Oral:
Children: 10-20 mg/kg/day (maximum: 400 mg)
Adults: 400 mg once daily
Product Availability Not available in U.S.
Dosage Forms - Canada
Tablet, sustained release, oral:
Bezalip® SR: 400 mg

Bezalip® SR (Can) *see* bezafibrate *(Canada only) on page 133*
BG 9273 *see* alefacept *on page 44*
BI-1356 *see* linagliptin *on page 539*
Biafine® *see* emollients *on page 328*
Biaxin® *see* clarithromycin *on page 215*
Biaxin® XL *see* clarithromycin *on page 215*

bicalutamide (bye ka LOO ta mide)

Medication Safety Issues
Sound-alike/look-alike issues:
Casodex® may be confused with Kapidex [DSC]
International issues:
Casodex [U.S., Canada, and multiple international markets] may be confused with Capadex brand name for propoxyphene/acetaminophen [Australia, New Zealand]
Synonyms CDX; ICI-176334
U.S. Brand Names Casodex®
Canadian Brand Names Apo-Bicalutamide®; Ava-Bicalutamide; Casodex®; CO Bicalutamide; Dom-Bicalutamide; JAMP-Bicalutamide; Mylan-Bicalutamide; Novo-Bicalutamide; PHL-Bicalutamide; PMS-Bicalutamide; PRO-Bicalutamide; ratio-Bicalutamide; Sandoz-Bicalutamide
Therapeutic Category Androgen
Use Treatment of metastatic prostate cancer (in combination with an LHRH agonist)
General Dosage Range Oral: *Adults:* 50 mg once daily
Dosage Forms
Tablet, oral: 50 mg
Casodex®: 50 mg

Bicillin® L-A *see* penicillin G benzathine *on page 702*
Bicillin® C-R *see* penicillin G benzathine and penicillin G procaine *on page 702*
Bicillin® C-R 900/300 *see* penicillin G benzathine and penicillin G procaine *on page 702*
BiCNU® *see* carmustine *on page 178*
Bidex®-400 [OTC] *see* guaifenesin *on page 433*
BiDil® *see* isosorbide dinitrate and hydralazine *on page 505*
BIG-IV *see* botulism immune globulin (intravenous-human) *on page 140*
Biltricide® *see* praziquantel *on page 753*

bimatoprost (bi MAT oh prost)

U.S. Brand Names Latisse®; Lumigan®
Canadian Brand Names Latisse®; Lumigan®; Lumigan® RC

Therapeutic Category Ophthalmic Agent, Miscellaneous

Use Reduction of intraocular pressure (IOP) in patients with open-angle glaucoma or ocular hypertension; hypotrichosis treatment of the eyelashes

General Dosage Range

Ophthalmic: *Adults:* Instill 1 drop into affected eye(s) once daily

Ophthalmic, topical: *Adults:* Place 1 drop on applicator and apply evenly along the skin of the upper eyelid at base of eyelashes once daily

Dosage Forms

Solution, ophthalmic:

Latisse®: 0.03% (3 mL)

Lumigan®: 0.01% (2.5 mL, 5 mL, 7.5 mL); 0.03% (2.5 mL, 5 mL, 7.5 mL)

Binosto™ *see* alendronate *on page* 45
Bio-D-Mulsion® [OTC] *see* cholecalciferol *on page* 205
Bio-D-Mulsion Forte® [OTC] *see* cholecalciferol *on page* 205
Bio-Amitriptyline (Can) *see* amitriptyline *on page* 64
Biobase™ (Can) *see* alcohol (ethyl) *on page* 43
Biobase-G™ (Can) *see* alcohol (ethyl) *on page* 43
Bio-Diazepam (Can) *see* diazepam *on page* 277
Bio-Furosemide (Can) *see* furosemide *on page* 412
BioGlo™ *see* fluorescein *on page* 393
Bio-Hydrochlorothiazide (Can) *see* hydrochlorothiazide *on page* 452
Bionect® *see* hyaluronate and derivatives *on page* 450
Bioniche Promethazine (Can) *see* promethazine *on page* 763
Bion® Tears [OTC] *see* artificial tears *on page* 93
Bio-Oxazepam (Can) *see* oxazepam *on page* 676
BioQuin® Durules™ (Can) *see* quinidine *on page* 782
Biotene® Moisturizing Mouth Spray [OTC] *see* saliva substitute *on page* 819
Biotene® Oral Balance® [OTC] *see* saliva substitute *on page* 819
BioThrax® *see* anthrax vaccine, adsorbed *on page* 77
Biphentin® (Can) *see* methylphenidate *on page* 590
bird flu vaccine *see* influenza virus vaccine (H5N1) *on page* 482
Bisac-Evac™ [OTC] *see* bisacodyl *on page* 134

bisacodyl (bis a KOE dil)

Medication Safety Issues

Sound-alike/look-alike issues:

Doxidan® may be confused with doxepin

Dulcolax® (bisacodyl) may be confused with Dulcolax® (docusate)

U.S. Brand Names Alophen® [OTC]; Bisac-Evac™ [OTC]; Biscolax™ [OTC]; Correctol® Tablets [OTC]; Dacodyl™ [OTC]; Doxidan® [OTC]; Dulcolax® [OTC]; ex-lax® Ultra [OTC]; Femilax™ [OTC]; Fleet® Bisacodyl [OTC]; Fleet® Stimulant Laxative [OTC]; Veracolate® [OTC]

Canadian Brand Names Apo-Bisacodyl® [OTC]; Bisacodyl-Odan [OTC]; Bisacolax [OTC]; Carter's Little Pills® [OTC]; Codulax [OTC]; Dulcolax® [OTC]; PMS-Bisacodyl [OTC]; ratio-Bisacodyl [OTC]; Silver Bullet Suppository [OTC]; Soflax [OTC]; The Magic Bullett [OTC]; Woman's Laxative [OTC]

Therapeutic Category Laxative

Use Treatment of constipation; colonic evacuation prior to procedures or examination

General Dosage Range

Oral:

Children >6 years: 5-10 mg (0.3 mg/kg) once daily

Adults: 5-15 mg as a single dose (maximum: 30 mg)

Rectal:

Children <2 years: 5 mg as a single dose

Children ≥2 years and Adults: 10 mg as a single dose

Dosage Forms

Solution, rectal:

Fleet® Bisacodyl [OTC]: 10 mg/30 mL (37 mL)

Suppository, rectal: 10 mg (12s, 50s, 100s, 500s)
Bisac-Evac™ [OTC]: 10 mg (8s, 12s, 50s, 100s, 500s, 1000s)
Biscolax™ [OTC]: 10 mg (12s, 100s)
Dulcolax® [OTC]: 10 mg (4s, 8s, 16s, 28s, 50s)
Tablet, oral: 5 mg, 10 mg
Tablet, delayed release, oral: 5 mg
Doxidan® [OTC]: 5 mg
Fleet® Stimulant Laxative [OTC]: 5 mg
Tablet, enteric coated, oral: 5 mg
Alophen® [OTC]: 5 mg
Bisac-Evac™ [OTC]: 5 mg
Correctol® Tablets [OTC]: 5 mg
Dacodyl™ [OTC]: 5 mg
Dulcolax® [OTC]: 5 mg
ex-lax® Ultra [OTC]: 5 mg
Femilax™ [OTC]: 5 mg
Veracolate® [OTC]: 5 mg

bisacodyl and polyethylene glycol-electrolyte solution *see* polyethylene glycol-electrolyte solution and bisacodyl *on page 739*

Bisacodyl-Odan [OTC] (Can) *see* bisacodyl *on page 134*

Bisacolax [OTC] (Can) *see* bisacodyl *on page 134*

bis(chloroethyl) nitrosourea *see* carmustine *on page 178*

bis-chloronitrosourea *see* carmustine *on page 178*

Biscolax™ [OTC] *see* bisacodyl *on page 134*

Bismatrol [OTC] *see* bismuth *on page 135*

Bismatrol Maximum Strength [OTC] *see* bismuth *on page 135*

bismuth (BIZ muth)

Medication Safety Issues

Sound-alike/look-alike issues:
Kaopectate® may be confused with Kayexalate®

Other safety concerns:
Maalox® Total Relief® is a different formulation than other Maalox® liquid antacid products which contain aluminum hydroxide, magnesium hydroxide, and simethicone.
Canadian formulation of Kaopectate® does not contain bismuth; the active ingredient in the Canadian formulation is attapulgite.

Synonyms bismuth subsalicylate; pink bismuth

U.S. Brand Names Bismatrol Maximum Strength [OTC]; Bismatrol [OTC]; Diotame [OTC]; Kao-Tin [OTC]; Kaopectate® Extra Strength [OTC]; Kaopectate® [OTC]; Peptic Relief [OTC]; Pepto Relief [OTC]; Pepto-Bismol® Maximum Strength [OTC]; Pepto-Bismol® [OTC]

Therapeutic Category Antidiarrheal

Use Subsalicylate formulation: Symptomatic treatment of mild, nonspecific diarrhea; control of traveler's diarrhea (enterotoxigenic *Escherichia coli*); as part of a multidrug regimen for *H. pylori* eradication to reduce the risk of duodenal ulcer recurrence

General Dosage Range Oral:
Subsalicylate based on 262 mg/5 mL liquid or 262 mg tablet (diarrhea):
Children 3-6 years: 1/3 tablet **or** 5 mL every 30 minutes to 1 hour as needed (maximum: 8 doses/day)
Children 6-9 years: 2/3 tablet **or** 10 mL every 30 minutes to 1 hour as needed (maximum: 8 doses/day)
Children 9-12 years: 1 tablet **or** 15 mL every 30 minutes to 1 hour as needed (maximum: 8 doses/day)
Subsalicylate based on 262 mg/15 mL liquid or 262 mg tablet:
Children >12 years: Diarrhea: 2 tablets **or** 30 mL every 30 minutes to 1 hour as needed (maximum: 8 doses/day)
Adults:
Diarrhea: 2 tablets **or** 30 mL every 30 minutes to 1 hour as needed (maximum: 8 doses/day)
H. pylori eradication: 524 mg 4 times/day

Dosage Forms

Caplet, oral:
Pepto-Bismol® [OTC]: 262 mg

Liquid, oral: 262 mg/15 mL (120 mL, 237 mL, 240 mL, 360 mL, 480 mL); 525 mg/15 mL (240 mL, 360 mL)
Bismatrol [OTC]: 262 mg/15 mL (240 mL)
Bismatrol Maximum Strength [OTC]: 525 mg/15 mL (240 mL)
Diotame [OTC]: 262 mg/15 mL (30 mL)
Kao-Tin [OTC]: 262 mg/15 mL (240 mL, 473 mL)
Kaopectate® [OTC]: 262 mg/15 mL (177 mL, 236 mL, 354 mL)
Kaopectate® Extra Strength [OTC]: 525 mg/15 mL (236 mL)
Peptic Relief [OTC]: 262 mg/15 mL (237 mL)
Pepto-Bismol® [OTC]: 262 mg/15 mL (120 mL, 240 mL, 360 mL, 480 mL)
Pepto-Bismol® Maximum Strength [OTC]: 525 mg/15 mL (120 mL, 240 mL, 360 mL)
Suspension, oral: 262 mg/15 mL (30 mL)
Tablet, chewable, oral: 262 mg
Bismatrol [OTC]: 262 mg
Diotame [OTC]: 262 mg
Peptic Relief [OTC]: 262 mg
Pepto Relief [OTC]: 262 mg
Pepto-Bismol® [OTC]: 262 mg

bismuth, metronidazole, and tetracycline

(BIZ muth, me troe NI da zole, & tet ra SYE kleen)

Synonyms bismuth subcitrate potassium, tetracycline, and metronidazole; bismuth subsalicylate, tetracycline, and metronidazole; metronidazole, bismuth subcitrate potassium, and tetracycline; metronidazole, bismuth subsalicylate, and tetracycline; tetracycline, metronidazole, and bismuth subcitrate potassium; tetracycline, metronidazole, and bismuth subsalicylate

U.S. Brand Names Helidac®; Pylera™

Therapeutic Category Antidiarrheal

Use As part of a multidrug regimen for *H. pylori* eradication to reduce the risk of duodenal ulcer recurrence in combination with an H_2 agonist (Helidac®) or omeprazole (Pylera™)

General Dosage Range Oral: *Adults:*
Helidac®: 2 bismuth subsalicylate 262.4 mg tablets, 1 metronidazole 250 mg tablet, and 1 tetracycline 500 mg capsule 4 times/day at meals and bedtime
Pylera™: 3 capsules 4 times/day after meals and at bedtime

Dosage Forms

Capsule:
Pylera™: Bismuth subcitrate potassium 140 mg, metronidazole 125 mg, and tetracycline hydrochloride 125 mg

Combination package:
Helidac® [each package contains 14 blister cards (2-week supply); each card contains the following]:
Tablet, chewable: Bismuth subsalicylate]: 262.4 mg (8s)
Tablet: Metronidazole: 250 mg (4s)
Capsule: Tetracycline: 500 mg (4s)

bismuth subcitrate potassium, tetracycline, and metronidazole *see* bismuth, metronidazole, and tetracycline *on page* 136

bismuth subsalicylate *see* bismuth *on page* 135

bismuth subsalicylate, tetracycline, and metronidazole *see* bismuth, metronidazole, and tetracycline *on page* 136

bisoprolol

(bis OH proe lol)

Medication Safety Issues

Sound-alike/look-alike issues:
Zebeta® may be confused with DiaBeta®, Zetia®

Synonyms bisoprolol fumarate

U.S. Brand Names Zebeta®

Canadian Brand Names Apo-Bisoprolol®; Ava-Bisoprolol; Mylan-Bisoprolol; Novo-Bisoprolol; PHL-Bisoprolol; PMS-Bisoprolol; PRO-Bisoprolol; Sandoz-Bisoprolol

Therapeutic Category Beta-Adrenergic Blocker

Use Treatment of hypertension, alone or in combination with other agents

General Dosage Range Dosage adjustment recommended in patients with renal impairment
Oral: *Adults and Elderly:* Initial: 2.5-5 mg once daily; Maintenance: 2.5-20 mg once daily

Dosage Forms

Tablet, oral: 5 mg, 10 mg

Zebeta®: 5 mg, 10 mg

bisoprolol and hydrochlorothiazide (bis OH proe lol & hye droe klor oh THYE a zide)

Medication Safety Issues

Sound-alike/look-alike issues:

Ziac® may be confused with Tiazac®, Zerit®

Synonyms bisoprolol fumarate and hydrochlorothiazide; hydrochlorothiazide and bisoprolol

U.S. Brand Names Ziac®

Canadian Brand Names Ziac®

Therapeutic Category Antihypertensive Agent, Combination

Use Treatment of hypertension

General Dosage Range Oral: *Adults:* Initial: Bisoprolol 2.5 mg and hydrochlorothiazide 6.25 mg once daily; Maintenance: Bisoprolol 2.5-20 mg and hydrochlorothiazide 6.25-12.5 mg once daily; Maximum dose (manufacturer recommended): Bisoprolol 20 mg and hydrochlorothiazide 12.5 mg once daily

Dosage Forms

Tablet, oral: 2.5/6.25: Bisoprolol 2.5 mg and hydrochlorothiazide 6.25 mg; 5/6.25: Bisoprolol 5 mg and hydrochlorothiazide 6.25 mg; 10/6.25: Bisoprolol 10 mg and hydrochlorothiazide 6.25 mg

Ziac®: 2.5/6.25: Bisoprolol 2.5 mg and hydrochlorothiazide 6.25 mg; 5/6.25: Bisoprolol 5 mg and hydrochlorothiazide 6.25 mg; 10/6.25: Bisoprolol 10 mg and hydrochlorothiazide 6.25 mg

bisoprolol fumarate *see* bisoprolol *on page* 136

bisoprolol fumarate and hydrochlorothiazide *see* bisoprolol and hydrochlorothiazide *on page* 137

bis-POM PMEA *see* adefovir *on page* 37

bistropamide *see* tropicamide *on page* 924

bivalent human papillomavirus vaccine *see* papillomavirus (types 16, 18) vaccine (human, recombinant) *on page* 691

bivalirudin (bye VAL i roo din)

Medication Safety Issues

High alert medication:

The Institute for Safe Medication Practices (ISMP) includes this medication among its list of drugs which have a heightened risk of causing significant patient harm when used in error.

Synonyms hirulog

U.S. Brand Names Angiomax®

Canadian Brand Names Angiomax®

Therapeutic Category Anticoagulant (Other)

Use Anticoagulant used in conjunction with aspirin for patients with unstable angina undergoing percutaneous transluminal coronary angioplasty (PTCA) or percutaneous coronary intervention (PCI) with provisional glycoprotein IIb/IIIa inhibitor; anticoagulant used in conjunction with aspirin for patients undergoing PCI with (or at risk of) heparin-induced thrombocytopenia (HIT) / thrombosis syndrome (HITTS)

Canadian labeling: Additional uses (not in U.S. labeling): In conjunction with aspirin for treatment of patients with ST-elevation myocardial infarction (STEMI) undergoing primary PCI; anticoagulant with or without aspirin in patients undergoing cardiac surgery with (or at risk of) heparin-induced thrombocytopenia (HIT) / thrombosis syndrome (HITTS)

General Dosage Range

I.V.: *Adults:* Bolus: 0.75 mg/kg; may repeat at 0.3 mg/kg if necessary; Infusion: 1.75 mg/kg/hour for duration of procedure and up to 4 hours postprocedure if needed; after 4 hours may continue 0.2 mg/kg/hour for up to 20 hours if needed

Dosage adjustment recommended in patients with renal impairment

Dosage Forms

Injection, powder for reconstitution:

Angiomax®: 250 mg

Bi-Zets [OTC] *see* benzocaine *on page* 121

BL4162A *see* anagrelide *on page* 74

Black Draught® [OTC] *see* senna *on page* 829

black widow spider species antivenin *see* antivenin *(Latrodectus mactans) on page 81*
black widow spider species antivenom *see* antivenin *(Latrodectus mactans) on page 81*
Blenoxane *see* bleomycin *on page 138*
Blenoxane® (Can) *see* bleomycin *on page 138*
bleo *see* bleomycin *on page 138*

bleomycin (blee oh MYE sin)

Medication Safety Issues

Sound-alike/look-alike issues:

Bleomycin may be confused with Cleocin®

High alert medication:

This medication is in a class the Institute for Safe Medication Practices (ISMP) includes among its list of drugs which have a heightened risk of causing significant patient harm when used in error.

Synonyms Blenoxane; bleo; bleomycin sulfate; BLM

Canadian Brand Names Blenoxane®; Bleomycin Injection, USP

Therapeutic Category Antineoplastic Agent

Use Treatment of squamous cell carcinomas of the head and neck, penis, cervix, or vulva, testicular carcinoma, Hodgkin lymphoma, and non-Hodgkin lymphoma; sclerosing agent for malignant pleural effusion

General Dosage Range Dosage adjustment recommended in patients with renal impairment or who develop toxicities.

I.V.: *Adults:* Dosage varies greatly depending on indication

Intrapleural: *Adults:* 60 units as a single instillation

Dosage Forms

Injection, powder for reconstitution: 15 units, 30 units

Bleomycin Injection, USP (Can) *see* bleomycin *on page 138*
bleomycin sulfate *see* bleomycin *on page 138*
Bleph®-10 *see* sulfacetamide (ophthalmic) *on page 858*
Bleph 10 DPS (Can) *see* sulfacetamide (ophthalmic) *on page 858*
Blephamide® *see* sulfacetamide and prednisolone *on page 859*
BLES (Can) *see* bovine lipid extract surfactant *(Canada only) on page 140*
Blis-To-Sol® [OTC] *see* tolnaftate *on page 904*
BLM *see* bleomycin *on page 138*
BMS-188667 *see* abatacept *on page 16*
BMS-224818 *see* belatacept *on page 118*
BMS-232632 *see* atazanavir *on page 98*
BMS-247550 *see* ixabepilone *on page 508*
BMS 337039 *see* aripiprazole *on page 90*
BMS-354825 *see* dasatinib *on page 256*
BMS-477118 *see* saxagliptin *on page 825*
B&O *see* belladonna and opium *on page 118*

boceprevir (boe SE pre vir)

Synonyms SCH503034

U.S. Brand Names Victrelis®

Canadian Brand Names Victrelis®

Therapeutic Category Antiviral Agent; Protease Inhibitor

Use Treatment of chronic hepatitis C (CHC) genotype 1 (in combination with peginterferon alfa and ribavirin) in adult patients with compensated liver disease (including cirrhosis) who were previously untreated or have failed prior therapy with peginterferon alfa and ribavirin therapy

General Dosage Range Oral: *Adults:* 800 mg 3 times/day

Dosage Forms

Capsule, oral:

Victrelis®: 200 mg

Boil-Ease® Pain Relieving [OTC] *see* benzocaine *on page 121*
BOL-303224-A *see* besifloxacin *on page 128*

Bonefos® (Can) *see* clodronate *(Canada only) on page 222*
Bonine® [OTC] [DSC] *see* meclizine *on page 566*
Boniva® *see* ibandronate *on page 468*
Bontril® (Can) *see* phendimetrazine *on page 711*
Bontril® PDM *see* phendimetrazine *on page 711*
Bontril® Slow-Release *see* phendimetrazine *on page 711*
Boostrix® *see* diphtheria and tetanus toxoids, and acellular pertussis vaccine *on page 298*

bortezomib (bore TEZ oh mib)

Medication Safety Issues

Sound-alike/look-alike issues:

Bortezomib may be confused with carfilzomib

High alert medication:

This medication is in a class the Institute for Safe Medication Practices (ISMP) includes among its list of drug classes which have a heightened risk of causing significant patient harm when used in error.

Administration issues:

The reconstituted concentrations for I.V. and SubQ administration are different; use caution when calculating the volume for each dose. The manufacturer provides stickers to facilitate identification of the route for reconstituted vials.

For I.V. or SubQ administration only. Intrathecal administration is contraindicated; inadvertent intrathecal administration has resulted in death. Bortezomib should **NOT** be prepared during the preparation of any intrathecal medications. After preparation, keep bortezomib in a location **away** from the separate storage location recommended for intrathecal medications. Bortezomib should **NOT** be delivered to the patient at the same time with any medications intended for intrathecal administration.

Synonyms LDP-341; MLN341; PS-341

U.S. Brand Names Velcade®

Canadian Brand Names Velcade®

Therapeutic Category Proteasome Inhibitor

Use Treatment of multiple myeloma; treatment of relapsed or refractory mantle cell lymphoma

General Dosage Range Dosage adjustment recommended in patients with hepatic impairment or who develop toxicities.

I.V., SubQ: *Adults:* Dosage varies greatly depending on indication

Dosage Forms

Injection, powder for reconstitution:

Velcade®: 3.5 mg

bosentan (boe SEN tan)

Medication Safety Issues

Sound-alike/look-alike issues:

Tracleer® may be confused with TriCor®

U.S. Brand Names Tracleer®

Canadian Brand Names CO Bosentan; Mylan-Bosentan; PMS-Bosentan; Sandoz-Bosentan; Tracleer®

Therapeutic Category Endothelin Antagonist

Use Treatment of pulmonary artery hypertension (PAH) (WHO Group I) in patients with NYHA Class II, III, or IV symptoms to improve exercise capacity and decrease the rate of clinical deterioration

General Dosage Range Dosage adjustment recommended in patients with hepatic impairment or on concomitant therapy

Oral:

Children >12 years and Adults <40 kg: Initial: 62.5 mg twice daily; Maintenance: 62.5 mg twice daily
Children >12 years and Adults ≥40 kg: Initial: 62.5 mg twice daily; Maintenance: 125 mg twice daily

Dosage Forms

Tablet, oral:

Tracleer®: 62.5 mg, 125 mg

Botox® *see* onabotulinumtoxinA *on page 667*
Botox® Cosmetic *see* onabotulinumtoxinA *on page 667*
botulinum toxin type A *see* abobotulinumtoxinA *on page 18*
botulinum toxin type A *see* incobotulinumtoxinA *on page 478*
botulinum toxin type A *see* onabotulinumtoxinA *on page 667*

botulinum toxin type B *see* rimabotulinumtoxinB *on page 802*

botulism immune globulin (intravenous-human)

(BOT yoo lism i MYUN GLOB you lin, in tra VEE nus, YU man)

Medication Safety Issues

Sound-alike/look-alike issues:

BabyBIG® may be confused with HBIG

Synonyms BIG-IV

U.S. Brand Names BabyBIG®

Therapeutic Category Immune Globulin

Use Treatment of infant botulism caused by toxin type A or B

General Dosage Range I.V.: *Infants <1 year:* 75 mg/kg as a single dose

Dosage Forms

Injection, powder for reconstitution [preservative free]:

BabyBIG®: ~100 mg

Boudreaux's® Butt Paste [OTC] *see* zinc oxide *on page 963*

bovine lipid extract surfactant *(Canada only)* (BOH vine LIP id EK strakt ser FAK tunt)

Canadian Brand Names BLES

Therapeutic Category Lung Surfactant

Use Treatment of neonatal respiratory distress syndrome (NRDS)

General Dosage Range Intratracheal: *Infants:* 5 mL/kg/dose (equals phospholipids 135 mg/kg/dose); may repeat if needed (maximum: 4 doses)

Product Availability Not available in U.S.

Dosage Forms - Canada

Suspension, intratracheal [preservative free]:

BLES®: Phospholipids 27 mg/mL (3 mL, 4 mL, 5 mL)

bovine lung surfactant *see* beractant *on page 128*

bovine lung surfactant *see* calfactant *on page 167*

BP 10-1 *see* sulfur and sulfacetamide *on page 862*

BP 50% *see* urea *on page 930*

BP Cleanser [OTC] *see* benzoyl peroxide *on page 124*

BP Cleansing Lotion [OTC] *see* benzoyl peroxide *on page 124*

BP Cleansing Wash *see* sulfur and sulfacetamide *on page 862*

BPO *see* benzoyl peroxide *on page 124*

BP Wash [OTC] *see* benzoyl peroxide *on page 124*

BRAF(V600E) kinase inhibitor RO5185426 *see* vemurafenib *on page 941*

BranchAmin® [DSC] *see* amino acid injection *on page 61*

Bravelle® *see* urofollitropin *on page 931*

brentuximab *see* brentuximab vedotin *on page 140*

brentuximab vedotin (bren TUX i mab ve DOE tin)

Medication Safety Issues

Sound-alike/look-alike issues:

Brentuximab may be confused with bendamustine, bevacizumab, rituximab

High alert medication:

This medication is in a class the Institute for Safe Medication Practices (ISMP) includes among its list of drug classes which have a heightened risk of causing significant patient harm when used in error.

Synonyms anti-CD30 ADC SGN-35; anti-CD30 antibody-drug conjugate SGN-35; antibody-drug conjugate SGN-35; brentuximab; SGN-35

U.S. Brand Names Adcetris™

Use

Treatment of Hodgkin lymphoma after failure of at least 2 prior chemotherapy regimens (in patients ineligible for transplant) or after stem cell transplant failure; treatment of systemic anaplastic large cell lymphoma (sALCL) after failure of at least 1 prior chemotherapy regimen

General Dosage Range Dosage adjustment recommended in patients who develop toxicities.

I.V.: *Adults:* 1.8 mg/kg every 3 weeks (maximum dose: 180 mg)

Dosage Forms

Injection, powder for reconstitution:

Adcetris™: 50 mg

Brethaire [DSC] *see* terbutaline *on page* 879

brethine *see* terbutaline *on page* 879

Brevibloc *see* esmolol *on page* 345

Brevibloc® (Can) *see* esmolol *on page* 345

Brevibloc® Premixed (Can) *see* esmolol *on page* 345

Brevicon® *see* ethinyl estradiol and norethindrone *on page* 359

Brevicon® 0.5/35 (Can) *see* ethinyl estradiol and norethindrone *on page* 359

Brevicon® 1/35 (Can) *see* ethinyl estradiol and norethindrone *on page* 359

Brevital® (Can) *see* methohexital *on page* 584

Brevital® Sodium *see* methohexital *on page* 584

Bricanyl [DSC] *see* terbutaline *on page* 879

Bricanyl® (Can) *see* terbutaline *on page* 879

Briellyn *see* ethinyl estradiol and norethindrone *on page* 359

Brilinta™ *see* ticagrelor *on page* 895

brimonidine (bri MOE ni deen)

Medication Safety Issues

Sound-alike/look-alike issues:

Brimonidine may be confused with bromocriptine

Synonyms brimonidine tartrate

U.S. Brand Names Alphagan® P

Canadian Brand Names Alphagan®; Apo-Brimonidine P®; Apo-Brimonidine®; PMS-Brimonidine Tartrate; ratio-Brimonidine; Sandoz-Brimonidine

Therapeutic Category $Alpha_2$ Agonist, Ophthalmic

Use Lowering of intraocular pressure (IOP) in patients with open-angle glaucoma or ocular hypertension

General Dosage Range Ophthalmic: *Children ≥2 years and Adults:* Instill 1 drop in affected eye(s) 3 times/day

Dosage Forms

Solution, ophthalmic: 0.15% (5 mL, 10 mL, 15 mL); 0.2% (5 mL, 10 mL, 15 mL)

Alphagan® P: 0.1% (5 mL, 10 mL, 15 mL); 0.15% (5 mL, 10 mL, 15 mL)

brimonidine and timolol (bri MOE ni deen & TIM oh lol)

Medication Safety Issues

Sound-alike/look-alike issues:

Combigan® may be confused with Combivent®, Comtan®

Synonyms brimonidine tartrate and timolol maleate; timolol and brimonidine

U.S. Brand Names Combigan®

Canadian Brand Names Combigan®

Therapeutic Category $Alpha_2$ Agonist, Ophthalmic; Beta-Blocker, Nonselective; Ophthalmic Agent, Antiglaucoma

Use Reduction of intraocular pressure (IOP) in patients with glaucoma or ocular hypertension

General Dosage Range Ophthalmic: *Children ≥2 years and Adults:* Instill 1 drop into affected eye(s) twice daily

Dosage Forms

Solution, ophthalmic [drops]:

Combigan®: Brimonidine 0.2% and timolol 0.5% (5 mL,10 mL)

Dosage Forms - Canada

Solution, ophthalmic [drops]:

Combigan®: Brimonidine 0.2% and timolol 0.5% (2.5 mL, 5 mL,10 mL)

brimonidine tartrate *see* brimonidine *on page* 141

brimonidine tartrate and timolol maleate *see* brimonidine and timolol *on page* 141

brinzolamide (brin ZOH la mide)

U.S. Brand Names Azopt®

Canadian Brand Names Azopt®

Therapeutic Category Carbonic Anhydrase Inhibitor

Use Treatment of elevated intraocular pressure in patients with ocular hypertension or open-angle glaucoma

General Dosage Range Ophthalmic: *Adults:* Instill 1 drop in affected eye(s) 3 times/day

Dosage Forms

Suspension, ophthalmic:

Azopt®: 1% (10 mL, 15 mL)

brinzolamide and timolol *(Canada only)* (brin ZOH la mide & TIM oh lol)

Synonyms brinzolamide and timolol maleate; timolol maleate and brinzolamide

Canadian Brand Names Azarga™

Therapeutic Category Beta-Adrenergic Blocker, Nonselective; Carbonic Anhydrase Inhibitor; Ophthalmic Agent, Antiglaucoma

Use Treatment of elevated intraocular pressure in patients with ocular hypertension or open-angle glaucoma

General Dosage Range Ophthalmic: *Adults:* Instill 1 drop twice daily

Product Availability Not available in U.S.

Dosage Forms - Canada

Solution, ophthalmic [drops]:

Azarga™: Brinzolamide 1% and timolol maleate 0.5% (5 mL)

brinzolamide and timolol maleate *see* brinzolamide and timolol *(Canada only) on page 142*

Brioschi® [OTC] *see* sodium bicarbonate *on page 840*

British anti-lewisite *see* dimercaprol *on page 290*

BRL 43694 *see* granisetron *on page 432*

Bromaline® [OTC] [DSC] *see* brompheniramine and pseudoephedrine *on page 144*

Bromaline® DM [OTC] *see* brompheniramine, pseudoephedrine, and dextromethorphan *on page 144*

Bromax [DSC] *see* brompheniramine *on page 143*

bromazepam *(Canada only)* (broe MA ze pam)

Medication Safety Issues

International issues:

Lexotan [multiple international markets] may be confused with Loxitane brand name for loxapine [U.S.]

Canadian Brand Names Apo-Bromazepam®; Lectopam®; Mylan-Bromazepam; Novo-Bromazepam; Nu-Bromazepam; PRO-Doc Limitee Bromazepam

Therapeutic Category Benzodiazepine; Sedative

Use Short-term, symptomatic treatment of anxiety

General Dosage Range Oral:

Adults: Initial: 6-18 mg/day in divided doses; Maintenance: 6-30 mg/day in divided doses

Elderly: Initial: 3 mg/day in divided doses

Product Availability Not available in U.S.

Dosage Forms - Canada

Tablet: 1.5 mg, 3 mg, 6 mg

Lectopam®: 3 mg, 6 mg

Bromday™ *see* bromfenac *on page 142*

Bromdex D *see* brompheniramine, pseudoephedrine, and dextromethorphan *on page 144*

Bromfed® DM *see* brompheniramine, pseudoephedrine, and dextromethorphan *on page 144*

bromfenac (BROME fen ak)

Synonyms bromfenac sodium

U.S. Brand Names Bromday™

Therapeutic Category Analgesic, Nonnarcotic; Nonsteroidal Antiinflammatory Drug (NSAID), Ophthalmic

Use Treatment of postoperative inflammation and reduction in ocular pain following cataract removal

General Dosage Range Ophthalmic: *Adults:* Instill 1 drop into affected eye(s) once daily

Dosage Forms

Solution, ophthalmic: 0.09% (2.5 mL, 5 mL)

Bromday™: 0.09% (1.7 mL)

bromfenac sodium *see* bromfenac *on page 142*

bromocriptine (broe moe KRIP teen)

Medication Safety Issues

Sound-alike/look-alike issues:

Bromocriptine may be confused with benztropine, brimonidine

Cycloset® may be confused with Glyset®

Parlodel® may be confused with pindolol, Provera®

Synonyms bromocriptine mesylate

U.S. Brand Names Cycloset®; Parlodel®; Parlodel® SnapTabs®

Canadian Brand Names Dom-Bromocriptine; PMS-Bromocriptine

Therapeutic Category Anti-Parkinson Agent (Dopamine Agonist); Ergot Alkaloid and Derivative

Use Treatment of hyperprolactinemia associated with amenorrhea with or without galactorrhea, infertility, or hypogonadism; treatment of prolactin-secreting adenomas; treatment of acromegaly; treatment of Parkinson disease

Cycloset®: Management of type 2 diabetes mellitus (noninsulin-dependent, NIDDM) as an adjunct to diet and exercise

General Dosage Range Oral:

Children 11-15 years: Initial: 1.25-2.5 mg daily; Maintenance: 2.5-10 mg/day

Children ≥16 years: Initial: 1.25-2.5 mg daily; Maintenance: 2.5-15 mg/day

Adults: Dosage varies greatly depending on indication

Dosage Forms

Capsule, oral: 5 mg

Parlodel®: 5 mg

Tablet, oral: 2.5 mg

Cycloset®: 0.8 mg

Parlodel® SnapTabs®: 2.5 mg

bromocriptine mesylate *see* bromocriptine *on page 143*

Bromphenex™ DM [OTC] *see* brompheniramine, pseudoephedrine, and dextromethorphan *on page 144*

brompheniramine (brome fen IR a meen)

Medication Safety Issues

BEERS Criteria medication:

This drug may be potentially inappropriate for use in geriatric patients (Quality of evidence - moderate; Strength of recommendation - strong).

Synonyms brompheniramine maleate; brompheniramine tannate

U.S. Brand Names Bromax [DSC]; J-Tan PD [OTC]; LoHist-12 [DSC]

Therapeutic Category Antihistamine

Use Symptomatic relief of perennial and seasonal allergic rhinitis, vasomotor rhinitis, and other respiratory allergies

General Dosage Range Oral:

Children 2 to <6 years: J-Tan PD: 1 mg (1 mL) every 4-6 hours (maximum: 6 mg [6 mL]/24 hours)

Children 6-12 years:

J-Tan PD: 2 mg (2 mL) every 4-6 hours (maximum: 12 mg [12 mL]/24 hours)

LoHist-12: One tablet every 12 hours (maximum: 2 tablets/day)

Children >12 years and Adults:

Bromax: One tablet twice daily

LoHist-12: 1-2 tablets every 12 hours (maximum: 4 tablets/day)

Dosage Forms

Liquid, oral:

J-Tan PD [OTC]: 1 mg/mL (30 mL)

brompheniramine and phenylephrine (brome fen IR a meen & fen il EF rin)

Synonyms brompheniramine maleate and phenylephrine hydrochloride; brompheniramine tannate and phenylephrine tannate; phenylephrine and brompheniramine

U.S. Brand Names BroveX™ PEB [OTC]; Dimaphen™ Children's Cold & Allergy [OTC]; Dimetapp® Children's Cold & Allergy [OTC]; Entre-B [OTC]; LoHist PEB [OTC]; Rynex PE; Vazobid-PD™ [OTC]

Therapeutic Category Alpha/Beta Agonist; Histamine H_1 Antagonist; Histamine H_1 Antagonist, First Generation

Use Temporary relief of upper respiratory conditions such as nasal congestion, runny nose, itchy/watery eyes, and sneezing due to the common cold, hay fever, or upper respiratory allergies

General Dosage Range Oral: *Children ≥2 years and Adults:* Dosage varies greatly depending on product.

Dosage Forms

Elixir, oral:

Dimaphen™ Children's Cold & Allergy [OTC]: Brompheniramine 1 mg and phenylephrine 2. 5 mg per 5 mL

Liquid, oral:

BroveX™ PEB [OTC], LoHist PEB [OTC]: Brompheniramine 4 mg and phenylephrine 10 mg per 5 mL

Dimetapp® Children's Cold & Allergy [OTC]: Brompheniramine 1 mg and phenylephrine 2.5 mg per 5 mL

Rynex PE: Brompheniramine 1 mg and phenylephrine 2.5 mg per 5 mL

Suspension, oral:

Entre-B [OTC]: Brompheniramine 6 mg and phenylephrine 10 mg per 5 mL

Vazobid-PD™ [OTC]: Brompheniramine 1.2 mg and phenylephrine 2 mg per 1 mL

brompheniramine and pseudoephedrine (brome fen IR a meen & soo doe e FED rin)

Synonyms brompheniramine maleate and pseudoephedrine hydrochloride; brompheniramine maleate and pseudoephedrine sulfate; pseudoephedrine and brompheniramine

U.S. Brand Names Bromaline® [OTC] [DSC]; Brotapp [OTC]; J-Tan D PD [OTC]; Lodrane® D [OTC]; LoHist PSB [OTC]; Q-Tapp Cold & Allergy [OTC]

Therapeutic Category Antihistamine/Decongestant Combination

Use Temporary relief of symptoms associated with seasonal and perennial allergic rhinitis, the common cold, or sinusitis

General Dosage Range Oral: *Children ≥2 years and Adults:* Dosage varies greatly depending on product

Dosage Forms

Capsule, oral:

Lodrane® D [OTC]: Brompheniramine 4 mg and pseudoephedrine 60 mg

Liquid, oral:

Brotapp [OTC]: Brompheniramine 1 mg and pseudoephedrine 15 mg per 5 mL

LoHist PSB [OTC]: Brompheniramine 4 mg and pseudoephedrine 20 mg per 5 mL

Q-Tapp Cold & Allergy [OTC]: Brompheniramine 1 mg and pseudoephedrine 15 mg per 5 mL

Liquid, oral [drops]:

J-Tan D PD: Brompheniramine maleate 1 mg and pseudoephedrine hydrochloride 7.5 mg per 1 mL (30 mL)

brompheniramine maleate *see* brompheniramine *on page* 143

brompheniramine maleate and phenylephrine hydrochloride *see* brompheniramine and phenylephrine *on page* 144

brompheniramine maleate and pseudoephedrine hydrochloride *see* brompheniramine and pseudoephedrine *on page* 144

brompheniramine maleate and pseudoephedrine sulfate *see* brompheniramine and pseudoephedrine *on page* 144

brompheniramine, pseudoephedrine, and dextromethorphan

(brome fen IR a meen, soo doe e FED rin, & deks troe meth OR fan)

Synonyms dextromethorphan hydrobromide, brompheniramine maleate, and pseudoephedrine hydrochloride; pseudoephedrine tannate, dextromethorphan tannate, and brompheniramine tannate

U.S. Brand Names Anaplex® DM; Bromaline® DM [OTC]; Bromdex D; Bromfed® DM; Bromphenex™ DM [OTC]; Brotapp-DM; LoHist PSB DM [OTC]; Myphetane DX [DSC]; Neo DM; PediaHist DM; Q-Tapp Cold & Cough [OTC]; Resperal-DM

Therapeutic Category Antihistamine; Cough Preparation; Decongestant

Use Relief of cough and upper respiratory symptoms (including nasal congestion) associated with allergy or the common cold

General Dosage Range Oral:

Children 2-6 years: Anaplex® DM: 1.25 mL every 4-6 hours (maximum: 4 doses/day)

Children 6-12 years:

Anaplex® DM: 2.5 mL every 4-6 hours (maximum: 4 doses/day)

Bromaline® DM: 10 mL every 4-6 hours (maximum: 4 doses/day)

Children >12 years and Adults:

Anaplex® DM: 5 mL every 4-6 hours (maximum: 4 doses/day)

Bromaline® DM: 20 mL every 4-6 hours (maximum: 4 doses/day)

Dosage Forms

Elixir, oral:

Bromaline® DM [OTC],Q-Tapp Cold & Cough [OTC]: Brompheniramine 1 mg, pseudoephedrine 15 mg, and dextromethorphan 5 mg per 5 mL

Liquid, oral:

Bromphenex™ DM [OTC]: Brompheniramine 4 mg, pseudoephedrine 60 mg, and dextromethorphan 30 mg per 5 mL

Brotapp-DM: Brompheniramine 1 mg, pseudoephedrine 15 mg, and dextromethorphan 5 mg per 5 mL

LoHist PSB DM [OTC]: Brompheniramine 4 mg, pseudoephedrine 20 mg, and dextromethorphan 20 mg per 5 mL

Q-Tapp Cold & Cough [OTC]: Brompheniramine maleate 1 mg, pseudoephedrine hydrochloride 15 mg, and dextromethorphan hydrobromide 5 mg per 5 mL

Solution, oral [drops]:

PediaHist DM: Brompheniramine 1 mg, pseudoephedrine 15 mg, and dextromethorphan 4 mg per 1 mL

Resperal-DM: Brompheniramine 1 mg, pseudoephedrine 12 mg, and dextromethorphan 5 mg per 1 mL

Syrup, oral:

Anaplex® DM, EndaCof-DM: Brompheniramine 4 mg, pseudoephedrine 60 mg, and dextromethorphan 30 mg per 5 mL

Bromatane DX, Neo DM: Brompheniramine 2 mg, pseudoephedrine 30 mg, and dextromethorphan 10 mg per 5 mL

Bromdex D: Brompheniramine 3 mg, pseudoephedrine 50 mg, and dextromethorphan 30 mg per 5 mL

brompheniramine tannate *see* brompheniramine *on page 143*

brompheniramine tannate and phenylephrine tannate *see* brompheniramine and phenylephrine *on page 144*

Brotapp [OTC] *see* brompheniramine and pseudoephedrine *on page 144*

Brotapp-DM *see* brompheniramine, pseudoephedrine, and dextromethorphan *on page 144*

Brovana® *see* arformoterol *on page 89*

BroveX™ PEB [OTC] *see* brompheniramine and phenylephrine *on page 144*

BSF208075 *see* ambrisentan *on page 58*

BSS® *see* balanced salt solution *on page 113*

BSS Plus® *see* balanced salt solution *on page 113*

BTX-A *see* onabotulinumtoxinA *on page 667*

B-type natriuretic peptide (human) *see* nesiritide *on page 636*

Budeprion XL® *see* bupropion *on page 150*

Budeprion SR® *see* bupropion *on page 150*

budesonide (systemic, oral inhalation) (byoo DES oh nide)

U.S. Brand Names Entocort® EC; Pulmicort Flexhaler®; Pulmicort Respules®

Canadian Brand Names Entocort®; Pulmicort® Turbuhaler®

Therapeutic Category Corticosteroid, Inhalant (Oral); Corticosteroid, Systemic

Use

Nebulization: Maintenance and prophylactic treatment of asthma

Oral capsule: Treatment of active Crohn disease (mild-to-moderate) involving the ileum and/or ascending colon; maintenance of remission (for up to 3 months) of Crohn disease (mild-to-moderate) involving the ileum and/or ascending colon

Oral inhalation: Maintenance and prophylactic treatment of asthma; includes patients who require oral corticosteroids and those who may benefit from systemic dose reduction/elimination

General Dosage Range

Inhalation:

Children ≥6 years: Initial: 180-360 mcg twice daily; Maintenance: 180 to >800 mcg/day in 2 divided doses

Adults: Initial: 180-720 mcg twice daily; Maintenance: 180-1440 mcg/day in 2 divided doses

Nebulization: *Children 12 months to 8 years:* 0.25-1 mg in 1-2 divided doses

Oral: *Adults:* Initial: 9 mg once daily; Maintenance: 6 mg once daily

Dosage Forms

Capsule, enteric coated, oral: 3 mg

Entocort® EC: 3 mg

Powder, for oral inhalation:

Pulmicort Flexhaler®: 90 mcg/inhalation (165 mg); 180 mcg/inhalation (225 mg)

Suspension, for nebulization: 0.25 mg/2 mL (30s); 0.5 mg/2 mL (30s)

Pulmicort Respules®: 0.25 mg/2 mL (30s); 0.5 mg/2 mL (30s); 1 mg/2 mL (30s)

Dosage Forms - Canada

Powder for oral inhalation:

Pulmicort® Turbuhaler®: 100 mcg/inhalation, 200 mcg/inhalation, 400 mcg/inhalation

budesonide (nasal) (byoo DES oh nide)

U.S. Brand Names Rhinocort Aqua®:

Canadian Brand Names Mylan-Budesonide AQ; Rhinocort® Aqua®; Rhinocort® Turbuhaler®

Therapeutic Category Corticosteroid, Nasal

Use Management of symptoms of seasonal or perennial rhinitis

Canadian labeling: Additional use (not in U.S. labeling): Prevention and treatment of nasal polyps

General Dosage Range Intranasal inhalation: *Children ≥6 years and Adults:* 64 mcg/day as a single 32 mcg spray in each nostril (maximum: 128 mcg/day [children <12 years]; 256 mcg/day [children ≥12 years and adults])

Dosage Forms

Suspension, intranasal:

Rhinocort Aqua®: 32 mcg/inhalation (8.6 g)

Dosage Forms - Canada

Powder for nasal inhalation:

Rhinocort® Turbuhaler®: 100 mcg/inhalation

Suspension, intranasal [spray]:

Rhinocort® Aqua®: 64 mcg/inhalation

budesonide and eformoterol *see* budesonide and formoterol *on page 146*

budesonide and formoterol (byoo DES oh nide & for MOH te rol)

Synonyms budesonide and eformoterol; eformoterol and budesonide; formoterol and budesonide; formoterol fumarate dihydrate and budesonide

U.S. Brand Names Symbicort®

Canadian Brand Names Symbicort®

Therapeutic Category $Beta_2$-Adrenergic Agonist, Long-Acting; Corticosteroid, Inhalant (Oral)

Use Treatment of asthma in patients ≥12 years of age where combination therapy is indicated; maintenance treatment of airflow obstruction associated with chronic obstructive pulmonary disease (COPD; including chronic bronchitis and emphysema)

General Dosage Range Inhalation:

Children 5-11 years: Symbicort® 80/4.5: Two inhalations twice daily (maximum: 4 inhalations/day)

Children ≥12 years: 2 inhalations once or twice daily (maximum: 4 inhalations/day)

Adults: 2 inhalations twice daily (maximum: 4 inhalations/day)

Dosage Forms

Aerosol for oral inhalation:

Symbicort® 80/4.5: Budesonide 80 mcg and formoterol fumarate dihydrate 4.5 mcg per actuation (6.9 g) [60 metered inhalations]; budesonide 80 mcg and formoterol fumarate dihydrate 4.5 mcg per actuation (10.2 g) [120 metered inhalations]

Symbicort® 160/4.5: Budesonide 160 mcg and formoterol fumarate dihydrate 4.5 mcg per actuation (6 g) [60 metered inhalations]; budesonide 160 mcg and formoterol fumarate dihydrate 4.5 mcg per actuation (10.2 g) [120 metered inhalations]

Dosage Forms - Canada

Powder for oral inhalation:

Symbicort® 100 Turbuhaler®: Budesonide 100 mcg and formoterol dihydrate 6 mcg per inhalation (available in 60 or 120 metered doses) [delivers ~80 mcg budesonide and 4.5 mcg formoterol per inhalation]

Symbicort® 200 Turbuhaler®: Budesonide 200 mcg and formoterol dihydrate 6 mcg per inhalation (available in 60 or 120 metered doses) [delivers ~160 mcg budesonide and 4.5 mcg formoterol per inhalation]

Buffasal [OTC] *see* aspirin *on page 96*

Bufferin® [OTC] *see* aspirin *on page 96*

Bufferin® Extra Strength [OTC] *see* aspirin *on page 96*

Buffinol [OTC] *see* aspirin *on page 96*

Bulk-K [OTC] *see* psyllium *on page 774*

bumetanide (byoo MET a nide)

Medication Safety Issues

Sound-alike/look-alike issues:

Bumetanide may be confused with Buminate®

Bumex® may be confused with Brevibloc®, Buprenex®

International issues:

Bumex [U.S.] may be confused with Permax brand name for pergolide [multiple international markets]

Synonyms Bumex

Canadian Brand Names Burinex®

Therapeutic Category Diuretic, Loop

Use Management of edema secondary to heart failure or hepatic or renal disease (including nephrotic syndrome)

General Dosage Range

I.M., I.V.:

Infants and Children: 0.015-0.1 mg/kg/dose every 6-24 hours (maximum: 10 mg/day)

Adults: 0.5-1 mg/dose; may repeat in 2-3 hours for up to 2 doses (maximum: 10 mg/day)

Oral:

Infants and Children: 0.015-0.1 mg/kg/dose every 6-24 hours (maximum: 10 mg/day)

Adults: 0.5-2 mg 1-2 times/day; may repeat in 4-5 hours for up to 2 doses (maximum: 10 mg/day)

Dosage Forms

Injection, solution: 0.25 mg/mL (2 mL, 4 mL, 10 mL)

Tablet, oral: 0.5 mg, 1 mg, 2 mg

Bumex *see* bumetanide *on page 147*

Buminate *see* albumin *on page 41*

Buminate-5% (Can) *see* albumin *on page 41*

Buminate-25% (Can) *see* albumin *on page 41*

Bupap *see* butalbital and acetaminophen *on page 154*

Buphenyl® *see* sodium phenylbutyrate *on page 845*

bupivacaine (byoo PIV a kane)

Medication Safety Issues

Sound-alike/look-alike issues:

Bupivacaine may be confused with mepivacaine, ropivacaine

Marcaine® may be confused with Narcan®

High alert medication:

The Institute for Safe Medication Practices (ISMP) includes this medication (epidural administration) among its list of drug classes which have a heightened risk of causing significant patient harm when used in error.

Synonyms bupivacaine hydrochloride

U.S. Brand Names Bupivacaine Spinal; Marcaine®; Marcaine® Spinal; Sensorcaine®; Sensorcaine®-MPF; Sensorcaine®-MPF Spinal

Canadian Brand Names Marcaine®; Sensorcaine®

Therapeutic Category Local Anesthetic

Use Local or regional anesthesia; spinal anesthesia; diagnostic and therapeutic procedures; obstetrical procedures (only 0.25% and 0.5% concentrations)

0.25%: Local infiltration, peripheral nerve block, sympathetic block, caudal or epidural block

0.5%: Peripheral nerve block, caudal and epidural block

0.75% **(not for obstetrical anesthesia)**: Retrobulbar block, epidural block. **Note:** Reserve for surgical procedures where a high degree of muscle relaxation and prolonged effect are necessary

General Dosage Range

Caudal block: *Children >12 years and Adults:* 15-30 mL of 0.25% or 0.5%

Epidural block: *Children >12 years and Adults:* 10-20 mL of 0.25% or 0.5% in 3-5 mL increments **or** 10-20 mL of 0.75% if high degree of muscle relaxation and prolonged effects needed

Infiltration (local): *Children >12 years and Adults:* 0.25% (maximum: 175 mg)

Nerve block: *Children >12 years and Adults:*

Peripheral: 5 mL of 0.25% or 0.5% (maximum: 400 mg/day)

Sympathetic: 20-50 mL of 0.25%

Retrobulbar anesthesia: *Children >12 years and Adults:* 2-4 mL of 0.75%

Spinal: *Adults:* Preservative free solution of 0.75% bupivacaine in 8.25% dextrose:

Cesarean section: 1-1.4 mL

Lower abdominal procedures: 1.6 mL

Lower extremity and perineal procedures: 1 mL

Normal vaginal delivery: 0.8 mL (higher doses may be required in some patients)

Dosage Forms

Injection, solution: 0.25% [2.5 mg/mL] (20 mL, 50 mL); 0.5% [5 mg/mL] (20 mL, 50 mL)

Marcaine®: 0.5% [5 mg/mL] (50 mL)

Sensorcaine®: 0.25% [2.5 mg/mL] (50 mL); 0.5% [5 mg/mL] (50 mL)

Injection, solution [preservative free]: 0.25% [2.5 mg/mL] (10 mL, 20 mL, 30 mL, 50 mL); 0.5% [5 mg/mL] (10 mL, 20 mL, 30 mL); 0.75% [7.5 mg/mL] (10 mL, 20 mL, 30 mL)

Marcaine®: 0.25% [2.5 mg/mL] (10 mL, 30 mL, 50 mL); 0.5% [5 mg/mL] (10 mL, 30 mL); 0.75% [7.5 mg/mL] (10 mL, 30 mL)

Sensorcaine®-MPF: 0.25% [2.5 mg/mL] (10 mL, 30 mL); 0.5% [5 mg/mL] (10 mL, 30 mL); 0.75% [7.5 mg/mL] (10 mL, 30 mL)

Injection, solution, premixed in $D_{8.25}W$ [preservative free]:

Bupivacaine Spinal: 0.75% [7.5 mg/mL] (2 mL)

Marcaine® Spinal: 0.75% [7.5 mg/mL] (2 mL)

Sensorcaine®-MPF Spinal: 0.75% [7.5 mg/mL] (2 mL)

bupivacaine and epinephrine (byoo PIV a kane & ep i NEF rin)

Medication Safety Issues

High alert medication:

The Institute for Safe Medication Practices (ISMP) includes this medication (epidural administration) among its list of drug classes which have a heightened risk of causing significant patient harm when used in error.

Synonyms epinephrine bitartrate and bupivacaine hydrochloride

U.S. Brand Names Marcaine® with Epinephrine; Sensorcaine® with Epinephrine; Sensorcaine®-MPF with Epinephrine; Vivacaine™

Canadian Brand Names Sensorcaine® with Epinephrine

Therapeutic Category Local Anesthetic

Use Local anesthetic (injectable) for peripheral nerve block, infiltration, sympathetic block, caudal or epidural block, retrobulbar block

General Dosage Range

Caudal block (preservative free): *Children >12 years and Adults:* 15-30 mL of 0.25% or 0.5%

Epidural block (preservative free): *Children >12 years and Adults:* 10-20 mL of 0.25% or 0.5% in 3-5 mL increments **or** 10-20 mL of 0.75% if high degree of muscle relaxation or prolonged effects needed

Infiltration (local): *Children >12 years and Adults:* 0.25% (maximum: 175 mg [bupivacaine])

Infiltration and nerve block (maxillary, mandibular): *Children >12 years and Adults:* 9 mg (1.8 mL) of bupivacaine as a 0.5% solution with epinephrine 1:200,000 per injection site; may repeat after 10 minutes if needed (maximum: 90 mg bupivacaine/appointment)

Nerve block: *Children >12 years and Adults:*

Peripheral: 5 mL of 0.25 or 0.5% (maximum: 400 mg/day [bupivacaine])

Sympathetic: 20-50 mL of 0.25%

Retrobulbar anesthesia: *Children >12 years and Adults:* 2-4 mL of 0.75%

Dosage Forms

Injection, solution [preservative free]: Bupivacaine 0.25% and epinephrine 1:200,000 (10 mL, 30 mL); bupivacaine 0.5% and epinephrine 1:200,000 (10 mL, 30 mL)

Marcaine® with Epinephrine: Bupivacaine 0.25% and epinephrine 1:200,000 (10 mL, 30 mL); bupivacaine 0.5% and epinephrine 1:200,000 (10 mL, 30 mL)

Sensorcaine® MPF with Epinephrine: Bupivacaine 0.25% and epinephrine 1:200,000 (10 mL, 30 mL); bupivacaine 0.5% and epinephrine 1:200,000 (10 mL, 30 mL); bupivacaine 0.75% and epinephrine 1:200,000 (30 mL)

Injection, solution: Bupivacaine 0.25% and epinephrine 1:200,000 (50 mL); bupivacaine 0.5% and epinephrine 1:200,000 (50 mL)

Marcaine® with Epinephrine, Sensorcaine® with Epinephrine: Bupivacaine 0.25% and epinephrine 1:200,000 (50 mL); bupivacaine 0.5% and epinephrine 1:200,000 (50 mL)

Injection, solution [for dental use]:

Marcaine® with Epinephrine, Vivacaine™: Bupivacaine 0.5% and epinephrine 1:200,000 (1.8 mL)

bupivacaine hydrochloride *see* bupivacaine *on page 147*

bupivacaine (liposomal) (byoo PIV a kane lye po SO mal)

Medication Safety Issues

Sound-alike/look-alike issues:

Bupivacaine may be confused with mepivacaine, ropivacaine

Bupivacaine liposomal may be confused with conventional bupivacaine

Bupivacaine liposomal may be confused with propofol due to similar white, milky appearance.

High alert medication:

The Institute for Safe Medication Practices (ISMP) includes this medication among its list of drug classes which have a heightened risk of causing significant patient harm when used in error.

Synonyms bupivacaine liposome; depoFoam bupivacaine; liposomal bupivacaine

U.S. Brand Names Exparel™

Therapeutic Category Analgesic, Nonopioid

Use Injected into the surgical site (eg, bunionectomy, hemorrhoidectomy) to provide postoperative analgesia

General Dosage Range Infiltration (local): *Adults:* 8 mL (106 mg) to 20 mL (266 mg) as a single dose (maximum total dose: 266 mg)

Dosage Forms

Injection, suspension [preservative free]:

Exparel™: 1.3% [13.3 mg/mL] (20 mL)

bupivacaine liposome *see* bupivacaine (liposomal) *on page 149*

Bupivacaine Spinal *see* bupivacaine *on page 147*

Buprenex® *see* buprenorphine *on page 149*

buprenorphine (byoo pre NOR feen)

Medication Safety Issues

Sound-alike/look-alike issues:

Buprenex® may be confused with Brevibloc®, Bumex®

High alert medication:

The Institute for Safe Medication Practices (ISMP) includes this medication among its list of drug classes which have a heightened risk of causing significant patient harm when used in error.

Synonyms buprenorphine hydrochloride

U.S. Brand Names Buprenex®; Butrans®; Subutex® [DSC]

Canadian Brand Names Buprenex®; Subutex®

Therapeutic Category Analgesic, Narcotic

Controlled Substance C-III

Use

Injection: Management of moderate-to-severe pain

Sublingual tablet: Treatment of opioid dependence

Transdermal patch: Management of moderate-to-severe chronic pain in patients requiring an around-the-clock opioid analgesic for an extended period of time

General Dosage Range Dosage adjustment recommended in patients with hepatic impairment.

I.M., I.V.:

Children 2-12 years: 2-6 **mcg**/kg every 4-6 hours

Children ≥13 years and Adults: Initial: 0.3 mg, may repeat once in 30-60 minutes then every 6-8 hours as needed; Maintenance: 0.15-0.6 mg every 4-8 hours as needed

Elderly: 0.15 mg every 6 hours

Sublingual: *Children ≥16 years and Adults:* Induction: 12-16 mg/day; Maintenance: 12-16 mg/day (target dose: 16 mg/day)

Transdermal: *Adults:* 5-20 **mcg**/hour applied once every 7 days (maximum: 20 **mcg**/hour once every 7 days)

Dosage Forms

Injection, solution: 0.3 mg/mL (1 mL)

Buprenex®: 0.3 mg/mL (1 mL)

Injection, solution [preservative free]: 0.3 mg/mL (1 mL)

Patch, transdermal:

Butrans®: 5 mcg/hr (4s); 10 mcg/hr (4s); 20 mcg/hr (4s)

Tablet, sublingual: 2 mg, 8 mg

buprenorphine and naloxone (byoo pre NOR feen & nal OKS one)

Medication Safety Issues

High alert medication:

The Institute for Safe Medication Practices (ISMP) includes this medication among its list of drug classes which have a heightened risk of causing significant patient harm when used in error.

Synonyms buprenorphine hydrochloride and naloxone hydrochloride dihydrate; naloxone and buprenorphine; naloxone hydrochloride dihydrate and buprenorphine hydrochloride

U.S. Brand Names Suboxone®

Canadian Brand Names Suboxone®

Therapeutic Category Analgesic, Narcotic

Controlled Substance C-III

Use Maintenance treatment for opioid dependence

General Dosage Range Sublingual: *Children ≥16 years and Adults:* 4-24 mg/day (target dose: 16 mg/day)

Dosage Forms

Film, sublingual:

Suboxone®: Buprenorphine 2 mg and naloxone 0.5 mg; buprenorphine 8 mg and naloxone 2 mg

Tablet, sublingual:

Suboxone®: Buprenorphine 2 mg and naloxone 0.5 mg; buprenorphine 8 mg and naloxone 2 mg

buprenorphine hydrochloride *see* buprenorphine *on page 149*

buprenorphine hydrochloride and naloxone hydrochloride dihydrate *see* buprenorphine and naloxone *on page 150*

Buproban® *see* bupropion *on page 150*

bupropion (byoo PROE pee on)

Medication Safety Issues

Sound-alike/look-alike issues:

Aplenzin™ may be confused with Albenza®, Relenza®

BuPROPion may be confused with busPIRone

Wellbutrin XL® may be confused with Wellbutrin SR®

Zyban® may be confused with Diovan®

Synonyms bupropion hydrobromide; bupropion hydrochloride

Tall-Man bu**PROP**ion

U.S. Brand Names Aplenzin™; Budeprion SR®; Budeprion XL®; Buproban®; Wellbutrin SR®; Wellbutrin XL®; Wellbutrin®; Zyban®

Canadian Brand Names Ava-Bupropion SR; Bupropion SR®; Novo-Bupropion SR; PMS-Bupropion SR; ratio-Bupropion SR; Sandoz-Bupropion SR; Wellbutrin® SR; Wellbutrin® XL; Zyban®

Therapeutic Category Antidepressant, Aminoketone

Use Treatment of major depressive disorder, including seasonal affective disorder (SAD); adjunct in smoking cessation

General Dosage Range Dosage adjustment recommended in patients with hepatic impairment

Oral:

Extended release: *Adults:*

Initial: Hydrochloride salt: 150 mg once daily; Maintenance: 300 mg once daily (maximum: 450 mg/day); Hydrobromide salt: 174-522 mg/day

Immediate release hydrochloride salt:

Adults: Initial: 100 mg twice daily; Maintenance: 100 mg 3 times/day (maximum: 450 mg/day)

Elderly: Initial: 37.5 mg twice daily, increase by 37.5-100 mg every 3-4 days as tolerated

Sustained release hydrochloride salt:

Adults: Initial: 150 mg once daily; Maintenance: 150 mg twice daily (maximum: 400 mg/day)

Elderly: Initial: 100 mg/day, increase by 37.5-100 mg every 3-4 days as tolerated

Dosage Forms

Tablet, oral: 75 mg, 100 mg

Wellbutrin®: 75 mg, 100 mg

Tablet, extended release, oral: 100 mg, 150 mg, 200 mg, 300 mg

Aplenzin™: 174 mg, 348 mg, 522 mg

Budeprion SR®: 100 mg, 150 mg

Budeprion XL®: 300 mg

Buproban®: 150 mg

Wellbutrin XL®: 150 mg, 300 mg

Tablet, sustained release, oral:

Wellbutrin SR®: 100 mg, 150 mg, 200 mg

Zyban®: 150 mg

bupropion hydrobromide *see* bupropion *on page 150*

bupropion hydrochloride *see* bupropion *on page 150*

Bupropion SR® (Can) *see* bupropion *on page 150*

Burinex® (Can) *see* bumetanide *on page 147*

Burn Jel® [OTC] *see* lidocaine (topical) *on page 535*

Burn Jel Plus [OTC] *see* lidocaine (topical) *on page 535*

Buscopan® (Can) *see* scopolamine (systemic) *on page 826*

buserelin acetate *see* buserelin *(Canada only) on page 151*

buserelin *(Canada only)* (BYOO se rel in)

Medication Safety Issues

Sound-alike/look-alike issues:

Suprefact® may be confused with Suprane®

Synonyms buserelin acetate

Canadian Brand Names Suprefact®; Suprefact® Depot

Therapeutic Category Luteinizing Hormone-Releasing Hormone Analog

Use Palliative treatment in patients with hormone-dependent advanced prostate cancer (stage D); treatment of endometriosis in women who do not require surgical intervention as first-line therapy (length of therapy is usually 6 months, but no longer than 9 months)

General Dosage Range

Intranasal: *Adults:* 400 mcg (200 mcg into each nostril) 3 times/day

SubQ: *Adults:*

Implants: 6.3 mg every 8 weeks **or** 9.45 mg every 12 weeks

Injection: Initial: 500 mcg every 8 hours for 7 days; maintenance: 200 mcg once daily

Product Availability Not available in U.S.

Dosage Forms - Canada

Implant, subcutaneous:

Suprefact® Depot: 6.3 mg, 9.45 mg

Injection, solution:

Suprefact®: 1 mg/mL (5.5 mL, 10 mL)

Solution, intranasal:

Suprefact®: 1mg/1mL (10 mL)

BuSpar *see* buspirone *on page 152*

BuSpar® (Can) *see* buspirone *on page 152*

buspirone (byoo SPYE rone)

Medication Safety Issues

Sound-alike/look-alike issues:

BusPIRone may be confused with buPROPion

Synonyms BuSpar; buspirone hydrochloride

Tall-Man bus**PIR**one

Canadian Brand Names Apo-Buspirone®; BuSpar®; Bustab®; Dom-Buspirone; Novo-Buspirone; Nu-Buspirone; PMS-Buspirone; Riva-Buspirone

Therapeutic Category Antianxiety Agent

Use Management of generalized anxiety disorder (GAD)

General Dosage Range Oral:

Children ≥6 years: Initial: 5 mg daily; Maintenance: Up to 60 mg/day in 2-3 divided doses

Adults: Initial: 7.5 mg twice daily; Maintenance: Up to 60 mg/day in 2 divided doses (target dose: 10-15 mg twice daily)

Elderly: Initial: 5 mg twice daily; Maintenance: 20-30 mg/day (maximum: 60 mg/day)

Dosage Forms

Tablet, oral: 5 mg, 7.5 mg, 10 mg, 15 mg, 30 mg

buspirone hydrochloride *see* buspirone *on page 152*

bussulfam *see* busulfan *on page 152*

Bustab® (Can) *see* buspirone *on page 152*

busulfan (byoo SUL fan)

Medication Safety Issues

Sound-alike/look-alike issues:

Myleran® may be confused with Alkeran®, Leukeran®, melphalan, Mylicon®

High alert medication:

This medication is in a class the Institute for Safe Medication Practices (ISMP) includes among its list of drug classes which have a heightened risk of causing significant patient harm when used in error.

Synonyms bussulfam; busulfanum; busulphan

U.S. Brand Names Busulfex®; Myleran®

Canadian Brand Names Busulfex®; Myleran®

Therapeutic Category Antineoplastic Agent

Use Palliative treatment of chronic myelogenous leukemia (CML) (oral); conditioning regimen prior to allogeneic hematopoietic progenitor cell transplantation (I.V.) for CML

General Dosage Range

I.V.:

Children ≤12 kg: **HSCT:** 1.1 mg/kg (actual body weight) every 6 hours for 16 doses

Children >12 kg: **HSCT:**0.8 mg/kg (actual body weight) every 6 hours for 16 doses

Adults: **HSCT:** 0.8 mg/kg every 6 hours for 16 doses (use ideal body weight or actual body weight, whichever is lower; use adjusted body weight if obese)

Oral: Dosage adjustment is recommended in patients who experience toxicity:

Children: Induction: 60 mcg/kg/day **or** 1.8 mg/m^2/day; Maintenance: Resume induction dose **or** 1-3 mg/day

Adults: Induction: 60 mcg/kg/day **or** 1.8 mg/m^2/day; usual range: 4-8 mg/day; Maintenance: Resume induction dose **or** 1-3 mg/day

Dosage Forms

Injection, solution:

Busulfex®: 6 mg/mL (10 mL)

Tablet, oral:

Myleran®: 2 mg

busulfanum *see* busulfan *on page 152*

Busulfex® *see* busulfan *on page 152*

busulphan *see* busulfan *on page 152*

butabarbital (byoo ta BAR bi tal)

Medication Safety Issues

Sound-alike/look-alike issues:

Butabarbital may be confused with butalbital

BEERS Criteria medication:

This drug may be potentially inappropriate for use in geriatric patients (Quality of evidence - high; Strength of recommendation - strong).

U.S. Brand Names Butisol Sodium®

Therapeutic Category Barbiturate

Controlled Substance C-III

Use Sedative; hypnotic

General Dosage Range Oral:

Children: 2-6 mg/kg preoperatively (maximum: 100 mg)

Adults: 15-30 mg 3-4 times/day **or** 50-100 mg as a single dose

Dosage Forms

Elixir, oral:

Butisol Sodium®: 30 mg/5 mL (480 mL)

Tablet, oral:

Butisol Sodium®: 30 mg, 50 mg

butalbital, acetaminophen, and caffeine

(byoo TAL bi tal, a seet a MIN oh fen, & KAF een)

Medication Safety Issues

Sound-alike/look-alike issues:

Fioricet® may be confused with Fiorinal®, Florinef®, Lorcet®, Percocet®

Repan® may be confused with Riopan®

Other safety concerns:

Duplicate therapy issues: This product contains acetaminophen, which may be a component of other combination products. Do not exceed the maximum recommended daily dose of acetaminophen.

Synonyms acetaminophen, butalbital, and caffeine

U.S. Brand Names Alagesic LQ; Anolor 300; Dolgic® Plus; Esgic-Plus™; Esgic®; Fioricet®; Margesic; Orbivan™; Repan®; Zebutal®

Therapeutic Category Barbiturate/Analgesic

Use Relief of the symptomatic complex of tension or muscle contraction headache

General Dosage Range Oral: *Adults:* 1-2 tablets/capsules or 15-30 mL every 4 hours (maximum: 6 tablets/capsules daily; 180 mL/day)

Dosage Forms

Capsule, oral:

Anolor 300, Esgic®, Margesic: Butalbital 50 mg, acetaminophen 325 mg, and caffeine 40 mg

Esgic-Plus™, Zebutal®: Butalbital 50 mg, acetaminophen 500 mg, and caffeine 40 mg

Orbivan™: Butalbital 50 mg, acetaminophen 300 mg, and caffeine 40 mg

Liquid, oral:

Alagesic LQ: Butalbital 50 mg, acetaminophen 325 mg, and caffeine 40 mg per 15 mL

Tablet, oral: Butalbital 50 mg, acetaminophen 325 mg, and caffeine 40 mg; butalbital 50 mg, acetaminophen 500 mg, and caffeine 40 mg

Dolgic® Plus: Butalbital 50 mg, acetaminophen 750 mg, and caffeine 40 mg

Esgic®, Fioricet®, Repan®: Butalbital 50 mg, acetaminophen 325 mg, and caffeine 40 mg

Esgic-Plus™: Butalbital 50 mg, acetaminophen 500 mg, and caffeine 40 mg

butalbital, acetaminophen, caffeine, and codeine

(byoo TAL bi tal, a seet a MIN oh fen, KAF een, & KOE deen)

Medication Safety Issues

Sound-alike/look-alike issues:

Fioricet® may be confused with Fiorinal®, Florinef®, Lorcet®, Percocet®

Phrenilin may be confused with Phenergan®

High alert medication:

The Institute for Safe Medication Practices (ISMP) includes this medication among its list of drug classes which have a heightened risk of causing significant patient harm when used in error.

Other safety concerns:

Duplicate therapy issues: This product contains acetaminophen, which may be a component of other combination products. Do not exceed the maximum recommended daily dose of acetaminophen.

Synonyms acetaminophen, caffeine, codeine, and butalbital; caffeine, acetaminophen, butalbital, and codeine; codeine, acetaminophen, butalbital, and caffeine

U.S. Brand Names Fioricet® with Codeine

Therapeutic Category Analgesic Combination (Opioid); Barbiturate

Controlled Substance C-III

Use Relief of symptoms of complex tension (muscle contraction) headache

General Dosage Range **Oral:** *Adults:* 1-2 capsules every 4 hours (maximum: 6 capsules/day)

Dosage Forms

Capsule: Butalbital 50 mg, acetaminophen 325 mg, caffeine 40 mg, and codeine 30 mg

Fioricet® with Codeine: Butalbital 50 mg, acetaminophen 325 mg, caffeine 40 mg, and codeine 30 mg

butalbital and acetaminophen (byoo TAL bi tal & a seet a MIN oh fen)

Medication Safety Issues

Other safety concerns:

Duplicate therapy issues: This product contains acetaminophen, which may be a component of other combination products. Do not exceed the maximum recommended daily dose of acetaminophen.

Synonyms acetaminophen and butalbital

U.S. Brand Names Bupap; Cephadyn [DSC]; Orviban® CF; Phrenilin® Forte; Phrenilin® [DSC]; Promacet; Sedapap®

Therapeutic Category Analgesic, Miscellaneous; Barbiturate

Use Relief of the symptomatic complex of tension or muscle contraction headache

General Dosage Range **Oral:** *Children ≥12 years and Adults:*

Butalbital 50 mg and acetaminophen 300-325 mg: 1-2 tablets every 4 hours as needed (maximum: 6 tablets/24 hours)

Butalbital 50 mg and acetaminophen 650 mg: One tablet/capsule every 4 hours as needed (maximum: 6 doses/24 hours)

Dosage Forms

Tablet, oral: Butalbital 50 mg and acetaminophen 325 mg

Bupap, Promacet, Sedapap®: Butalbital 50 mg and acetaminophen 650 mg

Orbivan® CF: Butalbital 50 mg and acetaminophen 300 mg

Capsule, oral:

Phrenilin® Forte: Butalbital 50 mg and acetaminophen 650 mg

butalbital, aspirin, and caffeine (byoo TAL bi tal, AS pir in, & KAF een)

Medication Safety Issues

Sound-alike/look-alike issues:

Fiorinal® may be confused with Fioricet®, Florical®, Florinef®

Synonyms aspirin, caffeine, and butalbital; butalbital compound

U.S. Brand Names Fiorinal®

Canadian Brand Names Fiorinal®

Therapeutic Category Barbiturate/Analgesic

Controlled Substance C-III

Use Relief of the symptomatic complex of tension or muscle contraction headache

General Dosage Range **Oral:** *Adults:* 1-2 tablets/capsules every 4 hours (maximum: 6 tablets/capsules daily)

Dosage Forms

Capsule: Butalbital 50 mg, aspirin 325 mg, and caffeine 40 mg

Fiorinal®: Butalbital 50 mg, aspirin 325 mg, and caffeine 40 mg

Tablet: Butalbital 50 mg, aspirin 325 mg, and caffeine 40 mg

butalbital, aspirin, caffeine, and codeine

(byoo TAL bi tal, AS pir in, KAF een, & KOE deen)

Medication Safety Issues

Sound-alike/look-alike issues:

Fiorinal® may be confused with Fioricet®, Florical®, Florinef®

High alert medication:

The Institute for Safe Medication Practices (ISMP) includes this medication among its list of drug classes which have a heightened risk of causing significant patient harm when used in error.

Synonyms aspirin, caffeine, codeine, and butalbital; butalbital compound and codeine; codeine and butalbital compound; codeine, butalbital, aspirin, and caffeine

U.S. Brand Names Ascomp® with Codeine; Fiorinal® with Codeine

Canadian Brand Names Fiorinal®-C 1/2; Fiorinal®-C 1/4; Tecnal C 1/2; Tecnal C 1/4

Therapeutic Category Analgesic, Narcotic; Barbiturate

Controlled Substance C-III

Use Relief of symptoms of complex tension (muscle contraction) headache

General Dosage Range Oral: *Adults:* 1-2 capsules every 4 hours as needed (maximum: 6 capsules/day)

Dosage Forms

Capsule: Butalbital 50 mg, aspirin 325 mg, caffeine 40 mg, and codeine 30 mg

Ascomp® with Codeine, Fiorinal® with Codeine: Butalbital 50 mg, aspirin 325 mg, caffeine 40 mg, and codeine 30 mg

butalbital compound *see* butalbital, aspirin, and caffeine *on page* 154

butalbital compound and codeine *see* butalbital, aspirin, caffeine, and codeine *on page* 155

butamben, tetracaine, and benzocaine *see* benzocaine, butamben, and tetracaine *on page* 123

butenafine (byoo TEN a feen)

Medication Safety Issues

Sound-alike/look-alike issues:

Lotrimin may be confused with Lotrisone®

Synonyms butenafine hydrochloride

U.S. Brand Names Lotrimin® ultra™ [OTC]; Mentax®

Therapeutic Category Antifungal Agent

Use Topical treatment of tinea pedis (athlete's foot), tinea cruris (jock itch), tinea corporis (ringworm), and tinea versicolor

General Dosage Range Topical: *Children >12 years and Adults:* Apply to affected area once or twice daily

Dosage Forms

Cream, topical:

Lotrimin® ultra™ [OTC]: 1% (12 g, 24 g)

Mentax®: 1% (15 g, 30 g)

butenafine hydrochloride *see* butenafine *on page* 155

Butisol Sodium® *see* butabarbital *on page* 153

butoconazole (byoo toe KOE na zole)

Synonyms butoconazole nitrate

U.S. Brand Names Gynazole-1® [DSC]

Canadian Brand Names Femstat® One; Gynazole-1®

Therapeutic Category Antifungal Agent

Use Local treatment of vulvovaginal candidiasis

General Dosage Range Intravaginal: *Adults:* Insert 1 applicatorful at bedtime

Dosage Forms

Cream, vaginal:

Gynazole-1®: 2% (5 g)

butoconazole nitrate *see* butoconazole *on page* 155

butorphanol (byoo TOR fa nole)

Medication Safety Issues

Sound-alike/look-alike issues:

Stadol may be confused with Haldol®, sotalol

High alert medication:

The Institute for Safe Medication Practices (ISMP) includes this medication among its list of drug classes which have a heightened risk of causing significant patient harm when used in error.

Synonyms butorphanol tartrate; Stadol

Canadian Brand Names Apo-Butorphanol®; PMS-Butorphanol

Therapeutic Category Analgesic, Narcotic

Controlled Substance C-IV

Use

Parenteral: Management of moderate-to-severe pain; preoperative medication; supplement to balanced anesthesia; management of pain during labor

Nasal spray: Management of moderate-to-severe pain, including migraine headache pain

General Dosage Range Dosage adjustment recommended in patients with hepatic or renal impairment

I.M.:

Adults: Initial: 2 mg, may repeat every 3-4 hours as needed; Usual range: 1-4 mg every 3-4 hours as needed **or** 2 mg prior to surgery

Elderly: Initial: 1/2 of the recommended dose, repeated dosing generally should be at least 6 hours apart

I.V.:

Adults: Initial: 1 mg, may repeat every 3-4 hours as needed; Usual range: 0.5-2 mg every 3-4 hours as needed **or** 2 mg and/or an incremental dose of 0.5-1 mg (up to 0.06 mg/kg) as supplement to surgery

Elderly: Initial: 1/2 of the recommended dose, repeated dosing generally should be at least 6 hours apart

Intranasal:

Adults: Initial: 1 spray (~1 mg) in 1 nostril, may repeat in 60-90 minutes, then repeat initial dose sequence in 3-4 hours after last dose as needed; may use initial dose of 1 spray in each nostril (2 mg) in patients who will remain recumbent

Elderly: Initial: Should not exceed 1 mg, may repeat after 90-120 minutes

Dosage Forms

Injection, solution: 1 mg/mL (1 mL); 2 mg/mL (1 mL, 2 mL, 10 mL)

Injection, solution [preservative free]: 1 mg/mL (1 mL); 2 mg/mL (1 mL, 2 mL)

Solution, intranasal: 10 mg/mL (2.5 mL)

butorphanol tartrate *see* butorphanol *on page 156*

Butrans® *see* buprenorphine *on page 149*

B vitamin combinations *see* vitamin B complex combinations *on page 950*

BW-430C *see* lamotrigine *on page 521*

BW524W91 *see* emtricitabine *on page 328*

Bydureon™ *see* exenatide *on page 369*

Byetta® *see* exenatide *on page 369*

Bystolic® *see* nebivolol *on page 631*

C1 esterase inhibitor *see* C1 inhibitor (human) *on page 156*

C1-INH *see* C1 inhibitor (human) *on page 156*

C1-inhibitor *see* C1 inhibitor (human) *on page 156*

C1INHRP *see* C1 inhibitor (human) *on page 156*

C2B8 monoclonal antibody *see* rituximab *on page 805*

2C4 antibody *see* pertuzumab *on page 710*

C7E3 *see* abciximab *on page 17*

C8-CCK *see* sincalide *on page 835*

311C90 *see* zolmitriptan *on page 966*

C225 *see* cetuximab *on page 192*

C1 inhibitor (human) (cee won in HIB i ter HYU man)

Synonyms C1 esterase inhibitor; C1-INH; C1-inhibitor; C1INHRP; human C1 inhibitor

U.S. Brand Names Berinert®; Cinryze®

Canadian Brand Names Berinert®

Therapeutic Category Blood Product Derivative

Use

Berinert®: Treatment of acute abdominal, facial, or laryngeal attacks of hereditary angioedema (HAE)
Cinryze®: Routine prophylaxis against angioedema attacks in patients with HAE

General Dosage Range **Oral:** *Adolescents and Adults:* Prophylaxis: 1000 units every 3-4 days **or** treatment: 20 units/kg

Dosage Forms

Injection, powder for reconstitution:
Berinert®: 500 units
Cinryze®: 500 units

cabazitaxel (ca baz i TAKS el)

Medication Safety Issues

High alert medication:
This medication is in a class the Institute for Safe Medication Practices (ISMP) includes among its list of drugs which have a heightened risk of causing significant patient harm when used in error.

Administration issues:
Cabazitaxel requires a two-step dilution process prior to administration.

Synonyms RPR-116258A; XRP6258

U.S. Brand Names Jevtana®

Canadian Brand Names Jevtana®

Use Treatment of hormone-refractory metastatic prostate cancer (in patients previously treated with a docetaxel-containing regimen)

General Dosage Range Dosage adjustment recommended in patients with hepatic impairment or who develop toxicities

I.V.: *Adults:* 25 mg/m^2 once every 3 weeks

Dosage Forms

Injection, solution:
Jevtana®: 40 mg/mL (1.5 mL)

cabergoline (ca BER goe leen)

Canadian Brand Names CO Cabergoline; Dostinex®

Therapeutic Category Ergot-like Derivative

Use Treatment of hyperprolactinemic disorders, either idiopathic or due to pituitary adenomas

Canadian labeling: Additional use (not in U.S. labeling): Prevention of the onset of physiological lactation in the puerperium when clinically indicated (eg, still born baby or neonatal death, conditions that interfere with suckling, severe acute or chronic mental illness). **Note:** Not indicated for suppression of established postpartum lactation.

General Dosage Range **Oral:** *Adults:* Initial: 0.25 mg twice weekly; Maintenance: Up to 1 mg twice weekly

Dosage Forms

Tablet, oral: 0.5 mg

Ca-DTPA *see* diethylene triamine penta-acetic acid *on page* 283
Caduet® *see* amlodipine and atorvastatin *on page* 66
CaEDTA *see* edetate CALCIUM disodium *on page* 323
Caelyx® (Can) *see* doxorubicin (liposomal) *on page* 314
Cafcit® *see* caffeine *on page* 157
CAFdA *see* clofarabine *on page* 222
Cafergor® (Can) *see* ergotamine and caffeine *on page* 340
Cafergot® *see* ergotamine and caffeine *on page* 340

caffeine (KAF een)

Synonyms caffeine and sodium benzoate; caffeine citrate; caffeine sodium benzoate; sodium benzoate and caffeine

U.S. Brand Names Cafcit®; Enerjets [OTC]; No Doz® Maximum Strength [OTC]; Vivarin® [OTC]

Therapeutic Category Stimulant

Use
Caffeine citrate: Treatment of idiopathic apnea of prematurity
Caffeine and sodium benzoate: Treatment of acute respiratory depression (not a preferred agent)
Caffeine [OTC labeling]: Restore mental alertness or wakefulness when experiencing fatigue

General Dosage Range

I.M. (caffeine and sodium benzoate):
Children: 8 mg/kg every 4 hours as needed
Adults: 250 mg as a single dose; may repeat as needed (maximum: 500 mg/dose; 2500 mg/day)

I.V.:
Neonates (caffeine citrate): Loading dose: 10-20 mg/kg; Maintenance: 5 mg/kg once daily
Children (caffeine and sodium benzoate): 8 mg/kg every 4 hours as needed
Adults (caffeine and sodium benzoate): 250 mg as a single dose; may repeat as needed (maximum: 500 mg/dose; 2500 mg/day) **or** 300-2000 mg (electroconvulsive therapy)

Oral:
Neonates (caffeine citrate): Loading dose: 10-20 mg/kg; Maintenance: 5 mg/kg once daily
Children ≥12 years and Adults: 100-200 mg every 3-4 hours as needed (OTC labeling)

SubQ (caffeine and sodium benzoate): *Children:* 8 mg/kg every 4 hours as needed

Dosage Forms

Caplet:
No Doz® Maximum Strength [OTC], Vivarin® [OTC]: 200 mg

Injection, solution [preservative free]: 20 mg/mL (3 mL)
Cafcit®: 20 mg/mL (3 mL)

Lozenge:
Enerjets® [OTC]: 75 mg

Solution, oral [preservative free]: 20 mg/mL (3 mL)
Cafcit®: 20 mg/mL

Tablet: 200 mg
Vivarin® [OTC]: 200 mg

caffeine, acetaminophen, and aspirin *see* acetaminophen, aspirin, and caffeine *on page* 26
caffeine, acetaminophen, butalbital, and codeine *see* butalbital, acetaminophen, caffeine, and codeine *on page* 153
caffeine and ergotamine *see* ergotamine and caffeine *on page* 340
caffeine and sodium benzoate *see* caffeine *on page* 157
caffeine, aspirin, and acetaminophen *see* acetaminophen, aspirin, and caffeine *on page* 26
caffeine citrate *see* caffeine *on page* 157
caffeine, dihydrocodeine, and acetaminophen *see* acetaminophen, caffeine, and dihydrocodeine *on page* 26
caffeine, orphenadrine, and aspirin *see* orphenadrine, aspirin, and caffeine *on page* 672
caffeine sodium benzoate *see* caffeine *on page* 157
Cal-C-Caps [OTC] *see* calcium citrate *on page* 164
Caladryl® Clear™ [OTC] *see* pramoxine *on page* 750

calamine (KAL a meen)

Synonyms calamine lotion

Therapeutic Category Topical Skin Product

Use Employed primarily as an astringent, protectant, and soothing agent for conditions such as poison ivy, poison oak, poison sumac, sunburn, insect bites, or minor skin irritations

General Dosage Range Topical: *Children and Adults:* Apply to affected area as often as needed

Dosage Forms

Suspension, topical: 8% (118 mL, 177 mL, 240 mL)

calamine lotion *see* calamine *on page* 158
Calan® *see* verapamil *on page* 942
Calan® SR *see* verapamil *on page* 942
Cal-Cee [OTC] *see* calcium citrate *on page* 164
Calci-Chew® [OTC] *see* calcium carbonate *on page* 161
Calciferol™ [OTC] *see* ergocalciferol *on page* 339
CalciFolic-D™ *see* vitamins (multiple/oral) *on page* 951

Calcijex® *see* calcitriol *on page 160*
Calcimar® (Can) *see* calcitonin *on page 159*
Calci-Mix® [OTC] *see* calcium carbonate *on page 161*
Calcionate [OTC] *see* calcium glubionate *on page 165*

calcipotriene (kal si POE try een)

U.S. Brand Names Calcitrene™; Dovonex®; Sorilux™
Canadian Brand Names Dovonex®
Therapeutic Category Antipsoriatic Agent
Use Treatment of plaque psoriasis (cream, foam, ointment); chronic, moderate-to-severe psoriasis of the scalp (solution)
General Dosage Range Topical: *Adults:* Cream, foam: Apply a thin film to affected area twice daily; Ointment: Apply a thin film to affected area 1-2 times daily; Solution: Apply to affected scalp twice daily
Dosage Forms
Aerosol, foam, topical:
Sorilux™: 0.005% (60 g, 120 g)
Cream, topical: 0.005% (60 g, 120 g)
Dovonex®: 0.005% (60 g, 120 g)
Ointment, topical:
Calcitrene™: 0.005% (60 g)
Solution, topical: 0.005% (60 mL)
Dovonex®: 0.005% (60 mL)

calcipotriene and betamethasone (kal si POE try een & bay ta METH a sone)

Synonyms betamethasone dipropionate and calcipotriene hydrate; calcipotriol and betamethasone dipropionate
U.S. Brand Names Taclonex Scalp®; Taclonex®
Canadian Brand Names Dovobet®; Xamiol®
Therapeutic Category Corticosteroid, Topical; Vitamin D Analog
Use Treatment of psoriasis vulgaris
General Dosage Range Topical: *Adults:* Apply to affected area once daily (maximum: 100 g/week)
Dosage Forms
Ointment, topical:
Taclonex®: Calcipotriene 0.005% and betamethasone 0.064% (60 g, 100 g)
Suspension, topical:
Taclonex Scalp®: Calcipotriene 0.005% and betamethasone 0.064%
Dosage Forms - Canada
Gel, topical:
Xamiol®: Calcipotriol 50 mcg/g and betamethasone 0.5 mg/g (30 g, 60 g, 2 x 60 g)
Ointment, topical:
Dovobet®: Calcipotriol 50 mcg/g and betamethasone 0.5 mg/g (30 g, 60 g, 120 g)

calcipotriol and betamethasone dipropionate *see* calcipotriene and betamethasone *on page 159*
Calcite-500 (Can) *see* calcium carbonate *on page 161*

calcitonin (kal si TOE nin)

Medication Safety Issues
Sound-alike/look-alike issues:
Calcitonin may be confused with calcitriol
Miacalcin® may be confused with Micatin®
Administration issues:
Calcitonin nasal spray is administered as a single spray into **one** nostril daily, using alternate nostrils each day.
Synonyms calcitonin (salmon)
U.S. Brand Names Fortical®; Miacalcin®
Canadian Brand Names Apo-Calcitonin®; Calcimar®; Caltine®; Miacalcin® NS; PRO-Calcitonin; Sandoz-Calcitonin
Therapeutic Category Polypeptide Hormone

Use Treatment of Paget disease of bone (osteitis deformans); adjunctive therapy for hypercalcemia; treatment of osteoporosis in women >5 years postmenopause

General Dosage Range

I.M., SubQ: *Adults:* Paget disease/osteoporosis: 50-100 units every 1-3 days; Hypercalcemia: 4-8 units/kg every 12 hours (maximum: 8 units/kg every 6 hours)

Intranasal: *Adults:* 200 units (1 spray) in one nostril daily

Dosage Forms

Injection, solution:

Miacalcin®: 200 units/mL (2 mL)

Solution, intranasal: 200 units/actuation (3.7 mL)

Fortical®: 200 units/actuation (3.7 mL)

Miacalcin®: 200 units/actuation (3.7 mL)

calcitonin (salmon) *see* calcitonin *on page* 159

Calcitrate [OTC] *see* calcium citrate *on page* 164

Cal-Citrate™ 225 [OTC] *see* calcium citrate *on page* 164

Calcitrene™ *see* calcipotriene *on page* 159

calcitriol (kal si TRYE ole)

Medication Safety Issues

Sound-alike/look-alike issues:

Calcitriol may be confused with alfacalcidol, Calciferol™, calcitonin, calcium carbonate, captopril, colestipol, paricalcitol, ropinirole

Administration issues:

Dosage is expressed in mcg (micrograms), **not** mg (milligrams); rare cases of acute overdose have been reported

Synonyms 1,25 dihydroxycholecalciferol

U.S. Brand Names Calcijex®; Rocaltrol®; Vectical®

Canadian Brand Names Calcijex®; Rocaltrol®

Therapeutic Category Vitamin D Analog

Use

Oral, injection: Management of hypocalcemia in patients on chronic renal dialysis; management of secondary hyperparathyroidism in patients with chronic kidney disease (CKD); management of hypocalcemia in hypoparathyroidism and pseudohypoparathyroidism

Topical: Management of mild-to-moderate plaque psoriasis

General Dosage Range Dosage adjustment recommended in patients who develop toxicities

I.V.: *Adults:* 0.5-4 mcg 3 times/week

Oral:

Children: 0.25-2 mcg/day **or** 0.01-0.015 mcg/kg/day (maximum: 0.5 mcg/day)

Adults: 0.25 mcg every other day to 2 mcg once daily

Topical: *Adults:* Apply to affected areas twice daily (maximum: 200 g/week)

Dosage Forms

Capsule, softgel, oral: 0.25 mcg, 0.5 mcg

Rocaltrol®: 0.25 mcg, 0.5 mcg

Injection, solution: 1 mcg/mL (1 mL)

Calcijex®: 1 mcg/mL (1 mL)

Ointment, topical:

Vectical®: 3 mcg/g (100 g)

Solution, oral: 1 mcg/mL (15 mL)

Rocaltrol®: 1 mcg/mL (15 mL)

calcium acetate (KAL see um AS e tate)

Medication Safety Issues

Sound-alike/look-alike issues:

PhosLo® may be confused with Phos-Flur®, ProSom

U.S. Brand Names Eliphos™; PhosLo®; Phoslyra™

Canadian Brand Names PhosLo®

Therapeutic Category Electrolyte Supplement, Oral

Use Control of hyperphosphatemia in end-stage renal failure; does not promote aluminum absorption

General Dosage Range Oral: *Adults:* Initial: 1334 mg with each meal; Maintenance: 2001-2668 mg with each meal

Dosage Forms

Gelcap, oral: 667 mg

PhosLo®: 667 mg

Solution, oral:

Phoslyra™: 667 mg/5 mL (473 mL)

Tablet, oral:

Eliphos™: 667 mg

calcium acetate and aluminum sulfate *see* aluminum sulfate and calcium acetate *on page* 57

calcium acetylhomotaurinate *see* acamprosate *on page* 18

calcium and vitamin D (KAL see um & VYE ta min dee)

Medication Safety Issues

Sound-alike/look-alike issues:

Os-Cal® may be confused with Asacol®

Synonyms vitamin D and calcium carbonate

U.S. Brand Names Cal-CYUM [OTC]; Caltrate® 600+D [OTC]; Caltrate® 600+Soy™ [OTC]; Caltrate® ColonHealth™ [OTC]; Chew-Cal [OTC]; Citracal® Maximum [OTC]; Citracal® Petites [OTC]; Citracal® Regular [OTC]; Liqua-Cal [OTC]; Os-Cal® 500+D [OTC]; Oysco 500+D [OTC]; Oysco D [OTC]; Oyst-Cal-D 500 [OTC]

Therapeutic Category Calcium Salt; Electrolyte Supplement, Oral; Vitamin, Fat Soluble

Use Dietary supplement, antacid

Dosage Forms

Caplet, oral:

Citracal® Maximum [OTC]: Calcium 315 mg and vitamin D 250 units

Capsule, softgel, oral: Calcium 500 mg and vitamin D 500 units; calcium 600 mg and vitamin D 100 units; calcium 600 mg and vitamin D 200 units

Liqua-Cal [OTC]: Calcium 600 mg and vitamin D 200 units

Tablet, oral: Calcium 250 mg and vitamin D 125 units; calcium 500 mg and vitamin D 125 units; calcium 500 mg and vitamin D 200 units; calcium 600 mg and vitamin D 125 units; calcium 600 mg and vitamin D 200 units

Caltrate® 600+D [OTC]: Calcium 600 mg and vitamin D 200 units

Caltrate® 600+Soy™ [OTC]: Calcium 600 mg and vitamin D 200 units

Caltrate® ColonHealth™ [OTC]: Calcium 600 mg and vitamin D 200 units

Citracal® Petites [OTC]: Calcium 200 mg and vitamin D 250 units

Citracal® Regular [OTC]: Calcium 250 mg and vitamin D 200 units

Oysco D [OTC]: Calcium 250 mg and vitamin D 125 units

Oysco 500+D [OTC]: Calcium 500 mg and vitamin D 200 units

Oyst-Cal-D 500 [OTC]: Calcium 500 mg and vitamin D 200 units

Tablet, chewable: Calcium 500 mg and vitamin D 100 units; calcium 600 mg and vitamin D 400 units

Os-Cal® 500+D [OTC]: Calcium 500 mg and vitamin D 400 units

Wafer, chewable:

Cal-CYUM [OTC]: Calcium 519 mg and vitamin D 150 units (50s)

Chew-Cal [OTC]: Calcium 333 mg and vitamin D 40 units (100s, 250s)

calcium carbonate (KAL see um KAR bun ate)

Medication Safety Issues

Sound-alike/look-alike issues:

Calcium carbonate may be confused with calcitriol

Florical® may be confused with Fiorinal®

Mylanta® may be confused with Mynatal®

Nephro-Calci® may be confused with Nephrocaps®

International issues:

Remegel [Hungary, Great Britain, and Ireland] may be confused with Renagel brand name for sevelamer [U.S., Canada, and multiple international markets]

Remegel: Brand name for calcium carbonate [Hungary, Great Britain, and Ireland], but also the brand name for aluminum hydroxide and magnesium carbonate [Netherlands]

Synonyms oscal

U.S. Brand Names Alcalak [OTC]; Alka-Mints® [OTC]; Cal-Gest® [OTC]; Cal-Mint [OTC]; Calci-Chew® [OTC]; Calci-Mix® [OTC]; Caltrate® 600 [OTC]; Children's Pepto [OTC]; Chooz® [OTC]; Florical® [OTC]; Maalox® Children's [OTC]; Maalox® Regular Strength [OTC]; Nephro-Calci® [OTC]; Nutralox® [OTC]; Oysco 500 [OTC]; Oystercal™ 500 [OTC]; Rolaids® Extra Strength [OTC]; Super Calcium 600 [OTC]; Titralac™ [OTC]; Tums® E-X [OTC]; Tums® Extra Strength Sugar Free [OTC]; Tums® Quickpak [OTC]; Tums® Smoothies™ [OTC]; Tums® Ultra [OTC]; Tums® [OTC]

Canadian Brand Names Apo-Cal®; Calcite-500; Caltrate®; Caltrate® Select; Os-Cal®; Tums Extra Strength; Tums Smoothies; Tums® Chews Extra Strength; Tums® Regular Strength; Tums® Ultra Strength

Therapeutic Category Antacid; Electrolyte Supplement, Oral

Use As an antacid; treatment and prevention of calcium deficiency or hyperphosphatemia (eg, osteoporosis, osteomalacia, mild/moderate renal insufficiency, hypoparathyroidism, postmenopausal osteoporosis, rickets); has been used to bind phosphate

General Dosage Range Oral:

Children <2 years: 45-65 mg/kg/day in 4 divided doses
Children 1-6 months: Adequate intake: 200 mg/day
Children 7-12 months: Adequate intake: 260 mg/day
Children 1-3 years: RDA: 700 mg/day
Children 2-5 years (24-47 lbs): Antacid: 161 mg (elemental calcium) as needed (maximum: 483 mg/day); Hypocalcemia: 45-65 mg/kg/day in 4 divided doses
Children 4-8 years: RDA: 1000 mg/day
Children 6-11 years (48-95 lbs): Antacid: 322 mg (elemental calcium) as needed (maximum: 966 mg/day); Hypocalcemia: 45-65 mg/kg/day in 4 divided doses
Children 9-18 years: RDA: 1300 mg/day
Children >11 years: 45-65 mg/kg/day in 4 divided doses
Adults 19-50 years: RDA: 1000 mg/day
Adults ≤51 years: Antacid: 1-2 tablets or 5-10 mL every 2 hours (maximum: 7000 mg/day); Hypocalcemia/dietary: 500-2000 mg/day in 2-4 divided doses
Adults ≥51 years, females: RDA: 1200 mg/day
Adults >51 years: Antacid: 1-2 tablets or 5-10 mL every 2 hours (maximum: 7000 mg/day); Hypocalcemia/dietary: 500-2000 mg/day in 2-4 divided doses; Osteoporosis: 1200 mg/day
Adults 51-70 years, males: RDA: 1000 mg/day
Adults >70 years, males: RDA: 1200 mg/day

Dosage Forms

Capsule, oral:
Calci-Mix® [OTC]: 1250 mg
Florical® [OTC]: 364 mg

Gum, chewing, oral:
Chooz® [OTC]: 500 mg (12s)

Powder, oral: (480 g)
Tums® Quickpak [OTC]: 1000 mg/packet (24s)

Suspension, oral: 1250 mg/5 mL (5 mL, 473 mL, 500 mL)

Tablet, oral: 648 mg, 650 mg, 1250 mg, 1500 mg
Caltrate® 600 [OTC]: 1500 mg
Florical® [OTC]: 364 mg
Nephro-Calci® [OTC]: 1500 mg
Oysco 500 [OTC]: 1250 mg
Oystercal™ 500 [OTC]: 1250 mg
Super Calcium 600 [OTC]: 1500 mg

Tablet, chewable, oral: 420 mg, 500 mg, 650 mg, 750 mg, 1250 mg
Alcalak [OTC]: 420 mg
Alka-Mints® [OTC]: 850 mg
Cal-Gest® [OTC]: 500 mg
Cal-Mint [OTC]: 650 mg
Calci-Chew® [OTC]: 1250 mg
Children's Pepto [OTC]: 400 mg
Maalox® Children's [OTC]: 400 mg
Maalox® Regular Strength [OTC]: 600 mg
Nutralox® [OTC]: 420 mg
Titralac™ [OTC]: 420 mg
Tums® [OTC]: 500 mg

Tums® E-X [OTC]: 750 mg
Tums® Extra Strength Sugar Free [OTC]: 750 mg
Tums® Smoothies™ [OTC]: 750 mg
Tums® Ultra [OTC]: 1000 mg

Tablet, softchew, oral:
Rolaids® Extra Strength [OTC]: 1177 mg

calcium carbonate and etidronate disodium *see* etidronate and calcium carbonate *(Canada only)* *on page 364*

calcium carbonate and magnesium hydroxide

(KAL see um KAR bun ate & mag NEE zhum hye DROKS ide)

Medication Safety Issues

Sound-alike/look-alike issues:
Mylanta® may be confused with Mynatal®

Synonyms magnesium hydroxide and calcium carbonate

U.S. Brand Names Mi-Acid™ Double Strength [OTC]; Mylanta® Gelcaps® [OTC]; Mylanta® Supreme [OTC]; Mylanta® Ultra [OTC]; Rolaids® Extra Strength [OTC]; Rolaids® [OTC]

Therapeutic Category Antacid

Use Hyperacidity

General Dosage Range Oral: *Adults:* 2-4 tablets between meals and at bedtime

Dosage Forms

Gelcap:
Mylanta® Gelcaps® [OTC]: Calcium carbonate 550 mg and magnesium hydroxide 125 mg

Liquid:
Mylanta® Supreme [OTC]: Calcium carbonate 400 mg and magnesium hydroxide 135 mg per 5 mL

Tablet, chewable: Calcium carbonate 550 mg and magnesium hydroxide 110 mg; calcium carbonate 675 mg and magnesium hydroxide 135 mg; calcium carbonate 700 mg and magnesium hydroxide 300 mg
Mi-Acid™ Double Strength [OTC], Mylanta® Ultra [OTC]: Calcium carbonate 700 mg and magnesium hydroxide 300 mg
Rolaids® [OTC]: Calcium carbonate 550 mg and magnesium hydroxide 110 mg
Rolaids® Extra Strength [OTC]: Calcium carbonate 675 mg and magnesium hydroxide 135 mg

calcium carbonate and simethicone (KAL see um KAR bun ate & sye METH i kone)

Medication Safety Issues

International issues:
Remegel Wind Relief [Great Britain] may be confused with Renagel brand name for sevelamer [U.S., Canada, and multiple international markets]

Synonyms simethicone and calcium carbonate

U.S. Brand Names Gas Ban™ [OTC]; Maalox® Advanced Maximum Strength [OTC]; Maalox® Junior Plus Antigas [OTC]; Titralac® Plus [OTC]

Therapeutic Category Antacid; Antiflatulent

Use Relief of acid indigestion, heartburn, bloating, pressure, and discomfort of gas

General Dosage Range Oral:

Children 6-11 years: Maalox® Junior Plus Antigas: Two tablets as symptoms occur or as directed by healthcare provider (maximum: 6 tablets/24 hours)

Children ≥12 years; Maalox® Advanced Maximum Strength: 1-2 tablets as symptoms occur or as directed by healthcare provider (maximum: 8 tablets/24 hours)

Adults: Maalox® Advanced Maximum Strength: 1-2 tablets as symptoms occur or as directed by healthcare provider (maximum: 8 tablets/24 hours); Titralac® Plus: Two tablets every 2-3 hours as needed (maximum: 19 tablets/24 hours)

Dosage Forms

Tablet, chewable:
Gas Ban™ [OTC]: Calcium carbonate 300 mg and simethicone 40 mg
Maalox® Advanced Maximum Strength [OTC]: Calcium carbonate 1000 mg and simethicone 60 mg
Maalox® Junior Plus Antigas [OTC]: Calcium carbonate 400 mg and simethicone 24 mg
Titralac® Plus [OTC]: Calcium carbonate 420 mg and simethicone 21 mg

calcium carbonate, folic acid, and magnesium carbonate *see* magnesium carbonate, calcium carbonate, and folic acid *on page 557*

calcium carbonate, magnesium hydroxide, and famotidine *see* famotidine, calcium carbonate, and magnesium hydroxide *on page 373*

calcium chloride (KAL see um KLOR ide)

Medication Safety Issues

Sound-alike/look-alike issues:

Calcium chloride may be confused with calcium gluconate

Administration issues:

Calcium chloride may be confused with calcium gluconate.

Confusion with the different intravenous salt forms of calcium has occurred. There is a threefold difference in the primary cation concentration between calcium chloride (in which 1 g = 14 mEq [270 mg] of elemental Ca++) and calcium gluconate (in which 1 g = 4.65 mEq [90 mg] of elemental Ca++).

Prescribers should specify which salt form is desired. Dosages should be expressed either as mEq, mg, or grams of the salt form.

Therapeutic Category Electrolyte Supplement, Oral

Use Treatment of hypocalcemia and conditions secondary to hypocalcemia (eg, tetany, seizures, arrhythmias); emergent treatment of severe hypermagnesemia

General Dosage Range I.V.: *Infants, Children, and Adults:* Dosage varies greatly depending on indication

Dosage Forms

Injection, solution: 10% (10 mL)

Injection, solution [preservative free]: 10% (10 mL)

calcium citrate (KAL see um SIT rate)

Medication Safety Issues

Sound-alike/look-alike issues:

Citracal® may be confused with Citrucel®

U.S. Brand Names Cal-C-Caps [OTC]; Cal-Cee [OTC]; Cal-Citrate™ 225 [OTC]; Calcitrate [OTC]

Canadian Brand Names Osteocit®

Therapeutic Category Electrolyte Supplement, Oral

Use Dietary supplement

General Dosage Range Oral:

Children 1-6 months: Adequate intake: 200 mg/day
Children 7-12 months: Adequate intake: 260 mg/day
Children 1-3 years: RDA: 700 mg/day
Children 4-8 years: RDA: 1000 mg/day
Children 9-18 years: RDA: 1300 mg/day
Adults: 500-2000 mg divided 2-4 times/day
Adults 19-50 years: RDA: 1000 mg/day
Adults ≥51 years, females: RDA: 1200 mg/day
Adults 51-70 years, males: RDA: 1000 mg/day
Adults >70 years, males: RDA: 1200 mg/day

Dosage Forms

Capsule, oral:

Cal-C-Caps [OTC]: Elemental calcium 180 mg
Cal-Citrate™ 225 [OTC]: Elemental calcium 225 mg

Granules, oral: (480 g)

Tablet, oral: Elemental calcium 250 mg

Cal-Cee [OTC]: Elemental calcium 250 mg
Calcitrate [OTC]: Elemental calcium 200 mg

calcium diethylene triamine penta-acetic acid (Ca-DTPA) *see* diethylene triamine penta-acetic acid *on page 283*

calcium disodium edetate *see* edetate CALCIUM disodium *on page 323*

calcium disodiumethylenediaminetetraacetic acid *see* edetate CALCIUM disodium *on page 323*

Calcium Disodium Versenate® *see* edetate CALCIUM disodium *on page 323*

calcium folinate *see* leucovorin calcium *on page 527*

calcium glubionate (KAL see um gloo BYE oh nate)

Medication Safety Issues

Sound-alike/look-alike issues:

Calcium glubionate may be confused with calcium gluconate

U.S. Brand Names Calcionate [OTC]

Therapeutic Category Electrolyte Supplement, Oral

Use Dietary supplement

General Dosage Range Oral:

Children 1-6 months: Adequate intake: 200 mg/day
Children 7-12 months: Adequate intake: 260 mg/day
Children 1-3 years: RDA: 700 mg/day
Children 4-8 years: RDA: 1000 mg/day
Children 9-18 years: RDA: 1300 mg/day
Adults 19-50 years: RDA: 1000 mg/day
Adults ≥51 years, females: RDA: 1200 mg/day
Adults 51-70 years, males: RDA: 1000 mg/day
Adults >70 years, males: RDA: 1200 mg/day

Dosage Forms

Syrup, oral:

Calcionate [OTC]: 1.8 g/5 mL (473 mL)

calcium gluconate (KAL see um GLOO koe nate)

Medication Safety Issues

Sound-alike/look-alike issues:

Calcium gluconate may be confused with calcium glubionate, cupric sulfate

Administration issues:

Calcium gluconate may be confused with calcium chloride.

Confusion with the different intravenous salt forms of calcium has occurred. There is a threefold difference in the primary cation concentration between calcium gluconate (in which 1 g = 4.65 mEq [90 mg] of elemental Ca++) and calcium chloride (in which 1 g = 14 mEq [270 mg] of elemental Ca++).

Prescribers should specify which salt form is desired. Dosages should be expressed either as mEq, mg, or grams of the salt form.

U.S. Brand Names Cal-G [OTC] [DSC]; Cal-GLU™ [OTC]

Therapeutic Category Electrolyte Supplement, Oral

Use

I.V.: Treatment of hypocalcemia and conditions secondary to hypocalcemia (eg, tetany, seizures, arrhythmias); treatment of cardiac disturbances secondary to hyperkalemia; adjunctive treatment of rickets, osteomalacia, and magnesium sulfate overdose; decrease capillary permeability in allergic conditions, nonthrombocytopenic purpura, and exudative dermatoses (eg, dermatitis herpetiformis, pruritus secondary to certain drugs)

Oral: Dietary calcium supplementation

General Dosage Range

I.V.: *Children and Adults:* Dosage varies greatly depending on indication

Oral:

Children 1-6 months: Adequate intake: 200 mg **elemental calcium** daily
Children 7-12 months: Adequate intake: 260 mg **elemental calcium** daily
Children 1-3 years: RDA: 700 mg **elemental calcium** daily
Children 4-8 years: RDA: 1000 mg **elemental calcium** daily
Children 9-18 years: RDA: 1300 mg **elemental calcium** daily
Adults 19-50 years: RDA: 1000 mg **elemental calcium** daily
Adults ≥51 years, females: RDA: 1200 mg **elemental calcium** daily
Adults 51-70 years, males: RDA: 1000 mg **elemental calcium** daily
Adults >70 years, males: RDA: 1200 mg **elemental calcium** daily

Dosage Forms

Capsule, oral:

Cal-GLU™ [OTC]: 515 mg

Injection, solution [preservative free]: 10% (10 mL, 50 mL, 100 mL, 200 mL)

Powder, oral: (480 g)

Tablet, oral: 500 mg, 648 mg

calcium lactate (KAL see um LAK tate)

Therapeutic Category Electrolyte Supplement, Oral

Use Treatment and prevention of calcium depletion

General Dosage Range Oral:

Children 1-6 months: Adequate intake: 200 mg/day
Children 7-12 months: Adequate intake: 260 mg/day
Children 1-3 years: RDA: 700 mg/day
Children 4-8 years: RDA: 1000 mg/day
Children 9-18 years: RDA: 1300 mg/day
Adults 19-50 years: RDA: 1000 mg/day
Adults ≥51 years, females: RDA: 1200 mg/day
Adults 51-70 years, males: RDA: 1000 mg/day
Adults >70 years, males: RDA: 1200 mg/day

Dosage Forms

Tablet, oral: 648 mg

calcium leucovorin *see* leucovorin calcium *on page 527*
calcium levoleucovorin *see* LEVOleucovorin *on page 532*
calcium pantothenate *see* pantothenic acid *on page 690*

calcium phosphate (tribasic) (KAL see um FOS fate tri BAY sik)

Synonyms tricalcium phosphate

U.S. Brand Names Posture® [OTC]

Therapeutic Category Electrolyte Supplement, Oral

Use Dietary supplement

General Dosage Range Oral:

Children 1-6 months: Adequate intake: 200 mg/day
Children 7-12 months: Adequate intake: 260 mg/day
Children 1-3 years: RDA: 700 mg/day
Children 4-8 years: RDA: 1000 mg/day
Children 9-18 years: RDA: 1300 mg/day
Adults: 2 tablets daily
Adults 19-50 years: RDA: 1000 mg/day
Adults ≥51 years, females: RDA: 1200 mg/day
Adults 51-70 years, males: RDA: 1000 mg/day
Adults >70 years, males: RDA: 1200 mg/day

Dosage Forms

Caplet:

Posture® [OTC]: Calcium 600 mg and phosphorus 280 mg

calcium polystyrene sulfonate *(Canada only)* (KAL see um pol i STI reen sul fo NATE)

Medication Safety Issues

Sound-alike/look-alike issues:

Calcium polystyrene sulfonate may be confused with sodium polystyrene sulfonate

Synonyms calcium polystyrene sulphonate

Canadian Brand Names Resonium Calcium®

Therapeutic Category Antidote

Use Treatment of hyperkalemia

General Dosage Range

Oral:

Children: 0.5-1 g/kg/day
Adults: 15 g 3-4 times/day

Rectal:

Children: 0.5-1 g/kg/day
Adults: 30 g once daily

Product Availability Not available in U.S.

Dosage Forms - Canada

Powder for suspension, oral/rectal:

Resonium Calcium®: 300 g

calcium polystyrene sulphonate *see* calcium polystyrene sulfonate *(Canada only) on page 166*
Cal-CYUM [OTC] *see* calcium and vitamin D *on page 161*
Caldecort® [OTC] *see* hydrocortisone (topical) *on page 457*
Caldolor® *see* ibuprofen *on page 468*

calfactant (kaf AKT ant)

Synonyms bovine lung surfactant

U.S. Brand Names Infasurf®

Therapeutic Category Lung Surfactant

Use Prevention of respiratory distress syndrome (RDS) in premature infants at high risk for RDS and for the treatment ("rescue") of premature infants who develop RDS

Prophylaxis: Therapy at birth with calfactant is indicated for premature infants <29 weeks of gestational age at significant risk for RDS. Should be administered as soon as possible, preferably within 30 minutes after birth.

Treatment: For infants ≤72 hours of age with RDS (confirmed by clinical and radiologic findings) and requiring endotracheal intubation.

General Dosage Range Intratracheal: *Premature infants:* 3 mL/kg (body weight at birth) every 12 hours for a total of 3 doses

Dosage Forms

Suspension, intratracheal [preservative free]:
Infasurf®: 35 mg phospholipids and 0.7 mg protein per mL (3 mL, 6 mL)

Cal-G [OTC] [DSC] *see* calcium gluconate *on page 165*
Cal-Gest® [OTC] *see* calcium carbonate *on page 161*
Cal-GLU™ [OTC] *see* calcium gluconate *on page 165*
Callergy Clear [OTC] *see* pramoxine *on page 750*
Cal-Mint [OTC] *see* calcium carbonate *on page 161*
Calmoseptine® [OTC] *see* menthol and zinc oxide (topical) *on page 574*
Calmylin with Codeine (Can) *see* guaifenesin, pseudoephedrine, and codeine *on page 437*
Caltine® (Can) *see* calcitonin *on page 159*
Caltrate® (Can) *see* calcium carbonate *on page 161*
Caltrate® 600 [OTC] *see* calcium carbonate *on page 161*
Caltrate® 600+D [OTC] *see* calcium and vitamin D *on page 161*
Caltrate® 600+Soy™ [OTC] *see* calcium and vitamin D *on page 161*
Caltrate® ColonHealth™ [OTC] *see* calcium and vitamin D *on page 161*
Caltrate® Select (Can) *see* calcium carbonate *on page 161*
Cambia™ *see* diclofenac (systemic) *on page 279*
Cambia® (Can) *see* diclofenac (systemic) *on page 279*
Camila® *see* norethindrone *on page 648*
Campath® [DSC] *see* alemtuzumab *on page 45*
campath-1H *see* alemtuzumab *on page 45*
Campho-Phenique® [OTC] *see* camphor and phenol *on page 167*

camphor and phenol (KAM for & FEE nole)

Synonyms phenol and camphor

U.S. Brand Names Campho-Phenique® [OTC]

Therapeutic Category Topical Skin Product

Use Relief of pain and itching associated with minor burns, sunburn, minor cuts, insect bites, minor skin irritation; temporary relief of pain from cold sores

General Dosage Range Topical: *Adults:* Apply 1-3 times/day

Dosage Forms

Gel, topical:
Campho-Phenique® [OTC]: Camphor 10.8% and phenol 4.7% (7 g, 14 g)

Liquid, topical: Camphor 10.8% and phenol 4.7% (45 mL)
Campho-Phenique® [OTC]: Camphor 10.8% and phenol 4.7% (22.5 mL, 45 mL)

camphorated tincture of opium (error-prone synonym) *see* paregoric *on page 692*

Campral® *see* acamprosate *on page* 18
Camptosar® *see* irinotecan *on page* 501
camptothecin-11 *see* irinotecan *on page* 501
camrese™ *see* ethinyl estradiol and levonorgestrel *on page* 357

canakinumab (can a KIN ue mab)

Synonyms ACZ885

U.S. Brand Names Ilaris®

Canadian Brand Names Ilaris™

Therapeutic Category Interleukin-1 Beta Inhibitor; Interleukin-1 Inhibitor; Monoclonal Antibody

Use Treatment of Cryopyrin-Associated Periodic Syndromes (CAPS), including familial cold autoinflammatory syndrome (FCAS) and Muckle-Wells syndrome (MWS)

General Dosage Range SubQ:

Children ≥4 years and 15-40 kg: 2-3 mg/kg every 8 weeks

Children ≥4 years and Adults >40 kg: 150 mg every 8 weeks

Dosage Forms

Injection, powder for reconstitution:

Ilaris®: 180 mg

Dosage Forms - Canada

Injection, powder for reconstitution:

Ilaris™: 150 mg

Canasa® *see* mesalamine *on page* 577
Cancidas® *see* caspofungin *on page* 180

candesartan (kan de SAR tan)

Medication Safety Issues

Sound-alike/look-alike issues:

Atacand® may be confused with antacid

Synonyms candesartan cilexetil

U.S. Brand Names Atacand®

Canadian Brand Names Apo-Candesartan; Atacand®; CO Candesartan; JAMP-Candesartan; Mylan-Candesartan; Sandoz-Candesartan; Teva-Candesartan

Therapeutic Category Angiotensin II Receptor Antagonist

Use Alone or in combination with other antihypertensive agents in treating hypertension; treatment of heart failure (NYHA class II-IV)

General Dosage Range Oral:

Children 1 to <6 years: Initial: 0.2 mg/kg/day in 1-2 divided doses; Maintenance: 0.05-0.4 mg/kg/day in 1-2 divided doses (maximum daily dose: 0.4 mg/kg/day)

Children 6 to <17 years: Initial: <50 kg: 4-8 mg/day in 1-2 divided doses; >50 kg: 8-16 mg/day in 1-2 divided doses; Maintenance: 2-32 mg/day in 1-2 divided doses (maximum daily dose: 32 mg/day)

Adults: Initial: 4-16 mg once daily; Maintenance: 4-32 mg/day in 1-2 divided doses

Dosage Forms

Tablet, oral:

Atacand®: 4 mg, 8 mg, 16 mg, 32 mg

candesartan and hydrochlorothiazide (kan de SAR tan & hye droe klor oh THYE a zide)

Synonyms candesartan cilexetil and hydrochlorothiazide; hydrochlorothiazide and candesartan

U.S. Brand Names Atacand HCT®

Canadian Brand Names Atacand® Plus

Therapeutic Category Antihypertensive Agent, Combination

Use Treatment of hypertension; combination product should not be used for initial therapy

General Dosage Range Oral: *Adults:* Candesartan 16-32 mg/day in 1-2 divided doses and hydrochlorothiazide 12.5-25 mg once daily

Dosage Forms

Tablet:

Atacand HCT®: 16/12.5: Candesartan 16 mg and hydrochlorothiazide 12.5 mg; 32/12.5: Candesartan 32 mg and hydrochlorothiazide 12.5 mg; 32/25: Candesartan 32 mg and hydrochlorothiazide 25 mg

candesartan cilexetil *see* candesartan *on page 168*

candesartan cilexetil and hydrochlorothiazide *see* candesartan and hydrochlorothiazide *on page 168*

Candida albicans (Monilia) (KAN dee da AL bi kans mo NIL ya)

Synonyms *Monilia* skin test

U.S. Brand Names Candin®

Therapeutic Category Diagnostic Agent

Use Screen for detection of nonresponsiveness to antigens in immunocompromised individuals

General Dosage Range Intradermal: *Children and Adults:* 0.1 mL

Dosage Forms

Injection, solution:

Candin®: 0.1 mL/dose (1 mL)

Candin® *see Candida albicans (Monilia) on page 169*

Candistatin® (Can) *see* nystatin (topical) *on page 657*

CanesOral® (Can) *see* fluconazole *on page 388*

Canesten® Topical (Can) *see* clotrimazole (topical) *on page 227*

Canesten® Vaginal (Can) *see* clotrimazole (topical) *on page 227*

Cankaid® [OTC] *see* carbamide peroxide *on page 173*

cannabidiol and tetrahydrocannabinol *see* tetrahydrocannabinol and cannabidiol *(Canada only) on page 884*

Canthacur-PS® (Can) *see* cantharidin, podophyllin resin, and salicylic acid *(Canada only) on page 169*

cantharidin, podophyllin, and salicylic acid *see* cantharidin, podophyllin resin, and salicylic acid *(Canada only) on page 169*

cantharidin, podophyllin resin, and salicylic acid *(Canada only)*

(kan THAR e din, po DOF fil um REZ in & sal i SIL ik AS id)

Synonyms cantharidin, podophyllin, and salicylic acid

Canadian Brand Names Canthacur-PS®; Cantharone® Plus

Therapeutic Category Keratolytic Agent

Use For removal of warts especially plantar, mosaic, and periungual; recommended for resistant and heavily keratinized warts; useful where painless application is desired. Canthacur-PS® is also indicated for removal of molluscum contagiosum.

General Dosage Range Topical: *Children ≥12 years and Adults:* Applied by physician only.

Product Availability Not available in the U.S.

Dosage Forms - Canada

Liquid:

Canthacur-PS®: Cantharidin 1%, podophyllin 5%, and salicylic acid 30% in a film-forming vehicle (7.5 mL)

Cantharone® Plus: Cantharidin 1%, podophyllin 2%, and salicylic acid 30% in a film-forming vehicle (7.5 mL)

Cantharone® Plus (Can) *see* cantharidin, podophyllin resin, and salicylic acid *(Canada only) on page 169*

Cantil® *see* mepenzolate *on page 574*

Capastat® Sulfate *see* capreomycin *on page 170*

CAPE *see* capecitabine *on page 170*

capecitabine (ka pe SITE a been)

Medication Safety Issues

Sound-alike/look-alike issues:

Xeloda® may be confused with Xenical®

High alert medication:

This medication is in a class the Institute for Safe Medication Practices (ISMP) includes among its list of drug classes which have a heightened risk of causing significant patient harm when used in error.

Synonyms CAPE

U.S. Brand Names Xeloda®

Canadian Brand Names Xeloda®

Therapeutic Category Antineoplastic Agent, Antimetabolite

Use Treatment of metastatic colorectal cancer; adjuvant therapy of Dukes C colon cancer; treatment of metastatic breast cancer

General Dosage Range Dosage adjustment recommended in patients with renal impairment or who develop toxicities

Oral: *Adults:* 1250 mg/m^2 twice daily for 2 weeks, every 21 days

Dosage Forms

Tablet, oral:

Xeloda®: 150 mg, 500 mg

Capex® *see* fluocinolone (topical) *on page* 392
Caphosol® *see* saliva substitute *on page* 819
Capital® and Codeine *see* acetaminophen and codeine *on page* 22
Capoten® (Can) *see* captopril *on page* 171
Caprelsa® *see* vandetanib *on page* 937

capreomycin (kap ree oh MYE sin)

Medication Safety Issues

Sound-alike/look-alike issues:

Capastat® may be confused with Cepastat®

Synonyms capreomycin sulfate

U.S. Brand Names Capastat® Sulfate

Therapeutic Category Antibiotic, Miscellaneous

Use Treatment of tuberculosis in conjunction with at least one other antituberculosis agent

General Dosage Range Dosage adjustment recommended in patients with renal impairment

I.M., I.V.: *Adults:* 1 g/day (maximum: 20 mg/kg/day) for 60-120 days, followed by 1 g 2-3 times/week

Dosage Forms

Injection, powder for reconstitution:

Capastat® Sulfate: 1 g

capreomycin sulfate *see* capreomycin *on page* 170

capsaicin (kap SAY sin)

Medication Safety Issues

Sound-alike/look-alike issues:

Zostrix® may be confused with Zestril®, Zovirax®

Synonyms NGX-4010

U.S. Brand Names Capzasin-HP® [OTC]; Capzasin-P® [OTC]; DiabetAid® Pain and Tingling Relief [OTC]; Qutenza™; Salonpas® Gel-Patch Hot [OTC]; Salonpas® Hot [OTC]; Trixaicin HP [OTC]; Trixaicin [OTC]; Zostrix® Diabetic Foot Pain [OTC]; Zostrix® [OTC]; Zostrix®-HP [OTC]

Canadian Brand Names Zostrix®; Zostrix® H.P.

Therapeutic Category Analgesic, Topical

Use

Topical patch (Qutenza™): Management of postherpetic neuralgia (PHN)

OTC labeling: Temporary treatment of minor pain associated with muscles and joints due to backache, strains, sprains, bruises, cramps, or arthritis; temporary relief of pain associated with diabetic neuropathy

General Dosage Range Topical:

Children ≥12 years: OTC labeling: Patch (Salonpas®-Hot): Apply patch to affected area up to 3-4 times/day

Adults: Patch (Qutenza™ [capsaicin 8%]): Apply patch to most painful area for 60 minutes (maximum: 4 patches in a single application); OTC products: Apply to affected area 3-4 times/day

Dosage Forms

Cream, topical: 0.025% (60 g)
- Capzasin-HP® [OTC]: 0.1% (42.5 g)
- Capzasin-P® [OTC]: 0.035% (42.5 g)
- Trixaicin [OTC]: 0.025% (60 g)
- Trixaicin HP [OTC]: 0.075% (60 g)
- Zostrix® [OTC]: 0.025% (60 g)
- Zostrix® Diabetic Foot Pain [OTC]: 0.075% (60 g)
- Zostrix®-HP [OTC]: 0.075% (60 g)

Gel, topical:
- Capzasin-P® [OTC]: 0.025% (42.5 g)

Liquid, topical:
- Capzasin-P® [OTC]: 0.15% (29.5 mL)

Lotion, topical:
- DiabetAid® Pain and Tingling Relief [OTC]: 0.025% (120 mL)

Patch, topical:
- Qutenza™: 8% (1s, 2s)
- Salonpas® Gel-Patch Hot [OTC]: 0.025% (3s, 6s)
- Salonpas® Hot [OTC]: 0.025% (1s)

captopril (KAP toe pril)

Medication Safety Issues

Sound-alike/look-alike issues:

Captopril may be confused with calcitriol, Capitrol®, carvedilol

International issues:

Acepril [Great Britain] may be confused with Accupril which is a brand name for quinapril in the U.S.

Acepril: Brand name for captopril [Great Britain], but also the brand name for enalapril [Hungary, Switzerland]; lisinopril [Malaysia]

Synonyms ACE

Canadian Brand Names Apo-Capto®; Capoten®; Dom-Captopril; Mylan-Captopril; Nu-Capto; PMS-Captopril; Teva-Captopril

Therapeutic Category Angiotensin-Converting Enzyme (ACE) Inhibitor

Use Management of hypertension; treatment of heart failure, left ventricular dysfunction after myocardial infarction, diabetic nephropathy

General Dosage Range Dosage adjustment recommended in patients with renal impairment

Oral:

Infants: Initial: 0.15-0.3 mg/kg/dose; Maximum: 6 mg/kg/day in 1-4 divided doses

Children: Initial: 0.3-0.5 mg/kg/dose; Maximum: 6 mg/kg/day in 2-4 divided doses

Older Children: Initial: 6.25-12.5 mg every 12-24 hours; Maximum: 6 mg/kg/day

Adolescents: Initial: 12.5-25 mg; Maximum: 450 mg/day

Adults: Initial: 6.25-25 mg 2-3 times/day; Maintenance: 25-450 mg/day in 2-3 divided doses

Dosage Forms

Tablet, oral: 12.5 mg, 25 mg, 50 mg, 100 mg

captopril and hydrochlorothiazide (KAP toe pril & hye droe klor oh THYE a zide)

Synonyms hydrochlorothiazide and captopril

Therapeutic Category Antihypertensive Agent, Combination

Use Management of hypertension

General Dosage Range Oral: *Adults:* Captopril 25-150 mg and hydrochlorothiazide 15-50 mg once daily

Dosage Forms

Tablet: 25/15: Captopril 25 mg and hydrochlorothiazide 15 mg; 25/25: Captopril 25 mg and hydrochlorothiazide 25 mg; 50/15: Captopril 50 mg and hydrochlorothiazide 15 mg; 50/25: Captopril 50 mg and hydrochlorothiazide 25 mg

Capzasin-HP® [OTC] *see* capsaicin *on page 170*

Capzasin-P® [OTC] *see* capsaicin *on page* 170
Carac® *see* fluorouracil (topical) *on page* 396
Carafate® *see* sucralfate *on page* 856

carbachol (KAR ba kole)

Medication Safety Issues

Sound-alike/look-alike issues:

Isopto® Carbachol may be confused with Isopto® Carpine

Synonyms carbacholine; carbamylcholine chloride

U.S. Brand Names Isopto® Carbachol; Miostat®

Canadian Brand Names Isopto® Carbachol; Miostat®

Therapeutic Category Cholinergic Agent

Use Lowers intraocular pressure in the treatment of glaucoma; cause miosis during surgery

General Dosage Range Ophthalmic: *Adults:* Instill 1-2 drops up to 3 times/day **or** 0.5 mL as a single dose

Dosage Forms

Solution, intraocular:

Miostat®: 0.01% (1.5 mL)

Solution, ophthalmic:

Isopto® Carbachol: 1.5% (15 mL); 3% (15 mL)

carbacholine *see* carbachol *on page* 172
Carbaglu® *see* carglumic acid *on page* 177

carbamazepine (kar ba MAZ e peen)

Medication Safety Issues

Sound-alike/look-alike issues:

CarBAMazepine may be confused with OXcarbazepine
Epitol® may be confused with Epinal®
TEGretol®, TEGretol®-XR may be confused with Mebaral®, Toprol-XL®, Toradol®, TRENtal®

BEERS Criteria medication:

This drug may be potentially inappropriate for use in geriatric patients (Quality of evidence - moderate; Strength of recommendation - strong).

Synonyms CBZ; SPD417

Tall-Man car**BAM**azepine

U.S. Brand Names Carbatrol®; Epitol®; Equetro®; TEGretol®; TEGretol®-XR

Canadian Brand Names Apo-Carbamazepine®; Dom-Carbamazepine; Mapezine®; Mylan-Carbamazepine CR; Nu-Carbamazepine; PMS-Carbamazepine; Sandoz-Carbamazepine; Taro-Carbamazepine Chewable; Tegretol®; Teva-Carbamazepine

Therapeutic Category Anticonvulsant

Use

Carbatrol®, Tegretol®, Tegretol®-XR: Partial seizures with complex symptomatology (psychomotor, temporal lobe), generalized tonic-clonic seizures (grand mal), mixed seizure patterns, trigeminal neuralgia

Equetro®: Acute manic and mixed episodes associated with bipolar 1 disorder

General Dosage Range Dosage adjustment recommended in patients with renal impairment.

Oral:

Extended release:

Capsules:

Children <12 years: Receiving ≥400 mg/day of carbamazepine may be converted to extended release capsules (Carbatrol®) using the same total daily dosage divided twice daily

Children 12-15 years: Initial: 400 mg/day; Maintenance: 800-1000 mg/day in 2 divided doses (maximum: 1000 mg/day)

Adolescents >15 years: Initial: 400 mg/day; Maintenance: 800-1200 mg/day in 2 divided doses (maximum: 1200 mg/day)

Adults: Bipolar disorder (Equetro®): Initial: 400 mg/day in 2 divided doses: Maintenance: Adjust by 200 mg daily increments (maximum: 1600 mg/day); Epilepsy: Initial: 400 mg/day; Maintenance: 800-1200 mg/day in 2 divided doses (maximum: 2400 mg/day)

Tablets:

Children 6-12 years: Initial: 200 mg/day; Maintenance: 400-800 mg/day in 2 divided doses (maximum: 1000 mg/day)

Children 12-15 years: Initial: 400 mg/day; Maintenance: 800-1000 mg/day in 2 divided doses (maximum: 1000 mg/day)

Adolescents >15 years and Adults: Initial: 400 mg/day; Maintenance: 800-1200 mg/day in 2 divided doses (maximum: 1200 mg/day)

Immediate release:

Children <6 years: Initial: 10-20 mg/kg/day in 2-3 divided doses (tablets) **or** 4 divided doses (suspension); Maintenance: Up to 35 mg/kg/day in 3-4 divided doses

Children 6-12 years: Initial: 200 mg/day in 2 divided doses (tablets) **or** 4 divided doses (suspension); Maintenance: 400-800 mg/day in 2-4 divided doses (maximum: 1000 mg/day)

Children 12-15 years: Initial: 400 mg/day in 2 divided doses (tablets) **or** 4 divided doses (suspension); Maintenance: 800-1000 mg/day in 3-4 divided doses (maximum: 1000 mg/day)

Adolescents >15 years: Initial: 400 mg/day in 2 divided doses (tablets) **or** 4 divided doses (suspension); Maintenance: 800-1200 mg/day in 3-4 divided doses (maximum: 1200 mg/day)

Adults: Epilepsy: Initial: 400 mg/day in 2 divided doses (tablets) **or** 4 divided doses (suspension); Maintenance: 800-1200 mg/day in 3-4 divided doses (maximum: 2400 mg/day); Trigeminal or glossopharyngeal neuralgia: Initial: 200 mg/day in 2 divided doses; Maintenance: 400-800 mg/day in 2 divided doses (maximum: 1200 mg/day)

Dosage Forms

Capsule, extended release, oral: 100 mg, 200 mg, 300 mg

Carbatrol®: 100 mg, 200 mg, 300 mg

Equetro®: 100 mg, 200 mg, 300 mg

Suspension, oral: 100 mg/5 mL (5 mL, 10 mL, 450 mL)

TEGretol®: 100 mg/5 mL (450 mL)

Tablet, oral: 200 mg

Epitol®: 200 mg

TEGretol®: 200 mg

Tablet, chewable, oral: 100 mg

TEGretol®: 100 mg

Tablet, extended release, oral: 200 mg, 400 mg

TEGretol®-XR: 100 mg, 200 mg, 400 mg

carbamide *see* urea *on page 930*

carbamide peroxide (KAR ba mide per OKS ide)

Synonyms urea peroxide

U.S. Brand Names Auraphene B® [OTC]; Auro® [OTC]; Cankaid® [OTC]; Debrox® [OTC]; E-R-O® [OTC]; Gly-Oxide® [OTC]; Murine® Ear Wax Removal Kit [OTC]; Murine® Ear [OTC]; Otix® [OTC]; Wax Away [OTC]

Therapeutic Category Antiinfective Agent, Oral; Otic Agent, Ceruminolytic

Use Relief of minor inflammation of gums, oral mucosal surfaces, and lips including canker sores and dental irritation; emulsify and disperse ear wax

General Dosage Range

Otic:

Children <12 years: Instill 1-5 drops twice daily

Children ≥12 years and Adults: Instill 5-10 drops twice daily

Topical (oral): *Children ≥2 years and Adults:* Apply several drops on affected area, expectorate after 2-3 minutes 4 times/day **or** place 10 drops on tongue, swish for several minutes, expectorate

Dosage Forms

Liquid, oral: 10% (60 mL)

Cankaid® [OTC]: 10% (15 mL)

Gly-Oxide® [OTC]: 10% (15 mL, 60 mL)

Solution, otic: 6.5% (15 mL)
Auraphene B® [OTC]: 6.5% (15 mL)
Auro® [OTC]: 6.5% (22.2 mL)
Debrox® [OTC]: 6.5% (15 mL, 30 mL)
E-R-O® [OTC]: 6.5% (15 mL)
Murine® Ear [OTC]: 6.5% (15 mL)
Murine® Ear Wax Removal Kit [OTC]: 6.5% (15 mL)
Otix® [OTC]: 6.5% (15 mL)
Wax Away [OTC]: 6.5% (15 mL)

carbamylcholine chloride *see* carbachol *on page 172*
Carbatrol® *see* carbamazepine *on page 172*

carbetocin *(Canada only)* (kar BE toe sin)

Medication Safety Issues
High alert medication:
The Institute for Safe Medication Practices (ISMP) includes oxytocin (carbetocin analog) among its list of drugs which have a heightened risk of causing significant patient harm when used in error.

Canadian Brand Names Duratocin™

Therapeutic Category Oxytocic Agent

Use Prevention of uterine atony and postpartum hemorrhage following elective cesarean section under anesthesia (epidural or spinal)

General Dosage Range I.V.: *Adults:* 100 mcg (single dose)

Product Availability Not available in U.S.

Dosage Forms - Canada
Injection, solution:
Duratocin™: 100 mcg/mL (1 mL)

carbidopa (kar bi DOE pa)

Medication Safety Issues
International issues:
Lodosyn [U.S.] may be confused with Lidosen brand name for lidocaine [Italy]

U.S. Brand Names Lodosyn®

Therapeutic Category Anti-Parkinson Agent (Dopamine Agonist)

Use Given with carbidopa-levodopa in the treatment of parkinsonism to enable a lower dosage of levodopa to be used and a more rapid response to be obtained and to decrease side effects; use with carbidopa-levodopa in patients requiring additional carbidopa; has no effect without levodopa

General Dosage Range Oral: *Adults:* 25 mg 3-4 times/day (maximum: 200 mg carbidopa/day)

Dosage Forms
Tablet, oral:
Lodosyn®: 25 mg

carbidopa and levodopa (kar bi DOE pa & lee voe DOE pa)

Medication Safety Issues
Sound-alike/look-alike issues:
Sinemet® may be confused with Serevent®
International issues:
Zimox: Brand name for carbidopa and levodopa [Greece], but also the brand name for amoxicillin [Italy]
Zimox [Greece] may be confused with Diamox which is a brand name for acetazolamide [Canada and multiple international markets]

Synonyms levodopa and carbidopa

U.S. Brand Names Parcopa®; Sinemet®; Sinemet® CR

Canadian Brand Names Apo-Levocarb®; Apo-Levocarb® CR; Dom-Levo-Carbidopa; Duodopa™; Levocarb CR; Nu-Levocarb; PRO-Levocarb; Sinemet®; Sinemet® CR; Teva-Levocarbidopa

Therapeutic Category Anti-Parkinson Agent (Dopamine Agonist)

Use Idiopathic Parkinson disease; postencephalitic parkinsonism; symptomatic parkinsonism

Duodopa™ intestinal gel: Canadian labeling (not available in U.S.): Treatment of advanced levodopa-responsive Parkinson disease in which severe motor symptoms are not controlled by other Parkinson agents

General Dosage Range Oral: *Adults:* Immediate release: Initial: Carbidopa 25 mg/levodopa 100 mg 3 times/day (maximum: 8 tablets of any strength/day **or** 200 mg of carbidopa and 2000 mg of levodopa); Controlled release: *Adults:* Initial: Carbidopa 50 mg/levodopa 200 mg 2 times/day, at intervals not <6 hours (maximum: 8 tablets/day)

Dosage Forms

Tablet: 10/100: Carbidopa 10 mg and levodopa 100 mg; 25/100: Carbidopa 25 mg and levodopa 100 mg; 25/250: Carbidopa 25 mg and levodopa 250 mg

Sinemet®:

10/100: Carbidopa 10 mg and levodopa 100 mg
25/100: Carbidopa 25 mg and levodopa 100 mg
25/250: Carbidopa 25 mg and levodopa 250 mg

Tablet, extended release: 25/100: Carbidopa 25 mg and levodopa 100 mg; 50/200: Carbidopa 50 mg and levodopa 200 mg

Tablet, orally disintegrating: 10/100: Carbidopa 10 mg and levodopa 100 mg; 25/100: Carbidopa 25 mg and levodopa 100 mg; 25/250: Carbidopa 25 mg and levodopa 250 mg

Parcopa®:

10/100: Carbidopa 10 mg and levodopa 100 mg [contains phenylalanine 3.4 mg/tablet; mint flavor]
25/100: Carbidopa 25 mg and levodopa 100 mg [contains phenylalanine 3.4 mg/tablet; mint flavor]
25/250: Carbidopa 25 mg and levodopa 250 mg [contains phenylalanine 8.4 mg/tablet; mint flavor]

Tablet, sustained release: 25/100: Carbidopa 25 mg and levodopa 100 mg; 50/200: Carbidopa 50 mg and levodopa 200 mg

Sinemet® CR:

25/100: Carbidopa 25 mg and levodopa 100 mg
50/200: Carbidopa 50 mg and levodopa 200 mg

Dosage Forms - Canada

Intestinal gel:

Duodopa™: Carbidopa 5 mg and levodopa 20 mg/1 mL (100 mL)

carbidopa, entacapone, and levodopa *see* levodopa, carbidopa, and entacapone *on page 531*

carbidopa, levodopa, and entacapone *see* levodopa, carbidopa, and entacapone *on page 531*

carbinoxamine (kar bi NOKS a meen)

Medication Safety Issues

BEERS Criteria medication:

This drug may be potentially inappropriate for use in geriatric patients (Quality of evidence - moderate; Strength of recommendation - strong).

Synonyms carbinoxamine maleate

U.S. Brand Names Arbinoxa™; Palgic®

Therapeutic Category Antihistamine

Use Seasonal and perennial allergic rhinitis; vasomotor rhinitis; allergic conjunctivitis; mild manifestations of urticaria and angioedema; dermatographism; adjunct therapy for anaphylactic reactions (after acute manifestations controlled)

General Dosage Range Oral:

Children 2-5 years: 0.2-0.4 mg/kg/day divided into 3-4 doses **or** 1-2 mg 3-4 times/day
Children 6-11 years: 2-4 mg 3-4 times/day
Adults: 4-8 mg 3-4 times/day

Dosage Forms

Solution, oral: 4 mg/5 mL (118 mL, 473 mL)

Arbinoxa™: 4 mg/5 mL (480 mL)
Palgic®: 4 mg/5 mL (480 mL)

Tablet, oral: 4 mg

Arbinoxa™: 4 mg
Palgic®: 4 mg

carbinoxamine maleate *see* carbinoxamine *on page 175*

Carbocaine® *see* mepivacaine *on page 575*

Carbocaine® 2% with Neo-Cobefrin® *see* mepivacaine and levonordefrin *on page 576*

carbolic acid *see* phenol *on page 713*

Carbolith™ (Can) *see* lithium *on page 544*

carboplatin (KAR boe pla tin)

Medication Safety Issues

Sound-alike/look-alike issues:

CARBOplatin may be confused with CISplatin, oxaliplatin

Paraplatin® may be confused with Platinol®

High alert medication:

This medication is in a class the Institute for Safe Medication Practices (ISMP) includes among its list of drug classes which have a heightened risk of causing significant patient harm when used in error.

BEERS Criteria medication:

This drug may be potentially inappropriate for use in geriatric patients (Quality of evidence - moderate; Strength of recommendation - strong).

Synonyms CBDCA; paraplatin

Tall-Man **CARBO**platin

Canadian Brand Names Carboplatin Injection; Carboplatin Injection - LIQ IV

Therapeutic Category Antineoplastic Agent

Use Initial treatment of advanced ovarian cancer in combination with other established chemotherapy agents; palliative treatment of recurrent ovarian cancer after prior chemotherapy, including cisplatin-based treatment

General Dosage Range Dosage adjustment recommended in renal impairment or who develop toxicities

I.V.: *Adults:* 300-360 mg/m^2 every 4 weeks **or** AUC of 4-6 (using Calvert formula)

Dosage Forms

Injection, solution [preservative free]: 10 mg/mL (5 mL, 15 mL, 45 mL, 60 mL)

Carboplatin Injection (Can) *see* carboplatin *on page 176*

Carboplatin Injection - LIQ IV (Can) *see* carboplatin *on page 176*

carboprost *see* carboprost tromethamine *on page 176*

carboprost tromethamine (KAR boe prost tro METH a meen)

Synonyms carboprost; prostaglandin F_2

U.S. Brand Names Hemabate®

Canadian Brand Names Hemabate®

Therapeutic Category Prostaglandin

Use Termination of pregnancy; treatment of refractory postpartum uterine bleeding

General Dosage Range I.M.: *Adults (females):* Abortion: 250 mcg at 1.5- to 3.5-hour intervals, a 500 mcg dose may be given if uterine response is not adequate after several 250 mcg doses (maximum total dose: 12 mg); Postpartum bleeding: 250 mcg; may repeat if needed (maximum total dose: 2 mg [8 doses])

Dosage Forms

Injection, solution:

Hemabate®: 250 mcg/mL (1 mL)

carbose D *see* carboxymethylcellulose *on page 176*

carboxymethylcellulose (kar boks ee meth il SEL yoo lose)

Medication Safety Issues

Sound-alike/look-alike issues:

Optive™ may be confused with Optivar®

Synonyms carbose D; carboxymethylcellulose sodium

U.S. Brand Names Optive™ [OTC]; Refresh Liquigel™ [OTC]; Refresh Plus® [OTC]; Refresh Tears® [OTC]; Tears Again® Night & Day™ [OTC]; Theratears® [OTC]

Canadian Brand Names Celluvisc™; Refresh Plus®; Refresh Tears®

Therapeutic Category Ophthalmic Agent, Miscellaneous

Use Artificial tear substitute

General Dosage Range Ophthalmic: *Adults:* Instill 1-2 drops into eye(s) 3-4 times/day

Dosage Forms

Gel, ophthalmic:

Tears Again® Night & Day™ [OTC]: 1.5% (3.5 g)

Liquid, ophthalmic:

Refresh Liquigel™ [OTC]: 1% (15 mL)

Solution, ophthalmic:
Optive™ [OTC]: 0.5% (15 mL, 30 mL)
Refresh Tears® [OTC]: 0.5% (15 mL)
Solution, ophthalmic [preservative free]:
Refresh Plus® [OTC]: 0.5% (0.4 mL)
Theratears® [OTC]: 0.25% (0.6 mL, 15 mL)

carboxymethylcellulose sodium *see* carboxymethylcellulose *on page* 176
Cardec™ DM [OTC] *see* chlorpheniramine, phenylephrine, and dextromethorphan *on page* 201
Cardene® I.V. *see* nicardipine *on page* 640
Cardene® SR *see* nicardipine *on page* 640
Cardizem® *see* diltiazem *on page* 288
Cardizem® CD *see* diltiazem *on page* 288
Cardizem® LA *see* diltiazem *on page* 288
Cardura® *see* doxazosin *on page* 311
Cardura-1™ (Can) *see* doxazosin *on page* 311
Cardura-2™ (Can) *see* doxazosin *on page* 311
Cardura-4™ (Can) *see* doxazosin *on page* 311
Cardura® XL *see* doxazosin *on page* 311

carfilzomib (kar FILZ oh mib)

Medication Safety Issues
Sound-alike/look-alike issues:
Carfilzomib may be confused with bortezomib
High alert medication:
This medication is in a class the Institute for Safe Medication Practices (ISMP) includes among its list of drug classes which have a heightened risk of causing significant patient harm when used in error.

Synonyms PR-171
U.S. Brand Names Kyprolis™
Therapeutic Category Antineoplastic Agent; Proteasome Inhibitor
Use Treatment of multiple myeloma in patients who have received at least 2 prior treatment regimens (including a proteasome inhibitor and an immunomodulator) with disease progression within 60 days after the most recent treatment
General Dosage Range Dosage adjustment recommended in patients who develop toxicities.
I.V.: *Adults:* 15-27 mg/m^2 on 2 consecutive days, each week for 3 weeks (days 1, 2, 8, 9, 15, and 16) of a 28-day treatment cycle
Dosage Forms
Injection, powder for reconstitution:
Kyprolis™: 60 mg

carglumic acid (kar GLU mik AS id)

Synonyms N-carbamoyl-L-glutamic acid; N-carbamylglutamate
U.S. Brand Names Carbaglu®
Therapeutic Category Antidote; Metabolic Alkalosis Agent; Urea Cycle Disorder (UCD) Treatment Agent
Use Adjunctive treatment of acute hyperammonemia and maintenance therapy of chronic hyperammonemia due to the deficiency of the hepatic enzyme N-acetylglutamate synthase (NAGS)
General Dosage Range Oral: *Children and Adults:* <100-250 mg/kg/day given in 2 or 4 divided doses
Dosage Forms
Tablet for solution, oral:
Carbaglu®: 200 mg

Carimune® NF *see* immune globulin *on page* 477
carisoprodate *see* carisoprodol *on page* 177

carisoprodol (kar eye soe PROE dole)

Medication Safety Issues
BEERS Criteria medication:
This drug may be potentially inappropriate for use in geriatric patients (Quality of evidence - moderate; Strength of recommendation - strong).

Synonyms carisoprodate; isobamate
U.S. Brand Names Soma®
Therapeutic Category Skeletal Muscle Relaxant
Controlled Substance C-IV
Use Short-term (2-3 weeks) treatment of acute musculoskeletal pain
General Dosage Range Oral: *Children ≥16 years and Adults:* 250-350 mg 3 times/day and at bedtime
Dosage Forms
Tablet, oral: 350 mg
Soma®: 250 mg, 350 mg

carisoprodol and aspirin (kar eye soe PROE dole & AS pir in)

Medication Safety Issues
BEERS Criteria medication:
This drug may be potentially inappropriate for use in geriatric patients (Quality of evidence - moderate; Strength of recommendation - strong).
Synonyms aspirin and carisoprodol; Soma Compound
Therapeutic Category Skeletal Muscle Relaxant
Controlled Substance C-IV
Use Relief of discomfort associated with acute, painful skeletal muscle conditions
General Dosage Range Oral: *Children ≥16 years and Adults:* 1-2 tablets 4 times/day (maximum: 8 tablets/24 hours)
Dosage Forms
Tablet: Carisoprodol 200 mg and aspirin 325 mg

carisoprodol, aspirin, and codeine (kar eye soe PROE dole, AS pir in, and KOE deen)

Medication Safety Issues
BEERS Criteria medication:
This drug may be potentially inappropriate for use in geriatric patients (Quality of evidence - moderate; Strength of recommendation - strong).
Synonyms aspirin, carisoprodol, and codeine; codeine, aspirin, and carisoprodol; soma compound w/ codeine
Therapeutic Category Skeletal Muscle Relaxant
Controlled Substance C-III
Use Skeletal muscle relaxant
General Dosage Range Oral: *Adults:* 1-2 tablets 4 times/day (maximum: 8 tablets/day)
Dosage Forms
Tablet: Carisoprodol 200 mg, aspirin 325 mg, and codeine 16 mg

Carmol® 10 [OTC] *see* urea *on page 930*
Carmol® 20 [OTC] *see* urea *on page 930*
Carmol® 40 *see* urea *on page 930*
Carmol® Deep Cleansing [OTC] *see* urea *on page 930*
Carmol-HC® *see* urea and hydrocortisone *on page 931*

carmustine (kar MUS teen)

Medication Safety Issues
Sound-alike/look-alike issues:
Carmustine may be confused with bendamustine, lomustine
High alert medication:
This medication is in a class the Institute for Safe Medication Practices (ISMP) includes among its list of drug classes which have a heightened risk of causing significant patient harm when used in error.
Synonyms BCNU; bis(chloroethyl) nitrosourea; bis-chloronitrosourea; carmustine polymer wafer; carmustinum; WR-139021
U.S. Brand Names BiCNU®; Gliadel®
Canadian Brand Names BiCNU®; Gliadel Wafer®
Therapeutic Category Antineoplastic Agent

Use

Injection: Treatment of brain tumors (glioblastoma, brainstem glioma, medulloblastoma, astrocytoma, ependymoma, and metastatic brain tumors), multiple myeloma, Hodgkin lymphoma (relapsed or refractory), non-Hodgkin lymphomas (relapsed or refractory)

Wafer (implant): Adjunct to surgery in patients with recurrent glioblastoma multiforme; adjunct to surgery and radiation in patients with newly-diagnosed high-grade malignant glioma

General Dosage Range Dosage adjustment recommended in patients with renal impairment or who develop toxicity.

I.V.: *Adults:* 150-200 mg/m^2 every 6-8 weeks **or** 75-100 mg/m^2/day for 2 days every 6-8 weeks

Implantation: *Adults:* 8 wafers placed in the resection cavity (total dose: 61.6 mg)

Dosage Forms

Injection, powder for reconstitution:

BiCNU®: 100 mg

Wafer, for implantation:

Gliadel®: 7.7 mg (8s)

carmustine polymer wafer *see* carmustine *on page 178*

carmustinum *see* carmustine *on page 178*

carnitine *see* levocarnitine *on page 530*

Carnitine-300 [OTC] *see* levocarnitine *on page 530*

Carnitor® *see* levocarnitine *on page 530*

Carnitor® SF *see* levocarnitine *on page 530*

Carrington® Antifungal [OTC] *see* miconazole (topical) *on page 599*

Carrington® Oral Wound Rinse [OTC] *see* maltodextrin *on page 561*

carteolol (ophthalmic) (KAR tee oh lole)

Medication Safety Issues

Sound-alike/look-alike issues:

Carteolol may be confused with carvedilol

Synonyms carteolol hydrochloride

Therapeutic Category Ophthalmic Agent, Antiglaucoma

Use Treatment of chronic open-angle glaucoma and intraocular hypertension

General Dosage Range Ophthalmic: *Adults:* Instill 1 drop in affected eye(s) twice daily

Dosage Forms

Solution, ophthalmic: 1% (5 mL, 10 mL, 15 mL)

carteolol hydrochloride *see* carteolol (ophthalmic) *on page 179*

Carter's Little Pills® [OTC] (Can) *see* bisacodyl *on page 134*

Cartia XT® *see* diltiazem *on page 288*

carvedilol (KAR ve dil ole)

Medication Safety Issues

Sound-alike/look-alike issues:

Carvedilol may be confused with atenolol, captopril, carbidopa, carteolol

Coreg® may be confused with Corgard®, Cortef®, Cozaar®

U.S. Brand Names Coreg CR®; Coreg®

Canadian Brand Names Apo-Carvedilol®; Ava-Carvedilol; Dom-Carvedilol; JAMP-Carvedilol; Mylan-Carvedilol; Novo-Carvedilol; PMS-Carvedilol; RAN™-Carvedilol; ratio-Carvedilol; ZYM-Carvedilol

Therapeutic Category Beta-Adrenergic Blocker

Use Mild-to-severe heart failure of ischemic or cardiomyopathic origin (usually in addition to standard therapy); left ventricular dysfunction following myocardial infarction (MI) (clinically stable with LVEF ≤40%); management of hypertension

General Dosage Range Oral: *Adults:* Immediate release: Initial: 3.125-6.25 mg twice daily; Maintenance: 6.25-50 mg twice daily (maximum: 50 mg/day [<85 kg]; 100 mg/day [>85 kg]); Extended release: Initial: 10 mg once daily; range: 10-80 mg once daily

Dosage Forms

Capsule, extended release, oral:

Coreg CR®: 10 mg, 20 mg, 40 mg, 80 mg

Tablet, oral: 3.125 mg, 6.25 mg, 12.5 mg, 25 mg

Coreg®: 3.125 mg, 6.25 mg, 12.5 mg, 25 mg

Casodex® *see* bicalutamide *on page 133*

caspofungin (kas poe FUN jin)

Synonyms caspofungin acetate

U.S. Brand Names Cancidas®

Canadian Brand Names Cancidas®

Therapeutic Category Antifungal Agent, Systemic

Use Treatment of invasive *Aspergillus* infections in patients who are refractory or intolerant of other therapy; treatment of candidemia and other *Candida* infections (intraabdominal abscesses, esophageal, peritonitis, pleural space); empirical treatment for presumed fungal infections in febrile neutropenic patient

General Dosage Range Dosage adjustment recommended in patients with hepatic impairment or on concomitant therapy

I.V.:

Children 3 months to 17 years: 70 mg/m^2 on day 1, subsequent dosing: 50-70 mg/m^2 once daily (maximum dose: 70 mg/day)

Adults: Initial: 70 mg on day 1; Subsequent dose: 50-70 mg once daily

Dosage Forms

Injection, powder for reconstitution:

Cancidas®: 50 mg, 70 mg

caspofungin acetate *see* caspofungin *on page 180*

Castellani Paint Modified [OTC] *see* phenol *on page 713*

castor oil (KAS tor oyl)

Synonyms oleum ricini

Therapeutic Category Laxative

Use Preparation for rectal or bowel examination or surgery; rarely used to relieve constipation; also applied to skin as emollient and protectant

General Dosage Range Oral:

Children 2-11 years: 5-15 mL as a single dose

Children ≥12 years and Adults: 15-60 mL as a single dose

Dosage Forms

Oil, oral: 100% (60 mL, 120 mL, 180 mL, 480 mL, 3840 mL)

castor oil, trypsin, and balsam Peru *see* trypsin, balsam Peru, and castor oil *on page 925*

Cataflam® *see* diclofenac (systemic) *on page 279*

Catapres® *see* clonidine *on page 224*

Catapres-TTS®-1 *see* clonidine *on page 224*

Catapres-TTS®-2 *see* clonidine *on page 224*

Catapres-TTS®-3 *see* clonidine *on page 224*

catechins *see* sinecatechins *on page 836*

Cathflo® Activase® *see* alteplase *on page 53*

Caverject® *see* alprostadil *on page 53*

Caverject Impulse® *see* alprostadil *on page 53*

CaviRinse™ *see* fluoride *on page 393*

Cayston® *see* aztreonam *on page 110*

Caziant® *see* ethinyl estradiol and desogestrel *on page 356*

CB-1348 *see* chlorambucil *on page 195*

CB7630 *see* abiraterone acetate *on page 17*

CBDCA *see* carboplatin *on page 176*

CBZ *see* carbamazepine *on page 172*

CC-5013 *see* lenalidomide *on page 525*

CCI-779 *see* temsirolimus *on page* 876
CCNU *see* lomustine *on page* 547
2-CdA *see* cladribine *on page* 215
CDB-2914 *see* ulipristal *on page* 928
CDCA *see* chenodiol *on page* 194
CDDP *see* cisplatin *on page* 213
CDP870 *see* certolizumab pegol *on page* 190
CDX *see* bicalutamide *on page* 133
CE *see* estrogens (conjugated/equine, systemic) *on page* 351
CE *see* estrogens (conjugated/equine, topical) *on page* 352
Ceclor® (Can) *see* cefaclor *on page* 181
Cedax® *see* ceftibuten *on page* 186
CEE *see* estrogens (conjugated/equine, systemic) *on page* 351
CEE *see* estrogens (conjugated/equine, topical) *on page* 352
CeeNU® *see* lomustine *on page* 547

cefaclor (SEF a klor)

Medication Safety Issues

Sound-alike/look-alike issues:

Cefaclor may be confused with cephalexin

Canadian Brand Names Apo-Cefaclor®; Ceclor®; Novo-Cefaclor; Nu-Cefaclor; PMS-Cefaclor

Therapeutic Category Cephalosporin (Second Generation)

Use Treatment of susceptible bacterial infections including otitis media, lower respiratory tract infections, acute exacerbations of chronic bronchitis, pharyngitis and tonsillitis, urinary tract infections, skin and skin structure infections

General Dosage Range Dosage adjustment recommended in patients with renal impairment

Oral:

Children >1 month: 20-40 mg/kg/day divided every 8-12 hours (maximum: 1 g/day)
Adults: 250-500 mg every 8 hours

Dosage Forms

Capsule, oral: 250 mg, 500 mg
Powder for suspension, oral: 125 mg/5 mL (75 mL, 150 mL); 250 mg/5 mL (75 mL, 150 mL); 375 mg/5 mL (50 mL, 100 mL)
Tablet, extended release, oral: 500 mg

cefadroxil (sef a DROKS il)

Synonyms cefadroxil monohydrate; Duricef

Canadian Brand Names Apo-Cefadroxil®; PRO-Cefadroxil; Teva-Cefadroxil

Therapeutic Category Cephalosporin (First Generation)

Use Treatment of susceptible bacterial infections, including those caused by group A beta-hemolytic *Streptococcus*

General Dosage Range Dosage adjustment recommended in patients with renal impairment

Oral:

Children: 30 mg/kg/day in 2 divided doses (maximum: 2 g/day)
Adults: 1-2 g/day in 2 divided doses

Dosage Forms

Capsule, oral: 500 mg
Powder for suspension, oral: 250 mg/5 mL (50 mL, 100 mL); 500 mg/5 mL (75 mL, 100 mL)
Tablet, oral: 1 g

cefadroxil monohydrate *see* cefadroxil *on page* 181

cefazolin (sef A zoe lin)

Medication Safety Issues

Sound-alike/look-alike issues:

CeFAZolin may be confused with cefoTEtan, cefOXitin, cefprozil, cefTAZidime, cefTRIAXone, cephalexin

Synonyms ancef; cefazolin sodium

Tall-Man ceFAZolin

Therapeutic Category Cephalosporin (First Generation)

Use Treatment of respiratory tract, skin, genital, urinary tract, biliary tract, bone and joint infections, and septicemia due to susceptible gram-positive cocci (except *Enterococcus*); some gram-negative bacilli including *E. coli*, *Proteus*, and *Klebsiella* may be susceptible; surgical prophylaxis

General Dosage Range Dosage adjustment recommended in patients with renal impairment

I.M., I.V.:

Children >1 month: 25-100 mg/kg/day divided every 6-8 hours (maximum: 6 g/day)

Adults: 250 mg to 1.5 g every 6-12 hours (maximum: 12 g/day)

Dosage Forms

Infusion, premixed iso-osmotic dextrose solution: 1 g (50 mL)

Injection, powder for reconstitution: 500 mg, 1 g, 2 g, 10 g, 20 g, 100 g, 300 g

cefazolin sodium *see* cefazolin *on page* *181*

cefdinir (SEF di ner)

Synonyms CFDN

U.S. Brand Names Omnicef® [DSC]

Therapeutic Category Cephalosporin (Third Generation)

Use Treatment of community-acquired pneumonia, acute exacerbations of chronic bronchitis, acute bacterial otitis media, acute maxillary sinusitis, pharyngitis/tonsillitis, and uncomplicated skin and skin structure infections.

General Dosage Range Dosage adjustment recommended in patients with renal impairment

Oral:

Children 6 months to 12 years: 14 mg/kg/day in 1-2 divided doses (maximum: 600 mg/day)

Children >12 years and Adults: 600 mg/day in 1-2 divided doses

Dosage Forms

Capsule, oral: 300 mg

Powder for suspension, oral: 125 mg/5 mL (60 mL, 100 mL); 250 mg/5 mL (60 mL, 100 mL)

cefditoren (sef de TOR en)

Medication Safety Issues

International issues:

Spectracef [U.S., Great Britain, Mexico, Portugal, Spain] may be confused with Spectrocef brand name for cefotaxime [Italy]

Synonyms cefditoren pivoxil

U.S. Brand Names Spectracef®

Therapeutic Category Antibiotic, Cephalosporin

Use Treatment of acute bacterial exacerbation of chronic bronchitis or community-acquired pneumonia (due to susceptible organisms including *Haemophilus influenzae*, *Haemophilus parainfluenzae*, *Streptococcus pneumoniae*-penicillin susceptible only, *Moraxella catarrhalis*); pharyngitis or tonsillitis (*Streptococcus pyogenes*); and uncomplicated skin and skin-structure infections (*Staphylococcus aureus* - not MRSA, *Streptococcus pyogenes*)

General Dosage Range Dosage adjustment recommended in patients with renal impairment

Oral: *Children ≥12 years and Adults:* 200-400 mg twice daily

Dosage Forms

Tablet, oral: 200 mg, 400 mg

Spectracef®: 200 mg, 400 mg

cefditoren pivoxil *see* cefditoren *on page* *182*

cefepime (SEF e pim)

Medication Safety Issues

Sound-alike/look-alike issues:

Cefepime may be confused with cefixime, cefTAZidime

Synonyms cefepime hydrochloride

U.S. Brand Names Maxipime® [DSC]

Canadian Brand Names Maxipime®

Therapeutic Category Cephalosporin (Fourth Generation)

Use Treatment of uncomplicated and complicated urinary tract infections, including pyelonephritis caused by *Escherichia coli, Klebsiella pneumoniae*, or *Proteus mirabilis*; monotherapy for febrile neutropenia; uncomplicated skin and skin structure infections caused by *Streptococcus pyogenes* or methicillin-susceptible staphylococci; moderate-to-severe pneumonia caused by *Streptococcus pneumoniae, Pseudomonas aeruginosa, Klebsiella pneumoniae*, or *Enterobacter* species; complicated intraabdominal infections (in combination with metronidazole) caused by *E. coli, P. aeruginosa, K. pneumoniae, Enterobacter* species, or *Bacteroides fragilis* against methicillin-susceptible staphylococci, *Enterobacter* sp, and many other gram-negative bacilli.

Children 2 months to 16 years: Empiric therapy of febrile neutropenia patients, uncomplicated skin/soft tissue infections, pneumonia, and uncomplicated/complicated urinary tract infections, including pyelonephritis.

General Dosage Range Dosage adjustment recommended in patients with renal impairment

I.M.:

Children ≥2 months: 50 mg/kg/dose every 12 hours

Adults: 500-1000 mg every 12 hours

I.V.:

Children ≥2 months: 50 mg/kg/dose every 8-12 hours

Adults: 1-2 g every 8-12 hours

Dosage Forms

Infusion, premixed iso-osmotic dextrose solution: 1 g (50 mL); 2 g (100 mL)

Injection, powder for reconstitution: 500 mg, 1 g, 2 g

cefepime hydrochloride *see* cefepime *on page* 182

cefotan *see* cefotetan *on page* 184

cefotaxime (sef oh TAKS eem)

Medication Safety Issues

Sound-alike/look-alike issues:

Cefotaxime may be confused with cefOXitin, cefuroxime

International issues:

Spectrocef [Italy] may be confused with Spectracef brand name for cefditoren [U.S., Great Britain, Mexico, Portugal, Spain]

Synonyms cefotaxime sodium

U.S. Brand Names Claforan®

Canadian Brand Names Cefotaxime Sodium For Injection; Claforan®

Therapeutic Category Cephalosporin (Third Generation)

Use Treatment of susceptible organisms in lower respiratory tract, skin and skin structure, bone and joint, urinary tract, intra-abdominal, gynecologic as well as bacteremia/septicemia, and documented or suspected central nervous system infections (eg, meningitis). Active against most gram-negative bacilli (not *Pseudomonas* spp) and gram-positive cocci (not enterococcus). Active against many penicillin-resistant pneumococci.

General Dosage Range Dosage adjustment recommended in patients with hepatic or renal impairment

I.M.:

Infants and Children 1 month to 12 years and <50 kg: 50-200 mg/kg/day in divided doses every 6-8 hours (maximum: 12 g/day)

Children ≥50 kg, Children >12 years, and Adults: 1-2 g every 4-12 hours **or** 0.5-1 g as a single dose

I.V.:

Infants and Children 1 month to 12 years and <50 kg: 50-200 mg/kg/day in divided doses every 6-8 hours (maximum: 12 g/day)

Children ≥50 kg, Children >12 years, and Adults: 1-2 g every 4-12 hours

Dosage Forms

Infusion, premixed iso-osmotic solution:

Claforan®: 1 g (50 mL); 2 g (50 mL)

Injection, powder for reconstitution: 500 mg, 1 g, 2 g, 10 g

Claforan®: 500 mg, 1 g, 2 g, 10 g

cefotaxime sodium *see* cefotaxime *on page* 183

Cefotaxime Sodium For Injection (Can) *see* cefotaxime *on page* 183

cefotetan (SEF oh tee tan)

Medication Safety Issues

Sound-alike/look-alike issues:

CefoTEtan may be confused with ceFAZolin, cefOXitin, cefTAZidime, Ceftin®, cefTRIAXone

Synonyms cefotan; cefotetan disodium

Tall-Man cefo**TE**tan

Therapeutic Category Antibiotic, Cephalosporin (Second Generation)

Use Surgical prophylaxis; intraabdominal infections and other mixed infections; respiratory tract, skin and skin structure, bone and joint, urinary tract and gynecologic as well as septicemia; active against gram-negative enteric bacilli including *E. coli*, *Klebsiella*, and *Proteus*; less active against staphylococci and streptococci than first generation cephalosporins, but active against anaerobes including *Bacteroides fragilis*

General Dosage Range Dosage adjustment recommended in patients with renal impairment

I.M.: *Adults:* 1-6 g/day divided every 12 hours **or** 1-2 g every 24 hours **or** 1-2 g prior to surgery

I.V.:

Adolescents: PID: 2 g every 12 hours

Adults: 1-6 g/day divided every 12 hours **or** 1-2 g every 24 hours **or** 1-2 g prior to surgery

Dosage Forms

Injection, powder for reconstitution: 1 g, 2 g, 10 g

cefotetan disodium *see* cefotetan *on page* 184

cefoxitin (se FOKS i tin)

Medication Safety Issues

Sound-alike/look-alike issues:

CefOXitin may be confused with ceFAZolin, cefotaxime, cefoTEtan, cefTAZidime, cefTRIAXone, Cytoxan

Mefoxin® may be confused with Lanoxin®

Synonyms cefoxitin sodium

Tall-Man cef**OX**itin

U.S. Brand Names Mefoxin®

Canadian Brand Names Cefoxitin For Injection

Therapeutic Category Cephalosporin (Second Generation)

Use Less active against staphylococci and streptococci than first generation cephalosporins, but active against anaerobes including *Bacteroides fragilis*; active against gram-negative enteric bacilli including *E. coli*, *Klebsiella*, and *Proteus*; used predominantly for respiratory tract, skin, bone and joint, urinary tract and gynecologic as well as septicemia; surgical prophylaxis; intraabdominal infections and other mixed infections; indicated for bacterial *Eikenella corrodens* infections

General Dosage Range Dosage adjustment recommended in patients with renal impairment

I.M.:

Children >3 months: 80-160 mg/kg/day divided every 4-6 hours (maximum: 12 g/day)

Adolescents: 80-160 mg/kg/day divided every 4-6 hours (maximum: 12 g/day) **or** 1-2 g prior to surgery

Adults: 1-2 g every 4-8 hours (maximum: 12 g/day) **or** 1-2 g prior to surgery

I.V.:

Children >3 months: 80-160 mg/kg/day divided every 4-6 hours (maximum: 12 g/day) **or** 30-40 mg/kg prior to surgery

Adolescents: 80-160 mg/kg/day divided every 4-6 hours (maximum: 12 g/day) **or** 1-2 g prior to surgery

Adults: 1-2 g every 4-8 hours (maximum: 12 g/day) **or** 1-2 g prior to surgery

Dosage Forms

Infusion, premixed iso-osmotic dextrose solution:

Mefoxin®: 1 g (50 mL); 2 g (50 mL)

Injection, powder for reconstitution: 1 g, 2 g, 10 g

Cefoxitin For Injection (Can) *see* cefoxitin *on page* 184

cefoxitin sodium *see* cefoxitin *on page* 184

cefpodoxime (sef pode OKS eem)

Medication Safety Issues

Sound-alike/look-alike issues:

Vantin may be confused with Ventolin®

Synonyms cefpodoxime proxetil; Vantin

Therapeutic Category Cephalosporin (Second Generation)

Use Treatment of susceptible acute, community-acquired pneumonia caused by *S. pneumoniae* or nonbeta-lactamase producing *H. influenzae*; acute uncomplicated gonorrhea caused by *N. gonorrhoeae*; uncomplicated skin and skin structure infections caused by *S. aureus* or *S. pyogenes*; acute otitis media caused by *S. pneumoniae*, *H. influenzae*, or *M. catarrhalis*; pharyngitis or tonsillitis; and uncomplicated urinary tract infections caused by *E. coli*, *Klebsiella*, and *Proteus*

General Dosage Range Dosage adjustment recommended in patients with renal impairment

Oral:

Children 2 months to 12 years: 10 mg/kg/day divided every 12 hours (maximum: 200 mg/dose)

Children ≥12 years and Adults: 100-400 mg every 12 hours **or** 200 mg as a single dose

Dosage Forms

Granules for suspension, oral: 50 mg/5 mL (50 mL, 100 mL); 100 mg/5 mL (50 mL, 100 mL)

Tablet, oral: 100 mg, 200 mg

cefpodoxime proxetil *see* cefpodoxime *on page 184*

cefprozil (sef PROE zil)

Medication Safety Issues

Sound-alike/look-alike issues:

Cefprozil may be confused with ceFAZolin, cefuroxime

Cefzil may be confused with Ceftin®

Synonyms Cefzil

Canadian Brand Names Apo-Cefprozil®; Auro-Cefprozil; Ava-Cefprozil; Cefzil®; RAN™-Cefprozil; Sandoz-Cefprozil

Therapeutic Category Cephalosporin (Second Generation)

Use Treatment of otitis media and infections involving the respiratory tract and skin and skin structure; active against methicillin-sensitive staphylococci, many streptococci, and various gram-negative bacilli including *E. coli*, some *Klebsiella*, *P. mirabilis*, *H. influenzae*, and *Moraxella*.

General Dosage Range Dosage adjustment recommended in patients with renal impairment

Oral:

Children 6 months to 2 years: 7.5-30 mg/kg/day divided every 12 hours

Children 2-12 years: 7.5-30 mg/kg/day divided every 12 hours **or** 20 mg/kg every 24 hours (maximum: 1 g/day)

Adolescents >12 years and Adults: 250-500 mg every 12 hours **or** 500 mg every 24 hours

Dosage Forms

Powder for suspension, oral: 125 mg/5 mL (50 mL, 75 mL, 100 mL); 250 mg/5 mL (50 mL, 75 mL, 100 mL)

Tablet, oral: 250 mg, 500 mg

ceftaroline fosamil (sef TAR oh leen FOS a mil)

Synonyms PPI-0903; PPI-0903M; T-91825; TAK-599

U.S. Brand Names Teflaro™

Therapeutic Category Antibiotic, Cephalosporin (Fifth Generation)

Use Treatment of acute bacterial skin and skin structure infections (ABSSSI) caused by susceptible isolates of *Staphylococcus aureus* (including methicillin-susceptible and -resistant isolates), *Streptococcus pyogenes, Streptococcus agalactiae, Escherichia coli, Klebsiella pneumoniae*, and *Klebsiella oxytoca,* and community-acquired pneumonia (CAP) caused by *Streptococcus pneumoniae* (including cases with concurrent bacteremia), *Staphylococcus aureus* (methicillin-susceptible isolates only), *Haemophilus influenzae, Klebsiella pneumoniae, Klebsiella oxytoca,* and *Escherichia coli*

General Dosage Range Dosage adjustment recommended in patients with renal impairment.

I.V.: *Adults:* 600 mg every 12 hours

Dosage Forms

Injection, powder for reconstitution:

Teflaro™: 600 mg

ceftazidime (SEF tay zi deem)

Medication Safety Issues

Sound-alike/look-alike issues:

CefTAZidime may be confused with ceFAZolin, cefepime, cefoTEtan, cefOXitin, cefTRIAXone

Ceptaz® may be confused with Septra®
Tazicef® may be confused with Tazidime®

International issues:

Ceftim [Portugual] and Ceftime [Thailand] brand names for ceftazidime may be confused with Ceftin brand name for cefuroxime [U.S., Canada]; Cefiton brand name for cefixime [Portugal]

Tall-Man cef**TAZ**idime

U.S. Brand Names Fortaz®; Tazicef®

Canadian Brand Names Ceftazidime For Injection; Fortaz®

Therapeutic Category Cephalosporin (Third Generation)

Use Treatment of documented susceptible *Pseudomonas aeruginosa* infection and infections due to other susceptible aerobic gram-negative organisms; empiric therapy of a febrile, granulocytopenic patient

General Dosage Range Dosage adjustment recommended in patients with renal impairment

I.M.: *Adults:* 500 mg to 2 g every 8-12 hours

I.V.:

Children 1 month to 12 years: 30-50 mg/kg every 8 hours (maximum: 6 g/day)
Children ≥12 years and Adults: 500 mg to 2 g every 8-12 hours (maximum: 6 g/day)

Dosage Forms

Infusion, premixed iso-osmotic solution:
Fortaz®: 1 g (50 mL); 2 g (50 mL)

Injection, powder for reconstitution: 1 g, 2 g, 6 g
Fortaz®: 500 mg, 1 g, 2 g, 6 g
Tazicef®: 1 g, 2 g, 6 g

Ceftazidime For Injection (Can) *see* ceftazidime *on page 185*

ceftibuten (sef TYE byoo ten)

Medication Safety Issues

Sound-alike/look-alike issues:
Cedax® may be confused with Cidex®

International issues:
Cedax [U.S. and multiple international markets] may be confused with Codex brand name for acetaminophen/codeine [Brazil] and *Saccharomyces boulardii* [Italy]

U.S. Brand Names Cedax®

Therapeutic Category Cephalosporin (Third Generation)

Use Treatment of acute exacerbations of chronic bronchitis, acute bacterial otitis media, and pharyngitis/tonsillitis

General Dosage Range Dosage adjustment recommended in patients with renal impairment

Oral:

Children 6 months to <12 years: 9 mg/kg/day (maximum: 400 mg/day)
Children ≥12 years and Adults: 400 mg once daily

Dosage Forms

Capsule, oral:
Cedax®: 400 mg

Powder for suspension, oral:
Cedax®: 90 mg/5 mL (60 mL, 90 mL, 120 mL); 180 mg/5 mL (30 mL, 60 mL)

Ceftin® *see* cefuroxime *on page 187*

ceftriaxone (sef trye AKS one)

Medication Safety Issues

Sound-alike/look-alike issues:
CefTRIAXone may be confused with CeFAZolin, cefoTEtan, cefOXitin, cefTAZidime, Cetraxal®
Rocephin® may be confused with Roferon®

Synonyms ceftriaxone sodium

Tall-Man cef**TRIAX**one

U.S. Brand Names Rocephin®

Canadian Brand Names Ceftriaxone for Injection; Ceftriaxone Sodium for Injection BP; Rocephin®

Therapeutic Category Cephalosporin (Third Generation)

Use Treatment of lower respiratory tract infections, acute bacterial otitis media, skin and skin structure infections, bone and joint infections, intraabdominal and urinary tract infections, pelvic inflammatory disease (PID), uncomplicated gonorrhea, bacterial septicemia, and meningitis; used in surgical prophylaxis

General Dosage Range Dosage adjustment recommended in patients with hepatic and renal impairment

I.M.:

Children: 50-100 mg/kg/day divided every 12-24 hours (maximum: 4 g/day) **or** 125 mg or 50 mg/kg as a single dose

Adults: 1-2 g every 12-24 hours **or** 125-250 mg as a single dose

I.V.:

Children: 50-100 mg/kg/day divided every 12-24 hours (maximum: 4 g/day)

Adults: 1-2 g every 12-24 hours

Dosage Forms

Infusion, premixed in D_5W: 1 g (50 mL); 2 g (50 mL)

Injection, powder for reconstitution: 250 mg, 500 mg, 1 g, 2 g, 10 g

Rocephin®: 500 mg, 1 g

Ceftriaxone for Injection (Can) *see* ceftriaxone *on page 186*

ceftriaxone sodium *see* ceftriaxone *on page 186*

Ceftriaxone Sodium for Injection BP (Can) *see* ceftriaxone *on page 186*

cefuroxime (se fyoor OKS eem)

Medication Safety Issues

Sound-alike/look-alike issues:

Cefuroxime may be confused with cefotaxime, cefprozil, deferoxamine

Ceftin® may be confused with Cefzil®, Cipro®

Zinacef® may be confused with Zithromax®

International issues:

Ceftin [U.S., Canada] may be confused with Cefiton brand name for cefixime [Portugal]; Ceftim brand name for ceftazidime [Portugal]; Ceftime brand name for ceftazidime [Thailand]

Synonyms cefuroxime axetil; cefuroxime sodium

U.S. Brand Names Ceftin®; Zinacef®

Canadian Brand Names Apo-Cefuroxime®; Auro-Cefuroxime; Ceftin®; Cefuroxime For Injection; PRO-Cefuroxime; ratio-Cefuroxime

Therapeutic Category Cephalosporin (Second Generation)

Use Treatment of infections caused by staphylococci, group B streptococci, *H. influenzae* (type A and B), *E. coli*, *Enterobacter*, *Salmonella*, and *Klebsiella*; treatment of susceptible infections of the upper and lower respiratory tract, otitis media, urinary tract, uncomplicated skin and soft tissue, bone and joint, sepsis, uncomplicated gonorrhea, and early Lyme disease; surgical prophylaxis

General Dosage Range Dosage adjustment recommended in patients with renal impairment

I.M., I.V.:

Children 3 months to 12 years: 75-150 mg/kg/day divided every 8 hours (maximum: 6 g/day)

Adolescents >12 years and Adults: 750 mg to 1.5 g every 6-8 hours (maximum: 6 g/day) **or** 1.5 g as a single dose

Oral:

Children 3 months to 12 years: 20-30 mg/kg/day in 2 divided doses **or** 125-250 mg every 12 hours (maximum: 1 g/day)

Adolescents >12 years and Adults: 125-500 mg every 12 hours **or** 1 g as a single dose

Dosage Forms

Infusion, premixed iso-osmotic solution:

Zinacef®: 750 mg (50 mL); 1.5 g (50 mL)

Injection, powder for reconstitution: 750 mg, 1.5 g, 7.5 g, 75 g

Zinacef®: 750 mg, 1.5 g, 7.5 g

Powder for suspension, oral: 125 mg/5 mL (100 mL); 250 mg/5 mL (50 mL, 100 mL)

Ceftin®: 125 mg/5 mL (100 mL); 250 mg/5 mL (50 mL, 100 mL)

Tablet, oral: 250 mg, 500 mg

Ceftin®: 250 mg, 500 mg

cefuroxime axetil *see* cefuroxime *on page 187*

Cefuroxime For Injection (Can) *see* cefuroxime *on page 187*

cefuroxime sodium *see* cefuroxime *on page 187*

Cefzil *see* cefprozil *on page* 185
Cefzil® (Can) *see* cefprozil *on page* 185
CeleBREX® *see* celecoxib *on page* 188
Celebrex® (Can) *see* celecoxib *on page* 188

celecoxib (se le KOKS ib)

Medication Safety Issues

Sound-alike/look-alike issues:

CeleBREX® may be confused with CeleXA®, Cerebyx®, Cervarix®, Clarinex®

U.S. Brand Names CeleBREX®

Canadian Brand Names Celebrex®

Therapeutic Category Nonsteroidal Antiinflammatory Drug (NSAID), COX-2 Selective

Use Relief of the signs and symptoms of osteoarthritis, ankylosing spondylitis, juvenile idiopathic arthritis (JIA), and rheumatoid arthritis; management of acute pain; treatment of primary dysmenorrhea

General Dosage Range Dosage adjustment recommended in patients with hepatic impairment

Oral:

Children ≥2 years and ≥10 kg to ≤25 kg: 50 mg twice daily
Children ≥2 years and >25 kg: 100 mg twice daily
Adults: 100-400 mg/day in 1-2 divided doses

Dosage Forms

Capsule, oral:

CeleBREX®: 50 mg, 100 mg, 200 mg, 400 mg

Celestone® *see* betamethasone *on page* 129
Celestone® Soluspan® *see* betamethasone *on page* 129
CeleXA® *see* citalopram *on page* 213
Celexa® (Can) *see* citalopram *on page* 213
CellCept® *see* mycophenolate *on page* 619
Cellugel® *see* hydroxypropyl methylcellulose *on page* 463

cellulose, oxidized regenerated (SEL yoo lose, OKS i dyzed re JEN er aye ted)

Synonyms absorbable cotton; oxidized regenerated cellulose

U.S. Brand Names Surgicel®; Surgicel® Fibrillar; Surgicel® NuKnit

Therapeutic Category Hemostatic Agent

Use Hemostatic; temporary packing for the control of capillary, venous, or small arterial hemorrhage

General Dosage Range **Topical:** *Adults:* Lay or hold firmly minimal amounts of the fabric strip on the bleeding site

Dosage Forms

Fabric, fibrous:

Surgicel® Fibrillar:
1" x 2" (10s)
2" x 4" (10s)
4" x 4" (10s)

Fabric, knitted:

Surgicel® NuKnit:
1" x 1" (24s)
1" x 3 1/2" (10s)
3" x 4" (24s)
6" x 9" (10s)

Fabric, sheer weave:

Surgicel®:
1/2" x 2" (24s)
2" x 3" (24s)
2" x 14" (24s)
4" x 8" (24s)

Celluvisc™ (Can) *see* carboxymethylcellulose *on page* 176
Celontin® *see* methsuximide *on page* 587
Celsentri™ (Can) *see* maraviroc *on page* 562

Cemill 500 [OTC] *see* ascorbic acid *on page* *94*
Cemill 1000 [OTC] *see* ascorbic acid *on page* *94*
Cenestin® *see* estrogens (conjugated A/synthetic) *on page* *351*
Cenestin (Can) *see* estrogens (conjugated A/synthetic) *on page* *351*
Centamin [OTC] *see* vitamins (multiple/oral) *on page* *951*
Centany® *see* mupirocin *on page* *618*
Centany® AT *see* mupirocin *on page* *618*
Centrum® [OTC] *see* vitamins (multiple/oral) *on page* *951*
Centrum Cardio® [OTC] *see* vitamins (multiple/oral) *on page* *951*
Centrum Kids® [OTC] *see* vitamins (multiple/pediatric) *on page* *952*
Centrum Performance® [OTC] *see* vitamins (multiple/oral) *on page* *951*
Centrum® Silver® [OTC] *see* vitamins (multiple/oral) *on page* *951*
Centrum® Silver® Ultra Men's [OTC] *see* vitamins (multiple/oral) *on page* *951*
Centrum® Silver® Ultra Women's [OTC] *see* vitamins (multiple/oral) *on page* *951*
Centrum® Ultra Men's [OTC] *see* vitamins (multiple/oral) *on page* *951*
Centrum® Ultra Women's [OTC] *see* vitamins (multiple/oral) *on page* *951*
***Centruroides* immune FAB2 (equine)** *see Centruroides* immune $F(ab')_2$ (equine) *on page* *189*

Centruroides immune $F(ab')_2$ (equine) (sen tra ROY dez i MYUN fab too E kwine)

Synonyms *Centruroides* immune FAB2 (equine); antivenin (*Centruroides*) immune $F(ab')_2$ (equine); antivenin scorpion; antivenom (*Centruroides*) immune $F(ab')_2$ (equine); antivenom scorpion; scorpion antivenin; scorpion antivenom

U.S. Brand Names Anascorp®

Therapeutic Category Antivenin

Use Treatment of scorpion envenomation

General Dosage Range

I.V.: *Children and Adults:* Initial: 3 vials (containing ≤360 mg total protein and ≥450 LD50 [mouse] neutralizing units); may administer additional vials in 1-vial increments every 30-60 minutes as needed.

Dosage Forms

Injection, powder for reconstitution:

Anascorp®: ≤120 mg total protein and ≥150 LD50 (mouse) neutralizing units

Cepacol® [OTC] *see* cetylpyridinium *on page* *192*
Cepacol® Fizzlers™ [OTC] *see* benzocaine *on page* *121*
Cepacol® Sore Throat [OTC] *see* benzocaine *on page* *121*
Cepacol® Sore Throat & Coating [OTC] *see* benzocaine *on page* *121*
Cepacol® Sore Throat Pain Relief [OTC] [DSC] *see* benzocaine *on page* *121*
Cepacol® Sore Throat Plus Coating Relief [OTC] *see* benzocaine *on page* *121*
Cepacol® Ultra Sore Throat [OTC] *see* benzocaine *on page* *121*
Cepastat® [OTC] *see* phenol *on page* *713*
Cepastat® Extra Strength [OTC] *see* phenol *on page* *713*
Cephadyn [DSC] *see* butalbital and acetaminophen *on page* *154*

cephalexin (sef a LEKS in)

Medication Safety Issues

Sound-alike/look-alike issues:

Cephalexin may be confused with cefaclor, ceFAZolin, ciprofloxacin
Keflex® may be confused with Keppra®, Valtrex®

Synonyms cephalexin monohydrate

U.S. Brand Names Keflex®

Canadian Brand Names Apo-Cephalex®; Dom-Cephalexin; Keflex®; Novo-Lexin; Nu-Cephalex; PMS-Cephalexin

Therapeutic Category Cephalosporin (First Generation)

Use Treatment of susceptible bacterial infections including respiratory tract infections, otitis media, skin and skin structure infections, bone infections, and genitourinary tract infections, including acute prostatitis; alternative therapy for acute infective endocarditis prophylaxis

General Dosage Range Dosage adjustment recommended in patients with renal impairment

Oral:

Children >1-15 years: 25-100 mg/kg/day divided every 6-12 hours (maximum: 4 g/day) **or** 50 mg/kg prior to procedure (maximum: 2 g)

Adolescents >15 years: 25-100 mg/kg/day divided every 6-12 hours (maximum: 4 g/day) **or** 50 mg/kg prior to procedure (maximum: 2 g) **or** 500 mg every 12 hours

Adults: 250-1000 mg every 6 hours **or** 500 mg every 12 hours (maximum: 4 g/day) **or** 2 g prior to procedure

Dosage Forms

Capsule, oral: 250 mg, 500 mg

Keflex®: 250 mg, 500 mg, 750 mg

Powder for suspension, oral: 125 mg/5 mL (100 mL, 200 mL); 250 mg/5 mL (100 mL, 200 mL)

Tablet, oral: 250 mg, 500 mg

cephalexin monohydrate *see* cephalexin *on page 189*

Ceprotin *see* protein C concentrate (human) *on page 769*

Cerebyx® (Can) *see* fosphenytoin *on page 409*

Cerefolin® NAC *see* methylfolate, methylcobalamin, and acetylcysteine *on page 590*

Ceretec™ *see* technetium Tc 99m exametazime *on page 871*

Cerezyme® *see* imiglucerase *on page 475*

Certain Dri® [OTC] *see* aluminum chloride hexahydrate *on page 55*

certolizumab pegol (cer to LIZ u mab PEG ol)

Synonyms CDP870

U.S. Brand Names Cimzia®

Canadian Brand Names Cimzia®

Therapeutic Category Gastrointestinal Agent, Miscellaneous; Tumor Necrosis Factor (TNF) Blocking Agent

Use Treatment of moderately- to severely-active Crohn disease in patients who have inadequate response to conventional therapy; moderately- to severely-active rheumatoid arthritis (as monotherapy or in combination with nonbiological disease-modifying antirheumatic drugs [DMARDS])

General Dosage Range SubQ: Adults: Initial: 400 mg, repeat dose 2 and 4 weeks after initial dose; Maintenance: 400 mg every 4 weeks **or** 200 mg every other week

Dosage Forms

Injection, powder for reconstitution [preservative free]:

Cimzia®: 200 mg

Injection, solution [preservative free]:

Cimzia®: 200 mg/mL (1 mL)

Cerubidine® *see* daunorubicin (conventional) *on page 256*

Cervarix® *see* papillomavirus (types 16, 18) vaccine (human, recombinant) *on page 691*

Cervidil® *see* dinoprostone *on page 291*

C.E.S. *see* estrogens (conjugated/equine, systemic) *on page 351*

C.E.S. *see* estrogens (conjugated/equine, topical) *on page 352*

C.E.S.® (Can) *see* estrogens (conjugated/equine, systemic) *on page 351*

Cetacaine® *see* benzocaine, butamben, and tetracaine *on page 123*

Cetafen® [OTC] *see* acetaminophen *on page 20*

Cetafen Cold® [OTC] *see* acetaminophen and phenylephrine *on page 24*

Cetafen® Extra [OTC] *see* acetaminophen *on page 20*

cetirizine (se TI ra zeen)

Medication Safety Issues

Sound-alike/look-alike issues:

ZyrTEC® may be confused with Lipitor®, Serax, Xanax®, Zantac®, Zerit®, Zocor®, ZyPREXA®, ZyrTEC-D®

ZyrTEC® (cetirizine) may be confused with ZyrTEC® Itchy Eye (ketotifen)

Synonyms cetirizine hydrochloride; P-071; UCB-P071

U.S. Brand Names All Day Allergy [OTC]; ZyrTEC® Allergy [OTC]; ZyrTEC® Children's Allergy [OTC]; ZyrTEC® Children's Hives Relief [OTC]

Canadian Brand Names Aller-Relief [OTC]; Apo-Cetirizine® [OTC]; Extra Strength Allergy Relief [OTC]; PMS-Cetirizine; Reactine [OTC]; Reactine™

Therapeutic Category Antihistamine

Use Perennial and seasonal allergic rhinitis and other allergic symptoms including urticaria; chronic idiopathic urticaria

General Dosage Range Dosage adjustment recommended in patients with hepatic or renal impairment

Oral:

Children 6-12 months: 2.5 mg once daily
Children 12 months to <2 years: 2.5 mg once or twice daily
Children 2-5 years: 2.5-5 mg/day in 1-2 divided doses
Children ≥6 years and Adults: 5-10 mg once daily
Elderly: Initial: 5 mg once daily

Dosage Forms

Capsule, liquid gel, oral:
ZyrTEC® Allergy [OTC]: 10 mg
Solution, oral: 5 mg/5 mL (5 mL)
Syrup, oral: 5 mg/5 mL (5 mL, 118 mL, 120 mL, 473 mL, 480 mL)
ZyrTEC® Children's Allergy [OTC]: 5 mg/5 mL (118 mL)
ZyrTEC® Children's Hives Relief [OTC]: 5 mg/5 mL (118 mL)
Tablet, oral: 5 mg, 10 mg
All Day Allergy [OTC]: 10 mg
ZyrTEC® Allergy [OTC]: 10 mg
Tablet, chewable, oral: 5 mg, 10 mg
All Day Allergy [OTC]: 5 mg, 10 mg
ZyrTEC® Children's Allergy [OTC]: 5 mg, 10 mg

cetirizine and pseudoephedrine (se TI ra zeen & soo doe e FED rin)

Medication Safety Issues

Sound-alike/look-alike issues:
ZyrTEC® may be confused with Lipitor®, Serax, Xanax®, Zantac®, Zocor®, Zyprexa®, Zyrtec-D®
ZyrTEC-D® may be confused with ZyrTEC®

Synonyms cetirizine hydrochloride and pseudoephedrine hydrochloride; pseudoephedrine hydrochloride and cetirizine hydrochloride

U.S. Brand Names ZyrTEC-D® Allergy & Congestion [OTC]

Canadian Brand Names Reactine® Allergy and Sinus

Therapeutic Category Antihistamine/Decongestant Combination

Use Treatment of symptoms of seasonal or perennial allergic rhinitis

General Dosage Range Dosage adjustment recommended in patients with hepatic or renal impairment

Oral: *Children ≥12 years:* 1 tablet twice daily (maximum: 2 tablets/day)

Dosage Forms

Tablet, extended release: Cetirizine hydrochloride 5 mg and pseudoephedrine hydrochloride 120 mg
ZyrTEC-D® Allergy & Congestion [OTC]: Cetirizine 5 mg and pseudoephedrine 120 mg

cetirizine hydrochloride *see* cetirizine *on page 190*
cetirizine hydrochloride and pseudoephedrine hydrochloride *see* cetirizine and pseudoephedrine *on page 191*
Cetraxal® *see* ciprofloxacin (otic) *on page 211*

cetrorelix (set roe REL iks)

Synonyms cetrorelix acetate

U.S. Brand Names Cetrotide®

Canadian Brand Names Cetrotide®

Therapeutic Category Antigonadotropic Agent

Use Inhibits premature luteinizing hormone (LH) surges in women undergoing controlled ovarian stimulation

General Dosage Range SubQ: *Adults (females):* 0.25 mg once daily **or** 3 mg as a single dose

Dosage Forms

Injection, powder for reconstitution:
Cetrotide®: 0.25 mg, 3 mg

cetrorelix acetate *see* cetrorelix *on page* 191
Cetrotide® *see* cetrorelix *on page* 191

cetuximab (se TUK see mab)

Medication Safety Issues
Sound-alike/look-alike issues:
Cetuximab may be confused with bevacizumab
Synonyms C225; IMC-C225; MOAB C225
U.S. Brand Names Erbitux®
Canadian Brand Names Erbitux®
Therapeutic Category Antineoplastic Agent, Monoclonal Antibody; Epidermal Growth Factor Receptor (EGFR) Inhibitor
Use Treatment of *KRAS* mutation-negative (wild-type), EGFR-expressing metastatic colorectal cancer (in combination with FOLFIRI [irinotecan, fluorouracil, and leucovorin] as first-line treatment, in combination with irinotecan [in patients refractory to irinotecan-based chemotherapy], or as a single agent in patients who have failed oxaliplatin and irinotecan based chemotherapy or who are intolerant to irinotecan); treatment of squamous cell cancer of the head and neck (as a single agent for recurrent or metastatic disease after platinum-based chemotherapy failure; in combination with radiation therapy as initial treatment of locally or regionally advanced disease; in combination with platinum and fluorouracil-based chemotherapy as first-line treatment of locoregional or metastatic disease)

Note: Cetuximab is not indicated for the treatment of *KRAS* mutation-positive colorectal cancer.
General Dosage Range Dosage adjustment recommended in patients who develop toxicities
I.V.: *Adults:* Loading dose: 400 mg/m^2; Maintenance: 250 mg/m^2 weekly
Dosage Forms
Injection, solution [preservative free]:
Erbitux®: 2 mg/mL (50 mL, 100 mL)

cetyl alcohol, glycerin, lanolin, mineral oil, and petrolatum *see* lanolin, cetyl alcohol, glycerin, petrolatum, and mineral oil *on page* 521

cetylpyridinium (SEE til peer i DI nee um)

Synonyms cetylpyridinium chloride; CPC
U.S. Brand Names Cepacol® [OTC]; DiabetAid Therapeutic Gingivitis Mouth Rinse [OTC] [DSC]
Therapeutic Category Local Anesthetic
Use Antiseptic to aid in the prevention and reduction of plaque and gingivitis, and to freshen breath
General Dosage Range Oral: *Children ≥6 years and Adults:* Rinse or gargle in mouth twice daily
Dosage Forms
Liquid, oral:
Cepacol® [OTC]: 0.05% (710 mL)

cetylpyridinium chloride *see* cetylpyridinium *on page* 192

cevimeline (se vi ME leen)

Medication Safety Issues
Sound-alike/look-alike issues:
Cevimeline may be confused with Savella®
Evoxac® may be confused with Eurax®
Synonyms cevimeline hydrochloride
U.S. Brand Names Evoxac®
Canadian Brand Names Evoxac®
Therapeutic Category Cholinergic Agent
Use Treatment of symptoms of dry mouth in patients with Sjögren syndrome
General Dosage Range Oral: *Adults:* 30 mg 3 times/day
Dosage Forms
Capsule, oral:
Evoxac®: 30 mg

cevimeline hydrochloride *see* cevimeline *on page* 192
CFDN *see* cefdinir *on page* 182

CG *see* chorionic gonadotropin (human) *on page 206*
CG5503 *see* tapentadol *on page 868*
C-Gel [OTC] *see* ascorbic acid *on page 94*
CGP 33101 *see* rufinamide *on page 814*
CGP-39393 *see* desirudin *on page 263*
CGP-42446 *see* zoledronic acid *on page 965*
CGP-57148B *see* imatinib *on page 474*
C-Gram [OTC] *see* ascorbic acid *on page 94*
CGS-20267 *see* letrozole *on page 526*
Champix® (Can) *see* varenicline *on page 938*
Chantix® *see* varenicline *on page 938*
Charac-25 [OTC] (Can) *see* charcoal, activated *on page 193*
Charac-50 [OTC] (Can) *see* charcoal, activated *on page 193*
Charactol-25 [OTC] (Can) *see* charcoal, activated *on page 193*
Charactol-50 [OTC] (Can) *see* charcoal, activated *on page 193*

charcoal, activated (CHAR kole AK tiv ay ted)

Medication Safety Issues

Sound-alike/look-alike issues:

Actidose® may be confused with Actos®

Synonyms activated carbon; activated charcoal; adsorbent charcoal; liquid antidote; medicinal carbon; medicinal charcoal

U.S. Brand Names Actidose® with Sorbitol [OTC]; Actidose®-Aqua [OTC]; Charcoal Plus® DS [OTC]; CharcoCaps® [OTC]; EZ-Char® [OTC]; Kerr Insta-Char® in Aqueous Base [OTC]; Kerr Insta-Char® in Sorbitol Base [OTC]; Requa® Activated Charcoal [OTC]

Canadian Brand Names Charac-25 [OTC]; Charac-50 [OTC]; Charactol-25 [OTC]; Charactol-50 [OTC]; Charcodote Susp [OTC]; Charcodote TFS [OTC]; Charcodote-Aqueous Sus; Premium Activated Charcoal [OTC]

Therapeutic Category Antidote

Use

Suspension: Activated charcoal is a nonabsorbable adsorbent that may be considered in the management of poisonings when gastrointestinal decontamination of drugs or chemicals is indicated (eg, presentation to a treatment facility within 1 hour of ingestion). Activated charcoal is generally an effective adsorbent of drugs and chemicals with a molecular weight range of 100-1000 daltons. Multidose activated charcoal may be considered if a patient has ingested a life-threatening amount of carbamazepine, dapsone, phenobarbital, quinine, or theophylline (Vale, 1999).

Capsules, tablets: Digestive aid

General Dosage Range Oral, NG:

Infants <1 year: Initial: 10-25 g; additional doses of 10-25 g can be given every 4 hours

Children 1-12 years: Initial: 25-50 g; additional doses of 10-25 g can be given every 4 hours

Children >12 years and Adults: Initial: 25-100 g; additional doses of 25-50 g can be given every 4 hours

Dosage Forms

Capsule, oral:

CharcoCaps® [OTC]: 260 mg

Pellets for suspension, oral:

EZ-Char® [OTC]: 25 g/bottle (1s)

Powder for suspension, oral: USP: 100% (30 g, 240 g)

Suspension, oral:

Actidose® with Sorbitol [OTC]: 25 g (120 mL); 50 g (240 mL)
Actidose®-Aqua [OTC]: 15 g (72 mL); 25 g (120 mL); 50 g (240 mL)
Kerr Insta-Char® in Aqueous Base [OTC]: 25 g (120 mL); 50 g (240 mL)
Kerr Insta-Char® in Sorbitol Base [OTC]: 25 g (120 mL); 50 g (240 mL)

Tablet, oral:

Requa® Activated Charcoal [OTC]: 250 mg

Tablet, enteric coated, oral:

Charcoal Plus® DS [OTC]: 250 mg

Charcoal Plus® DS [OTC] *see* charcoal, activated *on page 193*
CharcoCaps® [OTC] *see* charcoal, activated *on page 193*

Charcodote-Aqueous Sus (Can) *see* charcoal, activated *on page 193*
Charcodote Susp [OTC] (Can) *see* charcoal, activated *on page 193*
Charcodote TFS [OTC] (Can) *see* charcoal, activated *on page 193*
Chemet® *see* succimer *on page 855*
Chenodal™ *see* chenodiol *on page 194*
chenodeoxycholic acid *see* chenodiol *on page 194*

chenodiol (kee noe DYE ole)

Synonyms CDCA; chenodeoxycholic acid

U.S. Brand Names Chenodal™

Therapeutic Category Bile Acid

Use Oral dissolution of radiolucent cholesterol gallstones in selected patients as an alternative to surgery

General Dosage Range Oral: *Adults:* Initial: 250 mg twice daily; Maintenance: 13-16 mg/kg/day in 2 divided doses

Dosage Forms

Tablet, oral:

Chenodal™: 250 mg

Cheracol® D [OTC] *see* guaifenesin and dextromethorphan *on page 434*
Cheracol® Plus [OTC] *see* guaifenesin and dextromethorphan *on page 434*
Cheracol® Spray [OTC] *see* phenol *on page 713*
cheratussin *see* guaifenesin *on page 433*
Cheratussin® DAC *see* guaifenesin, pseudoephedrine, and codeine *on page 437*
Chew-C [OTC] *see* ascorbic acid *on page 94*
Chew-Cal [OTC] *see* calcium and vitamin D *on page 161*
CHG *see* chlorhexidine gluconate *on page 196*
chickenpox vaccine *see* varicella virus vaccine *on page 939*
Chiggerex® Plus [OTC] *see* benzocaine *on page 121*
ChiggerTox® [OTC] *see* benzocaine *on page 121*
Children's Advil® Cold (Can) *see* pseudoephedrine and ibuprofen *on page 773*
Children's Advil® Cold and Flu Multi-Symptom (Can) *see* ibuprofen, pseudoephedrine, and chlorpheniramine *on page 470*
Children's Nasal Decongestant [OTC] *see* pseudoephedrine *on page 771*
Children's Pepto [OTC] *see* calcium carbonate *on page 161*
children's vitamins *see* vitamins (multiple/pediatric) *on page 952*
Children's Motion Sickness Liquid [OTC] (Can) *see* dimenhydrinate *on page 289*
ChiRhoStim® *see* secretin *on page 827*
chloditan *see* mitotane *on page 607*
chlodithane *see* mitotane *on page 607*
chloral *see* chloral hydrate *on page 194*

chloral hydrate (KLOR al HYE drate)

Medication Safety Issues

High alert medication:

The Institute for Safe Medication Practices (ISMP) includes this medication among its list of drugs which have a heightened risk of causing significant patient harm when used in error.

BEERS Criteria medication:

This drug may be potentially inappropriate for use in geriatric patients (Quality of evidence - low; Strength of recommendation - strong).

Synonyms chloral; hydrated chloral; trichloroacetaldehyde monohydrate

U.S. Brand Names Somnote®

Canadian Brand Names PMS-Chloral Hydrate

Therapeutic Category Hypnotic, Miscellaneous

Controlled Substance C-IV

Use Short-term sedative and hypnotic (<2 weeks); sedative/hypnotic for diagnostic procedures; sedative prior to EEG evaluations

General Dosage Range Oral:
Children: Dosage varies greatly depending on indication
Adults: 250 mg 3 times/day **or** 500-1000 mg at bedtime or prior to procedure (maximum: 2 g/day)
Elderly: Hypnotic (oral): Initial: 250 mg at bedtime

Dosage Forms
Capsule, oral:
Somnote®: 500 mg

chlorambucil (klor AM byoo sil)

Medication Safety Issues
Sound-alike/look-alike issues:
Chlorambucil may be confused with Chloromycetin®
Leukeran® may be confused with Alkeran®, leucovorin, Leukine®, Myleran®
High alert medication:
This medication is in a class the Institute for Safe Medication Practices (ISMP) includes among its list of drug classes which have a heightened risk of causing significant patient harm when used in error.

Synonyms CB-1348; chlorambucilum; chloraminophene; chlorbutinum; WR-139013

U.S. Brand Names Leukeran®

Canadian Brand Names Leukeran®

Therapeutic Category Antineoplastic Agent

Use Management of chronic lymphocytic leukemia (CLL), Hodgkin lymphoma, non-Hodgkin lymphoma (NHL)

General Dosage Range Dosage adjustment recommended in patients with hepatic impairment or who develop toxicities
Oral: *Adults:* 0.1-0.2 mg/kg/day for 3-6 weeks **or** 0.4 mg/kg intermittently, biweekly, or monthly (may increase by 0.1 mg/kg/dose)

Dosage Forms
Tablet, oral:
Leukeran®: 2 mg

chlorambucilum *see* chlorambucil *on page 195*
chloraminophene *see* chlorambucil *on page 195*

chloramphenicol (klor am FEN i kole)

Medication Safety Issues
Sound-alike/look-alike issues:
Chloromycetin® may be confused with chlorambucil, Chlor-Trimeton®

Canadian Brand Names Chloromycetin®; Chloromycetin® Succinate; Diochloram®; Pentamycetin®

Therapeutic Category Antibiotic, Miscellaneous

Use Treatment of serious infections due to organisms resistant to other less toxic antibiotics or when its penetrability into the site of infection is clinically superior to other antibiotics to which the organism is sensitive; useful in infections caused by *Bacteroides*, *H. influenzae*, *Neisseria meningitidis*, *Salmonella*, and *Rickettsia*; active against many vancomycin-resistant enterococci

General Dosage Range I.V.: *Infants >30 days, Children, and Adults:* 50-100 mg/kg/day divided every 6 hours (maximum: 4 g/day)

Dosage Forms
Injection, powder for reconstitution: 1 g

ChloraPrep® [OTC] *see* chlorhexidine gluconate *on page 196*
ChloraPrep® Frepp® [OTC] *see* chlorhexidine gluconate *on page 196*
ChloraPrep® Sepp® [OTC] *see* chlorhexidine gluconate *on page 196*
Chlorascrub™ [OTC] *see* chlorhexidine gluconate *on page 196*
Chlorascrub™ Maxi [OTC] *see* chlorhexidine gluconate *on page 196*
Chloraseptic® Kids Sore Throat Spray [OTC] *see* phenol *on page 713*
Chloraseptic® Mouth Pain [OTC] *see* phenol *on page 713*
Chloraseptic® Sore Throat Gargle [OTC] *see* phenol *on page 713*
Chloraseptic® Sore Throat Spray [OTC] *see* phenol *on page 713*
chlorbutinum *see* chlorambucil *on page 195*

chlordiazepoxide (klor dye az e POKS ide)

Medication Safety Issues

Sound-alike/look-alike issues:

ChlordiazePOXIDE may be confused with chlorproMAZINE

Librium may be confused with Librax®

BEERS Criteria medication:

This drug may be potentially inappropriate for use in geriatric patients (Quality of evidence - high; Strength of recommendation - strong).

Synonyms Librium; methaminodiazepoxide hydrochloride

Tall-Man chlordiaze**POXIDE**

Therapeutic Category Benzodiazepine

Controlled Substance C-IV

Use Management of anxiety disorder or for the short-term relief of symptoms of anxiety; withdrawal symptoms of acute alcoholism; preoperative apprehension and anxiety

General Dosage Range Dosage adjustment recommended in patients with renal or hepatic impairment.

Oral:

Children ≥6 years: 10-30 mg/day in 2-4 divided doses

Adults: 15-100 mg/day in 3-4 divided doses

Elderly: 10-20 mg/day in 2-4 divided doses

Dosage Forms

Capsule, oral: 5 mg, 10 mg, 25 mg

chlordiazepoxide and amitriptyline hydrochloride *see* amitriptyline and chlordiazepoxide *on page 64*

chlordiazepoxide and clidinium *see* clidinium and chlordiazepoxide *on page 218*

chlorethazine *see* mechlorethamine *on page 566*

chlorethazine mustard *see* mechlorethamine *on page 566*

chlorhexidine and lidocaine *see* lidocaine and chlorhexidine *(Canada only) on page 537*

chlorhexidine gluconate (klor HEKS i deen GLOO koe nate)

Medication Safety Issues

Sound-alike/look-alike issues:

Peridex® may be confused with Precedex®

Synonyms 3M™ Avagard™ [OTC]; CHG

U.S. Brand Names Avagard™ [OTC]; Bactoshield® CHG [OTC]; Betasept® [OTC]; ChloraPrep® Frepp® [OTC]; ChloraPrep® Sepp® [OTC]; ChloraPrep® [OTC]; Chlorascrub™ Maxi [OTC]; Chlorascrub™ [OTC]; Dyna-Hex® [OTC]; Hibiclens® [OTC]; Hibistat® [OTC]; Operand® Chlorhexidine Gluconate [OTC]; Peridex®; periochip®; PerioGard® [OTC]

Canadian Brand Names Hibidil® 1:2000; ORO-Clense; Peridex® Oral Rinse

Therapeutic Category Antibiotic, Oral Rinse; Antibiotic, Topical

Use Skin cleanser for line placement, skin wounds, preoperative skin preparation; germicidal hand rinse; antibacterial dental rinse. Chlorhexidine is active against gram-positive and gram-negative organisms, facultative anaerobes, aerobes, and yeast. Chip, for periodontal pocket insertion: Reduces pocket depth in patients with adult periodontitis

Orphan drug: Peridex®: Oral mucositis with cytoreductive therapy when used for patients undergoing bone marrow transplant

General Dosage Range

Oral:

Periodontal chip: *Adults:* 1 chip is inserted into a periodontal pocket, repeat every 3 months in pockets with depth ≥5 mm (maximum: 8 chips/visit)

Rinse: *Adults:* Swish 15 mL in mouth, then expectorate twice daily

Topical:

Rinse/wash: *Adults:* Apply for 15 seconds and rinse

Sanitizer: *Adults:* Dispense 1 pumpful in each palm; repeat once

Scrub: *Adults:* Scrub 3 minutes and rinse, then wash for additional 3 minutes

Dosage Forms

Chip, for periodontal pocket insertion:
periochip®: 2.5 mg (20s)

Liquid, oral: 0.12% (15 mL, 473 mL, 475 mL, 480 mL)
Peridex®: 0.12% (118 mL, 473 mL, 1893 mL)
PerioGard® [OTC]: 0.12% (480 mL)

Liquid, topical:
Betasept® [OTC]: 4% (118 mL, 237 mL, 473 mL, 946 mL, 3840 mL)
Dyna-Hex® [OTC]: 2% (120 mL, 480 mL, 960 mL, 3840 mL); 4% (120 mL, 240 mL, 480 mL, 960 mL, 3840 mL)
Hibiclens® [OTC]: 4% (15 mL, 118 mL, 236 mL, 473 mL, 946 mL, 3840 mL)
Operand® Chlorhexidine Gluconate [OTC]: 4% (118 mL, 237 mL, 472 mL, 946 mL, 3785 mL)

Lotion, topical:
Avagard™ [OTC]: 1% (500 mL)

Solution, topical:
Bactoshield® CHG [OTC]: 2% (120 mL, 480 mL, 750 mL, 960 mL, 3840 mL); 4% (120 mL, 473 mL, 960 mL, 3840 mL)

Sponge, topical:
ChloraPrep® [OTC]: 2% (25s); 2% (25s); 2% (25s); 2% (25s); 2% (25s); 2% (25s); 2% (25s); 2% (25s)
ChloraPrep® Frepp® [OTC]: 2% (20s)
ChloraPrep® Sepp® [OTC]: 2% (200s)

Sponge/Brush, topical:
Bactoshield® CHG [OTC]: 4% (300s)

Swab, topical:
Chlorascrub™ [OTC]: 3.15% (100s)

Swabsticks, topical:
ChloraPrep® [OTC]: 2% (48s, 120s)
Chlorascrub™ [OTC]: 3.15% (50s)
Chlorascrub™ Maxi [OTC]: 3.15% (30s)

Wipe, topical:
Hibistat® [OTC]: 0.5% (50s)

Chlor Hist [OTC] *see* chlorpheniramine *on page 199*

chlormeprazine *see* prochlorperazine *on page 760*

2-chlorodeoxyadenosine *see* cladribine *on page 215*

chloroethane *see* ethyl chloride *on page 364*

Chloromag® *see* magnesium chloride *on page 557*

Chloromycetin® (Can) *see* chloramphenicol *on page 195*

Chloromycetin® Succinate (Can) *see* chloramphenicol *on page 195*

chlorophyll (KLOR oh fil)

Synonyms chlorophyllin

U.S. Brand Names Nullo® [OTC]

Therapeutic Category Gastrointestinal Agent, Miscellaneous

Use Control fecal odors in colostomy or ileostomy

General Dosage Range

Oral: *Children >12 years and Adults:* 100-200 mg/day in divided doses (maximum: 300 mg/day)

Ostomy: *Children >12 years and Adults:* Place 1-2 tablets in empty pouch each time it is reused or changed

Dosage Forms

Caplet, oral:
Nullo® [OTC]: Chlorophyllin copper complex 100 mg

chlorophyllin *see* chlorophyll *on page 197*

chloroprocaine (klor oh PROE kane)

Medication Safety Issues

Sound-alike/look-alike issues:

Nesacaine® may be confused with Neptazane™

High alert medication:

The Institute for Safe Medication Practices (ISMP) includes this medication (epidural administration) among its list of drug classes which have a heightened risk of causing significant patient harm when used in error.

Synonyms chloroprocaine hydrochloride

U.S. Brand Names Nesacaine®; Nesacaine®-MPF

Canadian Brand Names Nesacaine®-CE

Therapeutic Category Local Anesthetic

Use Infiltration anesthesia, peripheral nerve block, epidural anesthesia

General Dosage Range

Caudal block: *Adults:* Preservative-free: 2% or 3%: 15-25 mL; may repeat at 40-60 minute intervals

Infiltration and peripheral nerve block:

Children >3 years: Infiltration: Concentrations of 0.5-1% (maximum without epinephrine: 11 mg/kg); Nerve block: Concentrations of 1% to 1.5% (maximum without epinephrine: 11 mg/kg)

Adults: Dosage varies greatly depending on indication

Lumbar epidural block: *Adults:* Preservative-free: 2% or 3%: 2-2.5 mL per segment; Usual total volume: 15-25 mL, may repeat with doses that are 2-6 mL less than total initial dose every 40-50 minutes

Dosage Forms

Injection, solution:

Nesacaine®: 1% [10 mg/mL] (30 mL); 2% [20 mg/mL] (30 mL)

Injection, solution [preservative free]: 2% [20 mg/mL] (20 mL); 3% [30 mg/mL] (20 mL)

Nesacaine®-MPF: 2% [20 mg/mL] (20 mL); 3% [30 mg/mL] (20 mL)

chloroprocaine hydrochloride *see* chloroprocaine *on page 198*

chloroquine (KLOR oh kwin)

Medication Safety Issues

International issues:

Aralen [U.S., Mexico] may be confused with Paralen brand name for acetaminophen [Czech Republic]

Synonyms chloroquine phosphate

U.S. Brand Names Aralen®

Canadian Brand Names Aralen®; Novo-Chloroquine

Therapeutic Category Aminoquinoline (Antimalarial)

Use Suppression/chemoprophylaxis or treatment of acute malaria due to susceptible *Plasmodium malariae, P. vivax, P. ovale, P. falciparum*; extraintestinal amebiasis

General Dosage Range Dosage adjustment recommended in patients with renal impairment

Oral: *Children and Adults:* Dosage varies greatly depending on indication

Dosage Forms

Tablet, oral: 250 mg, 500 mg

Aralen®: 500 mg

chloroquine phosphate *see* chloroquine *on page 198*

chlorothiazide (klor oh THYE a zide)

Medication Safety Issues

International issues:

Diuril [U.S., Canada] may be confused with Duorol brand name for acetaminophen [Spain]

U.S. Brand Names Diuril®; Sodium Diuril®

Canadian Brand Names Diuril®

Therapeutic Category Diuretic, Thiazide

Use Management of mild-to-moderate hypertension; adjunctive treatment of edema

General Dosage Range
I.V.: *Adults:* 250-1000 mg once or twice daily (maximum: 1000 mg/day)
Oral:
Children <6 months: 10-30 mg/kg/day in 2 divided doses (maximum: 375 mg/day)
Children ≥6 months: 10-20 mg/kg/day in 1-2 divided doses (maximum: 375 mg/day)
Adults: 250-2000 mg/day in 1-2 divided doses (maximum: 1000 mg/day [CHF])

Dosage Forms
Injection, powder for reconstitution: 500 mg
Sodium Diuril®: 0.5 g
Suspension, oral:
Diuril®: 250 mg/5 mL (237 mL)
Tablet, oral: 250 mg, 500 mg

Chlorphen [OTC] *see* chlorpheniramine *on page 199*

Chlorphen-12™ [OTC] *see* chlorpheniramine *on page 199*

chlorpheniramine (klor fen IR a meen)

Medication Safety Issues
Sound-alike/look-alike issues:
Chlor-Trimeton® may be confused with Chloromycetin®
BEERS Criteria medication:
This drug may be potentially inappropriate for use in geriatric patients (Quality of evidence - moderate; Strength of recommendation - strong).

Synonyms chlorpheniramine maleate; CTM

U.S. Brand Names Aller-chlor® [OTC]; Allergy Relief [OTC]; Chlor Hist [OTC]; Chlor-Trimeton® Allergy [OTC]; Chlorphen [OTC]; Chlorphen-12™ [OTC]; ED Chlorped Jr [OTC]; Ed ChlorPed [OTC]; Ed-Chlortan [OTC]

Canadian Brand Names Chlor-Tripolon®; Novo-Pheniram

Therapeutic Category Antihistamine

Use Perennial and seasonal allergic rhinitis and other allergic symptoms including urticaria

General Dosage Range Oral: Chlorpheniramine maleate:
Immediate release:
Children 2-5 years: 1 mg every 4-6 hours (maximum: 6 mg/24 hours)
Children 6-11 years: 2 mg every 4-6 hours (maximum: 12 mg/24 hours)
Children ≥12 years and Adults: 4 mg every 4-6 hours (maximum: 24 mg/24 hours)
Extended release: *Children ≥12 years and Adults:* 12 mg every 12 hours (maximum: 24 mg/24 hours)

Dosage Forms
Liquid, oral:
Ed ChlorPed [OTC]: 2 mg/mL (60 mL)
Syrup, oral:
Aller-chlor® [OTC]: 2 mg/5 mL (118 mL)
ED Chlorped Jr [OTC]: 2 mg/5 mL (473 mL)
Tablet, oral: 4 mg
Aller-chlor® [OTC]: 4 mg
Allergy Relief [OTC]: 4 mg
Chlor Hist [OTC]: 4 mg
Chlor-Trimeton® Allergy [OTC]: 4 mg
Chlorphen [OTC]: 4 mg
Ed-Chlortan [OTC]: 4 mg
Tablet, extended release, oral:
Chlorphen-12™ [OTC]: 12 mg

chlorpheniramine and acetaminophen (klor fen IR a meen & a seet a MIN oh fen)

Medication Safety Issues
Other safety concerns:
Duplicate therapy issues: This product contains acetaminophen, which may be a component of other combination products. Do not exceed the maximum recommended daily dose of acetaminophen.

Synonyms acetaminophen and chlorpheniramine

U.S. Brand Names Coricidin HBP® Cold and Flu [OTC]

Therapeutic Category Antihistamine/Analgesic

Use Symptomatic relief of congestion, headache, aches and pains of colds and flu

General Dosage Range Oral: *Adults:* 2 tablets every 4 hours

Dosage Forms

Tablet:

Coricidin HBP® Cold and Flu [OTC]: Chlorpheniramine 2 mg and acetaminophen 325 mg

chlorpheniramine and dextromethorphan *see* dextromethorphan and chlorpheniramine *on page 273*

chlorpheniramine and phenylephrine (klor fen IR a meen & fen il EF rin)

Medication Safety Issues

Sound-alike/look-alike issues:

Rynatan® may be confused with Rynatuss®

Synonyms chlorpheniramine maleate and phenylephrine hydrochloride; phenylephrine and chlorpheniramine

U.S. Brand Names Ed ChlorPed D [OTC]; Ed-A-Hist™ [OTC]; LoHist [OTC]; Maxichlor PEH [OTC]; nasohist™ [OTC]; NoHist LQ [OTC]; NoHist [OTC]; Sudafed PE® Sinus + Allergy [OTC]; Triaminic® Children's Cold & Allergy [OTC]; Virdec [OTC]

Therapeutic Category Antihistamine/Decongestant Combination

Use Temporary relief of upper respiratory conditions such as nasal congestion, runny nose, and sneezing due to the common cold, hay fever, or allergic or vasomotor rhinitis

General Dosage Range Oral: *Children ≥2 years and Adults:* Dosage varies greatly depending on product

Dosage Forms

Liquid, oral:

Ed-A-Hist™ [OTC], NoHist LQ [OTC]: Chlorpheniramine 4 mg and phenylephrine 10 mg per 5 mL (473 mL)

Liquid, oral [drops]:

Ed ChlorPed D [OTC]: Chlorpheniramine 2 mg and phenylephrine 5 mg per 1 mL (60 mL)

LoHist [OTC]: Chlorpheniramine 1 mg and phenylephrine 2.5 mg per 1 mL (60 mL)

nasohist™ [OTC]: Chlorpheniramine 1 mg and phenylephrine 2 mg per 1 mL (30 mL)

Virdec [OTC]: Chlorpheniramine 1 mg and phenylephrine 3.5 mg per 1 mL (30 mL)

Syrup, oral:

Triaminic® Children's Cold & Allergy [OTC]: Chlorpheniramine 1 mg and phenylephrine 2.5 mg per 5 mL (118 mL)

Tablet, oral: Chlorpheniramine 4 mg and phenylephrine 10 mg

Ed-A-Hist™ [OTC], Nohist [OTC]: Chlorpheniramine 3 mg and phenylephrine 10 mg

Maxichlor PEH [OTC], Sudafed PE® Sinus + Allergy [OTC]: Chlorpheniramine 4 mg and phenylephrine 10 mg

chlorpheniramine and pseudoephedrine (klor fen IR a meen & soo doe e FED rin)

Medication Safety Issues

Sound-alike/look-alike issues:

Chlor-Trimeton® may be confused with Chloromycetin®

Sudafed® may be confused with Sufenta®

Synonyms Allerest; chlorpheniramine maleate and pseudoephedrine hydrochloride; chlorpheniramine tannate and pseudoephedrine tannate; pseudoephedrine and chlorpheniramine

U.S. Brand Names Dicel® Chewable [OTC]; LoHist-D [OTC]; Maxichlor PSE [OTC]; Neutrahist Pediatric [OTC]; SudoGest™ Sinus & Allergy [OTC]

Canadian Brand Names Triaminic® Cold & Allergy

Therapeutic Category Antihistamine/Decongestant Combination

Use Relief of nasal congestion associated with the common cold, hay fever, allergic rhinitis, and other allergies

General Dosage Range Oral: *Children ≥6 years and Adults:* Dosage varies greatly depending on product.

Dosage Forms

Liquid, oral:

LoHist-D [OTC]: Chlorpheniramine 2 mg and pseudoephedrine 30 mg per 5 mL (473 mL)

Liquid, oral [drops]:

Neutrahist Pediatric [OTC]: Chlorpheniramine 0.8 mg and pseudoephedrine 9 mg per 1 mL (30 mL)

Tablet, oral: Chlorpheniramine 4 mg and pseudoephedrine 60 mg

Maxichlor PSE [OTC], SudoGest™ Sinus & Allergy [OTC]: Chlorpheniramine 4 mg and pseudoephedrine 60 mg

Tablet, chewable, oral:

Dicel® Chewables [OTC]: Chlorpheniramine 2 mg and pseudoephedrine 30 mg

chlorpheniramine, dextromethorphan, and pseudoephedrine *see* chlorpheniramine, pseudoephedrine, and dextromethorphan *on page 202*

chlorpheniramine, dihydrocodeine, and pseudoephedrine *see* pseudoephedrine, dihydrocodeine, and chlorpheniramine *on page 773*

chlorpheniramine maleate *see* chlorpheniramine *on page 199*

chlorpheniramine maleate, acetaminophen, phenylephrine hydrochloride, and phenyltoloxamine citrate *see* acetaminophen, chlorpheniramine, phenylephrine, and phenyltoloxamine *on page 27*

chlorpheniramine maleate and dextromethorphan hydrobromide *see* dextromethorphan and chlorpheniramine *on page 273*

chlorpheniramine maleate and hydrocodone bitartrate *see* hydrocodone and chlorpheniramine *on page 455*

chlorpheniramine maleate and phenylephrine hydrochloride *see* chlorpheniramine and phenylephrine *on page 200*

chlorpheniramine maleate and pseudoephedrine hydrochloride *see* chlorpheniramine and pseudoephedrine *on page 200*

chlorpheniramine maleate, dihydrocodeine bitartrate, and phenylephrine hydrochloride *see* dihydrocodeine, chlorpheniramine, and phenylephrine *on page 287*

chlorpheniramine maleate, ibuprofen, and pseudoephedrine *see* ibuprofen, pseudoephedrine, and chlorpheniramine *on page 470*

chlorpheniramine maleate, pseudoephedrine hydrochloride, and dextromethorphan hydrobromide *see* chlorpheniramine, pseudoephedrine, and dextromethorphan *on page 202*

chlorpheniramine, phenylephrine, and dextromethorphan

(klor fen IR a meen, fen il EF rin, & deks troe meth OR fan)

Synonyms dextromethorphan, chlorpheniramine, and phenylephrine; phenylephrine, chlorpheniramine, and dextromethorphan

U.S. Brand Names Cardec™ DM [OTC]; Corfen-DM [OTC]; De-Chlor DM [OTC]; Ed A-Hist DM [OTC]; EndaCof [OTC]; Father John's® Plus [OTC]; Maxichlor PEH DM [OTC]; nasohist™ DM pediatric [OTC]; Neo DM [OTC]; NoHist DM [OTC]; PE-Hist-DM [OTC]; Virdec DM [OTC]

Therapeutic Category Antihistamine/Decongestant/Antitussive

Use Temporary relief of cough and upper respiratory symptoms associated with allergies or the common cold

General Dosage Range Oral: *Children ≥2 years and Adults:* Dosage varies greatly depending on product

Dosage Forms

Liquid, oral:

Corfen-DM [OTC], Ed A-Hist DM [OTC], NoHist DM [OTC]: Chlorpheniramine 4 mg, phenylephrine 10 mg, and dextromethorphan 15 mg per 5 mL

De-Chlor DM [OTC]: Chlorpheniramine 2 mg, phenylephrine 10 mg, and dextromethorphan 15 mg per 5 mL

Father John's® Plus [OTC]: Chlorpheniramine 2 mg, phenylephrine 5 mg, and dextromethorphan 5 mg per 15 mL

PE-Hist-DM [OTC]: Chlorpheniramine 2 mg, phenylephrine 5 mg, and dextromethorphan 15 mg per 5 mL

Liquid, oral [drops]:
Cardec™ DM [OTC], Virdec DM [OTC]: Chlorpheniramine 1 mg, phenylephrine 3.5 mg, and dextromethorphan 3 mg per 1 mL
EndaCof [OTC]: Chlorpheniramine 1 mg, phenylephrine 2.5 mg, and dextromethorphan 2.5 mg per 1 mL
nasohist™ DM pediatric [OTC]: Chlorpheniramine 1 mg, phenylephrine 2 mg, and dextromethorphan 3 mg per 1 mL
Neo DM [OTC]: Chlorpheniramine 0.75 mg, phenylephrine 1.75 mg, and dextromethorphan 2.75 mg per 1 mL

Tablet, oral: Chlorpheniramine 4 mg, phenylephrine 10 mg, and dextromethorphan 20 mg
Maxichlor PEH DM [OTC]: Chlorpheniramine 4 mg, phenylephrine 10 mg, and dextromethorphan 20 mg

chlorpheniramine, phenylephrine, and pyrilamine *see* chlorpheniramine, pyrilamine, and phenylephrine *on page 203*

chlorpheniramine, pseudoephedrine, and codeine

(klor fen IR a meen, soo doe e FED rin, & KOE deen)

Medication Safety Issues

High alert medication:
The Institute for Safe Medication Practices (ISMP) includes this medication among its list of drug classes which have a heightened risk of causing significant patient harm when used in error.

Synonyms codeine, chlorpheniramine, and pseudoephedrine; pseudoephedrine, chlorpheniramine, and codeine

U.S. Brand Names Phenylhistine DH [OTC]; Tricode® AR

Therapeutic Category Antihistamine/Decongestant/Antitussive

Controlled Substance C-V

Use Temporary relief of cough associated with minor throat or bronchial irritation or nasal congestion due to common cold, allergic rhinitis, or sinusitis

General Dosage Range Oral:
Children 6-11 years: 5 mL every 4 hours (maximum: 20 mL/24 hours)
Children ≥12 years and Adults: 10 mL every 4 hours (maximum: 40 mL/24 hours)

Dosage Forms

Elixir, oral:
Phenylhistine DH [OTC]: Chlorpheniramine 2 mg, pseudoephedrine 30 mg, and codeine 10 mg per 5 mL (120 mL, 480 mL)

Liquid, oral:
Tricode® AR: Chlorpheniramine 2 mg, pseudoephedrine 30 mg, and codeine 8 mg per 5 mL (473 mL)

chlorpheniramine, pseudoephedrine, and dextromethorphan

(klor fen IR a meen, soo doe e FED rin, & deks troe meth OR fan)

Synonyms chlorpheniramine maleate, pseudoephedrine hydrochloride, and dextromethorphan hydrobromide; chlorpheniramine tannate, pseudoephedrine tannate, and dextromethorphan tannate; chlorpheniramine, dextromethorphan, and pseudoephedrine; dexchlorpheniramine tannate, pseudoephedrine tannate, and dextromethorphan tannate; dextromethorphan, chlorpheniramine, and pseudoephedrine; pseudoephedrine, chlorpheniramine, and dextromethorphan

U.S. Brand Names Dicel® DM Chewables [OTC]; Kidkare Children's Cough/Cold [OTC]; M-END DM [OTC]; Maxichlor PSE DM [OTC]; Neutrahist PDX [OTC]; Pedia Relief™ Cough-Cold [OTC]; Pediatric Cough & Cold [OTC]; Rescon DM [OTC]

Therapeutic Category Antihistamine/Decongestant/Antitussive

Use Temporarily relieves nasal congestion, runny nose, cough, and sneezing due to the common cold, hay fever, or allergic rhinitis

General Dosage Range Oral: *Children ≥6 years and Adults:* Dosage varies greatly depending on product

Dosage Forms

Liquid, oral: Chlorpheniramine 1 mg, pseudoephedrine 15 mg, and dextromethorphan 5 mg per 5 mL
Kidkare Children's Cough/Cold [OTC], Pedia Relief™ [OTC], Pediatric Cough & Cold [OTC]: Chlorpheniramine 1 mg, pseudoephedrine 15 mg, and dextromethorphan 5 mg per 5 mL (120 mL)
Maxichlor PSE DM [OTC]: Chlorpheniramine 4 mg, pseudoephedrine 20 mg, and dextromethorphan 20 mg per 5 mL (473 mL)
M-END DM [OTC]: Chlorpheniramine 2 mg, pseudoephedrine 15 mg, and dextromethorphan 15 mg per 5 mL (30 mL)

Rescon DM [OTC]: Chlorpheniramine 2 mg, pseudoephedrine 30 mg, and dextromethorphan 10 mg per 5 mL (120 mL, 480 mL)

Liquid, oral [drops]:

Neutrahist PDX: Chlorpheniramine 0.8 mg, pseudoephedrine 9 mg, and dextromethorphan 3 mg per 1 mL (30 mL)

Tablet, oral: Chlorpheniramine 4 mg, pseudoephedrine 60 mg, and dextromethorphan 20 mg

Maxichlor PSE DM: Chlorpheniramine 4 mg, pseudoephedrine 60 mg, and dextromethorphan 20 mg

Tablet, chewable, oral:

Dicel® DM Chewables [OTC]: Chlorpheniramine 2 mg, pseudoephedrine 30 mg, and dextromethorphan 10 mg

chlorpheniramine, pseudoephedrine, and hydrocodone *see* hydrocodone, chlorpheniramine, and pseudoephedrine *on page 457*

chlorpheniramine, pyrilamine, and phenylephrine

(klor fen IR a meen, pye RIL a meen, & fen il EF rin)

Synonyms chlorpheniramine, phenylephrine, and pyrilamine; phenylephrine, chlorpheniramine, and pyrilamine; pyrilamine, chlorpheniramine, and phenylephrine

U.S. Brand Names MyHist-PD [DSC]; Ru-Hist Forte [DSC]

Therapeutic Category Alpha/Beta Agonist; Histamine H_1 Antagonist; Histamine H_1 Antagonist, First Generation

Use Symptomatic relief of rhinitis and nasal congestion due to colds or allergy

General Dosage Range Oral: *Children ≥2 years and Adults:* Dosage varies greatly depending on product

chlorpheniramine tannate and pseudoephedrine tannate *see* chlorpheniramine and pseudoephedrine *on page 200*

chlorpheniramine tannate, pseudoephedrine tannate, and dextromethorphan tannate *see* chlorpheniramine, pseudoephedrine, and dextromethorphan *on page 202*

chlorpromazine (klor PROE ma zeen)

Medication Safety Issues

Sound-alike/look-alike issues:

ChlorproMAZINE may be confused with chlordiazePOXIDE, chlorproPAMIDE, clomiPRAMINE, prochlorperazine, promethazine

Thorazine may be confused with thiamine, thioridazine

BEERS Criteria medication:

This drug may be potentially inappropriate for use in geriatric patients (Quality of evidence - moderate; Strength of recommendation - strong).

Synonyms chlorpromazine hydrochloride; CPZ; Thorazine

Tall-Man chlorpro**MAZINE**

Canadian Brand Names Chlorpromazine Hydrochloride Inj; Teva-Chlorpromazine

Therapeutic Category Phenothiazine Derivative

Use Management of psychotic disorders (control of mania, treatment of schizophrenia); control of nausea and vomiting; relief of restlessness and apprehension before surgery; acute intermittent porphyria; adjunct in the treatment of tetanus; intractable hiccups; combativeness and/or explosive hyperexcitable behavior in children 1-12 years of age and in short-term treatment of hyperactive children

General Dosage Range

I.M., I.V.:

Children ≥6 months: 0.5-1 mg/kg every 6-8 hours (maximum: <5 years [<22.7 kg]: 40 mg/day; 5-12 years [22.7-45.5 kg]: 75 mg/day)

Adults: Initial: 25 mg; may repeat (25-50 mg) in 1-4 hours; Usual dose: 300-800 mg/day (maximum: 400 mg every 4-6 hours)

Oral:

Children ≥6 months: 0.5-1 mg/ kg every 4-6 hours as needed

Adults: Dosage varies greatly depending on indication

Dosage Forms

Injection, solution: 25 mg/mL (1 mL, 2 mL)

Tablet, oral: 10 mg, 25 mg, 50 mg, 100 mg, 200 mg

chlorpromazine hydrochloride *see* chlorpromazine *on page 203*

Chlorpromazine Hydrochloride Inj (Can) *see* chlorpromazine *on page 203*

chlorpropamide (klor PROE pa mide)

Medication Safety Issues

Sound-alike/look-alike issues:

ChlorproPAMIDE may be confused with chlorproMAZINE

Diabinese may be confused with DiaBeta®, Diamox®

High alert medication:

The Institute for Safe Medication Practices (ISMP) includes this medication among its list of drugs which have a heightened risk of causing significant patient harm when used in error.

BEERS Criteria medication:

This drug may be potentially inappropriate for use in geriatric patients (Quality of evidence - high; Strength of recommendation - strong).

Tall-Man chlorpro**PAMIDE**

Canadian Brand Names Apo-Chlorpropamide®

Therapeutic Category Antidiabetic Agent, Oral

Use Management of blood sugar in type 2 diabetes mellitus (noninsulin-dependent, NIDDM)

General Dosage Range Oral:

Adults: Initial: 250 mg/day; Maintenance: 100-500 mg/day (maximum: 750 mg/day)

Elderly: Initial: 100-125 mg/day

Dosage Forms

Tablet, oral: 100 mg, 250 mg

chlorthalidone (klor THAL i done)

Synonyms Hygroton

U.S. Brand Names Thalitone®

Canadian Brand Names Apo-Chlorthalidone®

Therapeutic Category Diuretic, Miscellaneous

Use Management of mild-to-moderate hypertension when used alone or in combination with other agents; treatment of edema associated with heart failure or nephrotic syndrome. Recent studies have found chlorthalidone effective in the treatment of isolated systolic hypertension in the elderly.

General Dosage Range Oral:

Adults: 12.5-100 mg/day **or** 100 mg 3 times/week (maximum: 200 mg/day)

Elderly: Initial: 12.5-25 mg/day or every other day

Dosage Forms

Tablet, oral: 25 mg, 50 mg

Thalitone®: 15 mg

chlorthalidone and atenolol *see* atenolol and chlorthalidone *on page 99*

chlorthalidone and azilsartan *see* azilsartan and chlorthalidone *on page 108*

chlorthalidone and clonidine *see* clonidine and chlorthalidone *on page 225*

Chlor-Trimeton® Allergy [OTC] *see* chlorpheniramine *on page 199*

Chlor-Tripolon® (Can) *see* chlorpheniramine *on page 199*

Chlor-Tripolon ND® (Can) *see* loratadine and pseudoephedrine *on page 550*

chlorzoxazone (klor ZOKS a zone)

Medication Safety Issues

BEERS Criteria medication:

This drug may be potentially inappropriate for use in geriatric patients (Quality of evidence - moderate; Strength of recommendation - strong).

U.S. Brand Names Lorzone™; Parafon Forte® DSC

Canadian Brand Names Parafon Forte®; Strifon Forte®

Therapeutic Category Skeletal Muscle Relaxant

Use Symptomatic treatment of muscle spasm and pain associated with acute musculoskeletal conditions

General Dosage Range Oral:

Children: 20 mg/kg/day **or** 600 mg/m^2/day in 3-4 divided doses

Adults: 250-750 mg 3-4 times/day

Elderly: Initial: 250 mg 2-4 times/day

Dosage Forms

Caplet, oral:

Parafon Forte® DSC: 500 mg

Tablet, oral: 500 mg

Lorzone™: 375 mg, 750 mg

cholecalciferol (kole e kal SI fer ole)

Medication Safety Issues

Sound-alike/look-alike issues:

Cholecalciferol may be confused with alfacalcidol, ergocalciferol

Administration issues:

Liquid vitamin D preparations have the potential for dosing errors when administered to infants. Droppers should be clearly marked to easily provide 400 international units. For products intended for infants, the FDA recommends that accompanying droppers deliver no more than 400 international units per dose.

Synonyms D_3

U.S. Brand Names Bio-D-Mulsion Forte® [OTC]; Bio-D-Mulsion® [OTC]; D-3 [OTC]; D3-50™ [OTC]; D3-5™ [OTC]; DDrops® Baby [OTC]; DDrops® Kids [OTC]; DDrops® [OTC]; Delta® D3 [OTC]; Enfamil® D-Vi-Sol™ [OTC]; Maximum D3® [OTC]; Vitamin D3 [OTC]

Canadian Brand Names D-Vi-Sol®

Therapeutic Category Vitamin D Analog

Use Dietary supplement, treatment of vitamin D deficiency, or prophylaxis of deficiency

General Dosage Range Oral:

Children 0-12 months: Adequate intake: 400 units/day

Children 1 year to Adults ≤70 years: RDA: 600 units/day

Elderly >70 years: RDA: 800 units/day

Dosage Forms

Capsule, oral: 5000 units

D-3 [OTC]: 1000 units

D3-50™ [OTC]: 50,000 units

D3-5™ [OTC]: 5000 units

Maximum D3® [OTC]: 10,000 units

Capsule, softgel, oral:

D-3 [OTC]: 2000 units

Solution, oral:

Bio-D-Mulsion Forte® [OTC]: 2000 units/drop (30 mL)

Bio-D-Mulsion® [OTC]: 400 units/drop (30 mL)

DDrops® [OTC]: 1000 units/drop (10 mL); 2000 units/drop (10 mL)

DDrops® Baby [OTC]: 400 units/drop (10 mL)

DDrops® Kids [OTC]: 400 units/drop (10 mL)

Enfamil® D-Vi-Sol™ [OTC]: 400 units/mL (50 mL)

Tablet, oral: 400 units, 1000 units

Delta® D3 [OTC]: 400 units

Vitamin D3 [OTC]: 1000 units

cholecalciferol and alendronate *see* alendronate and cholecalciferol *on page 45*

cholera and traveler's diarrhea vaccine *see* traveler's diarrhea and cholera vaccine *(Canada only) on page 911*

cholera vaccine *see* traveler's diarrhea and cholera vaccine *(Canada only) on page 911*

cholestyramine resin (koe LES teer a meen REZ in)

U.S. Brand Names Prevalite®; Questran®; Questran® Light

Canadian Brand Names Novo-Cholamine; Novo-Cholamine Light; Olestyr; PMS-Cholestyramine; Questran®; Questran® Light Sugar Free; ZYM-Cholestyramine-Light; ZYM-Cholestyramine-Regular

Therapeutic Category Bile Acid Sequestrant

Use Adjunct in the management of primary hypercholesterolemia; pruritus associated with elevated levels of bile acids; regression of arteriolosclerosis

General Dosage Range Oral: *Adults:* 4-24 g/day in 1-6 divided doses

Dosage Forms

Powder for suspension, oral: Cholestyramine resin 4 g/5 g of powder (210 g); Cholestyramine resin 4 g/5.7 g of powder (239.4 g); Cholestyramine resin 4 g/9 g of powder (378 g); Cholestyramine resin 4 g/5 g packet (60s); Cholestyramine resin 4 g/5.7 g packet (60s); Cholestyramine resin 4 g/9 g packet (60s)

Prevalite®: Cholestyramine resin 4 g/5.5 g of powder (231 g); Cholestyramine resin 4 g/5.5 g packet (42s, 60s)

Questran®: Cholestyramine resin 4 g/9 g of powder (378 g); Cholestyramine resin 4 g/9 g packet (60s)

Questran® Light: Cholestyramine resin 4 g/5 g of powder (210 g); Cholestyramine resin 4 g/5 g packet (60s)

Choletec® *see* technetium Tc 99m mebrofenin *on page 871*

choline fenofibrate *see* fenofibric acid *on page 376*

choline magnesium trisalicylate (KOE leen mag NEE zhum trye sa LIS i late)

Synonyms tricosal; Trilisate

Therapeutic Category Analgesic, Nonnarcotic; Nonsteroidal Antiinflammatory Drug (NSAID)

Use Management of osteoarthritis, rheumatoid arthritis, and other arthritis; acute painful shoulder

General Dosage Range Oral:

Children <37 kg: 50 mg/kg/day in 2 divided doses

Children ≥37 kg: 2250 mg/day in divided doses

Adults: 500 mg to 1.5 g 2-3 times/day **or** 3 g at bedtime

Elderly: 750 mg 3 times/day

Dosage Forms

Liquid, oral: 500 mg/5 mL (240 mL)

Cholografin® Meglumine *see* iodipamide meglumine *on page 494*

chondroitin sulfate and sodium hyaluronate *see* sodium chondroitin sulfate and sodium hyaluronate *on page 842*

Chooz® [OTC] *see* calcium carbonate *on page 161*

choriogonadotropin alfa *see* chorionic gonadotropin (recombinant) *on page 206*

Chorionic Gonadotropin for Injection (Can) *see* chorionic gonadotropin (human) *on page 206*

chorionic gonadotropin (human) (kor ee ON ik goe NAD oh troe pin, HYU man)

Synonyms CG; hCG

U.S. Brand Names Novarel®; Pregnyl®

Canadian Brand Names Chorionic Gonadotropin for Injection; Pregnyl®

Therapeutic Category Gonadotropin

Use Induces ovulation and pregnancy in anovulatory, infertile females; treatment of hypogonadotropic hypogonadism, prepubertal cryptorchidism; spermatogenesis induction with follitropin alfa

General Dosage Range I.M.:

Children: Dosage varies greatly depending on indication

Adults (females): 5000-10,000 units 1 day following last dose of menotropins

Adults (males): 1000-2000 units 2-3 times/week

Dosage Forms

Injection, powder for reconstitution: 10,000 units

Novarel®: 10,000 units

Pregnyl®: 10,000 units

chorionic gonadotropin (recombinant)

(kor ee ON ik goe NAD oh troe pin ree KOM be nant)

Synonyms choriogonadotropin alfa; r-hCG

U.S. Brand Names Ovidrel®

Canadian Brand Names Ovidrel®

Therapeutic Category Gonadotropin; Ovulation Stimulator

Use As part of an assisted reproductive technology (ART) program, induces ovulation in infertile females who have been pretreated with follicle-stimulating hormones (FSH); induces ovulation and pregnancy in infertile females when the cause of infertility is functional

General Dosage Range SubQ: *Adults (females):* 250 mcg given 1 day following last dose of follicle stimulating agent

Dosage Forms

Injection, solution:

Ovidrel®: 257.5 mcg/0.515 mL (0.515 mL)

chromic phosphate P 32 (KROME ik FOS fate pe THUR tee too)

Synonyms P32; phosphorus p32

U.S. Brand Names Phosphocol® P 32

Therapeutic Category Radiopharmaceutical

Use Treatment of peritoneal or pleural effusions caused by metastatic disease by intracavitary instillation; may be injected interstitially for the treatment of cancer

General Dosage Range Based on 70 kg patient:

Intraperitoneal instillation: *Adults:* 370-740 megabecquerels (10-20 millicuries)

Intrapleural instillation: *Adults:* 222-444 megabecquerels (6-12 millicuries)

Interstitial instillation: *Adults:* ~3.7-18.5 megabecquerels/g of tumor weight (0.1-0.5 millicuries/g)

Dosage Forms

Injection, suspension:

Phosphocol® P 32: 185 MBq (5mCi) per mL

chromium *see* trace elements *on page* 908

CI-1008 *see* pregabalin *on page* 756

Cialis® *see* tadalafil *on page* 866

ciclesonide (oral inhalation) (sye KLES oh nide)

U.S. Brand Names Alvesco®

Canadian Brand Names Alvesco®

Therapeutic Category Corticosteroid, Inhalant (Oral)

Use Prophylactic management of bronchial asthma

General Dosage Range Oral inhalation: *Children ≥12 years and Adults:* 80-320 mcg twice daily (maximum: 640 mcg/day)

Dosage Forms

Aerosol, for oral inhalation:

Alvesco®: 80 mcg/inhalation (6.1 g); 160 mcg/inhalation (6.1 g)

Dosage Forms - Canada

Aerosol for oral inhalation:

Alvesco®: 100 mcg/inhalation; 200 mcg/inhalation

ciclesonide (nasal) (sye KLES oh nide)

U.S. Brand Names Omnaris®; Zetonna™

Canadian Brand Names Omnaris®

Therapeutic Category Corticosteroid, Nasal

Use Management of seasonal and perennial allergic rhinitis

General Dosage Range Intranasal:

Omnaris®: *Children ≥6 years and Adults:* 2 sprays (50 mcg/spray) per nostril once daily (maximum: 200 mcg/day)

Zetonna™: *Children ≥12 years and Adults:* 1 spray (37 mcg/spray) per nostril once daily (maximum: 74 mcg/day)

Dosage Forms

Aerosol, intranasal:

Zetonna™: 37 mcg/inhalation (6.1 g)

Suspension, intranasal:

Omnaris®: 50 mcg/inhalation (12.5 g)

Ciclodan™ *see* ciclopirox *on page* 207

Ciclodan™ Kit *see* ciclopirox *on page* 207

ciclopirox (sye kloe PEER oks)

Synonyms ciclopirox olamine

U.S. Brand Names Ciclodan™; Ciclodan™ Kit; Loprox®; Pedipirox™ -4 Kit; Penlac®

Canadian Brand Names Apo-Ciclopirox®; Loprox®; Penlac®; Stieprox®; Taro-Ciclopirox

Therapeutic Category Antifungal Agent

Use

Cream/suspension: Treatment of tinea pedis (athlete's foot), tinea cruris (jock itch), tinea corporis (ringworm), cutaneous candidiasis, and tinea versicolor (pityriasis)

Gel: Treatment of tinea pedis (athlete's foot), tinea corporis (ringworm); seborrheic dermatitis of the scalp

Lacquer (solution): Topical treatment of mild-to-moderate onychomycosis of the fingernails and toenails due to *Trichophyton rubrum* (not involving the lunula) and the immediately-adjacent skin

Shampoo: Treatment of seborrheic dermatitis of the scalp

General Dosage Range Topical:

Cream/suspension: *Children >10 years and Adults:* Apply twice daily

Gel: *Children >16 years and Adults:* Apply twice daily

Lacquer: *Children ≥12 years and Adults:* Apply to adjacent skin and affected nails daily; remove with alcohol every 7 days

Shampoo: *Children >16 years and Adults:* Apply 5-10 mL to wet hair, lather, and leave in place ~3 minutes, rinse; repeat twice weekly (allow minimum of 3 days between applications)

Dosage Forms

Cream, topical: 0.77% (15 g, 30 g, 90 g)

Gel, topical: 0.77% (30 g, 45 g, 100 g)

Loprox®: 0.77% (30 g, 45 g, 100 g)

Shampoo, topical: 1% (120 mL)

Loprox®: 1% (120 mL)

Solution, topical: 8% (6.6 mL)

Ciclodan™: 8% (6.6 mL)

Ciclodan™ Kit: 8% (6.6 mL)

Pedipirox™ -4 Kit: 8% (1s)

Penlac®: 8% (6.6 mL)

Suspension, topical: 0.77% (30 mL, 60 mL)

ciclopirox olamine *see* ciclopirox *on page* 207

cidecin *see* daptomycin *on page* 254

cidofovir (si DOF o veer)

U.S. Brand Names Vistide®

Therapeutic Category Antiviral Agent

Use Treatment of cytomegalovirus (CMV) retinitis in patients with acquired immunodeficiency syndrome (AIDS). **Note:** Should be administered with probenecid.

General Dosage Range Dosage adjustment recommended in patients with renal impairment

I.V.: *Adults:* Induction: 5 mg/kg once weekly for 2 consecutive weeks; Maintenance: 5 mg/kg once every 2 weeks

Dosage Forms

Injection, solution [preservative free]:

Vistide®: 75 mg/mL (5 mL)

cilazapril *(Canada only)* (sye LAY za pril)

Synonyms cilazapril monohydrate

Canadian Brand Names Apo-Cilazapril®; CO Cilazapril; Inhibace®; Mylan-Cilazapril; Novo-Cilazapril; PHL-Cilazapril; PMS-Cilazapril

Therapeutic Category Angiotensin-Converting Enzyme (ACE) Inhibitor

Use Management of hypertension; treatment of heart failure

General Dosage Range Dosage adjustment recommended in patients with hepatic or renal impairment

Oral:

Adults: Initial: 0.5-2.5 mg once daily (maximum: 5 mg/day [CHF]; 10 mg/day [HTN])

Elderly: Initial: 0.5-1.25 mg once daily (maximum: 2.5 mg/day [CHF]; 10 mg/day [HTN])

Product Availability Not available in U.S.

Dosage Forms - Canada

Tablet:

Inhibace®, Novo-Cilazapril: 1 mg, 2.5 mg, 5 mg

cilazapril and hydrochlorothiazide *(Canada only)*

(sye LAY za pril & hye droe klor oh THYE a zide)

Synonyms cilazapril monohydrate and hydrochlorothiazide; hydrochlorothiazide and cilazapril

Canadian Brand Names Apo-Cilazapril®/Hctz; Inhibace® Plus; Novo-Cilazapril/HCTZ

Therapeutic Category Angiotensin-Converting Enzyme (ACE) Inhibitor

Use Treatment of mild-to-moderate hypertension; not indicated for initial treatment of hypertension

General Dosage Range Dosage adjustment recommended in hepatic impairment.

Oral: *Adults:* Dose is individualized; range: Cilazapril 2.5-10 mg/hydrochlorothiazide 6.25-25 mg/day

Product Availability Not available in U.S.

Dosage Forms - Canada

Tablet: 5/12.5: Cilazapril 5 mg and hydrochlorothiazide 12.5 mg

Inhibace® Plus 5/12.5: Cilazapril 5 mg and hydrochlorothiazide 12.5 mg

cilazapril monohydrate *see* cilazapril *(Canada only) on page 208*

cilazapril monohydrate and hydrochlorothiazide *see* cilazapril and hydrochlorothiazide *(Canada only) on page 209*

cilostazol (sil OH sta zol)

Medication Safety Issues

Sound-alike/look-alike issues:

Pletal® may be confused with Plendil®

Synonyms OPC-13013

U.S. Brand Names Pletal®

Therapeutic Category Platelet Aggregation Inhibitor

Use Symptomatic management of peripheral vascular disease, primarily intermittent claudication

General Dosage Range Dosage adjustment recommended in patients on concomitant therapy

Oral: *Adults:* 100 mg twice daily

Dosage Forms

Tablet, oral: 50 mg, 100 mg

Pletal®: 50 mg, 100 mg

Ciloxan® *see* ciprofloxacin (ophthalmic) *on page 211*

cimetidine (sye MET i deen)

Medication Safety Issues

Sound-alike/look-alike issues:

Cimetidine may be confused with simethicone

U.S. Brand Names Tagamet HB 200® [OTC]

Canadian Brand Names Apo-Cimetidine®; Dom-Cimetidine; Mylan-Cimetidine; Novo-Cimetidine; Nu-Cimet; PMS-Cimetidine

Therapeutic Category Histamine H_2 Antagonist

Use Short-term treatment of active duodenal ulcers and benign gastric ulcers; maintenance therapy of duodenal ulcer; treatment of gastric hypersecretory states; treatment of gastroesophageal reflux disease (GERD)

OTC labeling: Prevention or relief of heartburn, acid indigestion, or sour stomach

General Dosage Range Dosage adjustment recommended in patients with renal impaiment

Oral:

Children <12 years: 20-40 mg/kg/day divided every 6 hours

Children ≥12 years: 20-40 mg/kg/day divided every 6 hours **or** 200 mg 1-2 times/day [OTC]

Adults: 300-600 mg 4 times/day **or** 400-800 mg 1-2 times/day **or** 200 mg 1-2 times/day [OTC]

Dosage Forms

Solution, oral: 300 mg/5 mL (237 mL, 240 mL, 250 mL, 473 mL, 480 mL)

Tablet, oral: 200 mg, 300 mg, 400 mg, 800 mg

Tagamet HB 200® [OTC]: 200 mg

Cimzia® *see* certolizumab pegol *on page 190*

cinacalcet (sin a KAL cet)

Synonyms AMG 073; cinacalcet hydrochloride

U.S. Brand Names Sensipar®

Canadian Brand Names Sensipar®

Therapeutic Category Calcimimetic

Use Treatment of secondary hyperparathyroidism in patients with chronic kidney disease (CKD) on dialysis; treatment of hypercalcemia in patients with parathyroid carcinoma; treatment of severe hypercalcemia in patients with primary hyperparathyroidism who are unable to undergo parathyroidectomy

General Dosage Range Dosage adjustment recommended in patients on concomitant therapy or who develop toxicities

Oral: *Adults:* Initial: 30 mg once or twice daily; Maintenance: Increase dose incrementally every 2-4 weeks to normalize calcium levels or maintain iPTH level (maximum: 360 mg/day [parathyroid cancer, primary hyperparathyroidism]; 180 mg/day [secondary hyperparathyroidism])

Dosage Forms

Tablet, oral:

Sensipar®: 30 mg, 60 mg, 90 mg

cinacalcet hydrochloride *see* cinacalcet *on page 209*

Cinryze® *see* C1 inhibitor (human) *on page 156*

Cipralex® (Can) *see* escitalopram *on page 345*

Cipro® *see* ciprofloxacin (systemic) *on page 210*

Cipro® XL (Can) *see* ciprofloxacin (systemic) *on page 210*

Ciprodex® *see* ciprofloxacin and dexamethasone *on page 211*

ciprofloxacin (systemic) (sip roe FLOKS a sin)

Medication Safety Issues

Sound-alike/look-alike issues:

Ciprofloxacin may be confused with cephalexin

Cipro® may be confused with Ceftin®

Synonyms ciprofloxacin hydrochloride

U.S. Brand Names Cipro®; Cipro® I.V.

Canadian Brand Names Apo-Ciproflox®; Auro-Ciprofloxacin; Ciprofloxacin Injection; Ciprofloxacin Intravenous Infusion; Cipro®; Cipro® XL; CO Ciprofloxacin; Dom-Ciprofloxacin; JAMP-Ciprofloxacin; Mint-Ciprofloxacin; Mylan-Ciprofloxacin; Novo-Ciprofloxacin; PHL-Ciprofloxacin; PMS-Ciprofloxacin; PRO-Ciprofloxacin; RAN™-Ciprofloxacin; ratio-Ciprofloxacin; Riva-Ciprofloxacin; Sandoz-Ciprofloxacin; Taro-Ciprofloxacin

Therapeutic Category Antibiotic, Quinolone

Use

Children: Complicated urinary tract infections and pyelonephritis due to *E. coli*. **Note:** Although effective, ciprofloxacin is not the drug of first choice in children.

Children and Adults: To reduce incidence or progression of disease following exposure to aerolized *Bacillus anthracis*.

Adults: Treatment of the following infections when caused by susceptible bacteria: Urinary tract infections; acute uncomplicated cystitis in females; chronic bacterial prostatitis; lower respiratory tract infections (including acute exacerbations of chronic bronchitis); acute sinusitis; skin and skin structure infections; bone and joint infections; complicated intraabdominal infections (in combination with metronidazole); infectious diarrhea; typhoid fever due to *Salmonella typhi* (eradication of chronic typhoid carrier state has not been proven); uncomplicated cervical and urethra gonorrhea (due to *N. gonorrhoeae*); nosocomial pneumonia; empirical therapy for febrile neutropenic patients (in combination with piperacillin)

Note: As of April 2007, the CDC no longer recommends the use of fluoroquinolones for the treatment of gonococcal disease.

General Dosage Range Dosage adjustment recommended in patients with renal impairment

I.V.:

Children: 20-30 mg/kg/day divided every 12 hours (maximum: 800 mg/day)

Adults: 200-400 mg every 8-12 hours

Oral:

Extended release: *Adults:* 500-1000 mg every 24 hours

Immediate release:

Children: 20-30 mg/kg/day in 2 divided doses (maximum: 1.5 g/day)

Adults: 250-750 mg every 12 hours or 250 mg to 1 g as a single dose

Dosage Forms

Infusion, premixed in D_5W: 200 mg (100 mL); 400 mg (200 mL)
Cipro® I.V.: 400 mg (200 mL)
Infusion, premixed in D_5W [preservative free]: 200 mg (100 mL); 400 mg (200 mL)
Injection, solution: 10 mg/mL (20 mL, 40 mL, 120 mL)
Injection, solution [preservative free]: 10 mg/mL (20 mL, 40 mL)
Microcapsules for suspension, oral:
Cipro®: 250 mg/5 mL (100 mL); 500 mg/5 mL (100 mL)
Tablet, oral: 100 mg, 250 mg, 500 mg, 750 mg
Cipro®: 250 mg, 500 mg
Tablet, extended release, oral: 500 mg, 1000 mg

ciprofloxacin (ophthalmic) (sip roe FLOKS a sin)

Medication Safety Issues

Sound-alike/look-alike issues:
Ciprofloxacin may be confused with cephalexin
Ciloxan® may be confused with Cytoxan

Synonyms ciprofloxacin hydrochloride

U.S. Brand Names Ciloxan®

Canadian Brand Names Ciloxan®

Therapeutic Category Antibiotic, Ophthalmic; Antibiotic, Quinolone

Use Treatment of superficial ocular infections (corneal ulcers, conjunctivitis) due to susceptible strains

General Dosage Range Ophthalmic:

Ointment: *Children >2 years and Adults:* Apply a 1/2" ribbon into the conjunctival sac 3 times/day for the first 2 days, followed by a 1/2" ribbon applied twice daily

Solution: *Children >1 year and Adults:* Conjunctivitis: Instill 1-2 drops in eye(s) every 2 hours while awake for 2 days, then 1-2 drops every 4 hours while awake; Corneal ulcer: Instill 2 drops into affected eye every 15 minutes for the first 6 hours, then 2 drops every 30 minutes for the remainder of the first day; on day 2 instill 2 drops into the affected eye hourly; on days 3-14 instill 2 drops every 4 hours

Dosage Forms

Ointment, ophthalmic:
Ciloxan®: 3.33 mg/g (3.5 g)
Solution, ophthalmic: 3.5 mg/mL (2.5 mL, 5 mL, 10 mL)
Ciloxan®: 3.5 mg/mL (5 mL)

ciprofloxacin (otic) (sip roe FLOKS a sin)

Medication Safety Issues

Sound-alike/look-alike issues:
Cetraxal® may be confused with cefTRIAXone
Ciprofloxacin may be confused with cephalexin

Synonyms ciprofloxacin hydrochloride

U.S. Brand Names Cetraxal®

Therapeutic Category Antibiotic, Otic; Antibiotic, Quinolone

Use Treatment of acute otitis externa due to susceptible strains of *Pseudomonas aeruginosa* or *Staphylococcus aureus*

General Dosage Range Otic: *Children ≥1 year and Adults:* 0.5 mg (0.25 mL) every 12 hours

Dosage Forms

Solution, otic [preservative free]:
Cetraxal®: 0.5 mg/0.25 mL (14s)

ciprofloxacin and dexamethasone (sip roe FLOKS a sin & deks a METH a sone)

Synonyms ciprofloxacin hydrochloride and dexamethasone; dexamethasone and ciprofloxacin

U.S. Brand Names Ciprodex®

Canadian Brand Names Ciprodex®

Therapeutic Category Antibiotic/Corticosteroid, Otic

Use Treatment of acute otitis media in pediatric patients with tympanostomy tubes or acute otitis externa in children and adults

General Dosage Range Otic: *Children and Adults:* Instill 4 drops into affected ear(s) twice daily

Dosage Forms

Suspension, otic:

Ciprodex®: Ciprofloxacin 0.3% and dexamethasone 0.1% (7.5 mL)

ciprofloxacin and hydrocortisone (sip roe FLOKS a sin & hye droe KOR ti sone)

Synonyms ciprofloxacin hydrochloride and hydrocortisone; hydrocortisone and ciprofloxacin

U.S. Brand Names Cipro® HC

Canadian Brand Names Cipro® HC

Therapeutic Category Antibiotic/Corticosteroid, Otic

Use Treatment of acute otitis externa, sometimes known as "swimmer's ear"

General Dosage Range Otic: *Children >1 year and Adults:* 3 drops into affected ear(s) twice daily

Dosage Forms

Suspension, otic:

Cipro® HC: Ciprofloxacin 0.2% and hydrocortisone 1% (10 mL)

ciprofloxacin hydrochloride *see* ciprofloxacin (ophthalmic) *on page 211*

ciprofloxacin hydrochloride *see* ciprofloxacin (otic) *on page 211*

ciprofloxacin hydrochloride *see* ciprofloxacin (systemic) *on page 210*

ciprofloxacin hydrochloride and dexamethasone *see* ciprofloxacin and dexamethasone *on page 211*

ciprofloxacin hydrochloride and hydrocortisone *see* ciprofloxacin and hydrocortisone *on page 212*

Ciprofloxacin Injection (Can) *see* ciprofloxacin (systemic) *on page 210*

Ciprofloxacin Intravenous Infusion (Can) *see* ciprofloxacin (systemic) *on page 210*

Cipro® HC *see* ciprofloxacin and hydrocortisone *on page 212*

Cipro® I.V. *see* ciprofloxacin (systemic) *on page 210*

cisapride (SIS a pride)

Medication Safety Issues

Sound-alike/look-alike issues:

Propulsid® may be confused with propranolol

U.S. Brand Names Propulsid®

Therapeutic Category Gastrointestinal Agent, Prokinetic

Use Treatment of nocturnal symptoms of gastroesophageal reflux disease (GERD); has demonstrated effectiveness for gastroparesis, refractory constipation, and nonulcer dyspepsia

General Dosage Range

Oral:

Children: 0.15-0.3 mg/kg 3-4 times/day (maximum: 10 mg/dose)

Adults: Initial: 5-10 mg 4 times/day, may increase to 20 mg 4 times/day if needed

cisatracurium (sis a tra KYOO ree um)

Medication Safety Issues

Sound-alike/look-alike issues:

Nimbex® may be confused with Revex®

High alert medication:

The Institute for Safe Medication Practices (ISMP) includes this medication among its list of drugs which have a heightened risk of causing significant patient harm when used in error.

Other safety concerns:

United States Pharmacopeia (USP) 2006: The Interdisciplinary Safe Medication Use Expert Committee of the USP has recommended the following:

- Hospitals, clinics, and other practice sites should institute special safeguards in the storage, labeling, and use of these agents and should include these safeguards in staff orientation and competency training.
- Healthcare professionals should be on high alert (especially vigilant) whenever a neuromuscular-blocking agent (NMBA) is stocked, ordered, prepared, or administered.

Synonyms cisatracurium besylate

U.S. Brand Names Nimbex®

Canadian Brand Names Nimbex®

Therapeutic Category Skeletal Muscle Relaxant

Use Adjunct to general anesthesia to facilitate endotracheal intubation and to relax skeletal muscles during surgery; to facilitate mechanical ventilation in ICU patients; does not relieve pain or produce sedation

General Dosage Range I.V.:

Children 1-23 months: Intubating dose: 0.15 mg/kg

Children 2-12 years: Intubating dose: 0.1-0.15 mg/kg over 5-15 seconds; Infusion: Initial: 3 mcg/kg/minute; Maintenance: 1-2 mcg/kg/minute (surgery) **or** 0.5-10 mcg/kg/minute (ICU)

Children >12 years: Infusion: Initial: 3 mcg/kg/minute; Maintenance: 1-2 mcg/kg/minute (surgery) **or** 0.5-10 mcg/kg/minute (ICU)

Adults: Intubating dose: 0.1-0.2 mg/kg; Infusion: Initial: 3 mcg/kg/minute; Maintenance: 1-2 mcg/kg/minute (surgery) **or** 0.5-10 mcg/kg/minute (ICU)

Dosage Forms

Injection, solution: 2 mg/mL (5 mL, 10 mL); 10 mg/mL (20 mL)

Nimbex®: 2 mg/mL (5 mL, 10 mL); 10 mg/mL (20 mL)

cisatracurium besylate *see* cisatracurium *on page* 212

CIS-MDP™ *see* technetium Tc 99m medronate *on page* 872

cisplatin (SIS pla tin)

Medication Safety Issues

Sound-alike/look-alike issues:

CISplatin may be confused with CARBOplatin, oxaliplatin

High alert medication:

This medication is in a class the Institute for Safe Medication Practices (ISMP) includes among its list of drugs which have a heightened risk of causing significant patient harm when used in error.

BEERS Criteria medication:

This drug may be potentially inappropriate for use in geriatric patients (Quality of evidence - moderate; Strength of recommendation - strong).

Administration issues:

Doses >100 mg/m^2 once every 3-4 weeks are rarely used and should be verified with the prescriber.

Synonyms CDDP; Platinol; Platinol-AQ

Tall-Man **CIS**platin

Therapeutic Category Antineoplastic Agent

Use Treatment of advanced bladder cancer, metastatic testicular cancer, and metastatic ovarian cancer

General Dosage Range Dosage adjustment recommended in patients with renal impairment

I.V.: *Adults:* 50-70 mg/m^2 every 3-4 weeks **or** 75-100 mg/m^2/day every 4 weeks **or** 20 mg/m^2/day for 5 days every 3 weeks

Dosage Forms

Injection, solution [preservative free]: 1 mg/mL (50 mL, 100 mL, 200 mL)

***Cis*-retinoic acid** *see* isotretinoin *on page* 505

13-*cis*-retinoic acid *see* isotretinoin *on page* 505

13-*cis*-vitamin A acid *see* isotretinoin *on page* 505

citalopram (sye TAL oh pram)

Medication Safety Issues

Sound-alike/look-alike issues:

CeleXA® may be confused with CeleBREX®, Cerebyx®, Ranexa™, ZyPREXA®

BEERS Criteria medication:

This drug may be potentially inappropriate for use in geriatric patients (Quality of evidence - moderate; Strength of recommendation - strong).

Synonyms citalopram hydrobromide; nitalapram

U.S. Brand Names CeleXA®

Canadian Brand Names Apo-Citalopram®; Auro-Citalopram; Ava-Citalopram; Celexa®; Citalopram-Odan; CO Citalopram; CTP 30; Dom-Citalopram; JAMP-Citalopram; Manda-Citalopram; Mint-Citalopram; Mylan-Citalopram; PHL-Citalopram; PMS-Citalopram; Q-Citalopram; RAN™-Citalo; ratio-Citalopram; Riva-Citalopram; Sandoz-Citalopram; Septa-Citalopram; Teva-Citalopram

Therapeutic Category Antidepressant

Use Treatment of depression

General Dosage Range Dosage adjustment recommended in patients with hepatic impairment

Oral:

Adults (<60 years): Initial: 20 mg daily; Maintenance: 40 mg daily; Maximum: 40 mg daily

Adults (≥60 years): Initial: 20 mg/day; Maximum: 20 mg/day

Dosage Forms

Solution, oral: 10 mg/5 mL (240 mL)

Tablet, oral: 10 mg, 20 mg, 40 mg

CeleXA®: 10 mg, 20 mg, 40 mg

citalopram hydrobromide *see* citalopram *on page 213*

Citalopram-Odan (Can) *see* citalopram *on page 213*

Citanest® Plain (Can) *see* prilocaine *on page 757*

Citanest® Plain Dental *see* prilocaine *on page 757*

Citracal® Maximum [OTC] *see* calcium and vitamin D *on page 161*

Citracal® Petites [OTC] *see* calcium and vitamin D *on page 161*

Citracal® Regular [OTC] *see* calcium and vitamin D *on page 161*

CitraNatal™ 90 DHA *see* vitamins (multiple/prenatal) *on page 952*

CitraNatal™ Assure *see* vitamins (multiple/prenatal) *on page 952*

CitraNatal™ B-Calm *see* vitamins (multiple/prenatal) *on page 952*

CitraNatal™ DHA *see* vitamins (multiple/prenatal) *on page 952*

CitraNatal® Harmony™ *see* vitamins (multiple/prenatal) *on page 952*

CitraNatal™ Rx *see* vitamins (multiple/prenatal) *on page 952*

citrate of magnesia *see* magnesium citrate *on page 558*

citric acid and D-gluconic acid irrigant *see* citric acid, magnesium carbonate, and glucono-delta-lactone *on page 214*

citric acid and potassium citrate *see* potassium citrate and citric acid *on page 745*

citric acid bladder mixture *see* citric acid, magnesium carbonate, and glucono-delta-lactone *on page 214*

citric acid, magnesium carbonate, and glucono-delta-lactone

(SI trik AS id, mag NEE see um KAR bo nate, and GLOO kon o DEL ta LAK tone)

Medication Safety Issues

Sound-alike/look-alike issues:

Renacidin® may be confused with Remicade®

Synonyms citric acid and D-gluconic acid irrigant; citric acid bladder mixture; citric acid, magnesium hydroxycarbonate, D-gluconic acid, magnesium acid citrate, and calcium carbonate; hemiacidrin

U.S. Brand Names Renacidin®

Therapeutic Category Irrigating Solution

Use Prevention of formation of calcifications of indwelling urinary tract catheters; treatment of renal and bladder calculi of the apatite or struvite type

General Dosage Range Irrigation: *Adults:* 30-60 mL into catheter 2-3 times/day **or** 30 mL into bladder, retained for 30-60 minutes then drained 4-6 times **or** 60-120 mL/hour

Dosage Forms

Solution, irrigation:

Renacidin®: Citric acid 6.602 g, magnesium carbonate 3.177 g, glucono-delta-lactone 0.198 g per 100 mL (500 mL)

citric acid, magnesium hydroxycarbonate, D-gluconic acid, magnesium acid citrate, and calcium carbonate *see* citric acid, magnesium carbonate, and glucono-delta-lactone *on page 214*

citric acid, sodium citrate, and potassium citrate

(SIT rik AS id, SOW dee um SIT rate, & poe TASS ee um SIT rate)

Medication Safety Issues

Sound-alike/look-alike issues:

Polycitra may be confused with Bicitra

Synonyms Polycitra; potassium citrate, citric acid, and sodium citrate; sodium citrate, citric acid, and potassium citrate

U.S. Brand Names Cytra-3; Tricitrates

Therapeutic Category Alkalinizing Agent

Use Conditions where long-term maintenance of an alkaline urine is desirable as in control and dissolution of uric acid and cystine calculi of the urinary tract

General Dosage Range Oral:

Children: 5-15 mL after meals and at bedtime

Adults: 15-30 mL after meals and at bedtime

Dosage Forms

Solution, oral:

Cytra-3, Tricitrates: Citric acid 334 mg, sodium citrate 500 mg, and potassium citrate 550 mg per 5 mL

citric acid, sodium picosulfate, and magnesium oxide *see* sodium picosulfate, magnesium oxide, and citric acid *on page* 846

Citroma® [OTC] *see* magnesium citrate *on page* 558

Citro-Mag® (Can) *see* magnesium citrate *on page* 558

citrovorum factor *see* leucovorin calcium *on page* 527

Citrucel® [OTC] *see* methylcellulose *on page* 588

CL-118,532 *see* triptorelin *on page* 922

CI-719 *see* gemfibrozil *on page* 422

CL-184116 *see* porfimer *on page* 741

CL-232315 *see* mitoxantrone *on page* 608

cladribine (KLA dri been)

Medication Safety Issues

Sound-alike/look-alike issues:

Cladribine may be confused with clevidipine, clofarabine, fludarabine

Leustatin® may be confused with lovastatin

High alert medication:

This medication is in a class the Institute for Safe Medication Practices (ISMP) includes among its list of drug classes which have a heightened risk of causing significant patient harm when used in error.

Synonyms 2-CdA; 2-chlorodeoxyadenosine

U.S. Brand Names Leustatin® [DSC]

Therapeutic Category Antineoplastic Agent

Use Treatment of hairy cell leukemia

General Dosage Range Dosage adjustment recommended in patients with renal impairment

I.V.: *Adults:* Continuous infusion: 0.09 mg/kg/day for 7 days

Dosage Forms

Injection, solution [preservative free]: 1 mg/mL (10 mL)

Claforan® *see* cefotaxime *on page* 183

Claravis™ *see* isotretinoin *on page* 505

Clarifoam™ EF *see* sulfur and sulfacetamide *on page* 862

Clarinex® *see* desloratadine *on page* 263

Clarinex-D® 12 Hour *see* desloratadine and pseudoephedrine *on page* 263

Clarinex-D® 24 Hour *see* desloratadine and pseudoephedrine *on page* 263

Claris™ *see* sulfur and sulfacetamide *on page* 862

clarithromycin (kla RITH roe mye sin)

Medication Safety Issues

Sound-alike/look-alike issues:

Clarithromycin may be confused with Claritin®, clindamycin, erythromycin

U.S. Brand Names Biaxin®; Biaxin® XL

Canadian Brand Names Apo-Clarithromycin®; Ava-Clarithromycin; Biaxin®; Biaxin® XL; Dom-Clarithromycin; Mylan-Clarithromycin; PMS-Clarithromycin; RAN™-Clarithromycin; ratio-Clarithromycin; Riva-Clarithromycin; Sandoz-Clarithromycin

Therapeutic Category Antibiotic, Macrolide

Use

Children:

Acute maxillary sinusitis due to susceptible *H. influenzae, S. pneumoniae,* or *Moraxella catarrhalis*

Acute otitis media due to susceptible *H. influenzae*, *M. catarrhalis*, or *S. pneumoniae*

Community-acquired pneumonia due to susceptible *Mycoplasma pneumoniae*, *S. pneumoniae*, or *Chlamydia pneumoniae* (TWAR)
Disseminated mycobacterial infections due to *M. avium* or *M. intracellulare*
Pharyngitis/tonsillitis due to susceptible *S. pyogenes*
Prevention of disseminated mycobacterial infections due to MAC disease in patients with advanced HIV infection
Uncomplicated skin/skin structure infection due to susceptible *S. aureus, S. pyogenes,* or mycobacterial infections

Adults:
Pharyngitis/tonsillitis due to susceptible *S. pyogenes*
Acute maxillary sinusitis due to susceptible *H. influenzae, M. catarrhalis,* or *S. pneumoniae*
Acute exacerbation of chronic bronchitis due to susceptible *H. influenzae*, *H. parainfluenzae*, *M. catarrhalis*, or *S. pneumoniae*
Community-acquired pneumonia due to susceptible *H. influenzae, H. parainfluenzae, M. catarrhalis, Mycoplasma pneumoniae, S. pneumoniae,* or *Chlamydia pneumoniae* (TWAR)
Uncomplicated skin/skin structure infections due to susceptible *S. aureus, S. pyogenes*
Disseminated mycobacterial infections due to *M. avium* or *M. intracellulare*
Prevention of disseminated mycobacterial infections due to *M. avium* complex (MAC) disease (eg, patients with advanced HIV infection)
Duodenal ulcer disease due to *H. pylori* in regimens with other drugs including amoxicillin and lansoprazole or omeprazole, or in combination with omeprazole or ranitidine bismuth citrate (no longer marketed in the U.S.). **Note:** Regimens that contain clarithromycin as the single antimicrobial agent are more likely to be associated with the development of clarithromycin resistance.

General Dosage Range Dosage adjustment recommended in patients with renal impairment

Oral:
Extended release: *Adults:* 1000 mg once daily
Immediate release:
Children: 15 mg/kg/day divided every 12 hours (maximum: 1 g/day) **or** 15 mg/kg prior to procedure (maximum: 500 mg)
Adults: 250-500 mg every 8-12 hours **or** 500 mg prior to procedure

Dosage Forms

Granules for suspension, oral: 125 mg/5 mL (50 mL, 100 mL); 250 mg/5 mL (50 mL, 100 mL)
Biaxin®: 125 mg/5 mL (50 mL, 100 mL); 250 mg/5 mL (50 mL, 100 mL)
Tablet, oral: 250 mg, 500 mg
Biaxin®: 250 mg, 500 mg
Tablet, extended release, oral: 500 mg
Biaxin® XL: 500 mg

clarithromycin, amoxicillin, and omeprazole *see* omeprazole, clarithromycin, and amoxicillin *on page 666*

clarithromycin, lansoprazole, and amoxicillin *see* lansoprazole, amoxicillin, and clarithromycin *on page 523*

Claritin® (Can) *see* loratadine *on page 549*

Claritin® 24 Hour Allergy [OTC] *see* loratadine *on page 549*

Claritin-D® 12 Hour Allergy & Congestion [OTC] *see* loratadine and pseudoephedrine *on page 550*

Claritin-D® 24 Hour Allergy & Congestion [OTC] *see* loratadine and pseudoephedrine *on page 550*

Claritin® Allergic Decongestant (Can) *see* oxymetazoline (nasal) *on page 681*

Claritin® Children's Allergy [OTC] *see* loratadine *on page 549*

Claritin® Extra (Can) *see* loratadine and pseudoephedrine *on page 550*

Claritin™ Eye [OTC] *see* ketotifen (ophthalmic) *on page 514*

Claritin® Kids (Can) *see* loratadine *on page 549*

Claritin® Liberator (Can) *see* loratadine and pseudoephedrine *on page 550*

Claritin® Liqui-Gels® 24 Hour Allergy [OTC] *see* loratadine *on page 549*

Claritin® RediTabs® 24 Hour Allergy [OTC] *see* loratadine *on page 549*

Clarus™ (Can) *see* isotretinoin *on page 505*

Clasteon® (Can) *see* clodronate *(Canada only) on page 222*

clavulanic acid and amoxicillin *see* amoxicillin and clavulanate *on page 70*

Clavulin® (Can) *see* amoxicillin and clavulanate *on page 70*

Clean & Clear® advantage® 3-in-1 [OTC] *see* benzoyl peroxide *on page* 124
Clean & Clear® Advantage® Acne Cleanser [OTC] *see* salicylic acid *on page* 816
Clean & Clear® Advantage® Acne Spot Treatment [OTC] *see* salicylic acid *on page* 816
Clean & Clear® Advantage® Invisible Acne Patch [OTC] *see* salicylic acid *on page* 816
Clean & Clear® Advantage® Oil-Free Acne [OTC] *see* salicylic acid *on page* 816
Clean & Clear® Blackhead Clearing Daily Cleansing [OTC] *see* salicylic acid *on page* 816
Clean & Clear® Blackhead Clearing Scrub [OTC] *see* salicylic acid *on page* 816
Clean & Clear® continuous control® [OTC] *see* benzoyl peroxide *on page* 124
Clean & Clear® Deep Cleaning [OTC] *see* salicylic acid *on page* 816
Clean & Clear® Dual Action Moisturizer [OTC] *see* salicylic acid *on page* 816
Clean & Clear® Invisible Blemish Treatment [OTC] *see* salicylic acid *on page* 816
Clean & Clear® persa-gel® 10 [OTC] *see* benzoyl peroxide *on page* 124
Clear eyes® for Dry Eyes Plus ACR Relief [OTC] *see* naphazoline (ophthalmic) *on page* 627
Clear eyes® for Dry Eyes plus Redness Relief [OTC] *see* naphazoline (ophthalmic) *on page* 627
Clear eyes® Redness Relief [OTC] *see* naphazoline (ophthalmic) *on page* 627
Clear eyes® Seasonal Relief [OTC] *see* naphazoline (ophthalmic) *on page* 627
Clearskin [OTC] *see* benzoyl peroxide *on page* 124

clemastine (KLEM as teen)

Medication Safety Issues

BEERS Criteria medication:

This drug may be potentially inappropriate for use in geriatric patients (Quality of evidence - moderate; Strength of recommendation - strong).

Synonyms clemastine fumarate

U.S. Brand Names Tavist® Allergy [OTC]

Therapeutic Category Antihistamine

Use Perennial and seasonal allergic rhinitis and other allergic symptoms including urticaria

General Dosage Range Oral:

Children <6 years: 0.05 mg/kg/day (base) **or** 0.335-0.67 mg/day (fumarate) in 2-3 divided doses (maximum: 1.34 mg/day [fumarate] or 1 mg/day [base])

Children 6-12 years: 0.67-1.34 mg fumarate (0.5-1 mg base) twice daily (maximum: 4.02 mg/day [3 mg base])

Children ≥12 years and Adults: 1.34-2.68 mg fumarate (1-2 mg base) 2-3 times/day (maximum: 8.04 mg/day [6 mg base])

Dosage Forms

Syrup, oral: 0.67 mg/5 mL (120 mL)

Tablet, oral: 1.34 mg, 2.68 mg

Tavist® Allergy [OTC]: 1.34 mg

clemastine fumarate *see* clemastine *on page* 217
Clenia® *see* sulfur and sulfacetamide *on page* 862
Cleocin® *see* clindamycin (topical) *on page* 219
Cleocin HCl® *see* clindamycin (systemic) *on page* 218
Cleocin Pediatric® *see* clindamycin (systemic) *on page* 218
Cleocin Phosphate® *see* clindamycin (systemic) *on page* 218
Cleocin T® *see* clindamycin (topical) *on page* 219
Cleocin® Vaginal Ovule *see* clindamycin (topical) *on page* 219

clevidipine (klev ID i peen)

Medication Safety Issues

Sound-alike/look-alike issues:

Clevidipine may be confused with cladribine, clofarabine, clomiPRAMINE
Cleviprex® may be confused with Claravis™

Synonyms clevidipine butyrate

U.S. Brand Names Cleviprex®

Therapeutic Category Calcium Channel Blocker

Use Management of hypertension

General Dosage Range I.V.: *Adults:* Initial: 1-2 mg/hour; Usual maintenance: 4-6 mg/hour; Maximum: 21 mg/hour (1000 mL/24 hours)

Dosage Forms

Injection, emulsion:

Cleviprex®: 0.5 mg/mL (50 mL, 100 mL)

clevidipine butyrate *see* clevidipine *on page 217*

Cleviprex® *see* clevidipine *on page 217*

clidinium and chlordiazepoxide (kli DI nee um & klor dye az e POKS ide)

Medication Safety Issues

Sound-alike/look-alike issues:

Librax® may be confused with Librium

BEERS Criteria medication:

This drug may be inappropriate for use in geriatric patients (Quality of evidence: moderate [clidinium]/ high [chlordiazepoxide]; Strength of recommendation - strong).

Synonyms chlordiazepoxide and clidinium

U.S. Brand Names Librax®

Canadian Brand Names Apo-Chlorax®; Librax®

Therapeutic Category Anticholinergic Agent

Use Adjunct treatment of peptic ulcer; treatment of irritable bowel syndrome

General Dosage Range Oral: *Adults:* 1-2 capsules 3-4 times/day

Dosage Forms

Capsule: Clidinium 2.5 mg and chlordiazepoxide 5 mg

Librax®: Clidinium 2.5 mg and chlordiazepoxide 5 mg

Climara® *see* estradiol (systemic) *on page 347*

ClimaraPro® *see* estradiol and levonorgestrel *on page 349*

Clindagel® *see* clindamycin (topical) *on page 219*

ClindaMax® *see* clindamycin (topical) *on page 219*

clindamycin (systemic) (klin da MYE sin)

Medication Safety Issues

Sound-alike/look-alike issues:

Cleocin® may be confused with bleomycin, Clinoril®, Cubicin®, Lincocin®

Clindamycin may be confused with clarithromycin, Claritin®, vancomycin

Synonyms clindamycin hydrochloride; clindamycin palmitate

U.S. Brand Names Cleocin HCl®; Cleocin Pediatric®; Cleocin Phosphate®

Canadian Brand Names Apo-Clindamycin®; Ava-Clindamycin; Clindamycin Injection, USP; Clindamycine; Dalacin™ C; Mylan-Clindamycin; PMS-Clindamycin; Riva-Clindamycin; Teva-Clindamycin

Therapeutic Category Antibiotic, Lincosamide

Use Treatment of susceptible bacterial infections, mainly those caused by anaerobes, streptococci, pneumococci, and staphylococci; pelvic inflammatory disease (I.V.)

General Dosage Range

I.M., I.V.:

Children >1 month: 20-40 mg/kg/day in 3-4 divided doses

Adults: 1.2-2.7 g/day in 2-4 divided doses (maximum: 4.8 g/day)

Oral:

Children: 8-20 mg/kg/day as hydrochloride or 8-25 mg/kg/day as palmitate in 3-4 divided doses (minimum dose of palmitate: 37.5 mg 3 times/day)

Adults: 150-450 mg every 6-8 hours (maximum: 1.8 g/day)

Dosage Forms

Capsule, oral: 75 mg, 150 mg, 300 mg

Cleocin HCl®: 75 mg, 150 mg, 300 mg

Granules for solution, oral: 75 mg/5 mL (100 mL)

Cleocin Pediatric®: 75 mg/5 mL (100 mL)

Infusion, premixed in D_5W:

Cleocin Phosphate®: 300 mg (50 mL); 600 mg (50 mL); 900 mg (50 mL)

Injection, solution: 150 mg/mL (2 mL, 4 mL, 6 mL, 60 mL)

Cleocin Phosphate®: 150 mg/mL (2 mL, 4 mL, 6 mL, 60 mL)

clindamycin (topical) (klin da MYE sin)

Medication Safety Issues

Sound-alike/look-alike issues:

Cleocin® may be confused with bleomycin, Clinoril®, Cubicin®, Lincocin®
Clindamycin may be confused with clarithromycin, Claritin®, vancomycin

Synonyms clindamycin phosphate

U.S. Brand Names Cleocin T®; Cleocin®; Cleocin® Vaginal Ovule; Clindagel®; ClindaMax®; ClindaReach® [DSC]; Clindesse®; Evoclin®

Canadian Brand Names Clinda-T; Clindasol™; Clindets; Dalacin® T; Dalacin® Vaginal; Taro-Clindamycin

Therapeutic Category Antibiotic, Lincosamide; Topical Skin Product, Acne

Use Treatment of bacterial vaginosis (vaginal cream, vaginal suppository); topically in treatment of severe acne

General Dosage Range

Intravaginal: *Adults:* Insert 1 ovule or applicatorful once daily **or** 1 applicatorful as a single dose (Clindesse®)

Topical: *Children ≥12 years and Adults:* Apply once or twice daily

Dosage Forms

Aerosol, foam, topical: 1% (50 g, 100 g)
Evoclin®: 1% (50 g, 100 g)
Cream, vaginal: 2% (40 g)
Cleocin®: 2% (40 g)
Clindesse®: 2% (5 g)
Gel, topical: 1% (30 g, 60 g)
Cleocin T®: 1% (30 g, 60 g)
Clindagel®: 1% (40 mL, 75 mL)
ClindaMax®: 1% (30 g, 60 g)
Lotion, topical: 1% (60 mL)
Cleocin T®: 1% (60 mL)
ClindaMax®: 1% (60 mL)
Pledget, topical: 1% (60s, 69s)
Cleocin T®: 1% (60s)
Solution, topical: 1% (30 mL, 60 mL)
Cleocin T®: 1% (30 mL, 60 mL)
Suppository, vaginal:
Cleocin® Vaginal Ovule: 100 mg (3s)

clindamycin and benzoyl peroxide (klin da MYE sin & BEN zoe il peer OKS ide)

Synonyms benzoyl peroxide and clindamycin; clindamycin phosphate and benzoyl peroxide

U.S. Brand Names Acanya®; BenzaClin®; Duac®

Canadian Brand Names BenzaClin®; Clindoxyl

Therapeutic Category Topical Skin Product; Topical Skin Product, Acne

Use Topical treatment of acne vulgaris

General Dosage Range Topical: *Children ≥12 years and Adults:* Apply once daily (Acanya®, Duac®) **or** twice daily (BenzaClin®) to affected areas

Dosage Forms

Gel, topical: Clindamycin 1% and benzoyl peroxide 5% (50 g); Clindamycin phosphate 1.2% and benzoyl peroxide 5% (45 g)
Acanya®: Clindamycin 1.2% and benzoyl peroxide 2.5% (50 g)
BenzaClin®: Clindamycin 1% and benzoyl peroxide 5% (25 g, 35 g, 50 g)
Duac®: Clindamycin 1.2% and benzoyl peroxide 5% (45 g)

clindamycin and tretinoin (klin da MYE sin & TRET i noyn)

Synonyms clindamycin phosphate and tretinoin; tretinoin and clindamycin

U.S. Brand Names Veltin™; Ziana®

Therapeutic Category Acne Products; Retinoic Acid Derivative; Topical Skin Product; Topical Skin Product, Acne

Use Treatment of acne vulgaris

General Dosage Range Topical: *Children ≥12 years and Adults:* Apply pea-size amount to entire face once daily at bedtime

Dosage Forms

Gel, topical:

Veltin™: Clindamycin phosphate 1.2% and tretinoin 0.025% (30 g, 60 g)

Ziana®: Clindamycin phosphate 1.2% and tretinoin 0.025% (30 g, 60 g)

Clindamycine (Can) *see* clindamycin (systemic) *on page 218*

clindamycin hydrochloride *see* clindamycin (systemic) *on page 218*

Clindamycin Injection, USP (Can) *see* clindamycin (systemic) *on page 218*

clindamycin palmitate *see* clindamycin (systemic) *on page 218*

clindamycin phosphate *see* clindamycin (topical) *on page 219*

clindamycin phosphate and benzoyl peroxide *see* clindamycin and benzoyl peroxide *on page 219*

clindamycin phosphate and tretinoin *see* clindamycin and tretinoin *on page 219*

ClindaReach® [DSC] *see* clindamycin (topical) *on page 219*

Clindasol™ (Can) *see* clindamycin (topical) *on page 219*

Clinda-T (Can) *see* clindamycin (topical) *on page 219*

Clindesse® *see* clindamycin (topical) *on page 219*

Clindets (Can) *see* clindamycin (topical) *on page 219*

Clindoxyl (Can) *see* clindamycin and benzoyl peroxide *on page 219*

Clinisol® *see* amino acid injection *on page 61*

Clinoril® *see* sulindac *on page 862*

Clinpro™ 5000 *see* fluoride *on page 393*

clioquinol and flumethasone *(Canada only)* (klye ok KWIN ole & floo METH a sone)

Synonyms flumethasone and clioquinol; iodochlorhydroxyquin and flumethasone

Canadian Brand Names Locacorten® Vioform®

Therapeutic Category Antibiotic, Topical; Corticosteroid, Topical

Use

Otic solution: Treatment of otitis externa; otomycosis due to *Aspergillus niger*

Topical cream: Treatment of corticosteroid-responsive dermatoses complicated by infection with bacterial and/or fungal agents

General Dosage Range

Otic: *Children >2 years and Adults:* Instill 2-3 drops into affected ear(s) 2 times/day

Topical: *Children >2 years and Adults:* Apply a thin layer to affected area 2-3 times/day

Product Availability Not available in U.S.

Dosage Forms - Canada

Cream, topical:

Locacorten® Vioform®: Clioquinol 3% and flumethasone 0.02% (15 g, 50 g)

Solution, otic:

Locacorten® Vioform®: Clioquinol 1% and flumethasone 0.02% (10 mL)

clobazam (KLOE ba zam)

Medication Safety Issues

Sound-alike/look-alike issues:

Clobazam may be confused with clonazePAM

U.S. Brand Names Onfi™

Canadian Brand Names Apo-Clobazam®; Clobazam-10; Dom-Clobazam; Frisium®; Novo-Clobazam; PMS-Clobazam

Therapeutic Category Anticonvulsant; Antidepressant

Controlled Substance C-IV

Use Adjunctive treatment of seizures associated with Lennox-Gastaut syndrome

Canadian labeling: Adjunctive treatment of epilepsy

General Dosage Range Dosage adjustment recommended in patients with hepatic impairment or CYP2C19 poor metabolizers.

Oral: *Children ≥2 years and Adults:* Initial: 5-10 mg/day; Maintenance: Up to 40 mg/day

Dosage Forms

Tablet, oral:

Onfi™: 5 mg, 10 mg, 20 mg

Dosage Forms - Canada

Tablet:

Alti-Clobazam, Apo-Clobazam®, Clobazam-10, Dom-Clobazam, Frisium®, Novo-Clobazam, PMS-Clobazam, ratio-Clobazam: 10 mg

Clobazam-10 (Can) *see* clobazam *on page* *220*

clobetasol (kloe BAY ta sol)

Medication Safety Issues

International issues:

Clobex [U.S., Canada, and multiple international markets] may be confused with Codex brand name for *Saccharomyces boulardii* [Italy]

Cloderm: Brand name for clobetasol [China, India, Malaysia, Singapore, Thailand], but also brand name for alclometasone [Indonesia]; clocortolone [U.S., Canada]; clotrimazole [Germany]

Synonyms clobetasol propionate

U.S. Brand Names Clobex®; Cormax®; Olux-E™; Olux®; Temovate E®; Temovate®

Canadian Brand Names Clobex®; Dermovate®; Mylan-Clobetasol Cream; Mylan-Clobetasol Ointment; Mylan-Clobetasol Scalp Application; Novo-Clobetasol; PMS-Clobetasol; ratio-Clobetasol; Taro-Clobetasol

Therapeutic Category Corticosteroid, Topical

Use Short-term relief of inflammation of moderate-to-severe corticosteroid-responsive dermatoses (very high potency topical corticosteroid)

General Dosage Range Topical:

Children ≥12 years: Apply to affected area twice daily (maximum: 50 g/week; 50 mL/week)

Adults: Apply to affected area twice daily **or** apply shampoo to dry scalp once daily (maximum: 50 g/week; 50 mL/week)

Dosage Forms

Aerosol, foam, topical: 0.05% (50 g, 100 g)

Olux-E™: 0.05% (50 g, 100 g)

Olux®: 0.05% (50 g, 100 g)

Cream, topical: 0.05% (15 g, 30 g, 45 g, 60 g)

Temovate E®: 0.05% (60 g)

Temovate®: 0.05% (30 g, 60 g)

Gel, topical: 0.05% (15 g, 30 g, 60 g)

Temovate®: 0.05% (60 g)

Lotion, topical: 0.05% (59 mL, 118 mL)

Clobex®: 0.05% (30 mL, 59 mL, 118 mL)

Ointment, topical: 0.05% (15 g, 30 g, 45 g, 60 g)

Temovate®: 0.05% (15 g, 30 g)

Shampoo, topical: 0.05% (118 mL)

Clobex®: 0.05% (118 mL)

Solution, topical: 0.05% (25 mL, 50 mL)

Clobex®: 0.05% (59 mL, 125 mL)

Cormax®: 0.05% (50 mL)

Temovate®: 0.05% (50 mL)

clobetasol propionate *see* clobetasol *on page* *221*
Clobex® *see* clobetasol *on page* *221*

clocortolone (kloe KOR toe lone)

Medication Safety Issues

International issues:

Cloderm: Brand name for clocortolone [U.S., Canada], but also brand name for alclometasone [Indonesia]; clobetasol [China, India, Malaysia, Singapore, Thailand]; clotrimazole [Germany]

Synonyms clocortolone pivalate

U.S. Brand Names Cloderm®

Canadian Brand Names Cloderm®

Therapeutic Category Corticosteroid, Topical

Use Inflammation of corticosteroid-responsive dermatoses (intermediate-potency topical corticosteroid)
General Dosage Range Topical: *Adults:* Apply sparingly to affected area 1-4 times/day
Dosage Forms
Cream, topical:
Cloderm®: 0.1% (30 g, 45 g, 75 g, 90 g)

clocortolone pivalate *see* clocortolone *on page 221*
Cloderm® *see* clocortolone *on page 221*

clodronate *(Canada only)* (KLOE droh nate)

Synonyms clodronate disodium
Canadian Brand Names Bonefos®; Clasteon®
Therapeutic Category Bisphosphonate Derivative
Use Management of hypercalcemia of malignancy; management of osteolysis due to bone metastases of malignancy
General Dosage Range Dosage adjustment recommended in patients with renal impairment
I.V.: *Adults:* 1500 mg as single dose (Clasteon®) **or** 300 mg/day (Clasteon®, Bonefos®); Maximum therapy: 10 days (Clasteon®); 7 days (Bonefos®)
Oral: *Adults:* 1600-2400 mg/day in 1-2 divided doses (maximum: 3200 mg/day)
Product Availability Not available in U.S.
Dosage Forms - Canada
Capsule, oral:
Bonefos®, Clasteon®: 400 mg
Injection, solution:
Bonefos®: 60 mg/mL (5 mL)
Clasteon®; 30 mg/mL (10 mL)

clodronate disodium *see* clodronate *(Canada only) on page 222*

clofarabine (klo FARE a been)

Medication Safety Issues
Sound-alike/look-alike issues:
Clofarabine may be confused with cladribine, clevidipine, cytarabine, nelarabine
High alert medication:
This medication is in a class the Institute for Safe Medication Practices (ISMP) includes among its list of drug classes which have a heightened risk of causing significant patient harm when used in error.
Synonyms CAFdA; clofarex
U.S. Brand Names Clolar®
Therapeutic Category Antineoplastic Agent, Antimetabolite (Purine Antagonist)
Use Treatment of relapsed or refractory acute lymphoblastic leukemia (ALL) in children (ages 1-21 years)
General Dosage Range Dosage adjustment recommended in patients who develop toxicities
I.V.: *Children >1 year and Adults ≤21 years:* 52 mg/m²/day days 1 through 5; repeat every 2-6 weeks
Dosage Forms
Injection, solution [preservative free]:
Clolar®: 1 mg/mL (20 mL)

clofarex *see* clofarabine *on page 222*
Clolar® *see* clofarabine *on page 222*
Clomid® *see* clomiphene *on page 222*

clomiphene (KLOE mi feen)

Medication Safety Issues
Sound-alike/look-alike issues:
ClomiPHENE may be confused with clomiPRAMINE, clonidine
Clomid® may be confused with clonidine
Serophene® may be confused with Sarafem®
Synonyms clomiphene citrate
Tall-Man clomi**PHENE**
U.S. Brand Names Clomid®; Serophene®
Canadian Brand Names Clomid®; Serophene®

Therapeutic Category Ovulation Stimulator

Use Treatment of ovulatory failure in patients desiring pregnancy

General Dosage Range Oral: *Adults (females):* First course: 50 mg/day for 5 days; Second course (if needed): 100 mg/day for 5 days

Dosage Forms

Tablet, oral: 50 mg

Clomid®: 50 mg

Serophene®: 50 mg

clomiphene citrate *see* clomiphene *on page* 222

clomipramine (kloe MI pra meen)

Medication Safety Issues

Sound-alike/look-alike issues:

ClomiPRAMINE may be confused with chlorproMAZINE, clevidipine, clomiPHENE, desipramine, Norpramin®

Anafranil® may be confused with alfentanil, enalapril, nafarelin

BEERS Criteria medication:

This drug may be potentially inappropriate for use in geriatric patients (Quality of evidence - high [moderate for SIADH]; Strength of recommendation - strong).

Synonyms clomipramine hydrochloride

Tall-Man clomi**PRAMINE**

U.S. Brand Names Anafranil®

Canadian Brand Names Anafranil®; Apo-Clomipramine®; CO Clomipramine; Dom-Clomipramine; Novo-Clomipramine

Therapeutic Category Antidepressant, Tricyclic (Tertiary Amine)

Use Treatment of obsessive-compulsive disorder (OCD)

General Dosage Range Oral:

Children ≥10 years: Initial: 25 mg/day; Maintenance: Up to 3 mg/kg/day (maximum: 200 mg/day)

Adults: Initial: 25 mg/day; Maintenance: Up to 250 mg/day

Dosage Forms

Capsule, oral: 25 mg, 50 mg, 75 mg

Anafranil®: 25 mg, 50 mg, 75 mg

clomipramine hydrochloride *see* clomipramine *on page* 223

Clonapam (Can) *see* clonazepam *on page* 223

clonazepam (kloe NA ze pam)

Medication Safety Issues

Sound-alike/look-alike issues:

ClonazePAM may be confused with clobazam, cloNIDine, clorazepate, cloZAPine, LORazepam

KlonoPIN® may be confused with cloNIDine, clorazepate, cloZAPine, LORazepam

BEERS Criteria medication:

This drug may be potentially inappropriate for use in geriatric patients (Quality of evidence - high; Strength of recommendation - strong).

Tall-Man clonaze**PAM**

U.S. Brand Names KlonoPIN®

Canadian Brand Names Apo-Clonazepam®; Clonapam; CO Clonazepam; Dom-Clonazepam; Mylan-Clonazepam; Novo-Clonazepam; Nu-Clonazepam; PHL-Clonazepam; PMS-Clonazepam; PRO-Clonazepam; ratio-Clonazepam; Riva-Clonazepam; Rivotril®; Sandoz-Clonazepam; ZYM-Clonazepam

Therapeutic Category Benzodiazepine

Controlled Substance C-IV

Use Alone or as an adjunct in the treatment of petit mal variant (Lennox-Gastaut), akinetic, and myoclonic seizures; petit mal (absence) seizures unresponsive to succimides; panic disorder with or without agoraphobia

General Dosage Range Oral:

Children <10 years or <30 kg: Initial: 0.01-0.03 mg/kg/day in 2-3 divided doses (maximum: 0.05 mg/kg/day); Maintenance: 0.1-0.2 mg/kg/day in 3 divided doses (maximum: 0.2 mg/kg/day)

Children ≥10 years or ≥30 kg and Adults: Panic disorders: Initial: 0.25 mg twice daily; Maintenance: 1-4 mg/day in 2 divided doses; Seizure disorders: Initial: Up to 1.5 mg/day in 3 divided doses; Maintenance: 0.05-2 mg/kg/day (maximum: 20 mg/day)

Dosage Forms

Tablet, oral: 0.5 mg, 1 mg, 2 mg

KlonoPIN®: 0.5 mg, 1 mg, 2 mg

Tablet, orally disintegrating, oral: 0.125 mg, 0.25 mg, 0.5 mg, 1 mg, 2 mg

clonidine (KLON i deen)

Medication Safety Issues

Sound-alike/look-alike issues:

CloNIDine may be confused with Clomid®, clomiPHENE, clonazePAM, cloZAPine, KlonoPIN®, quiNIDine

Catapres® may be confused with Cataflam®, Combipres

High alert medication:

The Institute for Safe Medication Practices (ISMP) includes this medication (epidural administration) among its list of drug classes which have a heightened risk of causing significant patient harm when used in error.

BEERS Criteria medication:

This drug may be potentially inappropriate for use in geriatric patients (Quality of evidence - low; Strength of recommendation - strong).

Administration issues:

Use caution when interpreting dosing information. Pediatric dose for epidural infusion expressed as mcg/kg/**hour**.

Other safety concerns:

Transdermal patch may contain conducting metal (eg, aluminum); remove patch prior to MRI. Errors have occurred when the inactive, optional adhesive cover has been applied instead of the active clonidine-containing patch.

Synonyms clonidine hydrochloride

Tall-Man cloNIDine

U.S. Brand Names Catapres-TTS®-1; Catapres-TTS®-2; Catapres-TTS®-3; Catapres®; Duraclon®; Kapvay®; Nexiclon™ XR

Canadian Brand Names Apo-Clonidine®; Catapres®; Dixarit®; Dom-Clonidine; Novo-Clonidine; Nu-Clonidine

Therapeutic Category Alpha-Adrenergic Agonist

Use

Oral:

Immediate release: Management of hypertension (monotherapy or as adjunctive therapy)

Extended release:

Kapvay™: Treatment of attention-deficit/hyperactivity disorder (ADHD) (monotherapy or as adjunctive therapy)

Nexiclon™ XR: Management of hypertension (monotherapy or as adjunctive therapy)

Epidural (Duraclon®): For continuous epidural administration as adjunctive therapy with opioids for treatment of severe cancer pain in patients tolerant to or unresponsive to opioids alone; epidural clonidine is generally more effective for neuropathic pain and less effective (or possibly ineffective) for somatic or visceral pain

Transdermal patch: Management of hypertension (monotherapy or as adjunctive therapy)

General Dosage Range Note: Dosing is expressed as the salt (clonidine hydrochloride) unless otherwise noted.

Epidural:

Children: Initial: 0.5 mcg/kg/**hour**

Adults: Initial: 30 mcg/hour; Maintenance: Up to 40 mcg/hour

Oral, immediate release:

Adults: Initial: 0.1 mg twice daily; Maintenance: 0.1-0.8 mg/day in 2 divided doses (maximum: 2.4 mg/day)

Elderly: Initial: 0.1 mg once daily

Oral, extended release:

Children ≥6 years: (Kapvay™): Initial: 0.1 mg at bedtime; maximum: 0.4 mg/day [ADHD use]

Adults (Nexiclon™ XR): Initial: 0.17 mg clonidine base once daily at bedtime; maintenance: 0.17-0.52 mg/day clonidine base once daily (maximum: 0.52 mg/day clonidine base) [antihypertensive]

Transdermal: *Adults:* Initial: 0.1 mg/24 hour patch applied once every 7 days; Maintenance: 0.1-0.3 mg/24 hour patch applied once every 7 days (maximum: 0.6 mg/24 hours)

Dosage Forms

Injection, solution [preservative free]: 100 mcg/mL (10 mL); 500 mcg/mL (10 mL)
Duraclon®: 100 mcg/mL (10 mL); 500 mcg/mL (10 mL)

Patch, transdermal: 0.1 mg/24 hours (4s); 0.2 mg/24 hours (4s); 0.3 mg/24 hours (4s)
Catapres-TTS®-1: 0.1 mg/24 hours (4s)
Catapres-TTS®-2: 0.2 mg/24 hours (4s)
Catapres-TTS®-3: 0.3 mg/24 hours (4s)

Suspension, extended release, oral:
Nexiclon™ XR: 0.09 mg/mL (118 mL)

Tablet, oral: 0.1 mg, 0.2 mg, 0.3 mg
Catapres®: 0.1 mg, 0.2 mg, 0.3 mg

Tablet, extended release, oral:
Kapvay®: 0.1 mg, 0.2 mg, 0.1 mg AM dose, 0.2 mg PM dose
Nexiclon™ XR: 0.17 mg

clonidine and chlorthalidone (KLON i deen & klor THAL i done)

Medication Safety Issues

Sound-alike/look-alike issues:
Combipres may be confused with Catapres®

Synonyms chlorthalidone and clonidine; Combipres

U.S. Brand Names Clorpres®

Therapeutic Category Antihypertensive Agent, Combination

Use Management of mild-to-moderate hypertension

General Dosage Range Oral: *Adults:* 1 tablet (clonidine 0.1-0.3 mg/chlorthalidone 15 mg/tablet) 1-2 times/day (maximum: clonidine 0.6 mg; chlorthalidone 30 mg)

Dosage Forms

Tablet:
Clorpres®: 0.1: Clonidine 0.1 mg and chlorthalidone 15 mg; 0.2: Clonidine 0.2 mg and chlorthalidone 15 mg; 0.3: Clonidine 0.3 mg and chlorthalidone 15 mg

clonidine hydrochloride *see* clonidine *on page 224*

clopidogrel (kloh PID oh grel)

Medication Safety Issues

Sound-alike/look-alike issues:
Plavix® may be confused with Elavil®, Paxil®, Pradax™ (Canada), Pradaxa®

Synonyms clopidogrel bisulfate

U.S. Brand Names Plavix®

Canadian Brand Names Apo-Clopidogrel®; CO Clopidogrel; Mylan-Clopidogrel; Plavix®; PMS-Clopidogrel; Sandoz-Clopidogrel; Teva-Clopidogrel

Therapeutic Category Antiplatelet Agent

Use Reduces rate of atherothrombotic events (myocardial infarction, stroke, vascular deaths) in patients with recent MI or stroke, or established peripheral arterial disease; reduces rate of atherothrombotic events in patients with unstable angina (UA) or non-ST-segment elevation MI (NSTEMI) managed medically or with percutaneous coronary intervention (PCI) (with or without stent) or CABG; reduces rate of death and atherothrombotic events in patients with ST-segment elevation MI (STEMI) managed medically

Canadian labeling: Additional use (not in U.S. labeling): Prevention of atherothrombotic and thromboembolic events, including stroke, in patients with atrial fibrillation with at least 1 risk factor for vascular events who are not suitable for treatment with an anticoagulant and are at a low risk for bleeding.

General Dosage Range Oral: *Adults:* Loading dose: 300 mg (maximum: 600 mg); Maintenance: 75 mg once daily

Dosage Forms

Tablet, oral: 75 mg, 300 mg
Plavix®: 75 mg, 300 mg

clopidogrel bisulfate *see* clopidogrel *on page 225*
Clopixol® (Can) *see* zuclopenthixol *(Canada only) on page 969*

Clopixol-Acuphase® (Can) *see* zuclopenthixol *(Canada only) on page 969*
Clopixol® Depot (Can) *see* zuclopenthixol *(Canada only) on page 969*

clorazepate (klor AZ e pate)

Medication Safety Issues

Sound-alike/look-alike issues:

Clorazepate may be confused with clofibrate, clonazepam, KlonoPIN®

BEERS Criteria medication:

This drug may be potentially inappropriate for use in geriatric patients (Quality of evidence - high; Strength of recommendation - strong).

Synonyms clorazepate dipotassium

U.S. Brand Names Tranxene® T-Tab®

Canadian Brand Names Apo-Clorazepate®; Novo-Clopate

Therapeutic Category Anticonvulsant; Benzodiazepine

Controlled Substance C-IV

Use Treatment of generalized anxiety disorder; management of ethanol withdrawal; adjunct anticonvulsant in management of partial seizures

General Dosage Range Oral:

Children 9-12 years: Initial: 3.75-7.5 mg twice daily; Maintenance: Up to 60 mg/day in 2-3 divided doses
Children >12 years: Initial: Up to 7.5 mg 2-3 times/day; Maintenance: Up to 90 mg/day
Adults: Initial: 7.5-15 mg 2-4 times/day; Maintenance: Up to 90 mg/day
Elderly: Anxiety: 7.5 mg 1-2 times/day

Dosage Forms

Tablet, oral: 3.75 mg, 7.5 mg, 15 mg
Tranxene® T-Tab®: 3.75 mg, 7.5 mg, 15 mg

clorazepate dipotassium *see* clorazepate *on page 226*
Clorpactin® WCS-90 [OTC] *see* oxychlorosene *on page 678*
Clorpres® *see* clonidine and chlorthalidone *on page 225*
Clotrimaderm (Can) *see* clotrimazole (topical) *on page 227*

clotrimazole (oral) (kloe TRIM a zole)

Medication Safety Issues

Sound-alike/look-alike issues:

Clotrimazole may be confused with co-trimoxazole
Mycelex may be confused with Myoflex®

International issues:

Cloderm: Brand name for clotrimazole [Germany], but also brand name for alclomethasone [Indonesia]; clobetasol [China, India, Malaysia, Singapore, Thailand]; clocortolone [U.S., Canada]

Canesten [multiple international markets] may be confused with Canesten Bifonazol Comp brand name for bifonazole/urea [Austria]; Canesten Extra brand name for bifonazole [China, Germany]; Canesten Extra Nagelset brand name for bifonazole/urea [Denmark]; Canesten Fluconazole brand name for fluconazole [New Zealand]; Canesten Oasis brand name for sodium citrate [Great Britain]; Canesten Once Daily brand name for bifonazole [Australia]; Canesten Oral brand name for fluconazole [United Kingdom]; Cenestin brand name for estrogens (conjugated A/synthetic) [U.S., Canada]

Mycelex: Brand name for clotrimazole [U.S.] may be confused with Mucolex brand name for bromhexine [Malaysia]; carbocisteine [Thailand]

Synonyms Mycelex

Therapeutic Category Antifungal Agent, Oral Nonabsorbed

Use Treatment of susceptible fungal infections, including oropharyngeal candidiasis; limited data suggest that clotrimazole troches may be effective for prophylaxis against oropharyngeal candidiasis in neutropenic patients

General Dosage Range Oral: *Children >3 years and Adults:* Prophylaxis: 10 mg 3 times/day; Treatment: 10 mg 5 times/day

Dosage Forms

Troche, oral: 10 mg

clotrimazole (topical) (kloe TRIM a zole)

Medication Safety Issues

Sound-alike/look-alike issues:

Clotrimazole may be confused with co-trimoxazole

Lotrimin® may be confused with Lotrisone®

International issues:

Cloderm: Brand name for clotrimazole [Germany], but also brand name for alclomethasone [Indonesia]; clobetasol [China, India, Malaysia, Singapore, Thailand]; clocortolone [U.S., Canada]

Canesten: Brand name for clotrimazole [multiple international markets] may be confused with Canesten Bifonazol Comp brand name for bifonazole/urea [Austria]; Canesten Extra brand name for bifonazole [China, Germany]; Canesten Extra Nagelset brand name for bifonazole/urea [Denmark]; Canesten Fluconazole brand name for fluconazole [New Zealand]; Canesten Oasis brand name for sodium citrate [Great Britain]; Canesten Once Daily brand name for bifonazole [Australia]; Canesten Oral brand name for fluconazole [United Kingdom]; Cenestin® brand name for estrogens (conjugated A/synthetic) [U.S., Canada]

U.S. Brand Names Anti-Fungal™ [OTC]; Cruex® [OTC]; Gyne-Lotrimin® 3 [OTC]; Gyne-Lotrimin® 7 [OTC]; Lotrimin® AF Athlete's Foot [OTC]; Lotrimin® AF for Her [OTC]; Lotrimin® AF Jock Itch [OTC]

Canadian Brand Names Canesten® Topical; Canesten® Vaginal; Clotrimaderm; Trivagizole-3®

Therapeutic Category Antifungal Agent, Topical; Antifungal Agent, Vaginal

Use Treatment of susceptible fungal infections, including dermatophytoses, superficial mycoses, and cutaneous candidiasis, as well as vulvovaginal candidiasis

General Dosage Range

Intravaginal: *Children >12 years and Adults:* Cream: Insert 1 applicatorful once daily

Topical: *Children >3 years and Adults:* Apply twice daily

Dosage Forms

Cream, topical: 1% (15 g, 30 g, 45 g)

Anti-Fungal™ [OTC]: 1% (113 g)

Cruex® [OTC]: 1% (15 g)

Lotrimin® AF Athlete's Foot [OTC]: 1% (12 g)

Lotrimin® AF for Her [OTC]: 1% (24 g)

Lotrimin® AF Jock Itch [OTC]: 1% (12 g)

Cream, vaginal: 1% (45 g); 2% (21 g)

Gyne-Lotrimin® 7 [OTC]: 1% (45 g)

Gyne-Lotrimin® 3 [OTC]: 2% (21 g)

Solution, topical: 1% (10 mL, 30 mL)

clotrimazole and betamethasone *see* betamethasone and clotrimazole *on page 130*

cloxacillin *(Canada only)* (kloks a SIL in)

Synonyms cloxacillin sodium

Canadian Brand Names Apo-Cloxi®; Novo-Cloxin; Nu-Cloxi

Therapeutic Category Penicillin

Use Treatment of bacterial infections including endocarditis, pneumonia, bone and joint infections, skin and soft-tissue infections, and sepsis that are caused by susceptible strains of penicillinase-producing staphylococci. **Note:** Exhibits good activity against *Staphylococcus aureus*; has activity against many streptococci, but is less active than penicillin and is generally not used in clinical practice to treat streptococcal infections.

General Dosage Range I.M., I.V., oral:

Children ≤20 kg: 25-50 mg/kg/day in divided doses every 6 hours

Children >20 kg and Adults: 250-500 mg every 6 hours

Product Availability Not available in U.S.

Dosage Forms - Canada

Capsule, oral: 250 mg, 500 mg

Injection, powder for reconstitution: 250 mg, 500 mg, 1000 mg, 2000 mg

Powder for suspension, oral: 125 mg/5 mL

cloxacillin sodium *see* cloxacillin *(Canada only) on page 227*

clozapine (KLOE za peen)

Medication Safety Issues

Sound-alike/look-alike issues:

CloZAPine may be confused with clonazePAM, cloNIDine, KlonoPIN®

Clozaril® may be confused with Clinoril®, Colazal®

BEERS Criteria medication:

This drug may be potentially inappropriate for use in geriatric patients (Quality of evidence - moderate; Strength of recommendation - strong).

Tall-Man cloZAPine

U.S. Brand Names Clozaril®; FazaClo®

Canadian Brand Names Apo-Clozapine®; Clozaril®; Gen-Clozapine

Therapeutic Category Antipsychotic Agent, Dibenzodiazepine

Use Treatment-refractory schizophrenia; to reduce risk of recurrent suicidal behavior in schizophrenia or schizoaffective disorder

General Dosage Range Dosage adjustment recommended in patients who develop toxicities

Oral: *Adults:* Initial: 12.5 mg once or twice daily; Maintenance: 12.5-900 mg/day (maximum: 900 mg/day)

Dosage Forms

Tablet, oral: 25 mg, 50 mg, 100 mg, 200 mg

Clozaril®: 25 mg, 100 mg

Tablet, orally disintegrating, oral: 12.5 mg, 25 mg, 100 mg

FazaClo®: 12.5 mg, 25 mg, 100 mg, 150 mg, 200 mg

Clozaril® *see* clozapine *on page* 228

CMA-676 *see* gemtuzumab ozogamicin *on page* 423

C-met/hepatocyte growth factor receptor tyrosine kinase inhibitor PF-02341066 *see* crizotinib *on page* 240

C-met/HGFR tyrosine kinase inhibitor PF-02341066 *see* crizotinib *on page* 240

CMV-IGIV *see* cytomegalovirus immune globulin (intravenous-human) *on page* 249

CNJ-016® *see* vaccinia immune globulin (intravenous) *on page* 933

CNTO-148 *see* golimumab *on page* 431

CNTO 1275 *see* ustekinumab *on page* 932

CoActifed® (Can) *see* triprolidine, pseudoephedrine, and codeine *(Canada only) on page* 922

coagulant complex inhibitor *see* antiinhibitor coagulant complex *on page* 79

coagulation factor I *see* fibrinogen concentrate (human) *on page* 382

coagulation factor VIIa *see* factor VIIa (recombinant) *on page* 371

CO Alendronate (Can) *see* alendronate *on page* 45

coal tar (KOLE tar)

Medication Safety Issues

International issues:

Pentrax [U.S., Canada, Great Britain, Ireland] may be confused with Permax brand name for pergolide [multiple international markets]

Synonyms crude coal tar; LCD; pix carbonis

U.S. Brand Names Balnetar® [OTC]; Betatar Gel® [OTC]; Cutar® [OTC]; Denorex® Therapeutic Protection 2-in-1 Shampoo + Conditioner [OTC]; Denorex® Therapeutic Protection [OTC]; DHS® Tar [OTC]; DHS™ Tar Gel [OTC]; Exorex® Penetrating Emulsion #2 [OTC]; Exorex® Penetrating Emulsion [OTC]; ionil-T® Plus [OTC]; ionil-T® [OTC]; MG217® Medicated Tar Extra Strength [OTC]; MG217® Medicated Tar Intensive Strength [OTC]; MG217® Medicated Tar [OTC]; Neutrogena® T/Gel® Extra Strength [OTC]; Neutrogena® T/Gel® Stubborn Itch Control [OTC]; Neutrogena® T/Gel® [OTC]; Oxipor® VHC [OTC]; Pentrax® [OTC]; Scytera™ [OTC]; Tera-Gel™ [OTC]; Thera-Gel [OTC]; Zetar® [OTC]

Canadian Brand Names Doak Oil Forte [OTC]; Doak Oil [OTC]; Emorex Gel [OTC]; Neuotrogena T/Gel Therapeutic Shampoo [OTC]; Odans Liquor Carbonis Detergens [OTC]; Pentrax Gold Shampoo [OTC]; Pentrax Tar Shampoo [OTC]; Psoriasin [OTC]; T/Gel Therapeutic Shampoo Extra Strength [OTC]; Targel® [OTC]; Tersa Tar Shp [OTC]

Therapeutic Category Antipsoriatic Agent; Antiseborrheic Agent, Topical

Use Topically for controlling dandruff, seborrheic dermatitis, or psoriasis

General Dosage Range Topical: *Adults:*
Bath: Add 60-90 mL (5-20%) or 15-25 mL (30%) to bath water, soak 5-20 minutes, use once daily to every 3 days
Scalp: Apply to lesions 3-12 hours before each shampoo
Shampoo: Rub into wet hair, rinse, repeat leaving on 5 minutes; apply twice weekly for 2 weeks then once weekly
Skin: Apply to affected areas 1-4 times/day, decrease to 2-3 times/week once condition controlled
Soap: Use on affected areas instead of regular soap

Dosage Forms

Aerosol, foam, topical:
Scytera™ [OTC]: Coal tar solution 10% (100 g)

Emulsion, topical:
Cutar® [OTC]: Coal tar solution 7.5% (180 mL, 3840 mL)
Exorex® Penetrating Emulsion [OTC]: Coal tar 1% (100 mL, 250 mL)
Exorex® Penetrating Emulsion #2 [OTC]: Coal tar 2% (100 mL, 250 mL)

Gel, topical:
DHS™ Tar Gel [OTC]: Solubilized coal tar extract 2.9% (240 mL)
Thera-Gel [OTC]: 0.5% (255 mL)

Lotion, topical:
MG217® Medicated Tar [OTC]: Coal tar solution 5% (120 mL)
Oxipor® VHC [OTC]: Coal tar solution 25% (56 mL, 120 mL)

Oil, topical:
Balnetar® [OTC]: Coal tar 2.5% (221 mL)

Ointment, topical:
MG217® Medicated Tar Intensive Strength [OTC]: Coal tar solution 10% (107 g)

Shampoo, topical:
Betatar Gel® [OTC]: Coal tar solution 12.5% (480 mL)
Denorex® Therapeutic Protection [OTC]: Coal tar solution 12.5% (118 mL, 240 mL, 300 mL)
DHS® Tar [OTC]: Solubilized coal tar extract 2.9% (120 mL, 240 mL, 480 mL)
ionil-T® [OTC]: Coal tar 1% (240 mL, 480 mL, 960 mL)
ionil-T® Plus [OTC]: Coal tar 2% (240 mL)
MG217® Medicated Tar Extra Strength [OTC]: Coal tar solution 15% (120 mL, 240 mL)
Neutrogena® T/Gel® [OTC]: Solubilized coal tar extract 2% (130 mL, 255 mL, 480 mL)
Neutrogena® T/Gel® Extra Strength [OTC]: Solubilized coal tar extract 4% (177 mL)
Neutrogena® T/Gel® Stubborn Itch Control [OTC]: Coal tar extract 2% (130 mL)
Pentrax® [OTC]: Coal tar 5% (236 mL)
Tera-Gel™ [OTC]: Solubilized coal tar extract 2% (120 mL, 255 mL)
Zetar® [OTC]: Coal tar 1% (177 mL)

Shampoo/Conditioner, topical:
Denorex® Therapeutic Protection 2-in-1 Shampoo + Conditioner [OTC]: Coal tar solution 12.5% (120 mL, 240 mL, 300 mL)

Solution, topical: 20% (473 mL)

coal tar and salicylic acid (KOLE tar & sal i SIL ik AS id)

Synonyms salicylic acid and coal tar

U.S. Brand Names Tarsum® [OTC]; X-Seb T® Pearl [OTC]; X-Seb T® Plus [OTC]

Canadian Brand Names Sebcur/T®

Therapeutic Category Antipsoriatic Agent; Antiseborrheic Agent, Topical

Use Relief of symptoms of seborrheal dermatitis, dandruff, and psoriasis

General Dosage Range Topical:
Gel: *Adults:* Apply to plaques, leave on up to 1 hour then rinse
Shampoo: *Adults:* Apply to wet hair, massage into scalp then rinse

Dosage Forms

Gel [shampoo]: Coal tar solution 10% [equivalent to coal tar 2%] and salicylic acid (120 mL, 240 mL)
Tarsum® [OTC]: Coal tar solution 10% [equivalent to coal tar 2%] and salicylic acid (120 mL, 240 mL)

Shampoo, topical: Coal tar solution 10% [equivalent to coal tar 2%] and salicylic acid (120 mL, 240 mL)
X-Seb T® Pearl [OTC], X-Seb T® Plus [OTC]: Coal tar solution 10% [equivalent to coal tar 2%] and salicylic acid (120 mL, 240 mL)

CO Amlodipine (Can) *see* amlodipine *on page* 65

Coartem® *see* artemether and lumefantrine *on page* 92

CO Atenolol (Can) *see* atenolol *on page 99*
CO Atorvastatin (Can) *see* atorvastatin *on page 100*
CO Azithromycin (Can) *see* azithromycin (systemic) *on page 108*
CO Betahistine (Can) *see* betahistine *(Canada only) on page 129*
CO Bicalutamide (Can) *see* bicalutamide *on page 133*
CO Bosentan (Can) *see* bosentan *on page 139*
CO Cabergoline (Can) *see* cabergoline *on page 157*

cocaine (koe KANE)

Synonyms cocaine hydrochloride
Therapeutic Category Local Anesthetic
Controlled Substance C-II
Use Topical anesthesia (and vasoconstriction) for mucous membranes
General Dosage Range **Topical:** *Adults:* Maximum total dose: 3 mg/kg **or** 200 mg (1% to 10% concentration)
Dosage Forms
Powder, for prescription compounding: USP: 100% (5 g, 25 g)
Solution, topical: 4% (4 mL, 10 mL); 10% (4 mL)

cocaine hydrochloride *see* cocaine *on page 230*
CO Candesartan (Can) *see* candesartan *on page 168*
CO Cilazapril (Can) *see* cilazapril *(Canada only) on page 208*
CO Ciprofloxacin (Can) *see* ciprofloxacin (systemic) *on page 210*
CO Citalopram (Can) *see* citalopram *on page 213*
CO Clomipramine (Can) *see* clomipramine *on page 223*
CO Clonazepam (Can) *see* clonazepam *on page 223*
CO Clopidogrel (Can) *see* clopidogrel *on page 225*
Codar® D *see* pseudoephedrine and codeine *on page 772*
Codar® GF *see* guaifenesin and codeine *on page 434*

codeine (KOE deen)

Medication Safety Issues
Sound-alike/look-alike issues:
Codeine may be confused with Cardene®, Cordran®, iodine, Lodine
High alert medication:
The Institute for Safe Medication Practices (ISMP) includes this medication among its list of drug classes which have a heightened risk of causing significant patient harm when used in error.
Synonyms codeine phosphate; codeine sulfate; methylmorphine
Canadian Brand Names Codeine Contin®; PMS-Codeine; ratio-Codeine
Therapeutic Category Analgesic, Narcotic; Antitussive
Controlled Substance C-II
Use Management of mild-to-moderately-severe pain
General Dosage Range Dosage adjustment recommended in patients with renal and hepatic impairment
Oral: *Adults:* Initial: 15-60 mg every 4 hours as needed; maximum total daily dose: 360 mg/day
Dosage Forms
Powder, for prescription compounding: USP: 100% (10 g, 25 g)
Solution, oral: 30 mg/5 mL (500 mL)
Tablet, oral: 15 mg, 30 mg, 60 mg
Dosage Forms - Canada
Tablet, controlled release:
Codeine Contin®: 50 mg, 100 mg, 150 mg, 200 mg

codeine, acetaminophen, butalbital, and caffeine *see* butalbital, acetaminophen, caffeine, and codeine *on page 153*
codeine and acetaminophen *see* acetaminophen and codeine *on page 22*
codeine and butalbital compound *see* butalbital, aspirin, caffeine, and codeine *on page 155*
codeine and guaifenesin *see* guaifenesin and codeine *on page 434*
codeine and promethazine *see* promethazine and codeine *on page 764*

codeine and pseudoephedrine *see* pseudoephedrine and codeine *on page 772*
codeine, aspirin, and carisoprodol *see* carisoprodol, aspirin, and codeine *on page 178*
codeine, butalbital, aspirin, and caffeine *see* butalbital, aspirin, caffeine, and codeine *on page 155*
codeine, chlorpheniramine, and pseudoephedrine *see* chlorpheniramine, pseudoephedrine, and codeine *on page 202*
Codeine Contin® (Can) *see* codeine *on page 230*
codeine, doxylamine, and acetaminophen *see* acetaminophen, codeine, and doxylamine *(Canada only) on page 27*
codeine, guaifenesin, and pseudoephedrine *see* guaifenesin, pseudoephedrine, and codeine *on page 437*
codeine, phenylephrine, and promethazine *see* promethazine, phenylephrine, and codeine *on page 765*
codeine phosphate *see* codeine *on page 230*
codeine phosphate and pseudoephedrine hydrochloride *see* pseudoephedrine and codeine *on page 772*
codeine, pseudoephedrine, and triprolidine *see* triprolidine, pseudoephedrine, and codeine *(Canada only) on page 922*
codeine sulfate *see* codeine *on page 230*
codeine, triprolidine, and pseudoephedrine *see* triprolidine, pseudoephedrine, and codeine *(Canada only) on page 922*
CO Diltiazem CD (Can) *see* diltiazem *on page 288*
CO Diltiazem T (Can) *see* diltiazem *on page 288*
Codituss DM [OTC] *see* phenylephrine, pyrilamine, and dextromethorphan *on page 718*
cod liver oil *see* vitamin A and vitamin D (topical) *on page 949*
Codulax [OTC] (Can) *see* bisacodyl *on page 134*
CO Enalapril (Can) *see* enalapril *on page 330*
CO Etidrocal (Can) *see* etidronate and calcium carbonate *(Canada only) on page 364*
Co-Etidronate (Can) *see* etidronate *on page 364*
CO Famciclovir (Can) *see* famciclovir *on page 372*
CO Finasteride (Can) *see* finasteride *on page 384*
CO Fluconazole (Can) *see* fluconazole *on page 388*
CO Fluoxetine (Can) *see* fluoxetine *on page 396*
CO Gabapentin (Can) *see* gabapentin *on page 413*
Cogentin® *see* benztropine *on page 126*
CO Glimepiride (Can) *see* glimepiride *on page 426*
CO Ipra-Sal (Can) *see* ipratropium and albuterol *on page 499*
CO Irbesartan (Can) *see* irbesartan *on page 500*
CO Irbesartan HCT (Can) *see* irbesartan and hydrochlorothiazide *on page 501*
Colace® [OTC] *see* docusate *on page 304*
Colace® (Can) *see* docusate *on page 304*
CO Latanoprost (Can) *see* latanoprost *on page 524*
Colax-C® (Can) *see* docusate *on page 304*
Colazal® *see* balsalazide *on page 114*
ColBenemid *see* colchicine and probenecid *on page 232*

colchicine (KOL chi seen)

Medication Safety Issues
Sound-alike/look-alike issues:
Colchicine may be confused with Cortrosyn®
U.S. Brand Names Colcrys®
Canadian Brand Names Jamp-Colchicine
Therapeutic Category Antigout Agent
Use Prevention and treatment of acute gout flares; treatment of familial Mediterranean fever (FMF)
General Dosage Range Dosage adjustment recommended in patients with renal impairment or on concomitant therapy

Oral:
Children 4-6 years: 0.3-1.8 mg/day in 1-2 divided doses
Children 6-12 years: 0.9-1.8 mg/day in 1-2 divided doses
Children 12-16 years: 1.2-2.4 mg/day in 1-2 divided doses
Children >16 years and Adults: 0.6-2.4 mg/day in 1-2 divided doses **or** Initial: 1.2 mg; repeat with 0.6 mg in 1 hour (maximum total therapy: 1.8 mg)

Dosage Forms
Tablet, oral:
Colcrys®: 0.6 mg

Dosage Forms - Canada
Tablet, oral: 1 mg [scored]

colchicine and probenecid (KOL chi seen & proe BEN e sid)

Synonyms ColBenemid; probenecid and colchicine

Therapeutic Category Antigout Agent

Use Treatment of chronic gouty arthritis when complicated by frequent, recurrent acute attacks of gout

General Dosage Range Dosage adjustment recommended in patients with renal impairment
Oral: *Adults:* Initial: One tablet daily; Maintenance: 1 tablet twice daily

Dosage Forms
Tablet: Colchicine 0.5 mg and probenecid 0.5 g

Colcrys® *see* colchicine *on page* 231
Cold Control PE [OTC] *see* acetaminophen, diphenhydramine, and phenylephrine *on page* 29
Coldcough PD *see* dihydrocodeine, chlorpheniramine, and phenylephrine *on page* 287

colesevelam (koh le SEV a lam)

U.S. Brand Names Welchol®

Canadian Brand Names Welchol®

Therapeutic Category Antihyperlipidemic Agent, Miscellaneous; Bile Acid Sequestrant

Use Management of elevated LDL in primary hypercholesterolemia (Fredrickson type IIa) when used alone or in combination with an HMG-CoA reductase inhibitor; management of heterozygous familial hypercholesterolemia (heFH) in adolescent patients (males and postmenarchal females 10-17 years of age) when used alone or in combination with an HMG-CoA reductase inhibitor, in patients who after an adequate trial of dietary therapy have LDL-C ≥190 mg/dL or LDL-C ≥160 mg/dL with positive family history of premature cardiovascular disease (CVD) or with two or more CVD risk factors; improve glycemic control in type 2 diabetes mellitus (noninsulin-dependent, NIDDM) in conjunction with diet, exercise, and insulin or oral antidiabetic agents

General Dosage Range Oral: *Children 10-17 years (males and postmenarchal females) and Adults:* 3.75 g/day in 1-2 divided doses

Dosage Forms
Granules for suspension, oral:
Welchol®: 3.75 g/packet (30s)
Tablet, oral:
Welchol®: 625 mg

Colestid® *see* colestipol *on page* 232
Colestid® Flavored *see* colestipol *on page* 232

colestipol (koe LES ti pole)

Medication Safety Issues
Sound-alike/look-alike issues:
Colestipol may be confused with calcitriol

Synonyms colestipol hydrochloride

U.S. Brand Names Colestid®; Colestid® Flavored

Canadian Brand Names Colestid®

Therapeutic Category Antihyperlipidemic Agent, Miscellaneous

Use Adjunct in management of primary hypercholesterolemia

General Dosage Range Oral: *Adults:* Granules: Initial: 5 g 1-2 times/day; Maintenance: 5-30 g/day once or in divided doses; Tablets: Initial: 2 g 1-2 times/day; Maintenance: 2-16 g/day once or in divided doses

Dosage Forms

Granules for suspension, oral: 5 g/scoop (500 g); 5 g/packet (30s, 90s)

Colestid®: 5 g/scoop (300 g, 500 g); 5 g/packet (30s, 90s)

Colestid® Flavored: 5 g/scoop (450 g); 5 g/packet (60s)

Tablet, oral: 1 g

Colestid®: 1 g

colestipol hydrochloride *see* colestipol *on page* *232*

CO Levetiracetam (Can) *see* levetiracetam *on page* *528*

CO Lisinopril (Can) *see* lisinopril *on page* *544*

colistimethate (koe lis ti METH ate)

Medication Safety Issues

Other safety concerns:

Due to the potential for dosing errors, it is recommended that prescriptions for colistimethate be expressed as colistin base only.

Synonyms colistimethate sodium; colistin methanesulfonate; colistin sulfomethate; pentasodium colistin methanesulfonate; polymyxin E

U.S. Brand Names Coly-Mycin® M

Canadian Brand Names Coly-Mycin® M

Therapeutic Category Antibiotic, Miscellaneous

Use Treatment of infections due to sensitive strains of certain gram-negative bacilli which are resistant to other antibacterials or in patients allergic to other antibacterials

General Dosage Range Dosage adjustment recommended in patients with renal impairment

I.M., I.V.: *Children and Adults:* 2.5-5 mg/kg/day **colistin base** in 2-4 divided doses

Dosage Forms

Injection, powder for reconstitution: colistin 150 mg

Coly-Mycin® M: colistin 150 mg

colistimethate sodium *see* colistimethate *on page* *233*

colistin, hydrocortisone, neomycin, and thonzonium *see* neomycin, colistin, hydrocortisone, and thonzonium *on page* *633*

colistin methanesulfonate *see* colistimethate *on page* *233*

colistin sulfomethate *see* colistimethate *on page* *233*

collagen *see* collagen hemostat *on page* *234*

collagen absorbable hemostat *see* collagen hemostat *on page* *234*

collagenase (systemic) (KOL la je nase)

Medication Safety Issues

Sound-alike/look-alike issues:

Collagenase clostridium histolyticum (Xiaflex®) may be confused with topical collagenase formulation (ie, Santyl®)

Xiaflex® may be confused with Zanaflex®

Synonyms collagenase clostridium histolyticum

U.S. Brand Names Xiaflex®

Therapeutic Category Enzyme

Use Treatment of Dupuytren contracture with a palpable cord

General Dosage Range **Intralesional:** *Adults:* 0.58 mg per cord

Dosage Forms

Injection, powder for reconstitution:

Xiaflex®: 0.9 mg

collagenase (topical) (KOL la je nase)

Medication Safety Issues

Sound-alike/look-alike issues:

Topical collagenase formulation (Santyl®) may be confused with the injectable collagenase clostridium histolyticum (Xiaflex®)

U.S. Brand Names Santyl®

Canadian Brand Names Santyl®

Therapeutic Category Enzyme

Use Promotes debridement of necrotic tissue in dermal ulcers and severe burns

General Dosage Range Topical: *Children and Adults:* Apply once daily

Dosage Forms

Ointment, topical:

Santyl®: 250 units/g (30 g)

collagenase clostridium histolyticum *see* collagenase (systemic) *on page* 233

collagen hemostat (KOL la jen HEE moe stat)

Medication Safety Issues

Sound-alike/look-alike issues:

Avitene® may be confused with Ativan®

Other safety concerns:

Over 100 reports of paralysis or other neural deficits have been received by the FDA, attributable to collagen hemostat-associated neuronal impingement

Synonyms collagen; collagen absorbable hemostat; MCH; microfibrillar collagen hemostat

U.S. Brand Names Avitene®; Avitene® Flour; Avitene® Ultrafoam™; EndoAvitene®; Helistat®; Helitene®; Instat™ MCH; SyringeAvitene™

Therapeutic Category Hemostatic Agent

Use Adjunct to hemostasis when control of bleeding by ligature is ineffective or impractical

General Dosage Range Topical: *Adults:* Apply dry directly to source of bleeding; remove excess material after ~10-15 minutes

Dosage Forms

Powder, topical:

Avitene® Flour: (0.5 g, 1 g, 5 g)
Helitene®: (0.5 g, 1 g)
Instat™ MCH: (0.5 g, 1 g)
SyringeAvitene™: (1 g)

Sheet, topical:

Avitene®: (1s, 6s)
EndoAvitene®: (6s)

Sponge, topical:

Avitene® Ultrafoam™: (6s)
Helistat®: (10s, 18s)

Colocort® *see* hydrocortisone (topical) *on page* 457
CO Losartan (Can) *see* losartan *on page* 551
CO Lovastatin (Can) *see* lovastatin *on page* 553
Coly-Mycin® M *see* colistimethate *on page* 233
Coly-Mycin® S *see* neomycin, colistin, hydrocortisone, and thonzonium *on page* 633
Colyte® *see* polyethylene glycol-electrolyte solution *on page* 738
Colyte™ (Can) *see* polyethylene glycol-electrolyte solution *on page* 738
Combantrin™ (Can) *see* pyrantel pamoate *on page* 775
Combigan® *see* brimonidine and timolol *on page* 141
CombiPatch® *see* estradiol and norethindrone *on page* 349
Combipres *see* clonidine and chlorthalidone *on page* 225
Combivent® *see* ipratropium and albuterol *on page* 499
Combivent® Respimat® *see* ipratropium and albuterol *on page* 499
Combivent UDV (Can) *see* ipratropium and albuterol *on page* 499
Combivir® *see* lamivudine and zidovudine *on page* 520
CO Meloxicam (Can) *see* meloxicam *on page* 569
CO Memantine (Can) *see* memantine *on page* 570
CO Metformin (Can) *see* metformin *on page* 579
CO Mirtazapine (Can) *see* mirtazapine *on page* 606
Commit® [OTC] *see* nicotine *on page* 640
Compazine *see* prochlorperazine *on page* 760
Complera™ *see* emtricitabine, rilpivirine, and tenofovir *on page* 329

Compound 347™ *see* enflurane *on page* 331
compound E *see* cortisone *on page* 238
compound F *see* hydrocortisone (systemic) *on page* 457
compound F *see* hydrocortisone (topical) *on page* 457
compound S *see* zidovudine *on page* 961
compound S, abacavir, and lamivudine *see* abacavir, lamivudine, and zidovudine *on page* 16
Compound W® [OTC] *see* salicylic acid *on page* 816
Compound W® One Step Invisible Strip [OTC] *see* salicylic acid *on page* 816
Compound W® One-Step Wart Remover [OTC] *see* salicylic acid *on page* 816
Compound W® One Step Wart Remover for Feet [OTC] *see* salicylic acid *on page* 816
Compound W® One-Step Wart Remover for Kids [OTC] *see* salicylic acid *on page* 816
Compoz® [OTC] *see* diphenhydramine (systemic) *on page* 292
Compro® *see* prochlorperazine *on page* 760
Comtan® *see* entacapone *on page* 333
Comtrex® Maximum Strength, Non-Drowsy Cold & Cough [OTC] *see* acetaminophen, dextromethorphan, and phenylephrine *on page* 28
Comvax® *see Haemophilus* B conjugate and hepatitis B vaccine *on page* 439
CO Mycophenolate (Can) *see* mycophenolate *on page* 619
Concept DHA™ *see* vitamins (multiple/prenatal) *on page* 952
Concept OB™ *see* vitamins (multiple/prenatal) *on page* 952
Conceptrol® [OTC] *see* nonoxynol 9 *on page* 647
Concerta® *see* methylphenidate *on page* 590
Condyline™ (Can) *see* podofilox *on page* 735
Condylox® *see* podofilox *on page* 735
Congest (Can) *see* estrogens (conjugated/equine, systemic) *on page* 351
Congestac® [OTC] *see* guaifenesin and pseudoephedrine *on page* 436

conivaptan (koe NYE vap tan)

Synonyms conivaptan hydrochloride; YM087

U.S. Brand Names Vaprisol®

Therapeutic Category Vasopressin Antagonist

Use Treatment of euvolemic and hypervolemic hyponatremia in hospitalized patients

General Dosage Range Dosage adjustment recommended in patients with hepatic impairment

I.V.: *Adults:* Loading dose: 20 mg bolus, followed by 20 mg as continuous infusion over 24 hours; Maintenance: 20-40 mg/day as a continuous infusion over 24 hours (maximum therapy: 4 days)

Dosage Forms

Infusion, premixed in D_5W:
Vaprisol®: 20 mg (100 mL)

conivaptan hydrochloride *see* conivaptan *on page* 235
conjugated estrogen *see* estrogens (conjugated/equine, systemic) *on page* 351
conjugated estrogen *see* estrogens (conjugated/equine, topical) *on page* 352
CO Norfloxacin (Can) *see* norfloxacin *on page* 649
Conray® *see* iothalamate meglumine *on page* 497
Conray® 30 *see* iothalamate meglumine *on page* 497
Conray® 43 *see* iothalamate meglumine *on page* 497
Constulose *see* lactulose *on page* 519
Contac® Cold 12 Hour Relief Non Drowsy (Can) *see* pseudoephedrine *on page* 771
Contac® Cold and Sore Throat, Non Drowsy, Extra Strength (Can) *see* acetaminophen and pseudoephedrine *on page* 25
Contac® Cold-Chest Congestion, Non Drowsy, Regular Strength (Can) *see* guaifenesin and pseudoephedrine *on page* 436
Contac® Cold + Flu Maximum Strength Non-Drowsy [OTC] *see* acetaminophen and phenylephrine *on page* 24
Contac® Cold + Flu Maximum Strength Non-Drowsy [OTC] *see* pseudoephedrine *on page* 771
continuous renal replacement therapy *see* electrolyte solution, renal replacement *on page* 325

copper (KOP er)

Medication Safety Issues

Sound-alike/look-alike issues:

Cupric sulfate may be confused with calcium gluconate

Synonyms cupric chloride; cupric chloride dihydrate

Therapeutic Category Trace Element, Parenteral

Use Supplement to intravenous solutions given for total parenteral nutrition (TPN) to maintain copper serum levels and to prevent depletion of endogenous stores and subsequent deficiency symptoms

General Dosage Range I.V. (as a parenteral nutrition component):

Infants and Children: 20 mcg/kg/day

Adults: 0.3-1.5 mg/day

Dosage Forms

Injection, solution [preservative free]: 0.4 mg/mL (10 mL)

Corlopam® *see* fenoldopam *on page 376*
Cormax® *see* clobetasol *on page 221*
CO Ropinirole (Can) *see* ropinirole *on page 810*
CO Rosuvastatin (Can) *see* rosuvastatin *on page 812*
Correctol® [OTC] *see* docusate *on page 304*
Correctol® Tablets [OTC] *see* bisacodyl *on page 134*
Cortaid® Advanced [OTC] *see* hydrocortisone (topical) *on page 457*
Cortaid® Intensive Therapy [OTC] *see* hydrocortisone (topical) *on page 457*
Cortaid® Maximum Strength [OTC] *see* hydrocortisone (topical) *on page 457*
Cortamed® (Can) *see* hydrocortisone (topical) *on page 457*
Cortef® *see* hydrocortisone (systemic) *on page 457*
Cortenema® *see* hydrocortisone (topical) *on page 457*
CortiCool® [OTC] *see* hydrocortisone (topical) *on page 457*

corticorelin (kor ti koe REL in)

Medication Safety Issues

Sound-alike/look-alike issues:

Acthrel® may be confused with Acthar
Corticorelin may be confused with corticotropin, cosyntropin, or Cortrosyn®

Synonyms corticorelin ovine triflutate; human corticotrophin-releasing hormone, analogue; ovine corticotrophin-releasing hormone (oCRH)

U.S. Brand Names Acthrel®

Therapeutic Category Diagnostic Agent, ACTH-Dependent Hypercortisolism

Use Diagnostic test used in adrenocorticotropic hormone (ACTH)-dependent Cushing syndrome to differentiate between pituitary and ectopic production of ACTH

General Dosage Range I.V.: *Adults:* 1 mcg/kg

Dosage Forms

Injection, powder for reconstitution:

Acthrel®: 100 mcg

corticorelin ovine triflutate *see* corticorelin *on page 237*

corticotropin (kor ti koe TROE pin)

Medication Safety Issues

Sound-alike/look-alike issues:

Corticotropin may be confused with corticorelin, cosyntropin

Synonyms ACTH; Acthar; adrenocorticotropic hormone; corticotropin, repository

U.S. Brand Names H.P. Acthar®

Therapeutic Category Adrenal Corticosteroid

Use Acute exacerbations of multiple sclerosis; infantile spasms; adjunctive therapy for exacerbations/acute episodes of rheumatic disorders (psoriatic arthritis, rheumatoid arthritis, juvenile idiopathic arthritis [JIA], ankylosing spondylitis); exacerbations or maintenance therapy for collagen diseases (systemic lupus erythematosus, systemic dermatomyositis); severe erythema multiforme; Stevens-Johnson syndrome; serum sickness; severe acute/chronic allergic and inflammatory ophthalmic disease (keratitis, iritis, iridocyclitis, diffuse posterior uveitis and choroiditis, optic neuritis, chorioretinitis, anterior segment inflammation); symptomatic sarcoidosis; to induce diuresis for remission of proteinuria in patients with nephrotic syndrome without idiopathic uremia or due to lupus erythematosus

General Dosage Range

I.M.:

Children <2 years: 75 units/m^2/dose twice daily (infantile spasms) followed by gradual downward titration of dose

Children >2 years: 40-80 units every 24-72 hours

Adults: 80-120 units/day for 2-3 weeks (MS) **or** 40-80 units every 24-72 hours (indications other than MS)

SubQ:

Children >2 years: 40-80 units every 24-72 hours

Adults: 80-120 units/day for 2-3 weeks (MS) **or** 40-80 units every 24-72 hours (indications other than MS)

Dosage Forms
Injection, gel:
H.P. Acthar®: 80 units/mL (5 mL)

corticotropin, repository *see* corticotropin *on page 237*
Cortifoam® *see* hydrocortisone (topical) *on page 457*
Cortifoam™ (Can) *see* hydrocortisone (topical) *on page 457*
Cortimyxin® (Can) *see* neomycin, polymyxin B, and hydrocortisone *on page 634*
cortisol *see* hydrocortisone (systemic) *on page 457*
cortisol *see* hydrocortisone (topical) *on page 457*

cortisone (KOR ti sone)

Medication Safety Issues
Sound-alike/look-alike issues:
Cortisone may be confused with Cardizem®, Cortizone®

Synonyms compound E; cortisone acetate
Therapeutic Category Adrenal Corticosteroid
Use Management of adrenocortical insufficiency
General Dosage Range Oral:
Children: 0.5-10 mg/kg/day **or** 20-300 mg/m^2/day divided every 6-8 hours
Adults: 25-300 mg /day divided every 12-24 hours

Dosage Forms
Tablet, oral: 25 mg

cortisone acetate *see* cortisone *on page 238*
Cortisporin® *see* neomycin, polymyxin B, and hydrocortisone *on page 634*
Cortisporin® Ointment *see* bacitracin, neomycin, polymyxin B, and hydrocortisone *on page 112*
Cortisporin® Otic (Can) *see* neomycin, polymyxin B, and hydrocortisone *on page 634*
Cortisporin®-TC *see* neomycin, colistin, hydrocortisone, and thonzonium *on page 633*
Cortisporin® Topical Ointment (Can) *see* bacitracin, neomycin, polymyxin B, and hydrocortisone *on page 112*
Cortizone-10® Hydratensive Healing [OTC] *see* hydrocortisone (topical) *on page 457*
Cortizone-10® Hydratensive Soothing [OTC] *see* hydrocortisone (topical) *on page 457*
Cortizone-10® Intensive Healing Eczema [OTC] *see* hydrocortisone (topical) *on page 457*
Cortizone-10® Maximum Strength [OTC] *see* hydrocortisone (topical) *on page 457*
Cortizone-10® Maximum Strength Cooling Relief [OTC] *see* hydrocortisone (topical) *on page 457*
Cortizone-10® Maximum Strength Easy Relief [OTC] *see* hydrocortisone (topical) *on page 457*
Cortizone-10® Maximum Strength Intensive Healing Formula [OTC] *see* hydrocortisone (topical) *on page 457*
Cortizone-10® Plus Maximum Strength [OTC] *see* hydrocortisone (topical) *on page 457*
Cortomycin *see* neomycin, polymyxin B, and hydrocortisone *on page 634*
Cortrosyn™ *see* cosyntropin *on page 239*
Corvert® *see* ibutilide *on page 471*
Corzide® *see* nadolol and bendroflumethiazide *on page 624*
CO Sertraline (Can) *see* sertraline *on page 831*
CO Simvastatin (Can) *see* simvastatin *on page 835*
Cosmegen® *see* dactinomycin *on page 251*
Cosopt® *see* dorzolamide and timolol *on page 310*
Cosopt® PF *see* dorzolamide and timolol *on page 310*
Cosopt® Preservative Free (Can) *see* dorzolamide and timolol *on page 310*
CO Sotalol (Can) *see* sotalol *on page 851*
CO Sumatriptan (Can) *see* sumatriptan *on page 863*

cosyntropin (koe sin TROE pin)

Medication Safety Issues

Sound-alike/look-alike issues:

Cortrosyn® may be confused with colchicine, corticorelin, corticotropin, Cotazym®
Cosyntropin may be confused with corticorelin, corticotropin

Synonyms Synacthen; tetracosactide

U.S. Brand Names Cortrosyn™

Canadian Brand Names Cortrosyn™; Synacthen® Depot

Therapeutic Category Diagnostic Agent

Use Diagnostic test to differentiate primary adrenal from secondary (pituitary) adrenocortical insufficiency

Synacthen® Depot (Canadian availability): Additional indications: Treatment of various disease states (eg, collagen, dermatologic, endocrine, ocular, hemolytic). Consult manufacturer labeling for detailed list.

General Dosage Range I.M., I.V.:

Children ≤2 years: 0.125 mg
Children >2 years and Adults: 0.25 mg

Dosage Forms

Injection, powder for reconstitution: 0.25 mg
Cortrosyn™: 0.25 mg

Injection, solution [preservative free]: 0.25 mg/mL (1 mL)

Dosage Forms - Canada

Injection, suspension:
Synacthen® Depot: 1 mg/mL (1 mL)

Cotazym® (Can) *see* pancrelipase *on page* 687
CO Temazepam (Can) *see* temazepam *on page* 875
CO Terbinafine (Can) *see* terbinafine (systemic) *on page* 878
CO Topiramate (Can) *see* topiramate *on page* 906
Cotridin *see* triprolidine, pseudoephedrine, and codeine *(Canada only) on page* 922
co-trimoxazole *see* sulfamethoxazole and trimethoprim *on page* 860
Coumadin® *see* warfarin *on page* 954
CO Valacyclovir (Can) *see* valacyclovir *on page* 933
CO Valsartan (Can) *see* valsartan *on page* 935
Covan® (Can) *see* triprolidine, pseudoephedrine, and codeine *(Canada only) on page* 922
Covaryx® *see* estrogens (esterified) and methyltestosterone *on page* 353
Covaryx® H.S. *see* estrogens (esterified) and methyltestosterone *on page* 353
CO Venlafaxine XR (Can) *see* venlafaxine *on page* 942
Covera® (Can) *see* verapamil *on page* 942
Covera-HS® [DSC] *see* verapamil *on page* 942
Covera-HS® (Can) *see* verapamil *on page* 942
Coversyl® (Can) *see* perindopril erbumine *on page* 709
Coversyl® Plus (Can) *see* perindopril erbumine and indapamide *(Canada only) on page* 709
Coversyl® Plus HD (Can) *see* perindopril erbumine and indapamide *(Canada only) on page* 709
Coversyl® Plus LD (Can) *see* perindopril erbumine and indapamide *(Canada only) on page* 709
co-vidarabine *see* pentostatin *on page* 707
coviracil *see* emtricitabine *on page* 328
Cozaar® *see* losartan *on page* 551
CO Zopiclone (Can) *see* zopiclone *(Canada only) on page* 967
CP358774 *see* erlotinib *on page* 341
CPC *see* cetylpyridinium *on page* 192
CPM *see* cyclophosphamide *on page* 244
CPT-11 *see* irinotecan *on page* 501
CPZ *see* chlorpromazine *on page* 203
13-CRA *see* isotretinoin *on page* 505
Cramp Tabs [OTC] *see* acetaminophen and pamabrom *on page* 24
Crantex® [DSC] *see* guaifenesin and phenylephrine *on page* 435

Creomulsion® Adult Formula [OTC] *see* dextromethorphan *on page* 272
Creomulsion® for Children [OTC] *see* dextromethorphan *on page* 272
Creon® *see* pancrelipase *on page* 687
Creo-Terpin® [OTC] *see* dextromethorphan *on page* 272
Crestor® *see* rosuvastatin *on page* 812
Cresylate™ *see* m-cresyl acetate *on page* 564
Crinone® *see* progesterone *on page* 762
Critic-Aid® Clear AF [OTC] *see* miconazole (topical) *on page* 599
Critic-Aid Skin Care® [OTC] *see* zinc oxide *on page* 963
Crixivan® *see* indinavir *on page* 479

crizotinib (kriz OH ti nib)

Medication Safety Issues

Sound-alike/look-alike issues:

Crizotinib may be confused with erlotinib, gefitinib

High alert medication:

This medication is in a class the Institute for Safe Medication Practices (ISMP) includes among its list of drug classes which have a heightened risk of causing significant patient harm when used in error.

Synonyms C-met/hepatocyte growth factor receptor tyrosine kinase inhibitor PF-02341066; C-met/HGFR tyrosine kinase inhibitor PF-02341066; MET tyrosine kinase inhibitor PF-02341066; PF-02341066

U.S. Brand Names Xalkori®

Canadian Brand Names Xalkori™

Therapeutic Category Antineoplastic Agent, Anaplastic Lymphoma Kinase Inhibitor; Antineoplastic Agent, Tyrosine Kinase Inhibitor

Use Treatment of locally advanced or metastatic nonsmall cell lung cancer (NSCLC) that is anaplastic lymphoma kinase (ALK) positive (as detected by an approved test)

General Dosage Range Dosage adjustment recommended in patients who develop toxicities.

Oral: *Adults:* 250 mg twice daily

Dosage Forms

Capsule, oral:

Xalkori®: 200 mg, 250 mg

CroFab® *see* crotalidae polyvalent immune FAB (ovine) *on page* 241
Crolom *see* cromolyn (ophthalmic) *on page* 241
cromoglycic acid *see* cromolyn (nasal) *on page* 241
cromoglycic acid *see* cromolyn (ophthalmic) *on page* 241
cromoglycic acid *see* cromolyn (systemic, oral inhalation) *on page* 240

cromolyn (systemic, oral inhalation) (KROE moe lin)

Synonyms cromoglycic acid; cromolyn sodium; disodium cromoglycate; DSCG

U.S. Brand Names Gastrocrom®

Canadian Brand Names Nalcrom®; Nu-Cromolyn; PMS-Sodium Cromoglycate

Therapeutic Category Mast Cell Stabilizer

Use

Inhalation: May be used as an adjunct in the prophylaxis of allergic disorders, including asthma; prevention of exercise-induced bronchospasm

Oral: Systemic mastocytosis

General Dosage Range

Inhalation: Nebulization: *Children ≥2 years and Adults:* Initial: 20 mg 4 times/day; Maintenance: 20 mg 3-4 times/day **or** 20 mg prior to exercise or allergen exposure

Oral:

Children 2-12 years: 100 mg 4 times/day (maximum: 40 mg/kg/day)
Children >12 years and Adults: 200 mg 4 times/day (maximum: 40 mg/kg/day)

Dosage Forms

Solution, for nebulization: 20 mg/2 mL (60s, 120s)

Solution, oral [preservative free]: 100 mg/5 mL (96s)

Gastrocrom®: 100 mg/5 mL (96s)

cromolyn (nasal) (KROE moe lin)

Medication Safety Issues

Sound-alike/look-alike issues:

NasalCrom® may be confused with Nasacort®, Nasalide®

Synonyms cromoglycic acid; cromolyn sodium; disodium cromoglycate; DSCG

U.S. Brand Names NasalCrom® [OTC]

Canadian Brand Names Apo-Cromolyn Nasal Spray® [OTC]; Rhinaris-CS Anti-Allergic Nasal Mist

Therapeutic Category Mast Cell Stabilizer

Use Prevention and treatment of seasonal and perennial allergic rhinitis

General Dosage Range Intranasal: *Children ≥2 years and Adults:* Instill 1 spray in each nostril 3-4 times/ day

Dosage Forms

Solution, intranasal: 40 mg/mL (26 mL)

NasalCrom® [OTC]: 40 mg/mL (13 mL)

cromolyn (ophthalmic) (KROE moe lin)

Synonyms Crolom; cromoglycic acid; cromolyn sodium; disodium cromoglycate; DSCG

Canadian Brand Names Opticrom®

Therapeutic Category Mast Cell Stabilizer

Use Treatment of vernal keratoconjunctivitis, vernal conjunctivitis, and vernal keratitis

General Dosage Range Ophthalmic: *Adults:* 1-2 drops in each eye 4-6 times/day

Dosage Forms

Solution, ophthalmic: 4% (10 mL)

cromolyn sodium *see* cromolyn (nasal) *on page 241*

cromolyn sodium *see* cromolyn (ophthalmic) *on page 241*

cromolyn sodium *see* cromolyn (systemic, oral inhalation) *on page 240*

crotalidae polyvalent immune FAB (ovine)

(kroe TAL ih die pol i VAY lent i MYUN fab (oh vine))

Synonyms antivenin (crotalidae) polyvalent, FAB (ovine); antivenom (crotalidae) polyvalent, FAB (ovine); crotaline antivenin, polyvalent, FAB (ovine); crotaline antivenom, polyvalent, FAB (ovine); FabAV, FAB (ovine); North American antisnake-bite serum, FAB (ovine); snake antivenin, FAB (ovine); snake antivenom, FAB (ovine)

U.S. Brand Names CroFab®

Therapeutic Category Antivenin

Use Management of patients with North American crotalid envenomations (eg, rattlesnakes [*Crotalus*, *Sistrurus*], copperheads, and cottonmouth/water moccasins [*Agkistrodon*])

General Dosage Range I.V.: *Children and Adults:* Initial dose: 4-6 vials, may repeat with 4-6 vials; Maintenance dose: Administer 2 vials every 6 hours for up to 18 hours

Dosage Forms

Injection, powder for reconstitution:

CroFab®: Derived from *Crotalus adamanteus, C. atrox, C. scutulatus*, and *Agkistrodon piscivorus* snake venoms

crotaline antivenin, polyvalent, FAB (ovine) *see* crotalidae polyvalent immune FAB (ovine) *on page 241*

crotaline antivenom, polyvalent, FAB (ovine) *see* crotalidae polyvalent immune FAB (ovine) *on page 241*

crotamiton (kroe TAM i tonn)

Medication Safety Issues

Sound-alike/look-alike issues:

Eurax® may be confused with Efudex®, Eulexin, Evoxac®, Serax, Urex

International issues:

Eurax [U.S., Canada, and multiple international markets] may be confused with Urex brand name for furosemide [Australia, China,Turkey] and methenamine [U.S., Canada]

U.S. Brand Names Eurax®

Canadian Brand Names Eurax Cream

Therapeutic Category Scabicides/Pediculicides

Use Treatment of scabies (*Sarcoptes scabiei*) and symptomatic treatment of pruritus

General Dosage Range Topical: *Children and Adults:* Pruritus: Massage into affected areas as needed; Scabies: Apply a thin layer from the neck to the toes, repeat in 24 hours; take a cleansing bath 48 hours after final application, may repeat after 7-10 days

Dosage Forms

Cream, topical:
Eurax®: 10% (60 g)

Lotion, topical:
Eurax®: 10% (60 mL, 480 mL)

cyanocobalamin (sye an oh koe BAL a min)

Synonyms vitamin B_{12}

U.S. Brand Names Ener-B® [OTC]; Nascobal®; Twelve Resin-K [OTC]

Therapeutic Category Vitamin, Water Soluble

Use Treatment of pernicious anemia; vitamin B_{12} deficiency due to dietary deficiencies or malabsorption diseases, inadequate secretion of intrinsic factor, and inadequate utilization of B_{12} (eg, during neoplastic treatment); increased B_{12} requirements due to pregnancy, thyrotoxicosis, hemorrhage, malignancy, liver or kidney disease

General Dosage Range

I.M., SubQ: *Children and Adults:* Dosage varies greatly depending on indication
Intranasal: *Adults:* Nascobal®: 500 mcg in one nostril once weekly
Oral: *Adults:* 250-2000 mcg/day

Dosage Forms

Injection, solution: 1000 mcg/mL (1 mL, 10 mL, 30 mL)
Lozenge, oral: 50 mcg (100s); 100 mcg (100s); 250 mcg (100s, 250s); 500 mcg (100s, 250s)
Lozenge, sublingual: 500 mcg (100s)
Solution, intranasal:
Nascobal®: 500 mcg/spray (2.3 mL)
Tablet, for buccal application/oral/sublingual:
Twelve Resin-K [OTC]: 1000 mcg
Tablet, oral: 50 mcg, 100 mcg, 250 mcg, 500 mcg, 1000 mcg
Ener-B® [OTC]: 100 mcg, 500 mcg, 1000 mcg
Tablet, sublingual: 1000 mcg, 2500 mcg, 5000 mcg
Tablet, timed release, oral: 1000 mcg
Ener-B® [OTC]: 1500 mcg

cyanocobalamin, folic acid, and pyridoxine *see* folic acid, cyanocobalamin, and pyridoxine *on page 404*
Cyclafem™ 1/35 *see* ethinyl estradiol and norethindrone *on page 359*
Cyclafem™ 7/7/7 *see* ethinyl estradiol and norethindrone *on page 359*
Cyclen® (Can) *see* ethinyl estradiol and norgestimate *on page 361*
Cyclessa® *see* ethinyl estradiol and desogestrel *on page 356*

cyclobenzaprine (sye kloe BEN za preen)

Medication Safety Issues

Sound-alike/look-alike issues:
Cyclobenzaprine may be confused with cycloSERINE, cyproheptadine
Flexeril® may be confused with Floxin®

BEERS Criteria medication:
This drug may be potentially inappropriate for use in geriatric patients (Quality of evidence - moderate; Strength of recommendation - strong).

International issues:
Flexin: Brand name for cyclobenzaprine [Chile], but also the brand name for diclofenac [Argentina] and orphenadrine [Israel]
Flexin [Chile] may be confused with Floxin brand name for flunarizine [Thailand], norfloxacin [South Africa], ofloxacin [U.S., Canada], and perfloxacin [Philippines]; Fluoxine brand name for fluoxetine [Thailand]

Synonyms cyclobenzaprine hydrochloride

U.S. Brand Names Amrix®; Fexmid®; Flexeril®

Canadian Brand Names Apo-Cyclobenzaprine®; Auro-Cyclobenzaprine; Ava-Cyclobenzaprine; Dom-Cyclobenzaprine; JAMP-Cyclobenzaprine; Mylan-Cyclobenzaprine; Novo-Cycloprine; Nu-Cyclobenzaprine; PHL-Cyclobenzaprine; PMS-Cyclobenzaprine; Q-Cyclobenzaprine; ratio-Cyclobenzaprine; Riva-Cycloprine; ZYM-Cyclobenzaprine

Therapeutic Category Skeletal Muscle Relaxant

Use Treatment of muscle spasm associated with acute, painful musculoskeletal conditions

General Dosage Range Dosage adjustment recommended in patients with hepatic impairment

Oral capsule, extended release: *Adults:* Usual: 15 mg once daily (maximum: 30 mg once daily)
Oral tablet, immediate release:
Children ≥15 years and Adults: Initial: 5 mg 3 times/day; Maintenance: 5-10 mg 3 times/day
Elderly: Initial: 5 mg

Dosage Forms

Capsule, extended release, oral: 15 mg, 30 mg
Amrix®: 15 mg, 30 mg
Tablet, oral: 5 mg, 7.5 mg, 10 mg
Fexmid®: 7.5 mg
Flexeril®: 5 mg, 10 mg

cyclobenzaprine hydrochloride *see* cyclobenzaprine *on page 243*
Cyclocort® (Can) *see* amcinonide *on page 59*
Cyclogyl® *see* cyclopentolate *on page 244*
Cyclomen® (Can) *see* danazol *on page 253*
Cyclomydril® *see* cyclopentolate and phenylephrine *on page 244*

cyclopentolate (sye kloe PEN toe late)

Synonyms cyclopentolate hydrochloride

U.S. Brand Names AK-Pentolate™; Cyclogyl®; Cylate™ [DSC]

Canadian Brand Names AK Pentolate Oph Soln; Cyclogyl®; Diopentolate®; Minims Cyclopentolate; PMS-Cyclopentolate

Therapeutic Category Anticholinergic Agent

Use Diagnostic procedures requiring mydriasis and cycloplegia

General Dosage Range Ophthalmic:

Children: Instill 1 drop of 0.5%, 1%, or 2% in eye followed by 1 drop of 0.5% or 1% in 5 minutes, if necessary

Adults: Instill 1 drop of 1% followed by another drop in 5 minutes; 2% solution in heavily pigmented iris

Dosage Forms

Solution, ophthalmic: 1% (2 mL, 5 mL, 15 mL); 2% (2 mL, 5 mL, 15 mL)

AK-Pentolate™: 1% (2 mL, 15 mL)

Cyclogyl®: 0.5% (15 mL); 1% (2 mL, 5 mL, 15 mL); 2% (2 mL, 5 mL, 15 mL)

cyclopentolate and phenylephrine (sye kloe PEN toe late & fen il EF rin)

Synonyms phenylephrine and cyclopentolate

U.S. Brand Names Cyclomydril®

Therapeutic Category Anticholinergic/Adrenergic Agonist

Use Induce mydriasis greater than that produced with cyclopentolate HCl alone

General Dosage Range Ophthalmic: *Children and Adults:* Instill 1 drop into eyes every 5-10 minutes, for up to 3 doses

Dosage Forms

Solution, ophthalmic:

Cyclomydril®: Cyclopentolate 0.2% and phenylephrine 1% (2 mL, 5 mL)

cyclopentolate hydrochloride *see* cyclopentolate *on page* *244*

cyclophosphamide (sye kloe FOS fa mide)

Medication Safety Issues

Sound-alike/look-alike issues:

Cyclophosphamide may be confused with cycloSPORINE, ifosfamide

Cytoxan may be confused with cefOXitin, Ciloxan®, cytarabine, CytoGam®, Cytosar®, Cytosar-U, Cytotec®

High alert medication:

This medication is in a class the Institute for Safe Medication Practices (ISMP) includes among its list of drugs which have a heightened risk of causing significant patient harm when used in error.

Synonyms CPM; CTX; CYT; Cytoxan; neosar

Canadian Brand Names Procytox®

Therapeutic Category Antineoplastic Agent

Use

Oncology-related uses: Treatment of Hodgkin lymphoma, non-Hodgkin lymphoma (including Burkitt lymphoma), chronic lymphocytic leukemia (CLL), chronic myelocytic leukemia (CML), acute myelocytic leukemia (AML), acute lymphocytic leukemia (ALL), mycosis fungoides, multiple myeloma, neuroblastoma, retinoblastoma; breast cancer; ovarian adenocarcinoma

Nononcology uses: Treatment of refractory nephrotic syndrome in children

General Dosage Range Dosage adjustment recommended in patients with hepatic or renal impairment

I.V.: *Children and Adults:* Dosage varies greatly depending on indication

Oral: *Children and Adults:* 1-5 mg/kg/day

Dosage Forms

Injection, powder for reconstitution: 500 mg, 1 g, 2 g

Tablet, oral: 25 mg, 50 mg

cycloserine (sye kloe SER een)

Medication Safety Issues

Sound-alike/look-alike issues:

CycloSERINE may be confused with cyclobenzaprine, cycloSPORINE

Tall-Man cyclo**SERINE**

U.S. Brand Names Seromycin®

Therapeutic Category Antibiotic, Miscellaneous

Use Adjunctive treatment in pulmonary or extrapulmonary tuberculosis

General Dosage Range Dosage adjustment recommended in patients with renal impairment

Oral:

Children: 10-20 mg/kg/day in 2 divided doses (maximum: 1000 mg/day)

Adults: Initial: 250 mg every 12 hours for 14 days; Maintenance: 500-1000 mg/day in 2 divided doses

Dosage Forms

Capsule, oral:

Seromycin®: 250 mg

Cycloset® *see* bromocriptine *on page 143*

cyclosporin A *see* cyclosporine (ophthalmic) *on page 246*

cyclosporin A *see* cyclosporine (systemic) *on page 245*

cyclosporine (systemic) (SYE kloe spor een)

Medication Safety Issues

Sound-alike/look-alike issues:

CycloSPORINE may be confused with cyclophosphamide, Cyklokapron®, cycloSERINE

CycloSPORINE modified (Neoral®, Gengraf®) may be confused with cycloSPORINE non-modified (SandIMMUNE®)

Gengraf® may be confused with Prograf®

Neoral® may be confused with Neurontin®, Nizoral®

SandIMMUNE® may be confused with SandoSTATIN®

Synonyms CsA; CyA; cyclosporin A

Tall-Man cyclo**SPORINE**

U.S. Brand Names Gengraf®; Neoral®; SandIMMUNE®

Canadian Brand Names Apo-Cyclosporine®; Neoral®; Rhoxal-cyclosporine; Sandimmune® I.V.; Sandoz-Cyclosporine

Therapeutic Category Immunosuppressant Agent

Use Prophylaxis of organ rejection in kidney, liver, and heart transplants, has been used with azathioprine and/or corticosteroids; severe, active rheumatoid arthritis (RA) not responsive to methotrexate alone; severe, recalcitrant plaque psoriasis in nonimmunocompromised adults unresponsive to or unable to tolerate other systemic therapy

General Dosage Range Dosage adjustment recommended in patients with renal impairment

I.V. (non-modified): *Children and Adults:* Initial dose: 5-6 mg/kg/day or one-third of the oral dose as a single dose; Maintenance: 3-7.5 mg/kg/day in 2-3 divided doses or give as continuous infusion over 24 hours

Oral:

Modified:

Children and Adults: Transplant: Heart: 7 ± 3 mg/kg/day in 2 divided doses; Liver: 8 ± 4 mg/kg/day in 2 divided doses; Renal: 9 ± 3 mg/kg/day in 2 divided doses

Adults: Initial: 2.5 mg/kg/day in 2 divided doses; Maintenance: Up to 4 mg/kg/day

Non-modified: *Children and Adults:* Initial: 10-14 mg/kg/day for 1-2 weeks; Maintenance: Taper by 5% per week to 3-10 mg/kg/day

Dosage Forms

Capsule, oral: 100 mg

Gengraf®: 25 mg, 100 mg

Capsule, softgel, oral: 25 mg, 50 mg, 100 mg

Neoral®: 25 mg, 100 mg

SandIMMUNE®: 25 mg, 100 mg

Injection, solution: 50 mg/mL (5 mL)

SandIMMUNE®: 50 mg/mL (5 mL)

Solution, oral: 100 mg/mL (50 mL)

Gengraf®: 100 mg/mL (50 mL)

Neoral®: 100 mg/mL (50 mL)

SandIMMUNE®: 100 mg/mL (50 mL)

cyclosporine (ophthalmic) (SYE kloe spor een)

Medication Safety Issues

Sound-alike/look-alike issues:

CycloSPORINE may be confused with cyclophosphamide, Cyklokapron®, cycloSERINE

Synonyms CsA; CyA; cyclosporin A

Tall-Man cyclo**SPORINE**

U.S. Brand Names Restasis®

Canadian Brand Names Restasis®

Therapeutic Category Immunosuppressant Agent

Use Increase tear production when suppressed tear production is presumed to be due to keratoconjunctivitis sicca-associated ocular inflammation (in patients not already using topical antiinflammatory drugs or punctal plugs)

General Dosage Range Ophthalmic (Restasis®): *Children ≥16 years and Adults:* Instill 1 drop in each eye every 12 hours

Dosage Forms

Emulsion, ophthalmic [preservative free]:

Restasis®: 0.05% (0.4 mL)

Cyestra-35 (Can) *see* cyproterone and ethinyl estradiol *(Canada only) on page 247*
Cyklokapron® *see* tranexamic acid *on page 910*
Cylate™ [DSC] *see* cyclopentolate *on page 244*
Cymbalta® *see* duloxetine *on page 319*

cyproheptadine (si proe HEP ta deen)

Medication Safety Issues

Sound-alike/look-alike issues:

Cyproheptadine may be confused with cyclobenzaprine
Periactin may be confused with Percodan®, Persantine®

BEERS Criteria medication:

This drug may be potentially inappropriate for use in geriatric patients (Quality of evidence - moderate; Strength of recommendation - strong).

International issues:

Periactin brand name for cyproheptadine [U.S., multiple international markets] may be confused with Perative brand name for an enteral nutrition preparation [multiple international markets] and brand name for ketoconazole [Argentina]

Synonyms cyproheptadine hydrochloride; Periactin

Canadian Brand Names Euro-Cyproheptadine; PMS-Cyproheptadine

Therapeutic Category Antihistamine

Use Perennial and seasonal allergic rhinitis and other allergic symptoms including urticaria

General Dosage Range

Oral:

Children 2-6 years: 2 mg every 8-12 hours (not to exceed 12 mg/day)
Children 7-14 years: 4 mg every 8-12 hours (not to exceed 16 mg/day)
Adults: 4-20 mg/day divided every 8 hours (not to exceed 0.5 mg/kg/day)

Dosage Forms

Syrup, oral: 2 mg/5 mL (473 mL, 480 mL)
Tablet, oral: 4 mg

cyproheptadine hydrochloride *see* cyproheptadine *on page 246*

cyproterone *(Canada only)* (sye PROE ter one)

Synonyms cyproterone acetate; SH 714

Canadian Brand Names Androcur®; Androcur® Depot; Novo-Cyproterone

Therapeutic Category Antiandrogen; Progestin

Use Palliative treatment of advanced prostate cancer

General Dosage Range

I.M.: *Adults (males):* 300 mg (3 mL) once weekly **or** every 2 weeks
Oral: *Adults (males):* 100-300 mg daily in 2-3 divided doses

Product Availability Not available in U.S.

Dosage Forms - Canada

Injection, solution: 100 mg/mL (3 mL)

Androcur® Depot: 100 mg/mL (3 mL)

Tablet: 50 mg

Androcur®, Apo-Cyproterone®, Gen-Cyproterone: 50 mg

cyproterone and ethinyl estradiol *(Canada only)*

(sye PROE ter one & ETH in il es tra DYE ole)

Synonyms ethinyl estradiol and cyproterone acetate

Canadian Brand Names Cyestra-35; Diane-35®; Novo-Cyproterone/Ethinyl Estradiol

Therapeutic Category Acne Products; Estrogen and Androgen Combination

Use Treatment of females with severe acne, unresponsive to oral antibiotics and other therapies, with associated symptoms of androgenization (including mild hirsutism or seborrhea). **Should not be used solely for contraception;** however, will provide reliable contraception if taken as recommended for approved indications.

General Dosage Range Oral: *Adults (females):* 1 tablet daily

Product Availability Not available in U.S.

Dosage Forms - Canada

Tablet, oral:

Diane-35: Cyproterone 2 mg and ethinyl estradiol 0.035 mg (21s)

cyproterone acetate *see* cyproterone *(Canada only) on page* 246
Cystadane® *see* betaine *on page* 129
Cystagon® *see* cysteamine *on page* 247

cysteamine (sis TEE a meen)

Synonyms cysteamine bitartrate

U.S. Brand Names Cystagon®

Therapeutic Category Urinary Tract Product

Use Treatment of nephropathic cystinosis

General Dosage Range Oral:

Children <12 years: Initial: 1/4 to 1/6 of maintenance dose; Maintenance: 1.3 g/m^2/day **or** 60 mg/kg/day in 4 divided doses (maximum dose: 1.95 g/m^2/day; 90 mg/kg/day)

Children ≥12 years and Adults >110 lbs: Initial: 1/4 to 1/6 of maintenance dose; Maintenance: 2 g/day in 4 divided doses (maximum: 1.95 g/m^2/day; 90 mg/kg/day)

Dosage Forms

Capsule, oral:

Cystagon®: 50 mg, 150 mg

cysteamine bitartrate *see* cysteamine *on page* 247

cysteine (SIS te een)

Synonyms cysteine hydrochloride

Therapeutic Category Nutritional Supplement

Use Supplement to crystalline amino acid solutions, in particular the specialized pediatric formulas (eg, Aminosyn® PF, TrophAmine®) to meet the intravenous amino acid nutritional requirements of infants receiving parenteral nutrition (PN)

General Dosage Range I.V.: *Infants:* Added as a fixed ratio to crystalline amino acid solution: 40 mg cysteine per g of amino acids; dosage will vary with the daily amino acid dosage; weight-based doses of cysteine (~70-160 mg/kg/day) have also been added directly to the daily parenteral nutrition solution

Dosage Forms

Capsule, oral: 500 mg

Injection, solution: 50 mg/mL (10 mL, 50 mL)

cysteine hydrochloride *see* cysteine *on page* 247
Cystistat® (Can) *see* hyaluronate and derivatives *on page* 450
Cysto-Conray™ II *see* iothalamate meglumine *on page* 497
Cystografin® *see* diatrizoate meglumine *on page* 276
Cystografin® Dilute *see* diatrizoate meglumine *on page* 276
Cysview™ *see* hexaminolevulinate *on page* 447

CYT *see* cyclophosphamide *on page 244*
cytarabine *see* cytarabine (conventional) *on page 248*

cytarabine (conventional) (sye TARE a been con VEN sha nal)

Medication Safety Issues

Sound-alike/look-alike issues:

Cytarabine may be confused with clofarabine, Cytosar®, Cytoxan, vidarabine
Cytarabine (conventional) may be confused with cytarabine liposomal
Cytosar-U may be confused with cytarabine, Cytovene®, Cytoxan, Neosar

High alert medication:

This medication is in a class the Institute for Safe Medication Practices (ISMP) includes among its list of drugs classes which have a heightened risk of causing significant patient harm when used in error.

Administration issues:

Intrathecal medication safety: The American Society of Clinical Oncology (ASCO)/Oncology Nursing Society (ONS) chemotherapy administration safety standards (Jacobson, 2009) encourage the following safety measures for intrathecal chemotherapy:

- Intrathecal medication should not be prepared during the preparation of any other agents
- After preparation, store in an isolated location or container clearly marked with a label identifying as "intrathecal" use only
- Delivery to the patient should only be with other medications also intended for administration into the central nervous system

Synonyms ara-C; arabinosylcytosine; conventional cytarabine; cytarabine; cytarabine hydrochloride; Cytosar-U; cytosine arabinosine hydrochloride

Canadian Brand Names Cytosar®

Therapeutic Category Antineoplastic Agent

Use Remission induction in acute myeloid leukemia (AML), treatment of acute lymphocytic leukemia (ALL) and chronic myelocytic leukemia (CML; blast phase); prophylaxis and treatment of meningeal leukemia

General Dosage Range Dosage adjustment recommended in patients with hepatic or renal impairment

I.V.: *Children and Adults:* AML Induction: 100-200 mg/m^2/day for 7 days

Dosage Forms

Injection, powder for reconstitution: 100 mg, 500 mg, 1 g, 2 g
Injection, solution: 20 mg/mL (25 mL)
Injection, solution [preservative free]: 20 mg/mL (5 mL, 50 mL); 100 mg/mL (20 mL)

cytarabine (liposomal) (sye TARE a been lye po SO mal)

Medication Safety Issues

Sound-alike/look-alike issues:

Cytarabine may be confused with clofarabine, Cytosar®, Cytoxan, vidarabine
Cytarabine liposomal may be confused with conventional cytarabine

High alert medication:

This medication is in a class the Institute for Safe Medication Practices (ISMP) includes among its list of drug classes which have a heightened risk of causing significant patient harm when used in error.

Administration issues:

Intrathecal medication safety: The American Society of Clinical Oncology (ASCO)/Oncology Nursing Society (ONS) chemotherapy administration safety standards (Jacobson, 2009) encourage the following safety measures for intrathecal chemotherapy:

- Intrathecal medication should not be prepared during the preparation of any other agents
- After preparation, store in an isolated location or container clearly marked with a label identifying as "intrathecal" use only
- Delivery to the patient should only be with other medications also intended for administration into the central nervous system

Synonyms cytarabine lipid complex; cytarabine liposome; DepoFoam-Encapsulated Cytarabine; DTC 101; liposomal cytarabine

U.S. Brand Names DepoCyt®

Canadian Brand Names DepoCyt®

Therapeutic Category Antineoplastic Agent, Antimetabolite (Purine)

Use Treatment of lymphomatous meningitis

General Dosage Range Dosage adjustment recommended in patients who develop toxicities

I.T.: *Adults:* Induction: 50 mg every 14 days for a total of 2 doses (weeks 1 and 3); Consolidation: 50 mg every 14 days for 3 doses (weeks 5, 7, and 9), followed by 50 mg at week 13; Maintenance: 50 mg every 28 days for 4 doses (weeks 17, 21, 25, and 29)

Dosage Forms

Injection, suspension, intrathecal [preservative free]:
DepoCyt®: 10 mg/mL (5 mL)

cytarabine hydrochloride *see* cytarabine (conventional) *on page 248*

cytarabine lipid complex *see* cytarabine (liposomal) *on page 248*

cytarabine liposome *see* cytarabine (liposomal) *on page 248*

CytoGam® *see* cytomegalovirus immune globulin (intravenous-human) *on page 249*

cytomegalovirus immune globulin (intravenous-human)

(sye toe meg a low VYE rus i MYUN GLOB yoo lin in tra VEE nus HYU man)

Medication Safety Issues

Sound-alike/look-alike issues:
CytoGam® may be confused with Cytoxan, Gamimune® N

Synonyms CMV-IGIV

U.S. Brand Names CytoGam®

Canadian Brand Names CytoGam®

Therapeutic Category Immune Globulin

Use Prophylaxis of cytomegalovirus (CMV) disease associated with kidney, lung, liver, pancreas, and heart transplants; concomitant use with ganciclovir should be considered in organ transplants (other than kidney) from CMV seropositive donors to CMV seronegative recipients

General Dosage Range I.V.: *Adults:* Initial: 150 mg/kg with 72 hours of transplant; 2-, 4-, 6- and 8 weeks after transplant: 100 mg/kg (kidney) **or** 150 mg/kg (liver, lung, pancreas, heart); 12 and 16 weeks after transplant: 50 mg/kg (kidney) **or** 100 mg/kg (liver, lung, pancreas, heart)

Dosage Forms

Injection, solution [preservative free]:
CytoGam®: 50 mg (± 10 mg)/mL (50 mL)

Cytomel® *see* liothyronine *on page 541*

Cytosar® (Can) *see* cytarabine (conventional) *on page 248*

Cytosar-U *see* cytarabine (conventional) *on page 248*

cytosine arabinosine hydrochloride *see* cytarabine (conventional) *on page 248*

cytostasan *see* bendamustine *on page 120*

Cytotec® *see* misoprostol *on page 606*

Cytovene® (Can) *see* ganciclovir (systemic) *on page 418*

Cytovene®-IV *see* ganciclovir (systemic) *on page 418*

Cytoxan *see* cyclophosphamide *on page 244*

Cytra-3 *see* citric acid, sodium citrate, and potassium citrate *on page 214*

Cytra-K *see* potassium citrate and citric acid *on page 745*

D2 *see* ergocalciferol *on page 339*

D2E7 *see* adalimumab *on page 36*

D_3 *see* cholecalciferol *on page 205*

D-3 [OTC] *see* cholecalciferol *on page 205*

D3-5™ [OTC] *see* cholecalciferol *on page 205*

D3-50™ [OTC] *see* cholecalciferol *on page 205*

D-3-mercaptovaline *see* penicillamine *on page 701*

d4T *see* stavudine *on page 853*

D_5W *see* dextrose *on page 275*

$D_{10}W$ *see* dextrose *on page 275*

$D_{25}W$ *see* dextrose *on page 275*

$D_{30}W$ *see* dextrose *on page 275*

$D_{40}W$ *see* dextrose *on page 275*

$D_{50}W$ *see* dextrose *on page 275*

$D_{60}W$ *see* dextrose *on page 275*

$D_{70}W$ *see* dextrose *on page* 275
D1694 *see* raltitrexed *(Canada only) on page* 786
D-23129 *see* ezogabine *on page* 370
DAB_{389}IL-2 *see* denileukin diftitox *on page* 260
DAB389 interleukin-2 *see* denileukin diftitox *on page* 260

dabigatran etexilate (da BIG a tran ett EX ill ate)

Medication Safety Issues

Sound-alike/look-alike issues:

Pradaxa® may be confused with Plavix®

Pradax™ (Canada) may be confused with Plavix®

High alert medication:

The Institute for Safe Medication Practices (ISMP) includes this medication among its list of drug classes which have a heightened risk of causing significant patient harm when used in error.

BEERS Criteria medication:

This drug may be potentially inappropriate for use in geriatric patients (Quality of evidence - moderate; Strength of recommendation - weak).

Synonyms dabigatran etexilate mesilate

U.S. Brand Names Pradaxa®

Canadian Brand Names Pradax™

Therapeutic Category Anticoagulant, Thrombin Inhibitor

Use Prevention of stroke and systemic embolism in patients with nonvalvular atrial fibrillation

2011 ACCF/AHA/HRS atrial fibrillation guidelines: Not recommended for patients with coexisting prosthetic heart valve or hemodynamically significant valve disease, severe renal failure (Cl_{cr} <15 mL/minute), or advanced liver disease (impaired baseline clotting function)

Canadian labeling: Additional uses (not in U.S. labeling): Postoperative thromboprophylaxis in patients who have undergone total hip or knee replacement procedures

General Dosage Range Dosage adjustment recommended in patients with renal impairment or patients on concomitant therapy.

Oral: *Adults:* 150 mg twice daily

Dosage Forms

Capsule, oral:

Pradaxa®: 75 mg, 150 mg

Dosage Forms - Canada

Capsule, oral:

Pradax™: 75 mg, 110 mg, 150 mg

dabigatran etexilate mesilate *see* dabigatran etexilate *on page* 250
DABIL2 *see* denileukin diftitox *on page* 260

dacarbazine (da KAR ba zeen)

Medication Safety Issues

Sound-alike/look-alike issues:

Dacarbazine may be confused with procarbazine

High alert medication:

This medication is in a class the Institute for Safe Medication Practices (ISMP) includes among its list of drugs which have a heightened risk of causing significant patient harm when used in error.

Synonyms DIC; dimethyl triazeno imidazole carboxamide; DTIC; DTIC-dome; imidazole carboxamide; imidazole carboxamide dimethyltriazene; WR-139007

Canadian Brand Names Dacarbazine for Injection

Therapeutic Category Antineoplastic Agent

Use Treatment of malignant melanoma, Hodgkin disease

General Dosage Range Dosage adjustment recommended in patients with renal impairment

I.V.:

Children: 375 mg/m^2 on days 1 and 15, repeat every 28 days

Adults: 375 mg/m^2 days 1 and 15 every 4 weeks **or** 250 mg/m^2 days 1-5 every 3 weeks

Dosage Forms

Injection, powder for reconstitution: 100 mg, 200 mg

Dacarbazine for Injection (Can) *see* dacarbazine *on page 250*
Dacodyl™ [OTC] *see* bisacodyl *on page 134*
Dacogen® *see* decitabine *on page 258*
DACT *see* dactinomycin *on page 251*

dactinomycin (dak ti noe MYE sin)

Medication Safety Issues

Sound-alike/look-alike issues:

DACTINomycin may be confused with Dacogen®, DAPTOmycin, DAUNOrubicin
Actinomycin may be confused with achromycin

High alert medication:

This medication is in a class the Institute for Safe Medication Practices (ISMP) includes among its list of drug classes which have a heightened risk of causing significant patient harm when used in error.

Synonyms ACT-D; actinomycin; actinomycin CI; actinomycin D; DACT

Tall-Man DACTINomycin

U.S. Brand Names Cosmegen®

Canadian Brand Names Cosmegen®

Therapeutic Category Antineoplastic Agent

Use Treatment of Wilms tumor, childhood rhabdomyosarcoma, Ewing sarcoma, metastatic testicular tumors (nonseminomatous), gestational trophoblastic neoplasm; regional perfusion (palliative or adjunctive) of locally recurrent or locoregional solid tumors (sarcomas, carcinomas, and adenocarcinomas)

General Dosage Range

I.V.:

Children >6 months: 15 mcg/kg/day **or** 400-600 mcg/m^2/day for 5 days every 3-6 weeks
Adults: 12-15 mcg/kg/day **or** 400-600 mcg/m^2/day for 5 days every 3-6 weeks **or** 1000 mcg/m^2 on day 1 **or** 500 mcg/dose days 1 and 2

Regional perfusion: *Adults:* Lower extremity or pelvis: 50 mcg/kg; Upper extremity: 35 mcg/kg

Dosage Forms

Injection, powder for reconstitution: 0.5 mg
Cosmegen®: 0.5 mg

Dairyaid® (Can) *see* lactase *on page 517*
Dakin's Solution *see* sodium hypochlorite solution *on page 842*
Dalacin™ C (Can) *see* clindamycin (systemic) *on page 218*
Dalacin® T (Can) *see* clindamycin (topical) *on page 219*
Dalacin® Vaginal (Can) *see* clindamycin (topical) *on page 219*

dalfampridine (dal FAM pri deen)

Medication Safety Issues

Sound-alike/look-alike issues:

Ampyra™ may be confused with anakinra
Dalfampridine may be confused with delavirdine, desipramine
Dalfampridine (U.S.) and fampridine (Canada) are different generic names for the same chemical entity (4-aminopyridine)

Synonyms 4-aminopyridine; 4-AP; EL-970; fampridine; fampridine-SR

U.S. Brand Names Ampyra™

Canadian Brand Names Fampyra™

Therapeutic Category Potassium Channel Blocker

Use Treatment to improve walking in multiple sclerosis (MS) patients

General Dosage Range Oral: Extended release: *Adults:* 10 mg every 12 hours

Dosage Forms

Tablet, extended release, oral:
Ampyra™: 10 mg

Dosage Forms - Canada

Tablet, extended release, oral:
Fampyra™: 10 mg

dalfopristin and quinupristin *see* quinupristin and dalfopristin *on page 783*

Daliresp® *see* roflumilast *on page* 809
Dalmane® (Can) *see* flurazepam *on page* 398
d-Alpha Gems™ [OTC] *see* vitamin E *on page* 950
***d*-alpha tocopherol** *see* vitamin E *on page* 950

dalteparin (dal TE pa rin)

Medication Safety Issues

High alert medication:

The Institute for Safe Medication Practices (ISMP) includes this medication among its list of drugs which have a heightened risk of causing significant patient harm when used in error.

National Patient Safety Goals:

The Joint Commission (TJC) requires healthcare organizations that provide anticoagulant therapy to have a process in place to reduce the risk of anticoagulant-associated patient harm. Patients receiving anticoagulants should receive individualized care through a defined process that includes standardized ordering, dispensing, administration, monitoring, and education. This does not apply to routine short-term use of anticoagulants for prevention of venous thromboembolism when the expectation is that the patient's laboratory values will remain within or close to normal values (NPSG.03.05.01).

Synonyms dalteparin sodium

U.S. Brand Names Fragmin®

Canadian Brand Names Fragmin®

Therapeutic Category Anticoagulant (Other)

Use Prevention of deep vein thrombosis (DVT) which may lead to pulmonary embolism, in patients requiring abdominal surgery who are at risk for thromboembolism complications (eg, patients >40 years of age, obesity, patients with malignancy, history of DVT or pulmonary embolism, and surgical procedures requiring general anesthesia and lasting >30 minutes); prevention of DVT in patients undergoing hip-replacement surgery; patients immobile during an acute illness; prevention of ischemic complications in patients with unstable angina or non-Q-wave myocardial infarction on concurrent aspirin therapy; in patients with cancer, extended treatment (6 months) of acute symptomatic venous thromboembolism (DVT and/or PE) to reduce the recurrence of venous thromboembolism

Canadian labeling: Additional use (unlabeled use in U.S.): Treatment of acute DVT; prevention of venous thromboembolism (VTE) in patients at risk of VTE undergoing general surgery; anticoagulant in extracorporeal circuit during hemodialysis and hemofiltration

General Dosage Range SubQ: *Adults:* Prophylaxis: 2500-5000 units daily; Treatment: 120 units/kg every 12 hours (maximum: 10,000 units/dose) **or** ~150-200 units/kg (maximum: 18,000 units/dose) once daily

Dosage Forms

Injection, solution:

Fragmin®: 25,000 anti-Xa units/mL (3.8 mL)

Injection, solution [preservative free]:

Fragmin®: 10,000 anti-Xa units/mL (1 mL); 2500 anti-Xa units/0.2 mL (0.2 mL); 5000 anti-Xa units/0.2 mL (0.2 mL); 7500 anti-Xa units/0.3 mL (0.3 mL); 12,500 anti-Xa units/0.5 mL (0.5 mL); 15,000 anti-Xa units/0.6 mL (0.6 mL); 18,000 anti-Xa units/0.72 mL (0.72 mL)

dalteparin sodium *see* dalteparin *on page* 252

danaparoid *(Canada only)* (da NAP a roid)

Medication Safety Issues

Sound-alike/look-alike issues:

Orgaran® may be confused with argatroban

Synonyms danaparoid sodium

Canadian Brand Names Orgaran®

Therapeutic Category Anticoagulant (Other)

Use Prevention of postoperative deep vein thrombosis (DVT) following orthopedic or major abdominal and thoracic surgery; prevention of DVT in patients with confirmed diagnosis of non-hemorrhagic stroke; management of heparin-induced thrombocytopenia (HIT)

General Dosage Range Dosage adjustment recommended in patients with renal impairment

SubQ:

Children: 10 units/kg every 12 hours
Adults: Dosage varies greatly depending on indication

I.V.:

Children: Initial bolus: 30 units/kg; maintenance: 1.2-4 units/kg/hour

Adults: Dosage varies greatly depending on indication

Product Availability Not available in U.S.

Dosage Forms - Canada

Injection, solution:

Orgaran®: 750 anti-Xa units/0.6 mL (0.6 mL)

danaparoid sodium *see* danaparoid *(Canada only) on page* *252*

danazol (DA na zole)

Medication Safety Issues

Sound-alike/look-alike issues:

Danazol may be confused with Dantrium®

Synonyms Danocrine

Canadian Brand Names Cyclomen®

Therapeutic Category Androgen

Use Treatment of endometriosis, fibrocystic breast disease, and hereditary angioedema

General Dosage Range Oral:

Adults (females): 100-800 mg/day in 2 divided doses

Adults (females/males): Hereditary angioedema: Initial: 200 mg 2-3 times/day; after favorable response decrease dosage by 50% or less

Dosage Forms

Capsule, oral: 50 mg, 100 mg, 200 mg

Dandrex *see* selenium sulfide *on page* *828*

Danocrine *see* danazol *on page* *253*

Dantrium® *see* dantrolene *on page* *253*

dantrolene (DAN troe leen)

Medication Safety Issues

Sound-alike/look-alike issues:

Dantrium® may be confused with danazol, Daraprim®

Revonto® may be confused with Revatio®

Synonyms dantrolene sodium

U.S. Brand Names Dantrium®; Revonto®

Canadian Brand Names Dantrium®

Therapeutic Category Skeletal Muscle Relaxant

Use Treatment of spasticity associated with upper motor neuron disorders (eg, spinal cord injury, stroke, cerebral palsy, or multiple sclerosis); management of malignant hyperthermia (MH); prevention of malignant hyperthermia in susceptible individuals (preoperative/postoperative administration)

Note: Dantrolene prophylaxis is not recommended for most MH-susceptible patients, provided nontriggering anesthetics are used and an adequate supply of dantrolene is available.

General Dosage Range

I.V.: *Children and Adults:* 1-2.5 mg/kg; may repeat up to cumulative dose of 10 mg/kg **or** 2.5 mg/kg as a single dose

Oral:

Children: 4-8 mg/kg/day in 4 divided doses **or** 0.5-2 mg/kg/dose 1-4 times daily (maximum: 400 mg daily)

Adults: 4-8 mg/kg/day in 4 divided doses **or** 25-100 mg 1-4 times daily (maximum: 400 mg daily)

Dosage Forms

Capsule, oral: 25 mg, 50 mg, 100 mg

Dantrium®: 25 mg, 50 mg, 100 mg

Injection, powder for reconstitution:

Dantrium®: 20 mg

Revonto®: 20 mg

dantrolene sodium *see* dantrolene *on page* *253*

dapcin *see* daptomycin *on page* *254*

dapsone (systemic) (DAP sone)

Medication Safety Issues

Sound-alike/look-alike issues:

Dapsone may be confused with Diprosone®

Synonyms diaminodiphenylsulfone

Therapeutic Category Antibiotic, Miscellaneous

Use Treatment of leprosy and dermatitis herpetiformis (infections caused by *Mycobacterium leprae*)

General Dosage Range Oral:

Children: 1-2 mg/kg once daily (maximum: 100 mg/day)

Adults: 50-300 mg once daily

Dosage Forms

Tablet, oral: 25 mg, 100 mg

dapsone (topical) (DAP sone)

Medication Safety Issues

Sound-alike/look-alike issues:

Dapsone may be confused with Diprosone®

Synonyms diaminodiphenylsulfone

U.S. Brand Names Aczone®

Canadian Brand Names Aczone™

Therapeutic Category Topical Skin Product, Acne

Use Topical treatment of acne vulgaris

General Dosage Range Topical: *Children ≥12 years and Adults:* Apply pea-sized amount (approximately) in thin layer to affected areas twice daily

Dosage Forms

Gel, topical:

Aczone®: 5% (30 g, 60 g)

Daptacel® *see* diphtheria and tetanus toxoids, and acellular pertussis vaccine *on page 298*

daptomycin (DAP toe mye sin)

Medication Safety Issues

Sound-alike/look-alike issues:

Cubicin® may be confused with Cleocin®

DAPTOmycin may be confused with DACTINomycin

Synonyms cidecin; dapcin; LY146032

Tall-Man DAPTOmycin

U.S. Brand Names Cubicin®

Canadian Brand Names Cubicin®

Therapeutic Category Antibiotic, Cyclic Lipopeptide

Use Treatment of complicated skin and skin structure infections caused by susceptible aerobic gram-positive organisms; *Staphylococcus aureus* bacteremia, including right-sided native valve infective endocarditis caused by MSSA or MRSA

General Dosage Range Dosage adjustment recommended in patients with renal impairment

I.V.: *Adults:* 4-6 mg/kg once daily

Dosage Forms

Injection, powder for reconstitution:

Cubicin®: 500 mg

Daraprim® *see* pyrimethamine *on page 778*

darbepoetin alfa (dar be POE e tin AL fa)

Medication Safety Issues

Sound-alike/look-alike issues:

Aranesp® may be confused with Aralast, Aricept®

Darbepoetin alfa may be confused with dalteparin, epoetin alfa, epoetin beta

Synonyms erythropoiesis-stimulating agent (ESA); erythropoiesis-stimulating protein; NESP; novel erythropoiesis-stimulating protein

U.S. Brand Names Aranesp®; Aranesp® SingleJect®

Canadian Brand Names Aranesp®

Therapeutic Category Colony-Stimulating Factor; Growth Factor; Recombinant Human Erythropoietin

Use Treatment of anemia due to concurrent myelosuppressive chemotherapy in patients with cancer (nonmyeloid malignancies) receiving chemotherapy (palliative intent) for a planned minimum of 2 additional months of chemotherapy; treatment of anemia due to chronic kidney disease (including patients on dialysis and not on dialysis)

Note: Darbepoetin is **not** indicated for use under the following conditions:

- Cancer patients receiving hormonal therapy, therapeutic biologic products, or radiation therapy unless also receiving concurrent myelosuppressive chemotherapy
- Cancer patients receiving myelosuppressive chemotherapy when the expected outcome is curative
- As a substitute for RBC transfusion in patients requiring immediate correction of anemia

Note: In clinical trials, darbepoetin has not demonstrated improved quality of life, fatigue, or well-being.

General Dosage Range

I.V.:

Children 1-18 years: 6.25-200 mcg/week

Adults: 0.45 mcg/kg once weekly **or** every 4 weeks **or** 0.75 mcg/kg once every 2 weeks **or** 6.25-200 mcg/week

SubQ:

Children 1-18 years: 6.25-200 mcg/week

Adults: 0.45-4.5 mcg/kg/week **or** 0.45 mcg/kg every 4 weeks **or** 0.75 mcg/kg once every 2 weeks **or** 500 mcg once every 3 weeks **or** 6.25-200 mcg/week

Dosage Forms

Injection, solution [preservative free]:

Aranesp®: 25 mcg/mL (1 mL); 40 mcg/mL (1 mL); 60 mcg/mL (1 mL); 100 mcg/mL (1 mL); 150 mcg/0.75 mL (0.75 mL); 200 mcg/mL (1 mL); 300 mcg/mL (1 mL)

Aranesp® SingleJect®: 25 mcg/0.42 mL (0.42 mL); 40 mcg/0.4 mL (0.4 mL); 60 mcg/0.3 mL (0.3 mL); 100 mcg/0.5 mL (0.5 mL); 150 mcg/0.3 mL (0.3 mL); 200 mcg/0.4 mL (0.4 mL); 300 mcg/0.6 mL (0.6 mL); 500 mcg/mL (1 mL)

darifenacin (dar i FEN a sin)

Medication Safety Issues

BEERS Criteria medication:

This drug may be potentially inappropriate for use in geriatric patients (Quality of evidence - varies based on comorbidity; Strength of recommendation - varies based on comorbidity)

Synonyms darifenacin hydrobromide; UK-88,525

U.S. Brand Names Enablex®

Canadian Brand Names Enablex®

Therapeutic Category Anticholinergic Agent

Use Management of symptoms of bladder overactivity (urge incontinence, urgency, and frequency)

General Dosage Range Dosage adjustment recommended in patients with hepatic impairment or on concomitant therapy

Oral: *Adults:* Initial: 7.5 mg once daily; Maintenance: 7.5-15 mg once daily

Dosage Forms

Tablet, extended release, oral:

Enablex®: 7.5 mg, 15 mg

darifenacin hydrobromide *see* darifenacin *on page* 255

darunavir (dar OO na veer)

Synonyms darunavir ethanolate; DRV; TMC-114

U.S. Brand Names Prezista®

Canadian Brand Names Prezista®

Therapeutic Category Antiretroviral Agent, Protease Inhibitor

Use Treatment of HIV-1 infections in combination with ritonavir and other antiretroviral agents

General Dosage Range Dosage adjustment recommended in patients on concomitant therapy or who develop toxicities.

Oral:
Children ≥3 years and ≥10 kg to <15 kg: Darunavir: 10 mg/kg twice daily; Ritonavir 1.5 mg/kg twice daily
Children ≥3 years and ≥15 kg to <30 kg: Darunavir: 375 mg twice daily; Ritonavir: 50 mg twice daily
Children ≥3 years and ≥30 kg to <40 kg: Darunavir: 450 mg twice daily; Ritonavir: 60 mg twice daily
Children ≥3 years and ≥40 kg: Darunavir: 600 mg twice daily; Ritonavir: 100 mg twice daily
Adults: Darunavir: 600 mg twice daily; Ritonavir: 100 mg twice daily **or** Darunavir: 800 mg once daily; Ritonavir: 100 mg once daily

Product Availability Prezista® 100 mg/mL oral suspension: FDA approved December 2011; availability expected in the second quarter of 2012

Dosage Forms
Tablet, oral:
Prezista®: 75 mg, 150 mg, 400 mg, 600 mg

Dosage Forms - Canada
Tablet:
Prezista®: 300 mg, 400 mg, 600 mg

darunavir ethanolate *see* darunavir *on page* 255

dasatinib (da SA ti nib)

Medication Safety Issues
Sound-alike/look-alike issues:
Dasatinib may be confused with bosutinib, imatinib, nilotinib, SUNItinib, vandetanib
High alert medication:
This medication is in a class the Institute for Safe Medication Practices (ISMP) includes among its list of drug classes which have a heightened risk of causing significant patient harm when used in error.

Synonyms BMS-354825
U.S. Brand Names Sprycel®
Canadian Brand Names Sprycel®
Therapeutic Category Antineoplastic Agent, Tyrosine Kinase Inhibitor
Use Treatment of chronic myelogenous leukemia (CML) in chronic, accelerated or blast (myeloid or lymphoid) phase resistant or intolerant to prior therapy (including imatinib); treatment of newly-diagnosed Philadelphia chromosome-positive (Ph+) CML in chronic phase; treatment of Philadelphia chromosome-positive (Ph+) acute lymphoblastic leukemia (ALL) resistant or intolerant to prior therapy
General Dosage Range Dosage adjustment recommended in patients on concomitant therapy or who develop toxicities
Oral: *Adults:* 100-180 mg once daily

Dosage Forms
Tablet, oral:
Sprycel®: 20 mg, 50 mg, 70 mg, 100 mg

DaTSCAN *see* ioflupane I 123 *on page* 495
DaTscan™ *see* ioflupane I 123 *on page* 495
daunomycin *see* daunorubicin (conventional) *on page* 256
DAUNOrubicin citrate *see* daunorubicin (liposomal) *on page* 257
DAUNOrubicin citrate (liposomal) *see* daunorubicin (liposomal) *on page* 257
DAUNOrubicin citrate liposome *see* daunorubicin (liposomal) *on page* 257

daunorubicin (conventional) (daw noe ROO bi sin con VEN sha nal)

Medication Safety Issues
Sound-alike/look-alike issues:
DAUNOrubicin may be confused with DACTINomycin, DOXOrubicin, DOXOrubicin liposomal, epirubicin, IDArubicin, valrubicin
Conventional formulation (Cerubidine®, DAUNOrubicin hydrochloride) may be confused with the liposomal formulation (DaunoXome®)
High alert medication:
The Institute for Safe Medication Practices (ISMP) includes this medication among its list of drug classes which have a heightened risk of causing significant patient harm when used in error.

Synonyms conventional daunomycin; daunomycin; DAUNOrubicin hydrochloride; rubidomycin hydrochloride
Tall-Man **DAUNO**rubicin (conventional)

U.S. Brand Names Cerubidine®
Canadian Brand Names Cerubidine®
Therapeutic Category Antineoplastic Agent
Use Treatment of acute lymphocytic leukemia (ALL) and acute myeloid leukemia (AML)
General Dosage Range Dosage adjustment recommended in patients with hepatic or renal impairment
I.V.:
Children <2 years or BSA <0.5 m²: 1 mg/kg/dose per protocol with frequency dependent on regimen employed (maximum cumulative dose: 10 mg/kg)
Children ≥2 years and BSA ≥0.5 m²: 25 mg/m² on day 1 every week for 4 cycles **or** 30-60 mg/m²/day for 3 days (maximum cumulative dose: 300 mg/m²)
Adults <60 years: 30-60 mg/m²/day for 2-3 days (maximum cumulative dose: 550 mg/m²; 400 mg/m² with chest irradiation)
Adults ≥60 years: 30 mg/m²/day for 2-3 days (maximum cumulative dose: 550 mg/m²; 400 mg/m² with chest irradiation)
Dosage Forms
Injection, powder for reconstitution: 20 mg
Cerubidine®: 20 mg
Injection, solution [preservative free]: 5 mg/mL (4 mL, 10 mL)

DAUNOrubicin hydrochloride *see* daunorubicin (conventional) *on page 256*

daunorubicin (liposomal) (daw noe ROO bi sin lye po SO mal)

Medication Safety Issues
Sound-alike/look-alike issues:
DAUNOrubicin liposomal may be confused with DACTINomycin, DOXOrubicin, DOXOrubicin liposomal, epirubicin, IDArubicin, valrubicin
Liposomal formulation (DaunoXome®) may be confused with the conventional formulation (Cerubidine®, Rubex®)
High alert medication:
The Institute for Safe Medication Practices (ISMP) includes this medication among its list of drug classes which have a heightened risk of causing significant patient harm when used in error.
Synonyms DAUNOrubicin citrate; DAUNOrubicin citrate (liposomal); DAUNOrubicin citrate liposome; liposomal DAUNOrubicin; NSC-697732
Tall-Man DAUNOrubicin (liposomal)
U.S. Brand Names DaunoXome®
Therapeutic Category Antineoplastic Agent
Use First-line treatment of advanced HIV-associated Kaposi sarcoma (KS)
General Dosage Range Dosage adjustment recommended in patients with hepatic or renal impairment
I.V.: *Adults:* 40 mg/m² every 2 weeks
Dosage Forms
Injection, solution [preservative free]:
DaunoXome®: 2 mg/mL (25 mL)

DaunoXome® *see* daunorubicin (liposomal) *on page 257*
Daxas™ (Can) *see* roflumilast *on page 809*
1-Day™ [OTC] *see* tioconazole *on page 898*
Daypro® *see* oxaprozin *on page 675*
Daytrana® *see* methylphenidate *on page 590*
dCF *see* pentostatin *on page 707*
DDAVP® *see* desmopressin *on page 264*
DDAVP® Melt (Can) *see* desmopressin *on page 264*
ddI *see* didanosine *on page 282*
DDrops® [OTC] *see* cholecalciferol *on page 205*
DDrops® Baby [OTC] *see* cholecalciferol *on page 205*
DDrops® Kids [OTC] *see* cholecalciferol *on page 205*
1-deamino-8-D-arginine vasopressin *see* desmopressin *on page 264*
Debrox® [OTC] *see* carbamide peroxide *on page 173*
Decadron *see* dexamethasone (systemic) *on page 266*

Decavac® [DSC] *see* diphtheria and tetanus toxoids *on page 295*

De-Chlor DM [OTC] *see* chlorpheniramine, phenylephrine, and dextromethorphan *on page 201*

decitabine (de SYE ta been)

Medication Safety Issues

Sound-alike/look-alike issues:

Dacogen® may be confused with DACTINomycin

High alert medication:

This medication is in a class the Institute for Safe Medication Practices (ISMP) includes among its list of drug classes which have a heightened risk of causing significant patient harm when used in error.

Synonyms 5-Aza-2'-deoxycytidine; 5-Aza-dCyd; deoxyazacytidine; dezocitidine

U.S. Brand Names Dacogen®

Therapeutic Category Antineoplastic Agent, Antimetabolite (Pyrimidine)

Use Treatment of myelodysplastic syndrome (MDS)

General Dosage Range Dosage adjustment recommended in patients who develop toxicities

I.V.: *Adults:* 15 mg/m^2 every 8 hours for 3 days every 6 weeks **or** 20 mg/m^2 daily for 5 days every 28 days

Dosage Forms

Injection, powder for reconstitution:

Dacogen®: 50 mg

Declomycin *see* demeclocycline *on page 260*

Deep Sea [OTC] *see* sodium chloride *on page 840*

deferasirox (de FER a sir ox)

Medication Safety Issues

Sound-alike/look-alike issues:

Deferasirox may be confused with deferiprone, deferoxamine

Synonyms ICL670

U.S. Brand Names Exjade®

Canadian Brand Names Exjade®

Therapeutic Category Antidote; Chelating Agent

Use Treatment of chronic iron overload due to blood transfusions (transfusional hemosiderosis)

General Dosage Range Dosage adjustment recommended in patients with renal or hepatic impairment or on concomitant therapy

Oral: *Children ≥2 years and Adults:* Initial: 20 mg/kg once daily; Maintenance: 20-30 mg/kg once daily (maximum dose: 40 mg/kg/day)

Dosage Forms

Tablet for suspension, oral:

Exjade®: 125 mg, 250 mg, 500 mg

deferiprone (de FER i prone)

Medication Safety Issues

Sound-alike/look-alike issues:

Deferiprone may be confused with deferoxamine, deferasirox

Synonyms APO-066

U.S. Brand Names Ferriprox®

Therapeutic Category Chelating Agent

Use Treatment of transfusional iron overload due to thalassemia syndromes with inadequate response to other chelation therapy

General Dosage Range Oral: *Adults:* 25-33 mg/kg 3 times/day (maximum: 99 mg/kg/day)

Dosage Forms

Tablet, oral:

Ferriprox®: 500 mg

deferoxamine (de fer OKS a meen)

Medication Safety Issues

Sound-alike/look-alike issues:

Deferoxamine may be confused with cefuroxime, deferasirox, deferiprone

Desferal® may be confused with desflurane, Desyrel®, Dexferrum®

International issues:

Desferal [U.S., Canada, and multiple international markets] may be confused with Deseril brand name for methysergide [Australia, Belgium, Great Britain, Netherlands]; Disophrol brand name for dexbrompheniramine and pseudoephedrine [Czech Republic, Poland, Turkey]

Synonyms deferoxamine mesylate; desferrioxamine; DFM

U.S. Brand Names Desferal®

Canadian Brand Names Desferal®; PMS-Deferoxamine

Therapeutic Category Antidote

Use Adjunct in the treatment of acute iron intoxication; treatment of chronic iron overload secondary to multiple transfusions

Canadian labeling (unlabeled use in the U.S.): Diagnosis of aluminum overload; treatment of chronic aluminum overload in patients with end-stage renal failure undergoing maintenance dialysis

General Dosage Range Dosage adjustment recommended in patients with renal impairment

I.M.: *Adults:* Initial: 1000 mg, followed by 500 mg every 4 hours for 2 doses; Maintenance: 500 mg every 4-12 hours **or** 500-1000 mg once daily (maximum: 6000 mg/day)

I.V.:

Children ≥3 years: 20-40 mg/kg/day 5-7 days per week; dose should not exceed 40 mg/kg/day until growth has ceased

Adults: Initial: 1000 mg, followed by 500 mg every 4 hours for 2 doses; Maintenance: 500 mg every 4-12 hours (maximum: 6000 mg/day) **or** 40-50 mg/kg/day (maximum: 60 mg/kg/day) 5-7 days per week

SubQ:

Children ≥3 years: 20-40 mg/kg/day (maximum: 1000-2000 mg/day)

Adults: 1000-2000 mg/day **or** 20-40 mg/kg/day

Dosage Forms

Injection, powder for reconstitution: 500 mg, 2 g

Desferal®: 500 mg, 2 g

deferoxamine mesylate *see* deferoxamine *on page* 258

Definity® *see* perflutren lipid microspheres *on page* 708

degarelix (deg a REL ix)

Medication Safety Issues

Sound-alike/look-alike issues:

Degarelix may be confused with cetrorelix, ganirelix

Synonyms degarelix acetate; FE200486

U.S. Brand Names Firmagon®

Canadian Brand Names Firmagon®

Therapeutic Category Antineoplastic Agent, Gonadotropin-Releasing Hormone Antagonist; Gonadotropin Releasing Hormone Antagonist

Use Treatment of advanced prostate cancer

General Dosage Range SubQ: *Adults:* Loading dose: 240 mg; Maintenance dose: 80 mg every 28 days

Dosage Forms

Injection, powder for reconstitution:

Firmagon®: 80 mg, 120 mg

degarelix acetate *see* degarelix *on page* 259

Dehydral® (Can) *see* methenamine *on page* 582

dehydrobenzperidol *see* droperidol *on page* 317

Delatestryl® *see* testosterone *on page* 881

delavirdine (de la VIR deen)

Medication Safety Issues

Sound-alike/look-alike issues:

Delavirdine may be confused with dalfampridine

Synonyms DLV; U-90152S

U.S. Brand Names Rescriptor®

Canadian Brand Names Rescriptor®

Therapeutic Category Antiviral Agent
Use Treatment of HIV-1 infection in combination with at least two additional antiretroviral agents
General Dosage Range **Oral:** *Children ≥16 years and Adults:* 400 mg 3 times/day
Dosage Forms
Tablet, oral:
Rescriptor®: 100 mg, 200 mg

Delestrogen® *see* estradiol (systemic) *on page 347*
Delfen® [OTC] *see* nonoxynol 9 *on page 647*
Delsym® [OTC] *see* dextromethorphan *on page 272*
delta-9-tetrahydro-cannabinol *see* dronabinol *on page 316*
delta-9-tetrahydrocannabinol and cannabinol *see* tetrahydrocannabinol and cannabidiol *(Canada only) on page 884*
delta-9 THC *see* dronabinol *on page 316*
deltacortisone *see* prednisone *on page 755*
Delta® D3 [OTC] *see* cholecalciferol *on page 205*
deltadehydrocortisone *see* prednisone *on page 755*
Demadex® *see* torsemide *on page 907*

demeclocycline (dem e kloe SYE kleen)

Synonyms Declomycin; demeclocycline hydrochloride; demethylchlortetracycline
Therapeutic Category Tetracycline Derivative
Use Treatment of susceptible bacterial infections (eg, acne, urinary tract infections, respiratory infections) caused by both gram-negative and gram-positive organisms
Note: Use of demeclocycline as an antibacterial agent is uncommon; alternative tetracycline agents (eg, doxycycline, minocycline, tetracycline) are generally preferred.
General Dosage Range Dosage adjustment recommended in patients with renal and hepatic impairment
Oral:
Children >8 years: 7-13 mg/kg/day (maximum: 600 mg/day) divided every 6-12 hours
Adults: 600 mg/day in 2 or 4 divided doses
Dosage Forms
Tablet, oral: 150 mg, 300 mg

demeclocycline hydrochloride *see* demeclocycline *on page 260*
Demerol® *see* meperidine *on page 574*
4-demethoxydaunorubicin *see* idarubicin *on page 472*
demethylchlortetracycline *see* demeclocycline *on page 260*
Demser® *see* metyrosine *on page 598*
Demulen® 30 (Can) *see* ethinyl estradiol and ethynodiol diacetate *on page 357*
Denavir® *see* penciclovir *on page 701*

denileukin diftitox (de ni LOO kin DIF ti toks)

Medication Safety Issues
High alert medication:
The Institute for Safe Medication Practices (ISMP) includes this medication among its list of drug classes which have a heightened risk of causing significant patient harm when used in error.
Synonyms DAB389 interleukin-2; DAB_{389}IL-2; DABIL2
U.S. Brand Names ONTAK®
Therapeutic Category Antineoplastic Agent, Miscellaneous
Use Treatment of persistent or recurrent cutaneous T-cell lymphoma (CTCL) whose malignant cells express the CD25 component of the IL-2 receptor
General Dosage Range Dosage adjustment recommended in patients who develop toxicities
I.V.: *Adults:* 9 or 18 mcg/kg/day days 1-5 every 21 days
Dosage Forms
Injection, solution:
ONTAK®: 150 mcg/mL (2 mL)

Denorex® Extra Strength Protection [OTC] *see* salicylic acid *on page 816*
Denorex® Extra Strength Protection 2-in-1 [OTC] *see* salicylic acid *on page 816*

Denorex® Therapeutic Protection [OTC] *see* coal tar *on page* 228
Denorex® Therapeutic Protection 2-in-1 Shampoo + Conditioner [OTC] *see* coal tar *on page* 228

denosumab (den OH sue mab)

Medication Safety Issues
Other safety concerns:
Duplicate therapy issues: Prolia® contains denosumab, which is the same ingredient contained in Xgeva®; patients receiving Xgeva® should not be treated with Prolia®

Synonyms AMG-162

U.S. Brand Names Prolia™; Xgeva®

Canadian Brand Names Prolia®; Xgeva®

Therapeutic Category Monoclonal Antibody

Use Treatment of osteoporosis in postmenopausal women at high risk for fracture; treatment of bone loss in men receiving androgen deprivation therapy (ADT) for nonmetastatic prostate cancer; treatment of bone loss in women receiving aromatase inhibitor (AI) therapy for breast cancer; prevention of skeletal-related events (eg, fracture, spinal cord compression, bone pain requiring surgery/radiation therapy) in patients with bone metastases from solid tumors

General Dosage Range SubQ: *Adults:* Prolia®: 60 mg every 6 months; Xgeva®: 120 mg every 4 weeks

Dosage Forms
Injection, solution [preservative free]:
Prolia™: 60 mg/mL (1 mL)
Xgeva®: 70 mg/mL (1.7 mL)

Denta 5000 Plus™ *see* fluoride *on page* 393
DentaGel™ *see* fluoride *on page* 393
Dentapaine [OTC] *see* benzocaine *on page* 121
Dent's Extra Strength Toothache Gum [OTC] *see* benzocaine *on page* 121
deodorized tincture of opium (error-prone synonym) *see* opium tincture *on page* 669
deoxyazacytidine *see* decitabine *on page* 258
2′-deoxycoformycin *see* pentostatin *on page* 707
deoxycoformycin *see* pentostatin *on page* 707
Depacon® *see* valproic acid *on page* 934
Depakene® *see* valproic acid *on page* 934
Depakote® *see* divalproex *on page* 302
Depakote® ER *see* divalproex *on page* 302
Depakote® Sprinkle *see* divalproex *on page* 302
Depen® *see* penicillamine *on page* 701
Deplin® *see* methylfolate *on page* 589
DepoCyt® *see* cytarabine (liposomal) *on page* 248
DepoDur® *see* morphine (liposomal) *on page* 614
Depo®-Estradiol *see* estradiol (systemic) *on page* 347
depoFoam bupivacaine *see* bupivacaine (liposomal) *on page* 149
DepoFoam-Encapsulated Cytarabine *see* cytarabine (liposomal) *on page* 248
Depo-Medrol® *see* methylprednisolone *on page* 591
Depo-Prevera® (Can) *see* medroxyprogesterone *on page* 567
Depo-Provera® *see* medroxyprogesterone *on page* 567
Depo-Provera® Contraceptive *see* medroxyprogesterone *on page* 567
depo-subQ provera 104® *see* medroxyprogesterone *on page* 567
Depotest® 100 (Can) *see* testosterone *on page* 881
Depo®-Testosterone *see* testosterone *on page* 881
deprenyl *see* selegiline *on page* 828
depsipeptide *see* romidepsin *on page* 809
DermaFungal [OTC] *see* miconazole (topical) *on page* 599
Dermagran® [OTC] *see* aluminum hydroxide *on page* 55
Dermagran® AF [OTC] *see* miconazole (topical) *on page* 599

Dermamycin® [OTC] *see* diphenhydramine (topical) *on page* 293
Dermarest® Eczema Medicated [OTC] *see* hydrocortisone (topical) *on page* 457
Dermarest® Eczema Medicated Moisturizer [OTC] *see* pramoxine *on page* 750
Dermarest® Psoriasis Medicated Moisturizer [OTC] *see* salicylic acid *on page* 816
Dermarest® Psoriasis Medicated Scalp Treatment [OTC] *see* salicylic acid *on page* 816
Dermarest® Psoriasis Medicated Shampoo/Conditioner [OTC] *see* salicylic acid *on page* 816
Dermarest® Psoriasis Medicated Skin Treatment [OTC] *see* salicylic acid *on page* 816
Dermarest® Psoriasis Overnight Treatment [OTC] *see* salicylic acid *on page* 816
Derma-Smoothe/FS® *see* fluocinolone (topical) *on page* 392
Dermatop® *see* prednicarbate *on page* 753
Dermazene® *see* iodoquinol and hydrocortisone *on page* 495
DermaZinc™ [OTC] *see* pyrithione zinc *on page* 779
Dermazole (Can) *see* miconazole (topical) *on page* 599
Dermoplast® Antibacterial [OTC] *see* benzocaine *on page* 121
Dermoplast® Pain Relieving [OTC] *see* benzocaine *on page* 121
DermOtic® *see* fluocinolone (otic) *on page* 391
Dermovate® (Can) *see* clobetasol *on page* 221
Desferal® *see* deferoxamine *on page* 258
desferrioxamine *see* deferoxamine *on page* 258

desflurane (DES flure ane)

Medication Safety Issues

Sound-alike/look-alike issues:

Desflurane may be confused with Desferal®

High alert medication:

The Institute for Safe Medication Practices (ISMP) includes this medication among its list of drug classes which have a heightened risk of causing significant patient harm when used in error.

U.S. Brand Names Suprane®

Canadian Brand Names Suprane®

Therapeutic Category General Anesthetic

Use Induction and/or maintenance of general anesthesia in adults; maintenance of anesthesia in intubated children; **Note:** Use of desflurane for induction of general anesthesia is not recommended due to its irritant properties and unpleasant odor which causes coughing, breath holding, laryngospasm, oxygen desaturation, increased secretions, hypertension, and tachycardia.

General Dosage Range Inhalation:

Children (intubated): 5.2% to 10% to maintain surgical levels of anesthesia

Adults: 2.5% to 8.5% to maintain surgical levels of anesthesia

Dosage Forms

Liquid, for inhalation:

Suprane®: 100% (240 mL)

desiccated thyroid *see* thyroid, desiccated *on page* 893

desipramine (des IP ra meen)

Medication Safety Issues

Sound-alike/look-alike issues:

Desipramine may be confused with clomiPRAMINE, dalfampridine, diphenhydrAMINE, disopyramide, imipramine, nortriptyline

Norpramin® may be confused with clomiPRAMINE, imipramine, Normodyne®, Norpace®, nortriptyline, Tenormin®

BEERS Criteria medication:

This drug may be potentially inappropriate for use in geriatric patients (SIADH: Quality of evidence - moderate; Strength of recommendation - strong).

International issues:

Norpramin: Brand name for desipramine [U.S., Canada], but also the brand name for enalapril/hydrochlorothiazide [Portugal]; omeprazole [Spain]

Synonyms desipramine hydrochloride; desmethylimipramine hydrochloride

U.S. Brand Names Norpramin®

Canadian Brand Names Dom-Desipramine; Novo-Desipramine; Nu-Desipramine; PMS-Desipramine

Therapeutic Category Antidepressant, Tricyclic (Secondary Amine)

Use Treatment of depression

General Dosage Range Oral:

Adolescents: 25-100 mg/day in single or divided doses (maximum: 150 mg/day)
Adults: 100-200 mg/day in single or divided doses (maximum: 300 mg/day)
Elderly: 25-100 mg/day in single or divided doses (maximum: 150 mg/day)

Dosage Forms

Tablet, oral: 10 mg, 25 mg, 50 mg, 75 mg, 100 mg, 150 mg
Norpramin®: 10 mg, 25 mg, 50 mg, 75 mg, 100 mg, 150 mg

desipramine hydrochloride *see* desipramine *on page* 262

desirudin (des i ROO din)

Medication Safety Issues

High alert medication:

The Institute for Safe Medication Practices (ISMP) includes this medication among its list of drugs which have a heightened risk of causing significant patient harm when used in error.

Synonyms CGP-39393; desulfato-hirudin; desulfatohirudin; desulphatohirudin; r-hirudin; recombinant desulfatohirudin; recombinant hirudin

U.S. Brand Names Iprivask®

Therapeutic Category Anticoagulant, Thrombin Inhibitor

Use Prophylaxis of deep vein thrombosis (DVT) in patients undergoing surgery for hip replacement

General Dosage Range Dosage adjustment recommended in patients with renal impairment

SubQ: *Adults:* 15 mg every 12 hours

Dosage Forms

Injection, powder for reconstitution [preservative free]:
Iprivask®: 15 mg

Desitin® [OTC] *see* zinc oxide *on page* 963

Desitin® Creamy [OTC] *see* zinc oxide *on page* 963

desloratadine (des lor AT a deen)

Medication Safety Issues

Sound-alike/look-alike issues:

Clarinex® may be confused with Celebrex®

U.S. Brand Names Clarinex®

Canadian Brand Names Aerius®; Aerius® Kids; Desloratadine Allergy Control

Therapeutic Category Antihistamine, Nonsedating

Use Relief of nasal and nonnasal symptoms of seasonal allergic rhinitis (SAR) and perennial allergic rhinitis (PAR); treatment of chronic idiopathic urticaria (CIU)

General Dosage Range Dosage adjustment recommended in adult patients with hepatic or renal impairment. Dosage not established in children with hepatic or renal impairment.

Oral:

Children 6-11 months: 1 mg once daily
Children 1-5 years: 1.25 mg once daily
Children 6-11 years: 2.5 mg once daily
Children ≥12 years and Adults: 5 mg once daily

Dosage Forms

Syrup, oral:
Clarinex®: 0.5 mg/mL (480 mL)

Tablet, oral: 5 mg
Clarinex®: 5 mg

Tablet, orally disintegrating, oral:
Clarinex®: 2.5 mg, 5 mg

Desloratadine Allergy Control (Can) *see* desloratadine *on page* 263

desloratadine and pseudoephedrine (des lor AT a deen & soo doe e FED rin)

Synonyms pseudoephedrine and desloratadine

U.S. Brand Names Clarinex-D® 12 Hour; Clarinex-D® 24 Hour

Therapeutic Category Antihistamine/Decongestant Combination, Nonsedating

Use Relief of nasal and non-nasal symptoms of seasonal allergic rhinitis

General Dosage Range Dosage adjustment recommended in patients with renal impairment.

Oral: *Children ≥12 years and Adults:* 12-hour formulation: 1 tablet twice daily; 24-hour formulation: 1 tablet once daily

Dosage Forms

Tablet, variable release:

Clarinex-D® 12 Hour: Desloratadine 2.5 mg [immediate release] and pseudoephedrine 120 mg [extended release]

Clarinex-D® 24 Hour: Desloratadine 5 mg [immediate release] and pseudoephedrine 240 mg [extended release]

desmethylimipramine hydrochloride *see* desipramine *on page* 262

desmopressin (des moe PRES in)

Synonyms 1-deamino-8-D-arginine vasopressin; desmopressin acetate

U.S. Brand Names DDAVP®; Stimate®

Canadian Brand Names Apo-Desmopressin®; DDAVP®; DDAVP® Melt; Minirin®; Novo-Desmopressin; Octostim®; PMS-Desmopressin

Therapeutic Category Vasopressin Analog, Synthetic

Use

Injection: Treatment of diabetes insipidus; maintenance of hemostasis and control of bleeding in hemophilia A with factor VIII coagulant activity levels >5% and mild-to-moderate classic von Willebrand disease (type 1) with factor VIII coagulant activity levels >5%

Nasal solutions (DDAVP® Nasal Spray and DDAVP® Rhinal Tube): Treatment of central diabetes insipidus

Nasal spray (Stimate®): Maintenance of hemostasis and control of bleeding in hemophilia A with factor VIII coagulant activity levels >5% and mild-to-moderate classic von Willebrand disease (type 1) with factor VIII coagulant activity levels >5%

Tablet: Treatment of central diabetes insipidus, temporary polyuria and polydipsia following pituitary surgery or head trauma, primary nocturnal enuresis

General Dosage Range

I.V.:

Infants and Children ≥3 months: 0.3 mcg/kg as a single dose, may repeat dose if needed

Adults: 2-4 mcg/day in 2 divided doses **or** one-tenth (1/10) of the intranasal maintenance dose **or** 0.3 mcg/kg as a single dose

Intranasal:

Infants 3-11 months: Initial: 5 mcg/day (0.05 mL/day) in 1-2 divided doses; Maintenance: 5-30 mcg/day (0.05-0.3 mL/day) in 1-2 divided doses

Children 12 months to 12 years: Initial: 5 mcg/day (0.05 mL/day) in 1-2 divided doses; Maintenance: 5-30 mcg/day (0.05-0.3 mL/day) in 1-2 divided doses **or** 150 mcg (1 spray of high concentration) as a single dose

Children >12 years and Adults <50 kg: 10-40 mcg/day (0.1-0.4 mL) in 1-3 divided doses **or** 150 mcg (1 spray of high concentration spray) as a single dose

Children >12 years and Adults ≥50 kg: 10-40 mcg/day in 1-3 divided doses **or** 300 mcg (1 spray each nostril of high concentration spray) as a single dose

Oral:

Children 4-5 years: Initial: 0.05 mg twice daily; Maintenance: 0.1-1.2 mg/day in 2-3 divided doses

Children ≥6 years: Initial: 0.05 mg twice daily **or** 0.2 mg at bedtime; Maintenance: 0.1-1.2 mg/day in 2-3 divided doses **or** 0.2-0.6 mg at bedtime

Adults: 0.2-0.6 mg at bedtime **or** 0.1-1.2 mg/day in 2-3 divided doses

SubQ: *Adults:* 2-4 mcg/day in 2 divided doses **or** one-tenth (1/10) of the intranasal maintenance dose

Dosage Forms

Injection, solution: 4 mcg/mL (1 mL, 10 mL)

DDAVP®: 4 mcg/mL (1 mL, 10 mL)

Solution, intranasal: 0.1 mg/mL (2.5 mL, 5 mL)

DDAVP®: 0.1 mg/mL (2.5 mL, 5 mL)

Stimate®: 1.5 mg/mL (2.5 mL)

Tablet, oral: 0.1 mg, 0.2 mg

DDAVP®: 0.1 mg, 0.2 mg

Dosage Forms - Canada

Tablet, sublingual:

DDAVP® Melt: 60 mcg, 120 mcg, 240 mcg

desmopressin acetate *see* desmopressin *on page 264*

Desocort® (Can) *see* desonide *on page 265*

Desogen® *see* ethinyl estradiol and desogestrel *on page 356*

desogestrel and ethinyl estradiol *see* ethinyl estradiol and desogestrel *on page 356*

Desonate® *see* desonide *on page 265*

desonide (DES oh nide)

U.S. Brand Names Desonate®; DesOwen®; LoKara™; Verdeso®

Canadian Brand Names Desocort®; PMS-Desonide; Tridesilon; Verdeso™

Therapeutic Category Corticosteroid, Topical

Use Treatment of inflammatory and pruritic manifestations of corticosteroid responsive dermatosis (low-to-medium potency corticosteroid); mild-to-moderate atopic dermatitis

General Dosage Range Topical:

Children ≥3 months: Foam, gel: Apply 2 times/day sparingly

Adults: Apply 2-3 times/day sparingly

Dosage Forms

Aerosol, foam, topical:

Verdeso®: 0.05% (50 g, 100 g)

Cream, topical: 0.05% (15 g, 60 g)

DesOwen®: 0.05% (60 g)

Gel, topical:

Desonate®: 0.05% (60 g)

Lotion, topical: 0.05% (59 mL, 60 mL, 118 mL)

DesOwen®: 0.05% (60 mL, 120 mL)

LoKara™: 0.05% (59 mL, 118 mL)

Ointment, topical: 0.05% (15 g, 60 g)

DesOwen® *see* desonide *on page 265*

Desoxicream (Can) *see* desoximetasone *on page 265*

desoximetasone (des oks i MET a sone)

Medication Safety Issues

Sound-alike/look-alike issues:

Desoximetasone may be confused with dexamethasone

Topicort® may be confused with Topic®

U.S. Brand Names Topicort®; Topicort® LP

Canadian Brand Names Desoxicream; Topicort®; Topicort® Gel; Topicort® Mild; Topicort® Ointment

Therapeutic Category Corticosteroid, Topical

Use Relieves inflammation and pruritic symptoms of corticosteroid-responsive dermatosis

General Dosage Range Topical: *Children and Adults:* Apply a thin film to affected area twice daily

Dosage Forms

Cream, topical: 0.05% (15 g, 60 g); 0.25% (15 g, 60 g, 100 g)

Topicort®: 0.25% (15 g, 60 g)

Topicort® LP: 0.05% (15 g, 60 g)

Gel, topical: 0.05% (15 g, 60 g)

Topicort®: 0.05% (15 g, 60 g)

Ointment, topical: 0.05% (60 g); 0.25% (15 g, 60 g)

Topicort®: 0.25% (15 g, 60 g)

desoxyephedrine hydrochloride *see* methamphetamine *on page 581*

Desoxyn® *see* methamphetamine *on page 581*

desoxyphenobarbital *see* primidone *on page 758*

Desquam-X® (Can) *see* benzoyl peroxide *on page 124*

Desquam-X® 5 [OTC] *see* benzoyl peroxide *on page 124*

Desquam-X® 10 [OTC] *see* benzoyl peroxide *on page 124*

desulfato-hirudin *see* desirudin *on page 263*

desulphatohirudin *see* desirudin *on page* 263

desvenlafaxine (des ven la FAX een)

Medication Safety Issues

BEERS Criteria medication:

This drug may be potentially inappropriate for use in geriatric patients (Quality of evidence - moderate; Strength of recommendation - strong).

Synonyms O-desmethylvenlafaxine; ODV

U.S. Brand Names Pristiq®

Canadian Brand Names Pristiq®

Therapeutic Category Antidepressant, Serotonin/Norepinephrine Reuptake Inhibitor

Use Treatment of major depressive disorder

General Dosage Range Dosage adjustment recommended in patients with hepatic or renal impairment

Oral: *Adults:* Initial: 50 mg once daily

Dosage Forms

Tablet, extended release, oral:

Pristiq®: 50 mg, 100 mg

Desyrel *see* trazodone *on page* 912

Detane® [OTC] *see* benzocaine *on page* 121

detemir insulin *see* insulin detemir *on page* 486

Detrol® *see* tolterodine *on page* 905

Detrol® LA *see* tolterodine *on page* 905

detryptoreline *see* triptorelin *on page* 922

Dex4® [OTC] *see* dextrose *on page* 275

dexamethasone (systemic) (deks a METH a sone)

Medication Safety Issues

Sound-alike/look-alike issues:

Dexamethasone may be confused with desoximetasone, dextroamphetamine

Decadron® may be confused with Percodan®

Synonyms Decadron; dexamethasone sodium phosphate

U.S. Brand Names Baycadron™; Dexamethasone Intensol™; DexPak® 10 Day TaperPak®; DexPak® 13 Day TaperPak®; DexPak® 6 Day TaperPak®

Canadian Brand Names Apo-Dexamethasone®; Dexasone®; Dom-Dexamethasone; PHL-Dexamethasone; PMS-Dexamethasone; PRO-Dexamethasone; ratio-Dexamethasone

Therapeutic Category Antiemetic; Antiinflammatory Agent; Corticosteroid, Systemic

Use Primarily as an antiinflammatory or immunosuppressant agent in the treatment of a variety of diseases including those of allergic, dermatologic, endocrine, hematologic, inflammatory, neoplastic, nervous system, renal, respiratory, rheumatic, and autoimmune origin; may be used in management of cerebral edema, chronic swelling, as a diagnostic agent, diagnosis of Cushing syndrome, antiemetic

General Dosage Range

I.M.:

Children: 0.03-2 mg/kg/day or 0.6-10 mg/m^2/day divided every 6-12 hours

Adults: 0.75-9 mg/day or 0.03-2 mg/kg/day or 0.6-0.75 mg/m^2/day in divided doses every 6-12 hours **or** 4 mg every 4-6 hours

I.V.:

Children: 0.03-2 mg/kg/day or 0.6-10 mg/m^2/day divided every 6-12 hours **or** 10 mg/m^2/dose every 12-24 hours on days of chemotherapy

Adults: Dosage varies greatly depending on indication

Intra-articular, intralesional, or soft tissue: *Adults:* 0.4-6 mg/day

Oral:

Children: 0.03-2 mg/kg/day or 0.6-10 mg/m^2/day divided every 6-12 hours

Adults: Dosage varies greatly depending on indication

Dosage Forms

Elixir, oral: 0.5 mg/5 mL (237 mL)

Baycadron™: 0.5 mg/5 mL (237 mL)

Injection, solution: 4 mg/mL (1 mL, 5 mL, 30 mL); 10 mg/mL (1 mL, 10 mL)

Injection, solution [preservative free]: 10 mg/mL (1 mL)

Solution, oral: 0.5 mg/5 mL (240 mL, 500 mL)
Dexamethasone Intensol™: 1 mg/mL (30 mL)
Tablet, oral: 0.5 mg, 0.75 mg, 1 mg, 1.5 mg, 2 mg, 4 mg, 6 mg
DexPak® 6 Day TaperPak®: 1.5 mg
DexPak® 10 Day TaperPak®: 1.5 mg
DexPak® 13 Day TaperPak®: 1.5 mg

dexamethasone (ophthalmic) (deks a METH a sone)

Medication Safety Issues

Sound-alike/look-alike issues:

Dexamethasone may be confused with desoximetasone, dextroamphetamine
Maxidex® may be confused with Maxzide®

Synonyms dexamethasone sodium phosphate

U.S. Brand Names Maxidex®; Ozurdex®

Canadian Brand Names Diodex®; Maxidex®; Ozurdex®

Therapeutic Category Antiinflammatory Agent, Ophthalmic; Corticosteroid, Ophthalmic

Use Management of steroid-responsive inflammatory conditions such as allergic conjunctivitis, iritis, or cyclitis; symptomatic treatment of corneal injury from chemical, radiation, or thermal burns, or penetration of foreign bodies. The ophthalmic solution is also indicated for otic use to treat steroid-responsive inflammatory conditions of the external auditory meatus.

Ophthalmic intravitreal implant (Ozurdex®): Treatment of macular edema following branch retinal vein occlusion (BRVO) or central retinal vein occlusion (CRVO); treatment of noninfective uveitis

General Dosage Range

Intravitreal: *Adults:* 0.7 mg implant in affected eye

Ophthalmic:

Adults:

Solution: Instill 1-2 drops into conjunctival sac every hour during the day and every other hour during the night; gradually reduce dose to 1 drop every 4 hours, then to 3-4 times/day

Suspension: Instill 1-2 drops up to 4-6 times/day or hourly in severe cases

Otic: *Adults:* Initial: Instill 3-4 drops of the solution into the aural canal 2-3 times a day; reduce dose gradually. Alternately, pack the aural canal with a gauze wick saturated with the solution; remove from the ear after 12-24 hours.

Dosage Forms

Implant, intravitreal:
Ozurdex®: 0.7 mg (1s)
Solution, ophthalmic: 0.1% (5 mL)
Suspension, ophthalmic:
Maxidex®: 0.1% (5 mL)

dexamethasone and ciprofloxacin *see* ciprofloxacin and dexamethasone *on page 211*

dexamethasone and tobramycin *see* tobramycin and dexamethasone *on page 902*

Dexamethasone Intensol™ *see* dexamethasone (systemic) *on page 266*

dexamethasone, neomycin, and polymyxin B *see* neomycin, polymyxin B, and dexamethasone *on page 634*

dexamethasone sodium phosphate *see* dexamethasone (ophthalmic) *on page 267*

dexamethasone sodium phosphate *see* dexamethasone (systemic) *on page 266*

Dexasone® (Can) *see* dexamethasone (systemic) *on page 266*

dexchlorpheniramine (deks klor fen EER a meen)

Medication Safety Issues

BEERS Criteria medication:

This drug may be potentially inappropriate for use in geriatric patients (Quality of evidence - moderate; Strength of recommendation - strong).

Synonyms dexchlorpheniramine maleate

Therapeutic Category Antihistamine

Use Perennial and seasonal allergic rhinitis and other allergic symptoms including urticaria

General Dosage Range Oral:
Regular release:
Children 2-5 years: 0.5 mg every 4-6 hours
Children 6-11 years: 1 mg every 4-6 hours
Adults: 2 mg every 4-6 hours
Timed release:
Children 6-11 years: 4 mg at bedtime
Adults: 4-6 mg at bedtime **or** every 8-10 hours

Dosage Forms
Syrup, oral: 2 mg/5 mL (473 mL)

dexchlorpheniramine maleate *see* dexchlorpheniramine *on page 267*

dexchlorpheniramine tannate, pseudoephedrine tannate, and dextromethorphan tannate *see* chlorpheniramine, pseudoephedrine, and dextromethorphan *on page 202*

Dexedrine® (Can) *see* dextroamphetamine *on page 270*

Dexedrine® Spansule® *see* dextroamphetamine *on page 270*

Dexferrum® *see* iron dextran complex *on page 501*

Dexilant™ *see* dexlansoprazole *on page 268*

Dexiron™ (Can) *see* iron dextran complex *on page 501*

dexlansoprazole (deks lan SOE pra zole)

Medication Safety Issues
Sound-alike/look-alike issues:
Dexlansoprazole may be confused with aripiprazole, lansoprazole
Kapidex [DSC] may be confused with Casodex®, Kadian®
International issues:
Kapidex [DSC] may be confused with Capadex which is a brand name for propoxyphene/acetaminophen combination product [Australia, New Zealand]

Synonyms Kapidex; TAK-390MR

U.S. Brand Names Dexilant™

Canadian Brand Names Dexilant™

Therapeutic Category Proton Pump Inhibitor; Substituted Benzimidazole

Use Short-term (4 weeks) treatment of heartburn associated with nonerosive GERD; short-term (up to 8 weeks) treatment of all grades of erosive esophagitis; to maintain healing of erosive esophagitis for up to 6 months

General Dosage Range Dosage adjustment recommended in patients with hepatic impairment
Oral: *Adults:* 30-60 mg once daily

Dosage Forms
Capsule, delayed release, oral:
Dexilant™: 30 mg, 60 mg

dexmedetomidine (deks MED e toe mi deen)

Medication Safety Issues
Sound-alike/look-alike issues:
Precedex® may be confused with Peridex®
High alert medication:
The Institute for Safe Medication Practices (ISMP) includes this medication among its list of drug classes which have a heightened risk of causing significant patient harm when used in error.
Administration issues:
Errors have occurred due to misinterpretation of dosing information; use caution. Maintenance dose expressed as mcg/kg/**hour**.

Synonyms dexmedetomidine hydrochloride

U.S. Brand Names Precedex®

Canadian Brand Names Precedex®

Therapeutic Category Alpha-Adrenergic Agonist - Central-Acting (Alpha$_2$-Agonists); Sedative

Use Sedation of initially intubated and mechanically ventilated patients during treatment in an intensive care setting; sedation prior to and/or during surgical or other procedures of nonintubated patients

General Dosage Range I.V.: *Adults:* Loading infusion: 0.5-1 mcg/kg; Maintenance infusion: 0.2-1 mcg/kg/**hour**

Dosage Forms
Injection, solution [preservative free]:
Precedex®: 100 mcg/mL (2 mL)

dexmedetomidine hydrochloride *see* dexmedetomidine *on page* 268

dexmethylphenidate (dex meth il FEN i date)

Medication Safety Issues
Sound-alike/look-alike issues:
Dexmethylphenidate may be confused with methadone
Focalin® may be confused with Folotyn®

Synonyms dexmethylphenidate hydrochloride

U.S. Brand Names Focalin XR®; Focalin®

Therapeutic Category Central Nervous System Stimulant, Nonamphetamine

Controlled Substance C-II

Use Treatment of attention-deficit/hyperactivity disorder (ADHD)

General Dosage Range Oral:
Extended release:
Children ≥6 years: Initial: 5 mg once daily; Maintenance: Up to 30 mg/day
Adults: Initial: 10 mg once daily; Maintenance: Up to 40 mg/day
Immediate release: *Children ≥6 years and Adults:* Initial: 2.5 mg twice daily; Maintenance: Up to 20 mg/day in 2 divided doses (at least 4 hours apart)

Dosage Forms
Capsule, extended release, oral:
Focalin XR®: 5 mg, 10 mg, 15 mg, 20 mg, 25 mg, 30 mg, 35 mg, 40 mg
Tablet, oral: 2.5 mg, 5 mg, 10 mg
Focalin®: 2.5 mg, 5 mg, 10 mg

dexmethylphenidate hydrochloride *see* dexmethylphenidate *on page* 269
DexPak® 6 Day TaperPak® *see* dexamethasone (systemic) *on page* 266
DexPak® 10 Day TaperPak® *see* dexamethasone (systemic) *on page* 266
DexPak® 13 Day TaperPak® *see* dexamethasone (systemic) *on page* 266

dexpanthenol (deks PAN the nole)

Synonyms pantothenyl alcohol

Therapeutic Category Gastrointestinal Agent, Stimulant

Use Prophylactic use to minimize paralytic ileus; treatment of postoperative distention; topical to relieve itching and to aid healing of minor dermatoses

General Dosage Range I.M.: *Adults:* Initial: 250-500 mg; repeat in 2 hours, followed by doses every 6 hours if needed

Dosage Forms
Injection, solution [preservative free]: 250 mg/mL (2 mL)

dexrazoxane (deks ray ZOKS ane)

Medication Safety Issues
Sound-alike/look-alike issues:
Zinecard® may be confused with Gemzar®

Synonyms ICRF-187

U.S. Brand Names Totect®; Zinecard®

Canadian Brand Names Zinecard®

Therapeutic Category Cardiovascular Agent, Other

Use
Zinecard®: Reduction of the incidence and severity of cardiomyopathy associated with doxorubicin administration in women with metastatic breast cancer who have received a cumulative doxorubicin dose of 300 mg/m^2 and who would benefit from continuing therapy with doxorubicin. (Not recommended for use with initial doxorubicin therapy.)
Totect®: Treatment of anthracycline-induced extravasation.

General Dosage Range Dosage adjustment recommended in patients with renal impairment and hepatic impairment

I.V.: *Adults:* A 10:1 ratio of dexrazoxane:doxorubicin (dexrazoxane 500 mg/m^2:doxorubicin 50 mg/m^2) (prevention of cardiomyopathy) **or** 1000 mg/m^2 on days 1 and 2 (maximum dose: 2000 mg), followed by 500 mg/m^2 on day 3 (maximum dose: 1000 mg) (anthracycline-induced extravasation)

Dosage Forms

Injection, powder for reconstitution: 250 mg, 500 mg

Totect®: 500 mg

Zinecard®: 250 mg, 500 mg

dextran (DEKS tran)

Medication Safety Issues

Sound-alike/look-alike issues:

Dextran may be confused with Dexedrine®

Synonyms 10% LMD; dextran 40; dextran, low molecular weight

U.S. Brand Names LMD®

Therapeutic Category Plasma Volume Expander

Use Blood volume expander used in treatment of shock or impending shock when blood or blood products are not available; also used as a priming fluid in pump oxygenators during cardiopulmonary bypass and for prophylaxis of venous thrombosis and pulmonary embolism in surgical procedures associated with a high risk of thromboembolic complications

General Dosage Range I.V.:

Dextran 40:

Children: Infuse 10 mL/kg as rapidly as possible (maximum: 20 mL/kg/day for the first 24 hours; 10 mL/kg/day thereafter); therapy should not be continued beyond 5 days

Adults: Infuse 500-1000 mL (~10 mL/kg) as rapidly as possible (maximum: 20 mL/kg/day for first 24 hours; 10 mL/kg/day thereafter); (5 days total therapy) **or** 50-100 g on the day of surgery, then 50 g (4 mL/minute) every 2-3 days during the period of risk

Dosage Forms

Infusion, premixed in D_5W:

LMD®: 10% Dextran 40 (500 mL)

Infusion, premixed in NS:

LMD®: 10% Dextran 40 (500 mL)

dextran 40 *see* dextran *on page* 270

dextran, low molecular weight *see* dextran *on page* 270

dextrin *see* wheat dextrin *on page* 955

dextrmethorphan, pyrilamine, and phenylephrine *see* phenylephrine, pyrilamine, and dextromethorphan *on page* 718

dextroamphetamine (deks troe am FET a meen)

Medication Safety Issues

Sound-alike/look-alike issues:

Dexedrine® may be confused with dextran, Excedrin®

Dextroamphetamine may be confused with dexamethasone

Synonyms dextroamphetamine sulfate

U.S. Brand Names Dexedrine® Spansule®; ProCentra®

Canadian Brand Names Dexedrine®

Therapeutic Category Amphetamine

Controlled Substance C-II

Use Narcolepsy; attention-deficit/hyperactivity disorder (ADHD)

General Dosage Range Oral:

Children 3-5 years: Initial: 2.5 mg once daily; Maintenance: 0.1-0.5 mg/kg once daily (maximum: 40 mg/day)

Children 6-12 years: Initial: 5 mg once or twice daily; Maintenance: 5-20 mg (0.1-0.5 mg/kg) once daily (maximum: 40 mg [ADHD]: 60 mg [narcolepsy])

Children >12 years: Initial: 5-10 mg/day in 1-2 divided doses; Maximum: Up to 40 mg/day [ADHD] or 60 mg/day [narcolepsy]

Adults: Initial: 10 mg once daily; Maximum: Up to 60 mg/day

Dosage Forms

Capsule, extended release, oral: 5 mg, 10 mg, 15 mg

Capsule, sustained release, oral:

Dexedrine® Spansule®: 5 mg, 10 mg, 15 mg

Solution, oral:

ProCentra®: 5 mg/5 mL (480 mL)

Tablet, oral: 5 mg, 10 mg

dextroamphetamine and amphetamine (deks troe am FET a meen & am FET a meen)

Medication Safety Issues

Sound-alike/look-alike issues:

Adderall® may be confused with Inderal®

Synonyms amphetamine and dextroamphetamine

U.S. Brand Names Adderall XR®; Adderall®

Canadian Brand Names Adderall XR®

Therapeutic Category Amphetamine

Controlled Substance C-II

Use Attention-deficit/hyperactivity disorder (ADHD); narcolepsy

General Dosage Range Oral:

Extended release:

Children 6-12 years: Initial: 5-10 mg once daily; Maintenance: Up to 30 mg/day

Adolescents 13-17 years: Initial: 10 mg once daily; Maintenance: 10-20 mg once daily (maximum: 60 mg/day)

Adults: 20 mg once daily (maximum: 60 mg/day)

Immediate release:

Children 3-5 years: Initial: 2.5 mg once daily; Maintenance: Up to 40 mg/day in 1-3 divided doses

Children 6-12 years: Initial: 5 mg once or twice daily; Maintenance: Up to 40 mg/day [ADHD] or 60 mg/day [narcolepsy] in 1-3 divided doses

Children >12 years and Adults: Initial: 5-10 mg in 1-2 divided doses; Maintenance: Up to 40 mg/day [ADHD] or 60 mg/day [narcolepsy] in 1-3 divided doses

Dosage Forms

Capsule, extended release, oral:

5 mg [dextroamphetamine sulfate 1.25 mg, dextroamphetamine saccharate 1.25 mg, amphetamine aspartate monohydrate 1.25 mg, amphetamine sulfate 1.25 mg]

10 mg [dextroamphetamine sulfate 2.5 mg, dextroamphetamine saccharate 2.5 mg, amphetamine aspartate monohydrate 2.5 mg, amphetamine sulfate 2.5 mg]

15 mg [dextroamphetamine sulfate 3.75 mg, dextroamphetamine saccharate 3.75 mg, amphetamine aspartate monohydrate 3.75 mg, amphetamine sulfate 3.75 mg]

20 mg [dextroamphetamine sulfate 5 mg, dextroamphetamine saccharate 5 mg, amphetamine aspartate monohydrate 5 mg, amphetamine sulfate 5 mg]

25 mg [dextroamphetamine sulfate 6.25 mg, dextroamphetamine saccharate 6.25 mg, amphetamine aspartate monohydrate 6.25 mg, amphetamine sulfate 6.25 mg]

30 mg [dextroamphetamine sulfate 7.5 mg, dextroamphetamine saccharate 7.5 mg, amphetamine aspartate monohydrate 7.5 mg, amphetamine sulfate 7.5 mg]

Adderall XR®:

5 mg [dextroamphetamine 1.25 mg, dextroamphetamine saccharate 1.25 mg, amphetamine aspartate monohydrate 1.25 mg, amphetamine sulfate 1.25 mg]

10 mg [dextroamphetamine sulfate 2.5 mg, dextroamphetamine saccharate 2.5 mg, amphetamine aspartate monohydrate 2.5 mg, amphetamine sulfate 2.5 mg]

15 mg [dextroamphetamine sulfate 3.75 mg, dextroamphetamine saccharate 3.75 mg, amphetamine aspartate monohydrate 3.75 mg, amphetamine sulfate 3.75 mg]

20 mg [dextroamphetamine sulfate 5 mg, dextroamphetamine saccharate 5 mg, amphetamine aspartate monohydrate 5 mg, amphetamine sulfate 5 mg]

25 mg [dextroamphetamine sulfate 6.25 mg, dextroamphetamine saccharate 6.25 mg, amphetamine aspartate monohydrate 6.25 mg, amphetamine sulfate 6.25 mg]

30 mg [dextroamphetamine sulfate 7.5 mg, dextroamphetamine saccharate 7.5 mg, amphetamine aspartate monohydrate 7.5 mg, amphetamine sulfate 7.5 mg]

Tablet, oral: 5 mg, 7.5 mg, 10 mg, 12.5 mg, 15 mg, 20 mg, 30 mg
5 mg [dextroamphetamine sulfate 1.25 mg, dextroamphetamine saccharate 1.25 mg, amphetamine aspartate monohydrate 1.25 mg, amphetamine sulfate 1.25 mg]
7.5 mg [dextroamphetamine sulfate 1.875 mg, dextroamphetamine saccharate 1.875 mg, amphetamine aspartate monohydrate 1.875 mg, amphetamine sulfate 1.875 mg]
10 mg [dextroamphetamine sulfate 2.5 mg, dextroamphetamine saccharate 2.5 mg, amphetamine aspartate monohydrate 2.5 mg, amphetamine sulfate 2.5 mg]
12.5 mg [dextroamphetamine sulfate 3.125 mg, dextroamphetamine saccharate 3.125 mg, amphetamine aspartate monohydrate 3.125 mg, amphetamine sulfate 3.125 mg]
15 mg [dextroamphetamine sulfate 3.75 mg, dextroamphetamine saccharate 3.75 mg, amphetamine aspartate monohydrate 3.75 mg, amphetamine sulfate 3.75 mg]
20 mg [dextroamphetamine sulfate 5 mg, dextroamphetamine saccharate 5 mg, amphetamine aspartate monohydrate 5 mg, amphetamine sulfate 5 mg]
30 mg [dextroamphetamine sulfate 7.5 mg, dextroamphetamine saccharate 7.5 mg, amphetamine aspartate monohydrate 7.5 mg, amphetamine sulfate 7.5 mg]
Adderall®:
5 mg [dextroamphetamine sulfate 1.25 mg, dextroamphetamine saccharate 1.25 mg, amphetamine aspartate monohydrate 1.25 mg, amphetamine sulfate 1.25 mg]
7.5 mg [dextroamphetamine sulfate 1.875 mg, dextroamphetamine saccharate 1.875 mg, amphetamine aspartate monohydrate 1.875 mg, amphetamine sulfate 1.875 mg]
10 mg [dextroamphetamine sulfate 2.5 mg, dextroamphetamine saccharate 2.5 mg, amphetamine aspartate monohydrate 2.5 mg, amphetamine sulfate 2.5 mg]
12.5 mg [dextroamphetamine sulfate 3.125 mg, dextroamphetamine saccharate 3.125 mg, amphetamine aspartate monohydrate 3.125 mg, amphetamine sulfate 3.125 mg]
15 mg [dextroamphetamine sulfate 3.75 mg, dextroamphetamine saccharate 3.75 mg, amphetamine aspartate monohydrate 3.75 mg, amphetamine sulfate 3.75 mg]
20 mg [dextroamphetamine sulfate 5 mg, dextroamphetamine saccharate 5 mg, amphetamine aspartate monohydrate 5 mg, amphetamine sulfate 5 mg]
30 mg [dextroamphetamine sulfate 7.5 mg, dextroamphetamine saccharate 7.5 mg, amphetamine aspartate monohydrate 7.5 mg, amphetamine sulfate 7.5 mg]

dextroamphetamine sulfate *see* dextroamphetamine *on page* 270

dextromethorphan (deks troe meth OR fan)

Medication Safety Issues

Sound-alike/look-alike issues:
Benylin® may be confused with Benadryl®, Ventolin®
Delsym® may be confused with Delfen®, Desyrel

U.S. Brand Names Creo-Terpin® [OTC]; Creomulsion® Adult Formula [OTC]; Creomulsion® for Children [OTC]; Delsym® [OTC]; Father John's® [OTC]; Hold® DM [OTC]; Nycoff [OTC]; PediaCare® Children's Long-Acting Cough [OTC]; Robafen Cough [OTC]; Robitussin® Children's Cough Long-Acting [OTC]; Robitussin® Cough Long Acting [OTC] [DSC]; Robitussin® CoughGels™ Long-Acting [OTC] [DSC]; Robitussin® Lingering Cold Long-Acting Cough [OTC]; Robitussin® Lingering Cold Long-Acting CoughGels® [OTC]; Scot-Tussin® Diabetes [OTC]; Silphen-DM [OTC]; Triaminic Thin Strips® Children's Long Acting Cough [OTC]; Triaminic® Children's Cough Long Acting [OTC]; Trocal® [OTC] [DSC]; Vicks® 44® Cough Relief [OTC]; Vicks® DayQuil® Cough [OTC]; Vicks® Nature Fusion™ Cough [OTC]

Therapeutic Category Antitussive

Use Symptomatic relief of coughs caused by the common cold or inhaled irritants

General Dosage Range Oral:
Extended release:
Children 4-6 years: 15 mg twice daily (maximum: 30 mg/day)
Children 6-12 years: 30 mg twice daily (maximum: 60 mg/day)
Children >12 years and Adults: 60 mg twice daily (maximum: 120 mg/day)
Immediate release:
Children 4-6 years: 2.5-7.5 mg every 4-8 hours (maximum: 30 mg/day)
Children 6-12 years: 5-10 mg every 4 hours **or** 15 mg every 6-8 hours (maximum: 60 mg/day)
Children >12 years and Adults: 10-20 mg every 4 hours **or** 30 mg every 6-8 hours (maximum: 120 mg/day)

Dosage Forms

Capsule, liquid filled, oral:
Robafen Cough [OTC]: 15 mg
Robitussin® Lingering Cold Long-Acting CoughGels® [OTC]: 15 mg

Liquid, oral:
Creo-Terpin® [OTC]: 10 mg/15 mL (120 mL)
Scot-Tussin® Diabetes [OTC]: 10 mg/5 mL (118 mL)
Vicks® 44® Cough Relief [OTC]: 10 mg/5 mL (120 mL)
Vicks® Nature Fusion™ Cough [OTC]: 30 mg/30 mL (240 mL)

Lozenge, oral:
Hold® DM [OTC]: 5 mg (10s)

Solution, oral:
PediaCare® Children's Long-Acting Cough [OTC]: 7.5 mg/5 mL (118 mL)
Vicks® DayQuil® Cough [OTC]: 15 mg/15 mL (177 mL, 295 mL)

Strip, orally disintegrating, oral:
Triaminic Thin Strips® Children's Long Acting Cough [OTC]: 7.5 mg (14s, 16s)

Suspension, extended release, oral:
Delsym® [OTC]: Dextromethorphan polistirex [equivalent to dextromethorphan hydrobromide] 30 mg/5 mL (89 mL, 148 mL)

Syrup, oral:
Creomulsion® Adult Formula [OTC]: 20 mg/15 mL (120 mL)
Creomulsion® for Children [OTC]: 5 mg/5 mL (120 mL)
Father John's® [OTC]: 10 mg/5 mL (118 mL, 236 mL)
Robitussin® Children's Cough Long-Acting [OTC]: 7.5 mg/5 mL (118 mL)
Robitussin® Lingering Cold Long-Acting Cough [OTC]: 15 mg/5 mL (118 mL)
Silphen-DM [OTC]: 10 mg/5 mL (120 mL)
Triaminic® Children's Cough Long Acting [OTC]: 7.5 mg/5 mL (118 mL)

Tablet, oral:
Nycoff [OTC]: 15 mg

dextromethorphan and chlorpheniramine (deks troe meth OR fan & klor fen IR a meen)

Synonyms chlorpheniramine and dextromethorphan; chlorpheniramine maleate and dextromethorphan hydrobromide; dextromethorphan hydrobromide and chlorpheniramine maleate

U.S. Brand Names Coricidin® HBP Cough & Cold [OTC]; Dimetapp® Children's Long Acting Cough Plus Cold [OTC]; Robitussin® Children's Cough & Cold Long-Acting [OTC]; Robitussin® Cough & Cold Long-Acting [OTC] [DSC]; Scot-Tussin® DM Maximum Strength [OTC]; Triaminic® Children's Softchews® Cough & Runny Nose [OTC]

Therapeutic Category Antitussive; Histamine H_1 Antagonist; Histamine H_1 Antagonist, First Generation

Use Symptomatic relief of runny nose, sneezing, itchy/watery eyes, cough, and other upper respiratory symptoms associated with hay fever, common cold, or upper respiratory allergies

General Dosage Range Oral:

Children 6-11 years: Dextromethorphan 10-15 mg and chlorpheniramine 2 mg every 4-6 hours as needed (maximum: 60 mg dextromethorphan and 10 mg chlorpheniramine/24 hours)

Children ≥12 years and Adults: Dextromethorphan 30 mg and chlorpheniramine 4 mg every 6 hours as needed (maximum: 120 mg dextromethorphan and 16 mg chlorpheniramine/24 hours)

Dosage Forms

Syrup:
Dimetapp® Children's Long Acting Cough Plus Cold [OTC]: Dextromethorphan 7.5 mg and chlorpheniramine 1 mg per 5 mL (118 mL)
Robitussin® Children's Cough and Cold Long-Acting [OTC]: Dextromethorphan 15 mg and chlorpheniramine 2 mg per 5 mL (118 mL)
Scot-Tussin® DM Maximum Strength [OTC]: Dextromethorphan 15 mg and chlorpheniramine 2 mg per 5 mL (118 mL)

Tablet:
Coricidin® HBP Cough and Cold [OTC]: Dextromethorphan 30 mg and chlorpheniramine 4 mg

Tablet, softchew:
Triaminic® Children's Softchews® Cough & Runny Nose [OTC]: Dextromethorphan 5 mg and chlorpheniramine 1 mg

dextromethorphan and guaifenesin *see* guaifenesin and dextromethorphan *on page* 434

dextromethorphan and phenylephrine (deks troe meth OR fan & fen il EF rin)

Synonyms dextromethorphan hydrobromide and phenylephrine hydrochloride; phenylephrine and dextromethorphan

U.S. Brand Names PediaCare® Children's Multi-Symptom Cold [OTC]; Safetussin® CD [OTC]; Sudafed PE® Children's Cold & Cough [OTC]; Triaminic Thin Strips® Children's Day Time Cold & Cough [OTC]; Triaminic® Day Time Cold & Cough [OTC]

Therapeutic Category Antitussive; Decongestant

Use Temporary relief of symptoms of hay fever, the common cold, and upper respiratory allergies including sinus/nasal congestion, minor bronchial/throat irritation, and cough

General Dosage Range Oral:

Children ≥4-12 years: Dosage varies greatly depending on product

Children ≥12 years and Adults: Safetussin® CD: 10 mL every 6 hours as needed (maximum: 40 mL/24 hours)

Dosage Forms

Liquid, oral:

Sudafed PE® Children's Cold + Cough [OTC]: Dextromethorphan 5 mg and phenylephrine 2.5 mg per 5 mL (118 mL)

Strip, orally disintegrating:

Triaminic Thin Strips® Children's Day Time Cold & Cough [OTC]: Dextromethorphan bromide 5 mg and phenylephrine 2.5 mg (14s, 16s, 48s)

Syrup:

PediaCare® Children's Multi-Symptom Cold [OTC], Triaminic® Day Time Cold & Cough [OTC]: Dextromethorphan 5 mg and phenylephrine 2.5 mg per 5 mL

Safetussin® CD [OTC]: Dextromethorphan 15 mg and phenylephrine 2.5 mg per 5 mL

dextromethorphan and promethazine *see* promethazine and dextromethorphan *on page 764*

dextromethorphan and pseudoephedrine *see* pseudoephedrine and dextromethorphan *on page 772*

dextromethorphan and quinidine (deks troe meth OR fan & KWIN i deen)

Synonyms dextromethorphan hydrobromide and quinidine sulfate; quinidine and dextromethorphan

U.S. Brand Names Nuedexta™

Canadian Brand Names Nuedexta™

Therapeutic Category Antiarrhythmic Agent, Class Ia; N-Methyl-D-Aspartate Receptor Antagonist

Use Treatment of pseudobulbar affect (PBA)

General Dosage Range

Oral: *Adults:* Initial: Once capsule once daily for 7 days; Maintenance: One capsule twice daily

Dosage Forms

Capsule, oral:

Nuedexta™: Dextromethorphan hydrobromide 20 mg and quinidine sulfate 10 mg

dextromethorphan, chlorpheniramine, and phenylephrine *see* chlorpheniramine, phenylephrine, and dextromethorphan *on page 201*

dextromethorphan, chlorpheniramine, and pseudoephedrine *see* chlorpheniramine, pseudoephedrine, and dextromethorphan *on page 202*

dextromethorphan, guaifenesin, and pseudoephedrine *see* guaifenesin, pseudoephedrine, and dextromethorphan *on page 437*

dextromethorphan hydrobromide, acetaminophen, and doxylamine succinate *see* acetaminophen, dextromethorphan, and doxylamine *on page 27*

dextromethorphan hydrobromide, acetaminophen, and phenylephrine hydrochloride *see* acetaminophen, dextromethorphan, and phenylephrine *on page 28*

dextromethorphan hydrobromide and chlorpheniramine maleate *see* dextromethorphan and chlorpheniramine *on page 273*

dextromethorphan hydrobromide and phenylephrine hydrochloride *see* dextromethorphan and phenylephrine *on page 273*

dextromethorphan hydrobromide and quinidine sulfate *see* dextromethorphan and quinidine *on page 274*

dextromethorphan hydrobromide, brompheniramine maleate, and pseudoephedrine hydrochloride *see* brompheniramine, pseudoephedrine, and dextromethorphan *on page 144*

dextromethorphan hydrobromide, guaifenesin, and phenylephrine hydrochloride *see* guaifenesin, dextromethorphan, and phenylephrine *on page 437*

dextrose (DEKS trose)

Medication Safety Issues

Sound-alike/look-alike issues:

Glutose™ may be confused with Glutofac®

High alert medication:

The Institute for Safe Medication Practices (ISMP) includes this medication (hypertonic solutions ≥20%) among its list of drugs which have a heightened risk of causing significant patient harm when used in error.

Other safety concerns:

Inappropriate use of low sodium or sodium-free intravenous fluids (eg D_5W, hypotonic saline) in pediatric patients can lead to significant morbidity and mortality due to hyponatremia (ISMP, 2009).

Synonyms anhydrous glucose; $D_{10}W$; $D_{25}W$; $D_{30}W$; $D_{40}W$; $D_{50}W$; D_5W; $D_{60}W$; $D_{70}W$; dextrose monohydrate; glucose; glucose monohydrate; glycosum

U.S. Brand Names BD™ Glucose [OTC]; Dex4® [OTC]; Enfamil® Glucose [OTC]; GlucoBurst® [OTC]; Glutol™ [OTC]; Glutose 15™ [OTC]; Glutose 45™ [OTC]; Insta-Glucose® [OTC]; Similac® Glucose [OTC]

Therapeutic Category Antidote, Hypoglycemia; Intravenous Nutritional Therapy

Use

Oral: Treatment of hypoglycemia

5% and 10% solutions: Peripheral infusion to provide calories and fluid replacement

25% (hypertonic) solution: Treatment of acute symptomatic episodes of hypoglycemia in infants and children to restore depressed blood glucose levels; adjunctive treatment of hyperkalemia when combined with insulin

50% (hypertonic) solution: Treatment of insulin-induced hypoglycemia (hyperinsulinemia or insulin shock) and adjunctive treatment of hyperkalemia in adolescents and adults

≥10% solutions: Infusion after admixture with amino acids for nutritional support

General Dosage Range

I.V.:

Infants ≤6 months: 0.25-1 g/kg/dose (maximum: 25 g/dose)

Children >6 months to 12 years: 0.5-1 g/kg/dose (maximum: 25 g/dose)

Adolescents and and Adults: 10-50 g/dose

Oral: *Children >2 years and and Adults:* 10-20 g as a single dose, may repeat if needed

Dosage Forms

Gel, oral:

Dex4® [OTC]: 40% (38 g)

GlucoBurst® [OTC]: 40% (37.5 g)

Glutose 15™ [OTC]: 40% (37.5 g)

Glutose 45™ [OTC]: 40% (112.5 g)

Insta-Glucose® [OTC]: 40% (31 g)

Infusion: 5% (25 mL, 50 mL, 100 mL, 150 mL, 250 mL, 500 mL, 1000 mL); 10% (150 mL, 250 mL, 500 mL, 1000 mL); 20% (500 mL, 1000 mL); 30% (500 mL, 1000 mL); 40% (500 mL, 1000 mL); 50% (50 mL, 500 mL, 1000 mL, 2000 mL, 5000 mL); 70% (250 mL, 500 mL, 1000 mL, 2000 mL)

Injection, solution: 25% (10 mL); 50% (50 mL)

Liquid, oral:

Dex4® [OTC]: 15 g/60 mL (60 mL)

Solution, oral:

Enfamil® Glucose [OTC]: 5% (89 mL); 10% (89 mL)

Glutol™ [OTC]: 55% (180 mL)

Similac® Glucose [OTC]: 5% (59 mL); 10% (59 mL)

Tablet, chewable, oral: 4 g

BD™ Glucose [OTC]: 5 g

Dex4® [OTC]: 4 g

GlucoBurst® [OTC]: 5 g

dextrose, levulose and phosphoric acid *see* fructose, dextrose, and phosphoric acid *on page 411*

dextrose monohydrate *see* dextrose *on page 275*

Dex-Tuss *see* guaifenesin and codeine *on page 434*

dezocitidine *see* decitabine *on page 258*

dFdC *see* gemcitabine *on page 422*

dFdCyd *see* gemcitabine *on page 422*

diatrizoate meglumine (dye a tri ZOE ate MEG loo meen)

Medication Safety Issues

High alert medication:

The Institute for Safe Medication Practices (ISMP) includes this medication among its list of drugs which have a heightened risk of causing significant patient harm when used in error.

U.S. Brand Names Cystografin®; Cystografin® Dilute

Therapeutic Category Iodinated Contrast Media; Radiological/Contrast Media, Ionic

Use

Solution for instillation: Retrograde cystourethrography; retrograde or ascending pyelography

Solution for injection: Arthrography, cerebral angiography, direct cholangiography, discography, drip infusion pyelography, excretory urography, peripheral arteriography, splenoportography, venography; contrast enhancement of computed tomographic head and body imaging

Dosage Forms

Solution, for instillation:

Cystografin®: 30% (100 mL, 300 mL)

Cystografin® Dilute: 18% (300 mL)

diatrizoate meglumine and diatrizoate sodium

(dye a tri ZOE ate MEG loo meen & dye a tri ZOE ate SOW dee um)

Medication Safety Issues

High alert medication:

The Institute for Safe Medication Practices (ISMP) includes this medication among its list of drug classes which have a heightened risk of causing significant patient harm when used in error.

Synonyms diatrizoate sodium and diatrizoate meglumine; Gastroview

U.S. Brand Names Gastrografin®; MD-76®R; MD-Gastroview®

Therapeutic Category Iodinated Contrast Media; Radiological/Contrast Media, Ionic

Use

Oral/rectal: Examination of GI tract; adjunct to contrast enhancement in computed tomography of the torso

Injection: Angiocardiography, aortography, central venography, cerebral angiography, cholangiography, digital arteriography, excretory urography, nephrotomography, peripheral angiography, peripheral arteriography, renal arteriography, renal venography, splenoportography, visceral arteriography; contrast enhancement of computed tomographic imaging

General Dosage Range

Oral:

Children <5 years: 30 mL, dilute 1:1 (if <10 kg or debilitated, dilute 1:3)

Children 5-10 years: 60 mL, dilute 1:1 (if <10 kg or debilitated, dilute 1:3)

Adults: 30-90 mL **or** 25-77 mL in 1000 mL tap water

Rectal:

Children <5 years: Dilute 1:5 in tap water

Children ≥5 years: Dilute 90 mL in 500 mL tap water

Adults: Dilute 240 mL in 1000 mL tap water

Dosage Forms

Solution, injection:

MD-76®R: Diatrizoate meglumine 660 mg and diatrizoate sodium 100 mg per 1 mL (50 mL, 100 mL, 200 mL)

Solution, oral/rectal:

Gastrografin®: Diatrizoate meglumine 660 mg and diatrizoate sodium 100 mg per 1 mL

MD-Gastroview®: Diatrizoate meglumine 660 mg and diatrizoate sodium 100 mg per 1 mL

diatrizoate meglumine and iodipamide meglumine

(dye a tri ZOE ate MEG loo meen & eye oh DI pa mide MEG loo meen)

Medication Safety Issues

High alert medication:

The Institute for Safe Medication Practices (ISMP) includes this medication among its list of drug classes which have a heightened risk of causing significant patient harm when used in error.

Synonyms iodipamide meglumine and diatrizoate meglumine

U.S. Brand Names Sinografin®

Therapeutic Category Iodinated Contrast Media; Radiological/Contrast Media, Ionic

Use Hysterosalpingography

General Dosage Range **Intrauterine:** *Adults:* Usual dose: 3-4 mL; Total dosage range: 1.5-10 mL

Dosage Forms

Injection, solution [for intrauterine instillation]:

Sinografin®: Diatrizoate meglumine 524 mg and iodipamide meglumine 268 mg per mL (10 mL)

diatrizoate sodium and diatrizoate meglumine *see* diatrizoate meglumine and diatrizoate sodium *on page* 277

Diatx®Zn *see* vitamins (multiple/oral) *on page* 951

Diazemuls® (Can) *see* diazepam *on page* 277

diazepam (dye AZ e pam)

Medication Safety Issues

Sound-alike/look-alike issues:

Diazepam may be confused with diazoxide, diltiazem, Ditropan, LORazepam

Valium® may be confused with Valcyte®

BEERS Criteria medication:

This drug may be potentially inappropriate for use in geriatric patients (Quality of evidence - high; Strength of recommendation - strong).

U.S. Brand Names Diastat®; Diastat® AcuDial™; Diazepam Intensol™; Valium®

Canadian Brand Names Apo-Diazepam®; Bio-Diazepam; Diastat®; Diazemuls®; Diazepam Auto Injector; Diazepam Injection USP; Novo-Dipam; PMS-Diazepam; Valium®

Therapeutic Category Benzodiazepine

Controlled Substance C-IV

Use Management of anxiety disorders, ethanol withdrawal symptoms; skeletal muscle relaxant; treatment of convulsive disorders; preoperative or preprocedural sedation and amnesia

Rectal gel: Management of selected, refractory epilepsy patients on stable regimens of antiepileptic drugs requiring intermittent use of diazepam to control episodes of increased seizure activity

General Dosage Range

I.M.: *Children >30 days and Adults:* Dosage varies greatly depending on indication

I.V.: *Children >30 days and Adults:* Dosage varies greatly depending on indication

Oral:

Children: 0.12-1 mg/kg/day divided every 6-8 hours **or** 0.2-0.3 mg/kg (maximum: 10 mg) prior to procedures

Adolescents: 0.12-0.8 mg/kg/day divided every 6-8 hours **or** 10 mg prior to procedures

Adults: Dosage varies greatly depending on indication

Rectal:

Gel:

Children 2-5 years: Initial: 0.5 mg/kg (maximum dose: 20 mg); may repeat in 4-12 hours if needed

Children 6-11 years: Initial: 0.3 mg/kg (maximum dose: 20 mg); may repeat in 4-12 hours if needed

Children ≥12 years and Adults: Initial: 0.2 mg/kg (maximum dose: 20 mg); may repeat in 4-12 hours if needed

Dosage Forms

Gel, rectal: 10 mg (2 mL); 20 mg (4 mL); 5 mg/mL (0.5 mL)

Diastat®: 5 mg/mL (0.5 mL)

Diastat® AcuDial™: 10 mg (2 mL); 20 mg (4 mL)

Injection, solution: 5 mg/mL (2 mL, 10 mL)

Solution, oral: 5 mg/5 mL (5 mL, 500 mL)

Diazepam Intensol™: 5 mg/mL (30 mL)

Tablet, oral: 2 mg, 5 mg, 10 mg

Valium®: 2 mg, 5 mg, 10 mg

Diazepam Auto Injector (Can) *see* diazepam *on page* 277

Diazepam Injection USP (Can) *see* diazepam *on page* 277

Diazepam Intensol™ *see* diazepam *on page* 277

diazoxide (dye az OKS ide)

Medication Safety Issues

Sound-alike/look-alike issues:

Diazoxide may be confused with diazepam, Dyazide®

U.S. Brand Names Proglycem®

Canadian Brand Names Proglycem®

Therapeutic Category Antihypertensive Agent; Antihypoglycemic Agent

Use Hypoglycemia related to islet cell adenoma, carcinoma, hyperplasia, or adenomatosis; nesidioblastosis; leucine sensitivity; extrapancreatic malignancy

General Dosage Range Oral:

Infants: 8-15 mg/kg/day in divided doses every 8-12 hours

Children and Adults: 3-8 mg/kg/day in divided doses every 8-12 hours

Dosage Forms

Suspension, oral:

Proglycem®: 50 mg/mL (30 mL)

Dosage Forms - Canada

Capsule, oral:

Proglycem®: 50 mg

Dibenzyline® *see* phenoxybenzamine *on page* 714

dibucaine (DYE byoo kane)

U.S. Brand Names Nupercainal® [OTC]

Therapeutic Category Local Anesthetic

Use Fast, temporary relief of pain and itching due to hemorrhoids, minor burns

General Dosage Range Topical:

Children: Apply to affected areas (maximum 7.5 g/24 hour period)

Adults: Apply to affected areas (maximum: 30 g/24 hour period)

Dosage Forms

Ointment, topical: 1% [10 mg/g] (30 g, 454 g)

Nupercainal® [OTC]: 1% [10 mg/g] (30 g, 60 g)

DIC *see* dacarbazine *on page 250*

Dicel® Chewable [OTC] *see* chlorpheniramine and pseudoephedrine *on page 200*

Dicel® DM Chewables [OTC] *see* chlorpheniramine, pseudoephedrine, and dextromethorphan *on page 202*

Dicetel® (Can) *see* pinaverium *(Canada only) on page 724*

dichloralphenazone, acetaminophen, and isometheptene *see* acetaminophen, isometheptene, and dichloralphenazone *on page 30*

dichloralphenazone, isometheptene, and acetaminophen *see* acetaminophen, isometheptene, and dichloralphenazone *on page 30*

Dickinson's® Witch Hazel [OTC] *see* witch hazel *on page 956*

Dickinson's® Witch Hazel Astringent Cleanser [OTC] *see* witch hazel *on page 956*

Dickinson's® Witch Hazel Cleansing Astringent [OTC] *see* witch hazel *on page 956*

Diclectin® (Can) *see* doxylamine and pyridoxine *(Canada only) on page 316*

diclofenac (systemic) (dye KLOE fen ak)

Medication Safety Issues

Sound-alike/look-alike issues:

Diclofenac may be confused with Diflucan®

Cataflam® may be confused with Catapres®

Voltaren may be confused with traMADol, Ultram®, Verelan®

BEERS Criteria medication:

This drug may be potentially inappropriate for use in geriatric patients (Quality of evidence - moderate; Strength of recommendation - strong).

International issues:

Diclofenac may be confused with Duphalac brand name for lactulose [multiple international markets]

Flexin: Brand name for diclofenac [Argentina], but also the brand name for cyclobenzaprine [Chile] and orphenadrine [Israel]

Flexin [Argentina] may be confused with Floxin brand name for flunarizine [Thailand], norfloxacin [South Africa], ofloxacin [U.S., Canada], and perfloxacin [Philippines]

Synonyms diclofenac potassium; diclofenac sodium; Voltaren

U.S. Brand Names Cambia™; Cataflam®; Voltaren®-XR; Zipsor®

Canadian Brand Names Apo-Diclo Rapide®; Apo-Diclo®; Apo-Diclo® SR®; Ava-Diclofenac; Ava-Diclofenac SR; Cambia®; Cataflam®; Diclofenac ECT; Diclofenac Sodium; Diclofenac Sodium SR; Diclofenac SR; Dom-Diclofenac; Dom-Diclofenac SR; NTP-Diclofenac; NTP-Diclofenac SR; Nu-Diclo; Nu-Diclo-SR; PMS-Diclofenac; PMS-Diclofenac SR; PMS-Diclofenac-K; PRO-Diclo-Rapide; Sandoz-Diclofenac; Sandoz-Diclofenac Rapide; Sandoz-Diclofenac SR; Teva-Diclofenac; Teva-Diclofenac K; Teva-Diclofenac SR; Voltaren Rapide®; Voltaren SR®; Voltaren®

Therapeutic Category Nonsteroidal Antiinflammatory Drug (NSAID)

Use

Capsule: Relief of mild-to-moderate acute pain

Immediate-release tablet: Relief of mild-to-moderate pain; primary dysmenorrhea; acute and chronic treatment of rheumatoid arthritis, osteoarthritis

Delayed-release tablet: Acute and chronic treatment of rheumatoid arthritis, osteoarthritis, ankylosing spondylitis

Extended-release tablet: Chronic treatment of osteoarthritis, rheumatoid arthritis

Oral solution: Treatment of acute migraine with or without aura

Suppository (CAN; not available in U.S.): Symptomatic treatment of rheumatoid arthritis and osteoarthritis (including degenerative joint disease of hip)

General Dosage Range Oral:
Immediate release capsule: *Adults:* 100 mg/day in 4 divided doses
Immediate release tablet: *Adults:* 100-200 mg/day in 2-4 divided doses
Delayed release tablet: *Adults:* 100-200 mg/day in 2-5 divided doses
Extended release tablet: *Adults:* 100-200 mg/day
Oral solution: *Adults:* 50 mg once

Dosage Forms
Capsule, liquid filled, oral:
Zipsor®: 25 mg
Powder for solution, oral:
Cambia™: 50 mg/packet (1s)
Tablet, oral: 50 mg
Cataflam®: 50 mg
Tablet, delayed release, enteric coated, oral: 25 mg, 50 mg, 75 mg
Tablet, extended release, oral: 100 mg
Voltaren®-XR: 100 mg

Dosage Forms - Canada
Suppository:
Voltaren®: 50 mg, 100mg

diclofenac (ophthalmic) (dye KLOE fen ak)

Medication Safety Issues
Sound-alike/look-alike issues:
Diclofenac may be confused with Diflucan®
International Issues:
Diclofenac may be confused with Duphalac brand name for lactulose [multiple international markets]
Flexin: Brand name for diclofenac [Argentina], but also the brand name for cyclobenzaprine [Chile] and orphenadrine [Israel]
Flexin [Argentina] may be confused with Floxin brand name for flunarizine [Thailand], norfloxacin [South Africa], ofloxacin [U.S., Canada], and pefloxacin [Philippines]

Synonyms diclofenac sodium

U.S. Brand Names Voltaren Ophthalmic®

Canadian Brand Names Voltaren Ophtha®

Therapeutic Category Nonsteroidal Antiinflammatory Drug (NSAID), Ophthalmic

Use Treatment of postoperative inflammation following cataract extraction; temporary relief of pain and photophobia in patients undergoing corneal refractive surgery

General Dosage Range Ophthalmic: *Adults:* 1-2 drops into affected eye 4 times/day

Dosage Forms
Solution, ophthalmic: 0.1% (2.5 mL, 5 mL)
Voltaren Ophthalmic®: 0.1% (2.5 mL, 5 mL)

diclofenac (topical) (dye KLOE fen ak)

Medication Safety Issues
Sound-alike/look-alike issues:
Diclofenac may be confused with Diflucan®
Voltaren® may be confused with traMADol, Ultram®, Verelan®
Other safety concerns:
Transdermal patch (Flector®) contains conducting metal (eg, aluminum); remove patch prior to MRI.
International issues:
Diclofenac may be confused with Duphalac brand name for lactulose [multiple international markets]
Flexin: Brand name for diclofenac [Argentina], but also the brand name for cyclobenzaprine [Chile] and orphenadrine [Israel]
Flexin [Argentina] may be confused with Floxin brand name for flunarizine [Thailand], norfloxacin [South Africa], ofloxacin [U.S., Canada], and perfloxacin [Philippines]

Synonyms diclofenac diethylamine [CAN]; diclofenac epolamine; diclofenac sodium

U.S. Brand Names Flector®; Pennsaid®; Solaraze®; Voltaren® Gel

Canadian Brand Names Pennsaid®; Voltaren® Emulgel™

Therapeutic Category Nonsteroidal Antiinflammatory Drug (NSAID), Topical

Use

Topical gel 1%: Relief of osteoarthritis pain in joints amenable to topical therapy (eg, ankle, elbow, foot, hand, knee, wrist)

Canadian labeling (not in U.S. labeling): Relief of pain associated with acute, localized joint/muscle injuries (eg, sports injuries, strains) in patients ≥16 years of age

Topical gel 3%: Actinic keratosis (AK) in conjunction with sun avoidance

Topical patch: Acute pain due to minor strains, sprains, and contusions

Topical solution: Relief of osteoarthritis pain of the knee

General Dosage Range Topical: *Adults:*

1% gel: Apply 2-4 g to affected joint 4 times/day (maximum: 16 g/day single joint of lower extremity, 8 g/day single joint of upper extremity); Maximum total body dose of 1% gel should not exceed 32 g per day.

3% gel: Apply to lesion area twice daily

Patch: Apply 1 patch twice daily

Solution: Apply 40 drops to each affected knee 4 times/day

Dosage Forms

Gel, topical:

Solaraze®: 3% (100 g)

Voltaren® Gel: 1% (100 g)

Patch, transdermal:

Flector®: 1.3% (30s)

Solution, topical:

Pennsaid®: 1.5% (150 mL)

Dosage Forms - Canada

Gel, topical:

Voltaren® Emulgel™: 1.16% (20 g, 50 g, 100 g)

Solution, topical:

Pennsaid®: 1.5% (15 ml, 30 mL, 60 mL, 120 mL)

diclofenac and misoprostol (dye KLOE fen ak & mye soe PROST ole)

Synonyms misoprostol and diclofenac

U.S. Brand Names Arthrotec®

Canadian Brand Names Arthrotec®

Therapeutic Category Analgesic, Nonnarcotic; Prostaglandin

Use Treatment of osteoarthritis and rheumatoid arthritis in patients at high risk for NSAID-induced gastric and duodenal ulceration

General Dosage Range Oral: *Adults:* Arthrotec® 50: One tablet 2-4 times/day; Arthrotec® 75: One tablet twice daily

Dosage Forms

Tablet, oral:

Arthrotec® 50: Diclofenac 50 mg and misoprostol 200 mcg

Arthrotec® 75: Diclofenac 75 mg and misoprostol 200 mcg

diclofenac diethylamine [CAN] *see* diclofenac (topical) *on page* 280

Diclofenac ECT (Can) *see* diclofenac (systemic) *on page* 279

diclofenac epolamine *see* diclofenac (topical) *on page* 280

diclofenac potassium *see* diclofenac (systemic) *on page* 279

diclofenac sodium *see* diclofenac (ophthalmic) *on page* 280

diclofenac sodium *see* diclofenac (systemic) *on page* 279

diclofenac sodium *see* diclofenac (topical) *on page* 280

Diclofenac Sodium (Can) *see* diclofenac (systemic) *on page* 279

Diclofenac Sodium SR (Can) *see* diclofenac (systemic) *on page* 279

Diclofenac SR (Can) *see* diclofenac (systemic) *on page* 279

dicloxacillin (dye kloks a SIL in)

Synonyms dicloxacillin sodium

Therapeutic Category Penicillin

Use Treatment of systemic infections such as pneumonia, skin and soft tissue infections, and osteomyelitis caused by penicillinase-producing staphylococci

General Dosage Range Oral:
Children <40 kg: 12.5-100 mg/kg/day divided every 6 hours
Children >40 kg: 125-250 mg every 6 hours
Adults: 125-1000 mg every 6-8 hours

Dosage Forms
Capsule, oral: 250 mg, 500 mg

dicloxacillin sodium *see* dicloxacillin *on page* 281

dicyclomine (dye SYE kloe meen)

Medication Safety Issues
Sound-alike/look-alike issues:
Dicyclomine may be confused with diphenhydrAMINE, doxycycline, dyclonine
Bentyl® may be confused with Aventyl®, Benadryl®, Bontril®, Cantil®, Proventil®, TRENtal®
BEERS Criteria medication:
This drug may be potentially inappropriate for use in geriatric patients (Quality of evidence - moderate; Strength of recommendation - strong).

Synonyms dicyclomine hydrochloride; dicycloverine hydrochloride

U.S. Brand Names Bentyl®

Canadian Brand Names Bentylol®; Dicyclomine Hydrochloride Injection; Formulex®; Jamp-Dicyclomine; Protylol; Riva-Dicyclomine

Therapeutic Category Anticholinergic Agent

Use Treatment of functional bowel/irritable bowel syndrome

General Dosage Range
I.M.: *Adults:* 80 mg/day in 4 divided doses
Oral:
Adults: Initial: 20 mg 4 times/day; Maintenance: Up to 160 mg/day in 4 divided doses
Elderly: Initial: 10-20 mg 4 times/day

Dosage Forms
Capsule, oral: 10 mg
Bentyl®: 10 mg
Injection, solution: 10 mg/mL (2 mL)
Bentyl®: 10 mg/mL (2 mL)
Syrup, oral: 10 mg/5 mL (473 mL)
Bentyl®: 10 mg/5 mL (480 mL)
Tablet, oral: 20 mg
Bentyl®: 20 mg

dicyclomine hydrochloride *see* dicyclomine *on page* 282
Dicyclomine Hydrochloride Injection (Can) *see* dicyclomine *on page* 282
dicycloverine hydrochloride *see* dicyclomine *on page* 282
Di-Dak-Sol *see* sodium hypochlorite solution *on page* 842

didanosine (dye DAN oh seen)

Medication Safety Issues
Sound-alike/look-alike issues:
Videx® may be confused with Lidex®

Synonyms ddI; dideoxyinosine

U.S. Brand Names Videx®; Videx® EC

Canadian Brand Names Videx®; Videx® EC

Therapeutic Category Antiviral Agent

Use Treatment of HIV infection; always to be used in combination with at least two other antiretroviral agents

General Dosage Range Dosage adjustment recommended in patients with renal impairment
Oral:
Delayed release:
Children ≥6 years and 20 kg to <25 kg: 200 mg once daily
Children ≥6 years and 25 kg to <60 kg and Adults <60 kg: 250 mg once daily
Children and Adults ≥60 kg: 400 mg once daily

Pediatric powder for oral solution (Videx®):
Infants 2 weeks to 8 months: 100 mg/m^2 twice daily
Children >8 months to 18 years: 120 mg/m^2 twice daily
Adolescents and Adults <60 kg: 125 mg twice daily **or** 250 mg once daily
Adolescents and Adults ≥60 kg: 200 mg twice daily **or** 400 mg once daily

Dosage Forms
Capsule, delayed release, enteric coated beadlets, oral: 125 mg, 200 mg, 250 mg, 400 mg
Videx® EC: 125 mg, 200 mg, 250 mg, 400 mg
Capsule, delayed release, enteric coated pellets, oral: 200 mg, 250 mg, 400 mg
Powder for solution, oral:
Videx®: 2 g/bottle, 4 g/bottle

dideoxyinosine *see* didanosine *on page* 282
Didrex® *see* benzphetamine *on page* 126
Didrocal® (Can) *see* etidronate and calcium carbonate *(Canada only) on page* 364
Didronel® *see* etidronate *on page* 364
dienogest and estradiol *see* estradiol and dienogest *on page* 349

dienogest *(Canada only)* (dye EN oh jest)

Medication Safety Issues
Sound-alike/look-alike issues:
Visanne® may be confused with Vyvanse®
Canadian Brand Names Visanne®
Therapeutic Category Antiandrogen
Use Management of pelvic pain associated with endometriosis
General Dosage Range Oral: *Adult females:* 2 mg once daily
Product Availability Not available in the U.S.
Dosage Forms - Canada
Tablet, oral:
Visanne®: 2 mg

diethylene triamine penta-acetic acid
(dye ETH i leen TRYE a meen PEN ta a SEE tik AS id)

Synonyms calcium diethylene triamine penta-acetic acid (Ca-DTPA); diethylenetriamine pentaacetic acid; DTPA; pentetate calcium trisodium; pentetate zinc trisodium; trisodium calcium diethylenetriaminepentaacetate (Ca-DTPA); zinc diethylene triamine penta-acetic acid (Zn-DTPA); zinc diethylenetriamine-pentaacetate (Zn-DTPA)
U.S. Brand Names Ca-DTPA; Zn-DTPA
Therapeutic Category Antidote
Use Treatment of known or suspected internal contamination with plutonium, americium, or curium
General Dosage Range
I.V.:
Children <12 years: Initial: Ca-DTPA: 14 mg/kg/day (maximum dose: 1 g/day); Maintenance: Zn-DTPA: 14 mg/kg/day (maximum: 1 g/day)
Children ≥12 years and Adults: Ca-DTPA: 1 g/day; Zn-DTPA: 1 g/day
Inhalation: *Children ≥12 years and Adults:* Ca-DTPA: 1 g/day; Zn-DTPA: 1 g/day
Dosage Forms
Injection, solution:
Ca-DTPA: 200 mg/mL (5 mL)
Zn-DTPA: 200 mg/mL (5 mL)

diethylenetriamine pentaacetic acid *see* diethylene triamine penta-acetic acid *on page* 283

diethylpropion (dye eth il PROE pee on)

Synonyms amfepramone; diethylpropion hydrochloride
Canadian Brand Names Tenuate®; Tenuate® Dospan®
Therapeutic Category Anorexiant
Controlled Substance C-IV

Use Short-term (few weeks) adjunct in the management of exogenous obesity

Pharmacotherapy for weight loss is recommended only for obese patients with a body mass index ≥30 kg/m^2, or ≥27 kg/m^2 in the presence of other risk factors such as hypertension, diabetes, and/or dyslipidemia or a high waist circumference; therapy should be used in conjunction with a comprehensive weight management program.

General Dosage Range Oral:
Controlled release: *Children >16 years and Adults:* 75 mg at midmorning
Immediate release: *Children >16 years and Adults:* 25 mg 3 times/day

Dosage Forms
Tablet, oral: 25 mg
Tablet, controlled release, oral: 75 mg

diethylpropion hydrochloride *see* diethylpropion *on page* 283

difenoxin and atropine (dye fen OKS in & A troe peen)

Synonyms atropine and difenoxin
U.S. Brand Names Motofen®
Therapeutic Category Antidiarrheal
Controlled Substance C-IV
Use Treatment of diarrhea
General Dosage Range Oral: *Adults:* 2 tablets (each tablet contains difenoxin hydrochloride 1 mg and atropine sulfate 0.025 mg) initially, then 1 tablet after each loose stool (maximum: 8 tablets/day)
Dosage Forms
Tablet, oral:
Motofen®: Difenoxin 1 mg and atropine 0.025 mg

Differin® *see* adapalene *on page* 36
Differin® XP (Can) *see* adapalene *on page* 36
Dificid™ *see* fidaxomicin *on page* 383
Difil-G® 400 *see* dyphylline and guaifenesin *on page* 321
difimicin *see* fidaxomicin *on page* 383

diflorasone (dye FLOR a sone)

Medication Safety Issues
International issues:
Florone [Germany, Greece] may be confused with Flogene brand name for piroxicam [Brazil]
Synonyms diflorasone diacetate
U.S. Brand Names ApexiCon® E; ApexiCon™
Therapeutic Category Corticosteroid, Topical
Use Relieves inflammation and pruritic symptoms of corticosteroid-responsive dermatosis (high- to very-high potency topical corticosteroid)
General Dosage Range Topical: *Adults:* Cream: Apply 2-4 times/day; Ointment: Apply 1-3 times/day
Dosage Forms
Cream, topical: 0.05% (15 g, 30 g, 60 g)
ApexiCon® E: 0.05% (30 g, 60 g)
Ointment, topical: 0.05% (15 g, 30 g, 60 g)
ApexiCon™: 0.05% (30 g, 60 g)

diflorasone diacetate *see* diflorasone *on page* 284
Diflucan® *see* fluconazole *on page* 388

diflunisal (dye FLOO ni sal)

Medication Safety Issues
BEERS Criteria medication:
This drug may be potentially inappropriate for use in geriatric patients (Quality of evidence - moderate; Strength of recommendation - strong).
Synonyms Dolobid
Canadian Brand Names Apo-Diflunisal®; Novo-Diflunisal; Nu-Diflunisal
Therapeutic Category Analgesic, Nonnarcotic; Nonsteroidal Antiinflammatory Drug (NSAID)

Use Management of inflammatory disorders usually including rheumatoid arthritis and osteoarthritis; can be used as an analgesic for treatment of mild-to-moderate pain

General Dosage Range Dosage adjustment recommended in patients with renal impairment

Oral: *Adults:* 250-500 mg every 8-12 hours (maximum: 1.5 g/day)

Dosage Forms

Tablet, oral: 500 mg

difluorodeoxycytidine hydrochlorothiazide *see* gemcitabine *on page* 422

difluprednate (dye floo PRED nate)

Medication Safety Issues

Sound-alike/look-alike issues:

Durezol® may be confused with Durasal™

U.S. Brand Names Durezol®

Therapeutic Category Corticosteroid, Ophthalmic

Use Treatment of inflammation and pain following ocular surgery; treatment of endogenous anterior uveitis

General Dosage Range **Ophthalmic:** *Adults:* Instill 1 drop in affected eye(s) 2-4 times/day (ocular surgery) **or** 4 times/day for 14 days (uveitis); taper to discontinue

Dosage Forms

Emulsion, ophthalmic:

Durezol®: 0.05% (5 mL)

Digibar™ 190 *see* barium *on page* 114

Digibind *see* digoxin immune Fab *on page* 286

DigiFab® *see* digoxin immune Fab *on page* 286

digitalis *see* digoxin *on page* 285

digoxin (di JOKS in)

Medication Safety Issues

Sound-alike/look-alike issues:

Digoxin may be confused with Desoxyn®, doxepin

Lanoxin® may be confused with Lasix®, levothyroxine, Levoxyl®, Levsinex®, Lomotil®, Mefoxin®, naloxone, Xanax®

High alert medication:

The Institute for Safe Medication Practices (ISMP) includes this medication among its list of drugs which have a heightened risk of causing significant patient harm when used in error.

BEERS Criteria medication:

This drug may be potentially inappropriate for use in geriatric patients (Quality of evidence - moderate; Strength of recommendation - strong).

International issues:

Lanoxin [U.S., Canada, and multiple international markets] may be confused with Limoxin brand name for ambroxol [Indonesia] and amoxicillin [Mexico]

Synonyms digitalis

U.S. Brand Names Lanoxin®

Canadian Brand Names Apo-Digoxin®; Digoxin Injection CSD; Lanoxin®; Pediatric Digoxin CSD; PMS-Digoxin; Toloxin®

Therapeutic Category Antiarrhythmic Agent, Miscellaneous; Cardiac Glycoside

Use Treatment of mild-to-moderate (or stage C as recommended by the ACCF/AHA) heart failure (HF); atrial fibrillation (rate-control)

Note: In treatment of atrial fibrillation (AF), use is not considered first-line unless AF coexistent with heart failure or in sedentary patients (Fuster, 2006).

General Dosage Range Dosage adjustment recommended in patients with renal impairment

I.M., I.V.:

Preterm infants: Digitalizing dose: 15-25 mcg/kg; Maintenance: 4-6 mcg/kg/day in divided doses every 12 hours

Full-term infants: Digitalizing dose: 20-30 mcg/kg; Maintenance: 5-8 mcg/kg/day in divided doses every 12 hours

Children 1 month to 2 years: Digitalizing dose: 30-50 mcg/kg; Maintenance: 7.5-12 mcg/kg/day in divided doses every 12 hours

Children 2-5 years: Digitalizing dose: 25-35 mcg/kg; Maintenance: 6-9 mcg/kg/day in divided doses every 12 hours
Children 5-10 years: Digitalizing dose: 15-30 mcg/kg; Maintenance: 4-8 mcg/kg/day in divided doses every 12 hours
Children >10 years: Digitalizing dose: 8-12 mcg/kg; Maintenance: 2-3 mcg/kg once daily
Adults: Digitalizing dose: 0.5-1 mg; Maintenance: 0.1-0.4 mg once daily

Oral:
Preterm infants: Digitalizing dose: 20-30 mcg/kg; Maintenance: 5-7.5 mcg/kg/day in divided doses every 12 hours
Full-term infants: Digitalizing dose: 25-35 mcg/kg; Maintenance: 6-10 mcg/kg/day in divided doses every 12 hours
Children 1 month to 2 years: Digitalizing dose: 35-60 mcg/kg; Maintenance: 10-15 mcg/kg/day in divided doses every 12 hours
Children 2-5 years: Digitalizing dose: 30-40 mcg/kg; Maintenance: 7.5-10 mcg/kg/day in divided doses every 12 hours
Children 5-10 years: Digitalizing dose: 20-35 mcg/kg; Maintenance: 5-10 mcg/kg/day in divided doses every 12 hours
Children >10 years: Digitalizing dose: 10-15 mcg/kg; Maintenance: 2.5-5 mcg/kg once daily
Adults: Digitalizing dose: 0.75-1.5 mg; Maintenance: 0.125-0.5 mg once daily

Dosage Forms
Injection, solution: 250 mcg/mL (1 mL, 2 mL)
Lanoxin®: 100 mcg/mL (1 mL); 250 mcg/mL (2 mL)
Solution, oral: 50 mcg/mL (2.5 mL, 5 mL, 60 mL)
Tablet, oral: 125 mcg, 250 mcg
Lanoxin®: 125 mcg, 250 mcg

Dosage Forms - Canada
Tablet, oral:
Apo-Digoxin®: 62.5 mcg, 125 mcg, 250 mcg

digoxin immune Fab (di JOKS in i MYUN fab)

Synonyms antidigoxin fab fragments, ovine; Digibind
U.S. Brand Names DigiFab®
Canadian Brand Names DigiFab®
Therapeutic Category Antidote
Use Treatment of life-threatening or potentially life-threatening digoxin intoxication, including:

- acute digoxin ingestion (ie, >10 mg in adults; >0.1 mg/kg or >4 mg in children; ingestions resulting in serum concentrations >10 ng/mL)
- chronic ingestions leading to steady-state digoxin concentrations >6 ng/mL in adults or >4 ng/mL in children
- manifestations of digoxin toxicity due to overdose (eg, life-threatening ventricular arrhythmias, progressive bradycardia, second- or third-degree heart block not responsive to atropine, serum potassium >5.5 mEq/L in adults or >6 mEq/L in children)

General Dosage Range I.V.:
Acute ingestion of known amount: *Children and Adults:* Digoxin Immune Fab Dose (vials) = Total body load (mg) / (0.5)
Based on steady-state digoxin concentration:
Infants and Children ≤20 kg: Digoxin Immune Fab Dose (mg) = [(serum digoxin concentration [ng/mL] x weight [kg]) / 100] x (digoxin immune Fab amount per vial [mg/vial])
Note: Digoxin immune Fab amount per vial: 40 mg/vial.
Children >20 kg and Adults: Digoxin Immune Fab Dose (vials) = (serum digoxin concentration [ng/mL] x weight [kg]) / 100
Amount ingested and blood level unknown:
Children ≤20 kg: Acute toxicity: 20 vials total in 2 divided doses; Chronic toxicity: 1 vial may be sufficient
Children >20 kg and Adults: Acute toxicity: 20 vials total in 2 divided doses; Chronic toxicity: 6 vials

Dosage Forms
Injection, powder for reconstitution:
DigiFab®: 40 mg

Digoxin Injection CSD (Can) *see* digoxin *on page* 285
dihematoporphyrin ether *see* porfimer *on page* 741
dihydroartemisinin hemisuccinate sodium *see* artesunate *on page* 92

dihydrocodeine, aspirin, and caffeine (dye hye droe KOE deen, AS pir in, & KAF een)

Medication Safety Issues

Sound-alike/look-alike issues:

Synalgos®-DC may be confused with Synagis®

High alert medication:

The Institute for Safe Medication Practices (ISMP) includes this medication among its list of drug classes which have a heightened risk of causing significant patient harm when used in error.

Synonyms dihydrocodeine compound

U.S. Brand Names Synalgos®-DC

Therapeutic Category Analgesic, Narcotic

Controlled Substance C-III

Use Management of mild-to-moderate pain that requires relaxation

General Dosage Range Oral: *Adults:* 1-2 capsules every 4-6 hours as needed

Dosage Forms

Capsule, oral:

Synalgos®-DC: Dihydrocodeine 16 mg, aspirin 356.4 mg, and caffeine 30 mg

dihydrocodeine bitartrate, acetaminophen, and caffeine *see* acetaminophen, caffeine, and dihydrocodeine *on page 26*

dihydrocodeine bitartrate, pseudoephedrine hydrochloride, and chlorpheniramine maleate *see* pseudoephedrine, dihydrocodeine, and chlorpheniramine *on page 773*

dihydrocodeine, chlorpheniramine, and phenylephrine

(dye hye droe KOE deen, klor fen IR a meen, & fen il EF rin)

Medication Safety Issues

High alert medication:

The Institute for Safe Medication Practices (ISMP) includes this medication among its list of drug classes which have a heightened risk of causing significant patient harm when used in error.

Synonyms chlorpheniramine maleate, dihydrocodeine bitartrate, and phenylephrine hydrochloride; phenylephrine, chlorpheniramine, and dihydrocodeine

U.S. Brand Names Coldcough PD; DiHydro-PE [OTC]; Novahistine DH; Tusscough DHC™

Therapeutic Category Antihistamine; Antihistamine/Decongestant/Antitussive; Antitussive; Decongestant

Controlled Substance C-III; C-V

Use Symptomatic relief of cough and congestion associated with the upper respiratory tract

General Dosage Range

Oral:

Children 2-6 years: Novahistine DH: 1.25-2.5 mL every 4-6 hours as needed (maximum: 10 mL/day)

Children 6-12 years: Novahistine DH: 2.5-5 mL every 4-6 hours as needed (maximum: 20 mL/day)

Children >12 years and Adults: Novahistine DH: 5-10 mL every 4-6 hours as needed (maximum: 40 mL/day)

Dosage Forms

Liquid, oral:

Novahistine DH: Dihydrocodeine 7.5 mg, chlorpheniramine 2 mg and phenylephrine 5 mg per 5 mL

Syrup, oral:

Coldcough PD, DiHydro-PE [OTC]: Dihydrocodeine 3 mg, chlorpheniramine 2 mg, and phenylephrine 7.5 mg per 5 mL

Tusscough DHC™: Dihydrocodeine 3 mg, chlorpheniramine 5 mg, and phenylephrine 20 mg per 5 mL

dihydrocodeine compound *see* dihydrocodeine, aspirin, and caffeine *on page 287*

DiHydro-CP *see* pseudoephedrine, dihydrocodeine, and chlorpheniramine *on page 773*

dihydroergotamine (dye hye droe er GOT a meen)

Synonyms DHE; dihydroergotamine mesylate

U.S. Brand Names D.H.E. 45®; Migranal®

Canadian Brand Names Migranal®

Therapeutic Category Ergot Alkaloid and Derivative

Use Treatment of migraine headache with or without aura; injection also indicated for treatment of cluster headaches

General Dosage Range

I.M., SubQ: *Adults:* 1 mg initially, may repeat hourly up to 3 mg total (maximum: 6 mg/week)

I.V.: *Adults:* 1 mg initially, may repeat hourly up to 2 mg total (maximum: 6 mg/week)

Intranasal: *Adults:* 1 spray (0.5 mg) in each nostril initially, may repeat after 15 minutes up to 4 sprays total (maximum: 6 sprays/24 hours; 8 sprays/week)

Dosage Forms

Injection, solution: 1 mg/mL (1 mL)

D.H.E. 45®: 1 mg/mL (1 mL)

Solution, intranasal:

Migranal®: 4 mg/mL (1 mL)

dihydroergotamine mesylate *see* dihydroergotamine *on page 287*

dihydroergotoxine *see* ergoloid mesylates *on page 340*

dihydrogenated ergot alkaloids *see* ergoloid mesylates *on page 340*

dihydrohydroxycodeinone *see* oxycodone *on page 678*

dihydromorphinone *see* hydromorphone *on page 460*

DiHydro-PE [OTC] *see* dihydrocodeine, chlorpheniramine, and phenylephrine *on page 287*

dihydroqinghaosu hemisuccinate sodium *see* artesunate *on page 92*

dihydroxyanthracenedione *see* mitoxantrone *on page 608*

dihydroxyanthracenedione dihydrochloride *see* mitoxantrone *on page 608*

1,25 dihydroxycholecalciferol *see* calcitriol *on page 160*

dihydroxydeoxynorvinkaleukoblastine *see* vinorelbine *on page 947*

dihydroxypropyl theophylline *see* dyphylline *on page 321*

diiodohydroxyquin *see* iodoquinol *on page 494*

Dilacor XR® *see* diltiazem *on page 288*

Dilantin® *see* phenytoin *on page 719*

Dilantin-125® *see* phenytoin *on page 719*

Dilatrate®-SR *see* isosorbide dinitrate *on page 504*

Dilaudid® *see* hydromorphone *on page 460*

Dilaudid-HP® *see* hydromorphone *on page 460*

Dilaudid-HP-Plus® (Can) *see* hydromorphone *on page 460*

Dilaudid® Sterile Powder (Can) *see* hydromorphone *on page 460*

Dilaudid-XP® (Can) *see* hydromorphone *on page 460*

Dilt-CD *see* diltiazem *on page 288*

Diltia XT® *see* diltiazem *on page 288*

diltiazem (dil TYE a zem)

Medication Safety Issues

Sound-alike/look-alike issues:

Cardizem® may be confused with Cardene®, Cardene SR®, Cardizem CD®, Cardizem SR®, cortisone

Cartia XT® may be confused with Procardia XL®

Diltiazem may be confused with Calan®, diazepam, Dilantin®

Tiazac® may be confused with Tigan®, Tiazac® XC [CAN], Ziac®

High alert medication:

The Institute for Safe Medication Practices (ISMP) includes this medication (I.V. formulation) among its list of drug classes which have a heightened risk of causing significant patient harm when used in error.

Administration issues:

Significant differences exist between oral and I.V. dosing. Use caution when converting from one route of administration to another.

International issues:

Cardizem [U.S., Canada, and multiple international markets] may be confused with Cardem brand name for celiprolol [Spain]

Cartia XT [U.S.] may be confused with Cartia brand name for aspirin [multiple international markets]

Dilacor XR [U.S.] may be confused with Dilacor brand name for verapamil [Brazil]

Dipen [Greece] may be confused with Depen brand name for penicillamine [U.S.]; Depin brand name for nifedipine [India]; Depon brand name for acetaminophen [Greece]

Tiazac: Brand name for diltiazem [U.S, Canada], but also the brand name for pioglitazone [Chile]

Synonyms diltiazem hydrochloride

U.S. Brand Names Cardizem®; Cardizem® CD; Cardizem® LA; Cartia XT®; Dilacor XR®; Dilt-CD; Dilt-XR; Diltia XT®; Diltzac; Matzim™ LA; Taztia XT®; Tiazac®

Canadian Brand Names Apo-Diltiaz CD®; Apo-Diltiaz SR®; Apo-Diltiaz TZ®; Apo-Diltiaz®; Apo-Diltiaz® Injectable; Ava-Diltiazem; Cardizem® CD; CO Diltiazem CD; CO Diltiazem T; Diltiazem HCl ER®; Diltiazem Hydrochloride Injection; Diltiazem TZ; Diltiazem-CD; Nu-Diltiaz; Nu-Diltiaz-CD; PMS-Diltiazem CD; ratio-Diltiazem CD; Sandoz-Diltiazem CD; Sandoz-Diltiazem T; Teva-Diltiazem; Teva-Diltiazem CD; Teva-Diltiazem HCL ER Capsules; Tiazac®; Tiazac® XC

Therapeutic Category Calcium Channel Blocker

Use

Oral: Essential hypertension; chronic stable angina or angina from coronary artery spasm

Injection: Control of rapid ventricular rate in patients with atrial fibrillation or atrial flutter; conversion of paroxysmal supraventricular tachycardia (PSVT)

General Dosage Range

I.V.: *Adults:* Bolus: 0.25 mg/kg, may repeat 0.35 mg/kg after 15 minutes; Infusion: 5-15 mg/hour

Oral:

Extended release: *Adults:* Initial: 120-240 mg once daily **or** 60-120 mg twice daily; Maintenance: 120-540 mg once daily **or** 240-360 mg/day in 2 divided doses

Immediate release: *Adults:* Initial: 30 mg 4 times/day; Maintenance: 120-320 mg/day in divided doses

Dosage Forms

Capsule, extended release, oral: 60 mg, 90 mg, 120 mg, 180 mg, 240 mg, 300 mg, 360 mg, 420 mg

Cardizem® CD: 120 mg, 180 mg, 240 mg, 300 mg, 360 mg

Cartia XT®: 120 mg, 180 mg, 240 mg, 300 mg

Dilacor XR®: 240 mg

Dilt-CD: 120 mg, 180 mg, 240 mg, 300 mg

Dilt-XR: 120 mg, 180 mg, 240 mg

Diltia XT®: 120 mg, 180 mg, 240 mg

Diltzac: 120 mg, 180 mg, 240 mg, 300 mg, 360 mg

Taztia XT®: 120 mg, 180 mg, 240 mg, 300 mg, 360 mg

Tiazac®: 120 mg, 180 mg, 240 mg, 300 mg, 360 mg, 420 mg

Injection, powder for reconstitution: 100 mg

Injection, solution: 5 mg/mL (5 mL, 10 mL, 25 mL)

Tablet, oral: 30 mg, 60 mg, 90 mg, 120 mg

Cardizem®: 30 mg, 60 mg, 90 mg, 120 mg

Tablet, extended release, oral:

Cardizem® LA: 120 mg, 180 mg, 240 mg, 300 mg, 360 mg, 420 mg

Matzim™ LA: 180 mg, 240 mg, 300 mg, 360 mg, 420 mg

Dosage Forms - Canada

Tablet, extended release:

Tiazac® XC: 120 mg, 180 mg, 240 mg, 300 mg, 360 mg

Diltiazem-CD (Can) *see* diltiazem *on page 288*

Diltiazem HCl ER® (Can) *see* diltiazem *on page 288*

diltiazem hydrochloride *see* diltiazem *on page 288*

Diltiazem Hydrochloride Injection (Can) *see* diltiazem *on page 288*

Diltiazem TZ (Can) *see* diltiazem *on page 288*

Dilt-XR *see* diltiazem *on page 288*

Diltzac *see* diltiazem *on page 288*

Dimaphen™ Children's Cold & Allergy [OTC] *see* brompheniramine and phenylephrine *on page 144*

dimenhydrinate (dye men HYE dri nate)

Medication Safety Issues

Sound-alike/look-alike issues:

DimenhyDRINATE may be confused with diphenhydrAMINE

BEERS Criteria medication:

This drug may be potentially inappropriate for use in geriatric patients (Quality of evidence - varies based on comorbidity; Strength of recommendation - varies based on comorbidity)

Tall-Man dimenhy**DRINATE**

U.S. Brand Names Dramamine® for kids [OTC]; Dramamine® [OTC]; Driminate [OTC]; TripTone® [OTC]

Canadian Brand Names Apo-Dimenhydrinate® [OTC]; Children's Motion Sickness Liquid [OTC]; Dimenhydrinate Injection; Dinate® [OTC]; Gravol IM; Gravol® [OTC]; Jamp-Dimenhydrinate [OTC]; Nauseatol [OTC]; Novo-Dimenate [OTC]; PMS-Dimenhydrinate [OTC]; Sandoz-Dimenhydrinate [OTC]; Travel Tabs [OTC]

Therapeutic Category Antihistamine

Use Treatment and prevention of nausea, vertigo, and vomiting associated with motion sickness

General Dosage Range

Oral:

Children 2-5 years: 12.5-25 mg every 6-8 hours (maximum: 75 mg/day)

Children 6-12 years: 25-50 mg every 6-8 hours (maximum: 150 mg/day)

I.M.:

Children: 1.25 mg/kg **or** 37.5 mg/m^2 4 times/day (maximum: 300 mg/day)

Adults: 50-100 mg every 4 hours

I.V.: *Adults:* 50-100 mg every 4 hours

Dosage Forms

Injection, solution: 50 mg/mL (1 mL)

Tablet, oral: 50 mg

Dramamine® [OTC]: 50 mg

Driminate [OTC]: 50 mg

TripTone® [OTC]: 50 mg

Tablet, chewable, oral:

Dramamine® [OTC]: 50 mg

Dramamine® for kids [OTC]: 25 mg

Dimenhydrinate Injection (Can) *see* dimenhydrinate *on page 289*

dimercaprol (dye mer KAP role)

Synonyms 2,3-dimercapto-1-propanol; 2,3-dimercaptopropan-1-Ol; 2,3-dimercaptopropanol; BAL; British anti-lewisite; dithioglycerol

U.S. Brand Names BAL in Oil®

Therapeutic Category Chelating Agent

Use Antidote to gold, arsenic (except arsine), or acute mercury poisoning (except nonalkyl mercury); adjunct to edetate CALCIUM disodium in acute lead poisoning

General Dosage Range I.M.: *Children and Adults:* Dosage varies greatly depending on indication

Dosage Forms

Injection, oil:

BAL in Oil®: 100 mg/mL (3 mL)

2,3-dimercapto-1-propanol *see* dimercaprol *on page 290*

2,3-dimercaptopropan-1-Ol *see* dimercaprol *on page 290*

2,3-dimercaptopropanol *see* dimercaprol *on page 290*

Dimetapp® Children's Cold & Allergy [OTC] *see* brompheniramine and phenylephrine *on page 144*

Dimetapp® Children's Long Acting Cough Plus Cold [OTC] *see* dextromethorphan and chlorpheniramine *on page 273*

Dimetapp® Children's Nighttime Cold & Congestion [OTC] *see* diphenhydramine and phenylephrine *on page 294*

dimethyl sulfoxide (dye meth il sul FOKS ide)

Synonyms DMSO

U.S. Brand Names Rimso-50®

Canadian Brand Names Dimethyl Sulfoxide Irrigation, USP; Kemsol®; Rimso-50®

Therapeutic Category Urinary Tract Product

Use Symptomatic relief of interstitial cystitis

General Dosage Range Bladder instillation: *Adults:* Instill 50 mL and allow to remain for 15 minutes, may repeat every 1-2 weeks

Dosage Forms

Solution, intravesical:

Rimso-50®: 50% (50 mL)

Dimethyl Sulfoxide Irrigation, USP (Can) *see* dimethyl sulfoxide *on page* 290
dimethyl triazeno imidazole carboxamide *see* dacarbazine *on page* 250
Dinate® [OTC] (Can) *see* dimenhydrinate *on page* 289

dinoprostone (dye noe PROST one)

Medication Safety Issues

International issues:

Cervidil brand name for dinoprostone [U.S., Canada, Australia, New Zealand], but also the brand name for gemeprost [Italy]

Synonyms PGE_2; prostaglandin E_2

U.S. Brand Names Cervidil®; Prepidil®; Prostin E2®

Canadian Brand Names Cervidil®; Prepidil®; Prostin E_2®

Therapeutic Category Prostaglandin

Use

Endocervical gel: Promote cervical ripening in patients at or near term in whom there is a medical or obstetrical indication for the induction of labor

Suppositories: Terminate pregnancy from 12th through 20th week of gestation; evacuate uterus in cases of missed abortion or intrauterine fetal death up to 28 weeks of gestation; manage benign hydatidiform mole (nonmetastatic gestational trophoblastic disease)

Vaginal insert: Initiation and/or continuation of cervical ripening in patients at or near term in whom there is a medical or obstetrical indication for the induction of labor

General Dosage Range

Endocervical: *Children (females of reproductive age) and Adults (females):* 0.5 mg; may repeat every 6 hours if needed. Maximum cumulative dose: 1.5 mg/24 hours

Intravaginal: *Children (females of reproductive age) and Adults (females):* Insert: 10 mg; remove at onset of active labor or after 12 hours; Suppository: 20 mg every 3-5 hours until abortion occurs

Dosage Forms

Gel, endocervical:

Prepidil®: 0.5 mg/3 g (3 g)

Insert, vaginal:

Cervidil®: 10 mg (1s)

Suppository, vaginal:

Prostin E2®: 20 mg (5s)

Diocaine® (Can) *see* proparacaine *on page* 766
Diocarpine (Can) *see* pilocarpine (ophthalmic) *on page* 723
Diochloram® (Can) *see* chloramphenicol *on page* 195
Diocto [OTC] *see* docusate *on page* 304
dioctyl calcium sulfosuccinate *see* docusate *on page* 304
dioctyl sodium sulfosuccinate *see* docusate *on page* 304
Diodex® (Can) *see* dexamethasone (ophthalmic) *on page* 267
Diodoquin® (Can) *see* iodoquinol *on page* 494
Diogent® (Can) *see* gentamicin (ophthalmic) *on page* 424
Diomycin® (Can) *see* erythromycin (ophthalmic) *on page* 343
Dionephrine® (Can) *see* phenylephrine (ophthalmic) *on page* 716
Diopentolate® (Can) *see* cyclopentolate *on page* 244
Diopred® (Can) *see* prednisolone (ophthalmic) *on page* 754
Dioptic's Atropine Solution (Can) *see* atropine *on page* 102
Dioptimyd® (Can) *see* sulfacetamide and prednisolone *on page* 859
Dioptrol® (Can) *see* neomycin, polymyxin B, and dexamethasone *on page* 634
Diosulf™ (Can) *see* sulfacetamide (ophthalmic) *on page* 858
Diotame [OTC] *see* bismuth *on page* 135
Diotrope® (Can) *see* tropicamide *on page* 924
Diovan® *see* valsartan *on page* 935
Diovan HCT® *see* valsartan and hydrochlorothiazide *on page* 936
Diovol® (Can) *see* aluminum hydroxide and magnesium hydroxide *on page* 56
Diovol® Ex (Can) *see* aluminum hydroxide and magnesium hydroxide *on page* 56

Diovol Plus® (Can) *see* aluminum hydroxide, magnesium hydroxide, and simethicone *on page* 56
Dipentum® *see* olsalazine *on page* 664
Diphen [OTC] *see* diphenhydramine (systemic) *on page* 292
Diphenhist® [OTC] *see* diphenhydramine (systemic) *on page* 292

diphenhydramine (systemic) (dye fen HYE dra meen)

Medication Safety Issues

Sound-alike/look-alike issues:

DiphenhydrAMINE may be confused with desipramine, dicyclomine, dimenhyDRINATE
Benadryl® may be confused with benazepril, Bentyl®, Benylin®, Caladryl®

BEERS Criteria medication:

This drug may be potentially inappropriate for use in geriatric patients (Quality of evidence - moderate; Strength of recommendation - strong).

International issues:

Sominex brand name for diphenhydramine [U.S., Canada], but also the brand name for promethazine [Great Britain]; valerian [Chile]

Synonyms diphenhydramine citrate; diphenhydramine hydrochloride; diphenhydramine tannate

Tall-Man diphenhydr**AMINE**

U.S. Brand Names Aler-Cap [OTC]; Aler-Dryl [OTC]; Aler-Tab [OTC]; AllerMax® [OTC]; Altaryl [OTC]; Anti-Hist [OTC]; Banophen™ [OTC]; Benadryl® Allergy Quick Dissolve [OTC]; Benadryl® Allergy [OTC]; Benadryl® Children's Allergy FastMelt® [OTC]; Benadryl® Children's Allergy Perfect Measure™ [OTC]; Benadryl® Children's Allergy [OTC]; Benadryl® Children's Dye Free Allergy [OTC]; Benadryl® Dye-Free Allergy [OTC]; Compoz® [OTC]; Diphen [OTC]; Diphenhist® [OTC]; Geri-Dryl; Histaprin [OTC]; Nytol® Quick Caps [OTC]; Nytol® Quick Gels [OTC]; PediaCare® Children's Allergy [OTC]; PediaCare® Children's NightTime Cough [OTC]; Q-dryl [OTC]; Quenalin [OTC]; Siladryl Allergy [OTC]; Silphen [OTC]; Simply Sleep® [OTC]; Sleep-ettes D [OTC]; Sleep-Tabs [OTC]; Sleepinal® [OTC]; Sominex® Maximum Strength [OTC]; Sominex® [OTC]; Theraflu® Thin Strips® Multi Symptom [OTC]; Triaminic Thin Strips® Children's Cough & Runny Nose [OTC]; Twilite® [OTC]; Unisom® SleepGels® Maximum Strength [OTC]; Unisom® SleepMelts™ [OTC]; Vicks® ZzzQuil™ [OTC]

Canadian Brand Names Allerdryl®; Allernix; Benadryl®; Nytol®; Nytol® Extra Strength; PMS-Diphenhydramine; Simply Sleep®; Sominex®

Therapeutic Category Histamine H_1 Antagonist; Histamine H_1 Antagonist, First Generation

Use Symptomatic relief of allergic symptoms caused by histamine release including nasal allergies and allergic dermatosis; adjunct to epinephrine in the treatment of anaphylaxis; nighttime sleep aid; prevention or treatment of motion sickness; antitussive; management of parkinsonian syndrome including drug-induced extrapyramidal symptoms

General Dosage Range

I.M., I.V.:

Children: 5 mg/kg/day **or** 150 mg/m^2/day in divided every 6-8 hours (maximum: 300 mg/day)
Adults: 10-100 per dose (maximum: 400 mg/day)
Elderly: Initial: 25 mg 2-3 times/day

Oral:

Children 2 to <6 years: 5 mg/kg/day **or** 150 mg/m^2/day in divided every 6-8 hours (maximum: 300 mg/day) **or** 6.25 mg every 4-6 hours (maximum: 37.5 mg/day)
Children 6 to <12 years: 5 mg/kg/day **or** 150 mg/m^2/day in divided every 6-8 hours (maximum: 300 mg/day) **or** 12.5-25 mg every 4-6 hours (maximum: 150 mg/day)
Children ≥12 years: 5 mg/kg/day **or** 150 mg/m^2/day in divided doses every 6-8 hours **or** 25-50 mg every 4-6 hours (maximum: 300 mg/day) **or** 50 mg at bedtime
Adults: 25-50 mg every 4-6 hours (maximum: 400 mg/day) **or** 50 mg at bedtime
Elderly: Initial: 25 mg 2-3 times/day

Dosage Forms

Caplet, oral:

Aler-Dryl [OTC]: 50 mg
AllerMax® [OTC]: 50 mg
Anti-Hist [OTC]: 25 mg
Compoz® [OTC]: 50 mg
Histaprin [OTC]: 25 mg
Nytol® Quick Caps [OTC]: 25 mg
Simply Sleep® [OTC]: 25 mg
Sleep-ettes D [OTC]: 50 mg

Sominex® Maximum Strength [OTC]: 50 mg
Twilite® [OTC]: 50 mg

Capsule, oral: 25 mg, 50 mg
Aler-Cap [OTC]: 25 mg
Banophen™ [OTC]: 25 mg
Benadryl® Allergy [OTC]: 25 mg
Diphen [OTC]: 25 mg
Diphenhist® [OTC]: 25 mg
Q-dryl [OTC]: 25 mg
Sleepinal® [OTC]: 50 mg

Capsule, liquid filled, oral:
Vicks® ZzzQuil™ [OTC]: 25 mg

Capsule, softgel, oral:
Benadryl® Dye-Free Allergy [OTC]: 25 mg
Compoz® [OTC]: 50 mg
Nytol® Quick Gels [OTC]: 50 mg
Unisom® SleepGels® Maximum Strength [OTC]: 50 mg

Captab, oral:
Diphenhist® [OTC]: 25 mg

Elixir, oral:
Altaryl [OTC]: 12.5 mg/5 mL (480 mL, 3840 mL)
Banophen™ [OTC]: 12.5 mg/5 mL (120 mL, 480 mL)

Injection, solution: 50 mg/mL (1 mL, 10 mL)

Injection, solution [preservative free]: 50 mg/mL (1 mL)

Liquid, oral:
AllerMax® [OTC]: 12.5 mg/5 mL (120 mL)
Benadryl® Children's Allergy [OTC]: 12.5 mg/5 mL (118 mL, 236 mL)
Benadryl® Children's Allergy Perfect Measure™ [OTC]: 12.5 mg/5 mL (5 mL)
Benadryl® Children's Dye Free Allergy [OTC]: 12.5 mg/5 mL (118 mL)
Siladryl Allergy [OTC]: 12.5 mg/5 mL (118 mL, 237 mL, 473 mL)
Vicks® ZzzQuil™ [OTC]: 50 mg/30 mL (177 mL, 354 mL)

Solution, oral: 12.5 mg/5 mL (5 mL, 10 mL, 20 mL)
Diphenhist® [OTC]: 12.5 mg/5 mL (118 mL, 473 mL)
Q-dryl [OTC]: 12.5 mg/5 mL (120 mL, 240 mL, 480 mL)

Strip, orally disintegrating, oral:
Benadryl® Allergy Quick Dissolve [OTC]: 25 mg (10s)
Theraflu® Thin Strips® Multi Symptom [OTC]: 25 mg (12s, 24s)
Triaminic Thin Strips® Children's Cough & Runny Nose [OTC]: 12.5 mg (14s)

Syrup, oral:
PediaCare® Children's Allergy [OTC]: 12.5 mg/5 mL (118 mL)
PediaCare® Children's NightTime Cough [OTC]: 12.5 mg/5 mL (118 mL)
Quenalin [OTC]: 12.5 mg/5 mL (118 mL)
Silphen [OTC]: 12.5 mg/5 mL (118 mL, 237 mL, 473 mL)

Tablet, oral: 25 mg, 50 mg
Aler-Tab [OTC]: 25 mg
Banophen™ [OTC]: 25 mg
Benadryl® Allergy [OTC]: 25 mg
Geri-Dryl: 25 mg
Sleep-Tabs [OTC]: 25 mg
Sominex® [OTC]: 25 mg

Tablet, orally dissolving, oral:
Benadryl® Children's Allergy FastMelt® [OTC]: 12.5 mg
Unisom® SleepMelts™ [OTC]: 25 mg

diphenhydramine (topical) (dye fen HYE dra meen)

Medication Safety Issues

Sound-alike/look-alike issues:
DiphenhydrAMINE may be confused with desipramine, dicyclomine, dimenhyDRINATE
Benadryl® may be confused with benazepril, Bentyl®, Benylin®, Caladryl®

Administration issues:

Institute for Safe Medication Practices (ISMP) has reported cases of patients mistakenly *swallowing* Benadryl® Itch Stopping [OTC] gel intended for topical application. Unclear labeling and similar packaging of the topical gel in containers resembling an oral liquid are factors believed to be contributing to the administration errors. The topical gel contains camphor which can be toxic if swallowed. ISMP has requested the manufacturer to make the necessary changes to prevent further confusion.

Synonyms diphenhydramine hydrochloride

Tall-Man diphenhydr**AMINE**

U.S. Brand Names Banophen™ Anti-Itch [OTC]; Benadryl® Extra Strength Itch Stopping [OTC]; Benadryl® Itch Relief Extra Strength [OTC]; Benadryl® Itch Stopping Extra Strength [OTC]; Benadryl® Itch Stopping [OTC]; Dermamycin® [OTC]

Canadian Brand Names Benadryl® Cream; Benadryl® Itch Relief Stick; Benadryl® Spray

Therapeutic Category Histamine H_1 Antagonist; Histamine H_1 Antagonist, First Generation; Topical Skin Product

Use Topically for relief of pain and itching associated with insect bites, minor cuts and burns, or rashes due to poison ivy, poison oak, and poison sumac

General Dosage Range Topical: *Children ≥2 years and Adults:* Apply 1% or 2% up to 3-4 times/day

Dosage Forms

Cream, topical: 2% (30 g)

Banophen™ Anti-Itch [OTC]: 2% (28.4 g)

Benadryl® Itch Stopping [OTC]: 1% (14.2 g, 28.3 g)

Benadryl® Itch Stopping Extra Strength [OTC]: 2% (14.2 g)

Dermamycin® [OTC]: 2% (28 g)

Gel, topical:

Benadryl® Extra Strength Itch Stopping [OTC]: 2% (120 mL)

Liquid, topical:

Benadryl® Itch Relief Extra Strength [OTC]: 2% (14 mL)

Benadryl® Itch Stopping Extra Strength [OTC]: 2% (59 mL)

Dermamycin® [OTC]: 2% (60 mL)

diphenhydramine and acetaminophen *see* acetaminophen and diphenhydramine *on page* 23

diphenhydramine and ASA *see* aspirin and diphenhydramine *on page* 97

diphenhydramine and aspirin *see* aspirin and diphenhydramine *on page* 97

diphenhydramine and phenylephrine (dye fen HYE dra meen & fen il EF rin)

Synonyms diphenhydramine hydrochloride and phenylephrine hydrochloride; diphenhydramine tannate and phenylephrine tannate; phenylephrine and diphenhydramine; phenylephrine hydrochloride and diphenhydramine hydrochloride; phenylephrine tannate and diphenhydramine tannate

U.S. Brand Names Aldex® CT; Benadryl-D® Allergy & Sinus [OTC]; Benadryl-D® Children's Allergy & Sinus [OTC]; Dimetapp® Children's Nighttime Cold & Congestion [OTC]; Robitussin® Night Time Cough & Cold [OTC] [DSC]; Triaminic® Children's Night Time Cold & Cough [OTC]; Triaminic® Children's Thin Strips® Night Time Cold & Cough [OTC]

Therapeutic Category Alpha/Beta Agonist; Histamine H_1 Antagonist; Histamine H_1 Antagonist, First Generation

Use Temporary relief of symptoms of allergic rhinitis, sinusitis, and other upper respiratory conditions, including sinus/nasal congestion, sneezing, stuffy/runny nose, itchy/watery eyes, and cough

General Dosage Range Oral:

Children 6-11 years: Aldex® CT: 1/2 to 1 tablet every 6 hours; OTC labeling: 5-10 mL or 1 strip every 4 hours as needed (maximum: 6 doses/24 hours)

Children ≥12 years and Adults: Aldex® CT: 1-2 tablets every 6 hours; OTC labeling: 10-20 mL every 4 hours as needed or 1 tablet every 4 hours as needed (maximum: 6 doses/24 hours)

Dosage Forms

Liquid, oral:

Benadryl-D® Children's Allergy & Sinus [OTC]: Diphenhydramine 12.5 mg and phenylephrine 5 mg per 5 mL (118 mL)

Strip, orally disintegrating:

Triaminic® Children's Thin Strips® Night Time Cold & Cough [OTC]: Diphenhydramine 12.5 mg and phenylephrine 5 mg

Syrup, oral:

Dimetapp® Children's Nighttime Cold and Congestion [OTC]: Diphenhydramine 6.25 mg and phenylephrine 2.5 mg per 5 mL (120 mL)

Triaminic® Children's Night Time Cold & Cough [OTC]: Diphenhydramine 6.25 mg and phenylephrine 2.5 mg per 5 mL (118 mL)

Tablet, oral:

Benadryl-D® Allergy & Sinus [OTC]: Diphenhydramine 25 mg and phenylephrine 10 mg

Tablet, chewable, oral:

Aldex® CT: Diphenhydramine 12.5 mg and phenylephrine 5 mg

diphenhydramine citrate *see* diphenhydramine (systemic) *on page 292*

diphenhydramine citrate and aspirin *see* aspirin and diphenhydramine *on page 97*

diphenhydramine hydrochloride *see* diphenhydramine (systemic) *on page 292*

diphenhydramine hydrochloride *see* diphenhydramine (topical) *on page 293*

diphenhydramine hydrochloride and phenylephrine hydrochloride *see* diphenhydramine and phenylephrine *on page 294*

diphenhydramine, phenylephrine hydrochloride, and acetaminophen *see* acetaminophen, diphenhydramine, and phenylephrine *on page 29*

diphenhydramine tannate *see* diphenhydramine (systemic) *on page 292*

diphenhydramine tannate and phenylephrine tannate *see* diphenhydramine and phenylephrine *on page 294*

diphenoxylate and atropine (dye fen OKS i late & A troe peen)

Medication Safety Issues

Sound-alike/look-alike issues:

Lomotil® may be confused with LaMICtal®, LamISIL®, lamoTRIgine, Lanoxin®, Lasix®, loperamide

International issues:

Lomotil [U.S., Canada, and multiple international markets] may be confused with Ludiomil brand name for maprotiline [multiple international markets]

Lomotil: Brand name for diphenoxylate [U.S., Canada, and multiple international markets], but also the brand name for loperamide [Mexico, Philippines]

Synonyms atropine and diphenoxylate

U.S. Brand Names Lomotil®

Canadian Brand Names Lomotil®

Therapeutic Category Antidiarrheal

Controlled Substance C-V

Use Treatment of diarrhea

General Dosage Range Oral:

Children 2-12 years: Initial: Diphenoxylate 0.3-0.4 mg/kg/day in 4 divided doses (maximum: 10 mg/day); Maintenance: Reduce as needed, may be as low as 25% of the initial daily dose

Adults: Initial: Diphenoxylate 5 mg 4 times/day (maximum: 20 mg/day); Maintenance: Reduce as needed, may be as low as 5 mg/day

Dosage Forms

Solution, oral: Diphenoxylate 2.5 mg and atropine 0.025 mg per 5 mL

Tablet, oral: Diphenoxylate 2.5 mg and atropine 0.025 mg

diphenylhydantoin *see* phenytoin *on page 719*

diphtheria and tetanus toxoids (dif THEER ee a & TET a nus TOKS oyds)

Medication Safety Issues

Sound-alike/look-alike issues:

Diphtheria and Tetanus Toxoids (Td) may be confused with tuberculin purified protein derivative (PPD)

Pediatric diphtheria and tetanus (DT) may be confused with adult tetanus and diphtheria (Td)

Synonyms DT; Td; tetanus and diphtheria toxoid

U.S. Brand Names Decavac® [DSC]; Tenivac™

Canadian Brand Names Td Adsorbed

Therapeutic Category Toxoid

Use

Diphtheria and tetanus toxoids adsorbed for pediatric use (DT): Infants and children through 6 years of age: Active immunization against diphtheria and tetanus when pertussis vaccine is contraindicated

Tetanus and diphtheria toxoids adsorbed for adult use (Td) (Decavac®, Tenivac™): Children ≥7 years of age and Adults: Active immunization against diphtheria and tetanus; tetanus prophylaxis in wound management

The Advisory Committee on Immunization Practices (ACIP) recommends routine vaccination for the following:

- Adults and children ≥7 years should receive a booster dose of Td every 10 years; may substitute a single Td booster dose with Tdap
- Children 7-10 years of age, adults, and the elderly (≥65 years) who are wounded in bombings or similar mass casualty events who have penetrating injuries or nonintact skin exposure and who cannot confirm receipt of a tetanus booster within the previous 5 years, may also receive a single dose of Td; children ≥11 years and adults may also receive Td if Tdap is unavailable

General Dosage Range I.M.:

DT: *Children 6 weeks to <7 years:* Primary immunization: 0.5 mL per dose, total of 5 doses

Td: *Children ≥7 years and Adults:* Primary immunization: Two 0.5 mL doses 4-8 weeks apart, followed by third 0.5 mL dose 6-8 months later, total of 3 doses; Booster immunization: 0.5 mL every 10 years

Dosage Forms

Injection, suspension [Td, adult; preservative free]: Diphtheria 2 Lf units and tetanus 2 Lf units per 0.5 mL (0.5 mL)

Tenivac™: Diphtheria 2 Lf units and tetanus 5 Lf units per 0.5 mL (0.5 mL)

Injection, suspension [DT, pediatric; preservative free]: Diphtheria 25 Lf units and tetanus 5 Lf units per 0.5 mL (0.5 mL)

diphtheria and tetanus toxoids, acellular pertussis and *Haemophilus influenzae* b conjugate vaccine

(dif THEER ee a & TET a nus TOKS oyds, ay CEL yoo lar per TUS sis & hem OF fi lus in floo EN za bee KON joo gate vak SEEN)

Synonyms *Haemophilus influenzae* b conjugate vaccine and diphtheria, tetanus toxoids, and acellular pertussis vaccine; DTaP/Hib

U.S. Brand Names TriHIBit® [DSC]

Therapeutic Category Toxoid; Vaccine, Inactivated Bacteria

Use Active immunization of children 15-18 months of age for prevention of diphtheria, tetanus, pertussis, and invasive disease caused by *H. influenzae* type b

The Advisory Committee on Immunization Practices (ACIP) recommends the use of TriHIBit® for the fourth dose of the diphtheria, tetanus, pertussis, and *Haemophilus* vaccine series. Whenever feasible, the same manufacturer should be used to provide the pertussis component; however, vaccination should not be deferred if a specific brand is not known or is not available.

General Dosage Range I.M.: *Children 15-18 months:* 0.5 mL

Dosage Forms

Injection, suspension [preservative free]:

TriHIBit®: Diphtheria 6.7 Lf units, tetanus 5 Lf units, acellular pertussis antigens [inactivated pertussis toxin 23.4 mcg, filamentous hemagglutinin 23.4 mcg], and *Haemophilus* b capsular polysaccharide 10 mcg [bound to tetanus toxoid 24 mcg] per 0.5 mL (0.5 mL) [Tripedia® vaccine used to reconstitute ActHIB® forms TriHIBit®]

diphtheria and tetanus toxoids, acellular pertussis, and poliovirus vaccine

(dif THEER ee a & TET a nus TOKS oyds, ay CEL yoo lar per TUS sis & POE lee oh VYE rus vak SEEN)

Medication Safety Issues

Sound-alike/look-alike issues:

Adacel® (trade name for Diphtheria and Tetanus Toxoids, and Acellular Pertussis Vaccine) should not be confused with Adacel®-Polio (trade name for Diphtheria and Tetanus Toxoids, Acellular Pertussis, and Poliovirus Vaccine in Canada)

Synonyms diphtheria and tetanus toxoids and acellular pertussis adsorbed, and inactivated poliovirus vaccine combined; diphtheria, tetanus toxoids, acellular pertussis (DTaP); DTaP-IPV; poliovirus, inactivated (IPV)

U.S. Brand Names Kinrix®

Canadian Brand Names Adacel®-Polio

Therapeutic Category Vaccine, Inactivated

Use Kinrix®: Active immunization against diphtheria, tetanus, pertussis, and poliomyelitis, used as the fifth dose in the DTaP series and the 4th dose in the IPV series

The Advisory Committee on Immunization Practices (ACIP) recommends routine vaccination for use as the fifth dose in the DTaP series and the fourth dose in the IPV series in children who received DTaP (Infanrix®) and/or DTaP-Hepatitis B-IPV (Pediarix®) as the first 3 doses and DTaP (Infanrix®) as the fourth dose. Whenever feasible, the same manufacturer should be used to provide the pertussis component; however, vaccination should not be deferred if a specific brand is not known or is not available.

Adacel®-Polio (Canadian availability): Active booster immunization against diphtheria, tetanus, pertussis, and poliomyelitis; alternative to fifth dose of DTaP-IPV; May be used for wound management when a tetanus toxoid-containing vaccine is needed for wound management [refer to current National Advisory Committee on Immunization (NACI) guidelines]

General Dosage Range I.M.: *Children 4-6 years:* 0.5 mL

Dosage Forms

Injection, suspension [preservative free]:

Kinrix®: Diphtheria toxoid 25 Lf, tetanus toxoid 10 Lf, acellular pertussis antigens [inactivated pertussis toxin 25 mcg, filamentous hemagglutinin 25 mcg, pertactin 8 mcg], type 1 poliovirus 40 D-antigen units, type 2 poliovirus 8 D-antigen units, and type 3 poliovirus 32 D-antigen units per 0.5 mL (0.5 mL)

Dosage Forms - Canada

Injection, suspension [preservative free]:

Adacel®-Polio: Diphtheria toxoid 2 Lf, tetanus toxoid 5 Lf, acellular pertussis antigens [inactivated pertussis toxoid 2.5 mcg, filamentous hemagglutinin 5 mcg, pertactin 3 mcg, types 2 and 3 fimbriae 5 mcg], type 1 poliovirus 40 D-antigen units, type 2 poliovirus 8 D-antigen units, and type 3 poliovirus 32 D-antigen units per 0.5 mL (0.5 mL)

diphtheria and tetanus toxoids, acellular pertussis, hepatitis B (recombinant), poliovirus (inactivated), and *Haemophilus influenzae* B conjugate (adsorbed) vaccine

(dif THEER ee a & TET a nus TOKS oyds, ay CEL yoo lar per TUS sis, hep a TYE tis bee ree KOM be nant, POE lee oh VYE rus in ak ti VAY ted, & hem OF fi lus in floo EN za bee KON joo gate ad SORBED vak SEEN)

Medication Safety Issues

Sound-alike/look-alike issues:

Infanrix Hexa™ may be confused with Infanrix®

Synonyms diphtheria and tetanus toxoids and acellular pertussis, hepatitis B (recombinant), inactivated poliovirus vaccine, and *Haemophilus influenzae* type B combined; DTaP-HepB-IPV-Hib

Canadian Brand Names Infanrix Hexa™

Therapeutic Category Vaccine, Inactivated (Bacterial, Viral)

Use Active primary immunization against diphtheria, tetanus, pertussis, hepatitis B, poliomyelitis and disease caused by *Haemophilus influenzae* type b in infants and children 6 weeks to 2 years of age; booster immunization (at 18 months) in infants who previously received a full primary vaccination course of each component of the vaccine

General Dosage Range I.M.: *Children 6 weeks to 2 years:* Primary immunization: 0.5 mL every 8 weeks for a total of 3 doses; booster dose: 0.5 mL

Product Availability Not available in U.S.

Dosage Forms - Canada

Injection, suspension:

Infanrix Hexa™: Diphtheria toxoid 25 Lf, tetanus toxoid 10 Lf, acellular pertussis antigens [inactivated pertussis toxin 25 mcg, filamentous hemagglutinin 25 mcg, pertactin 8 mcg], HBsAg 10 mcg, type 1 poliovirus 40 D antigen units, type 2 poliovirus 8 D antigen units and type 3 poliovirus 32 D antigen units, *Haemophilus* b capsular polysaccharide 10 mcg [bound to tetanus toxoid 20-40 mcg] per 0.5 mL (0.5 mL) [contains aluminum, neomycin sulfate (trace amounts), polymyxin B (trace amounts), polysorbate 20, polysorbate 80, and yeast protein ≤5%; Pediarix™ vaccine used to reconstitute Hib forms Infanrix Hexa™]

diphtheria and tetanus toxoids, acellular pertussis, poliovirus and *Haemophilus* b conjugate vaccine

(dif THEER ee a & TET a nus TOKS oyds ay CEL yoo lar per TUS sis POE lee oh VYE rus & hem OF fi lus bee KON joo gate vak SEEN)

Medication Safety Issues

Administration issues:

Pentacel® is supplied in two vials, one containing DTaP-IPV liquid and one containing Hib powder, which must be mixed together in order to administer the recommended vaccine components.

Synonyms *Haemophilus* B conjugate (Hib); *Haemophilus* B polysaccharide; diphtheria toxoid; diphtheria, tetanus toxoids, acellular pertussis (DTaP); DTaP-IPV/Hib; pertussis, acellular (adsorbed); poliovirus, inactivated (IPV); tetanus toxoid

U.S. Brand Names Pentacel®

Canadian Brand Names Pediacel®; Pentacel®

Therapeutic Category Vaccine, Inactivated

Use Active immunization against diphtheria, tetanus, pertussis, poliomyelitis, and invasive disease caused by *H. influenzae* type b in children 6 weeks through 4 years of age

Advisory Committee on Immunization Practices (ACIP) recommends that Pentacel® (DTaP-IPV/Hib) may be used to provide the recommended DTaP, IPV, and Hib immunization in children <5 years of age. Whenever feasible, the same manufacturer should be used to provide the pertussis component; however, vaccination should not be deferred if a specific brand is not known or is not available. The Hib component in Pentacel® contains a tetanus toxoid conjugate. A Hib vaccine containing the PRP-OMP conjugate (PedvaxHIB®) may provide a more rapid seroconversion following the first dose and may be preferable to use in certain populations (eg, American Indian or Alaska Native children).

General Dosage Range I.M.: *Children 6 weeks to ≤4 years:* 0.5 mL

Dosage Forms

Injection, suspension:

Pentacel®: Diphtheria toxoid 15 Lf, tetanus toxoid 5 Lf, acellular pertussis antigens, poliovirus, and *Haemophilus* b capsular polysaccharide 10 mcg per 0.5 mL (0.5 mL)

diphtheria and tetanus toxoids and acellular pertussis adsorbed, and inactivated poliovirus vaccine combined *see* diphtheria and tetanus toxoids, acellular pertussis, and poliovirus vaccine *on page 296*

diphtheria and tetanus toxoids and acellular pertussis adsorbed, hepatitis B (recombinant) and inactivated poliovirus vaccine combined *see* diphtheria, tetanus toxoids, acellular pertussis, hepatitis B (recombinant), and poliovirus (inactivated) vaccine *on page 300*

diphtheria and tetanus toxoids and acellular pertussis, hepatitis B (recombinant), inactivated poliovirus vaccine, and *Haemophilus influenzae* type B combined *see* diphtheria and tetanus toxoids, acellular pertussis, hepatitis B (recombinant), poliovirus (inactivated), and *Haemophilus influenzae* B conjugate (adsorbed) vaccine *on page 297*

diphtheria and tetanus toxoids, and acellular pertussis vaccine

(dif THEER ee a & TET a nus TOKS oyds & ay CEL yoo lar per TUS sis vak SEEN)

Medication Safety Issues

Sound-alike/look-alike issues:

Adacel® (Tdap) may be confused with Daptacel® (DTaP)

Tdap (Adacel®, Boostrix®) may be confused with DTaP (Daptacel®, Infanrix®, Tripedia)

Administration issues:

Carefully review product labeling to prevent inadvertent administration of Tdap when DTaP is indicated. Tdap contains lower amounts of diphtheria toxoid and some pertussis antigens than DTaP.

Tdap is not indicated for use in children <10 years of age

DTaP is not indicated for use in persons ≥7 years of age

Guidelines are available in case of inadvertent administration of these products; refer to ACIP recommendations, February 2006 available at http://www.cdc.gov/mmwr/preview/mmwrhtml/rr55e223a1.htm

Other safety concerns:

DTaP: Diphtheria and tetanus toxoids and acellular pertussis vaccine

DTP: Diphtheria and tetanus toxoids and pertussis vaccine (unspecified pertussis antigens)

DTwP: Diphtheria and tetanus toxoids and whole-cell pertussis vaccine (no longer available on U.S. market)

Tdap: Tetanus toxoid, reduced diphtheria toxoid, and acellular pertussis vaccine

Synonyms DTaP; Tdap; tetanus toxoid, reduced diphtheria toxoid, and acellular pertussis, adsorbed; Tripedia

U.S. Brand Names Adacel®; Boostrix®; Daptacel®; Infanrix®

Canadian Brand Names Adacel®; Boostrix®

Therapeutic Category Toxoid

Use

Daptacel®, Infanrix® (DTaP): Active immunization against diphtheria, tetanus, and pertussis from age 6 weeks through 6 years of age (prior to seventh birthday)

Adacel®, Boostrix® (Tdap): Active booster immunization against diphtheria, tetanus, and pertussis

The Advisory Committee on Immunization Practices (ACIP) recommends routine vaccination for the following:

Children 6 weeks to <7 years (DTaP):

- For primary immunization against diphtheria, tetanus and pertussis
- Pediatric patients who are wounded in bombings or similar mass casualty events and who have penetrating injuries or nonintact skin exposure, and have an uncertain vaccination history should receive a tetanus booster with DTaP (if no contraindications exist) (CDC, 57[RR6], 2008)

Children 7-10 years (Tdap):

- Children not fully vaccinated against pertussis should receive a single dose of Tdap (if no contraindications exist) (CDC, 60[1], 2011)
- Children never vaccinated against diphtheria, tetanus, or pertussis, or whose vaccination status is not known should receive a series of three vaccinations containing tetanus and diphtheria toxoids and the first dose should be with Tdap (CDC, 60[1], 2011)

Adolescents 11-18 years (Tdap):

- A single dose of Tdap as a booster dose in adolescents who have completed the recommended childhood DTaP vaccination series (preferred age of administration is 11-12 years) (CDC, 60[1], 2011)

Adolescents ≥11 years and Adults (Tdap):

- Persons wounded in bombings or similar mass casualty events and who cannot confirm receipt of a tetanus booster within the previous 5 years and who have penetrating injuries or nonintact skin exposure should receive a single dose of Tdap (CDC, 57 [RR6] 2008; CDC, 61[25], 2012)

Adults ≥19 years (including adults ≥65 years) (Tdap): A single dose of Tdap should be given to all patients who have not previously received Tdap. Following administration of Tdap, Td vaccine should be used for routine boosters. (CDC, 61[25], 2012). The following patients, who have not yet received Tdap or for whom vaccine status is not known, should receive a single dose of Tdap as soon as feasible:

- Pregnant (>20 weeks gestation) or postpartum women (CDC, 57[RR4], 2008; CDC, 60[41], 2011; CDC, 61[4], 2012
- Close contacts of children <12 months of age; Tdap should ideally be administered at least 2 weeks prior to beginning close contact (CDC, 55[RR17], 2006; CDC, 60[41], 2011; CDC, 61[4], 2012)
- Healthcare providers with direct patient contact (CDC, 55[RR17], 2006; CDC, 61[4], 2012)

Note: Tdap is currently recommended for a single dose only (all age groups) (CDC, 60[1], 2011; CDC, 61 [25], 2012)

General Dosage Range I.M.:

Children 6 weeks to <7 years: Primary immunization: 0.5 mL per dose, total of 5 doses

Children ≥10 years and Adults: Booster immunization: 0.5 mL as a single dose

Dosage Forms

Injection, suspension [Tdap, booster formulation]:

Adacel®: Diphtheria 2 Lf units, tetanus 5 Lf units, and acellular pertussis antigens per 0.5 mL (0.5 mL)

Boostrix®: Diphtheria 2.5 Lf units, tetanus 5 Lf units, and acellular pertussis antigens per 0.5 mL (0.5 mL)

Injection, suspension [DTaP, active immunization formulation]:

Daptacel®: Diphtheria 15 Lf units, tetanus 5 Lf units, and acellular pertussis antigens per 0.5 mL (0.5 mL)

Infanrix®: Diphtheria 25 Lf units, tetanus 10 Lf units, and acellular pertussis antigens per 0.5 mL (0.5 mL) [preservative free]

diphtheria antitoxin (dif THEER ee a an tee TOKS in)

Therapeutic Category Antitoxin

Use Treatment of diphtheria (neutralizes unbound toxin, available from CDC)

General Dosage Range I.M., I.V.: *Children and Adults:* 20,000-120,000 units

diphtheria, tetanus toxoids, acellular pertussis (DTaP) *see* diphtheria and tetanus toxoids, acellular pertussis, and poliovirus vaccine *on page 296*

diphtheria, tetanus toxoids, acellular pertussis (DTaP) *see* diphtheria and tetanus toxoids, acellular pertussis, poliovirus and *Haemophilus* b conjugate vaccine *on page 298*

diphtheria, tetanus toxoids, acellular pertussis, hepatitis B (recombinant), and poliovirus (inactivated) vaccine

(dif THEER ee a, TET a nus TOKS oyds, ay CEL yoo lar per TUS sis, hep a TYE tis bee ree KOM be nant, & POE lee oh VYE rus in ak ti VAY ted vak SEEN)

Synonyms diphtheria and tetanus toxoids and acellular pertussis adsorbed, hepatitis B (recombinant) and inactivated poliovirus vaccine combined; diphtheria, tetanus toxoids, acellular pertussis, hepatitis B (recombinant), and poliovirus vaccine; DTaP-HepB-IPV

U.S. Brand Names Pediarix®

Canadian Brand Names Pediarix®

Therapeutic Category Vaccine

Use Combination vaccine for the active immunization against diphtheria, tetanus, pertussis, hepatitis B virus (all known subtypes), and poliomyelitis (caused by poliovirus types 1, 2, and 3)

The Advisory Committee on Immunization Practices (ACIP) recommends Pediarix® for the following:

- Primary vaccination for DTaP, Hep B, and IPV in children at 2, 4, and 6 months of age.
- To complete the primary vaccination series in children who have received DTaP (Infanrix®) and who are scheduled to receive the other components of the vaccine. Whenever feasible, the same manufacturer should be used to provide the pertussis component; however, vaccination should not be deferred if a specific brand is not known or is not available. HepB and IPV from different manufacturers are interchangeable.

General Dosage Range I.M.: *Children 6 weeks to <7 years:* 0.5 mL/dose for a total of 3 doses

Dosage Forms

Injection, suspension [preservative free]:

Pediarix®: Diphtheria toxoid 25 Lf, tetanus toxoid 10 Lf, acellular pertussis antigens per 0.5 mL (0.5 mL)

diphtheria, tetanus toxoids, acellular pertussis, hepatitis B (recombinant), and poliovirus vaccine *see* diphtheria, tetanus toxoids, acellular pertussis, hepatitis B (recombinant), and poliovirus (inactivated) vaccine *on page 300*

diphtheria toxoid *see* diphtheria and tetanus toxoids, acellular pertussis, poliovirus and *Haemophilus* b conjugate vaccine *on page 298*

dipivalyl epinephrine *see* dipivefrin *on page 300*

dipivefrin (dye PI ve frin)

Synonyms dipivalyl epinephrine; dipivefrin hydrochloride; DPE

Canadian Brand Names Ophtho-Dipivefrin™; PMS-Dipivefrin; Propine®

Therapeutic Category Adrenergic Agonist Agent

Use Reduces elevated intraocular pressure in chronic open-angle glaucoma; also used to treat ocular hypertension, low tension, and secondary glaucomas

General Dosage Range Ophthalmic: *Adults:* Instill 1 drop every 12 hours

dipivefrin hydrochloride *see* dipivefrin *on page 300*

Diprivan® *see* propofol *on page 766*

Diprolene® *see* betamethasone *on page 129*

Diprolene® AF *see* betamethasone *on page 129*

Diprolene® Glycol (Can) *see* betamethasone *on page 129*

dipropylacetic acid *see* valproic acid *on page 934*

Diprosone® (Can) *see* betamethasone *on page 129*

dipyridamole (dye peer ID a mole)

Medication Safety Issues

Sound-alike/look-alike issues:

Dipyridamole may be confused with disopyramide

Persantine® may be confused with Periactin

BEERS Criteria medication:

This drug may be potentially inappropriate for use in geriatric patients (Quality of evidence - moderate; Strength of recommendation - strong).

International issues:

Persantine [U.S., Canada, Belgium, Denmark, France] may be confused with Permitil brand name for sildenafil [Argentina]

U.S. Brand Names Persantine®

Canadian Brand Names Apo-Dipyridamole FC®; Dipyridamole For Injection; Persantine®

Therapeutic Category Antiplatelet Agent; Vasodilator

Use

Oral: Used with warfarin to decrease thrombosis in patients after artificial heart valve replacement

I.V.: Diagnostic agent in CAD

General Dosage Range

I.V.: *Adults:* 0.14 mg/kg/minute for 4 minutes (maximum: 60 mg)

Oral: *Children ≥12 years and Adults:* 75-100 mg 4 times/day

Dosage Forms

Injection, solution: 5 mg/mL (2 mL, 10 mL)

Tablet, oral: 25 mg, 50 mg, 75 mg

Persantine®: 25 mg, 50 mg, 75 mg

dipyridamole and aspirin *see* aspirin and dipyridamole *on page* 98

Dipyridamole For Injection (Can) *see* dipyridamole *on page* 300

disalicylic acid *see* salsalate *on page* 820

DisCoVisc® *see* sodium chondroitin sulfate and sodium hyaluronate *on page* 842

disodium cromoglycate *see* cromolyn (nasal) *on page* 241

disodium cromoglycate *see* cromolyn (ophthalmic) *on page* 241

disodium cromoglycate *see* cromolyn (systemic, oral inhalation) *on page* 240

disodium thiosulfate pentahydrate *see* sodium thiosulfate *on page* 848

***d*-isoephedrine hydrochloride** *see* pseudoephedrine *on page* 771

disopyramide (dye soe PEER a mide)

Medication Safety Issues

Sound-alike/look-alike issues:

Disopyramide may be confused with desipramine, dipyridamole

Norpace® may be confused with Norpramin®

BEERS Criteria medication:

This drug may be potentially inappropriate for use in geriatric patients (Quality of evidence - low; Strength of recommendation - strong).

Synonyms disopyramide phosphate

U.S. Brand Names Norpace®; Norpace® CR

Canadian Brand Names Norpace®; Rythmodan®; Rythmodan®-LA

Therapeutic Category Antiarrhythmic Agent, Class I-A

Use Life-threatening ventricular arrhythmias (eg, sustained ventricular tachycardia)

General Dosage Range Dosage adjustment recommended in patients with hepatic or renal impairment

Oral:

Controlled release:

Adults <50 kg: 200 mg every 12 hours

Adults ≥50 kg: 300 mg every 12 hours

Immediate release:

Children <1 year: 10-30 mg/kg/day in 4 divided doses

Children 1-4 years: 10-20 mg/kg/day in 4 divided doses

Children 4-12 years: 10-15 mg/kg/day in 4 divided doses

Children 12-18 years: 6-15 mg/kg/day in 4 divided doses

Adults <50 kg: 100 mg every 6 hours

Adults ≥50 kg: 150 mg every 6 hours

Dosage Forms

Capsule, oral: 100 mg, 150 mg

Norpace®: 100 mg, 150 mg

Capsule, controlled release, oral:

Norpace® CR: 100 mg, 150 mg

disopyramide phosphate *see* disopyramide *on page* 301

disulfiram (dye SUL fi ram)

Medication Safety Issues

Sound-alike/look-alike issues:

Disulfiram may be confused with Diflucan®

U.S. Brand Names Antabuse®

Therapeutic Category Aldehyde Dehydrogenase Inhibitor Agent

Use Management of chronic alcoholism

General Dosage Range Oral: *Adults:* Initial: 500 mg once daily; Maintenance: 125-500 mg once daily (maximum: 500 mg/day)

Dosage Forms

Tablet, oral: 250 mg, 500 mg

Antabuse®: 250 mg, 500 mg

dithioglycerol *see* dimercaprol *on page* 290

dithranol *see* anthralin *on page* 76

Ditropan *see* oxybutynin *on page* 677

Ditropan XL® *see* oxybutynin *on page* 677

diurex® [OTC] *see* pamabrom *on page* 686

diurex® Aquagels® [OTC] *see* pamabrom *on page* 686

diurex® Maximum Relief [OTC] *see* pamabrom *on page* 686

Diuril® *see* chlorothiazide *on page* 198

divalproex (dye VAL proe ex)

Medication Safety Issues

Sound-alike/look-alike issues:

Depakote® may be confused with Depakene®, Depakote® ER, Senokot®

Depakote® ER may be confused with divalproex enteric coated

Synonyms divalproex sodium; valproate semisodium; valproic acid derivative

U.S. Brand Names Depakote®; Depakote® ER; Depakote® Sprinkle

Canadian Brand Names Apo-Divalproex®; Dom-Divalproex; Epival®; Mylan-Divalproex; Novo-Divalproex; Nu-Divalproex; PHL-Divalproex; PMS-Divalproex

Therapeutic Category Anticonvulsant, Miscellaneous; Antimanic Agent; Histone Deacetylase Inhibitor

Use Monotherapy and adjunctive therapy in the treatment of patients with complex partial seizures; monotherapy and adjunctive therapy of simple and complex absence seizures; adjunctive therapy in patients with multiple seizure types that include absence seizures

Depakote®, Depakote® ER: Mania associated with bipolar disorder; migraine prophylaxis

General Dosage Range Dosage adjustment recommended in patients with hepatic impairment

Oral:

Children and Adults: Simple and complex absence seizures: Initial: 15 mg/kg/day; Maintenance: Up to 60 mg/kg/day

Children ≥10 years and Adults: Complex partial seizures: Initial: 10-15 mg/kg/day in 1-3 divided doses; Maintenance: Up to 60 mg/kg/day

Children ≥16 years and Adults: Migraine prophylaxis: Depakote® ER: 500-1000 mg once daily; Depakote® 250 mg twice daily (maximum: 1000 mg/day)

Adults: Mania: Depakote®: Initial: 750 mg/day in divided doses; Depakote® ER: Initial: 25 mg/kg/day given once daily; Maintenance: Up to 60 mg/kg/day

Dosage Forms

Capsule, sprinkle, oral: 125 mg

Depakote® Sprinkle: 125 mg

Tablet, delayed release, oral: 125 mg, 250 mg, 500 mg
Depakote®: 125 mg, 250 mg, 500 mg
Tablet, extended release, oral: 250 mg, 500 mg
Depakote® ER: 250 mg, 500 mg

divalproex sodium *see* divalproex *on page 302*
Divigel® *see* estradiol (systemic) *on page 347*
Dixarit® (Can) *see* clonidine *on page 224*
5071-1DL(6) *see* megestrol *on page 569*
***dl*-alpha tocopherol** *see* vitamin E *on page 950*
DLV *see* delavirdine *on page 259*
4-DMDR *see* idarubicin *on page 472*
***D*-mannitol** *see* mannitol *on page 561*
DMSA *see* succimer *on page 855*
DMSA *see* technetium Tc 99m succimer *on page 872*
DMSO *see* dimethyl sulfoxide *on page 290*
D-Natural-5 [OTC] *see* vitamin A and vitamin D (systemic) *on page 949*
Doak Oil [OTC] (Can) *see* coal tar *on page 228*
Doak Oil Forte [OTC] (Can) *see* coal tar *on page 228*
Doan's® Extra Strength [OTC] *see* magnesium salicylate *on page 560*

dobutamine (doe BYOO ta meen)

Medication Safety Issues
Sound-alike/look-alike issues:
DOBUTamine may be confused with DOPamine
High alert medication:
The Institute for Safe Medication Practices (ISMP) includes this medication among its list of drugs which have a heightened risk of causing significant patient harm when used in error.

Synonyms dobutamine hydrochloride

Tall-Man DOBUTamine

Canadian Brand Names Dobutamine Injection, USP; Dobutrex®

Therapeutic Category Adrenergic Agonist Agent

Use Short-term management of patients with cardiac decompensation

General Dosage Range I.V.: *Children and Adults:* 2.5-20 mcg/kg/minute (maximum: 40 mcg/kg/minute)

Dosage Forms
Infusion, premixed in D_5W: 1 mg/mL (250 mL, 500 mL); 2 mg/mL (250 mL); 4 mg/mL (250 mL)
Injection, solution: 12.5 mg/mL (20 mL, 40 mL)

dobutamine hydrochloride *see* dobutamine *on page 303*
Dobutamine Injection, USP (Can) *see* dobutamine *on page 303*
Dobutrex® (Can) *see* dobutamine *on page 303*
Docefrez™ *see* docetaxel *on page 303*

docetaxel (doe se TAKS el)

Medication Safety Issues
Sound-alike/look-alike issues:
DOCEtaxel may confused with PACLitaxel
Taxotere® may be confused with Taxol®
High alert medication:
This medication is in a class the Institute for Safe Medication Practices (ISMP) includes among its list of drug classes which have a heightened risk of causing significant patient harm when used in error.
Administration issues:
Multiple concentrations: Docetaxel is available as a one-vial formulation at concentrations of 10 mg/mL (generic formulation) and 20 mg/mL (concentrate; Taxotere®), and as a lyophilized powder (Docefrez™) which is reconstituted (with provided diluent) to 20 mg/0.8 mL (20 mg vial) or 24 mg/mL (80 mg vial). Docetaxel was previously available as a two-vial formulation (a concentrated docetaxel solution vial and a diluent vial) resulting in a reconstituted concentration of 10 mg/mL. The two-vial formulation has been discontinued by the manufacturer. Admixture errors have occurred due to the availability of various docetaxel concentrations.

Synonyms RP-6976

Tall-Man DOCEtaxel

U.S. Brand Names Docefrez™; Taxotere®

Canadian Brand Names Docetaxel for Injection; Taxotere®

Therapeutic Category Antineoplastic Agent

Use Treatment of breast cancer (locally advanced/metastatic or adjuvant treatment of operable node-positive); locally-advanced or metastatic nonsmall cell lung cancer (NSCLC); hormone refractory, metastatic prostate cancer; advanced gastric adenocarcinoma; locally-advanced squamous cell head and neck cancer

General Dosage Range Dosage adjustment recommended in patients with hepatic impairment, on concomitant therapy, or who develop toxicities.

I.V.: *Adults:* 60-100 mg/m^2 every 3 weeks

Dosage Forms

Injection, powder for reconstitution:

Docefrez™: 20 mg, 80 mg

Injection, solution: 10 mg/mL (2 mL, 8 mL, 16 mL)

Taxotere®: 20 mg/mL (1 mL, 4 mL)

Docetaxel for Injection (Can) *see* docetaxel *on page* 303

docosanol (doe KOE san ole)

Synonyms *n*-docosanol; behenyl alcohol

U.S. Brand Names Abreva® [OTC]

Therapeutic Category Antiviral Agent, Topical

Use Treatment of herpes simplex of the face or lips

General Dosage Range Topical: *Children ≥12 years and Adults:* Apply 5 times/day to affected area

Dosage Forms

Cream, topical:

Abreva® [OTC]: 10% (2 g)

Doc-Q-Lace [OTC] *see* docusate *on page* 304

Doc-Q-Lax [OTC] *see* docusate and senna *on page* 305

docusate (DOK yoo sate)

Medication Safety Issues

Sound-alike/look-alike issues:

Colace® may be confused with Calan®, Cozaar®

Dulcolax® (docusate) may be confused with Dulcolax® (bisacodyl)

International issues:

Docusate may be confused with Doxinate brand name for doxylamine and pyridoxine [India]

Synonyms dioctyl calcium sulfosuccinate; dioctyl sodium sulfosuccinate; docusate calcium; docusate potassium; docusate sodium; DOSS; DSS

U.S. Brand Names Colace® [OTC]; Correctol® [OTC]; Diocto [OTC]; Doc-Q-Lace [OTC]; Docu-Soft [OTC]; DocuSoft S™ [OTC]; Dok™ [OTC]; DSS® [OTC]; Dulcolax® Stool Softener [OTC]; Dulcolax® [OTC]; Enemeez® Plus [OTC]; Enemeez® [OTC]; Fleet® Pedia-Lax™ Liquid Stool Softener [OTC]; Fleet® Sof-Lax® [OTC]; Kao-Tin [OTC]; Kaopectate® Stool Softener [OTC]; Phillips'® Liquid-Gels® [OTC]; Phillips'® Stool Softener Laxative [OTC]; Silace [OTC]

Canadian Brand Names Apo-Docusate-Sodium®; Colace®; Colax-C®; Novo-Docusate Calcium; Novo-Docusate Sodium; PMS-Docusate Calcium; PMS-Docusate Sodium; Regulex®; Selax®; Soflax™

Therapeutic Category Stool Softener

Use Stool softener in patients who should avoid straining during defecation and constipation associated with hard, dry stools; prophylaxis for straining (Valsalva) following myocardial infarction. A safe agent to be used in elderly; some evidence that doses <200 mg are ineffective; stool softeners are unnecessary if stool is well hydrated or "mushy" and soft; shown to be ineffective used long-term.

General Dosage Range

Oral:

Children <3 years: 10-40 mg/day in 1-4 divided doses
Children 3-6 years: 20-60 mg/day in 1-4 divided doses
Children 6-12 years: 40-150 mg/day in 1-4 divided doses
Adolescents and Adults: 50-500 mg/day in 1-4 divided doses

Rectal: *Older children and Adults:* Add 50-100 mg to enema fluid

Dosage Forms

Capsule, oral:
Colace® [OTC]: 50 mg, 100 mg
Doc-Q-Lace [OTC]: 100 mg

Capsule, liquid, oral:
DocuSoft S™ [OTC]: 100 mg

Capsule, softgel, oral: 50 mg, 100 mg, 240 mg, 250 mg
Correctol® [OTC]: 100 mg
Docu-Soft [OTC]: 100 mg
Dok™ [OTC]: 100 mg, 250 mg
DSS® [OTC]: 100 mg, 250 mg
Dulcolax® [OTC]: 100 mg
Dulcolax® Stool Softener [OTC]: 100 mg
Fleet® Sof-Lax® [OTC]: 100 mg
Kao-Tin [OTC]: 240 mg
Kaopectate® Stool Softener [OTC]: 240 mg
Phillips'® Liquid-Gels® [OTC]: 100 mg
Phillips'® Stool Softener Laxative [OTC]: 100 mg

Liquid, oral: 50 mg/5 mL (10 mL, 25 mL, 473 mL); 150 mg/15 mL (480 mL)
Diocto [OTC]: 150 mg/15 mL (473 mL)
Fleet® Pedia-Lax™ Liquid Stool Softener [OTC]: 50 mg/15 mL (118 mL)
Silace [OTC]: 150 mg/15 mL (473 mL)

Solution, rectal:
Enemeez® [OTC]: 283 mg/5 mL (5 mL)
Enemeez® Plus [OTC]: 283 mg/5 mL (5 mL)

Syrup, oral: 20 mg/5 mL (25 mL, 473 mL)
Colace® [OTC]: 60 mg/15 mL (473 mL)
Diocto [OTC]: 60 mg/15 mL (473 mL)
Doc-Q-Lace [OTC]: 60 mg/15 mL (480 mL)
Silace [OTC]: 60 mg/15 mL (480 mL)

Tablet, oral: 100 mg
Dok™ [OTC]: 100 mg

docusate and senna (DOK yoo sate & SEN na)

Medication Safety Issues

Sound-alike/look-alike issues:
Senokot® may be confused with Depakote®

Synonyms senna and docusate; senna-S

U.S. Brand Names Doc-Q-Lax [OTC]; Dok™ Plus [OTC]; Geri-Stool [OTC]; Peri-Colace® [OTC]; Senexon-S [OTC]; Senna Plus [OTC]; SennaLax-S [OTC]; Senokot-S® [OTC]; SenoSol™-SS [OTC]

Therapeutic Category Laxative, Stimulant; Stool Softener

Use Short-term treatment of constipation

General Dosage Range Oral:

Children 2-6 years: Initial: 4.3 mg sennosides plus 25 mg docusate (1/2 tablet) once daily (maximum: 1 tablet twice daily)

Children 6-12 years: Initial: 8.6 sennosides plus 50 mg docusate (1 tablet) once daily (maximum: 2 tablets twice daily)

Children ≥12 years and Adults: Initial: 2 tablets (17.2 mg sennosides plus 100 mg docusate) once daily (maximum: 4 tablets twice daily)

Dosage Forms

Tablet: Docusate 50 mg and sennosides 8.6 mg
Doc-Q-Lax [OTC], Dok™ Plus [OTC], Geri-Stool [OTC], Peri-Colace® [OTC], Senexon-S [OTC], SennaLax-S [OTC], Senna Plus [OTC], Senokot-S® [OTC], SenoSol™-SS [OTC]: Docusate 50 mg and sennosides 8.6 mg

docusate calcium *see* docusate *on page* 304
docusate potassium *see* docusate *on page* 304
docusate sodium *see* docusate *on page* 304
Docu-Soft [OTC] *see* docusate *on page* 304
DocuSoft S™ [OTC] *see* docusate *on page* 304

dofetilide (doe FET il ide)

Medication Safety Issues

Sound-alike/look-alike issues:

Dofetilide may be confused with defibrotide

U.S. Brand Names Tikosyn®

Canadian Brand Names Tikosyn®

Therapeutic Category Antiarrhythmic Agent, Class III

Use Maintenance of normal sinus rhythm in patients with chronic atrial fibrillation/atrial flutter of longer than 1-week duration who have been converted to normal sinus rhythm; conversion of atrial fibrillation and atrial flutter to normal sinus rhythm

General Dosage Range Dosage adjustment recommended in patients with renal impairment

Oral: *Adults:* Initial: 500 mcg twice daily; Maintenance: 125-500 mcg twice daily **or** 125 mcg once daily

Dosage Forms

Capsule, oral:

Tikosyn®: 125 mcg, 250 mcg, 500 mcg

Dofus [OTC] *see* Lactobacillus *on page* 518
Dok™ [OTC] *see* docusate *on page* 304
Dok™ Plus [OTC] *see* docusate and senna *on page* 305

dolasetron (dol A se tron)

Medication Safety Issues

Sound-alike/look-alike issues:

Anzemet® may be confused with Aldomet, Antivert®, Avandamet®

Dolasetron may be confused with granisetron, ondansetron, palonosetron

Synonyms dolasetron mesylate; MDL 73,147EF

U.S. Brand Names Anzemet®

Canadian Brand Names Anzemet®

Therapeutic Category Selective 5-HT_3 Receptor Antagonist

Use

U.S. labeling:

Injection: Prevention and treatment of postoperative nausea and vomiting

Oral: Prevention of nausea and vomiting associated with emetogenic cancer chemotherapy (initial and repeat courses); prevention of postoperative nausea and vomiting

Canadian labeling: Oral: Prevention of nausea and vomiting associated with emetogenic cancer chemotherapy (initial and repeat courses)

General Dosage Range

I.V.:

Children 2-16 years: 0.35 mg/kg as a single dose (maximum: 12.5 mg)

Adults: 12.5 mg or 100 mg as a single dose

Oral:

Children 2-16 years: 1.2-1.8 mg/kg as a single dose (maximum: 100 mg/dose)

Adults: 100 mg as single dose

Dosage Forms

Injection, solution:

Anzemet®: 20 mg/mL (0.625 mL, 5 mL, 25 mL)

Tablet, oral:

Anzemet®: 50 mg, 100 mg

dolasetron mesylate *see* dolasetron *on page* 306
Dolgic® Plus *see* butalbital, acetaminophen, and caffeine *on page* 153
Dolobid *see* diflunisal *on page* 284
Dolophine® *see* methadone *on page* 581

Dom-Mefenamic Acid (Can) *see* mefenamic acid *on page* 568
Dom-Meloxicam (Can) *see* meloxicam *on page* 569
Dom-Metformin (Can) *see* metformin *on page* 579
Dom-Methimazole (Can) *see* methimazole *on page* 583
Dom-Metoprolol-L (Can) *see* metoprolol *on page* 595
Dom-Metoprolol-B (Can) *see* metoprolol *on page* 595
Dom-Minocycline (Can) *see* minocycline *on page* 604
Dom-Mirtazapine (Can) *see* mirtazapine *on page* 606
Dom-Moclobemide (Can) *see* moclobemide *(Canada only) on page* 609
Dom-Nortriptyline (Can) *see* nortriptyline *on page* 650
Dom-Ondansetron (Can) *see* ondansetron *on page* 667
Dom-Oxybutynin (Can) *see* oxybutynin *on page* 677
Dom-Paroxetine (Can) *see* paroxetine *on page* 693

domperidone *(Canada only)* (dom PE ri done)

Medication Safety Issues

Sound-alike/look-alike issues:

Domperidone may be confused with iloperidone

Synonyms domperidone maleate

Canadian Brand Names Apo-Domperidone®; Dom-Domperidone; Mylan-Domperidone; Nu-Domperidone; PHL-Domperidone; PMS-Domperidone; RAN™-Domperidone; ratio-Domperidone; Teva-Domperidone

Therapeutic Category Dopamine Antagonist

Use Symptomatic management of upper GI motility disorders associated with chronic and subacute gastritis and diabetic gastroparesis; prevention of GI symptoms associated with use of dopamine-agonist anti-Parkinson agents

General Dosage Range Dosage adjustment recommended in patients with renal impairment

Oral: *Adults:* 10-20 mg 3-4 times/day

Product Availability Not available in U.S.

Dosage Forms - Canada

Tablet: 10 mg

Apo-Domperidone®, Dom-Domperidone, Novo-Domperidone, Nu-Domperidone, PHL-Domperidone, PMS-Domperidone, ratio-Domperidone: 10 mg

domperidone maleate *see* domperidone *(Canada only) on page* 308
Dom-Pindolol (Can) *see* pindolol *on page* 724
Dom-Pioglitazone (Can) *see* pioglitazone *on page* 725
Dom-Piroxicam (Can) *see* piroxicam *on page* 727
Dom-Pravastatin (Can) *see* pravastatin *on page* 752
Dom-Propranolol (Can) *see* propranolol *on page* 767
Dom-Quetiapine (Can) *see* quetiapine *on page* 781
Dom-Ramipril (Can) *see* ramipril *on page* 786
Dom-Ranitidine (Can) *see* ranitidine *on page* 788
Dom-Risedronate (Can) *see* risedronate *on page* 803
Dom-Risperidone (Can) *see* risperidone *on page* 803
Dom-Salbutamol (Can) *see* albuterol *on page* 41
Dom-Sertraline (Can) *see* sertraline *on page* 831
Dom-Simvastatin (Can) *see* simvastatin *on page* 835
Dom-Sotalol (Can) *see* sotalol *on page* 851
Dom-Sucralfate (Can) *see* sucralfate *on page* 856
Dom-Sumatriptan (Can) *see* sumatriptan *on page* 863
Dom-Temazepam (Can) *see* temazepam *on page* 875
Dom-Terazosin (Can) *see* terazosin *on page* 878
Dom-Terbinafine (Can) *see* terbinafine (systemic) *on page* 878
Dom-Tiaprofenic (Can) *see* tiaprofenic acid *(Canada only) on page* 895
Dom-Ticlopidine (Can) *see* ticlopidine *on page* 895

Dom-Timolol (Can) *see* timolol (ophthalmic) *on page 897*
Dom-Topiramate (Can) *see* topiramate *on page 906*
Dom-Trazodone (Can) *see* trazodone *on page 912*
Dom-Ursodiol C (Can) *see* ursodiol *on page 932*
DOM-Valacyclovir (Can) *see* valacyclovir *on page 933*
Dom-Verapamil SR (Can) *see* verapamil *on page 942*
Dom-Zopiclone (Can) *see* zopiclone *(Canada only) on page 967*

donepezil (doh NEP e zil)

Medication Safety Issues
Sound-alike/look-alike issues:
Aricept® may be confused with AcipHex®, Ascriptin®, and Azilect®
Synonyms E2020
U.S. Brand Names Aricept®; Aricept® ODT
Canadian Brand Names Aricept®; Aricept® RDT
Therapeutic Category Acetylcholinesterase Inhibitor; Cholinergic Agent
Use Treatment of mild, moderate, or severe dementia of the Alzheimer type
General Dosage Range Oral: *Adults:* 5 mg once daily; Maintenance: 5-23 mg once daily
Dosage Forms
Tablet, oral: 5 mg, 10 mg
Aricept®: 5 mg, 10 mg, 23 mg
Tablet, orally disintegrating, oral: 5 mg, 10 mg
Aricept® ODT: 5 mg, 10 mg

Donnatal® *see* hyoscyamine, atropine, scopolamine, and phenobarbital *on page 467*
Donnatal Extentabs® *see* hyoscyamine, atropine, scopolamine, and phenobarbital *on page 467*

dopamine (DOE pa meen)

Medication Safety Issues
Sound-alike/look-alike issues:
DOPamine may be confused with DOBUTamine, Dopram®
High alert medication:
The Institute for Safe Medication Practices (ISMP) includes this medication among its list of drugs which have a heightened risk of causing significant patient harm when used in error.
Synonyms dopamine hydrochloride; Intropin
Tall-Man DOPamine
Therapeutic Category Adrenergic Agonist Agent
Use Adjunct in the treatment of shock (eg, MI, open heart surgery, renal failure, cardiac decompensation) which persists after adequate fluid volume replacement
General Dosage Range I.V.:
Children: 1-20 mcg/kg/minute (maximum: 50 mcg/kg/minute)
Adults: 1-50 mcg/kg/minute
Dosage Forms
Infusion, premixed in D_5W: 0.8 mg/mL (250 mL, 500 mL); 1.6 mg/mL (250 mL, 500 mL); 3.2 mg/mL (250 mL)
Injection, solution: 40 mg/mL (5 mL, 10 mL); 80 mg/mL (5 mL, 10 mL); 160 mg/mL (5 mL)

dopamine hydrochloride *see* dopamine *on page 309*
Dopram® *see* doxapram *on page 311*
Doral® *see* quazepam *on page 780*
Doribax® *see* doripenem *on page 309*

doripenem (dore i PEN em)

Medication Safety Issues
Sound-alike/look-alike issues:
Doripenem may be confused with ertapenem
Doribax® may be confused with Zovirax®
Synonyms S-4661

U.S. Brand Names Doribax®

Canadian Brand Names Doribax®

Therapeutic Category Antibiotic, Carbapenem

Use Treatment of complicated intraabdominal infections and complicated urinary tract infections (including pyelonephritis) due to susceptible aerobic gram-positive, aerobic gram-negative (including *Pseudomonas aeruginosa*), and anaerobic bacteria

Canadian labeling: Additional use (not in U.S. labeling): Treatment of healthcare-associated pneumonia (including ventilator-associated pneumonia)

General Dosage Range Dosage adjustment recommended in patients with renal impairment

I.V.: *Adults:* 500 mg every 8 hours

Dosage Forms

Injection, powder for reconstitution:

Doribax®: 250 mg, 500 mg

dornase alfa (DOOR nase AL fa)

Synonyms recombinant human deoxyribonuclease; rhDNase

U.S. Brand Names Pulmozyme®

Canadian Brand Names Pulmozyme®

Therapeutic Category Enzyme

Use Management of cystic fibrosis patients to reduce the frequency of respiratory infections that require parenteral antibiotics in patients with FVC ≥40% of predicted; in conjunction with standard therapies, to improve pulmonary function in patients with cystic fibrosis

General Dosage Range **Inhalation:** *Children ≥3 months and Adults:* 2.5 mg once daily

Dosage Forms

Solution, for nebulization [preservative free]:

Pulmozyme®: 2.5 mg/2.5 mL (30s)

Doryx® *see* doxycycline *on page* 314

dorzolamide (dor ZOLE a mide)

Synonyms dorzolamide hydrochloride

U.S. Brand Names Trusopt®

Canadian Brand Names Sandoz-Dorzolamide; Trusopt®

Therapeutic Category Carbonic Anhydrase Inhibitor

Use Treatment of elevated intraocular pressure in patients with ocular hypertension or open-angle glaucoma

General Dosage Range **Ophthalmic:** *Children and Adults:* Instill 1 drop into affected eye(s) 3 times/day

Dosage Forms

Solution, ophthalmic: 2% (10 mL)

Trusopt®: 2% (10 mL)

Dosage Forms - Canada

Solution, ophthalmic [drops; preservative free]:

Trusopt®: 2% (0.2 mL)

dorzolamide and timolol (dor ZOLE a mide & TYE moe lole)

Synonyms timolol and dorzolamide

U.S. Brand Names Cosopt®; Cosopt® PF

Canadian Brand Names Apo-Dorzo-Timop; Cosopt®; Cosopt® Preservative Free; Sandoz-Dorzolamide/Timolol

Therapeutic Category Beta-Adrenergic Blocker; Carbonic Anhydrase Inhibitor

Use Treatment of elevated intraocular pressure in patients with ocular hypertension or open-angle glaucoma

General Dosage Range **Ophthalmic:** *Children ≥2 years and Adults:* Instill 1 drop into affected eye(s) twice daily

Dosage Forms

Solution, ophthalmic [drops]: Dorzolamide 2% and timolol 0.5% (10 mL)
Cosopt®: Dorzolamide 2% and timolol 0.5% (10 mL)

Solution, ophthalmic [drops, preservative free]:
Cosopt® PF: Dorzolamide 2% and timolol 0.5% (0.2 mL)

dorzolamide hydrochloride *see* dorzolamide *on page* 310

DOSS *see* docusate *on page* 304

Dostinex® (Can) *see* cabergoline *on page* 157

Double Tussin DM [OTC] *see* guaifenesin and dextromethorphan *on page* 434

Dovobet® (Can) *see* calcipotriene and betamethasone *on page* 159

Dovonex® *see* calcipotriene *on page* 159

doxapram (DOKS a pram)

Medication Safety Issues

Sound-alike/look-alike issues:
Doxapram may be confused with doxazosin, doxepin, DOXOrubicin
Dopram® may be confused with DOPamine

International issues:
Doxapram may be confused with Doxinate brand name for doxylamine and pyridoxine [Italy]

Synonyms doxapram hydrochloride

U.S. Brand Names Dopram®

Therapeutic Category Respiratory Stimulant

Use Respiratory and CNS stimulant for respiratory depression secondary to anesthesia, drug-induced CNS depression; acute hypercapnia secondary to COPD

General Dosage Range I.V.: *Adults:* 0.5-1 mg/kg every 5 minutes until response (maximum total dose: 2 mg/kg) **or** 1-5 mg/minute until response; should not be continued >2 hours (maximum total dose: 4 mg/kg; 3 g/day)

Dosage Forms

Injection, solution: 20 mg/mL (20 mL)
Dopram®: 20 mg/mL (20 mL)

doxapram hydrochloride *see* doxapram *on page* 311

doxazosin (doks AY zoe sin)

Medication Safety Issues

Sound-alike/look-alike issues:
Doxazosin may be confused with doxapram, doxepin, DOXOrubicin
Cardura® may be confused with Cardene®, Cordarone®, Cordran®, Coumadin®, K-Dur®, Ridaura®

BEERS Criteria medication:
This drug may be potentially inappropriate for use in geriatric patients (Quality of evidence - moderate; Strength of recommendation - strong).

Synonyms doxazosin mesylate

U.S. Brand Names Cardura®; Cardura® XL

Canadian Brand Names Alti-Doxazosin; Apo-Doxazosin®; Cardura-1™; Cardura-2™; Cardura-4™; Gen-Doxazosin; Mylan-Doxazosin; Novo-Doxazosin

Therapeutic Category Alpha-Adrenergic Blocking Agent

Use

Immediate release formulation: Treatment of hypertension as monotherapy or in conjunction with diuretics, ACE inhibitors, beta-blockers, or calcium antagonists

Immediate release and extended release formulations: Treatment of urinary outflow obstruction and/or obstructive and irritative symptoms associated with benign prostatic hyperplasia (BPH)

General Dosage Range Oral:

Extended release: *Adults:* Initial: 4 mg once daily; Maintenance: 4-8 mg/day (maximum: 8 mg/day)

Immediate release:

Adults: Initial: 1-4 mg once daily; Maintenance: 4-8 mg/day (maximum: 8 mg/day [BPH]; 16 mg/day [Hypertension])

Elderly: Initial: 0.5 mg once daily

Dosage Forms
Tablet, oral: 1 mg, 2 mg, 4 mg, 8 mg
Cardura®: 1 mg, 2 mg, 4 mg, 8 mg
Tablet, extended release, oral:
Cardura® XL: 4 mg, 8 mg

doxazosin mesylate *see* doxazosin *on page* 311

doxepin (systemic) (DOKS e pin)

Medication Safety Issues
Sound-alike/look-alike issues:
Doxepin may be confused with digoxin, doxapram, doxazosin, Doxidan®, doxycycline
SINEquan® may be confused with saquinavir, SEROquel®, Singulair®, Zonegran®
BEERS Criteria medication:
This drug may be potentially inappropriate for use in geriatric patients (Quality of evidence - high [moderate for SIADH]; Strength of recommendation - strong).
International issues:
Doxal [Finland] may be confused with Doxil brand name for doxorubicin (liposomal) [U.S., Israel]
Doxal brand name for doxepin [Finland] but also brand name for pyridoxine/thiamine [Brazil]

Synonyms doxepin hydrochloride

U.S. Brand Names Silenor®

Canadian Brand Names Apo-Doxepin®; Doxepine; Novo-Doxepin; Sinequan®

Therapeutic Category Antidepressant, Tricyclic (Tertiary Amine)

Use Depression; treatment of insomnia (with difficulty of sleep maintenance)

General Dosage Range Dosage adjustment recommended for oral route in patients with hepatic impairment
Oral:
Adults: Initial: 25-150 mg/day in 2-3 divided doses; Maintenance: Up to 300 mg/day in single (≤150 mg) or divided doses; 3-6 mg once daily prior to bedtime (insomnia)
Elderly: Initial: 10-25 mg at bedtime; Maintenance: Up to 75 mg at bedtime

Dosage Forms
Capsule, oral: 10 mg, 25 mg, 50 mg, 75 mg, 100 mg, 150 mg
Solution, oral: 10 mg/mL (118 mL, 120 mL)
Tablet, oral:
Silenor®: 3 mg, 6 mg

doxepin (topical) (DOKS e pin)

Medication Safety Issues
Sound-alike/look-alike issues:
Doxepin may be confused with digoxin, doxapram, doxazosin, Doxidan®, doxycycline
Zonalon® may be confused with Zone-A®
International issues:
Doxal [Finland] may be confused with Doxil brand name for doxorubicin (liposomal) [U.S., Israel]
Doxal brand name for doxepin [Finland] but also brand name for pyridoxine/thiamine [Brazil]

Synonyms doxepin hydrochloride

U.S. Brand Names Prudoxin™; Zonalon®

Canadian Brand Names Zonalon®

Therapeutic Category Topical Skin Product

Use Short-term (<8 days) management of moderate pruritus in adults with atopic dermatitis or lichen simplex chronicus

General Dosage Range
Dental: *Adults:* Apply 3-4 times/day
Topical: *Adults:* Apply a thin film 4 times/day (maximum total therapy: 8 days)

Dosage Forms
Cream, topical:
Prudoxin™: 5% (45 g)
Zonalon®: 5% (30 g, 45 g)

Doxepine (Can) *see* doxepin (systemic) *on page* 312
doxepin hydrochloride *see* doxepin (systemic) *on page* 312

doxepin hydrochloride *see* doxepin (topical) *on page* 312

doxercalciferol (doks er kal si fe FEER ole)

Synonyms 1α-hydroxyergocalciferol

U.S. Brand Names Hectorol®

Canadian Brand Names Hectorol®

Therapeutic Category Vitamin D Analog

Use Treatment of secondary hyperparathyroidism in patients with chronic kidney disease

General Dosage Range

I.V.: *Adults:* Initial: 4 mcg 3 times/week after dialysis; Maintenance: Up to 18 mcg/week

Oral:

Adults (dialysis patients): Initial: 10 mcg 3 times/week at dialysis; Maintenance: Up to 60 mcg/week

Adults (predialysis patients): Initial: 1 mcg/day; Maintenance: Up to 3.5 mcg/day

Dosage Forms

Capsule, softgel, oral:

Hectorol®: 0.5 mcg, 1 mcg, 2.5 mcg

Injection, solution:

Hectorol®: 2 mcg/mL (1 mL, 2 mL)

Doxidan® [OTC] *see* bisacodyl *on page* 134

Doxil® *see* doxorubicin (liposomal) *on page* 314

doxorubicin (doks oh ROO bi sin)

Medication Safety Issues

Sound-alike/look-alike issues:

DOXOrubicin may be confused with DACTINomycin, DAUNOrubicin, DAUNOrubicin liposomal, doxapram, doxazosin, DOXOrubicin liposomal, epirubicin, IDArubicin, valrubicin

Adriamycin PFS® may be confused with achromycin, Aredia®, Idamycin®

Conventional formulation (Adriamycin PFS®, Adriamycin RDF®) may be confused with the liposomal formulation (Doxil®)

High alert medication:

The Institute for Safe Medication Practices (ISMP) includes this medication among its list of drug classes which have a heightened risk of causing significant patient harm when used in error.

Administration issues:

Use caution when selecting product for preparation and dispensing; indications, dosages and adverse event profiles differ between conventional DOXOrubicin hydrochloride solution and DOXOrubicin liposomal. Both formulations are the same concentration. As a result, serious errors have occurred.

Other safety concerns:

ADR is an error-prone abbreviation

International issues:

Doxil® may be confused with Doxal® which is a brand name for doxepin in Finland, a brand name for doxycycline in Austria, and a brand name for pyridoxine/thiamine combination in Brazil

Rubex, a discontinued brand name for DOXOrubicin in the U.S, is a brand name for ascorbic acid in Ireland

Synonyms ADR (error-prone abbreviation); Adria; conventional doxorubicin; doxorubicin hydrochloride; hydroxydaunomycin hydrochloride; hydroxyldaunorubicin hydrochloride

Tall-Man DOXOrubicin

U.S. Brand Names Adriamycin®

Canadian Brand Names Adriamycin®; Doxorubicin Hydrochloride Injection

Therapeutic Category Antineoplastic Agent

Use Treatment of acute lymphocytic leukemia (ALL), acute myeloid leukemia (AML), Hodgkin disease, malignant lymphoma, soft tissue and bone sarcomas, thyroid cancer, small cell lung cancer, breast cancer, gastric cancer, ovarian cancer, bladder cancer, neuroblastoma, and Wilms tumor

General Dosage Range Dosage adjustment recommended in patients with hepatic impairment or who develop toxicities

I.V.: *Children and Adults:* Dosage varies greatly depending on indication

Dosage Forms

Injection, powder for reconstitution: 10 mg, 50 mg
Adriamycin®: 10 mg, 20 mg, 50 mg

Injection, solution [preservative free]: 2 mg/mL (5 mL, 10 mL, 25 mL, 75 mL, 100 mL)
Adriamycin®: 2 mg/mL (5 mL, 10 mL, 25 mL, 100 mL)

doxorubicin hydrochloride *see* doxorubicin *on page 313*

Doxorubicin Hydrochloride Injection (Can) *see* doxorubicin *on page 313*

DOXOrubicin hydrochloride (liposomal) *see* doxorubicin (liposomal) *on page 314*

DOXOrubicin hydrochloride liposome *see* doxorubicin (liposomal) *on page 314*

doxorubicin (liposomal) (doks oh ROO bi sin lye po SO mal)

Medication Safety Issues

Sound-alike/look-alike issues:

DOXOrubicin liposomal may be confused with DACTINomycin, DAUNOrubicin, DAUNOrubicin liposomal, doxapram, doxazosin, DOXOrubicin, epirubicin, IDArubicin, valrubicin

DOXOrubicin liposomal may be confused with DAUNOrubicin liposomal

Doxil® may be confused with Doxy 100™, Paxil®

Liposomal formulation (Doxil®) may be confused with the conventional formulation (Adriamycin PFS®, Adriamycin RDF®)

High alert medication:

This medication is in a class the Institute for Safe Medication Practices (ISMP) includes among its list of drug classes which have a heightened risk of causing significant patient harm when used in error.

Administration issues:

Use caution when selecting product for preparation and dispensing; indications, dosages and adverse event profiles differ between conventional DOXOrubicin hydrochloride solution and DOXOrubicin liposomal. Both formulations are the same concentration. As a result, serious errors have occurred. Liposomal formulation of doxorubicin should NOT be substituted for doxorubicin hydrochloride on a mg-per-mg basis.

International issues:

Doxil [U.S., Israel] may be confused with Doxal brand name for doxepin [Finland] and pyridoxine/thiamine [Brazil]

Synonyms DOXOrubicin hydrochloride (liposomal); DOXOrubicin hydrochloride liposome; Lipodox; liposomal DOXOrubicin; pegylated DOXOrubicin liposomal; pegylated liposomal DOXOrubicin

Tall-Man DOXOrubicin (liposomal)

U.S. Brand Names Doxil®

Canadian Brand Names Caelyx®; Myocet™

Therapeutic Category Antineoplastic Agent

Use Treatment of ovarian cancer (progressive or recurrent), multiple myeloma (after failure of at least 1 prior therapy), and AIDS-related Kaposi sarcoma (after failure of or intolerance to prior systemic therapy)

General Dosage Range Dosage adjustment recommended in patients with hepatic impairment or who develop toxicities

I.V.: *Adults:* 20-30 mg/m^2 every 3 weeks **or** 50 mg/m^2 every 4 weeks

Dosage Forms

Injection, solution:
Doxil®: 2 mg/mL (10 mL, 25 mL)

Doxy 100™ *see* doxycycline *on page 314*

Doxycin (Can) *see* doxycycline *on page 314*

doxycycline (doks i SYE kleen)

Medication Safety Issues

Sound-alike/look-alike issues:

Doxycycline may be confused with dicyclomine, doxepin, doxylamine

Doxy100™ may be confused with Doxil®

Monodox® may be confused with Maalox®

Oracea® may be confused with Orencia®

Vibramycin® may be confused with vancomycin, Vibativ™

Synonyms doxycycline calcium; doxycycline hyclate; doxycycline monohydrate

U.S. Brand Names Adoxa®; Alodox™; Doryx®; Doxy 100™; Monodox®; Ocudox™; Oracea®; Oraxyl™; Periostat®; Vibramycin®

Canadian Brand Names Apo-Doxy Tabs®; Apo-Doxy®; Dom-Doxycycline; Doxycin; Doxytab; Novo-Doxylin; Nu-Doxycycline; Periostat®; PHL-Doxycycline; PMS-Doxycycline; Vibra-Tabs®; Vibramycin®

Therapeutic Category Tetracycline Derivative

Use Principally in the treatment of infections caused by susceptible *Rickettsia*, *Chlamydia*, and *Mycoplasma*; alternative to mefloquine for malaria prophylaxis; treatment for syphilis, uncomplicated *Neisseria gonorrhoeae* (alternative agent), *Listeria*, *Actinomyces israelii*, and *Clostridium* infections in penicillin-allergic patients; used for community-acquired pneumonia and other common infections due to susceptible organisms; anthrax due to *Bacillus anthracis,* including inhalational anthrax (postexposure); treatment of infections caused by uncommon susceptible gram-negative and gram-positive organisms including *Borrelia recurrentis*, *Ureaplasma urealyticum*, *Haemophilus ducreyi*, *Yersinia pestis*, *Francisella tularensis*, *Vibrio cholerae*, *Campylobacter fetus*, *Brucella* spp, *Bartonella bacilliformis*, and *Klebsiella granulomatis,* Q fever, Lyme disease; treatment of inflammatory lesions associated with rosacea; intestinal amebiasis; severe acne

General Dosage Range

I.V.:

Children ≤8 years: 2.2 mg/kg every 12 hours

Children >8 years and ≤45 kg: 2-5 mg/kg/day in 1-2 divided doses (maximum: 200 mg/day)

Children >8 years and >45 kg and Adults: 100-200 mg/day in 1-2 divided doses

Oral:

Children ≤8 years: 2.2 mg/kg every 12 hours

Children >8 years and ≤45 kg: 2-5 mg/kg/day in 1-2 divided doses (maximum: 200 mg/day)

Children >8 years and >45 kg: 100-200 mg/day in 1-2 divided doses

Adults: 100-200 mg/day in 1-2 divided doses **or** 300 mg as a single dose **or** 40 mg/day in 1-2 divided doses

Dosage Forms

Capsule, oral: 50 mg, 75 mg, 100 mg, 150 mg

Adoxa®: 150 mg

Monodox®: 75 mg, 100 mg

Ocudox™: 50 mg

Oracea®: 40 mg [30 mg (immediate release) and 10 mg (delayed release)]

Oraxyl™: 20 mg

Vibramycin®: 100 mg

Injection, powder for reconstitution: 100 mg

Doxy 100™: 100 mg

Powder for suspension, oral:

Vibramycin®: 25 mg/5 mL (60 mL)

Syrup, oral:

Vibramycin®: 50 mg/5 mL (473 mL)

Tablet, oral: 20 mg, 50 mg, 75 mg, 100 mg, 150 mg

Alodox™: 20 mg

Periostat®: 20 mg

Tablet, delayed release coated beads, oral: 75 mg, 100 mg, 150 mg

Tablet, delayed release coated pellets, oral:

Doryx®: 150 mg

doxycycline calcium *see* doxycycline *on page 314*

doxycycline hyclate *see* doxycycline *on page 314*

doxycycline monohydrate *see* doxycycline *on page 314*

doxylamine (dox IL a meen)

Medication Safety Issues

Sound-alike/look-alike issues:

Doxylamine may be confused with doxycycline

BEERS Criteria medication:

This drug may be potentially inappropriate for use in geriatric patients (Quality of evidence - moderate; Strength of recommendation - strong).

Synonyms doxylamine succinate

U.S. Brand Names Aldex® AN

Canadian Brand Names Unisom®-2

Therapeutic Category Antihistamine

Use Treatment of short-term insomnia

General Dosage Range Oral: *Adults:* 1 tablet 30 minutes before bedtime

Dosage Forms

Tablet, chewable, oral:

Aldex® AN: 5 mg

doxylamine, acetaminophen, and dextromethorphan *see* acetaminophen, dextromethorphan, and doxylamine *on page* 27

doxylamine and pyridoxine *(Canada only)* (dox IL a meen & peer i DOX een)

Medication Safety Issues

Sound-alike/look-alike issues:

Doxylamine may be confused with doxycycline

Synonyms doxylamine succinate and pyridoxine hydrochloride; pyridoxine and doxylamine

Canadian Brand Names Diclectin®

Therapeutic Category Antihistamine; Vitamin

Use Treatment of pregnancy-associated nausea and vomiting

General Dosage Range Oral: *Adults:* 2 tablets (a total of doxylamine 20 mg and pyridoxine 20 mg) at bedtime; may increase by 1 tablet in the morning and/or afternoon in severe cases

Product Availability Not available in U.S.

Dosage Forms - Canada

Tablet, delayed release:

Diclectin®: Doxylamine 10 mg and pyridoxine 10 mg

doxylamine succinate *see* doxylamine *on page* 315

doxylamine succinate and pyridoxine hydrochloride *see* doxylamine and pyridoxine *(Canada only) on page* 316

doxylamine succinate, codeine phosphate, and acetaminophen *see* acetaminophen, codeine, and doxylamine *(Canada only) on page* 27

Doxytab (Can) *see* doxycycline *on page* 314

DPA *see* valproic acid *on page* 934

DPE *see* dipivefrin *on page* 300

D-penicillamine *see* penicillamine *on page* 701

DPH *see* phenytoin *on page* 719

DPM™ [OTC] *see* urea *on page* 930

Dramamine® [OTC] *see* dimenhydrinate *on page* 289

Dramamine® for kids [OTC] *see* dimenhydrinate *on page* 289

Dramamine® Less Drowsy Formula [OTC] *see* meclizine *on page* 566

DRAXIMAGE® DTPA *see* technetium Tc 99m diethylene triamine penta-acetic acid *on page* 871

DRAXIMAGE® Gluceptate *see* technetium Tc 99m gluceptate *on page* 871

DRAXIMAGE® MDP-25 *see* technetium Tc 99m medronate *on page* 872

Driminate [OTC] *see* dimenhydrinate *on page* 289

Drinkables® Fruits and Vegetables [OTC] *see* vitamins (multiple/oral) *on page* 951

Drinkables® MultiVitamins [OTC] *see* vitamins (multiple/oral) *on page* 951

Drisdol® *see* ergocalciferol *on page* 339

Dristan® [OTC] *see* oxymetazoline (nasal) *on page* 681

Dristan® Long Lasting Nasal (Can) *see* oxymetazoline (nasal) *on page* 681

Dristan® N.D. (Can) *see* acetaminophen and pseudoephedrine *on page* 25

Dristan® N.D., Extra Strength (Can) *see* acetaminophen and pseudoephedrine *on page* 25

Dritho-Creme® *see* anthralin *on page* 76

Dritho-Scalp® *see* anthralin *on page* 76

Drixoral® Nasal (Can) *see* oxymetazoline (nasal) *on page* 681

Drixoral® ND (Can) *see* pseudoephedrine *on page* 771

dronabinol (droe NAB i nol)

Medication Safety Issues

Sound-alike/look-alike issues:

Dronabinol may be confused with droperidol

Synonyms delta-9 THC; delta-9-tetrahydro-cannabinol; tetrahydrocannabinol; THC

Canadian Brand Names Marinol®

Therapeutic Category Antiemetic

Controlled Substance C-III

Use Chemotherapy-associated nausea and vomiting refractory to other antiemetic(s); AIDS-related anorexia

General Dosage Range Oral:

Children: Initial: 5 mg/m^2 as a single dose; Maintenance: 5 mg/m^2/dose every 2-4 hours for a total of 4-6 doses/day (maximum: 15 mg/m^2/dose)

Adults: Initial: 5 mg/m^2 as a single dose; Maintenance: 5 mg/m^2/dose every 2-4 hours for a total of 4-6 doses/day (maximum: 15 mg/m^2/dose) **or** Initial: 2.5 mg twice daily; Maintenance: Titrate up to 20 mg/day in 2 divided doses

Dosage Forms

Capsule, soft gelatin, oral: 2.5 mg, 5 mg, 10 mg

dronedarone (droe NE da rone)

Medication Safety Issues

BEERS Criteria medication:

This drug may be potentially inappropriate for use in geriatric patients (Quality of evidence - moderate/ high; Strength of recommendation - strong).

Synonyms dronedarone hydrochloride; SR33589

U.S. Brand Names Multaq®

Canadian Brand Names Multaq®

Therapeutic Category Antiarrhythmic Agent, Miscellaneous

Use To reduce the risk of hospitalization for atrial fibrillation (AF) in patients in sinus rhythm with a history of paroxysmal or persistent AF

General Dosage Range Oral: *Adults:* 400 mg twice daily

Dosage Forms

Tablet, oral:

Multaq®: 400 mg

dronedarone hydrochloride *see* dronedarone *on page 317*

droperidol (droe PER i dole)

Medication Safety Issues

Sound-alike/look-alike issues:

Droperidol may be confused with dronabinol

Synonyms dehydrobenzperidol

Canadian Brand Names Droperidol Injection, USP

Therapeutic Category Antiemetic; Antipsychotic Agent, Butyrophenone

Use Prevention and/or treatment of nausea and vomiting from surgical and diagnostic procedures

General Dosage Range I.M., I.V.:

Children 2-12 years: Maximum: 0.1 mg/kg; additional doses may be repeated

Adults: Maximum initial dose: 2.5 mg; additional doses of 1.25 mg may be administered

Dosage Forms

Injection, solution: 2.5 mg/mL (2 mL)

Injection, solution [preservative free]: 2.5 mg/mL (2 mL)

Droperidol Injection, USP (Can) *see* droperidol *on page 317*

drospirenone and estradiol (droh SPYE re none & es tra DYE ole)

Medication Safety Issues

BEERS Criteria medication:

This drug may be potentially inappropriate for use in geriatric patients (Quality of evidence - high [oral and transdermal patch]; Strength of recommendation - strong [oral and transdermal patch]).

Synonyms E2 and DRSP; estradiol and drospirenone

U.S. Brand Names Angeliq®

Canadian Brand Names Angeliq®

Therapeutic Category Estrogen and Progestin Combination

Use Treatment of moderate-to-severe vasomotor symptoms associated with menopause; treatment of vulvar and vaginal atrophy associated with menopause

General Dosage Range Oral: *Adults (females):* 1 tablet daily

Product Availability Angeliq® (drospirenone 0.25 mg and estradiol 0.5 mg) tablets: FDA approved March 2012; anticipated availability currently undetermined

Dosage Forms

Tablet:

Angeliq®: Drospirenone 0.5 mg and estradiol 1 mg

drospirenone and ethinyl estradiol *see* ethinyl estradiol and drospirenone *on page* 356

drospirenone, ethinyl estradiol, and levomefolate calcium *see* ethinyl estradiol, drospirenone, and levomefolate *on page* 363

drotrecogin alfa (activated) (dro TRE coe jin AL fa ak ti VAY ted)

Medication Safety Issues

Administration issues:

Use caution when interpreting dosing information. Maintenance dose expressed as mcg/kg/**hour**.

Synonyms activated protein C, human, recombinant; drotrecogin alfa, activated; protein C (activated), human, recombinant; rhAPC

U.S. Brand Names Xigris® [DSC]

Canadian Brand Names Xigris®

Therapeutic Category Protein C (Activated)

Use Reduction of mortality from severe sepsis (associated with organ dysfunction) in adults at high risk of death (eg, APACHE II score ≥25)

Note: As of October, 2011, drotrecogin alfa has been withdrawn from the market (worldwide).

General Dosage Range I.V.: *Adults:* 24 mcg/kg/**hour** for 96 hours

Product Availability No longer available; withdrawn from the market (worldwide) as of October 25, 2011.

drotrecogin alfa, activated *see* drotrecogin alfa (activated) *on page* 318

Droxia® *see* hydroxyurea *on page* 464

Dr. Scholl's® Callus Removers [OTC] *see* salicylic acid *on page* 816

Dr. Scholl's® Clear Away® One Step Wart Remover [OTC] *see* salicylic acid *on page* 816

Dr. Scholl's® Clear Away® Plantar Wart Remover For Feet [OTC] *see* salicylic acid *on page* 816

Dr. Scholl's® Clear Away® Wart Remover [OTC] *see* salicylic acid *on page* 816

Dr. Scholl's® Clear Away® Wart Remover Fast-Acting [OTC] *see* salicylic acid *on page* 816

Dr. Scholl's® Clear Away® Wart Remover Invisible Strips [OTC] *see* salicylic acid *on page* 816

Dr. Scholl's® Corn/Callus Remover [OTC] *see* salicylic acid *on page* 816

Dr. Scholl's® Corn Removers [OTC] *see* salicylic acid *on page* 816

Dr. Scholl's® Extra-Thick Callus Removers [OTC] *see* salicylic acid *on page* 816

Dr. Scholl's® Extra Thick Corn Removers [OTC] *see* salicylic acid *on page* 816

Dr. Scholl's® For Her Corn Removers [OTC] *see* salicylic acid *on page* 816

Dr. Scholl's® OneStep Callus Removers [OTC] *see* salicylic acid *on page* 816

Dr. Scholl's® OneStep Corn Removers [OTC] *see* salicylic acid *on page* 816

Dr. Scholl's® Small Corn Removers [OTC] *see* salicylic acid *on page* 816

Dr. Scholl's® Ultra-Thin Corn Removers [OTC] *see* salicylic acid *on page* 816

DRV *see* darunavir *on page* 255

Drysol™ *see* aluminum chloride hexahydrate *on page* 55

DSCG *see* cromolyn (nasal) *on page* 241

DSCG *see* cromolyn (ophthalmic) *on page* 241

DSCG *see* cromolyn (systemic, oral inhalation) *on page* 240

DSS *see* docusate *on page* 304

DSS® [OTC] *see* docusate *on page* 304

DT *see* diphtheria and tetanus toxoids *on page* 295

DTaP *see* diphtheria and tetanus toxoids, and acellular pertussis vaccine *on page* 298

DTaP-HepB-IPV *see* diphtheria, tetanus toxoids, acellular pertussis, hepatitis B (recombinant), and poliovirus (inactivated) vaccine *on page 300*

DTaP-HepB-IPV-Hib *see* diphtheria and tetanus toxoids, acellular pertussis, hepatitis B (recombinant), poliovirus (inactivated), and *Haemophilus influenzae* B conjugate (adsorbed) vaccine *on page 297*

DTaP/Hib *see* diphtheria and tetanus toxoids, acellular pertussis and *Haemophilus influenzae* b conjugate vaccine *on page 296*

DTaP-IPV *see* diphtheria and tetanus toxoids, acellular pertussis, and poliovirus vaccine *on page 296*

DTaP-IPV/Hib *see* diphtheria and tetanus toxoids, acellular pertussis, poliovirus and *Haemophilus* b conjugate vaccine *on page 298*

DTC 101 *see* cytarabine (liposomal) *on page 248*

DTIC *see* dacarbazine *on page 250*

DTIC-dome *see* dacarbazine *on page 250*

DTO (error-prone abbreviation) *see* opium tincture *on page 669*

DTPA *see* diethylene triamine penta-acetic acid *on page 283*

DTPA *see* pentetate indium disodium in 111 *on page 706*

D-Trp(6)-LHRH *see* triptorelin *on page 922*

Duac® *see* clindamycin and benzoyl peroxide *on page 219*

Duet® *see* vitamins (multiple/prenatal) *on page 952*

Duetact™ *see* pioglitazone and glimepiride *on page 725*

Duet® Balanced DHA[ec] *see* vitamins (multiple/prenatal) *on page 952*

Duexis® *see* ibuprofen and famotidine *on page 470*

Dukoral® (Can) *see* traveler's diarrhea and cholera vaccine *(Canada only) on page 911*

Dulcolax® [OTC] *see* bisacodyl *on page 134*

Dulcolax® [OTC] *see* docusate *on page 304*

Dulcolax Balance® [OTC] *see* polyethylene glycol 3350 *on page 737*

Dulcolax® Stool Softener [OTC] *see* docusate *on page 304*

Dulera® *see* mometasone and formoterol *on page 611*

Dull-C® [OTC] *see* ascorbic acid *on page 94*

duloxetine (doo LOX e teen)

Medication Safety Issues

Sound-alike/look-alike issues:

Cymbalta® may be confused with Symbyax®
DULoxetine may be confused with FLUoxetine

BEERS Criteria medication:

This drug may be potentially inappropriate for use in geriatric patients (Quality of evidence - moderate; Strength of recommendation - strong).

Synonyms (+)-(*S*)-*N*-methyl-γ-(1-naphthyloxy)-2-thiophenepropylamine hydrochloride; duloxetine hydrochloride; LY248686

Tall-Man **DUL**oxetine

U.S. Brand Names Cymbalta®

Canadian Brand Names Cymbalta®

Therapeutic Category Antidepressant, Serotonin/Norepinephrine Reuptake Inhibitor

Use Acute and maintenance treatment of major depressive disorder (MDD); treatment of generalized anxiety disorder (GAD); management of diabetic peripheral neuropathic pain (DPNP); management of fibromyalgia (FM); chronic musculoskeletal pain (eg, chronic low back pain, osteoarthritis)

General Dosage Range Oral:

Adults: 30-60 mg/day in 1-2 divided doses (maximum: 120 mg/day)
Elderly: Initial: 20 mg 1-2 times/day

Dosage Forms

Capsule, delayed release, enteric coated pellets, oral:
Cymbalta®: 20 mg, 30 mg, 60 mg

duloxetine hydrochloride *see* duloxetine *on page 319*

Duodopa™ (Can) *see* carbidopa and levodopa *on page 174*

Duodote™ *see* atropine and pralidoxime *on page 103*

DuoFilm® [OTC] *see* salicylic acid *on page 816*

Duofilm® (Can) *see* salicylic acid *on page 816*
Duoforte® 27 (Can) *see* salicylic acid *on page 816*
DuoNeb® *see* ipratropium and albuterol *on page 499*
DuoTrav™ (Can) *see* travoprost and timolol *(Canada only) on page 912*
Duovent® UDV (Can) *see* ipratropium and fenoterol *(Canada only) on page 500*
DuP 753 *see* losartan *on page 551*
Duraclon® *see* clonidine *on page 224*
Duragesic® *see* fentanyl *on page 377*
Duragesic® MAT (Can) *see* fentanyl *on page 377*
Duralith® (Can) *see* lithium *on page 544*
Duramist Plus [OTC] *see* oxymetazoline (nasal) *on page 681*
Duramorph *see* morphine (systemic) *on page 612*
Duratocin™ (Can) *see* carbetocin *(Canada only) on page 174*
Durela™ (Can) *see* tramadol *on page 909*
Durezol® *see* difluprednate *on page 285*
Duricef *see* cefadroxil *on page 181*
Durolane® (Can) *see* hyaluronate and derivatives *on page 450*

dutasteride (doo TAS teer ide)

U.S. Brand Names Avodart®
Canadian Brand Names Avodart®
Therapeutic Category Antineoplastic Agent, Anthracenedione
Use Treatment of symptomatic benign prostatic hyperplasia (BPH) as monotherapy or combination therapy with tamsulosin
General Dosage Range Oral: *Adults (males):* 0.5 mg once daily
Dosage Forms
Capsule, softgel, oral:
Avodart®: 0.5 mg

dutasteride and tamsulosin (doo TAS teer ide & tam SOO loe sin)

Synonyms tamsulosin and dutasteride; tamsulosin hydrochloride and dutasteride
U.S. Brand Names Jalyn™
Therapeutic Category 5 Alpha-Reductase Inhibitor; Alpha$_1$ Blocker
Use Treatment of symptomatic benign prostatic hyperplasia (BPH)
General Dosage Range Oral: *Adults (males):* 1 capsule (0.5 mg dutasteride/0.4 mg tamsulosin) once daily
Dosage Forms
Capsule, oral:
Jalyn™: Dutasteride 0.5 mg and tamsulosin hydrochloride 0.4 mg

Dutoprol™ *see* metoprolol and hydrochlorothiazide *on page 595*
Duvoid® (Can) *see* bethanechol *on page 131*
D-Vi-Sol® (Can) *see* cholecalciferol *on page 205*
DW286 *see* gemifloxacin *on page 422*
DX-88 *see* ecallantide *on page 321*
Dyazide® *see* hydrochlorothiazide and triamterene *on page 453*

dyclonine (DYE kloe neen)

Medication Safety Issues
Sound-alike/look-alike issues:
Dyclonine may be confused with dicyclomine
Synonyms dyclonine hydrochloride
U.S. Brand Names Sucrets® Children's [OTC]; Sucrets® Maximum Strength [OTC]; Sucrets® Regular Strength [OTC]
Therapeutic Category Local Anesthetic
Use Temporary relief of pain associated with oral mucosa

General Dosage Range Oral: Lozenge: *Children ≥2 years and Adults:* One lozenge every 2 hours as needed (maximum: 10 lozenges/day)

Dosage Forms

Lozenge, oral:

Sucrets® Children's [OTC]: 1.2 mg (18s)
Sucrets® Maximum Strength [OTC]: 3 mg (18s)
Sucrets® Regular Strength [OTC]: 2 mg (18s)

dyclonine hydrochloride *see* dyclonine *on page 320*
Dymista™ *see* azelastine and fluticasone *on page 108*
Dynacin® *see* minocycline *on page 604*
DynaCirc CR® [DSC] *see* isradipine *on page 506*
Dyna-Hex® [OTC] *see* chlorhexidine gluconate *on page 196*

dyphylline (DYE fi lin)

Synonyms dihydroxypropyl theophylline

U.S. Brand Names Lufyllin®

Therapeutic Category Theophylline Derivative

Use Bronchodilator in reversible airway obstruction due to asthma, chronic bronchitis, or emphysema

General Dosage Range Oral: *Adults:* Up to 15 mg/kg 4 times daily

Dosage Forms

Tablet, oral:

Lufyllin®: 200 mg, 400 mg

dyphylline and guaifenesin (DYE fi lin & gwye FEN e sin)

Synonyms guaifenesin and dyphylline

U.S. Brand Names Difil-G® 400

Therapeutic Category Expectorant; Theophylline Derivative

Use Treatment of bronchial asthma and reversible bronchospasm associated with chronic bronchitis and emphysema

General Dosage Range Oral: *Adults:* Dyphylline 200 mg and guaifenesin 400 mg: One tablet 3-4 times daily (maximum: 2 tablets 3-4 times daily)

Dosage Forms

Tablet, oral:

Difil-G® 400: Dyphylline 200 mg and guaifenesin 400 mg

Dyrenium® *see* triamterene *on page 917*
Dysport™ *see* abobotulinumtoxinA *on page 18*
E2 and DRSP *see* drospirenone and estradiol *on page 317*
7E3 *see* abciximab *on page 17*
E2020 *see* donepezil *on page 309*
E 2080 *see* rufinamide *on page 814*
E7389 *see* eribulin *on page 341*
EACA *see* aminocaproic acid *on page 61*
Ebixa® (Can) *see* memantine *on page 570*

ecallantide (e KAL lan tide)

Synonyms DX-88

U.S. Brand Names Kalbitor®

Therapeutic Category Kallikrein Inhibitor

Use Treatment of acute attacks of hereditary angioedema (HAE)

General Dosage Range SubQ: *Children ≥16 years and Adults:* 30 mg; may repeat once (maximum: 60 mg/24 hours)

Dosage Forms

Injection, solution [preservative free]:

Kalbitor®: 10 mg/mL (1 mL)

echothiophate iodide (ek oh THYE oh fate EYE oh dide)

Synonyms ecostigmine iodide

U.S. Brand Names Phospholine Iodide®

Therapeutic Category Cholinesterase Inhibitor

Use Used as miotic in treatment of chronic, open-angle glaucoma; may be useful in specific cases of angle-closure glaucoma (postiridectomy or where surgery refused/contraindicated); postcataract surgery-related glaucoma; accommodative esotropia

General Dosage Range Ophthalmic:

Children: Diagnosis: Instill 1 drop of (0.125%) into both eyes at bedtime for 2-3 weeks; Treatment: Instill 1 drop of 0.06% once daily **or** 0.125% every other day (maximum: 0.125% daily)

Adults: Initial: 1 drop (0.03%) twice daily; Maintenance: 1 dose daily or every other day

Dosage Forms

Powder for reconstitution, ophthalmic:

Phospholine Iodide®: 6.25 mg (5 mL)

EC-Naprosyn® *see* naproxen *on page 628*

***E. coli* asparaginase** *see* asparaginase (*E. coli*) *on page 95*

econazole (e KONE a zole)

Synonyms econazole nitrate

Therapeutic Category Antifungal Agent

Use Topical treatment of tinea pedis (athlete's foot), tinea cruris (jock itch), tinea corporis (ringworm), tinea versicolor, and cutaneous candidiasis

General Dosage Range Topical: *Children and Adults:* Apply sufficient quantity once or twice daily

Dosage Forms

Cream, topical: 1% (15 g, 30 g, 85 g)

econazole nitrate *see* econazole *on page 322*

Econopred *see* prednisolone (ophthalmic) *on page 754*

ecostigmine iodide *see* echothiophate iodide *on page 322*

Ecotrin® [OTC] *see* aspirin *on page 96*

Ecotrin® Arthritis Strength [OTC] *see* aspirin *on page 96*

Ecotrin® Low Strength [OTC] *see* aspirin *on page 96*

Ectosone (Can) *see* betamethasone *on page 129*

eculizumab (e kue LIZ oo mab)

Synonyms h5G1.1; monoclonal antibody 5G1.1; monoclonal antibody anti-C5

U.S. Brand Names Soliris®

Canadian Brand Names Soliris®

Therapeutic Category Monoclonal Antibody; Monoclonal Antibody, Complement Inhibitor

Use Treatment of paroxysmal nocturnal hemoglobinuria (PNH) to reduce hemolysis; treatment of atypical hemolytic uremic syndrome (aHUS) to inhibit complement-mediated thrombotic microangiopathy

Note: Not indicated for the treatment of hemolytic uremic syndrome related to Shiga toxin *E. coli* (STEC-HUS)

General Dosage Range I.V.:

Children 5 kg to <10 kg: Induction: 300 mg weekly for 1 dose; Maintenance: 300 mg at week 2, then 300 mg every 3 weeks

Children 10 kg to <20 kg: Induction: 600 mg weekly for 1 dose; Maintenance: 300 mg at week 2, then 300 mg every 2 weeks

Children 20 kg to <30 kg: Induction: 600 mg weekly for 2 doses; Maintenance: 600 mg at week 3, then 600 mg every 2 weeks

Children 30 kg to <40 kg: Induction: 600 mg weekly for 2 doses; Maintenance: 900 mg at week 3, then 900 mg every 2 weeks

Children ≥40 kg: Induction: 900 mg weekly for 4 doses; Maintenance: 1200 mg at week 5, then 1200 mg every 2 weeks

Adults: aHUS: Induction: 900 mg weekly for 4 doses; Maintenance: 1200 mg at week 5, then 1200 mg every 2 weeks **or** PNH: Induction: 600 mg weekly for 4 doses; Maintenance: 900 mg at week 5, then 900 mg every 2 weeks

Dosage Forms

Injection, solution [preservative free]:

Soliris®: 10 mg/mL (30 mL)

Ed-A-Hist™ [OTC] *see* chlorpheniramine and phenylephrine *on page 200*

Ed A-Hist DM [OTC] *see* chlorpheniramine, phenylephrine, and dextromethorphan *on page 201*

edarbi™ *see* azilsartan *on page 108*

edarbyclor™ *see* azilsartan and chlorthalidone *on page 108*

Ed ChlorPed [OTC] *see* chlorpheniramine *on page 199*

Ed ChlorPed D [OTC] *see* chlorpheniramine and phenylephrine *on page 200*

ED Chlorped Jr [OTC] *see* chlorpheniramine *on page 199*

Ed-Chlortan [OTC] *see* chlorpheniramine *on page 199*

Edecrin® *see* ethacrynic acid *on page 355*

edetate CALCIUM disodium (ED e tate KAL see um dye SOW dee um)

Medication Safety Issues

Sound-alike look-alike issues:

To avoid potentially serious errors, the abbreviation "EDTA" should **never** be used.

Edetate CALCIUM disodium (CaEDTA) may be confused with edetate disodium (Na_2EDTA) (not commercially available in the U.S. or Canada). CDC recommends that edetate disodium should **never** be used for chelation therapy in children. Fatal hypocalcemia may result if edetate disodium is used for chelation therapy instead of edetate calcium disodium. ISMP recommends confirming the diagnosis to help distinguish between the two drugs prior to dispensing and/or administering either drug.

Edetate CALCIUM disodium may be confused with etomidate

Synonyms CaEDTA; calcium disodium edetate; calcium disodiumethylenediaminetetraacetic acid; edetate disodium CALCIUM; EDTA (CALCIUM disodium) (error-prone abbreviation)

U.S. Brand Names Calcium Disodium Versenate®

Therapeutic Category Chelating Agent

Use Treatment of symptomatic acute and chronic lead poisoning

General Dosage Range Dosage adjustment recommended in patients with renal impairment

I.M., I.V.: *Children and Adults:* 1000-1500 mg/m^2/day (25-75 mg/kg/day)

Dosage Forms

Injection, solution:

Calcium Disodium Versenate®: 200 mg/mL (2.5 mL)

edetate disodium CALCIUM *see* edetate CALCIUM disodium *on page 323*

Edex® *see* alprostadil *on page 53*

Edluar™ *see* zolpidem *on page 966*

edrophonium (ed roe FOE nee um)

Synonyms edrophonium chloride

U.S. Brand Names Enlon®

Canadian Brand Names Enlon®; Tensilon®

Therapeutic Category Cholinergic Agent

Use Diagnosis of myasthenia gravis; differentiation of cholinergic crises from myasthenia crises; reversal of nondepolarizing neuromuscular blockers

General Dosage Range

I.M.:

Infants: 0.5-1 mg

Children ≤34 kg: 1 mg

Children >34 kg: 5 mg

Adults: 10 mg, followed by 2 mg if no response

I.V.:

Infants: 0.1 mg, followed by 0.4 mg if no response (maximum total dose: 0.5 mg)

Children ≤34 kg: 0.04 mg/kg as single dose or followed by 0.16 mg/kg if no response **or** 1 mg, followed by 1mg every 30-45 seconds if no response (maximum total dose: 5 mg)

Children >34 kg: 0.04 mg/kg as single dose or followed by 0.16 mg/kg if no response **or** 2 mg, followed by 1 mg every 30-45 seconds if no response (maximum total dose: 10 mg)

Adults: 2 mg test dose, followed by 8 mg if no response **or** 1-10 mg as a single dose **or** 10 mg every 5-10 minutes up to 40 mg **or** 1 mg; may repeat after 1 minute

Dosage Forms

Injection, solution:

Enlon®: 10 mg/mL (15 mL)

edrophonium and atropine (ed roe FOE nee um & A troe peen)

Synonyms atropine sulfate and edrophonium chloride; edrophonium chloride and atropine sulfate

U.S. Brand Names Enlon-Plus®

Therapeutic Category Anticholinergic Agent; Antidote; Cholinergic Agonist

Use Reversal of nondepolarizing neuromuscular blockers; adjunct treatment of respiratory depression caused by curare overdose

General Dosage Range I.V.: *Adults:* 0.05-0.1 mL/kg (0.5-1 mg/kg of edrophonium and 0.007-0.014 mg/kg of atropine)

Dosage Forms

Injection, solution:

Enlon-Plus®: Edrophonium 10 mg/mL and atropine 0.14 mg/mL (5 mL, 15 mL)

edrophonium chloride *see* edrophonium *on page 323*

edrophonium chloride and atropine sulfate *see* edrophonium and atropine *on page 324*

ED-SPAZ *see* hyoscyamine *on page 465*

EDTA (CALCIUM disodium) (error-prone abbreviation) *see* edetate CALCIUM disodium *on page 323*

Edurant™ *see* rilpivirine *on page 801*

EEMT™ *see* estrogens (esterified) and methyltestosterone *on page 353*

EEMT™ HS *see* estrogens (esterified) and methyltestosterone *on page 353*

E.E.S.® *see* erythromycin (systemic) *on page 342*

EES® (Can) *see* erythromycin (systemic) *on page 342*

efavirenz (e FAV e renz)

U.S. Brand Names Sustiva®

Canadian Brand Names Sustiva®

Therapeutic Category Antiretroviral Agent, Nonnucleoside Reverse Transcriptase Inhibitor (NNRTI)

Use Treatment of HIV-1 infections in combination with at least two other antiretroviral agents

General Dosage Range Dosage adjustment recommended in patients on concomitant therapy

Oral:

Children ≥3 years and 10 kg to <15 kg: 200 mg once daily
Children ≥3 years and 15 kg to <20 kg: 250 mg once daily
Children ≥3 years and 20 kg to <25 kg: 300 mg once daily
Children ≥3 years and 25 kg to <32.5 kg: 350 mg once daily
Children ≥3 years and 32.5 kg to <40 kg: 400 mg once daily
Children ≥3 years and ≥40 kg and Adults: 600 mg once daily

Dosage Forms

Capsule, oral:

Sustiva®: 50 mg, 200 mg

Tablet, oral:

Sustiva®: 600 mg

efavirenz, emtricitabine, and tenofovir

(e FAV e renz, em trye SYE ta been, & te NOE fo veer)

Synonyms emtricitabine, efavirenz, and tenofovir; FTC, TDF, and EFV; tenofovir disoproxil fumarate, efavirenz, and emtricitabine

U.S. Brand Names Atripla®

Canadian Brand Names Atripla®

Therapeutic Category Antiretroviral Agent, Nonnucleoside Reverse Transcriptase Inhibitor (NNRTI); Antiretroviral Agent, Nucleoside Reverse Transcriptase Inhibitor (NRTI); Antiretroviral Agent, Reverse Transcriptase Inhibitor (Nucleotide)

Use Treatment of HIV infection

General Dosage Range Oral: *Children ≥12 years and ≥40 kg, Adolescents, and Adults:* 1 tablet (efavirenz 600 mg/emtricitabine 200 mg/tenofovir 300 mg) once daily

Dosage Forms

Tablet:

Atripla®: Efavirenz 600 mg, emtricitabine 200 mg, and tenofovir disoproxil fumarate 300 mg

Effer-K® *see* potassium bicarbonate and potassium citrate *on page 743*

Effexor® *see* venlafaxine *on page 942*

Effexor XR® *see* venlafaxine *on page 942*

Effient® *see* prasugrel *on page 752*

eflornithine (ee FLOR ni theen)

Medication Safety Issues

Sound-alike/look-alike issues:

Vaniqa® may be confused with Viagra®

Synonyms DFMO; eflornithine hydrochloride

U.S. Brand Names Vaniqa®

Canadian Brand Names Vaniqa®

Therapeutic Category Antiprotozoal; Topical Skin Product

Use Cream: Females ≥12 years: Reduce unwanted hair from face and adjacent areas under the chin

Orphan status: Injection: Treatment of meningoencephalitic stage of *Trypanosoma brucei gambiense* infection (sleeping sickness)

General Dosage Range Dosage adjustment recommended in patients with renal impairment

I.V.: *Adults:* 100 mg/kg/dose every 6 hours

Topical: *Children and Adults:* Apply thin layer to affected areas twice daily

Dosage Forms

Cream, topical:

Vaniqa®: 13.9% (30 g)

eflornithine hydrochloride *see* eflornithine *on page 325*

eformoterol and budesonide *see* budesonide and formoterol *on page 146*

Efudex® *see* fluorouracil (topical) *on page 396*

E-Gem® [OTC] *see* vitamin E *on page 950*

E-Gem® Lip Care [OTC] *see* vitamin E *on page 950*

E-Gems® [OTC] *see* vitamin E *on page 950*

E-Gems® Elite [OTC] *see* vitamin E *on page 950*

E-Gems® Plus [OTC] *see* vitamin E *on page 950*

Egrifta® *see* tesamorelin *on page 881*

EHDP *see* etidronate *on page 364*

EL-970 *see* dalfampridine *on page 251*

Elaprase® *see* idursulfase *on page 472*

Elavil *see* amitriptyline *on page 64*

Eldepryl® *see* selegiline *on page 828*

Eldopaque® [OTC] *see* hydroquinone *on page 461*

Eldopaque® (Can) *see* hydroquinone *on page 461*

Eldopaque Forte® *see* hydroquinone *on page 461*

Eldoquin® [OTC] *see* hydroquinone *on page 461*

Eldoquin® (Can) *see* hydroquinone *on page 461*

Eldoquin Forte® *see* hydroquinone *on page 461*

electrolyte lavage solution *see* polyethylene glycol-electrolyte solution *on page 738*

electrolyte lavage solution *see* polyethylene glycol-electrolyte solution and bisacodyl *on page 739*

electrolyte solution, renal replacement

(ee LEK trow lite soe LOO shun REE nil ree PLASE ment)

Medication Safety Issues

High alert medication:

The Institute for Safe Medication Practices (ISMP) includes this medication among its list of drug classes which have a heightened risk of causing significant patient harm when used in error.

Synonyms continuous renal replacement therapy; CRRT; renal replacement solution

U.S. Brand Names Normocarb HF® 25; Normocarb HF® 35; PrismaSol

Therapeutic Category Alkalinizing Agent; Electrolyte Supplement

Use Used as a replacement solution to replenish water, correct electrolytes, and adjust acid-base balance depleted by hemofiltration or hemodiafiltration (continuous renal replacement therapy [CRRT]); drug poisoning when CRRT is used to remove filterable substances

General Dosage Range **Continuous renal replacement circuit:** *Children and Adults:*

Pre- or post-filter: Volume of solution administered depends upon the patient's fluid balance, target fluid balance, body weight, and amount of fluid removed during hemofiltration process.

Post-filter replacement: Volume infused/hour should not be greater than 1/3 of blood flow rate (eg, blood flow rate 100 mL/minute [6000 mL/hour]; post-filter replacement rate ≤2000 mL/hour)

Dosage Forms

Injection, solution [concentrate; preservative free]:

Normocarb HF® 25: Bicarbonate 25 mEq/L, chloride 116.5 mEq/L, magnesium 1.5 mEq/L, sodium 140 mEq/L (240 mL) [strength represents final solution after mixing; when diluted as directed, makes 3240 mL of infusate]

Normocarb HF® 35: Bicarbonate 35 mEq/L, chloride 106.5 mEq/L, magnesium 1.5 mEq/L, sodium 140 mEq/L (240 mL) [strength represents final solution after mixing; when diluted as directed, makes 3240 mL of infusate]

Injection, solution [preservative free]:

PrismaSol B22GK 2/0: Bicarbonate 22 mEq/L, chloride 118.5 mEq/L, dextrose 100 mg/dL, lactate 3 mEq/L, magnesium 1.5 mEq/L, potassium 2 mEq/L, sodium 140 mEq/L (5000 mL) [strength represents final solution after mixing]

PrismaSol BGK 2/0: Bicarbonate 32 mEq/L, chloride 108 mEq/L, dextrose 100 mg/dL, lactate 3 mEq/L, magnesium 1 mEq/L, potassium 2 mEq/L, sodium 140 mEq/L (5000 mL) [strength represents final solution after mixing]

PrismaSol BGK 2/3.5: Bicarbonate 32 mEq/L, calcium 3.5 mEq/L, chloride 111.5 mEq/L, dextrose 100 mg/dL, lactate 3 mEq/L, magnesium 1 mEq/L, potassium 2 mEq/L, sodium 140 mEq/L (5000 mL) [strength represents final solution after mixing]

PrismaSol BGK 4/0/1.2: Bicarbonate 32 mEq/L, chloride 110.2 mEq/L, dextrose 100 mg/dL, lactate 3 mEq/L, magnesium 1.2 mEq/L, potassium 4 mEq/L, sodium 140 mEq/L (5000 mL) [strength represents final solution after mixing]

PrismaSol BGK 4/2.5: Bicarbonate 32 mEq/L, calcium 2.5 mEq/L, chloride 113 mEq/L, dextrose 100 mg/dL, lactate 3 mEq/L, magnesium 1.5 mEq/L, potassium 4 mEq/L, sodium 140 mEq/L (5000 mL) [strength represents final solution after mixing]

PrismaSol BK 0/0/1.2: Bicarbonate 32 mEq/L, chloride 106.2 mEq/L, lactate 3 mEq/L, magnesium 1.2 mEq/L, sodium 140 mEq/L (5000 mL) [strength represents final solution after mixing]

Elelyso™ *see* taliglucerase alfa *on page* *867*
Elestat® *see* epinastine *on page* *334*
Elestrin® *see* estradiol (systemic) *on page* *347*
Eletone® *see* emollients *on page* *328*

eletriptan (el e TRIP tan)

Synonyms eletriptan hydrobromide

U.S. Brand Names Relpax®

Canadian Brand Names Relpax®

Therapeutic Category Serotonin 5-$HT_{1B,\ 1D}$ Receptor Agonist

Use Acute treatment of migraine, with or without aura

General Dosage Range **Oral:** *Adults:* 20-40 mg as a single dose, may repeat (maximum: 80 mg/day)

Dosage Forms

Tablet, oral:

Relpax®: 20 mg, 40 mg

eletriptan hydrobromide *see* eletriptan *on page* *326*
Elidel® *see* pimecrolimus *on page* *723*
Eligard® *see* leuprolide *on page* *527*
Elimite *see* permethrin *on page* *709*
Eliphos™ *see* calcium acetate *on page* *160*
Eliquis™ (Can) *see* apixaban *(Canada only) on page* *81*
Elitek® *see* rasburicase *on page* *789*

Elixophyllin® Elixir *see* theophylline *on page 888*
ella® *see* ulipristal *on page 928*
Ellence® *see* epirubicin *on page 336*
Elmiron® *see* pentosan polysulfate sodium *on page 707*
Elocom® (Can) *see* mometasone (topical) *on page 610*
Elocon® *see* mometasone (topical) *on page 610*
Eloxatin® *see* oxaliplatin *on page 674*
Elspar® *see* asparaginase (*E. coli*) *on page 95*
Eltor® (Can) *see* pseudoephedrine *on page 771*

eltrombopag (el TROM boe pag)

Synonyms eltrombopag olamine; Revolade®; SB-497115; SB-497115-GR

U.S. Brand Names Promacta®

Canadian Brand Names Revolade™

Therapeutic Category Colony Stimulating Factor; Thrombopoietic Agent

Use Treatment of thrombocytopenia in patients with chronic immune (idiopathic) thrombocytopenic purpura (ITP) at risk for bleeding who have had insufficient response to corticosteroids, immune globulin, or splenectomy

General Dosage Range Dosage adjustment recommended in patients with hepatic impairment, of East-Asian ethnicity, or who develop toxicities

Oral: *Adults:* 50 mg once daily (maximum: 75 mg/day)

Product Availability

Promacta® 12.5 mg tablets (new strength): FDA approved December 2011; expected availability currently unknown.

Product labeling for Promacta® has also been updated to include dosage adjustment recommendations utilizing the new 12.5 mg strength.

Dosage Forms

Tablet, oral:

Promacta®: 25 mg, 50 mg, 75 mg

eltrombopag olamine *see* eltrombopag *on page 327*
Eltroxin® (Can) *see* levothyroxine *on page 533*
Emadine® *see* emedastine *on page 327*
Embeda™ *see* morphine and naltrexone *on page 614*
Emcyt® *see* estramustine *on page 350*
EMD 68843 *see* vilazodone *on page 945*

emedastine (em e DAS teen)

Synonyms emedastine difumarate

U.S. Brand Names Emadine®

Therapeutic Category Antihistamine, H_1 Blocker, Ophthalmic

Use Treatment of allergic conjunctivitis

General Dosage Range Ophthalmic: *Children ≥3 years and Adults:* Instill 1 drop in affected eye up to 4 times/day

Dosage Forms

Solution, ophthalmic:

Emadine®: 0.05% (5 mL)

emedastine difumarate *see* emedastine *on page 327*
Emend® *see* aprepitant *on page 88*
Emend® IV (Can) *see* fosaprepitant *on page 408*
Emend® for Injection *see* fosaprepitant *on page 408*
Emetrol® [OTC] *see* fructose, dextrose, and phosphoric acid *on page 411*
EMLA® *see* lidocaine and prilocaine *on page 538*
Emo-Cort® (Can) *see* hydrocortisone (topical) *on page 457*
emollient cream *see* emollients *on page 328*
emollient foam *see* emollients *on page 328*

emollient lotion *see* emollients *on page 328*

emollients (ee MOL ee ents)

Medication Safety Issues

International issues:

Biafine: Topical emulsion [U.S.], but also a brand name for trolamine [multiple international markets]

Synonyms emollient cream; emollient foam; emollient lotion

U.S. Brand Names Atopiclair®; Atrapro™ Antipruritic; Aurstat®; Biafine®; Eletone®; EpiCeram® Skin Barrier; HylatopicPlus™; HylatopicPlus™ -Aurstat [DSC]; Hylatopic™; Mimyx®; Neosalus®; Normlshield®; Promiseb™; PruClair™; PruMyx™; PruTect™; PR™ Cream; Tropazone™

Therapeutic Category Skin and Mucous Membrane Agent, Miscellaneous; Topical Skin Product

Use Counteract dryness and itchy skin; lubricate and moisturize skin; aid in protection and healing of superficial wounds, burns, and minor abrasions; relief of itching, burning, and pain experienced with various types of dermatoses (including atopic dermatitis, allergic contact dermatitis, and radiation dermatitis); dermal donor and graft site management

General Dosage Range Topical: *Adults:* Apply to affected area 2-3 times daily

Dosage Forms

Aerosol, foam, topical:

HylatopicPlus™: (100 g, 150 g)
Hylatopic™: (100 g)
Neosalus®: (70 g, 200 g)

Cream, topical:

Atopiclair®: (100 g)
Eletone®: (100 g)
HylatopicPlus™: (100 g)
Neosalus®: (100 g, 180 g)
Normlshield®: (120 g)
Promiseb™: (30 g)
PruClair™: (100 g)
PR™ Cream: (56.7 g)
Tropazone™: (120 g)

Cream, topical [preservative free]:

Mimyx®: (140 g)
PruMyx™: (140 g)

Emulsion, topical:

Biafine®: (45 g, 90 g)
EpiCeram® Skin Barrier: (50 g, 90 g, 100 g)
PruTect™: (45 g, 90 g)

Gel, topical:

Atrapro™ Antipruritic: (113 g)
Aurstat®: (225 mL)

Lotion, topical:

Neosalus®: (236 mL)
Tropazone™: (140 g)

Emoquette™ *see* ethinyl estradiol and desogestrel *on page 356*

Emorex Gel [OTC] (Can) *see* coal tar *on page 228*

Emsam® *see* selegiline *on page 828*

emtricitabine (em trye SYE ta been)

Synonyms BW524W91; coviracil; FTC

U.S. Brand Names Emtriva®

Canadian Brand Names Emtriva®

Therapeutic Category Antiretroviral Agent, Nucleoside Reverse Transcriptase Inhibitor (NRTI)

Use Treatment of HIV infection in combination with at least two other antiretroviral agents

General Dosage Range Dosage adjustment recommended in patients with renal impairment

Oral:

Capsule: *Children 3 months to 17 years and >33 kg and Adults:* 200 mg once daily

Solution:
Children <3 months: 3 mg/kg/day
Children 3 months to 17 years: 6 mg/kg once daily (maximum: 240 mg/day)
Adults: 240 mg once daily

Dosage Forms

Capsule, oral:
Emtriva®: 200 mg

Solution, oral:
Emtriva®: 10 mg/mL (170 mL)

emtricitabine and tenofovir (em trye SYE ta been & te NOE fo veer)

Synonyms tenofovir and emtricitabine

U.S. Brand Names Truvada®

Canadian Brand Names Truvada®

Therapeutic Category Antiretroviral Agent, Nucleoside Reverse Transcriptase Inhibitor (NRTI); Antiretroviral Agent, Reverse Transcriptase Inhibitor (Nucleotide)

Use

Treatment of HIV-1 infection in combination with other antiretroviral agents in adults and pediatric patients ≥12 years of age

Preexposure prophylaxis (PrEP) for prevention of HIV-1 infection in adults who are at high risk for acquiring HIV

High risk individuals include those with partners known to be HIV-1 infected or who engage in sexual activity within a high prevalence area or social network, and one or more of the following:
- Inconsistent or no condom use
- Diagnosis of sexually-transmitted infections
- Exchange of sex for commodities
- Use of illicit drugs or alcohol dependence
- Incarceration
- Partner of unknown HIV-1 status with any of the above risk factors

When prescribing PrEP health care providers **MUST**:
- Include PrEP as part of a comprehensive prevention strategy because PrEP alone is not always effective in preventing HIV-1 infection
- Counsel all uninfected patients to strictly adhere to the dosing schedule, because adherence was strongly correlated with effectiveness in clinical trials
- Confirm a negative HIV-1 test prior to starting PrEP; if a candidate has acute viral infection symptoms and unprotected exposure events <1 month prior, delay PrEP for at least 1 month and retest HIV-1 status or use an Food and Drug Administration (FDA) test approved for HIV-1 diagnosis, including acute or primary HIV-1 infection
- Retest for HIV-1 infection at least every 3 months while the patient receives PrEP

General Dosage Range Dosage adjustment recommended in patients with renal impairment

Oral: *Children ≥12 (and >35 kg), Adolescents (≥35 kg), and Adults:* 1 tablet (emtricitabine 200 mg and tenofovir 300 mg) once daily

Dosage Forms

Tablet:
Truvada®: Emtricitabine 200 mg and tenofovir 300 mg

emtricitabine, efavirenz, and tenofovir *see* efavirenz, emtricitabine, and tenofovir *on page 324*

emtricitabine, rilpivirine, and tenofovir

(em trye SYE ta been, ril pi VIR een, & te NOE fo veer)

Synonyms FTC/RPV/TDF; rilpivirine, emtricitabine, and tenofovir; tenofovir disoproxil fumarate, rilpivirine, and emtricitabine; tenofovir, emtricitabine, and rilpivirine

U.S. Brand Names Complera™

Canadian Brand Names Complera™

Therapeutic Category Antiretroviral Agent, Reverse Transcriptase Inhibitor (Non-nucleoside); Antiretroviral Agent, Reverse Transcriptase Inhibitor (Nucleoside); Antiretroviral Agent, Reverse Transcriptase Inhibitor (Nucleotide)

Use Treatment of human immunodeficiency virus type 1 (HIV-1) infection in antiretroviral treatment-naive adult patients

General Dosage Range Oral: *Adults:* One tablet once daily

Dosage Forms

Tablet, oral:

Complera™: Emtricitabine 200 mg, rilpivirine 25 mg, and tenofovir 300 mg

Emtriva® *see* emtricitabine *on page* 328

ENA 713 *see* rivastigmine *on page* 806

Enablex® *see* darifenacin *on page* 255

enalapril (e NAL a pril)

Medication Safety Issues

Sound-alike/look-alike issues:

Enalapril may be confused with Anafranil®, Elavil®, Eldepryl®, ramipril

Administration issues:

Significant differences exist between oral and I.V. dosing. Use caution when converting from one route of administration to another.

International issues:

Acepril [Hungary, Switzerland] may be confused with Accupril which is a brand name for quinapril [U.S., Canada, multiple international markets]

Acepril: Brand name for enalapril [Hungary, Switzerland], but also brand name for captopril [Great Britain]; lisinopril [Malaysia]

Synonyms enalapril maleate

U.S. Brand Names Vasotec®

Canadian Brand Names Apo-Enalapril®; CO Enalapril; Mylan-Enalapril; Novo-Enalapril; PMS-Enalapril; PRO-Enalapril; RAN™-Enalapril; ratio-Enalapril; Riva-Enalapril; Sandoz-Enalapril; Sig-Enalapril; Taro-Enalapril; Teva-Enalapril; Vasotec®

Therapeutic Category Angiotensin-Converting Enzyme (ACE) Inhibitor

Use Treatment of hypertension; treatment of symptomatic heart failure; treatment of asymptomatic left ventricular dysfunction

General Dosage Range Dosage adjustment recommended in patients with renal impairment.

Oral:

Children 1 month to 17 years: Initial: 0.08 mg/kg/day (up to 5 mg) in 1-2 divided doses; Maintenance: Up to 0.58 mg/kg (40 mg)

Adults: Initial: 2.5-5 mg/day in 1-2 divided doses; Maintenance: 2.5-40 mg/day in 1-2 divided doses

Dosage Forms

Tablet, oral: 2.5 mg, 5 mg, 10 mg, 20 mg

Vasotec®: 2.5 mg, 5 mg, 10 mg, 20 mg

enalapril and hydrochlorothiazide (e NAL a pril & hye droe klor oh THYE a zide)

Medication Safety Issues

International issues:

Norpramin: Brand name for enalapril/hydrochlorothiazide [Portugal], but also the brand name for desipramine [U.S., Canada]; omeprazole [Spain]

Synonyms enalapril maleate and hydrochlorothiazide; hydrochlorothiazide and enalapril

U.S. Brand Names Vaseretic®

Canadian Brand Names Vaseretic®

Therapeutic Category Antihypertensive Agent, Combination

Use Treatment of hypertension

General Dosage Range Oral: *Adults:* Enalapril 5-10 mg and hydrochlorothiazide 12.5-25 mg once daily (maximum: 40 mg/day [enalapril]; 50 mg/day [hydrochlorothiazide])

Dosage Forms

Tablet: 5/12.5: Enalapril 5 mg and hydrochlorothiazide 12.5 mg; 10/25: Enalapril 10 mg and hydrochlorothiazide 25 mg

Vaseretic®: 10/25: enalapril 10 mg and hydrochlorothiazide 25 mg

enalaprilat (en AL a pril at)

Medication Safety Issues

Administration issues:

Significant differences exist between oral and I.V. dosing. Use caution when converting from one route of administration to another.

Canadian Brand Names Vasotec® I.V

Therapeutic Category Angiotensin-Converting Enzyme (ACE) Inhibitor

Use Treatment of hypertension when oral therapy is not practical

General Dosage Range Dosage adjustment recommended in patients with renal impairment.

I.V.: *Adults:* 0.625-5 mg every 6 hours

Dosage Forms

Injection, solution: 1.25 mg/mL (1 mL, 2 mL)

enalapril maleate *see* enalapril *on page* 330

enalapril maleate and hydrochlorothiazide *see* enalapril and hydrochlorothiazide *on page* 330

Enbrel® *see* etanercept *on page* 354

Enbrel® SureClick® *see* etanercept *on page* 354

Encare® [OTC] *see* nonoxynol 9 *on page* 647

Encora® *see* vitamins (multiple/oral) *on page* 951

EndaCof [OTC] *see* chlorpheniramine, phenylephrine, and dextromethorphan *on page* 201

EndaCof-DC *see* pseudoephedrine and codeine *on page* 772

EndoAvitene® *see* collagen hemostat *on page* 234

Endocet® *see* oxycodone and acetaminophen *on page* 679

Endodan® *see* oxycodone and aspirin *on page* 680

Endometrin® *see* progesterone *on page* 762

Enduron *see* methyclothiazide *on page* 587

Enemeez® [OTC] *see* docusate *on page* 304

Enemeez® Plus [OTC] *see* docusate *on page* 304

Ener-B® [OTC] *see* cyanocobalamin *on page* 242

Enerjets [OTC] *see* caffeine *on page* 157

Enfamil® D-Vi-Sol™ [OTC] *see* cholecalciferol *on page* 205

Enfamil® Glucose [OTC] *see* dextrose *on page* 275

enflurane (EN floo rane)

Medication Safety Issues

Sound-alike/look-alike issues:

Enflurane may be confused with isoflurane

High alert medication:

The Institute for Safe Medication Practices (ISMP) includes this medication among its list of drug classes which have a heightened risk of causing significant patient harm when used in error.

U.S. Brand Names Compound 347™

Therapeutic Category General Anesthetic

Use Maintenance of general anesthesia

Note: Use for induction of general anesthesia is an FDA-labeled indication; however, it is not recommended clinically due to its irritant properties and unpleasant odor which causes breath-holding and coughing. In addition, other labeled indications that are not routinely used and/or recommended clinically include use as analgesia during vaginal delivery and use as an adjunct to other general anesthetic agents during Cesarean section delivery.

General Dosage Range Inhalation: *Adults:* Maintenance: 0.5% to 3% (maximum concentration: 3%)

Dosage Forms

Liquid, for inhalation:

Compound 347™: >99.9% (250 mL)

enfuvirtide (en FYOO vir tide)

Synonyms T-20

U.S. Brand Names Fuzeon®

Canadian Brand Names Fuzeon®

Therapeutic Category Antiretroviral Agent, Fusion Protein Inhibitor

Use Treatment of HIV-1 infection in combination with other antiretroviral agents in treatment-experienced patients with evidence of HIV-1 replication despite ongoing antiretroviral therapy

General Dosage Range Dosage adjustment recommended in patients with renal impairment

SubQ:

Children 6-16 years: 2 mg/kg twice daily (maximum: 90 mg/dose)

Adolescents ≥16 years and Adults: 90 mg twice daily

Dosage Forms

Injection, powder for reconstitution [preservative free]:

Fuzeon®: 108 mg

ENG *see* etonogestrel *on page 366*

Engerix-B® *see* hepatitis B vaccine (recombinant) *on page 445*

Engerix-B® and Havrix® *see* hepatitis A and hepatitis B recombinant vaccine *on page 444*

enhanced-potency inactivated poliovirus vaccine *see* poliovirus vaccine (inactivated) *on page 736*

Enjuvia™ *see* estrogens (conjugated B/synthetic) *on page 351*

Enlon® *see* edrophonium *on page 323*

Enlon-Plus® *see* edrophonium and atropine *on page 324*

enoxaparin (ee noks a PA rin)

Medication Safety Issues

Sound-alike/look-alike issues:

Lovenox® may be confused with Lasix®, Levaquin®, Lotronex®, Protonix®

High alert medication:

The Institute for Safe Medication Practices (ISMP) includes this medication among its list of drugs which have a heightened risk of causing significant patient harm when used in error.

National Patient Safety Goals:

The Joint Commission (TJC) requires healthcare organizations that provide anticoagulant therapy to have a process in place to reduce the risk of anticoagulant-associated patient harm. Patients receiving anticoagulants should receive individualized care through a defined process that includes standardized ordering, dispensing, administration, monitoring and education. This does not apply to routine short-term use of anticoagulants for prevention of venous thromboembolism when the expectation is that the patient's laboratory values will remain within or close to normal values (NPSG.03.05.01).

Synonyms enoxaparin sodium

U.S. Brand Names Lovenox®

Canadian Brand Names Enoxaparin Injection; Lovenox®; Lovenox® HP

Therapeutic Category Anticoagulant (Other)

Use

Acute coronary syndromes: Unstable angina (UA), non-ST-elevation (NSTEMI), and ST-elevation myocardial infarction (STEMI)

DVT prophylaxis: Following hip or knee replacement surgery, abdominal surgery, or in medical patients with severely-restricted mobility during acute illness who are at risk for thromboembolic complications

DVT treatment (acute): Inpatient treatment (patients with and without pulmonary embolism) and outpatient treatment (patients without pulmonary embolism)

Note: High-risk patients include those with one or more of the following risk factors: >40 years of age, obesity, general anesthesia lasting >30 minutes, malignancy, history of deep vein thrombosis or pulmonary embolism

General Dosage Range Dosage adjustment recommended in patients with renal impairment

SubQ: *Adults:* Prophylaxis: 30 mg every 12 hours **or** 40 mg once daily; Treatment: 1 mg/kg every 12 hours **or** 1.5 mg/kg once daily

STEMI indication only:

<75 years: 30 mg I.V. bolus plus 1 mg/kg SubQ every 12 hours

≥75 years: 0.75 mg/kg SubQ every 12 hours

Dosage Forms

Injection, solution: 100 mg/mL (3 mL)

Lovenox®: 100 mg/mL (3 mL)

Injection, solution [preservative free]: 30 mg/0.3 mL (0.3 mL); 40 mg/0.4 mL (0.4 mL); 60 mg/0.6 mL (0.6 mL); 80 mg/0.8 mL (0.8 mL); 100 mg/mL (1 mL); 120 mg/0.8 mL (0.8 mL); 150 mg/mL (1 mL)

Lovenox®: 30 mg/0.3 mL (0.3 mL); 40 mg/0.4 mL (0.4 mL); 60 mg/0.6 mL (0.6 mL); 80 mg/0.8 mL (0.8 mL); 100 mg/mL (1 mL); 120 mg/0.8 mL (0.8 mL); 150 mg/mL (1 mL)

Enoxaparin Injection (Can) *see* enoxaparin *on page 332*

enoxaparin sodium *see* enoxaparin *on page* 332

Enpresse® *see* ethinyl estradiol and levonorgestrel *on page* 357

entacapone (en TA ka pone)

U.S. Brand Names Comtan®

Canadian Brand Names Comtan®; Sandoz-Entacapone; Teva-Entacapone

Therapeutic Category Anti-Parkinson Agent; Reverse COMT Inhibitor

Use Adjunct to levodopa/carbidopa therapy in patients with idiopathic Parkinson disease who experience "wearing-off" symptoms at the end of a dosing interval

General Dosage Range **Oral:** *Adults:* 200 mg with each dose of levodopa/carbidopa (maximum: 1600 mg/day)

Dosage Forms

Tablet, oral:

Comtan®: 200 mg

entacapone, carbidopa, and levodopa *see* levodopa, carbidopa, and entacapone *on page* 531

entecavir (en TE ka veer)

U.S. Brand Names Baraclude®

Canadian Brand Names Baraclude®

Therapeutic Category Antiretroviral Agent, Reverse Transcriptase Inhibitor (Nucleoside)

Use Treatment of chronic hepatitis B infection, with compensated or decompensated liver disease, in adults with evidence of active viral replication and either evidence of persistent transaminase elevations or histologically-active disease

General Dosage Range Dosage adjustment recommended in patients with renal impairment.

Oral: *Adolescents ≥16 years and Adults:* 0.5-1 mg once daily

Dosage Forms

Solution, oral:

Baraclude®: 0.05 mg/mL (210 mL)

Tablet, oral:

Baraclude®: 0.5 mg, 1 mg

Entereg® *see* alvimopan *on page* 57

Entero-H™ *see* barium *on page* 114

enterotoxigenic *Escherichia coli* and *Vibrio cholera* vaccine *see* traveler's diarrhea and cholera vaccine *(Canada only) on page* 911

Entero Vu™ *see* barium *on page* 114

Entero VU™ 24% *see* barium *on page* 114

Entertainer's Secret® [OTC] *see* saliva substitute *on page* 819

Entex® LA (Can) *see* guaifenesin and pseudoephedrine *on page* 436

Entocort® (Can) *see* budesonide (systemic, oral inhalation) *on page* 145

Entocort® EC *see* budesonide (systemic, oral inhalation) *on page* 145

Entre-B [OTC] *see* brompheniramine and phenylephrine *on page* 144

Entrophen® (Can) *see* aspirin *on page* 96

Entsol® [OTC] *see* sodium chloride *on page* 840

Enulose *see* lactulose *on page* 519

Eovist® *see* gadoxetate *on page* 417

EPEG *see* etoposide *on page* 366

ephedrine (systemic) (e FED rin)

Medication Safety Issues

Sound-alike/look-alike issues:

EPHEDrine may be confused with Epifrin®, EPINEPHrine

Synonyms ephedrine sulfate

Tall-Man ePHEDrine

Therapeutic Category Alpha/Beta Agonist

Use Treatment of nasal congestion, anesthesia-induced hypotension

General Dosage Range

I.V.:

Children: 0.2-0.3 mg/kg/dose every 4-6 hours

Adults: 5-25 mg/dose; repeat after 5-10 minutes as needed, then every 3-4 hours (maximum: 150 mg/day)

Oral: *Children ≥12 years and Adults:* 12.5-50 mg every 4 hours as needed (maximum: 150 mg/day)

Dosage Forms

Capsule, oral: 25 mg

Injection, solution [preservative free]: 50 mg/mL (1 mL)

ephedrine sulfate *see* ephedrine (systemic) *on page* 333

EpiCeram® Skin Barrier *see* emollients *on page* 328

Epi-Clenz™ [OTC] *see* alcohol (ethyl) *on page* 43

epidoxorubicin *see* epirubicin *on page* 336

Epiduo® *see* adapalene and benzoyl peroxide *on page* 36

Epi E-Z Pen® (Can) *see* epinephrine (systemic, oral inhalation) *on page* 334

Epiflur™ *see* fluoride *on page* 393

Epifoam® *see* pramoxine and hydrocortisone *on page* 751

Epiklor™ *see* potassium chloride *on page* 744

Epiklor™/25 *see* potassium chloride *on page* 744

epinastine (ep i NAS teen)

Synonyms epinastine hydrochloride

U.S. Brand Names Elestat®

Therapeutic Category Antihistamine, H_1 Blocker, Ophthalmic

Use Treatment of allergic conjunctivitis

General Dosage Range Ophthalmic: *Children ≥2 years and Adults:* Instill 1 drop into each eye twice daily

Dosage Forms

Solution, ophthalmic: 0.05% (5 mL)

Elestat®: 0.05% (5 mL)

epinastine hydrochloride *see* epinastine *on page* 334

epinephrine (systemic, oral inhalation) (ep i NEF rin)

Medication Safety Issues

Sound-alike/look-alike issues:

EPINEPHrine may be confused with ePHEDrine

Epifrin® may be confused with ephedrine, EpiPen®

High alert medication:

The Institute for Safe Medication Practices (ISMP) includes this medication among its list of drugs which have a heightened risk of causing significant patient harm when used in error.

Administration issues:

Medication errors have occurred due to confusion with epinephrine products expressed as ratio strengths (eg, 1:1000 vs 1:10,000).

Epinephrine 1:1000 = 1 mg/mL and is most commonly used I.M.

Epinephrine 1:10,000 = 0.1 mg/mL and is used I.V.

Medication errors have occurred when topical epinephrine 1 mg/mL (1:1000) has been inadvertently injected. Vials of injectable and topical epinephrine look very similar. Epinephrine should always be appropriately labeled with the intended administration.

International issues:

EpiPen [U.S., Canada, and multiple international markets] may be confused with Epigen brand name for glycyrrhizinic acid [Argentina, Mexico, Russia] and Epopen brand name for epoetin alfa [Spain]

Synonyms adrenaline; epinephrine bitartrate; epinephrine hydrochloride; racemic epinephrine; racepinephrine

Tall-Man EPINEPHrine

U.S. Brand Names Adrenalin®; Asthmanefrin™ [OTC]; EpiPen 2-Pak®; EpiPen Jr 2-Pak®; Primatene® Mist [OTC] [DSC]; S2® [OTC]; Twinject®

Canadian Brand Names Adrenalin®; Epi E-Z Pen®; EpiPen®; EpiPen® Jr; Twinject®

Therapeutic Category Alpha/Beta Agonist

Use Treatment of bronchospasms, bronchial asthma, viral croup, anaphylactic reactions, cardiac arrest; added to local anesthetics to decrease systemic absorption of intraspinal and local anesthetics and increase duration of action; decrease superficial hemorrhage

General Dosage Range

I.M.:

Adults: 0.3-0.5 mg (**1:1000** [1 mg/mL] solution) every 15-20 minutes

EpiPen® Jr., Twinject®: *Children 15-29 kg:* 0.15 mg as single dose; may repeat if needed

EpiPen®, Twinject®: *Children ≥30 kg and Adults:* 0.3 mg as single dose; may repeat if needed

Inhalation: *Children ≥4 years and Adults:* 1 inhalation; may repeat once after 1 minute, then do not use again for at least 3 hours

I.V. (**1:10,000** [0.1 mg/mL] solution):

Children: 0.01 mg/kg kg (maximum single dose: 1 mg) every 3-5 minutes as needed **or** 0.1-1 mcg/kg/minute as a continuous infusion **or** 0.01 mg/kg every 20 minutes (hypersensitivity reaction)

Adults: 1 mg every 3-5 minutes (up to 0.2 mg/kg) **or** 1-10 mcg/minute as a continuous infusion

Nebulization (S2® Racepinephrine, OTC):

Children <4 years: Jet nebulizer: 0.05 mL/kg (maximum dose: 0.5 mL) diluted in 3 mL NS up to every 2 hours

Children ≥4 years and Adults:

Hand-bulb nebulizer: Add 0.5 mL (~10 drops) to nebulizer; 1-3 inhalations up to every 3 hours if needed

Jet nebulizer: Add 0.5 mL (~10 drops) to nebulizer and dilute with 3 mL of NS. Administer over ~15 minutes every 3-4 hours as needed.

SubQ:

Children: 0.01 mg/kg (**1:1000** [1 mg/mL] solution) every 20 minutes for 3 doses or as condition requires (maximum: 0.3 mg/dose)

Adults: 0.3-0.5 mg (**1:1000** [1 mg/mL] solution) every 15-20 minutes for 3 doses or as condition requires

EpiPen® Jr, Twinject®: *Children 15-29 kg:* 0.15 mg as single dose; may repeat if needed

EpiPen®, Twinject®: *Children ≥30 kg and Adults:* 0.3 mg as single dose; may repeat if needed

Product Availability Auvi-Q™: FDA approved August 2012; anticipated availability currently unknown. Consult prescribing information for additional information.

Dosage Forms

Injection, solution: 0.1 mg/mL (10 mL); 1 mg/mL (1 mL, 30 mL)

Adrenalin®: 1 mg/mL (1 mL, 30 mL)

EpiPen 2-Pak®: 0.3 mg/0.3 mL (2 mL)

EpiPen Jr 2-Pak®: 0.15 mg/0.3 mL (2 mL)

Twinject®: 0.15 mg/0.15 mL (1.1 mL); 0.3 mg/0.3 mL (1.1 mL)

Injection, solution [preservative free]: 1 mg/mL (1 mL)

Solution, for oral inhalation [preservative free]:

Asthmanefrin™ [OTC]: Racepinephrine 2.25% (0.5 mL)

S2® [OTC]: Racepinephrine 2.25% (0.5 mL)

epinephrine (nasal) (ep i NEF rin)

Medication Safety Issues

Sound-alike/look-alike issues:

EPINEPHrine may be confused with ePHEDrine

Synonyms adrenaline; epinephrine hydrochloride

Tall-Man EPINEPHrine

U.S. Brand Names Adrenalin®

Canadian Brand Names Adrenalin®

Therapeutic Category Alpha/Beta Agonist

Use Treatment of nasal congestion

General Dosage Range Intranasal: *Children ≥6 years and Adults:* Apply **1:1000** (1 mg/mL) solution locally as drops, spray, or with sterile swab

Dosage Forms

Solution, intranasal:

Adrenalin®: 1 mg/mL (30 mL)

epinephrine and articaine hydrochloride *see* articaine and epinephrine *on page* 92

epinephrine and chlorpheniramine (ep i NEF rin & klor fen IR a meen)

Synonyms insect sting kit

U.S. Brand Names Ana-Kit®

Therapeutic Category Antidote

Use Anaphylaxis emergency treatment of insect bites or stings by the sensitive patient that may occur within minutes of insect sting or exposure to an allergic substance

General Dosage Range

I.M., SubQ: Epinephrine (1:1000):

Children <2 years: 0.05-0.1 mL
Children 2-6 years: 0.15 mL
Children 6-12 years: 0.2 mL
Children >12 years and Adults: 0.3 mL

Oral: Chlorpheniramine (2 mg/tablet):

Children <6 years: 1 tablet
Children 6-12 years: 2 tablets
Children >12 years and Adults: 4 tablets

Dosage Forms

Kit:

Ana-Kit®: Epinephrine 1:1000 (1 mL), chlorpheniramine chewable tablet 2 mg (4), sterile alcohol pads (2), tourniquet (1)

epinephrine and lidocaine *see* lidocaine and epinephrine *on page 537*
epinephrine bitartrate *see* epinephrine (systemic, oral inhalation) *on page 334*
epinephrine bitartrate and bupivacaine hydrochloride *see* bupivacaine and epinephrine *on page 148*
epinephrine hydrochloride *see* epinephrine (nasal) *on page 335*
epinephrine hydrochloride *see* epinephrine (systemic, oral inhalation) *on page 334*
EpiPen® (Can) *see* epinephrine (systemic, oral inhalation) *on page 334*
EpiPen 2-Pak® *see* epinephrine (systemic, oral inhalation) *on page 334*
EpiPen® Jr (Can) *see* epinephrine (systemic, oral inhalation) *on page 334*
EpiPen Jr 2-Pak® *see* epinephrine (systemic, oral inhalation) *on page 334*
epipodophyllotoxin *see* etoposide *on page 366*
epipodophyllotoxin *see* etoposide phosphate *on page 366*
EpiQuin® Micro *see* hydroquinone *on page 461*

epirubicin (ep i ROO bi sin)

Medication Safety Issues

Sound-alike/look-alike issues:

EPIrubicin may be confused with DOXOrubicin, DAUNOrubicin, eriBULin, idarubicin

International issues:

Ellence [U.S.] may be confused with Elase brand name for dornase alfa [Chile, France, Malaysia]

High alert medication:

This drug is in a class the Institute for Safe Medication Practices (ISMP) includes among its list of drug classes which have a heightened risk of causing significant patient harm when used in error.

Synonyms epidoxorubicin; epirubicin hydrochloride; pidorubicin; pidorubicin hydrochloride

Tall-Man EPIrubicin

U.S. Brand Names Ellence®

Canadian Brand Names Ellence®; Epirubicin for Injection; Epirubicin Hydrochloride Injection; Pharmorubicin®

Therapeutic Category Antineoplastic Agent, Anthracycline; Antineoplastic Agent, Antibiotic

Use Adjuvant therapy component for primary breast cancer

General Dosage Range Dosage adjustment recommended in patients with hepatic or renal impairment or who develop toxicities

I.V.: *Adults:* 100 mg/m^2 on day 1 every 3 weeks **or** 60 mg/m^2 on days 1 and 8 every 4 weeks

Dosage Forms

Injection, powder for reconstitution: 50 mg

Injection, solution [preservative free]: 2 mg/mL (5 mL, 25 mL, 75 mL, 100 mL)

Ellence®: 2 mg/mL (25 mL, 100 mL)

Epirubicin for Injection (Can) *see* epirubicin *on page 336*
epirubicin hydrochloride *see* epirubicin *on page 336*

Epirubicin Hydrochloride Injection (Can) *see* epirubicin *on page* 336
Epitol® *see* carbamazepine *on page* 172
Epival® (Can) *see* divalproex *on page* 302
Epival® I.V. (Can) *see* valproic acid *on page* 934
Epivir® *see* lamivudine *on page* 520
Epivir-HBV® *see* lamivudine *on page* 520

eplerenone (e PLER en one)

Medication Safety Issues

Sound-alike/look-alike issues:

Inspra™ may be confused with Spiriva®

U.S. Brand Names Inspra™

Therapeutic Category Antihypertensive Agent; Selective Aldosterone Blocker

Use Treatment of hypertension (may be used alone or in combination with other antihypertensive agents); treatment of heart failure (HF) following acute MI

General Dosage Range Dosage adjustment recommended in patients on concomitant therapy or based on potassium concentrations

Oral: *Adults:* Initial: 25-50 mg once daily; Maintenance: 50 mg once or twice daily (maximum: 100 mg/day)

Dosage Forms

Tablet, oral: 25 mg, 50 mg

Inspra™: 25 mg, 50 mg

EPO *see* epoetin alfa *on page* 337

epoetin alfa (e POE e tin AL fa)

Medication Safety Issues

Sound-alike/look-alike issues:

Epoetin alfa may be confused with darbepoetin alfa, epoetin beta

Epogen® may be confused with Neupogen®

International issues:

Epopen [Spain] may be confused with EpiPen brand name for epinephrine [U.S., Canada, and multiple international markets]

Synonyms *r*HuEPO; *r*HuEPO-α; EPO; erythropoiesis-stimulating agent (ESA); erythropoietin

U.S. Brand Names Epogen®; Procrit®

Canadian Brand Names Eprex®

Therapeutic Category Colony-Stimulating Factor

Use Treatment of anemia due to concurrent myelosuppressive chemotherapy in patients with cancer (nonmyeloid malignancies) receiving chemotherapy (palliative intent) for a planned minimum of 2 additional months of chemotherapy; treatment of anemia due to chronic kidney disease (including patients on dialysis and not on dialysis) to decrease the need for RBC transfusion; treatment of anemia associated with HIV (zidovudine) therapy when endogenous erythropoietin levels ≤500 mUnits/mL; reduction of allogeneic RBC transfusion for elective, noncardiac, nonvascular surgery when perioperative hemoglobin is >10 to ≤13 g/dL and there is a high risk for blood loss

Note: Epoetin is **not** indicated for use under the following conditions:

- Cancer patients receiving hormonal therapy, therapeutic biologic products, or radiation therapy unless also receiving concurrent myelosuppressive chemotherapy
- Cancer patients receiving myelosuppressive chemotherapy when the expected outcome is curative
- Surgery patients who are willing to donate autologous blood
- Surgery patients undergoing cardiac or vascular surgery
- As a substitute for RBC transfusion in patients requiring immediate correction of anemia

Note: In clinical trials (and one meta-analysis), epoetin has not demonstrated improved quality of life, fatigue, or well-being.

General Dosage Range I.V., SubQ: Children and Adults: Dosage varies greatly depending on indication

Dosage Forms

Injection, solution:

Epogen®: 10,000 units/mL (2 mL); 20,000 units/mL (1 mL)

Procrit®: 10,000 units/mL (2 mL); 20,000 units/mL (1 mL)

Injection, solution [preservative free]:

Epogen®: 2000 units/mL (1 mL); 3000 units/mL (1 mL); 4000 units/mL (1 mL); 10,000 units/mL (1 mL)

Procrit®: 2000 units/mL (1 mL); 3000 units/mL (1 mL); 4000 units/mL (1 mL); 10,000 units/mL (1 mL); 40,000 units/mL (1 mL)

Dosage Forms - Canada

Injection, solution [preservative free]:

Eprex®: 1000 units/0.5 mL (0.5 mL), 2000 units/0.5 mL (0.5 mL), 3000 units/0.3 mL (0.3 mL), 4000 units/0.4 mL (0.4 mL), 5000 units/0.5 mL (0.5 mL), 6000 units/0.6 mL (0.6 mL), 8000 units/0.8 mL (0.8 mL), 10,000 units/mL (1 mL), 20,000 units/0.5 mL (0.5 mL), 30,000 units/0.75 mL (0.75 mL), 40,000 units/mL (1 mL) [contains polysorbate 80; prefilled syringe, free of human serum albumin]

Epogen® *see* epoetin alfa *on page* 337

epoprostenol (e poe PROST en ole)

Medication Safety Issues

High alert medication:

The Institute for Safe Medication Practices (ISMP) includes this medication among its list of drugs which have a heightened risk of causing significant patient harm when used in error.

Synonyms epoprostenol sodium; PGI_2; PGX; prostacyclin

U.S. Brand Names Flolan®; Veletri®

Canadian Brand Names Flolan®

Therapeutic Category Platelet Inhibitor

Use Treatment of pulmonary arterial hypertension (PAH) (WHO Group I) in patients with NYHA Class III or IV symptoms to improve exercise capacity

General Dosage Range I.V.: *Adults:* Initial: 1-2 ng/kg/minute; increase dose in increments of 1-2 ng/kg/minute every 15 minutes until response

Dosage Forms

Injection, powder for reconstitution: 0.5 mg, 1.5 mg

Flolan®: 0.5 mg, 1.5 mg

Veletri®: 1.5 mg

epoprostenol sodium *see* epoprostenol *on page* 338

epothilone B lactam *see* ixabepilone *on page* 508

Eprex® (Can) *see* epoetin alfa *on page* 337

eprosartan (ep roe SAR tan)

U.S. Brand Names Teveten®

Canadian Brand Names Teveten®

Therapeutic Category Angiotensin II Receptor Antagonist

Use Treatment of hypertension; may be used alone or in combination with other antihypertensives

General Dosage Range Oral: *Adults:* Initial: 400-600 mg once daily; Maintenance: 400-800 mg/day in 1-2 divided doses

Dosage Forms

Tablet, oral: 600 mg

Teveten®: 400 mg, 600 mg

eprosartan and hydrochlorothiazide (ep roe SAR tan & hye droe klor oh THYE a zide)

Synonyms eprosartan mesylate and hydrochlorothiazide; hydrochlorothiazide and eprosartan

U.S. Brand Names Teveten® HCT

Canadian Brand Names Teveten® HCT; Teveten® Plus

Therapeutic Category Angiotensin II Antagonist Combination; Antihypertensive Agent, Combination; Diuretic, Thiazide

Use Treatment of hypertension (not indicated for initial treatment)

General Dosage Range Oral: *Adults:* Eprosartan 600 mg and hydrochlorothiazide 12.5-25 mg once daily

Dosage Forms

Tablet:

Teveten® HCT: 600 mg/12.5 mg: Eprosartan 600 mg and hydrochlorothiazide 12.5 mg; 600 mg/25 mg: Eprosartan 600 mg and hydrochlorothiazide 25 mg

eprosartan mesylate and hydrochlorothiazide *see* eprosartan and hydrochlorothiazide *on page 338*

epsilon aminocaproic acid *see* aminocaproic acid *on page 61*

epsom salts *see* magnesium sulfate *on page 560*

EPT *see* teniposide *on page 877*

eptacog alfa (activated) *see* factor VIIa (recombinant) *on page 371*

eptifibatide (ep TIF i ba tide)

Medication Safety Issues

High alert medication:

The Institute for Safe Medication Practices (ISMP) includes this medication among its list of drugs which have a heightened risk of causing significant patient harm when used in error.

Synonyms intrifiban

U.S. Brand Names Integrilin®

Canadian Brand Names Integrilin®

Therapeutic Category Antiplatelet Agent

Use Treatment of patients with acute coronary syndrome (unstable angina/non-ST-segment elevation myocardial infarction [UA/NSTEMI]), including patients who are to be managed medically and those undergoing percutaneous coronary intervention (PCI including angioplasty, intracoronary stenting)

General Dosage Range Dosage adjustment recommended in patients with renal impairment

I.V.: *Adults:* Bolus: 180 mcg/kg (maximum: 22.6 mg), repeat once for PCI; Infusion: 2 mcg/kg/minute (maximum: 15 mg/hour)

Dosage Forms

Injection, solution:

Integrilin®: 0.75 mg/mL (100 mL); 2 mg/mL (10 mL, 100 mL)

Epzicom® *see* abacavir and lamivudine *on page 16*

Equalactin® [OTC] *see* polycarbophil *on page 737*

Equalizer Gas Relief [OTC] *see* simethicone *on page 834*

Equanil *see* meprobamate *on page 576*

Equetro® *see* carbamazepine *on page 172*

ER-086526 *see* eribulin *on page 341*

Eraxis™ *see* anidulafungin *on page 76*

Erbitux® *see* cetuximab *on page 192*

ergocalciferol (er goe kal SIF e role)

Medication Safety Issues

Sound-alike/look-alike issues:

Calciferol™ may be confused with calcitriol

Drisdol® may be confused with Drysol™

Ergocalciferol may be confused with alfacalcidol, cholecalciferol

Administration issues:

Liquid vitamin D preparations have the potential for dosing errors when administered to infants. Droppers should be clearly marked to easily provide 400 international units. For products intended for infants, the FDA recommends that accompanying droppers deliver no more than 400 international units per dose.

Synonyms activated ergosterol; D2; viosterol; vitamin D2

U.S. Brand Names Calciferol™ [OTC]; Drisdol®; Drisdol® [OTC]

Canadian Brand Names Drisdol®; Ostoforte®

Therapeutic Category Vitamin D Analog

Use Treatment of refractory rickets, hypophosphatemia, hypoparathyroidism; dietary supplement

General Dosage Range Oral:

Children 0-12 months: Adequate intake: 400 units/day

Children 1 year to Adults ≤70 years: RDA: 600 units/day

Elderly >70 years: RDA: 800 units/day

Dosage Forms

Capsule, oral: 50,000 units

Drisdol®: 50,000 units

Capsule, softgel, oral: 50,000 units
Solution, oral: 8000 units/mL (60 mL)
Calciferol™ [OTC]: 8000 units/mL (60 mL)
Drisdol® [OTC]: 8000 units/mL (60 mL)
Tablet, oral: 400 units

ergoloid mesylates (ER goe loid MES i lates)

Medication Safety Issues
BEERS Criteria medication:
This drug may be potentially inappropriate for use in geriatric patients (Quality of evidence - high; Strength of recommendation - strong).

Synonyms dihydroergotoxine; dihydrogenated ergot alkaloids; Hydergine [DSC]

Canadian Brand Names Hydergine®

Therapeutic Category Ergot Alkaloid and Derivative

Use Treatment of cerebrovascular insufficiency in primary progressive dementia, Alzheimer dementia, and senile onset

General Dosage Range Oral: *Adults:* Initial: 1 mg 3 times/day; Maintenance: 3-12 mg/day in 3 divided doses

Dosage Forms
Tablet, oral: 1 mg

Ergomar® *see* ergotamine *on page 340*
ergometrine maleate *see* ergonovine *(Canada only) on page 340*

ergonovine *(Canada only)* (er goe NOE veen)

Synonyms ergometrine maleate; ergonovine maleate

Canadian Brand Names Ergonovine Maleate Injection

Therapeutic Category Ergot Alkaloid and Derivative

Use Prevention and treatment of postpartum and postabortion hemorrhage caused by uterine atony

General Dosage Range I.M., I.V.: *Adults:* 0.2 mg, may repeat in 2-4 hours if needed, up to maximum of 5 total doses

Product Availability Not available in the U.S.

Dosage Forms - Canada
Injection, solution: 0.25 mg/mL (1 mL)

ergonovine maleate *see* ergonovine *(Canada only) on page 340*
Ergonovine Maleate Injection (Can) *see* ergonovine *(Canada only) on page 340*

ergotamine (er GOT a meen)

Synonyms ergotamine tartrate

U.S. Brand Names Ergomar®

Therapeutic Category Ergot Alkaloid and Derivative

Use Abort or prevent vascular headaches, such as migraine, migraine variants, or so-called "histaminic cephalalgia"

General Dosage Range Sublingual: *Adults:* 1 tablet initially, then 1 tablet every 30 minutes if needed (maximum: 3 tablets/day; 5 tablets/week)

Dosage Forms
Tablet, sublingual:
Ergomar®: 2 mg

ergotamine and caffeine (er GOT a meen & KAF een)

Medication Safety Issues
Sound-alike/look-alike issues:
Cafergot® may be confused with Carafate®

Synonyms caffeine and ergotamine; ergotamine tartrate and caffeine

U.S. Brand Names Cafergot®; Migergot®

Canadian Brand Names Cafergor®

Therapeutic Category Antimigraine Agent; Ergot Derivative; Stimulant

Use Abort or prevent vascular headaches, such as migraine, migraine variants, or so-called "histaminic cephalalgia"

General Dosage Range

Oral: *Adults:* 2 tablets initially, then 1 tablet every 30 minutes as needed (maximum: 6 tablets/attack; 10 tablets/week)

Rectal: *Adults:* 1 suppository initially; may repeat after 1 hour if needed (maximum: 2 doses/attack; 5 doses/week)

Dosage Forms

Suppository, rectal:

Migergot®: Ergotamine tartrate 2 mg and caffeine 100 mg (12s)

Tablet, oral: Ergotamine tartrate 1 mg and caffeine 100 mg

Cafergot®: Ergotamine tartrate 1 mg and caffeine 100 mg

ergotamine tartrate *see* ergotamine *on page* 340

ergotamine tartrate and caffeine *see* ergotamine and caffeine *on page* 340

eribulin (er i BUE lin)

Medication Safety Issues

Sound-alike/look-alike issues:

EriBULin may be confused with EPIrubicin, erlotinib

High alert medication:

This medication is in a class the Institute for Safe Medication Practices (ISMP) includes among its list of drug classes which have a heightened risk of causing significant patient harm when used in error.

Synonyms B1939; E7389; ER-086526; eribulin mesylate; halichondrin B analog

Tall-Man eri**BUL**in

U.S. Brand Names Halaven™

Therapeutic Category Antineoplastic Agent, Antimicrotubular

Use Treatment of metastatic breast cancer in patients who have received at least 2 prior chemotherapy regimens

General Dosage Range Dosage adjustment recommended in patients with renal or hepatic impairment or who develop toxicities

I.V.: *Adults:* 1.4 mg/m^2/dose days 1 and 8 every 3 weeks

Dosage Forms

Injection, solution:

Halaven™: 0.5 mg/mL (2 mL)

eribulin mesylate *see* eribulin *on page* 341

Erivedge™ *see* vismodegib *on page* 948

erlotinib (er LOE tye nib)

Medication Safety Issues

Sound-alike/look-alike issues:

Erlotinib may be confused with crizotinib, eribulin, gefitinib, imatinib, SUNItinib, vandetanib

High alert medication:

This medication is in a class the Institute for Safe Medication Practices (ISMP) includes among its list of drug classes which have a heightened risk of causing significant patient harm when used in error.

Synonyms CP358774; erlotinib hydrochloride; OSI-774

U.S. Brand Names Tarceva®

Canadian Brand Names Tarceva®

Therapeutic Category Antineoplastic Agent, Tyrosine Kinase Inhibitor

Use Treatment of locally advanced or metastatic nonsmall cell lung cancer (NSCLC) refractory to at least 1 prior chemotherapy regimen (as monotherapy); maintenance treatment of locally advanced or metastatic NCSLC which has not progressed after 4-6 cycles of first line platinum-based chemotherapy; locally advanced, unresectable or metastatic pancreatic cancer (first-line therapy in combination with gemcitabine)

Canadian labeling: First-line treatment of locally advanced or metastatic nonsmall cell lung cancer (NSCLC) with known EGFR mutation (as monotherapy); treatment of locally advanced or metastatic NSCLC refractory to at least 1 prior chemotherapy regimen and positive or unknown EGFR status (as monotherapy); maintenance treatment of locally advanced or metastatic NCSLC which has not progressed after 4 cycles of first line platinum-based chemotherapy

General Dosage Range Dosage adjustment recommended in patients with hepatic impairment, on concomitant therapy, who smoke, or who develop toxicities
Oral: *Adults:* 100-150 mg/day

Dosage Forms
Tablet, oral:
Tarceva®: 25 mg, 100 mg, 150 mg

erlotinib hydrochloride *see* erlotinib *on page* 341
E-R-O® [OTC] *see* carbamide peroxide *on page* 173
Errin® *see* norethindrone *on page* 648
Ertaczo® *see* sertaconazole *on page* 830

ertapenem (er ta PEN em)

Medication Safety Issues
Sound-alike/look-alike issues:
Ertapenem may be confused with doripenem, imipenem, meropenem
INVanz® may be confused with AVINza®, I.V. vancomycin

Synonyms ertapenem sodium; L-749,345; MK0826

U.S. Brand Names INVanz®

Canadian Brand Names Invanz®

Therapeutic Category Antibiotic, Carbapenem

Use Treatment of the following moderate-to-severe infections: Complicated intraabdominal infections, complicated skin and skin structure infections (including diabetic foot infections without osteomyelitis, animal and human bites), complicated UTI (including pyelonephritis), acute pelvic infections (including postpartum endomyometritis, septic abortion, postsurgical gynecologic infections), and community-acquired pneumonia. Prophylaxis of surgical site infection following elective colorectal surgery. Antibacterial coverage includes aerobic gram-positive organisms, aerobic gram-negative organisms, and anaerobic organisms.

Note: Methicillin-resistant *Staphylococcus aureus, Enterococcus* spp, penicillin-resistant strains of *Streptococcus pneumoniae, Acinetobacter*, and *Pseudomonas aeruginosa*, are **resistant** to ertapenem while most extended-spectrum β-lactamase (ESBL)-producing bacteria remain sensitive to ertapenem.

General Dosage Range Dosage adjustment recommended in patients with renal impairment
I.M., I.V.:
Children 3 months to 12 years: 15 mg/kg twice daily (maximum: 1 g/day)
Adolescents ≥13 years and Adults: 1 g once daily or as single dose

Dosage Forms
Injection, powder for reconstitution:
INVanz®: 1 g

ertapenem sodium *see* ertapenem *on page* 342
Erwinase® (Can) *see* asparaginase (*Erwinia*) *on page* 96
Erwinaze™ *see* asparaginase (*Erwinia*) *on page* 96
Erwinia chrysanthemi *see* asparaginase (*Erwinia*) *on page* 96
Ery *see* erythromycin (topical) *on page* 343
Erybid™ (Can) *see* erythromycin (systemic) *on page* 342
Eryc® (Can) *see* erythromycin (systemic) *on page* 342
EryPed® *see* erythromycin (systemic) *on page* 342
Ery-Tab® *see* erythromycin (systemic) *on page* 342
Erythrocin® *see* erythromycin (systemic) *on page* 342
Erythrocin® Lactobionate-I.V. *see* erythromycin (systemic) *on page* 342

erythromycin (systemic) (er ith roe MYE sin)

Medication Safety Issues
Sound-alike/look-alike issues:
Erythromycin may be confused with azithromycin, clarithromycin
Eryc® may be confused with Emcyt®, Ery-Tab®

Synonyms erythromycin base; erythromycin ethylsuccinate; erythromycin lactobionate; erythromycin stearate

U.S. Brand Names E.E.S.®; Ery-Tab®; EryPed®; Erythro-RX; Erythrocin®; Erythrocin® Lactobionate-I.V.; PCE®

Canadian Brand Names Apo-Erythro Base®; Apo-Erythro E-C®; Apo-Erythro-ES®; Apo-Erythro-S®; EES®; Erybid™; Eryc®; Novo-Rythro Estolate; Novo-Rythro Ethylsuccinate; Nu-Erythromycin-S; PCE®

Therapeutic Category Antibiotic, Macrolide

Use Treatment of susceptible bacterial infections including *S. pyogenes*, some *S. pneumoniae,* some *S. aureus*, *M. pneumoniae*, *Legionella pneumophila*, diphtheria, pertussis, *Chlamydia*, erythrasma, *N. gonorrhoeae*, *E. histolytica*, syphilis and nongonococcal urethritis, and *Campylobacter* gastroenteritis; used in conjunction with neomycin for decontaminating the bowel

General Dosage Range

I.V.:

Children: 15-50 mg/kg/day divided every 6 hours (maximum: 4 g/day)

Adults: 15-20 mg/kg/day divided every 6 hours **or** 500 mg to 1 g every 6 hours or as a continuous infusion over 24 hours (maximum: 4 g/day)

Oral:

Children: 30-50 mg/kg/day in 2-4 divided doses (maximum base or stearate: 2 g/day; maximum ethylsuccinate: 3.2 g/day)

Adults: Base: 250-500 mg every 6-12 hours (maximum base or ethylsuccinate: 400-800 mg every 6-12 hours)

Dosage Forms

Capsule, delayed release, enteric coated pellets, oral: 250 mg

Granules for suspension, oral:

E.E.S.®: Erythromycin activity 200 mg/5 mL (100 mL, 200 mL)

Injection, powder for reconstitution:

Erythrocin® Lactobionate-I.V.: Erythromycin activity 500 mg

Powder, for prescription compounding:

Erythro-RX: USP: 100% (50 g)

Powder for suspension, oral:

EryPed®: Erythromycin activity 200 mg/5 mL (100 mL); Erythromycin activity 400 mg/5 mL (100 mL)

Tablet, oral: 250 mg, Erythromycin activity 400 mg, 500 mg

E.E.S.®: Erythromycin activity 400 mg

Erythrocin®: Erythromycin activity 250 mg, Erythromycin activity 500 mg

Tablet, delayed release, enteric coated, oral:

Ery-Tab®: 250 mg, 333 mg, 500 mg

Tablet, polymer coated particles, oral:

PCE®: 333 mg, 500 mg

erythromycin (ophthalmic) (er ith roe MYE sin)

Medication Safety Issues

Sound-alike/look-alike issues:

Erythromycin may be confused with azithromycin

Synonyms erythromycin base

U.S. Brand Names Ilotycin™

Canadian Brand Names Diomycin®; PMS-Erythromycin

Therapeutic Category Antibiotic, Macrolide; Antibiotic, Ophthalmic

Use Treatment of superficial eye infections involving the conjunctiva or cornea

General Dosage Range Ophthalmic: *Children and Adults:* Instill 1/2" (1.25 cm) 2-6 times/day

Dosage Forms

Ointment, ophthalmic: 0.5% (1 g, 3.5 g, 3.75 g)

Ilotycin™: 0.5% (1 g)

Ointment, ophthalmic [preservative free]: 0.5% (1 g, 3.5 g)

erythromycin (topical) (er ith roe MYE sin)

Medication Safety Issues

Sound-alike/look-alike issues:

Erythromycin may be confused with azithromycin, clarithromycin

U.S. Brand Names Akne-mycin®; Ery

Canadian Brand Names Sans Acne®

Therapeutic Category Acne Products; Antibiotic, Macrolide; Antibiotic, Topical; Topical Skin Product; Topical Skin Product, Acne

Use Treatment of acne vulgaris

General Dosage Range Topical: *Children and Adults:* Apply over the affected area twice daily

Dosage Forms

Gel, topical: 2% (30 g, 60 g)

Ointment, topical:

Akne-mycin®: 2% (25 g)

Pledget, topical: 2% (60s)

Ery: 2% (60s)

Solution, topical: 2% (60 mL)

Dosage Forms - Canada

Solution, topical:

Sans Acne®: 2% (60 mL)

erythromycin and benzoyl peroxide (er ith roe MYE sin & BEN zoe il per OKS ide)

Synonyms benzoyl peroxide and erythromycin

U.S. Brand Names Benzamycin®; Benzamycin® Pak

Canadian Brand Names Benzamycin®

Therapeutic Category Acne Products

Use Topical control of acne vulgaris

General Dosage Range Topical: *Adolescents ≥12 years and Adults:* Apply twice daily

Dosage Forms

Gel, topical: Erythromycin 30 mg and benzoyl peroxide 50 mg per g (23 g, 47g)

Benzamycin®: Erythromycin 30 mg and benzoyl peroxide 50 mg per g (47 g)

Benzamycin® Pak: Erythromycin 30 mg and benzoyl peroxide 50 mg per 0.8 g packet (60s)

erythromycin and sulfisoxazole (er ith roe MYE sin & sul fi SOKS a zole)

Medication Safety Issues

Sound-alike/look-alike issues:

Pediazole® may be confused with Pediapred®

Synonyms sulfisoxazole and erythromycin

U.S. Brand Names E.S.P.®

Canadian Brand Names Pediazole®

Therapeutic Category Macrolide (Antibiotic); Sulfonamide

Use Treatment of susceptible bacterial infections of the upper and lower respiratory tract, otitis media in children caused by susceptible strains of *Haemophilus influenzae*, and many other infections in patients allergic to penicillin

General Dosage Range Dosage adjustment recommended in patients with renal impaiment

Oral:

Children ≥2 months: 50 mg/kg/day erythromycin and 150 mg/kg/day sulfisoxazole in divided doses every 6 hours

Adults: 400 mg erythromycin and 1200 mg sulfisoxazole every 6 hours

Dosage Forms

Powder for oral suspension: Erythromycin 200 mg and sulfisoxazole 600 mg per 5 mL

E.S.P.®: Erythromycin 200 mg and sulfisoxazole 600 mg per 5 mL

erythromycin base *see* erythromycin (ophthalmic) *on page* *343*
erythromycin base *see* erythromycin (systemic) *on page* *342*
erythromycin ethylsuccinate *see* erythromycin (systemic) *on page* *342*
erythromycin lactobionate *see* erythromycin (systemic) *on page* *342*
erythromycin stearate *see* erythromycin (systemic) *on page* *342*
erythropoiesis-stimulating agent (ESA) *see* darbepoetin alfa *on page* *254*
erythropoiesis-stimulating agent (ESA) *see* epoetin alfa *on page* *337*
erythropoiesis-stimulating agent (ESA) *see* peginesatide *on page* *696*
erythropoiesis-stimulating protein *see* darbepoetin alfa *on page* *254*
erythropoietin *see* epoetin alfa *on page* *337*
Erythro-RX *see* erythromycin (systemic) *on page* *342*

escitalopram (es sye TAL oh pram)

Medication Safety Issues

Sound-alike/look-alike issues:

Lexapro® may be confused with Loxitane®

BEERS Criteria medication:

This drug may be potentially inappropriate for use in geriatric patients (Quality of evidence - moderate; Strength of recommendation - strong).

International issues:

Zavesca: Brand name for escitalopram [in multiple international markets; ISMP April 21, 2010], but also brand name for miglustat [Canada, U.S., and multiple international markets]

Synonyms escitalopram oxalate; Lu-26-054; S-citalopram

U.S. Brand Names Lexapro®

Canadian Brand Names Cipralex®

Therapeutic Category Antidepressant, Selective Serotonin Reuptake Inhibitor

Use Treatment of major depressive disorder; generalized anxiety disorders (GAD)

Canadian labeling: Additional use (not in U.S. labeling): Treatment of obsessive-compulsive disorder (OCD)

General Dosage Range Dosage adjustment recommended in patients with hepatic impairment

Oral:

Children ≥12 years and Adults: Initial: 10 mg once daily; Maintenance: 10-20 mg once daily

Elderly: 10 mg once daily

Dosage Forms

Solution, oral: 1 mg/mL (240 mL)

Lexapro®: 1 mg/mL (240 mL)

Tablet, oral: 5 mg, 10 mg, 20 mg

Lexapro®: 5 mg, 10 mg, 20 mg

Dosage Forms - Canada

Tablet:

Cipralex®: 10 mg, 20 mg

escitalopram oxalate *see* escitalopram *on page* 345

eserine salicylate *see* physostigmine *on page* 721

Esgic® *see* butalbital, acetaminophen, and caffeine *on page* 153

Esgic-Plus™ *see* butalbital, acetaminophen, and caffeine *on page* 153

Eskalith *see* lithium *on page* 544

esmolol (ES moe lol)

Medication Safety Issues

Sound-alike/look-alike issues:

Esmolol may be confused with Osmitrol®

Brevibloc® may be confused with Brevital®, Bumex®, Buprenex®

High alert medication:

The Institute for Safe Medication Practices (ISMP) includes this medication among its list of drugs which have a heightened risk of causing significant patient harm when used in error.

Synonyms esmolol hydrochloride

U.S. Brand Names Brevibloc

Canadian Brand Names Brevibloc®; Brevibloc® Premixed

Therapeutic Category Antiarrhythmic Agent, Class II; Beta-Adrenergic Blocker

Use Treatment of supraventricular tachycardia (SVT) and atrial fibrillation/flutter (control ventricular rate); treatment of intraoperative and postoperative tachycardia and/or hypertension; treatment of noncompensatory sinus tachycardia

General Dosage Range **I.V.:** *Adults:* Bolus: 80 mg **or** 500 mcg/kg; Infusion: 50-200 mcg/kg/minute (maximum: 300 mcg/kg/minute)

Dosage Forms

Infusion, premixed in NS [preservative free]:

Brevibloc: 2000 mg (100 mL); 2500 mg (250 mL)

Injection, solution [preservative free]: 10 mg/mL (10 mL)

Brevibloc: 10 mg/mL (10 mL)

esmolol hydrochloride *see* esmolol *on page* 345

esomeprazole (es oh ME pray zol)

Medication Safety Issues

Sound-alike/look-alike issues:

Esomeprazole may be confused with ARIPiprazole
NexIUM® may be confused with NexAVAR®

Synonyms esomeprazole magnesium; esomeprazole sodium

U.S. Brand Names NexIUM®; NexIUM® I.V.

Canadian Brand Names Apo-Esomeprazole®; Nexium®

Therapeutic Category Proton Pump Inhibitor

Use

Oral: Short-term (4-8 weeks) treatment of erosive esophagitis; maintaining symptom resolution and healing of erosive esophagitis; treatment of symptomatic gastroesophageal reflux disease (GERD); as part of a multidrug regimen for *Helicobacter pylori* eradication in patients with duodenal ulcer disease (active or history of within the past 5 years); prevention of gastric ulcers in patients at risk (age ≥60 years and/or history of gastric ulcer) associated with continuous NSAID therapy; long-term treatment of pathological hypersecretory conditions including Zollinger-Ellison syndrome

Canadian labeling: Additional use (not in U.S. labeling): Oral: Treatment of nonerosive reflux disease (NERD)

I.V.: Short-term (≤10 days) treatment of gastroesophageal reflux disease (GERD) when oral therapy is not possible or appropriate

General Dosage Range Dosage adjustment recommended in patients with hepatic impairment.

I.V.:

Children 1 month to <1 year: 0.5 mg/kg once daily
Children 1-17 years: <55 kg: 10 mg once daily; ≥55 kg: 20 mg once daily
Adults: 20-40 mg once daily

Oral:

Children 1 month to <1 year: 3-5 kg: 2.5 mg once daily; >5-7.5 kg: 5 mg once daily; >7.5 kg: 10 mg once daily
Children 1-11 years: <20 kg: 10 mg once daily; ≥20 kg: 10-20 mg once daily
Children 12-17 years: 20-40 mg once daily
Adults: 20-40 mg once daily **or** 80-240 mg/day in divided doses (hypersecretory conditions)

Dosage Forms

Capsule, delayed release, oral:
NexIUM®: 20 mg, 40 mg

Granules for suspension, delayed release, oral:
NexIUM®: 10 mg/packet (30s); 20 mg/packet (30s); 40 mg/packet (30s)

Injection, powder for reconstitution:
NexIUM® I.V.: 20 mg, 40 mg

Dosage Forms - Canada Note: Strength expressed as base.

Granules, for oral suspension, delayed release, as magnesium:
Nexium®: 10 mg/packet (28s)

Tablet, extended release, as magnesium:
Nexium®: 20 mg, 40 mg

esomeprazole and naproxen *see* naproxen and esomeprazole *on page* 629
esomeprazole magnesium *see* esomeprazole *on page* 346
esomeprazole sodium *see* esomeprazole *on page* 346
Esopho-Cat® *see* barium *on page* 114
Esoterica® Daytime [OTC] *see* hydroquinone *on page* 461
Esoterica® Nighttime [OTC] *see* hydroquinone *on page* 461
E.S.P.® *see* erythromycin and sulfisoxazole *on page* 344
Estalis® (Can) *see* estradiol and norethindrone *on page* 349
Estalis-Sequi® (Can) *see* estradiol and norethindrone *on page* 349

estazolam (es TA zoe lam)

Medication Safety Issues

Sound-alike/look-alike issues:

ProSom® may be confused with PhosLo®, Proscar®, PROzac®, Psorcon®

BEERS Criteria medication:

This drug may be potentially inappropriate for use in geriatric patients (Quality of evidence - high; Strength of recommendation - strong).

Synonyms ProSom

Therapeutic Category Benzodiazepine

Controlled Substance C-IV

Use Short-term management of insomnia

General Dosage Range Oral:

Adults: 0.5-2 mg at bedtime

Elderly: Initial: 0.5 mg at bedtime in small or debilitated patients

Dosage Forms

Tablet, oral: 1 mg, 2 mg

Ester-E™ [OTC] *see* vitamin E *on page 950*

esterified estrogen and methyltestosterone *see* estrogens (esterified) and methyltestosterone *on page 353*

esterified estrogens *see* estrogens (esterified) *on page 353*

Estrace® *see* estradiol (systemic) *on page 347*

Estrace® *see* estradiol (topical) *on page 348*

Estraderm® (Can) *see* estradiol (systemic) *on page 347*

estradiol *see* estradiol (systemic) *on page 347*

17β-estradiol *see* estradiol (topical) *on page 348*

estradiol (systemic) (es tra DYE ole)

Medication Safety Issues

Sound-alike/look-alike issues:

Alora® may be confused with Aldara®

Elestrin® may be confused with alosetron

BEERS Criteria medication:

This drug may be potentially inappropriate for use in geriatric patients (Quality of evidence - high [oral and transdermal patch]; Strength of recommendation - strong [oral and transdermal patch]).

Other safety issues:

Transdermal patch may contain conducting metal (eg, aluminum); remove patch prior to MRI.

International issues:

Vivelle: Brand name for estradiol [U.S. and multiple international markets, but also the brand name for ethinyl estradiol and norgestimate [Austria]

Synonyms estradiol; estradiol acetate; estradiol transdermal; estradiol valerate

U.S. Brand Names Alora®; Climara®; Delestrogen®; Depo®-Estradiol; Divigel®; Elestrin®; Estrace®; Estrasorb®; EstroGel®; Evamist®; Femring®; Femtrace®; Menostar®; Vivelle-Dot®

Canadian Brand Names Climara®; Depo®-Estradiol; Estraderm®; Estradot®; EstroGel®; Menostar®; Oesclim®; Sandoz-Estradiol Derm 100; Sandoz-Estradiol Derm 50; Sandoz-Estradiol Derm 75

Therapeutic Category Estrogen Derivative

Use Treatment of moderate-to-severe vasomotor symptoms associated with menopause; treatment of moderate-to-severe vulvar and vaginal atrophy associated with menopause; hypoestrogenism (due to hypogonadism, castration, or primary ovarian failure); advanced prostatic cancer (palliation); metastatic breast cancer (palliation) in men and postmenopausal women; postmenopausal osteoporosis (prophylaxis)

General Dosage Range

I.M.:

Cypionate:

Adults (females): Hypoestrogenism: 1.5-2 mg monthly

Adults (females): Menopause: 1-5 mg every 3-4 weeks

Valerate:

Adults (females): Menopause: 10-20 mg every 4 weeks

Adults (males): Prostate cancer: 30 mg or more every 1-2 weeks

Oral:
Adults (females):
Estrace®: Breast cancer: 10 mg 3 times/day; Hypoestrogenism: 1-2 mg/day; Menopause: 0.5-2 mg/day
Femtrace®: Menopause: 0.45-1.8 mg/day
Adults (males): Estrace®: Prostate cancer: 1-2 mg 3 times/day; Breast cancer: 10 mg 3 times/day
Intravaginal: *Adults (females):* (Femring®): 0.05-0.1 mg, leave in place for 3 months
Topical: *Adults (females):*
Emulsion (Estrasorb®): 3.48 g applied once daily in the morning
Gel: 1.25 g/day (EstroGel®) or 0.87-1.7 g/day (Elestrin®) or 0.25-1 g/day (Divigel®) applied at the same time each day
Spray (Evamist®): 1 spray (1.53 mg) per day; dosing range: 1-3 sprays/day
Transdermal: *Adults (females):*
Alora®, Estraderm®, Vivelle-Dot®: Apply twice weekly continuously or cyclically (3 weeks on, 1 week off)
Climara®: Apply once weekly continuously or cyclically (3 weeks on, 1 week off)
Menostar®: Apply once weekly continuously

Dosage Forms
Emulsion, topical:
Estrasorb®: 2.5 mg/g (56s)
Gel, topical:
Divigel®: 0.1% (30s)
Elestrin®: 0.06% (70 g)
EstroGel®: 0.06% (50 g)
Injection, oil: 10 mg/mL (5 mL); 20 mg/mL (5 mL); 40 mg/mL (5 mL)
Delestrogen®: 10 mg/mL (5 mL); 20 mg/mL (5 mL); 40 mg/mL (5 mL)
Depo®-Estradiol: 5 mg/mL (5 mL)
Patch, transdermal: 0.025 mg/24 hours (4s); 0.0375 mg/24 hours (4s); 0.05 mg/24 hours (4s); 0.06 mg/24 hours (4s); 0.075 mg/24 hours (4s); 0.1 mg/24 hours (4s)
Alora®: 0.025 mg/24 hours (8s); 0.05 mg/24 hours (8s); 0.075 mg/24 hours (8s); 0.1 mg/24 hours (8s)
Climara®: 0.025 mg/24 hours (4s); 0.0375 mg/24 hours (4s); 0.05 mg/24 hours (4s); 0.06 mg/24 hours (4s); 0.075 mg/24 hours (4s); 0.1 mg/24 hours (4s)
Menostar®: 0.014 mg/24 hours (4s)
Vivelle-Dot®: 0.025 mg/24 hours (24s); 0.0375 mg/24 hours (24s); 0.05 mg/24 hours (24s); 0.075 mg/24 hours (24s); 0.1 mg/24 hours (24s)
Ring, vaginal:
Femring®: 0.05 mg/24 hours (1s); 0.1 mg/24 hours (1s)
Solution, topical:
Evamist®: 1.53 mg/spray (8.1 mL)
Tablet, oral: 0.5 mg, 1 mg, 2 mg
Estrace®: 0.5 mg, 1 mg, 2 mg
Femtrace®: 0.9 mg

estradiol (topical) (es tra DYE ole)

Medication Safety Issues
BEERS Criteria medication:
This drug may be potentially inappropriate for use in geriatric patients (Quality of evidence - moderate [topical]; Strength of recommendation - weak [topical]).
International issues:
Estring [U.S., Canada, and multiple international markets] may be confused with Estrena [Finland]

Synonyms 17β-estradiol

U.S. Brand Names Estrace®; Estring®; Vagifem®

Canadian Brand Names Estrace®; Estring®; Vagifem®; Vagifem® 10

Therapeutic Category Estrogen Derivative

Use Treatment of moderate-to-severe vulvar and vaginal atrophy associated with menopause

General Dosage Range Intravaginal: *Adults (females):*
Cream: Initial: 2-4 g/day for 1-2 weeks, then 1/2 the initial dose for 1-2 weeks; Maintenance: 1 g 1-3 times/week
Ring: Estring®: Insert 2 mg, leave in place for 3 months
Tablet: Initial: Insert 1 tablet (10 mcg) once daily for 2 weeks; Maintenance: Insert 1 tablet twice weekly

Dosage Forms

Cream, vaginal:

Estrace®: 0.1 mg/g (42.5 g)

Ring, vaginal:

Estring®: 2 mg (1s)

Tablet, vaginal:

Vagifem®: 10 mcg

estradiol acetate *see* estradiol (systemic) *on page 347*

estradiol and dienogest (es tra DYE ole & dye EN oh jest)

Synonyms dienogest and estradiol; estradiol valerate and dienogest

U.S. Brand Names Natazia®

Therapeutic Category Contraceptive; Estrogen and Progestin Combination

Use Prevention of pregnancy; treatment of heavy menstrual bleeding

General Dosage Range Oral: *Children and Adults (females, postmenarche):* 1 tablet daily

Dosage Forms

Tablet, oral [four-phasic formulation]:

Natazia®:

Days 1-2: Estradiol valerate 3 mg [2 dark yellow tablets]
Days 3-7: Estradiol valerate 2 mg and dienogest 2 mg [5 medium red tablets]
Days 8-24: Estradiol valerate 2 mg and dienogest 3 mg [17 light yellow tablets]
Days 25-26: Estradiol valerate 1 mg [2 dark red tablets]
Days 27-28: 2 white inactive tablets (28s)

estradiol and drospirenone *see* drospirenone and estradiol *on page 317*

estradiol and levonorgestrel (es tra DYE ole & LEE voe nor jes trel)

Synonyms levonorgestrel and estradiol

U.S. Brand Names ClimaraPro®

Therapeutic Category Estrogen and Progestin Combination

Use Women with an intact uterus: Treatment of moderate-to-severe vasomotor symptoms associated with menopause; prevention of postmenopausal osteoporosis

General Dosage Range Transdermal: *Adults (females):* Apply 1 patch (estradiol 0.045 mg/levonorgestrel 0.015 mg) weekly

Dosage Forms

Patch, transdermal:

ClimaraPro®: Estradiol 0.045 mg and levonorgestrel 0.015 mg per 24 hours (4s)

estradiol and NGM *see* estradiol and norgestimate *on page 350*

estradiol and norethindrone (es tra DYE ole & nor eth IN drone)

Synonyms norethindrone and estradiol

U.S. Brand Names Activella®; CombiPatch®; Mimvey™

Canadian Brand Names Estalis-Sequi®; Estalis®

Therapeutic Category Estrogen and Progestin Combination

Use Women with an intact uterus:

Tablet: Treatment of moderate-to-severe vasomotor symptoms associated with menopause; treatment of vulvar and vaginal atrophy; prophylaxis for postmenopausal osteoporosis

Transdermal patch: Treatment of moderate-to-severe vasomotor symptoms associated with menopause; treatment of vulvar and vaginal atrophy; treatment of hypoestrogenism due to hypogonadism, castration, or primary ovarian failure

General Dosage Range

Oral: *Adults (females):* 1 tablet daily

Transdermal: *Adults (females):* Apply 1 patch twice weekly

Dosage Forms

Patch, transdermal:

CombiPatch®:

0.05/0.14: Estradiol 0.05 mg and norethindrone 0.14 mg per day (8s) [9 sq cm]
0.05/0.25: Estradiol 0.05 mg and norethindrone 0.25 mg per day (8s) [16 sq cm]

Tablet, oral: 0.5/0.1: Estradiol 0.5 mg and norethindrone acetate 0.1 mg (28s); Estradiol 1 mg and norethindrone acetate 0.5 mg (28s)
Activella® 0.5/0.1: Estradiol 0.5 mg and norethindrone acetate 0.1 mg (28s)
Activella® 1/0.5, Mimvey™: Estradiol 1 mg and norethindrone acetate 0.5 mg (28s)

Dosage Forms - Canada

Combination pack:
Estalis-Sequi® 140/50:
Patch, transdermal (Vivelle®): Estradiol 50 mcg per day (4s) [14.5 sq cm; total estradiol 4.33 mg]
Patch, transdermal (Estalis®): Norethindrone 140 mcg and estradiol 50 mcg per day (4s) [9 sq cm; total norethindrone 2.7 mg, total estradiol 0.62 mg]
Estalis-Sequi® 250/50:
Patch, transdermal (Vivelle®): Estradiol 50 mcg per day (4s) [14.5 sq cm; total estradiol 4.33 mg]
Patch, transdermal (Estalis®): Norethindrone 250 mcg and estradiol 50 mcg per day (4s) [16 sq cm; total norethindrone 4.8 mg, total estradiol 0.51 mg]

Patch, transdermal:
Estalis®:
140/50: Norethindrone 140 mcg and estradiol 50 mcg per day (8s) [9 sq cm; total norethindrone 2.7 mg, total estradiol 0.62 mg]
250/50 Norethindrone 250 mcg and estradiol 50 mcg per day (8s) [16 sq cm; total norethindrone 4.8 mg, total estradiol 0.51 mg]

estradiol and norgestimate (es tra DYE ole & nor JES ti mate)

Medication Safety Issues

BEERS Criteria medication:
This drug may be potentially inappropriate for use in geriatric patients (Quality of evidence - high [oral and transdermal patch]; Strength of recommendation - strong [oral and transdermal patch]).

Synonyms estradiol and NGM; norgestimate and estradiol; Ortho Prefest

U.S. Brand Names Prefest™

Therapeutic Category Estrogen and Progestin Combination

Use Women with an intact uterus: Treatment of moderate-to-severe vasomotor symptoms associated with menopause; treatment of atrophic vaginitis; prevention of osteoporosis

General Dosage Range Oral: *Adults (females):* 1 tablet of estradiol 1 mg once daily for 3 days, followed by 1 tablet of estradiol 1 mg and norgestimate 0.09 mg once daily for 3 days; repeat sequence continuously

Dosage Forms

Tablet, oral:
Prefest™: Estradiol 1 mg [15 peach tablets] and estradiol 1 mg and norgestimate 0.09 mg [15 white tablets]

estradiol transdermal *see* estradiol (systemic) *on page 347*

estradiol valerate *see* estradiol (systemic) *on page 347*

estradiol valerate and dienogest *see* estradiol and dienogest *on page 349*

Estradot® (Can) *see* estradiol (systemic) *on page 347*

Estragyn (Can) *see* estrogens (esterified) *on page 353*

estramustine (es tra MUS teen)

Medication Safety Issues

Sound-alike/look-alike issues:
Emcyt® may be confused with Eryc®
Estramustine may be confused with exemestane.

High alert medication:
The Institute for Safe Medication Practices (ISMP) includes this medication among its list of drug classes which have a heightened risk of causing significant patient harm when used in error.

Synonyms estramustine phosphate; estramustine phosphate sodium; NSC-89199

U.S. Brand Names Emcyt®

Canadian Brand Names Emcyt®

Therapeutic Category Antineoplastic Agent

Use Palliative treatment of progressive or metastatic prostate cancer

General Dosage Range Oral: *Adults (males):* 14 mg/kg/day (range: 10-16 mg/kg/day) in 3 or 4 divided doses

Dosage Forms

Capsule, oral:

Emcyt®: 140 mg

estramustine phosphate *see* estramustine *on page 350*

estramustine phosphate sodium *see* estramustine *on page 350*

Estrasorb® *see* estradiol (systemic) *on page 347*

Estratab® (Can) *see* estrogens (esterified) *on page 353*

Estring® *see* estradiol (topical) *on page 348*

EstroGel® *see* estradiol (systemic) *on page 347*

estrogenic substances, conjugated *see* estrogens (conjugated/equine, systemic) *on page 351*

estrogenic substances, conjugated *see* estrogens (conjugated/equine, topical) *on page 352*

estrogens (conjugated A/synthetic) (ES troe jenz, KON joo gate ed, aye, sin THET ik)

Medication Safety Issues

Sound-alike/look-alike issues:

Cenestin® may be confused with Senexon®

BEERS Criteria medication:

This drug may be potentially inappropriate for use in geriatric patients (Quality of evidence - high; Strength of recommendation - strong).

International issues:

Cenestin [U.S., Canada] may be confused with Canesten which is a brand name for clotrimazole [multiple international markets]

U.S. Brand Names Cenestin®

Canadian Brand Names Cenestin

Therapeutic Category Estrogen Derivative

Use Treatment of moderate-to-severe vasomotor symptoms of menopause; treatment of vulvar and vaginal atrophy

General Dosage Range Oral: *Adults (females):* 0.3-1.25 mg once daily

Dosage Forms

Tablet, oral:

Cenestin®: 0.3 mg, 0.45 mg, 0.625 mg, 0.9 mg, 1.25 mg

estrogens (conjugated B/synthetic) (ES troe jenz, KON joo gate ed, bee, sin THET ik)

Medication Safety Issues

Sound-alike/look-alike issues:

Enjuvia™ may be confused with Januvia®

BEERS Criteria medication:

This drug may be potentially inappropriate for use in geriatric patients (Quality of evidence - high; Strength of recommendation - strong).

U.S. Brand Names Enjuvia™

Therapeutic Category Estrogen Derivative

Use Treatment of moderate-to-severe vasomotor symptoms of menopause; treatment of vulvar and vaginal atrophy associated with menopause; treatment of moderate-to-severe vaginal dryness and pain with intercourse associated with menopause

General Dosage Range Oral: *Adults (females):* 0.3-1.25 mg once daily

Dosage Forms

Tablet, oral:

Enjuvia™: 0.3 mg, 0.45 mg, 0.625 mg, 0.9 mg, 1.25 mg

estrogens (conjugated/equine, systemic) (ES troe jenz KON joo gate ed, EE kwine)

Medication Safety Issues

Sound-alike/look-alike issues:

Premarin® may be confused with Primaxin®, Provera®, Remeron®

BEERS Criteria medication:

This drug may be potentially inappropriate for use in geriatric patients (Quality of evidence - high [oral]; Strength of recommendation - strong [oral]).

Synonyms C.E.S.; CE; CEE; conjugated estrogen; estrogenic substances, conjugated

U.S. Brand Names Premarin®

Canadian Brand Names C.E.S.®; Congest; PMS-Conjugated Estrogens C.S.D.; Premarin®

Therapeutic Category Estrogen Derivative

Use Treatment of moderate-to-severe vasomotor symptoms associated with menopause; treatment of vulvar and vaginal atrophy due to menopause; hypoestrogenism (due to hypogonadism, castration, or primary ovarian failure); prostatic cancer (palliation); breast cancer (palliation); postmenopausal osteoporosis (prophylaxis); abnormal uterine bleeding

General Dosage Range

I.M., I.V.: *Children (postmenarche) and Adults (females):* Abnormal uterine bleeding: 25 mg, may repeat in 6-12 hours if needed

Oral:

Adolescents and Adult (females): 0.3-1.25 mg daily or cyclically **or** 10 mg 3 times/day [breast cancer]

Adults (males): Breast cancer: 10 mg 3 times/day; Prostate cancer: 1.25-2.5 mg 3 times/day

Dosage Forms

Injection, powder for reconstitution:

Premarin®: 25 mg

Tablet, oral:

Premarin®: 0.3 mg, 0.45 mg, 0.625 mg, 0.9 mg, 1.25 mg

estrogens (conjugated/equine, topical) (ES troe jenz KON joo gate ed, EE kwine)

Medication Safety Issues

Sound-alike/look-alike issues:

Premarin® may be confused with Primaxin®, Provera®, Remeron®

BEERS Criteria medication:

This drug may be potentially inappropriate for use in geriatric patients (Quality of evidence - moderate [topical]; Strength of recommendation - weak [topical]).

Synonyms C.E.S.; CE; CEE; conjugated estrogen; estrogenic substances, conjugated

U.S. Brand Names Premarin®

Canadian Brand Names Premarin®

Therapeutic Category Estrogen Derivative

Use Treatment of atrophic vaginitis and kraurosis vulvae; moderate-to-severe dyspareunia (pain during intercourse) due to vaginal/vulvar atrophy of menopause

General Dosage Range Intravaginal: *Adults (females):*

Atrophic vaginitis, kraurosis vulvae: 0.5-2 g/day given cyclically

Moderate-to-severe dyspareunia due to menopause: 0.5 g twice weekly (eg, Monday and Thursday) **or** once daily cyclically

Dosage Forms

Cream, vaginal:

Premarin®: 0.625 mg/g (30 g)

estrogens (conjugated/equine) and medroxyprogesterone

(ES troe jenz KON joo gate ed/EE kwine & me DROKS ee proe JES te rone)

Medication Safety Issues

BEERS Criteria medication:

This drug may be potentially inappropriate for use in geriatric patients (Quality of evidence - high [oral]; Strength of recommendation - strong [oral]).

Synonyms medroxyprogesterone and estrogens (conjugated); MPA and estrogens (conjugated)

U.S. Brand Names Premphase®; Prempro®

Canadian Brand Names Premphase®; Premplus®; Prempro®

Therapeutic Category Estrogen and Progestin Combination

Use Women with an intact uterus: Treatment of moderate-to-severe vasomotor symptoms associated with menopause; treatment of moderate-to-severe vulvar and vaginal atrophy due to menopause; postmenopausal osteoporosis (prophylaxis)

General Dosage Range Oral: *Adults (females):* Prempro®: Conjugated estrogen 0.3-0.625 mg/mPA 1.5-5 mg once daily **or** Premphase®: One 0.625 mg tablet daily on days 1 through 14 and 1 conjugated estrogen 0.625 mg/mPA 5 mg tablet daily on days 15 through 28

Dosage Forms

Tablet:

Premphase® [therapy pack contains two separate tablet formulations]: Conjugated estrogens 0.625 mg [14 maroon tablets] and conjugated estrogen 0.625 mg/medroxyprogesterone 5 mg [14 light blue tablets] (28s)

Prempro®:

0.3/1.5: Conjugated estrogens 0.3 mg and medroxyprogesterone 1.5 mg (28s)
0.45/1.5: Conjugated estrogens 0.45 mg and medroxyprogesterone 1.5 mg (28s)
0.625/2.5: Conjugated estrogens 0.625 mg and medroxyprogesterone 2.5 mg (28s)
0.625/5: Conjugated estrogens 0.625 mg and medroxyprogesterone 5 mg (28s)

estrogens (esterified) (ES troe jenz, es TER i fied)

Medication Safety Issues

BEERS Criteria medication:

This drug may be potentially inappropriate for use in geriatric patients (Quality of evidence - high [oral]; Strength of recommendation - strong [oral]).

Synonyms esterified estrogens

U.S. Brand Names Menest®

Canadian Brand Names Estragyn; Estratab®; Menest®

Therapeutic Category Estrogen Derivative

Use Treatment of moderate-to-severe vasomotor symptoms associated with menopause; treatment of moderate-to-severe vulvar and vaginal atrophy associated with menopause; hypoestrogenism (due to hypogonadism, castration, or primary ovarian failure); advanced prostatic cancer (palliation), metastatic breast cancer (palliation) in men and postmenopausal women

General Dosage Range

Oral:

Adults (females): Hypogonadism: 2.5-7.5 mg/day for 20 days followed by a 10-day rest, repeat until response; Castration or ovarian failure: 1.25 mg/day, cyclically; Menopause 0.3-1.25 mg/day given cyclically; Breast cancer: 10 mg 3 times/day

Adults (males): Breast cancer: 10 mg 3 times/day; Prostate cancer: 1.25-2.5 mg 3 times/day

Dosage Forms

Tablet, oral:

Menest®: 0.3 mg, 0.625 mg, 1.25 mg, 2.5 mg

estrogens (esterified) and methyltestosterone
(ES troe jenz es TER i fied & meth il tes TOS te rone)

Medication Safety Issues

Sound-alike/look-alike issues:

Estratest® may be confused with Eskalith®, Estratab®, Estratest® H.S.
Estratest® H.S. may be confused with Eskalith®, Estratab®, Estratest®

Synonyms esterified estrogen and methyltestosterone; methyltestosterone and esterified estrogen

U.S. Brand Names Covaryx®; Covaryx® H.S.; EEMT™; EEMT™ HS

Therapeutic Category Estrogen and Androgen Combination

Use Treatment of moderate-to-severe vasomotor symptoms associated with menopause not improved by estrogens alone

General Dosage Range Oral: *Adults (females):* Usual dosage range (based on esterified estrogen component): 0.625-1.25 mg every day for 3 weeks and then discontinued for 1 week off

Dosage Forms

Tablet: Esterified estrogen 0.625 mg and methyltestosterone 1.25 mg; esterified estrogens 1.25 mg and methyltestosterone 2.5 mg

Covaryx® H.S., EEMT™ HS: Esterified estrogen 0.625 mg and methyltestosterone 1.25 mg
Covaryx®, EEMT™: Esterified estrogen 1.25 mg and methyltestosterone 2.5 mg

estropipate (ES troe pih pate)

Medication Safety Issues

BEERS Criteria medication:

This drug may be potentially inappropriate for use in geriatric patients (Quality of evidence - high [oral]; Strength of recommendation - strong [oral]).

Synonyms Ortho Est; piperazine estrone sulfate

Canadian Brand Names Ogen®

Therapeutic Category Estrogen Derivative

Use Treatment of moderate-to-severe vasomotor symptoms associated with menopause; treatment of vulvar and vaginal atrophy; hypoestrogenism (due to hypogonadism, castration, or primary ovarian failure); osteoporosis (prophylaxis)

General Dosage Range Dosage adjustment recommended in patients with hepatic impairment

Oral: *Adults (females):* 0.75-6 mg once daily or cyclically [menopause] **or** 1.5-9 mg for the first 3 weeks, followed by a rest period of 8-10 days [hypoestrogenism] **or** 0.75 mg for 25 days of a 31 day cycle [osteoporosis]

Dosage Forms

Tablet, oral: 0.75 mg, 1.5 mg, 3 mg

Estrostep® Fe *see* ethinyl estradiol and norethindrone *on page* 359

eszopiclone (es zoe PIK lone)

Medication Safety Issues

Sound-alike/look-alike issues:

Lunesta® may be confused with Neulasta®

BEERS Criteria medication:

This drug may be potentially inappropriate for use in geriatric patients (Quality of evidence - moderate; Strength of recommendation - strong).

U.S. Brand Names Lunesta®

Therapeutic Category Hypnotic, Miscellaneous

Controlled Substance C-IV

Use Treatment of insomnia

General Dosage Range Dosage adjustment recommended in patients with hepatic impairment or on concomitant therapy

Oral:

Adults: Initial: 1-2 mg immediately before bedtime (maximum: 3 mg/day)

Elderly: Maximum: 2 mg/day

Dosage Forms

Tablet, oral:

Lunesta®: 1 mg, 2 mg, 3 mg

etanercept (et a NER sept)

Medication Safety Issues

Sound-alike/look-alike issues:

Enbrel® may be confused with Levbid®

U.S. Brand Names Enbrel®; Enbrel® SureClick®

Canadian Brand Names Enbrel®

Therapeutic Category Antirheumatic, Disease Modifying

Use Treatment of moderately- to severely-active rheumatoid arthritis (RA); moderately- to severely-active polyarticular juvenile idiopathic arthritis (JIA); psoriatic arthritis; active ankylosing spondylitis (AS); moderate-to-severe chronic plaque psoriasis

General Dosage Range SubQ:

Children 2-17 years: 0.8 mg/kg (maximum: 50 mg) once weekly **or** 0.4 mg/kg (maximum: 25 mg) twice weekly

Adults: 50 mg once weekly **or** 25-50 mg twice weekly

Dosage Forms

Injection, powder for reconstitution [preservative free]:

Enbrel®: 25 mg

Injection, solution [preservative free]:

Enbrel®: 50 mg/mL (0.51 mL, 0.98 mL)

Enbrel® SureClick®: 50 mg/mL (0.98 mL)

ethacrynate sodium *see* ethacrynic acid *on page* 355

ethacrynic acid (eth a KRIN ik AS id)

Medication Safety Issues

Sound-alike/look-alike issues:

Edecrin® may be confused with Eulexin, Ecotrin®

Synonyms ethacrynate sodium

U.S. Brand Names Edecrin®; Sodium Edecrin®

Canadian Brand Names Edecrin®; Sodium Edecrin®

Therapeutic Category Diuretic, Loop

Use Management of edema associated with congestive heart failure; hepatic cirrhosis or renal disease; short-term management of ascites due to malignancy, idiopathic edema, and lymphedema

General Dosage Range

I.V.: *Adults:* 0.5-1 mg/kg/dose (maximum: 100 mg/dose)

Oral:

Children: 1-3 mg/kg/day

Adults: 50-400 mg/day in 1-2 divided doses

Elderly: Initial: 25-50 mg/day

Dosage Forms

Injection, powder for reconstitution:

Sodium Edecrin®: 50 mg

Tablet, oral:

Edecrin®: 25 mg

ethambutol (e THAM byoo tole)

Medication Safety Issues

Sound-alike/look-alike issues:

Myambutol® may be confused with Nembutal®

Synonyms ethambutol hydrochloride

U.S. Brand Names Myambutol®

Canadian Brand Names Etibi®

Therapeutic Category Antimycobacterial Agent

Use Treatment of pulmonary tuberculosis in conjunction with other antituberculosis agents

General Dosage Range Dosage adjustment recommended in patients with renal impairment

Oral:

Children: 15-20 mg/kg/day (maximum: 1 g/day) **or** 50 mg/kg twice weekly (maximum: 2.5 g/dose)

Adults: Daily therapy: 1.5-2.5 g/kg/day (maximum dose: 1.5-2.5 g); 3 times/week DOT: 25-30 mg/kg/dose (maximum dose: 2.4 g/dose); Twice weekly DOT: 50 mg/kg/dose (maximum dose: 4 g/dose)

Dosage Forms

Tablet, oral: 100 mg, 400 mg

Myambutol®: 100 mg, 400 mg

ethambutol hydrochloride *see* ethambutol *on page* 355

Ethamolin® *see* ethanolamine oleate *on page* 355

ethanoic acid *see* acetic acid *on page* 31

ethanol *see* alcohol (ethyl) *on page* 43

ethanolamine oleate (ETH a nol a meen OH lee ate)

Medication Safety Issues

Sound-alike/look-alike issues:

Ethamolin® may be confused with ethanol

Synonyms monoethanolamine

U.S. Brand Names Ethamolin®

Therapeutic Category Sclerosing Agent

Use Orphan drug: Sclerosing agent used for bleeding esophageal varices

General Dosage Range Injection: *Adults:* 1.5-5 mL per varix (maximum: 20 mL total)

Dosage Forms

Injection, solution:

Ethamolin®: 5% (2 mL)

etherified starch *see* tetrastarch *on page 885*

ethinyl estradiol and cyproterone acetate *see* cyproterone and ethinyl estradiol *(Canada only) on page 247*

ethinyl estradiol and desogestrel (ETH in il es tra DYE ole & des oh JES trel)

Medication Safety Issues

Sound-alike/look-alike issues:

Apri® may be confused with Apriso™

Ortho-Cept® may be confused with Ortho-Cyclen®

Synonyms desogestrel and ethinyl estradiol

U.S. Brand Names Apri®; Azurette™; Caziant®; Cyclessa®; Desogen®; Emoquette™; Kariva®; Mircette®; Ortho-Cept®; Reclipsen®; Velivet™; Viorele

Canadian Brand Names Cyclessa®; Linessa®; Marvelon®; Ortho-Cept®

Therapeutic Category Contraceptive, Oral

Use Prevention of pregnancy

General Dosage Range Oral: *Children and Adults (females, postmenarche):* 1 tablet daily

Dosage Forms

Tablet, oral [low dose formulation]:

Azurette™:

Day 1-21: Ethinyl estradiol 0.02 mg and desogestrel 0.15 mg [21 white tablets]

Day 22-23: 2 inactive green tablets

Day 24-28: Ethinyl estradiol 0.01 mg [5 blue tablets] (28s)

Kariva®:

Day 1-21: Ethinyl estradiol 0.02 mg and desogestrel 0.15 mg [21 white tablets]

Day 22-23: 2 inactive light green tablets

Day 24-28: Ethinyl estradiol 0.01 mg [5 light blue tablets] (28s)

Mircette®, Viorele:

Day 1-21: Ethinyl estradiol 0.02 mg and desogestrel 0.15 mg [21 white tablets]

Day 22-23: 2 inactive green tablets

Day 24-28: Ethinyl estradiol 0.01 mg [5 yellow tablets] (28s)

Tablet, oral [monophasic formulation]:

Apri® 28: Ethinyl estradiol 0.03 mg and desogestrel 0.15 mg [21 rose tablets and 7 white inactive tablets] (28s)

Desogen®, Reclipsen®: Ethinyl estradiol 0.03 mg and desogestrel 0.15 mg [21 white tablets and 7 green inactive tablets] (28s)

Emoquette™: Ethinyl estradiol 0.03 mg and desogestrel 0.15 mg [21 white tablets and 7 light green inactive tablets] (28s)

Ortho-Cept® 28: Ethinyl estradiol 0.03 mg and desogestrel 0.15 mg [21 light orange tablets and 7 green inactive tablets] (28s)

Tablet, oral [triphasic formulation]:

Caziant®:

Day 1-7: Ethinyl estradiol 0.025 mg and desogestrel 0.1 mg [7 white tablets]

Day 8-14: Ethinyl estradiol 0.025 mg and desogestrel 0.125 mg [7 light blue tablets]

Day 15-21: Ethinyl estradiol 0.025 mg and desogestrel 0.15 mg [7 blue tablets]

Day 22-28: 7 green inactive tablets (28s)

Cyclessa®:

Day 1-7: Ethinyl estradiol 0.025 mg and desogestrel 0.1 mg [7 light yellow tablets]

Day 8-14: Ethinyl estradiol 0.025 mg and desogestrel 0.125 mg [7 orange tablets]

Day 15-21: Ethinyl estradiol 0.025 mg and desogestrel 0.15 mg [7 red tablets]

Day 22-28: 7 green inactive tablets (28s)

Velivet™:

Day 1-7: Ethinyl estradiol 0.025 mg and desogestrel 0.1 mg [7 beige tablets]

Day 8-14: Ethinyl estradiol 0.025 mg and desogestrel 0.125 mg [7 orange tablets]

Day 15-21: Ethinyl estradiol 0.025 mg and desogestrel 0.15 mg [7 pink tablets]

Day 22-28: 7 white inactive tablets (28s)

ethinyl estradiol and drospirenone (ETH in il es tra DYE ole & droh SPYE re none)

Medication Safety Issues

Sound-alike/look-alike issues:

Yaz® may be confused with Beyaz™, Yasmin®

Synonyms drospirenone and ethinyl estradiol

U.S. Brand Names Gianvi™; Loryna™; Ocella™; Syeda™; Vestura™; Yasmin®; Yaz®; Zarah®

Canadian Brand Names Yasmin®; Yaz®

Therapeutic Category Contraceptive, Oral

Use Prevention of pregnancy; treatment of premenstrual dysphoric disorder (PMDD); treatment of acne

General Dosage Range Oral: *Children and Adults (females, postmenarche):* 1 tablet daily

Dosage Forms

Tablet, oral:

Gianvi™: Ethinyl estradiol 0.03 mg and drospirenone 3 mg [24 light pink active tablets and 4 white inactive tablets] (28s)

Loryna™: Ethinyl estradiol 0.02 mg and drospirenone 3 mg [24 peach active tablets and 4 white inactive tablets] (28s)

Ocella™, Syeda™, Yasmin®: Ethinyl estradiol 0.03 mg and drospirenone 3 mg [21 yellow active tablets and 7 white inactive tablets] (28s)

Vestura™: Ethinyl estradiol 0.02 mg and drospirenone 3 mg [24 pink active tablets and 4 peach inactive tablets] (28s)

Yaz®: Ethinyl estradiol 0.02 mg and drospirenone 3 mg [24 light pink active tablets and 4 white inactive tablets] (28s)

Zarah®: Ethinyl estradiol 0.03 mg and drospirenone 3 mg [21 blue active tablets and 7 peach inactive tablets] (28s)

ethinyl estradiol and ethynodiol diacetate

(ETH in il es tra DYE ole & e thye noe DYE ole dye AS e tate)

Medication Safety Issues

Sound-alike/look-alike issues:

Demulen® may be confused with Dalmane®, Demerol®

Synonyms ethynodiol diacetate and ethinyl estradiol

U.S. Brand Names Kelnor™; Zovia®

Canadian Brand Names Demulen® 30

Therapeutic Category Contraceptive, Oral

Use Prevention of pregnancy

General Dosage Range Oral: *Children and Adults (females, postmenarche):* 1 tablet daily

Dosage Forms

Tablet, oral [monophasic formulation]:

Kelnor™ 1/35: Ethinyl estradiol 0.035 mg and ethynodiol diacetate 1 mg [21 light yellow tablets and 7 white inactive tablets] (28s)

Zovia® 1/35-28: Ethinyl estradiol 0.035 mg and ethynodiol diacetate 1 mg [21 light pink tablets and 7 white inactive tablets] (28s)

Zovia® 1/50-28: Ethinyl estradiol 0.05 mg and ethynodiol diacetate 1 mg [21 pink tablets and 7 white inactive tablets] (28s)

ethinyl estradiol and etonogestrel (ETH in il es tra DYE ole & et oh noe JES trel)

Synonyms etonogestrel and ethinyl estradiol

U.S. Brand Names NuvaRing®

Canadian Brand Names NuvaRing®

Therapeutic Category Contraceptive, Oral; Estrogen and Progestin Combination

Use Prevention of pregnancy

General Dosage Range Vaginal: *Children and Adults (females, postmenarche):* Insert one ring and leave in place for 3 consecutive weeks, then remove for 1 week

Dosage Forms

Ring, vaginal:

NuvaRing®: Ethinyl estradiol 0.015 mg/day and etonogestrel 0.12 mg/day (3s) [3-week duration]

ethinyl estradiol and levonorgestrel (ETH in il es tra DYE ole & LEE voe nor jes trel)

Medication Safety Issues

Sound-alike/look-alike issues:

Nordette® may be confused with Nicorette®

Portia® may be confused with Potiga™

Seasonale® may be confused with Seasonique®

Tri-Levlen® may be confused with Trilafon®

Synonyms levonorgestrel and ethinyl estradiol

U.S. Brand Names Altavera™; Amethia™; Amethia™ Lo; Amethyst™; Aviane™; camrese™; Enpresse®; Introvale™; Jolessa™; Lessina®; Levora®; LoSeasonique®; Lutera®; Lybrel®; Marlissa; Myzilra™; Nordette® 28; Orsythia™; Portia®; Quasense®; Seasonale® [DSC]; Seasonique®; Sronyx®; Trivora®

Canadian Brand Names Alesse®; Aviane®; Min-Ovral®; Seasonale®; Triphasil®; Triquilar®

Therapeutic Category Contraceptive, Oral

Use Prevention of pregnancy; postcoital contraception

General Dosage Range Oral: *Children and Adults (females, postmenarche):* 1 tablet daily **or** 2 tablets as soon as possible (but within 72 hours of unprotected intercourse), followed by 2 tablets 12 hours later

Dosage Forms

Tablet, oral [low-dose formulation]:

Aviane™: Ethinyl estradiol 0.02 mg and levonorgestrel 0.1 mg [21 orange tablets and 7 light green inactive tablets] (28s)

Lessina®: Ethinyl estradiol 0.02 mg and levonorgestrel 0.1 mg [21 pink tablets and 7 white inactive tablets] (28s)

Lutera®, Sronyx®: Ethinyl estradiol 0.02 mg and levonorgestrel 0.1 mg [21 white tablets and 7 peach inactive tablets] (28s)

Orsythia™: Ethinyl estradiol 0.02 mg and levonorgestrel 0.1 mg [21 pink tablets and 7 light green inactive tablets] (28s)

Tablet, oral [monophasic formulation]:

Altavera™: Ethinyl estradiol 0.03 mg and levonorgestrel 0.15 mg [21 peach tablets and 7 white inactive tablets] (28s)

Levora®: Ethinyl estradiol 0.03 mg and levonorgestrel 0.15 mg [21 white tablets and 7 peach inactive tablets] (28s)

Marlissa: Ethinyl estradiol 0.03 mg and levonorgestrel 0.15 mg [21 light orange tablets and 7 pink inactive tablets] (28s)

Nordette® 28: Ethinyl estradiol 0.03 mg and levonorgestrel 0.15 mg [21 light orange tablets and 7 pink inactive tablets] (28s)

Portia® 28: Ethinyl estradiol 0.03 mg and levonorgestrel 0.15 mg [21 pink tablets and 7 white inactive tablets] (28s)

Tablet, oral [extended cycle regimen]: Ethinyl estradiol 0.02 mg and levonorgestrel 0.1 mg [84 tablets] and ethinyl estradiol 0.01 mg [7 tablets] (91s)

Amethia™:Ethinyl estradiol 0.03 mg and levonorgestrel 0.15 mg [84 white tablets] and ethinyl estradiol 0.01 mg [7 light blue tablets] (91s)

Amethia™ Lo: Ethinyl estradiol 0.02 mg and levonorgestrel 0.1 mg [84 white tablets] and ethinyl estradiol 0.01 mg [7 blue tablets] (91s)

camrese™: Ethinyl estradiol 0.03 mg and levonorgestrel 0.15 mg [84 light blue-green tablets] and ethinyl estradiol 0.01 mg [7 yellow tablets] (91s)

Introvale™: Ethinyl estradiol 0.03 mg and levonorgestrel 0.15 mg [84 peach tablets and 7 white inactive tablets] (91s)

Jolessa™: Ethinyl estradiol 0.03 mg and levonorgestrel 0.15 mg [84 pink tablets and 7 white inactive tablets] (91s)

LoSeasonique®: Ethinyl estradiol 0.02 mg and levonorgestrel 0.1 mg [84 orange tablets] and ethinyl estradiol 0.01 mg [7 yellow tablets] (91s)

Quasense®: Ethinyl estradiol 0.03 mg and levonorgestrel 0.15 mg] [84 white tablets and 7 peach inactive tablets] (91s)

Seasonique®: Ethinyl estradiol 0.03 mg and levonorgestrel 0.15 mg [84 light blue-green tablets] and ethinyl estradiol 0.01 mg [7 yellow tablets] (91s)

Tablet, oral [noncyclic regimen]:

Amethyst™: Ethinyl estradiol 0.02 mg and levonorgestrel 0.09 mg [28 white tablets] (28s)

Lybrel®: Ethinyl estradiol 0.02 mg and levonorgestrel 0.09 mg [28 yellow tablets] (28s)

Tablet, oral [triphasic formulation]:

Enpresse®:

Day 1-6: Ethinyl estradiol 0.03 mg and levonorgestrel 0.05 mg [6 pink tablets]

Day 7-11: Ethinyl estradiol 0.04 mg and levonorgestrel 0.075 mg [5 white tablets]

Day 12-21: Ethinyl estradiol 0.03 mg and levonorgestrel 0.125 mg [10 orange tablets]

Day 22-28: 7 light green inactive tablets (28s)

Myzilra™:
Day 1-6: Ethinyl estradiol 0.03 mg and levonorgestrel 0.05 mg [6 beige tablets]
Day 7-11: Ethinyl estradiol 0.04 mg and levonorgestrel 0.075 mg [5 white tablets]
Day 12-21: Ethinyl estradiol 0.03 mg and levonorgestrel 0.125 mg [10 light yellow tablets]
Day 22-28: 7 light green inactive tablets (28s)
Trivora®:
Day 1-6: Ethinyl estradiol 0.03 mg and levonorgestrel 0.05 mg [6 blue tablets]
Day 7-11: Ethinyl estradiol 0.04 mg and levonorgestrel 0.075 mg [5 white tablets]
Day 12-21: Ethinyl estradiol 0.03 mg and levonorgestrel 0.125 mg [10 pink tablets]
Day 22-28: 7 peach inactive tablets (28s)

ethinyl estradiol and NGM *see* ethinyl estradiol and norgestimate *on page 361*

ethinyl estradiol and norelgestromin (ETH in il es tra DYE ole & nor el JES troe min)

Synonyms norelgestromin and ethinyl estradiol

U.S. Brand Names Ortho Evra®

Canadian Brand Names Evra®

Therapeutic Category Contraceptive, Oral; Estrogen and Progestin Combination

Use Prevention of pregnancy

General Dosage Range Topical: *Children and Adults (females, postmenarche):* Apply one patch weekly for 3 weeks, followed by one week that is patch-free

Dosage Forms

Patch, transdermal:

Ortho Evra®: Ethinyl estradiol 0.75 mg and norelgestromin 6 mg [releases ethinyl estradiol 20 mcg and norelgestromin 150 mcg per day] (1s, 3s)

Dosage Forms - Canada

Patch, transdermal:

Evra®: Ethinyl estradiol 0.6 mg and norelgestromin 6 mg (1s, 3s)

ethinyl estradiol and norethindrone (ETH in il es tra DYE ole & nor eth IN drone)

Medication Safety Issues

Sound-alike/look-alike issues:

femhrt® may be confused with Femara®
Lo Loestrin™ Fe may be confused with Loestrin® Fe
Modicon® may be confused with Mylicon®
Norinyl® may be confused with Nardil®

Synonyms norethindrone acetate and ethinyl estradiol; Ortho Novum

U.S. Brand Names Alyacen 1/35; Alyacen 7/7/7; Aranelle®; Balziva™; Brevicon®; Briellyn; Cyclafem™ 1/35; Cyclafem™ 7/7/7; Estrostep® Fe; Femcon® Fe; femhrt®; femhrt® Lo; Generess™ Fe; Gildess® FE 1.5/30; Gildess® FE 1/20; Jevantique™ [DSC]; Jinteli™; Junel® 1.5/30; Junel® 1/20; Junel® Fe 1.5/30; Junel® Fe 1/20; Leena®; Lo Loestrin™ Fe; Loestrin® 21 1.5/30; Loestrin® 21 1/20; Loestrin® 24 Fe; Loestrin® Fe 1.5/30; Loestrin® Fe 1/20; Microgestin® 1.5/30; Microgestin® 1/20; Microgestin® Fe 1.5/30; Microgestin® Fe 1/20; Modicon®; Necon® 0.5/35; Necon® 1/35; Necon® 10/11; Necon® 7/7/7; Norinyl® 1+35; Nortrel® 0.5/35; Nortrel® 1/35; Nortrel® 7/7/7; Ortho-Novum® 1/35; Ortho-Novum® 7/7/7; Ovcon® 35; Ovcon® 50 [DSC]; Tilia™ Fe; Tri-Legest™ Fe; Tri-Norinyl®; Wymzya™ Fe; Zenchent Fe™; Zenchent™; Zeosa™

Canadian Brand Names Brevicon® 0.5/35; Brevicon® 1/35; FemHRT®; Loestrin™ 1.5/30; Minestrin™ 1/20; Ortho® 0.5/35; Ortho® 1/35; Ortho® 7/7/7; Select™ 1/35; Synphasic®

Therapeutic Category Contraceptive, Oral

Use Prevention of pregnancy; treatment of acne; moderate-to-severe vasomotor symptoms associated with menopause; prevention of osteoporosis (in women at significant risk only)

General Dosage Range Oral: *Children and Adults (females, postmenarche):* 1 tablet daily

Dosage Forms

Tablet, oral:

femhrt® 1/5: Ethinyl estradiol 0.005 mg and norethindrone acetate 1 mg [white tablets] (28s, 90s)
femhrt® Lo 0.5/2.5: Ethinyl estradiol 0.0025 mg and norethindrone acetate 0.5 mg [white tablets] (28s, 90s)

Tablet, oral [monophasic formulation]:
Alyacen 1/35: Ethinyl estradiol 0.035 mg and norethindrone 1 mg [21 peach tablets and 7 light green inactive tablets] (28s)
Balziva™: Ethinyl estradiol 0.035 mg and norethindrone 0.4 mg [21 light peach tablets and 7 white inactive tablets] (28s)
Brevicon®: Ethinyl estradiol 0.035 mg and norethindrone 0.5 mg [21 blue tablets and 7 orange inactive tablets] (28s)
Briellyn: Ethinyl estradiol 0.035 mg and norethindrone 0.4 mg [21 light peach tablets and 7 white-off-white inactive tablets] (28s)
Cyclafem™ 1/35: Ethinyl estradiol 0.035 mg and norethindrone 1 mg [21 pink tablets and 7 light green inactive tablets] (28s)
Gildess® FE 1/20: Ethinyl estradiol 0.02 mg and norethindrone acetate 1 mg [21 white tablets] and ferrous fumarate 75 mg [7 white-speckled brown tablets] (28s)
Gildess® FE 1.5/30: Ethinyl estradiol 0.03 mg and norethindrone acetate 1.5 mg [21 light green tablets] and ferrous fumarate 75 mg [7 white-speckled brown tablets] (28s)
Junel® 1/20: Ethinyl estradiol 0.02 mg and norethindrone acetate 1 mg [yellow tablets] (21s)
Junel® 1.5/30, Loestrin® 21 1.5/30: Ethinyl estradiol 0.03 mg and norethindrone acetate 1.5 mg [pink tablets] (21s)
Junel® Fe 1/20: Ethinyl estradiol 0.02 mg and norethindrone acetate 1 mg [21 yellow tablets] and ferrous fumarate 75 mg [7 brown tablets] (28s)
Junel® Fe 1.5/30, Loestrin® Fe 21 1.5/30: Ethinyl estradiol 0.03 mg and norethindrone acetate 1.5 mg [21 pink tablets] and ferrous fumarate 75 mg [7 brown tablets] (28s)
Loestrin® 21 1/20: Ethinyl estradiol 0.02 mg and norethindrone acetate 1 mg [light yellow tablets] (21s)
Lo Loestrin™ Fe: Ethinyl estradiol 0.01 mg and norethindrone acetate 1mg [24 blue tablets] and ethinyl estradiol 0.01 mg [2 white tablets] and ferrous fumarate 75 mg [2 brown tablets] (28s)
Loestrin® 24 Fe: Ethinyl estradiol 0.02 mg and norethindrone acetate 1 mg [24 white tablets] and ferrous fumarate 75 mg [4 brown tablets] (28s)
Loestrin® Fe 1/20: Ethinyl estradiol 0.02 mg and norethindrone acetate 1 mg [21 light yellow tablets] and ferrous fumarate 75 mg [7 brown tablets] (28s)
Loestrin® Fe 1.5/30: Ethinyl estradiol 0.03 mg and norethindrone acetate 1.5 mg [21 pink tablets] and ferrous fumarate 75 mg [7 brown tablets] (28s)
Microgestin® 1/20: Ethinyl estradiol 0.02 mg and norethindrone acetate 1 mg [white tablets] (21s)
Microgestin® 1.5/30: Ethinyl estradiol 0.03 mg and norethindrone acetate 1.5 mg [green tablets] (21s)
Microgestin® Fe 1/20: Ethinyl estradiol 0.02 mg and norethindrone acetate 1 mg [21 white tablets] and ferrous fumarate 75 mg [7 brown tablets] (28s)
Microgestin® Fe 1.5/30: Ethinyl estradiol 0.03 mg and norethindrone acetate 1.5 mg [21 green tablets] and ferrous fumarate 75 mg [7 brown tablets] (28s)
Modicon®: Ethinyl estradiol 0.035 mg and norethindrone 0.5 mg [21 white tablets and 7 green inactive tablets] (28s)
Necon® 0.5/35, Nortrel® 0.5/35: Ethinyl estradiol 0.035 mg and norethindrone 0.5 mg [21 light yellow tablets and 7 white inactive tablets] (28s)
Necon® 1/35: Ethinyl estradiol 0.035 mg and norethindrone 1 mg [21 dark yellow tablets and 7 white inactive tablets] (28s)
Norinyl® 1+35: Ethinyl estradiol 0.035 mg and norethindrone 1 mg [21 yellow-green tablets and 7 orange inactive tablets] (28s)
Nortrel® 1/35:
Ethinyl estradiol 0.035 mg and norethindrone 1 mg [yellow tablets] (21s)
Ethinyl estradiol 0.035 mg and norethindrone 1 mg [21 yellow tablets and 7 white inactive tablets] (28s)
Ortho-Novum® 1/35: Ethinyl estradiol 0.035 mg and norethindrone 1 mg [21 peach tablets and 7 green inactive tablets] (28s)
Ovcon® 35: Ethinyl estradiol 0.035 mg and norethindrone 0.4 mg [21 light peach tablets and 7 green inactive tablets] (28s)
Zenchent™: Ethinyl estradiol 0.035 mg and norethindrone 0.4 mg [21 orange tablets and 7 white inactive tablets] (28s)

Tablet, chewable, oral [monophasic formulation]: Ethinyl estradiol 0.035 mg and norethindrone 0.4 mg [21 tablets] and ferrous fumarate 75 mg [7 tablets] (28s)
Femcon® Fe, Wymzya™ Fe: Ethinyl estradiol 0.035 mg and norethindrone 0.4 mg [21 white tablets] and ferrous fumarate 75 mg [7 brown tablets] (28s)
Generess™ Fe: Ethinyl estradiol 0.025 mg and norethindrone 0.8 mg [24 light green tablets] and ferrous fumarate 75 mg [4 brown tablets] (28s)
Zenchent Fe™, Zeosa™: Ethinyl estradiol 0.035 mg and norethindrone 0.4 mg [21 light yellow tablets] and ferrous fumarate 75 mg [7 brown tablets] (28s)

Tablet, oral [biphasic formulation]:

Necon® 10/11:

Day 1-10: Ethinyl estradiol 0.035 mg and norethindrone 0.5 mg [10 light yellow tablets]
Day 11-21: Ethinyl estradiol 0.035 mg and norethindrone 1 mg [11 dark yellow tablets]
Day 22-28: 7 white inactive tablets (28s)

Tablet, oral [triphasic formulation]:

Alyacen 7/7/7:

Day 1-7: Ethinyl estradiol 0.035 mg and norethindrone 0.5 mg [7 white-off-white tablets]
Day 8-14: Ethinyl estradiol 0.035 mg and norethindrone 0.75 mg [7 light peach tablets]
Day 15-21: Ethinyl estradiol 0.035 mg and norethindrone 1 mg [7 peach tablets]
Day 22-28: 7 light green inactive tablets (28s)

Aranelle®:

Day 1-7: Ethinyl estradiol 0.035 mg and norethindrone 0.5 mg [7 light yellow tablets]
Day 8-16: Ethinyl estradiol 0.035 mg and norethindrone 1 mg [9 white tablets]
Day 17-21: Ethinyl estradiol 0.035 mg and norethindrone 0.5 mg [5 light yellow tablets]
Day 22-28: 7 peach inactive tablets (28s)

Cyclafem™ 7/7/7:

Day 1-7: Ethinyl estradiol 0.035 mg and norethindrone 0.5 mg [7 white tablets]
Day 8-14: Ethinyl estradiol 0.035 mg and norethindrone 0.75 mg [7 light pink tablets]
Day 15-21: Ethinyl estradiol 0.035 mg and norethindrone 1 mg [7 pink tablets]
Day 22-28: 7 light green inactive tablets (28s)

Estrostep® Fe, Tilia™ Fe:

Day 1-5: Ethinyl estradiol 0.02 mg and norethindrone acetate 1 mg [5 white triangular tablets]
Day 6-12: Ethinyl estradiol 0.03 mg and norethindrone acetate 1 mg [7 white square tablets]
Day 13-21: Ethinyl estradiol 0.035 mg and norethindrone acetate 1 mg [9 white round tablets]
Day 22-28: Ferrous fumarate 75 mg [7 brown tablets] (28s)

Leena®:

Day 1-7: Ethinyl estradiol 0.035 mg and norethindrone 0.5 mg [7 light blue tablets]
Day 8-16: Ethinyl estradiol 0.035 mg and norethindrone 1 mg [9 light yellow-green tablets]
Day 17-21: Ethinyl estradiol 0.035 mg and norethindrone 0.5 mg [5 light blue tablets]
Day 22-28: 7 orange inactive tablets (28s)

Necon® 7/7/7, Ortho-Novum® 7/7/7:

Day 1-7: Ethinyl estradiol 0.035 mg and norethindrone 0.5 mg [7 white tablets]
Day 8-14: Ethinyl estradiol 0.035 mg and norethindrone 0.75 mg [7 light peach tablets]
Day 15-21: Ethinyl estradiol 0.035 mg and norethindrone 1 mg [7 peach tablets]
Day 22-28: 7 green inactive tablets (28s)

Nortrel® 7/7/7:

Day 1-7: Ethinyl estradiol 0.035 mg and norethindrone 0.5 mg [7 light yellow tablets]
Day 8-14: Ethinyl estradiol 0.035 mg and norethindrone 0.75 mg [7 blue tablets]
Day 15-21: Ethinyl estradiol 0.035 mg and norethindrone 1 mg [7 peach tablets]
Day 22-28: 7 white inactive tablets (28s)

Tri-Legest™ Fe:

Day 1-5: Ethinyl estradiol 0.02 mg and norethindrone acetate 1 mg [5 light pink tablets]
Day 6-12: Ethinyl estradiol 0.03 mg and norethindrone acetate 1 mg [7 light yellow tablets]
Day 13-21: Ethinyl estradiol 0.035 mg and norethindrone acetate 1 mg [9 light blue tablets]
Day 22-28: Ferrous fumarate 75 mg [7 brown tablets] (28s)

Tri-Norinyl®:

Day 1-7: Ethinyl estradiol 0.035 mg and norethindrone 0.5 mg [7 blue tablets]
Day 8-16: Ethinyl estradiol 0.035 mg and norethindrone 1 mg [9 yellow-green tablets]
Day 17-21: Ethinyl estradiol 0.035 mg and norethindrone 0.5 mg [5 blue tablets]
Day 22-28: 7 orange inactive tablets (28s)

ethinyl estradiol and norgestimate (ETH in il es tra DYE ole & nor JES ti mate)

Medication Safety Issues

Sound-alike/look-alike issues:

Ortho-Cyclen® may be confused with Ortho-Cept®
Ortho Tri-Cyclen® may be confused with Ortho Tri-Cyclen® Lo

International issues:

Vivelle: Brand name for ethinyl estradiol/norgestimate [Austria], but also a brand name for estradiol [U.S. (discontinued), Belgium]

Synonyms ethinyl estradiol and NGM; norgestimate and ethinyl estradiol

U.S. Brand Names MonoNessa®; Ortho Tri-Cyclen®; Ortho Tri-Cyclen® Lo; Ortho-Cyclen®; Previfem®; Sprintec®; Tri-Previfem®; Tri-Sprintec®; TriNessa®

Canadian Brand Names Cyclen®; Tri-Cyclen®; Tri-Cyclen® Lo

Therapeutic Category Contraceptive, Oral

Use Prevention of pregnancy; treatment of acne

General Dosage Range Oral: *Children and Adults (females, postmenarche):* 1 tablet daily

Dosage Forms

Tablet, oral [monophasic formulation]:

MonoNessa®, Ortho-Cyclen®: Ethinyl estradiol 0.035 mg and norgestimate 0.25 mg [21 blue tablets and 7 dark green inactive tablets] (28s)

Previfem®: Ethinyl estradiol 0.035 mg and norgestimate 0.25 mg [21 blue tablets and 7 light green inactive tablets] (28s)

Sprintec®: Ethinyl estradiol 0.035 mg and norgestimate 0.25 mg [21 blue tablets and 7 white inactive tablets] (28s)

Tablet, oral [triphasic formulation]:

Ortho Tri-Cyclen®, TriNessa®:

Day 1-7: Ethinyl estradiol 0.035 mg and norgestimate 0.18 mg [7 white tablets]
Day 8-14: Ethinyl estradiol 0.035 mg and norgestimate 0.215 mg [7 light blue tablets]
Day 15-21: Ethinyl estradiol 0.035 mg and norgestimate 0.25 mg [7 blue tablets]
Day 22-28: 7 dark green inactive tablets (28s)

Tri-Previfem®::

Day 1-7: Ethinyl estradiol 0.035 mg and norgestimate 0.18 mg [7 white tablets]
Day 8-14: Ethinyl estradiol 0.035 mg and norgestimate 0.215 mg [7 light blue tablets]
Day 15-21: Ethinyl estradiol 0.035 mg and norgestimate 0.25 mg [7 blue tablets]
Day 22-28: 7 light green inactive tablets (28s)

Tri-Sprintec®:

Day 1-7: Ethinyl estradiol 0.035 mg and norgestimate 0.18 mg [7 gray tablets]
Day 8-14: Ethinyl estradiol 0.035 mg and norgestimate 0.215 mg [7 light blue tablets]
Day 15-21: Ethinyl estradiol 0.035 mg and norgestimate 0.25 mg [7 blue tablets]
Day 22-28: 7 white inactive tablets (28s)

Ortho Tri-Cyclen® Lo:

Day 1-7: Ethinyl estradiol 0.025 mg and norgestimate 0.18 mg [7 white tablets]
Day 8-14: Ethinyl estradiol 0.025 mg and norgestimate 0.215 mg [7 light blue tablets]
Day 15-21: Ethinyl estradiol 0.025 mg and norgestimate 0.25 mg [7 dark blue tablets]
Day 22-28: 7 dark green inactive tablets (28s)

ethinyl estradiol and norgestrel (ETH in il es tra DYE ole & nor JES trel)

Synonyms Lo Ovral; morning after pill; norgestrel and ethinyl estradiol

U.S. Brand Names Cryselle® 28; Lo/Ovral®-28; Low-Ogestrel®; Ogestrel®

Canadian Brand Names Lo-Femenal 21; Ovral®

Therapeutic Category Contraceptive, Oral

Use Prevention of pregnancy; postcoital contraceptive or "morning after" pill

General Dosage Range Oral: *Children and Adults (females, postmenarche):* 1 tablet daily **or** 2-4 tablets as single dose or in two divided doses (depending on formulation) within 72 hours of unprotected intercourse and 2-4 tablets 12 hours after first dose

Dosage Forms

Tablet, oral [monophasic formulation]: Ethinyl estradiol 0.03 mg and norgestrel 0.3 mg [21 tablets and 7 inactive tablets] (28s)

Cryselle® 28: Ethinyl estradiol 0.03 mg and norgestrel 0.3 mg [21 white tablets and 7 light green inactive tablets] (28s)

Low-Ogestrel®: Ethinyl estradiol 0.03 mg and norgestrel 0.3 mg [21 white tablets and 7 peach inactive tablets] (28s)

Lo/Ovral®-28: Ethinyl estradiol 0.03 mg and norgestrel 0.3 mg [21 white tablets and 7 pink inactive tablets] (28s)

Ogestrel®: Ethinyl estradiol 0.05 mg and norgestrel 0.5 mg [21 white tablets and 7 peach inactive tablets] (28s)

ethinyl estradiol, drospirenone, and levomefolate

(ETH in il es tra DYE ole, droh SPYE re none, & lee voe me FOE late)

Medication Safety Issues

Sound-alike/look-alike issues:

Beyaz™ may be confused with Yaz®

Synonyms drospirenone, ethinyl estradiol, and levomefolate calcium; ethinyl estradiol, drospirenone, and levomefolate calcium; levomefolate calcium, drospirenone, and ethinyl estradiol; levomefolate, drospirenone, and ethinyl estradiol

U.S. Brand Names Beyaz™; Safyral™

Therapeutic Category Contraceptive; Estrogen and Progestin Combination

Use Prevention of pregnancy; treatment of premenstrual dysphoric disorder (PMDD); treatment of acne; folate supplementation

General Dosage Range Oral: *Children ≥14 years and Adults:* 1 tablet daily

Dosage Forms

Tablet, oral:

Beyaz™: Ethinyl estradiol 0.02 mg, drospirenone 3 mg, and levomefolate calcium 0.451 mg [24 pink tablets] and levomefolate calcium 0.451 mg [4 light orange tablets] (28s)

Safyral™: Ethinyl estradiol 0.03 mg, drospirenone 3 mg, and levomefolate calcium 0.451 mg [21 orange tablets] and levomefolate calcium 0.451 mg [7 light orange tablets] (28s)

ethinyl estradiol, drospirenone, and levomefolate calcium *see* ethinyl estradiol, drospirenone, and levomefolate *on page 363*

ethiofos *see* amifostine *on page 59*

ethionamide (e thye on AM ide)

U.S. Brand Names Trecator®

Canadian Brand Names Trecator®

Therapeutic Category Antimycobacterial Agent

Use Treatment of tuberculosis and other mycobacterial diseases, in conjunction with other antituberculosis agents, when first-line agents have failed or resistance has been demonstrated

General Dosage Range Dosage adjustment recommended in patients with renal impairment

Oral:

Children: 15-20 mg/kg/day in 2-3 divided doses (maximum: 1 g/day)

Adults: 250-750 mg/day in 1-4 divided doses (maximum: 1 g/day)

Dosage Forms

Tablet, oral:

Trecator®: 250 mg

ethosuximide (eth oh SUKS i mide)

Medication Safety Issues

Sound-alike/look-alike issues:

Ethosuximide may be confused with methsuximide

Zarontin® may be confused with Neurontin®, Xalatan®, Zantac®, Zaroxolyn®

U.S. Brand Names Zarontin®

Canadian Brand Names Zarontin®

Therapeutic Category Anticonvulsant

Use Management of absence (petit mal) seizures

General Dosage Range Oral:

Children 3-6 years: Initial: 250 mg/day; Maintenance: 20 mg/kg/day (maximum: 1.5 g/day in divided doses)

Children ≥6 years: Initial: 500 mg/day; Maintenance: 20 mg/kg/day (maximum: 1.5 g/day in divided doses)

Adults: Initial: 500 mg/day (maximum: 1.5 g/day in divided doses)

Dosage Forms

Capsule, softgel, oral: 250 mg

Zarontin®: 250 mg

Solution, oral: 250 mg/5 mL (473 mL)

Zarontin®: 250 mg/5 mL (480 mL)

ethotoin (ETH oh toyn)

Synonyms ethylphenylhydantoin
U.S. Brand Names Peganone®
Therapeutic Category Hydantoin
Use Generalized tonic-clonic or complex-partial seizures
General Dosage Range Oral:
Children ≥1 year: Maximum initial dose: 750 mg/day; usual maintenance dose: 0.5-1 g/day; maximum dose: 3 g/day
Adults: Initial dose: ≤1 g/day; usual maintenance dose: 2-3 g/day
Dosage Forms
Tablet, oral:
Peganone®: 250 mg

ethoxynaphthamido penicillin sodium *see* nafcillin *on page 624*
ethyl alcohol *see* alcohol (ethyl) *on page 43*
ethyl aminobenzoate *see* benzocaine *on page 121*

ethyl chloride (ETH il KLOR ide)

Synonyms chloroethane
U.S. Brand Names Gebauer's Ethyl Chloride®
Therapeutic Category Local Anesthetic
Use Local anesthetic in minor operative procedures; control pain associated with injections, starting I.V. lines, and venipuncture; relieve pain caused by minor sport injury, bruises, myofascial and visceral pain syndromes
General Dosage Range Topical: *Adults:* Dosage varies greatly depending on indication
Dosage Forms
Aerosol, spray, topical:
Gebauer's Ethyl Chloride®: 100% (103.5 mL)

ethyl eicosapentaenoate *see* icosapent ethyl *on page 472*
ethyl-eicosapentaenoic acid *see* icosapent ethyl *on page 472*
ethyl-EPA *see* icosapent ethyl *on page 472*
ethyl esters of omega-3 fatty acids *see* omega-3-acid ethyl esters *on page 665*
ethyl icosapentate *see* icosapent ethyl *on page 472*
ethylphenylhydantoin *see* ethotoin *on page 364*
ethynodiol diacetate and ethinyl estradiol *see* ethinyl estradiol and ethynodiol diacetate *on page 357*
Ethyol® *see* amifostine *on page 59*
Etibi® (Can) *see* ethambutol *on page 355*

etidronate (e ti DROE nate)

Medication Safety Issues
Sound-alike/look-alike issues:
Etidronate may be confused with etomidate
Synonyms EHDP; etidronate disodium; sodium etidronate
U.S. Brand Names Didronel®
Canadian Brand Names Co-Etidronate; Mylan-Etidronate
Therapeutic Category Bisphosphonate Derivative
Use Symptomatic treatment of Paget disease; prevention and treatment of heterotopic ossification due to spinal cord injury or after total hip replacement
General Dosage Range Oral: *Adults:* 5-20 mg/kg/day
Dosage Forms
Tablet, oral: 200 mg, 400 mg
Didronel®: 400 mg

etidronate and calcium carbonate *(Canada only)*

(e ti DROE nate & KAL see um KAR bun ate)
Synonyms calcium carbonate and etidronate disodium; etidronate disodium and calcium

Canadian Brand Names CO Etidrocal; Didrocal®; Mylan-Eti-Cal Carepac; Novo-Etidronatecal

Therapeutic Category Bisphosphonate Derivative; Calcium Salt

Use Treatment and prevention of postmenopausal osteoporosis; prevention of corticosteroid-induced osteoporosis

General Dosage Range Oral: *Adults:* Etidronate disodium 400 mg once daily for 14 days, followed by calcium carbonate 1250 mg (500 mg elemental calcium) once daily for 76 days

Product Availability Not available in U.S.

Dosage Forms - Canada

Combination package [each package contains 5 blister cards (90-day supply)]:

Didrocal®:

Tablet, etidronate: 400 mg (14s) [first card (white tablets)]

Tablet, calcium: 1250 mg (76s) [remaining cards (blue tablets)]

etidronate disodium *see* etidronate *on page 364*

etidronate disodium and calcium *see* etidronate and calcium carbonate *(Canada only) on page 364*

etodolac (ee toe DOE lak)

Medication Safety Issues

Sound-alike/look-alike issues:

Lodine may be confused with codeine, iodine, Lopid®

BEERS Criteria medication:

This drug may be potentially inappropriate for use in geriatric patients (Quality of evidence - moderate; Strength of recommendation - strong).

Synonyms etodolic acid; Lodine

Canadian Brand Names Apo-Etodolac®; Utradol™

Therapeutic Category Analgesic, Nonnarcotic; Nonsteroidal Antiinflammatory Drug (NSAID)

Use Acute and long-term use in the management of signs and symptoms of osteoarthritis; rheumatoid arthritis and juvenile idiopathic arthritis (JIA); management of acute pain

General Dosage Range Oral:

Extended release:

Children 6-16 years and 20-30 kg: 400 mg once daily

Children 6-16 years and 31-45 kg: 600 mg once daily

Children 6-16 years and 46-60 kg: 800 mg once daily

Children 6-16 years and >60 kg: 1000 mg once daily

Adults: 400-1000 mg once daily

Regular release: *Adults:* 200-400 mg every 6-12 hours as needed **or** 500 mg 2 times/day (maximum: 1 g/day)

Dosage Forms

Capsule, oral: 200 mg, 300 mg

Tablet, oral: 400 mg, 500 mg

Tablet, extended release, oral: 400 mg, 500 mg, 600 mg

etodolic acid *see* etodolac *on page 365*

EtOH *see* alcohol (ethyl) *on page 43*

etomidate (e TOM i date)

Medication Safety Issues

Sound-alike/look-alike issues:

Etomidate may be confused with etidronate

High alert medication:

The Institute for Safe Medication Practices (ISMP) includes this medication among its list of drugs which have a heightened risk of causing significant patient harm when used in error.

U.S. Brand Names Amidate®

Canadian Brand Names Amidate®

Therapeutic Category General Anesthetic

Use Induction and maintenance of general anesthesia

General Dosage Range I.V.: *Children >10 years and Adults:* Induction: 0.2-0.6 mg/kg; Maintenance: 5-20 mcg/kg/minute

Dosage Forms

Injection, solution: 2 mg/mL (10 mL, 20 mL)

Amidate®: 2 mg/mL (10 mL, 20 mL)

etonogestrel (e toe noe JES trel)

Synonyms 3-keto-desogestrel; ENG

U.S. Brand Names Implanon®; Nexplanon®

Therapeutic Category Contraceptive; Progestin

Use Prevention of pregnancy; for use in women who request long-acting (up to 3 years) contraception

General Dosage Range Subdermal: *Adults (females, postmenarche):* Implant 1 rod for up to 3 years

Dosage Forms

Rod, subdermal:

Implanon®: 68 mg

Nexplanon®: 68 mg

etonogestrel and ethinyl estradiol *see* ethinyl estradiol and etonogestrel *on page 357*

ETOP *see* etoposide phosphate *on page 366*

Etopophos® *see* etoposide phosphate *on page 366*

etoposide (e toe POE side)

Medication Safety Issues

Sound-alike/look-alike issues:

Etoposide may be confused with teniposide

Etoposide may be confused with etoposide phosphate (a prodrug of etoposide which is rapidly converted in the plasma to etoposide)

VePesid may be confused with Versed

High alert medication:

This medication is in a class the Institute for Safe Medication Practices (ISMP) includes among its list of drug classes which have a heightened risk of causing significant patient harm when used in error.

Synonyms EPEG; epipodophyllotoxin; VePesid; VP-16; VP-16-213

U.S. Brand Names Toposar®

Canadian Brand Names Etoposide Injection USP; Vepesid™

Therapeutic Category Antineoplastic Agent

Use Treatment of refractory testicular tumors (injectable formulation); treatment of small cell lung cancer (SCLC)

Canadian labeling: Treatment of small cell lung cancer (SCLC; first- and second-line); treatment of nonsmall cell lung cancer (NSCLC); treatment of non-Hodgkin lymphomas (first-line); treatment of testicular cancer (first-line [injectable formulation] and refractory)

General Dosage Range Dosage adjustment recommended in patients with hepatic impairment, renal impairment, or who develop toxicities.

I.V., oral: *Adults:* Dosage varies greatly depending on indication

Dosage Forms

Capsule, softgel, oral: 50 mg

Injection, solution: 20 mg/mL (5 mL, 25 mL, 50 mL, 100 mL)

Toposar®: 20 mg/mL (5 mL, 25 mL, 50 mL)

etoposide phosphate (e toe POE side FOS fate)

Medication Safety Issues

Sound-alike/look-alike issues:

Etoposide phosphate may be confused with etoposide, teniposide

Etoposide phosphate is a prodrug of etoposide and is rapidly converted in the plasma to etoposide. To avoid confusion or dosing errors, **dosage should be expressed as the desired etoposide dose,** not as the etoposide phosphate dose (eg, etoposide phosphate equivalent to ____ mg etoposide).

High alert medication:

This medication is in a class the Institute for Safe Medication Practices (ISMP) includes among its list of drug classes which have a heightened risk of causing significant patient harm when used in error.

Synonyms epipodophyllotoxin; ETOP

U.S. Brand Names Etopophos®

Therapeutic Category Antineoplastic Agent

Use Treatment of refractory testicular tumors; treatment of small cell lung cancer

General Dosage Range Dosage adjustment recommended in patients with hepatic or renal impairment

I.V.: *Adults:* Dosage varies greatly depending on indication

Dosage Forms

Injection, powder for reconstitution:

Etopophos®: 100 mg

Etoposide Injection USP (Can) *see* etoposide *on page* 366

ETR *see* etravirine *on page* 367

etravirine (et ra VIR een)

Medication Safety Issues

International issues:

Etravirine [U.S. and multiple international markets] may be confused with ethaverine [multiple international markets]

Synonyms ETR; TMC125

U.S. Brand Names Intelence®

Canadian Brand Names Intelence®

Therapeutic Category Antiretroviral Agent, Nonnucleoside Reverse Transcriptase Inhibitor (NNRTI)

Use Treatment of HIV-1 infection in combination with at least two additional antiretroviral agents in treatment-experienced patients exhibiting viral replication with documented nonnucleoside reverse transcriptase inhibitor (NNRTI) resistance

General Dosage Range Oral:

Children ≥6 years and ≥16 kg to <20 kg: 100 mg twice daily

Children ≥6 years and ≥20 kg to <25 kg: 125 mg twice daily

Children ≥6 years and ≥25 kg to <30 kg: 150 mg twice daily

Children ≥6 years and ≥30 kg and Adults: 200 mg twice daily

Dosage Forms

Tablet, oral:

Intelence®: 25 mg, 100 mg, 200 mg

Euflex® (Can) *see* flutamide *on page* 399

Euflexxa® *see* hyaluronate and derivatives *on page* 450

Euglucon® (Can) *see* glyburide *on page* 428

Eulexin *see* flutamide *on page* 399

Eulexin® (Can) *see* flutamide *on page* 399

***Euphorbia peplus* derivative** *see* ingenol mebutate *on page* 484

Eurax® *see* crotamiton *on page* 241

Eurax Cream (Can) *see* crotamiton *on page* 241

Euro-Cyproheptadine (Can) *see* cyproheptadine *on page* 246

Euro-Lithium (Can) *see* lithium *on page* 544

eutectic mixture of lidocaine and tetracaine *see* lidocaine and tetracaine *on page* 539

Euthyrox (Can) *see* levothyroxine *on page* 533

Evac-U-Gen® [OTC] *see* senna *on page* 829

Evamist® *see* estradiol (systemic) *on page* 347

everolimus (e ver OH li mus)

Medication Safety Issues

Sound-alike/look-alike issues:

Everolimus may be confused with sirolimus, tacrolimus, temsirolimus

High alert medication:

This medication is in a class the Institute for Safe Medication Practices (ISMP) includes among its list of drug classes which have a heightened risk of causing significant patient harm when used in error.

Administration issues:

Tablets (Afinitor®, Zortress®) and tablets for oral suspension (Afinitor® Disperz) are not interchangeable; do not combine formulations to achieve desired dose.

Synonyms RAD001

U.S. Brand Names Afinitor®; Afinitor® Disperz; Zortress®

Canadian Brand Names Afinitor®

Therapeutic Category Antineoplastic Agent, mTOR Kinase Inhibitor; mTOR Kinase Inhibitor

Use

Afinitor®: Treatment of advanced hormone receptor-positive, HER2-negative breast cancer in postmenopausal women (in combination with exemestane and after letrozole or anastrozole failure); treatment of advanced renal cell cancer (RCC), after sunitinib or sorafenib failure; treatment of renal angiomyolipoma with tuberous sclerosis complex (TSC) not requiring immediate surgery; treatment of subependymal giant cell astrocytoma (SEGA) associated with TSC which requires intervention, but cannot be curatively resected; treatment of advanced, metastatic or unresectable pancreatic neuroendocrine tumors (PNET)

Afinitor® Disperz: Treatment of subependymal giant cell astrocytoma (SEGA) associated with TSC which requires intervention, but cannot be curatively resected

Zortress®: Prophylaxis of organ rejection in renal transplantation patients at low-moderate immunologic risk

General Dosage Range Dosage adjustment recommended in patients with hepatic impairment, on concomitant therapy, or who develop toxicities

Oral: *Children ≥1 year and Adults:* Dosage varies greatly depending on indication

Product Availability Afinitor Disperz (tablets for oral suspension): FDA approved August 2012; anticipated availability in November 2012. Consult prescribing information for additional information.

Dosage Forms

Tablet, oral:

Afinitor®: 2.5 mg, 5 mg, 7.5 mg, 10 mg

Zortress®: 0.25 mg, 0.5 mg, 0.75 mg

Everone® 200 (Can) *see* testosterone *on page* 881
Evicel™ *see* fibrin sealant *on page* 383
Evista® *see* raloxifene *on page* 785
Evithrom® *see* thrombin (topical) *on page* 893
Evoclin® *see* clindamycin (topical) *on page* 219
Evoxac® *see* cevimeline *on page* 192
Evra® (Can) *see* ethinyl estradiol and norelgestromin *on page* 359
Exactacain® *see* benzocaine, butamben, and tetracaine *on page* 123
Exalgo® *see* hydromorphone *on page* 460
Excedrin® Extra Strength [OTC] *see* acetaminophen, aspirin, and caffeine *on page* 26
Excedrin® Migraine [OTC] *see* acetaminophen, aspirin, and caffeine *on page* 26
Excedrin PM® [OTC] *see* acetaminophen and diphenhydramine *on page* 23
Excedrin® Sinus Headache [OTC] *see* acetaminophen and phenylephrine *on page* 24
Excedrin® Tension Headache [OTC] *see* acetaminophen *on page* 20
ExeFen-DMX *see* guaifenesin, pseudoephedrine, and dextromethorphan *on page* 437
ExeFen-IR *see* guaifenesin and pseudoephedrine *on page* 436
Exelderm® *see* sulconazole *on page* 858
Exelon® *see* rivastigmine *on page* 806

exemestane (ex e MES tane)

Medication Safety Issues

Sound-alike/look-alike issues:

Aromasin® may be confused with Arimidex®

Exemestane may be confused with estramustine.

U.S. Brand Names Aromasin®

Canadian Brand Names Aromasin®

Therapeutic Category Antineoplastic Agent, Miscellaneous

Use Treatment of advanced breast cancer in postmenopausal women whose disease has progressed following tamoxifen therapy; adjuvant treatment of postmenopausal estrogen receptor-positive early breast cancer following 2-3 years of tamoxifen (for a total of 5 years of adjuvant therapy)

General Dosage Range Dosage adjustment recommended in patients on concomitant therapy

Oral: *Adults (postmenopausal females):* 25 mg once daily

Dosage Forms
Tablet, oral: 25 mg
Aromasin®: 25 mg

exenatide (ex EN a tide)

Synonyms AC 2993; AC002993; exendin-4; LY2148568
U.S. Brand Names Bydureon™; Byetta®
Canadian Brand Names Byetta®
Therapeutic Category Antidiabetic Agent, Incretin Mimetic
Use Treatment of type 2 diabetes mellitus (noninsulin-dependent, NIDDM) to improve glycemic control

Canadian labeling: In conjunction with metformin and/or sulfonylurea for treatment of type 2 diabetes mellitus (noninsulin-dependent, NIDDM) to improve glycemic control

General Dosage Range **SubQ:** *Adults:*
Immediate release: Initial: 5 mcg twice daily; Maintenance: 5-10 mcg twice daily
Extended release: 2 mg once weekly

Dosage Forms
Injection, microspheres for suspension, extended release:
Bydureon™: 2 mg
Injection, solution:
Byetta®: 250 mcg/mL (1.2 mL, 2.4 mL)

exendin-4 *see* exenatide *on page 369*
Exforge® *see* amlodipine and valsartan *on page 67*
Exforge HCT® *see* amlodipine, valsartan, and hydrochlorothiazide *on page 68*
Exjade® *see* deferasirox *on page 258*
ex-lax® [OTC] *see* senna *on page 829*
ex-lax® Maximum Strength [OTC] *see* senna *on page 829*
ex-lax® Ultra [OTC] *see* bisacodyl *on page 134*
Exorex® Penetrating Emulsion [OTC] *see* coal tar *on page 228*
Exorex® Penetrating Emulsion #2 [OTC] *see* coal tar *on page 228*
Exparel™ *see* bupivacaine (liposomal) *on page 149*
Extavia® *see* interferon beta-1b *on page 492*
extended release epidural morphine *see* morphine (liposomal) *on page 614*
Extina® *see* ketoconazole (topical) *on page 512*
Extraneal *see* icodextrin *on page 471*
Extra Strength Allergy Relief [OTC] (Can) *see* cetirizine *on page 190*
EYE001 *see* pegaptanib *on page 695*
Eye-Stream® (Can) *see* balanced salt solution *on page 113*
Eylea™ *see* aflibercept (ophthalmic) *on page 38*
E-Z-Cat® *see* barium *on page 114*
E-Z Cat® Dry *see* barium *on page 114*
EZ-Char® [OTC] *see* charcoal, activated *on page 193*
E-Z-Disk™ *see* barium *on page 114*
E-Z-Dose™ with Liquid Polibar Plus® *see* barium *on page 114*

ezetimibe (ez ET i mibe)

Medication Safety Issues
Sound-alike/look-alike issues:
Ezetimibe may be confused with ezogabine
Zetia® may be confused with Zebeta®, Zestril®

U.S. Brand Names Zetia®
Canadian Brand Names Ezetrol®
Therapeutic Category Antilipemic Agent, 2-Azetidinone

Use Use in combination with dietary therapy for the treatment of primary hypercholesterolemia (as monotherapy or in combination with HMG-CoA reductase inhibitors); homozygous sitosterolemia; homozygous familial hypercholesterolemia (in combination with atorvastatin or simvastatin); mixed hyperlipidemia (in combination with fenofibrate)

General Dosage Range **Oral:** *Children ≥10 years and Adults:* 10 mg once daily

Dosage Forms

Tablet, oral:

Zetia®: 10 mg

ezetimibe and simvastatin (ez ET i mibe & SIM va stat in)

Medication Safety Issues

Sound-alike/look-alike issues:

Vytorin® may be confused with Vyvanse®

Synonyms simvastatin and ezetimibe

U.S. Brand Names Vytorin®

Therapeutic Category Antilipemic Agent, 2-Azetidinone

Use Used in combination with dietary modification for the treatment of primary hypercholesterolemia and homozygous familial hypercholesterolemia

General Dosage Range Dosage adjustment recommended in patients with renal impairment or on concomitant therapy

Oral: *Adults:* Ezetimibe 10 mg and simvastatin 10-40 mg once daily

Dosage Forms

Tablet:

Vytorin®:

10/10: Ezetimibe 10 mg and simvastatin 10 mg
10/20: Ezetimibe 10 mg and simvastatin 20 mg
10/40: Ezetimibe 10 mg and simvastatin 40 mg
10/80: Ezetimibe 10 mg and simvastatin 80 mg

Ezetrol® (Can) *see* ezetimibe *on page* 369
EZG *see* ezogabine *on page* 370
E-Z-HD™ *see* barium *on page* 114

ezogabine (e ZOG a been)

Medication Safety Issues

Sound-alike/look-alike issues:

Ezogabine may be confused with ezetimibe.
Potiga™ may be confused with Portia®

Synonyms D-23129; EZG; retigabine; RTG

U.S. Brand Names Potiga™

Therapeutic Category Anticonvulsant, Neuronal Potassium Channel Opener

Controlled Substance C-V

Use Adjuvant treatment of partial-onset seizures

General Dosage Range Dosage adjustment recommended in patients with renal impairment or hepatic impairment.

Oral:

Adults: Initial: 100 mg 3 times/day; Maintenance: 200-400 mg 3 times/day (maximum: 1200 mg/day)
Elderly: Initial: 50 mg 3 times/day; Maintenance: 250 mg 3 times/day (maximum: 750 mg/day)

Dosage Forms

Tablet, oral:

Potiga™: 50 mg, 200 mg, 300 mg, 400 mg

E-Z-Paque® *see* barium *on page* 114
E-Z-Paste® *see* barium *on page* 114
F_3T *see* trifluridine *on page* 919
FabAV, FAB (ovine) *see* crotalidae polyvalent immune FAB (ovine) *on page* 241
FaBB *see* folic acid, cyanocobalamin, and pyridoxine *on page* 404
Fabrazyme® *see* agalsidase beta *on page* 39
Factive® *see* gemifloxacin *on page* 422

factor VIIa (recombinant) (FAK ter SEV en aye ree KOM be nant)

Synonyms coagulation factor VIIa; eptacog alfa (activated); rFVIIa

U.S. Brand Names NovoSeven® RT

Canadian Brand Names Niastase®; Niastase® RT

Therapeutic Category Antihemophilic Agent; Blood Product Derivative

Use Treatment of bleeding episodes and prevention of bleeding in surgical interventions in patients with either hemophilia A or B with inhibitors to factor VIII or factor IX, acquired hemophilia, or congenital factor VII deficiency

General Dosage Range I.V.: *Children and Adults:* Dosage varies greatly depending on indication

Dosage Forms

Injection, powder for reconstitution [preservative free]:

NovoSeven® RT: 1 mg, 2 mg, 5 mg, 8 mg

factor VIII concentrate *see* antihemophilic factor/von Willebrand factor complex (human) *on page* 78

factor VIII (human) *see* antihemophilic factor (human) *on page* 78

factor VIII (human) *see* antihemophilic factor/von Willebrand factor complex (human) *on page* 78

factor VIII (recombinant) *see* antihemophilic factor (recombinant) *on page* 78

factor IX (FAK ter nyne)

Medication Safety Issues

Sound-alike/look-alike issues:

Factor IX may be confused with Factor IX Complex

Synonyms factor IX concentrate

U.S. Brand Names AlphaNine® SD; BeneFix®; Mononine®

Canadian Brand Names BeneFix®; Immunine® VH; Mononine®

Therapeutic Category Antihemophilic Agent

Use Prevention and control of bleeding in patients with factor IX deficiency (hemophilia B or Christmas disease)

NOTE: Contains either **nondetectable levels of factors II, VII, and X** (AlphaNine®, Mononine®) or **only factor IX** (BeneFIX®). Therefore, **NOT INDICATED** for replacement therapy of any other clotting factor besides factor IX or for reversal of anticoagulation due to either vitamin K antagonists or other anticoagulants (eg, dabigatran), hemophilia A patients with factor VIII inhibitors, or patients in a hemorrhagic state caused by reduced production of liver-dependent coagulation factors (eg, hepatitis, cirrhosis).

General Dosage Range I.V.: *Children and Adults:* Dosage varies greatly depending on indication

Dosage Forms

Injection, powder for reconstitution [recombinant]:

BeneFix®: ~250 units, ~500 units, ~1000 units, ~2000 units [exact potency labeled on each vial]

Injection, powder for reconstitution [human derived]:

AlphaNine® SD: ~500 units, ~1000 units, ~1500 units [exact potency labeled on each vial]

Mononine®: ~500 units, ~1000 units [exact potency labeled on each vial]

factor IX complex (human) (FAK ter nyne KOM pleks HYU man)

Medication Safety Issues

Sound-alike/look-alike issues:

Factor IX Complex may be confused with Factor IX

Synonyms PCC; prothrombin complex concentrate

U.S. Brand Names Bebulin® VH; Profilnine® SD

Therapeutic Category Antihemophilic Agent

Use Prevention and control of bleeding in patients with factor IX deficiency (hemophilia B or Christmas disease)

General Dosage Range I.V.: *Children and Adults:* Dosage varies greatly depending on indication

Dosage Forms

Injection, powder for reconstitution:

Bebulin® VH: Exact potency labeled on each vial

Profilnine® SD: ~500 units, ~1000 units, ~1500 units [exact potency labeled on each vial]

factor IX concentrate *see* factor IX *on page* 371

factor 13 *see* factor XIII concentrate (human) *on page* 372

factor XIII concentrate (human) (FAK ter THIR teen KON cen trate HYU man)

Medication Safety Issues

Sound-alike/look-alike issues:

Factor XIII may be confused with Factor VIII

Synonyms activated factor XIII; factor 13; FXIII

U.S. Brand Names Corifact®

Therapeutic Category Antihemophilic Agent; Blood Product Derivative

Use Prophylaxis against bleeding episodes in congenital factor XIII deficiency

General Dosage Range I.V.: *Children and Adults:* Initial: 40 units/kg; Maintenance: Varies depending on desired factor XIII trough levels

Dosage Forms

Injection, powder for reconstitution:

Corifact®: Exact potency labeled on each vial

famciclovir (fam SYE kloe veer)

Medication Safety Issues

Sound-alike/look-alike issues:

Famvir® may be confused with Femara®

U.S. Brand Names Famvir®

Canadian Brand Names Apo-Famciclovir®; Ava-Famciclovir; CO Famciclovir; Famvir®; PMS-Famciclovir; Sandoz-Famciclovir

Therapeutic Category Antiviral Agent

Use Treatment of acute herpes zoster (shingles) in immunocompetent patients; treatment and suppression of recurrent episodes of genital herpes in immunocompetent patients; treatment of herpes labialis (cold sores) in immunocompetent patients; treatment of recurrent orolabial/genital (mucocutaneous) herpes simplex in HIV-infected patients

General Dosage Range

Dosage adjustment recommended in patients with renal impairment

Oral: *Adults:* 250-1000 mg twice daily **or** 500 mg every 8 hours **or** 1500 mg once

Dosage Forms

Tablet, oral: 125 mg, 250 mg, 500 mg

Famvir®: 125 mg, 250 mg, 500 mg

famotidine (fa MOE ti deen)

Medication Safety Issues

Sound-alike/look-alike issues:

Famotidine may be confused with FLUoxetine, furosemide

U.S. Brand Names Heartburn Relief Maximum Strength [OTC]; Heartburn Relief [OTC]; Pepcid®; Pepcid® AC Maximum Strength [OTC]; Pepcid® AC [OTC]

Canadian Brand Names Acid Control; Apo-Famotidine®; Apo-Famotidine® Injectable; Famotidine Omega; Mylan-Famotidine; Novo-Famotidine; Nu-Famotidine; Pepcid®; Pepcid® AC; Pepcid® I.V.; Ulcidine

Therapeutic Category Histamine H_2 Antagonist

Use Maintenance therapy and treatment of duodenal ulcer; treatment of gastroesophageal reflux disease (GERD), active benign gastric ulcer; pathological hypersecretory conditions

OTC labeling: Relief of heartburn, acid indigestion, and sour stomach

General Dosage Range Dosage adjustment recommended in patients with renal impairment

I.V.:

Children 1-16 years: 0.25 mg/kg every 12 hours (maximum: 40 mg/day)

Adults: 20 mg every 12 hours

Oral:

Children <3 months: 0.5 mg/kg once daily

Children 3-12 months: 0.5 mg/kg twice daily

Children 1-11 years: 0.5-1 mg/kg/day in 1-2 divided doses (maximum: 80 mg/day)

Children 12-16 years: 0.5-1 mg/kg/day in 1-2 divided doses (maximum: 80 mg/day) **or** 10-20 mg every 12 hours (OTC dosing)

Adults: 20-40 mg/day in 1-2 divided doses **or** 20-160 mg every 6 hours [hypersecretory conditions]

Dosage Forms

Infusion, premixed in NS [preservative free]: 20 mg (50 mL)
Injection, solution: 10 mg/mL (4 mL, 20 mL, 50 mL)
Injection, solution [preservative free]: 10 mg/mL (2 mL)
Powder for suspension, oral: 40 mg/5 mL (50 mL)
Pepcid®: 40 mg/5 mL (50 mL)
Tablet, oral: 10 mg, 20 mg, 40 mg
Heartburn Relief [OTC]: 10 mg
Heartburn Relief Maximum Strength [OTC]: 20 mg
Pepcid®: 20 mg, 40 mg
Pepcid® AC [OTC]: 10 mg
Pepcid® AC Maximum Strength [OTC]: 20 mg
Tablet, chewable, oral:
Pepcid® AC Maximum Strength [OTC]: 20 mg

famotidine and ibuprofen *see* ibuprofen and famotidine *on page 470*

famotidine, calcium carbonate, and magnesium hydroxide

(fa MOE ti deen, KAL see um KAR bun ate, & mag NEE zhum hye DROKS ide)

Synonyms calcium carbonate, magnesium hydroxide, and famotidine; magnesium hydroxide, famotidine, and calcium carbonate

U.S. Brand Names Pepcid® Complete® [OTC]; Tums® Dual Action [OTC]

Canadian Brand Names Pepcid® Complete® [OTC]

Therapeutic Category Antacid; Histamine H_2 Antagonist

Use Relief of heartburn due to acid indigestion

General Dosage Range Oral: *Children ≥12 years and Adults:* 1 tablet (famotidine 10 mg/calcium carbonate 800 mg/magnesium hydroxide 165 mg) as needed (maximum: 2 tablets/day)

Dosage Forms

Tablet, chewable, oral:
Pepcid® Complete® [OTC], Tums® Dual Action [OTC]: Famotidine 10 mg, calcium carbonate 800 mg, and magnesium hydroxide 165 mg

Famotidine Omega (Can) *see* famotidine *on page 372*
fampridine *see* dalfampridine *on page 251*
fampridine-SR *see* dalfampridine *on page 251*
Fampyra™ (Can) *see* dalfampridine *on page 251*
Famvir® *see* famciclovir *on page 372*
Fanapt® *see* iloperidone *on page 473*
Fansidar® [DSC] *see* sulfadoxine and pyrimethamine *on page 860*
2F-ara-AMP *see* fludarabine *on page 389*
Fareston® *see* toremifene *on page 907*
Faslodex® *see* fulvestrant *on page 411*
Fasturtec® (Can) *see* rasburicase *on page 789*

fat emulsion (fat e MUL shun)

Medication Safety Issues

Sound-alike/look-alike issues:
Intralipid® may be confused with ViperSlide™ (lubricant used during atherectomy procedures)

Synonyms intravenous fat emulsion

U.S. Brand Names Intralipid®; Liposyn® III

Canadian Brand Names Intralipid®; Liposyn® II

Therapeutic Category Intravenous Nutritional Therapy

Use Source of calories and essential fatty acids for patients requiring parenteral nutrition of extended duration; prevention and treatment of essential fatty acid deficiency (EFAD)

General Dosage Range I.V.:
Infants: Initial: 1-2 g/kg/day; Maintenance: Up to 3 g/kg/day
Children: 1-2 g/kg/day; Maintenance: Up to 2-3 g/kg/day **or** 8% to 10% of caloric intake given 2-3 times weekly

Adolescents and Adults: Initial: 1 g/kg/day; Maintenance: Up to 2.5 g/kg/day **or** 8% to 10% of caloric intake given 2-3 times weekly

Dosage Forms

Injection, emulsion:

Intralipid®: 20% (100 mL, 250 mL, 500 mL, 1000 mL); 30% (500 mL)

Liposyn® III: 10% (250 mL, 500 mL); 20% (250 mL, 500 mL); 30% (500 mL)

Father John's® [OTC] *see* dextromethorphan *on page 272*

Father John's® Plus [OTC] *see* chlorpheniramine, phenylephrine, and dextromethorphan *on page 201*

FazaClo® *see* clozapine *on page 228*

5-FC *see* flucytosine *on page 389*

FC1157a *see* toremifene *on page 907*

[^{18}F]-FDG *see* fludeoxyglucose F 18 *on page 390*

FE200486 *see* degarelix *on page 259*

febuxostat (feb UX oh stat)

Synonyms TEI-6720; TMX-67

U.S. Brand Names Uloric®

Canadian Brand Names Uloric®

Therapeutic Category Xanthine Oxidase Inhibitor

Use Chronic management of hyperuricemia in patients with gout

General Dosage Range Oral: *Adults:* 40-80 mg once daily

Dosage Forms

Tablet, oral:

Uloric®: 40 mg, 80 mg

Feiba NF *see* antiinhibitor coagulant complex *on page 79*

Feiba VH [DSC] *see* antiinhibitor coagulant complex *on page 79*

felbamate (FEL ba mate)

U.S. Brand Names Felbatol®

Therapeutic Category Anticonvulsant

Use Monotherapy or adjunctive therapy in the treatment of partial seizures (with and without generalization); adjunctive therapy in the treatment of partial and generalized seizures associated with Lennox-Gastaut syndrome; not indicated for use as first-line treatment

General Dosage Range Dosage adjustment recommended in patients with renal impairment or on concomitant therapy

Oral:

Children 2-14 years: Initial: 15 mg/kg/day in divided doses 3 or 4 times/day; Maintenance: Up to 45 mg/kg/day in divided doses 3 or 4 times/day (maximum: 3600 mg/day)

Children >14 years and Adults: Initial: 1200 mg/day in divided doses 3 or 4 times/day; Maintenance: Up to 3600 mg/day in divided doses 3 or 4 times/day.

Dosage Forms

Suspension, oral: 600 mg/5 mL (240 mL, 473 mL)

Felbatol®: 600 mg/5 mL (240 mL, 960 mL)

Tablet, oral: 400 mg, 600 mg

Felbatol®: 400 mg, 600 mg

Felbatol® *see* felbamate *on page 374*

Feldene® *see* piroxicam *on page 727*

felodipine (fe LOE di peen)

Medication Safety Issues

Sound-alike/look-alike issues:

Plendil® may be confused with Isordil®, pindolol, Pletal®, PriLOSEC®, Prinivil®

Synonyms Plendil

Canadian Brand Names Plendil®; Renedil®; Sandoz-Felodipine

Therapeutic Category Calcium Channel Blocker

Use Treatment of hypertension

General Dosage Range Dosage adjustment recommended in patients with hepatic impairment

Oral:

Adults: Initial: 2.5-10 mg once daily; Maintenance: 2.5-20 mg once daily (maximum: 20 mg/day)
Elderly: Initial: 2.5 mg/day

Dosage Forms

Tablet, extended release, oral: 2.5 mg, 5 mg, 10 mg

felodipine and ramipril *see* ramipril and felodipine *(Canada only) on page 786*

Femara® *see* letrozole *on page 526*

Femcon® Fe *see* ethinyl estradiol and norethindrone *on page 359*

Femecal OB *see* vitamins (multiple/prenatal) *on page 952*

femhrt® *see* ethinyl estradiol and norethindrone *on page 359*

FemHRT® (Can) *see* ethinyl estradiol and norethindrone *on page 359*

femhrt® Lo *see* ethinyl estradiol and norethindrone *on page 359*

Femilax™ [OTC] *see* bisacodyl *on page 134*

Femiron® [OTC] *see* ferrous fumarate *on page 379*

Fem-Prin® [OTC] *see* acetaminophen, aspirin, and caffeine *on page 26*

Femring® *see* estradiol (systemic) *on page 347*

Femstat® One (Can) *see* butoconazole *on page 155*

Femtrace® *see* estradiol (systemic) *on page 347*

Fenesin DM IR [OTC] *see* guaifenesin and dextromethorphan *on page 434*

Fenesin IR [OTC] *see* guaifenesin *on page 433*

Fenesin PE IR *see* guaifenesin and phenylephrine *on page 435*

fenofibrate (fen oh FYE brate)

Medication Safety Issues

Sound-alike/look-alike issues:

TriCor® may be confused with Fibricor®, Tracleer®

Synonyms procetofene; proctofene

U.S. Brand Names Antara®; Fenoglide®; Lipofen®; Lofibra®; TriCor®; Triglide®

Canadian Brand Names Apo-Feno-Micro®; Apo-Feno-Super®; Apo-Fenofibrate®; Dom-Fenofibrate Micro; Feno-Micro-200; Fenofibrate Micro; Fenofibrate-S; Fenomax; Lipidil EZ®; Lipidil Micro®; Lipidil Supra®; Mylan-Fenofibrate Micro; Novo-Fenofibrate; Novo-Fenofibrate Micronized; Novo-Fenofibrate-S; Nu-Fenofibrate; PHL-Fenofibrate Micro; PHL-Fenofibrate Supra; PMS-Fenofibrate Micro; PRO-Feno-Super; ratio-Fenofibrate MC; Riva-Fenofibrate Micro; Sandoz-Fenofibrate S

Therapeutic Category Antihyperlipidemic Agent, Miscellaneous

Use Adjunct to dietary therapy for the treatment of adults with elevations of serum triglyceride levels (types IV and V hyperlipidemia); adjunct to dietary therapy for the reduction of low density lipoprotein cholesterol (LDL-C), total cholesterol (total-C), triglycerides, and apolipoprotein B (apo B), and to increase high density lipoprotein cholesterol (HDL-C) in adult patients with primary hypercholesterolemia or mixed dyslipidemia (Fredrickson types IIa and IIb)

General Dosage Range Dosage adjustment recommended in patients with renal impairment

Oral: *Adults and Elderly:* Dosage varies greatly depending on product

Dosage Forms

Capsule, oral: 67 mg, 134 mg, 200 mg

Antara®: 43 mg, 130 mg
Lipofen®: 50 mg, 150 mg
Lofibra®: 67 mg, 134 mg, 200 mg

Tablet, oral: 54 mg, 160 mg

Fenoglide®: 40 mg, 120 mg
Lofibra®: 54 mg, 160 mg
TriCor®: 48 mg, 145 mg
Triglide®: 50 mg, 160 mg

Fenofibrate Micro (Can) *see* fenofibrate *on page 375*

Fenofibrate-S (Can) *see* fenofibrate *on page 375*

fenofibric acid (fen oh FYE brik AS id)

Medication Safety Issues

Sound-alike/look-alike issues:

Fibricor® may be confused with Tricor®

TriLipix® may be confused with Trileptal®, TriLyte®

Synonyms ABT-335; choline fenofibrate

U.S. Brand Names Fibricor®; TriLipix®

Therapeutic Category Antilipemic Agent, Fibric Acid

Use Adjunct to dietary therapy for the treatment of severely elevated serum triglyceride levels; adjunct to dietary therapy for the reduction of low density lipoprotein cholesterol (LDL-C), total cholesterol (total-C), triglycerides, and apolipoprotein B (apo B) and to increase high density lipoprotein cholesterol (HDL-C) in patients with primary hypercholesterolemia or mixed dyslipidemia

TriLipix™ is also indicated as adjunct to dietary therapy concomitantly with a statin to reduce triglyceride levels and increase HDL-C levels in patients with mixed dyslipidemia and coronary heart disease (CHD) or at risk for CHD

General Dosage Range Dosage adjustment recommended in patients with renal impairment

Oral: *Adults:* Fibricor®: 35-105 mg once daily (maximum: 105 mg/day); TriLipix™: 45-135 mg once daily (maximum: 135 mg/day)

Dosage Forms

Capsule, delayed release, oral:

TriLipix®: 45 mg, 135 mg

Tablet, oral: 35 mg, 105 mg

Fibricor®: 35 mg, 105 mg

Fenoglide® *see* fenofibrate *on page* 375

fenoldopam (fe NOL doe pam)

Synonyms fenoldopam mesylate

U.S. Brand Names Corlopam®

Therapeutic Category Antihypertensive Agent

Use Treatment of severe hypertension (up to 48 hours in adults), including in patients with renal compromise; short-term (up to 4 hours) blood pressure reduction in pediatric patients

General Dosage Range I.V.:

Children: Initial: 0.2 mcg/kg/minute, may increase to 0.3-0.5 mcg/kg/minute every 20-30 minutes (maximum: 0.8 mcg/kg/minute)

Adults: Initial: 0.03-0.1 mcg/kg/minute, may increase in increments of 0.05-0.1 mcg/kg/minute every 15 minutes (maximum: 1.6 mcg/kg/minute)

Dosage Forms

Injection, solution: 10 mg/mL (1 mL, 2 mL)

Corlopam®: 10 mg/mL (1 mL, 2 mL)

fenoldopam mesylate *see* fenoldopam *on page* 376

Fenomax (Can) *see* fenofibrate *on page* 375

Feno-Micro-200 (Can) *see* fenofibrate *on page* 375

fenoprofen (fen oh PROE fen)

Medication Safety Issues

Sound-alike/look-alike issues:

Fenoprofen may be confused with flurbiprofen

BEERS Criteria medication:

This drug may be potentially inappropriate for use in geriatric patients (Quality of evidence - moderate; Strength of recommendation - strong).

Synonyms fenoprofen calcium

U.S. Brand Names Nalfon®

Canadian Brand Names Nalfon®

Therapeutic Category Analgesic, Nonnarcotic; Nonsteroidal Antiinflammatory Drug (NSAID)

Use Symptomatic treatment of acute and chronic rheumatoid arthritis and osteoarthritis; relief of mild-to-moderate pain

General Dosage Range Oral: *Adults:* 200 mg every 4-6 hours as needed **or** 300-600 mg 3-4 times/day (maximum: 3.2 g/day)

Dosage Forms

Capsule, oral:

Nalfon®: 200 mg, 400 mg

Tablet, oral: 600 mg

fenoprofen calcium *see* fenoprofen *on page 376*

fenoterol and ipratropium *see* ipratropium and fenoterol *(Canada only) on page 500*

fenoterol hydrobromide and ipratropium bromide *see* ipratropium and fenoterol *(Canada only) on page 500*

fentanyl (FEN ta nil)

Medication Safety Issues

Sound-alike/look-alike issues:

FentaNYL may be confused with alfentanil, SUFentanil

High alert medication:

The Institute for Safe Medication Practices (ISMP) includes this medication among its list of drug classes which have a heightened risk of causing significant patient harm when used in error.

Administration issues:

Fentanyl transdermal system patches: Leakage of fentanyl gel from the patch has been reported; patch may be less effective; do not use. Thoroughly wash any skin surfaces coming into direct contact with gel with water (do not use soap). May contain conducting metal (eg, aluminum); remove patch prior to MRI.

Other safety concerns:

Fentanyl transdermal system patches:

Dosing of transdermal fentanyl patches may be confusing. Transdermal fentanyl patches should always be prescribed in mcg/hour, not size. Patch dosage form of Duragesic®-12 actually delivers 12.5 mcg/hour of fentanyl. Use caution, as orders may be written as "Duragesic 12.5" which can be erroneously interpreted as a 125 mcg dose.

Patches should be stored and disposed of with care to avoid accidental exposure to children. The FDA has issued numerous safety advisories to warn users of the possible consequences (including hospitalization and death) of inappropriate storage or disposal of patches.

Abstral®, Actiq®, Fentora®, Onsolis®, and Subsys® are not interchangeable; do not substitute doses on a mcg-per-mcg basis.

Synonyms fentanyl citrate; fentanyl hydrochloride; fentanyl patch; OTFC (oral transmucosal fentanyl citrate)

Tall-Man fenta**NYL**

U.S. Brand Names Abstral®; Actiq®; Duragesic®; Fentora®; Lazanda®; Onsolis®; Subsys®

Canadian Brand Names Abstral™; Actiq®; Duragesic®; Duragesic® MAT; Fentanyl Citrate Injection, USP; Novo-Fentanyl; PMS-Fentanyl MTX; RAN™-Fentanyl Matrix Patch; RAN™-Fentanyl Transdermal System; ratio-Fentanyl

Therapeutic Category Analgesic, Narcotic; General Anesthetic

Controlled Substance C-II

Use

Injection: Relief of pain, preoperative medication, adjunct to general or regional anesthesia

Transdermal patch (eg, Duragesic®): Management of persistent moderate-to-severe chronic pain in opioid-tolerant patients when around-the clock analgesia is needed for an extended period of time

Transmucosal lozenge (eg, Actiq®), buccal tablet (Fentora®), buccal film (Onsolis®), nasal spray (Lazanda®), sublingual tablet (Abstral®), sublingual spray (Subsys®): Management of breakthrough cancer pain in opioid-tolerant patients

Note: "Opioid-tolerant" patients are defined as patients who are taking at least:

Oral morphine 60 mg/day, **or**

Transdermal fentanyl 25 mcg/hour, **or**

Oral oxycodone 30 mg/day, **or**

Oral hydromorphone 8 mg/day, **or**

Oral oxymorphone 25 mg/day, **or**

Equianalgesic dose of another opioid for at least 1 week

General Dosage Range

I.M.: *Adults:* 50-100 mcg/dose as a single dose

I.V.:

Children 2-12 years: 2-3 mcg/kg/dose every 1-2 hours

Children >12 years and Adults: 25-100 mcg as a single dose

Nasal: *Adults:* Initial 100 mcg; Maintenance dose range: 100-800 mcg; maximum single dose: 800 mcg; maximum frequency: 4 administrations/day

Transmucosal:

Buccal film (Onsolis™): *Adults:* Initial: 200 mcg; Maintenance dose range: 200-1200 mcg; maximum dose: 1200 mcg film; maximum frequency: 4 applications/day

Buccal tablet (Fentora®): *Adults:* Initial: 100 mcg; may repeat (maximum: 2 doses per breakthrough pain episode every 4 hours)

Lozenge (Actiq®): *Children ≥16 years and Adults:* Initial: 200 mcg; may repeat (maximum: 2 doses per breakthrough pain episode every 4 hours; maximum daily dose: 4 units/day)

Sublingual spray (Subsys®): Adults: Initial: 100 mcg; may repeat (maximum: 2 doses per breakthrough pain every 4 hours); maintenance dose range: 100-1600 mcg per breakthrough pain episode; maximum 4 breakthrough doses/day

Sublingual tablet (Abstral®): *Adults:* Initial: 100 mcg; may repeat (maximum: 2 doses per breakthrough pain episode every 2 hours); usual maximum: 800 mcg/dose

Transdermal: *Children ≥2 years and Adults:* 12.5-300 mcg/hour applied every 72 hours

Dosage Forms

Film, for buccal application:

Onsolis®: 200 mcg (30s); 400 mcg (30s); 600 mcg (30s); 800 mcg (30s); 1200 mcg (30s)

Injection, solution [preservative free]: 0.05 mg/mL (2 mL, 5 mL, 10 mL, 20 mL, 30 mL, 50 mL)

Liquid, sublingual, [spray]:

Subsys®: 100 mcg (30s); 200 mcg (30s); 400 mcg (30s); 600 mcg (30s); 800 mcg (30s)

Lozenge, oral: 200 mcg (30s); 400 mcg (30s); 600 mcg (30s); 800 mcg (30s); 1200 mcg (30s); 1600 mcg (30s)

Actiq®: 200 mcg (30s); 400 mcg (30s); 600 mcg (30s); 800 mcg (30s); 1200 mcg (30s); 1600 mcg (30s)

Patch, transdermal: 12 [delivers 12.5 mcg/hr] (5s); 25 [delivers 25 mcg/hr] (5s); 50 [delivers 50 mcg/hr] (5s); 75 [delivers 75 mcg/hr] (5s); 100 [delivers 100 mcg/hr] (5s)

Duragesic®: 12 [delivers 12.5 mcg/hr] (5s); 25 [delivers 25 mcg/hr] (5s); 50 [delivers 50 mcg/hr] (5s); 75 [delivers 75 mcg/hr] (5s); 100 [delivers 100 mcg/hr] (5s)

Powder, for prescription compounding: USP: 100% (1 g)

Solution, intranasal, as citrate [spray]:

Lazanda®: 100 mcg/spray (5 mL); 400 mcg/spray (5 mL) [delivers 8 metered sprays]

Tablet, for buccal application:

Fentora®: 100 mcg (28s); 200 mcg (28s); 400 mcg (28s); 600 mcg (28s); 800 mcg (28s)

Tablet, sublingual:

Abstral®: 100 mcg (12s, 32s); 200 mcg (12s, 32s); 300 mcg (12s, 32s); 400 mcg (12s, 32s); 600 mcg (32s); 800 mcg (32s)

Dosage Forms - Canada

Patch, transdermal, as base: 12 mcg/hr (5s); 25 mcg/hr (5s); 50 mcg/hr (5s); 75 mcg/hr (5s); 100 mcg/hr (5s)

Duragesic® MAT: 12 mcg/hr (5s); 25 mcg/hr (5s); 50 mcg/hr (5s); 75 mcg/hr (5s); 100 mcg/hr (5s)

fentanyl citrate *see* fentanyl *on page* 377
Fentanyl Citrate Injection, USP (Can) *see* fentanyl *on page* 377
fentanyl hydrochloride *see* fentanyl *on page* 377
fentanyl patch *see* fentanyl *on page* 377
Fentora® *see* fentanyl *on page* 377
Feosol® [OTC] *see* ferrous sulfate *on page* 380
Feraheme® *see* ferumoxytol *on page* 381
Ferate [OTC] *see* ferrous gluconate *on page* 380
Fergon® [OTC] *see* ferrous gluconate *on page* 380
Fer-In-Sol® [OTC] *see* ferrous sulfate *on page* 380
Fer-In-Sol® (Can) *see* ferrous sulfate *on page* 380
Fer-iron [OTC] *see* ferrous sulfate *on page* 380
Fermalac (Can) *see* Lactobacillus *on page* 518
Ferodan™ (Can) *see* ferrous sulfate *on page* 380

Ferretts® [OTC] *see* ferrous fumarate *on page* 379
Ferrex™ 150 [OTC] *see* polysaccharide-iron complex *on page* 740
Ferrex™ 150 Forte *see* polysaccharide-iron complex, vitamin B12, and folic acid *on page* 741
Ferrex™ 150 Forte Plus *see* polysaccharide-iron complex, vitamin B12, and folic acid *on page* 741
Ferrex™ 150 Plus [OTC] *see* polysaccharide-iron complex *on page* 740
ferric (III) hexacyanoferrate (II) *see* ferric hexacyanoferrate *on page* 379

ferric gluconate (FER ik GLOO koe nate)

Medication Safety Issues

Sound-alike/look-alike issues:

Ferric gluconate may be confused with ferumoxytol

Synonyms sodium ferric gluconate

U.S. Brand Names Ferrlecit®; Nulecit™ [DSC]

Canadian Brand Names Ferrlecit®

Therapeutic Category Iron Salt

Use Treatment of iron-deficiency anemia in patients undergoing hemodialysis in conjunction with erythropoietin therapy

General Dosage Range I.V.:

Children ≥6 years: 1.5 mg/kg of elemental iron per dialysis session (maximum: 125 mg/dose)

Adults: 125 mg of elemental iron per dialysis session

Dosage Forms

Injection, solution: Elemental iron 12.5 mg/mL (5 mL)

Ferrlecit®: Elemental iron 12.5 mg/mL (5 mL)

ferric hexacyanoferrate (FER ik hex a SYE an oh fer ate)

Synonyms ferric (III) hexacyanoferrate (II); insoluble prussian blue; prussian blue

U.S. Brand Names Radiogardase®

Therapeutic Category Antidote

Use Treatment of known or suspected internal contamination with radioactive cesium and/or radioactive or nonradioactive thallium

General Dosage Range Oral:

Children 2-12 years: 1 g 3 times/day

Children >12 years and Adults: 1-3 g 3 times/day

Dosage Forms

Capsule, oral:

Radiogardase®: 0.5 g

ferric subsulfate (FER ik sub SULL fate)

Synonyms monsel's solution

U.S. Brand Names AstrinGyn®

Therapeutic Category Hemostatic Agent

Use Hemostatic in minor surgical procedures

General Dosage Range Topical: *Adults:* Apply evenly to wound.

Dosage Forms

Solution, topical: (8 mL, 59 mL)

AstrinGyn®: (8 g)

Ferriprox® *see* deferiprone *on page* 258
Ferrlecit® *see* ferric gluconate *on page* 379
Ferrocite™ [OTC] *see* ferrous fumarate *on page* 379
Ferro-Sequels® [OTC] *see* ferrous fumarate *on page* 379

ferrous fumarate (FER us FYOO ma rate)

Synonyms iron fumarate

U.S. Brand Names Femiron® [OTC]; Ferretts® [OTC]; Ferro-Sequels® [OTC]; Ferrocite™ [OTC]; Hemocyte® [OTC]; Ircon® [OTC]

Canadian Brand Names Palafer®

Therapeutic Category Electrolyte Supplement, Oral

Use Prevention and treatment of iron-deficiency anemias

General Dosage Range Oral:

Children: 1-6 mg elemental iron/kg/day in 1-3 divided doses

Adults: 60 mg elemental iron 2-4 times/day

Dosage Forms

Tablet, oral: 324 mg

Femiron® [OTC]: 63 mg

Ferretts® [OTC]: 325 mg

Ferrocite™ [OTC]: 324 mg

Hemocyte® [OTC]: 324 mg

Ircon® [OTC]: 200 mg

Tablet, timed release, oral:

Ferro-Sequels® [OTC]: 150 mg

ferrous gluconate (FER us GLOO koe nate)

Synonyms iron gluconate

U.S. Brand Names Ferate [OTC]; Fergon® [OTC]

Canadian Brand Names Apo-Ferrous Gluconate®; Novo-Ferrogluc

Therapeutic Category Electrolyte Supplement, Oral

Use Prevention and treatment of iron-deficiency anemias

General Dosage Range Oral:

Children: 1-6 mg Fe/kg/day in 1-3 divided doses

Adults: 60 mg 1-4 times/day

Dosage Forms

Tablet, oral: 246 mg, 324 mg, 325 mg

Ferate [OTC]: 240 mg

Fergon® [OTC]: 240 mg

ferrous sulfate (FER us SUL fate)

Medication Safety Issues

Sound-alike/look-alike issues:

Feosol® may be confused with Fer-In-Sol®

Fer-In-Sol® may be confused with Feosol®

Slow FE® may be confused with Slow-K®

Administration issues:

Fer-In-Sol® (manufactured by Mead Johnson) and a limited number of generic products are available at a concentration of 15 mg/mL. However, many other generics and brand name products of ferrous sulfate oral liquid drops are available at a concentration of 15 mg/0.6 mL. Check concentration closely prior to dispensing. Prescriptions written in milliliters (mL) should be clarified.

Synonyms $FeSO_4$; iron sulfate

U.S. Brand Names Feosol® [OTC]; Fer-In-Sol® [OTC]; Fer-iron [OTC]; MyKidz Iron 10™ [OTC]; Slow FE® [OTC]; Slow Release [OTC]

Canadian Brand Names Apo-Ferrous Sulfate®; Fer-In-Sol®; Ferodan™

Therapeutic Category Electrolyte Supplement, Oral

Use Prevention and treatment of iron-deficiency anemias

General Dosage Range Oral:

Extended release: *Adults:* 250 mg 1-2 times/day

Immediate release:

Children: 1-6 mg Fe/kg/day in 1-3 divided doses (maximum: 15 mg/day [prophylaxis dosing])

Adults: 300 mg 1-4 times/day

Dosage Forms

Elixir, oral: 220 mg/5 mL (473 mL, 480 mL)

Liquid, oral: 300 mg/5 mL (5 mL); 75 mg/mL (50 mL)

Fer-In-Sol® [OTC]: 75 mg/mL (50 mL)

Fer-iron [OTC]: 75 mg/mL (50 mL)

Suspension, oral:

MyKidz Iron 10™ [OTC]: 75 mg/1.5 mL (118 mL)

Tablet, oral: 324 mg, 325 mg
Feosol® [OTC]: 200 mg
Tablet, enteric coated, oral: 324 mg, 325 mg
Tablet, extended release, oral: 140 mg
Tablet, slow release, oral: 160 mg
Slow FE® [OTC]: 142 mg
Slow Release [OTC]: 140 mg

Fertinorm® H.P. (Can) *see* urofollitropin *on page* 931

ferumoxytol (fer ue MOX i tol)

Medication Safety Issues
Sound-alike/look-alike issues:
Ferumoxytol may be confused with ferric gluconate, iron dextran complex, iron sucrose
U.S. Brand Names Feraheme®
Canadian Brand Names Feraheme®
Therapeutic Category Iron Salt
Use Treatment of iron-deficiency anemia in chronic kidney disease
General Dosage Range I.V.: *Adults:* 510 mg (17 mL) as a single dose; repeat once 3-8 days later
Dosage Forms
Injection, solution:
Feraheme®: Elemental iron 30 mg/mL (17 mL)

FESO *see* fesoterodine *on page* 381
$FeSO_4$ *see* ferrous sulfate *on page* 380

fesoterodine (fes oh TER oh deen)

Medication Safety Issues
Sound-alike/look-alike issues:
Fesoterodine may be confused with fexofenadine, tolterodine
BEERS Criteria medication:
This drug may be potentially inappropriate for use in geriatric patients (Quality of evidence - varies based on comorbidity; Strength of recommendation - varies based on comorbidity)
Synonyms FESO; fesoterodine fumarate
U.S. Brand Names Toviaz®
Therapeutic Category Anticholinergic Agent
Use Treatment of patients with an overactive bladder with symptoms of urinary frequency, urgency, or urge incontinence.
General Dosage Range Dosage adjustment recommended in patients with renal impairment or on concomitant therapy
Oral: *Adults:* 4-8 mg once daily
Dosage Forms
Tablet, extended release, oral:
Toviaz®: 4 mg, 8 mg

fesoterodine fumarate *see* fesoterodine *on page* 381
Feverall® [OTC] *see* acetaminophen *on page* 20
Fexmid® *see* cyclobenzaprine *on page* 243

fexofenadine (feks oh FEN a deen)

Medication Safety Issues
Sound-alike/look-alike issues:
Fexofenadine may be confused with fesoterodine
Allegra® may be confused with Viagra®
International issues:
Allegra [U.S, Canada, and multiple international markets] may be confused with Allegro brand name for fluticasone [Israel] and frovatriptan [Germany]
Synonyms fexofenadine hydrochloride
U.S. Brand Names Allegra®; Allegra® Allergy 12 Hour [OTC]; Allegra® Allergy 24 Hour [OTC]; Allegra® Children's Allergy ODT [OTC]; Allegra® Children's Allergy [OTC]

Canadian Brand Names Allegra®

Therapeutic Category Antihistamine

Use Relief of symptoms associated with seasonal allergic rhinitis; treatment of chronic idiopathic urticaria
OTC labeling: Relief of symptoms associated with allergic rhinitis

General Dosage Range Dosage adjustment recommended in patients with renal impairment

Oral:
Children 6 months to <2 years: 15 mg twice daily
Children 2-11 years: 30 mg twice daily
Children ≥12 years and Adults: 60 mg twice daily **or** 180 mg once daily

Dosage Forms

Suspension, oral:
Allegra®: 6 mg/mL (300 mL)
Allegra® Children's Allergy [OTC]: 6 mg/mL (120 mL)

Tablet, oral: 30 mg, 60 mg, 180 mg
Allegra® Allergy 12 Hour [OTC]: 60 mg
Allegra® Allergy 24 Hour [OTC]: 180 mg
Allegra® Children's Allergy [OTC]: 30 mg

Tablet, orally disintegrating, oral:
Allegra® Children's Allergy ODT [OTC]: 30 mg

fexofenadine and pseudoephedrine (feks oh FEN a deen & soo doe e FED rin)

Medication Safety Issues

Sound-alike/look-alike issues:
Allegra-D® may be confused with Viagra®

International issues:
Allegra-D [U.S, Canada, and multiple international markets] may be confused with Allegro brand name for fluticasone [Israel] and frovatriptan [Germany]

Synonyms pseudoephedrine and fexofenadine

U.S. Brand Names Allegra-D® 12 Hour; Allegra-D® 24 Hour

Canadian Brand Names Allegra-D®

Therapeutic Category Antihistamine/Decongestant Combination

Use Relief of symptoms associated with seasonal allergic rhinitis in adults and children ≥12 years of age

General Dosage Range Dosage adjustment recommended in patients with renal impairment

Oral: *Children ≥12 years and Adults:* 1 tablet (fexofenadine 60 mg/pseudoephedrine 120 mg) twice daily **or** 1 tablet (fexofenadine 180 mg/pseudoephedrine 240 mg) once daily

Dosage Forms

Tablet, extended release: Fexofenadine 60 mg [immediate release] and pseudoephedrine 120 mg [extended release]; fexofenadine 180 mg [immediate release] and pseudoephedrine 240 mg [extended release]
Allegra-D® 12 Hour: Fexofenadine 60 mg [immediate release] and pseudoephedrine 120 mg [extended release]
Allegra-D® 24 Hour: Fexofenadine 180 mg [immediate release] and pseudoephedrine 240 mg [extended release]

fexofenadine hydrochloride *see* fexofenadine *on page 381*
^{18F}fludeoxyglucose *see* fludeoxyglucose F 18 *on page 390*
Fiberall® [OTC] *see* psyllium *on page 774*
FiberCon® [OTC] *see* polycarbophil *on page 737*
Fiber-Lax [OTC] *see* polycarbophil *on page 737*
Fibertab [OTC] *see* polycarbophil *on page 737*
Fiber-Tabs™ [OTC] *see* polycarbophil *on page 737*
Fibricor® *see* fenofibric acid *on page 376*

fibrinogen concentrate (human) (fi BRIN o gin KON suhn trate HYU man)

Synonyms coagulation factor I

U.S. Brand Names RiaSTAP®

Therapeutic Category Blood Product Derivative

Use Treatment of acute bleeding episodes in patients with congenital fibrinogen deficiency (afibrinogenemia and hypofibrinogenemia)

General Dosage Range I.V.: *Children and Adults:* When baseline fibrinogen level is known: Dose (mg/kg) = [Target level (mg/dL) - measured level (mg/dL)] **divided by** 1.7 (mg/dL per mg/kg body weight) **or** when baseline fibrinogen level is not known: 70 mg/kg

Dosage Forms

Injection, powder for reconstitution:

RiaSTAP®: 900-1300 mg [contains albumin (human); exact potency labeled on vial]

fibrin sealant (FI brin SEEL ent)

Medication Safety Issues

Administration issues:

Serious and fatal air or gas embolisms have occurred during or after fibrin sealant application using air or gas pressurized spray devices, particularly when used improperly. Manufacturer directions should be followed closely to ensure safe use of spray devices.

Synonyms fibrin sealant (human); FS; FS VH S/D; Tisseel VH S/D

U.S. Brand Names Artiss; Evicel™; TachoSil®; Tisseel

Canadian Brand Names Tisseel

Therapeutic Category Hemostatic Agent

Use

Artiss: Aid in adhering autologous skin grafts in burn patients or tissue flaps during facial rhytidectomy surgery (facelift) (not indicated for hemostasis)

Evicel™: Adjunct to hemostasis in surgery when control of bleeding by conventional surgical techniques is ineffective or impractical

TachoSil®: Adjunct to hemostasis in cardiovascular surgery when control of bleeding by conventional surgical technique is ineffective or impractical

Tisseel: Adjunct to hemostasis in cardiopulmonary bypass surgery (including fully heparinized patients) and splenic injury (due to blunt or penetrating trauma to the abdomen) when the control of bleeding by conventional surgical techniques is ineffective or impractical; adjunctive sealant for closure of colostomies

General Dosage Range Topical: *Children >6 months and Adults:* Dosage varies greatly depending on product

Dosage Forms

Kit:

Artiss: Solution, topical: Fibrinogen 67-106 mg/mL and thrombin 2.5-6.5 units/mL (2 mL, 4 mL, 10 mL)

Tisseel: Powder for solution, topical: Fibrinogen 67-106 mg/mL and thrombin 400-625 units/mL (2 mL, 4 mL, 10 mL)

Tisseel: Solution, topical: Fibrinogen 67-106 mg/mL and thrombin 400-625 units/mL (2 mL, 4 mL, 10 mL)

Kit [preservative free]:

Evicel™: Solution, topical: Fibrinogen 55-85 mg/mL and thrombin 800-1200 units/mL (2 mL, 4 mL, 10 mL)

Patch, topical:

TachoSil®: Fibrinogen 3.6-7.4 mg/cm^2 and thrombin 1.3-2.7 units/cm^2 (1s, 2s)

fibrin sealant (human) *see* fibrin sealant *on page 383*

Fibro-XL [OTC] *see* psyllium *on page 774*

Fibro-Lax [OTC] *see* psyllium *on page 774*

fidaxomicin (fye DAX oh mye sin)

Synonyms difimicin; lipiarrmycin; OPT-80; PAR-101; tiacumicin B

U.S. Brand Names Dificid™

Canadian Brand Names Dificid™

Therapeutic Category Antibiotic, Macrolide

Use Treatment of *Clostridium difficile*-associated diarrhea (CDAD)

General Dosage Range No dosage adjustment recommended in patients with hepatic or renal impairment.

Oral: *Adults:* 200 mg twice daily

Dosage Forms

Tablet, oral:

Dificid™: 200 mg

filgrastim (fil GRA stim)

Medication Safety Issues

Sound-alike/look-alike issues:

Neupogen® may be confused with Epogen®, Neulasta®, Neumega®, Nutramigen®

International issues:

Neupogen [U.S., Canada, and multiple international markets] may be confused with Neupro brand name for rotigotine [multiple international markets]

Synonyms G-CSF; granulocyte colony stimulating factor

U.S. Brand Names Neupogen®

Canadian Brand Names Neupogen®

Therapeutic Category Colony-Stimulating Factor

Use

Cancer patients (nonmyeloid malignancies) receiving myelosuppressive chemotherapy to decrease the incidence of infection (febrile neutropenia) in regimens associated with a high incidence of neutropenia with fever

Acute myelogenous leukemia (AML) following induction or consolidation chemotherapy to shorten time to neutrophil recovery and reduce the duration of fever

Cancer patients (nonmyeloid malignancies) receiving bone marrow transplant to shorten the duration of neutropenia and neutropenia-related events (eg, neutropenic fever)

Peripheral stem cell transplantation to mobilize hematopoietic progenitor cells for apheresis collection

Severe chronic neutropenia (SCN; chronic administration) to reduce the incidence and duration of neutropenic complications (fever, infections, oropharyngeal ulcers) in symptomatic patients with congenital, cyclic, or idiopathic neutropenia

General Dosage Range

I.V.: *Children and Adults:* 5-10 mcg/kg/day

SubQ: *Children and Adults:* 5-10 mcg/kg/day **or** 6 mcg/kg twice daily

Product Availability

Tbo-filgrastim: FDA approved August 2012; availability anticipated November 2013.

Tbo-filgrastim is a short-acting recombinant form of G-CSF (biologically similar to Neupogen®), indicated to reduce the duration of severe neutropenia in patients with nonmyeloid malignancies.

Dosage Forms

Injection, solution [preservative free]:

Neupogen®: 300 mcg/mL (1 mL, 1.6 mL); 600 mcg/mL (0.5 mL, 0.8 mL)

Finacea® *see* azelaic acid *on page 107*

Finacea® Plus™ *see* azelaic acid *on page 107*

finasteride (fi NAS teer ide)

Medication Safety Issues

Sound-alike/look-alike issues:

Finasteride may be confused with furosemide

Proscar® may be confused with ProSom, Provera®, PROzac®

U.S. Brand Names Propecia®; Proscar®

Canadian Brand Names CO Finasteride; JAMP-Finasteride; Mylan-Finasteride; Novo-Finasteride; PMS-Finasteride; Propecia®; Proscar®; ratio-Finasteride; Sandoz-Finasteride; Teva-Finasteride

Therapeutic Category Antiandrogen

Use

Propecia®: Treatment of male pattern hair loss in **men only**. Safety and efficacy were demonstrated in men between 18-41 years of age.

Proscar®: Treatment of symptomatic benign prostatic hyperplasia (BPH); can be used in combination with an alpha-blocker, doxazosin

General Dosage Range Oral: *Adults:* 1 mg or 5 mg once daily

Dosage Forms

Tablet, oral: 5 mg

Propecia®: 1 mg

Proscar®: 5 mg

fingolimod (fin GOL i mod)

Synonyms FTY720

U.S. Brand Names Gilenya®

Canadian Brand Names Gilenya®

Therapeutic Category Sphingosine 1-Phosphate (S1P) Receptor Modulator

Use Treatment of relapsing forms of multiple sclerosis (MS) to reduce the frequency of clinical exacerbations and delay disability progression

General Dosage Range Oral: *Adults:* 0.5 mg once daily

Dosage Forms

Capsule, oral:

Gilenya®: 0.5 mg

Fioricet® *see* butalbital, acetaminophen, and caffeine *on page 153*

Fioricet® with Codeine *see* butalbital, acetaminophen, caffeine, and codeine *on page 153*

Fiorinal® *see* butalbital, aspirin, and caffeine *on page 154*

Fiorinal®-C 1/2 (Can) *see* butalbital, aspirin, caffeine, and codeine *on page 155*

Fiorinal®-C 1/4 (Can) *see* butalbital, aspirin, caffeine, and codeine *on page 155*

Fiorinal® with Codeine *see* butalbital, aspirin, caffeine, and codeine *on page 155*

Firazyr® *see* icatibant *on page 471*

Firmagon® *see* degarelix *on page 259*

First®-Lansoprazole *see* lansoprazole *on page 522*

First®-Omeprazole *see* omeprazole *on page 665*

First™-Progesterone VGS 25 *see* progesterone *on page 762*

First™-Progesterone VGS 50 *see* progesterone *on page 762*

First™-Progesterone VGS 100 *see* progesterone *on page 762*

First™-Progesterone VGS 200 *see* progesterone *on page 762*

First™-Progesterone VGS 400 *see* progesterone *on page 762*

First®-Testosterone *see* testosterone *on page 881*

First®-Testosterone MC *see* testosterone *on page 881*

fisalamine *see* mesalamine *on page 577*

fish oil *see* omega-3-acid ethyl esters *on page 665*

FK228 *see* romidepsin *on page 809*

FK506 *see* tacrolimus (systemic) *on page 865*

Flagyl® *see* metronidazole (systemic) *on page 596*

Flagyl® 375 *see* metronidazole (systemic) *on page 596*

Flagyl® ER *see* metronidazole (systemic) *on page 596*

Flagystatin® (Can) *see* metronidazole and nystatin *(Canada only) on page 597*

Flamazine® (Can) *see* silver sulfadiazine *on page 833*

Flarex® *see* fluorometholone *on page 395*

flavan *see* flavocoxid *on page 385*

flavocoxid (fla vo KOKS id)

Synonyms flavan; flavonoid

U.S. Brand Names Limbrel 250™; Limbrel 500™; Limbrel™ [DSC]

Therapeutic Category Antiinflammatory Agent

Use Clinical dietary management of the metabolic processes of osteoarthritis

General Dosage Range Oral: *Adults:* 250-500 mg every 12 hours

Dosage Forms

Capsule, oral:

Limbrel 250™: 250 mg

Limbrel 500™: 500 mg

flavonoid *see* flavocoxid *on page 385*

flavoxate (fla VOKS ate)

Medication Safety Issues

Sound-alike/look-alike issues:

FlavoxATE may be confused with fluvoxaMINE

BEERS Criteria medication:

This drug may be potentially inappropriate for use in geriatric patients (Quality of evidence - varies based on comorbidity; Strength of recommendation - varies based on comorbidity)

Synonyms flavoxate hydrochloride; Urispas

Tall-Man flavox**ATE**

Canadian Brand Names Apo-Flavoxate®; Urispas®

Therapeutic Category Antispasmodic Agent, Urinary

Use Antispasmodic to provide symptomatic relief of dysuria, nocturia, suprapubic pain, urgency, and incontinence due to detrusor instability and hyperreflexia in elderly with cystitis, urethritis, urethrocystitis, urethrotrigonitis, and prostatitis

General Dosage Range Oral: *Children >12 years and Adults:* 100-200 mg 3-4 times/day

Dosage Forms

Tablet, oral: 100 mg

flavoxate hydrochloride *see* flavoxate *on page 386*
Flebogamma® DIF *see* immune globulin *on page 477*

flecainide (fle KAY nide)

Medication Safety Issues

Sound-alike/look-alike issues:

Flecainide may be confused with fluconazole
Tambocor™ may be confused with Pamelor™, Temodar®, tamoxifen, Tamiflu®

BEERS Criteria medication:

This drug may be potentially inappropriate for use in geriatric patients (Quality of evidence - high; Strength of recommendation - strong).

Synonyms flecainide acetate

U.S. Brand Names Tambocor™

Canadian Brand Names Apo-Flecainide®; Tambocor™

Therapeutic Category Antiarrhythmic Agent, Class I-C

Use Prevention and suppression of documented life-threatening ventricular arrhythmias (eg, sustained ventricular tachycardia); controlling symptomatic, disabling supraventricular tachycardias in patients without structural heart disease in whom other agents fail

General Dosage Range Dosage adjustment recommended in patients with renal impairment

Oral:

Children: Initial: 3 mg/kg/day **or** 50-100 mg/m^2/day in 3 divided doses; Maintenance: 3-6 mg/kg/day **or** 100-150 mg/m^2/day in 3 divided doses (maximum: 11 mg/kg/day; 200 mg/m^2/day)

Adults: Initial: 50-100 mg every 12 hours; Maintenance: 100-400 mg/day in 2 divided doses (maximum: 400 mg/day)

Dosage Forms

Tablet, oral: 50 mg, 100 mg, 150 mg
Tambocor™: 50 mg, 100 mg, 150 mg

flecainide acetate *see* flecainide *on page 386*
Flector® *see* diclofenac (topical) *on page 280*
Fleet® Bisacodyl [OTC] *see* bisacodyl *on page 134*
Fleet® Enema [OTC] *see* sodium phosphates *on page 845*
Fleet Enema® (Can) *see* sodium phosphates *on page 845*
Fleet® Enema Extra® [OTC] *see* sodium phosphates *on page 845*
Fleet® Glycerin Suppositories [OTC] *see* glycerin *on page 429*
Fleet® Liquid Glycerin [OTC] *see* glycerin *on page 429*
Fleet® Pedia-Lax™ Chewable Tablet [OTC] *see* magnesium hydroxide *on page 558*
Fleet® Pedia-Lax™ Enema [OTC] *see* sodium phosphates *on page 845*
Fleet® Pedia-Lax™ Glycerin Suppositories [OTC] *see* glycerin *on page 429*
Fleet® Pedia-Lax™ Liquid Glycerin Suppositories [OTC] *see* glycerin *on page 429*

Fleet® Pedia-Lax™ Liquid Stool Softener [OTC] *see* docusate *on page 304*
Fleet® Pedia-Lax™ Quick Dissolve [OTC] *see* senna *on page 829*
Fleet® Sof-Lax® [OTC] *see* docusate *on page 304*
Fleet® Stimulant Laxative [OTC] *see* bisacodyl *on page 134*
Fletcher's® [OTC] *see* senna *on page 829*
Flexbumin 25% *see* albumin *on page 41*
Flexeril® *see* cyclobenzaprine *on page 243*
Flex-Power [OTC] *see* trolamine *on page 923*
Flintstones™ Complete [OTC] *see* vitamins (multiple/pediatric) *on page 952*
Flintstones™ Gummies [OTC] *see* vitamins (multiple/pediatric) *on page 952*
Flintstones™ Plus Bone Building Support [OTC] *see* vitamins (multiple/pediatric) *on page 952*
Flintstones™ Plus Bone Building Support Gummies [OTC] *see* vitamins (multiple/pediatric) *on page 952*
Flintstones™ Plus Immunity Support [OTC] *see* vitamins (multiple/pediatric) *on page 952*
Flintstones™ Plus Immunity Support Gummies [OTC] *see* vitamins (multiple/pediatric) *on page 952*
Flintstones™ Plus Iron [OTC] *see* vitamins (multiple/pediatric) *on page 952*
Flintstones™ Sour Gummies [OTC] *see* vitamins (multiple/pediatric) *on page 952*
floctafenina *see* floctafenine *(Canada only) on page 387*

floctafenine *(Canada only)* (flok ta FEN een)

Synonyms floctafenina; floctafeninum

Canadian Brand Names Apo-Floctafenine®

Therapeutic Category Nonsteroidal Antiinflammatory Drug (NSAID), Oral

Use Short-term management of acute, mild-to-moderate pain

General Dosage Range Dosage adjustment recommended in patients with renal impairment

Oral: *Adults:* 200-400 mg every 6-8 hours as needed (maximum: 1200 mg/day)

Product Availability Not available in U.S.

Dosage Forms - Canada

Tablet, oral:

Apo-Floctafenine®: 200 mg, 400 mg

floctafeninum *see* floctafenine *(Canada only) on page 387*
Flolan® *see* epoprostenol *on page 338*
Flomax® *see* tamsulosin *on page 868*
Flomax® CR (Can) *see* tamsulosin *on page 868*
Flonase® *see* fluticasone (nasal) *on page 400*
Flo-Pred™ *see* prednisolone (systemic) *on page 754*
Floranex™ [OTC] *see* Lactobacillus *on page 518*
Flora-Q™ [OTC] *see* Lactobacillus *on page 518*
Florastor® [OTC] *see Saccharomyces boulardii on page 815*
Florastor® Kids [OTC] *see Saccharomyces boulardii on page 815*
Florazole® ER (Can) *see* metronidazole (systemic) *on page 596*
Florbetapir 18F *see* florbetapir F18 *on page 387*
Florbetapir F-18 *see* florbetapir F18 *on page 387*

florbetapir F18 (flor BAY ta pir)

Synonyms Florbetapir 18F; Florbetapir F-18

U.S. Brand Names Amyvid™

Therapeutic Category Radiopharmaceutical

Use Radioactive agent for positron emission tomography (PET) imaging estimation of beta-amyloid neuritic plaque density in the brain of patients being evaluated for cognitive decline (eg, Alzheimer disease)

Product Availability Amyvid™: FDA approved April 2012; availability expected June 2012

Dosage Forms

Injection, solution:

Amyvid™: Florbetapir 0.1-19 mcg and F 18 500-1900 MBq (13.5-51 mCi) per 1 mL (10 mL, 30 mL, 50 mL)

Florical® [OTC] *see* calcium carbonate *on page 161*

Florinef *see* fludrocortisone *on page 390*

Florinef® (Can) *see* fludrocortisone *on page 390*

Flovent *see* fluticasone (oral inhalation) *on page 400*

Flovent® Diskus® *see* fluticasone (oral inhalation) *on page 400*

Flovent® HFA *see* fluticasone (oral inhalation) *on page 400*

Floxin Otic Singles *see* ofloxacin (otic) *on page 660*

floxuridine (floks YOOR i deen)

Medication Safety Issues

Sound-alike/look-alike issues:

Floxuridine may be confused with Fludara®, fludarabine

FUDR® may be confused with Fludara®

High alert medication:

This medication is in a class the Institute for Safe Medication Practices (ISMP) includes among its list of drug classes which have a heightened risk of causing significant patient harm when used in error.

Synonyms fluorodeoxyuridine; FUDR

Canadian Brand Names FUDR®

Therapeutic Category Antineoplastic Agent

Use Management of hepatic metastases of colorectal and gastric cancers

General Dosage Range Dosage adjustment recommended in patients with hepatic impairment

Intraarterial: *Adults:* 0.1-0.6 mg/kg/day

Dosage Forms

Injection, powder for reconstitution: 500 mg

Fluad™ (Can) *see* influenza virus vaccine (inactivated) *on page 482*

Fluanxol® (Can) *see* flupentixol *(Canada only) on page 397*

Fluanxol® Depot (Can) *see* flupentixol *(Canada only) on page 397*

Fluarix® *see* influenza virus vaccine (inactivated) *on page 482*

flubenisolone *see* betamethasone *on page 129*

Flucaine *see* proparacaine and fluorescein *on page 766*

fluconazole (floo KOE na zole)

Medication Safety Issues

Sound-alike/look-alike issues:

Fluconazole may be confused with flecainide, FLUoxetine, furosemide, itraconazole, voriconazole

Diflucan® may be confused with diclofenac, Diprivan®, disulfiram

International issues:

Canesten (oral capsules) [Great Britain] may be confused with Canesten brand name for clotrimazole (various dosage forms) [multiple international markets]; Cenestin brand name estrogens (conjugated A/synthetic) [U.S., Canada]

U.S. Brand Names Diflucan®

Canadian Brand Names Apo-Fluconazole®; CanesOral®; CO Fluconazole; Diflucan®; Dom-Fluconazole; Fluconazole Injection; Fluconazole Omega; Monicure; Mylan-Fluconazole; Novo-Fluconazole; PHL-Fluconazole; PMS-Fluconazole; PRO-Fluconazole; Riva-Fluconazole; Taro-Fluconazole; ZYM-Fluconazole

Therapeutic Category Antifungal Agent

Use Treatment of candidiasis (esophageal, oropharyngeal, peritoneal, urinary tract, vaginal); systemic candida infections (eg, candidemia, disseminated candidiasis, and pneumonia); cryptococcal meningitis; antifungal prophylaxis in allogeneic bone marrow transplant recipients

General Dosage Range Dosage adjustment recommended in patients with renal impairment

Oral, I.V.:

Children: Loading dose: 6-12 mg/kg/dose; maintenance: 3-12 mg/kg/dose once daily; duration and dosage depend on location and severity of infection

Adults: 150 mg once **or** Loading dose: 200-800 mg; maintenance: 200-800 mg once daily; duration and dosage depend on location and severity of infection

Dosage Forms

Infusion, premixed iso-osmotic dextrose solution: 200 mg (100 mL); 400 mg (200 mL)

Infusion, premixed iso-osmotic sodium chloride solution: 100 mg (50 mL); 200 mg (100 mL); 400 mg (200 mL)

Infusion, premixed iso-osmotic sodium chloride solution [preservative free]: 200 mg (100 mL); 400 mg (200 mL)

Powder for suspension, oral: 10 mg/mL (35 mL); 40 mg/mL (35 mL)

Diflucan®: 10 mg/mL (35 mL); 40 mg/mL (35 mL)

Tablet, oral: 50 mg, 100 mg, 150 mg, 200 mg

Diflucan®: 50 mg, 100 mg, 150 mg, 200 mg

Fluconazole Injection (Can) *see* fluconazole *on page* 388

Fluconazole Omega (Can) *see* fluconazole *on page* 388

flucytosine (floo SYE toe seen)

Medication Safety Issues

Sound-alike/look-alike issues:

Flucytosine may be confused with fluorouracil

Ancobon® may be confused with Oncovin

High alert medication:

The Institute for Safe Medication Practices (ISMP) includes this medication among its list of drugs which have a heightened risk of causing significant patient harm when used in error.

Synonyms 5-FC; 5-fluorocytosine; 5-flurocytosine

U.S. Brand Names Ancobon®

Canadian Brand Names Ancobon®

Therapeutic Category Antifungal Agent

Use Adjunctive treatment of systemic fungal infections (eg, septicemia, endocarditis, UTI, meningitis, or pulmonary) caused by susceptible strains of *Candida* or *Cryptococcus*

General Dosage Range Dosage adjustment recommended in patients with renal impairment

Oral: *Adults:* 50-150 mg/kg/day in divided doses every 6 hours

Dosage Forms

Capsule, oral: 250 mg, 500 mg

Ancobon®: 250 mg, 500 mg

Fludara® *see* fludarabine *on page* 389

fludarabine (floo DARE a been)

Medication Safety Issues

Sound-alike/look-alike issues:

Fludarabine may be confused with cladribine, floxuridine, Flumadine®

Fludara® may be confused with FUDR®

High alert medication:

This medication is in a class the Institute for Safe Medication Practices (ISMP) includes among its list of drug classes which have a heightened risk of causing significant patient harm when used in error.

Synonyms 2F-ara-AMP; fludarabine phosphate

U.S. Brand Names Fludara®; Oforta™ [DSC]

Canadian Brand Names Fludara®

Therapeutic Category Antineoplastic Agent

Use Treatment of progressive or refractory B-cell chronic lymphocytic leukemia (CLL)

Canadian labeling: Second-line treatment of chronic lymphocytic leukemia (CLL); second-line treatment of low-grade, refractory non-Hodgkin lymphoma (NHL)

General Dosage Range Dosage adjustment recommended in patients with renal impairment or who develop toxicities.

Oral: *Adults:* 40 mg/m^2/day for 5 days every 28 days

I.V.: *Adults:* 25 mg/m^2/day for 5 days every 28 days

Dosage Forms

Injection, powder for reconstitution: 50 mg

Fludara®: 50 mg

Injection, solution [preservative free]: 25 mg/mL (2 mL)

Dosage Forms - Canada

Tablet, oral:

Fludara®: 10 mg

fludarabine phosphate *see* fludarabine *on page 389*

fludeoxyglucose F 18 (floo de oks i GLOO kose ef AYE teen)

Medication Safety Issues

Other safety concerns:

Radiopharmaceutical: Use appropriate precaution for handling, disposal, and minimizing exposure to patients and healthcare personnel. Use under supervision of experienced personnel. Should be stored in original lead container or adequate radiation shield.

Synonyms ^{18F}fludeoxyglucose; fluorodeoxyglucose F18 injection; [^{18}F]-FDG

Therapeutic Category Radiopharmaceutical

Use Fluorinated deoxyglucose used in conjunction with positron emission tomography (PET) to detect areas in the brain with abnormal glucose metabolism linked with foci of epileptogenic seizures

fludrocortisone (floo droe KOR ti sone)

Medication Safety Issues

Sound-alike/look-alike issues:

Florinef® may be confused with Fioricet®, Fiorinal®

Synonyms 9α-fluorohydrocortisone acetate; Florinef; fludrocortisone acetate; fluohydrisone acetate; fluohydrocortisone acetate

Canadian Brand Names Florinef®

Therapeutic Category Adrenal Corticosteroid (Mineralocorticoid)

Use Partial replacement therapy for primary and secondary adrenocortical insufficiency in Addison disease; treatment of salt-losing adrenogenital syndrome

General Dosage Range Oral:

Children: 0.05-0.1 mg/day

Adults: 0.05-0.2 mg/day (range: 0.1 mg 3 times/week to 0.2 mg/day)

Dosage Forms

Tablet, oral: 0.1 mg

fludrocortisone acetate *see* fludrocortisone *on page 390*

FluLaval® *see* influenza virus vaccine (inactivated) *on page 482*

Flumadine® *see* rimantadine *on page 802*

flumazenil (FLOO may ze nil)

Medication Safety Issues

Sound-alike/look-alike issues:

Flumazenil may be confused with influenza virus vaccine

U.S. Brand Names Romazicon®

Canadian Brand Names Anexate®; Flumazenil Injection; Flumazenil Injection, USP; Romazicon®

Therapeutic Category Antidote

Use Benzodiazepine antagonist; reverses sedative effects of benzodiazepines used in conscious sedation and general anesthesia; treatment of benzodiazepine overdose

General Dosage Range I.V.:

Children: Initial: 0.01 mg/kg (maximum dose: 0.2 mg), may repeat 0.01 mg/kg (maximum dose: 0.2 mg) as needed (maximum cumulative total: 1 mg or 0.05 mg/kg, whichever is lower)

Adults: Benzodiazepine overdose: Initial: 0.2 mg, may repeat with 0.3 mg, then 0.5 mg (maximum cumulative total dose: 5 mg); Reversal of conscious sedation/general anesthesia: Initial: 0.2 mg, may repeat (maximum total dose: 1 mg)

Dosage Forms

Injection, solution: 0.1 mg/mL (5 mL, 10 mL)

Romazicon®: 0.1 mg/mL (5 mL)

Flumazenil Injection (Can) *see* flumazenil *on page 390*
Flumazenil Injection, USP (Can) *see* flumazenil *on page 390*
flumethasone and clioquinol *see* clioquinol and flumethasone *(Canada only) on page 220*
FluMist® *see* influenza virus vaccine (live/attenuated) *on page 484*

flunarizine *(Canada only)* (floo NAR i zeen)

Synonyms flunarizine hydrochloride
Canadian Brand Names Novo-Flunarizine
Therapeutic Category Calcium-Entry Blocker (Selective)
Use Prophylaxis of migraine (with and without aura)
General Dosage Range Oral: *Adults <65 years:* 10 mg once daily
Product Availability Not available in U.S.
Dosage Forms - Canada
Capsule, oral: 5 mg

flunarizine hydrochloride *see* flunarizine *(Canada only) on page 391*

flunisolide (nasal) (floo NISS oh lide)

Medication Safety Issues
Sound-alike/look-alike issues:
Flunisolide may be confused with Flumadine®, fluocinonide
Canadian Brand Names Apo-Flunisolide®; Nasalide®; Rhinalar®
Therapeutic Category Corticosteroid, Nasal
Use Seasonal or perennial rhinitis
General Dosage Range Intranasal:
Children 6-14 years: 1-2 sprays 2-3 times/day (maximum: 4 sprays/day in each nostril)
Children ≥15 years and Adults: 2 sprays twice daily (maximum: 8 sprays/day in each nostril)
Dosage Forms
Solution, intranasal: 25 mcg/actuation (25 mL); 29 mcg/actuation (25 mL)

fluocinolone (ophthalmic) (floo oh SIN oh lone)

Medication Safety Issues
Sound-alike/look-alike issues:
Fluocinolone may be confused with fluocinonide
Synonyms fluocinolone acetonide
U.S. Brand Names Retisert®
Therapeutic Category Corticosteroid, Ophthalmic
Use Treatment of chronic, noninfectious uveitis affecting the posterior segment of the eye
General Dosage Range Ocular implant: *Children ≥12 years and Adults:* One silicone-encased tablet (0.59 mg) is designed to release 0.6 mcg/day, decreasing over 30 days to a steady-state release rate of 0.3-0.4 mcg/day for 30 months
Dosage Forms
Implant, intravitreal:
Retisert®: 0.59 mg (1s)

fluocinolone (otic) (floo oh SIN oh lone)

Medication Safety Issues
Sound-alike/look-alike issues:
Fluocinolone may be confused with fluocinonide
Synonyms fluocinolone acetonide
U.S. Brand Names DermOtic®
Therapeutic Category Corticosteroid, Otic
Use Relief of chronic eczematous external otitis
General Dosage Range Otic: *Children ≥2 years and Adults:* 5 drops into affected ear twice daily
Dosage Forms
Oil, otic: 0.01% (20 mL)
DermOtic®: 0.01% (20 mL)

fluocinolone (topical) (floo oh SIN oh lone)

Medication Safety Issues

Sound-alike/look-alike issues:

Fluocinolone may be confused with fluocinonide

Synonyms fluocinolone acetonide

U.S. Brand Names Capex®; Derma-Smoothe/FS®

Canadian Brand Names Capex®; Derma-Smoothe/FS®; Synalar®

Therapeutic Category Corticosteroid, Topical

Use Relief of susceptible inflammatory dermatosis [low, medium corticosteroid]; dermatitis or psoriasis of the scalp; atopic dermatitis in adults and children ≥3 months of age

General Dosage Range Topical:

Children ≥3 months: Apply a thin layer to affected area 2-4 times/day

Adults: Body: Apply thin layer to affected area 2-4 times/day; Scalp: 1 ounce daily (Capex®) **or** massage into wet hair and leave on for at least 4 hours (Derma-Smoothe/FS®)

Dosage Forms

Cream, topical: 0.01% (15 g, 60 g); 0.025% (15 g, 60 g)

Oil, topical: 0.01% (118 mL)

Derma-Smoothe/FS®: 0.01% (120 mL)

Ointment, topical: 0.025% (15 g, 60 g)

Shampoo, topical:

Capex®: 0.01% (120 mL)

Solution, topical: 0.01% (60 mL)

fluocinolone acetonide *see* fluocinolone (ophthalmic) *on page* 391

fluocinolone acetonide *see* fluocinolone (otic) *on page* 391

fluocinolone acetonide *see* fluocinolone (topical) *on page* 392

fluocinolone, hydroquinone, and tretinoin

(floo oh SIN oh lone, HYE droe kwin one, & TRET i noyn)

Synonyms hydroquinone, fluocinolone acetonide, and tretinoin; tretinoin, fluocinolone acetonide, and hydroquinone

U.S. Brand Names Tri-Luma®

Therapeutic Category Corticosteroid, Topical; Depigmenting Agent; Retinoic Acid Derivative

Use Short-term treatment of moderate-to-severe melasma of the face

General Dosage Range Topical: *Adults:* Apply a thin film once daily to affected areas.

Dosage Forms

Cream, topical:

Tri-Luma®: Fluocinolone acetonide 0.01%, hydroquinone 4%, and tretinoin 0.05% (30 g)

fluocinonide (floo oh SIN oh nide)

Medication Safety Issues

Sound-alike/look-alike issues:

Fluocinonide may be confused with flunisolide, fluocinolone

Lidex® may be confused with Lasix®, Videx®

Synonyms Lidex

U.S. Brand Names Vanos®

Canadian Brand Names Lidemol®; Lidex®; Lyderm®; Tiamol®; Topactin; Topsyn®

Therapeutic Category Corticosteroid, Topical

Use Antiinflammatory, antipruritic; treatment of plaque-type psoriasis (up to 10% of body surface area) [high-potency topical corticosteroid]

General Dosage Range Topical:

Children <12 years: Apply thin layer of 0.05% cream to affected area 2-4 times/day

Children ≥12 years and Adults: Apply thin layer of 0.05% cream to affected area 2-4 times/day **or** apply a thin layer of 0.1% cream once or twice daily to affected area

Dosage Forms

Cream, topical:

Vanos®: 0.1% (30 g, 60 g, 120 g)

Cream, anhydrous, emollient, topical: 0.05% (15 g, 30 g, 60 g, 120 g)

Cream, aqueous, emollient, topical: 0.05% (15 g, 30 g, 60 g)
Gel, topical: 0.05% (15 g, 30 g, 60 g)
Ointment, topical: 0.05% (15 g, 30 g, 60 g)
Solution, topical: 0.05% (20 mL, 60 mL)

fluohydrisone acetate *see* fludrocortisone *on page 390*
fluohydrocortisone acetate *see* fludrocortisone *on page 390*
Fluorabon™ *see* fluoride *on page 393*
Fluor-A-Day® *see* fluoride *on page 393*
Fluor-A-Day (Can) *see* fluoride *on page 393*

fluorescein (FLURE e seen)

Synonyms fluorescein sodium; sodium fluorescein; soluble fluorescein

U.S. Brand Names AK-Fluor®; BioGlo™; Fluorescite®; Fluorets®; Ful-Glo®

Canadian Brand Names Fluorescite®

Therapeutic Category Diagnostic Agent

Use

Injection: Diagnostic aid in ophthalmic angiography and angioscopy
Topical: To stain the anterior segment of the eye for procedures (such as fitting contact lenses), disclosing corneal injury, and in applanation tonometry

General Dosage Range Dosage adjustment recommended in patients with renal impairment

I.V.:
Children: 3.5 mg/lb (7.7 mg/kg) as a single dose
Adults: 500-750 mg as a single dose

Ophthalmic: *Children and Adults:* Apply moistened strip until desired amount of staining obtained

Dosage Forms

Injection, solution: 10% (5 mL); 25% (2 mL)
AK-Fluor®: 10% (5 mL)
Injection, solution [preservative free]:
Fluorescite®: 10% (5 mL)
Strip, ophthalmic:
BioGlo™: 1 mg (100s, 300s)
Fluorets®: 1 mg (100s)
Ful-Glo®: 0.6 mg (300s); 1 mg (100s)

fluorescein and proparacaine *see* proparacaine and fluorescein *on page 766*
fluorescein sodium *see* fluorescein *on page 393*
Fluorescite® *see* fluorescein *on page 393*
Fluorets® *see* fluorescein *on page 393*

fluoride (FLOR ide)

Medication Safety Issues

Sound-alike/look-alike issues:
Phos-Flur® may be confused with PhosLo®
International issues:
Fluorex [France] may be confused with Flarex brand name for fluorometholone [U.S., Canada, and multiple international markets] and Fluarix brand name for influenza virus vaccine (inactivated) [U.S., and multiple international markets]

Synonyms acidulated phosphate fluoride; sodium fluoride; stannous fluoride

U.S. Brand Names Act® Kids [OTC]; Act® Restoring™ [OTC]; Act® Total Care™ [OTC]; Act® [OTC]; CaviRinse™; Clinpro™ 5000; ControlRx™; ControlRx™ Multi; Denta 5000 Plus™; DentaGel™; Epiflur™; Fluor-A-Day®; Fluorabon™; Fluorinse®; Fluoritab; Flura-Drops®; Gel-Kam® Rinse; Gel-Kam® [OTC]; Just For Kids™ [OTC]; Lozi-Flur™; NeutraCare®; NeutraGard® Advanced; Omni Gel™ [OTC]; OrthoWash™; PerioMed™; Phos-Flur®; Phos-Flur® Rinse [OTC]; PreviDent®; PreviDent® 5000 Booster; PreviDent® 5000 Dry Mouth; PreviDent® 5000 Plus®; PreviDent® 5000 Sensitive; StanGard® Perio; Stop®

Canadian Brand Names Fluor-A-Day

Therapeutic Category Mineral, Oral

Use Prevention of dental caries

General Dosage Range Oral:

Cream: *Children ≥6 years and Adults:* Brush on teeth once daily

Fluorinse®, PreviDent® rinse: *Children >6 years and Adults:* Once weekly, vigorously swish 5-10 mL (Fluorinse®) or 10 mL (PreviDent®) in mouth for 1 minute, then spit

Gel or Rinse:

Children 6-12 years: 5-10 mL rinse or apply to teeth and spit daily after brushing

Adults: 10 mL rinse or apply to teeth and spit daily after brushing

Lozenge: *Adults:* 1 daily

Lozenge/oral drops/tablets:

Fluoride content of drinking water <0.3 ppm:

Children 6 months to 3 years: 0.25 mg/day

Children 3-6 years: 0.5 mg/day

Children 6-16 years: 1 mg/day

Fluoride content of drinking water 0.3-0.6 ppm:

Children 3-6 years: 0.25 mg/day

Children 6-16 years: 0.5 mg/day

Dosage Forms

Cream, oral: 1.1% (51 g)

Denta 5000 Plus™: 1.1% (51 g)

PreviDent® 5000 Plus®: 1.1% (51 g)

Gel, oral:

PreviDent® 5000 Booster: 1.1% (100 mL, 106 mL)

PreviDent® 5000 Dry Mouth: 1.1% (100 mL)

PreviDent® 5000 Sensitive: 1.1% (100 mL)

Gel, topical: 1.1% (56 g)

DentaGel™: 1.1% (56 g)

Gel-Kam® [OTC]: 0.4% (129 g)

Just For Kids™ [OTC]: 0.4% (122 g)

NeutraCare®: 1.1% (60 g)

NeutraGard® Advanced: 1.1% (60 g)

Omni Gel™ [OTC]: 0.4% (122 g); 0.4% (122 g)

Phos-Flur®: 1.1% (51 g)

PreviDent®: 1.1% (56 g)

Stop®: 0.4% (120 g)

Liquid, oral:

Fluoritab: 0.125 mg/drop

Lozenge, oral:

Lozi-Flur™: 2.21 mg (90s)

Paste, oral:

Clinpro™ 5000: 1.1% (113 g)

ControlRx™: 1.1% (57 g)

ControlRx™ Multi: 1.1% (57 g)

Solution, oral: 1.1 mg/mL (50 mL); 0.2% (473 mL); 0.63% (300 mL)

Act® [OTC]: 0.05% (532 mL)

Act® Kids [OTC]: 0.05% (500 mL, 532 mL)

Act® Restoring™ [OTC]: 0.02% (1000 mL); 0.05% (532 mL)

Act® Total Care™ [OTC]: 0.02% (1000 mL); 0.05% (88 mL, 532 mL)

CaviRinse™: 0.2% (240 mL)

Fluor-A-Day®: 0.278 mg/drop (30 mL)

Fluorabon™: 0.55 mg/0.6 mL (60 mL)

Fluorinse®: 0.2% (480 mL)

Flura-Drops®: 0.55 mg/drop (24 mL)

Gel-Kam® Rinse: 0.63% (300 mL)

OrthoWash™: 0.044% (480 mL)

PerioMed™: 0.63% (284 mL)

Phos-Flur® Rinse [OTC]: 0.044% (473 mL, 500 mL)

PreviDent®: 0.2% (473 mL)

StanGard® Perio: 0.63% (284 mL)

Tablet, chewable, oral: 0.55 mg, 1.1 mg, 2.2 mg

Epiflur™: 0.55 mg, 1.1 mg, 2.2 mg

Fluor-A-Day®: 0.55 mg, 1.1 mg, 2.2 mg

Fluoritab: 1.1 mg, 2.2 mg

Fluorinse® *see* fluoride *on page* 393
Fluoritab *see* fluoride *on page* 393
5-fluorocytosine *see* flucytosine *on page* 389
fluorodeoxyglucose F18 injection *see* fludeoxyglucose F 18 *on page* 390
fluorodeoxyuridine *see* floxuridine *on page* 388
9α-fluorohydrocortisone acetate *see* fludrocortisone *on page* 390

fluorometholone (flure oh METH oh lone)

Medication Safety Issues

International issues:

Flarex [U.S., Canada, and multiple international markets] may be confused with Fluarix brand name for influenza virus vaccine (inactivated) [U.S. and multiple international markets] and Fluorex brand name for fluoride [France]

U.S. Brand Names Flarex®; FML Forte®; FML®

Canadian Brand Names Flarex®; FML Forte®; FML®; PMS-Fluorometholone

Therapeutic Category Adrenal Corticosteroid

Use Treatment of steroid-responsive inflammatory conditions of the eye

General Dosage Range Ophthalmic:

Ointment: *Children ≥2 years, Adolescents, and Adults:* Apply small amount (~1/2" ribbon) every 4 hours (initial: 24-48 hours) **or** 1-3 times daily

Suspension:

Children ≥2 years, Adolescents, and Adults (FML®, FML® Forte): Instill 1 drop every 4 hours (initial: 24-48 hours) **or** 1 drop 2-4 times daily

Adults (Flarex®): Instill 2 drops (initial: 24-48 hours) **or** 1-2 drops 2-4 times daily

Dosage Forms

Ointment, ophthalmic:

FML®: 0.1% (3.5 g)

Suspension, ophthalmic: 0.1% (5 mL, 10 mL, 15 mL)

Flarex®: 0.1% (5 mL)

FML Forte®: 0.25% (5 mL, 10 mL)

FML®: 0.1% (5 mL, 10 mL, 15 mL)

Fluoroplex® *see* fluorouracil (topical) *on page* 396
5-fluorouracil *see* fluorouracil (systemic) *on page* 395
5-fluorouracil *see* fluorouracil (topical) *on page* 396

fluorouracil (systemic) (flure oh YOOR a sil)

Medication Safety Issues

Sound-alike/look-alike issues:

Fluorouracil may be confused with flucytosine

High alert medication:

This medication is in a class the Institute for Safe Medication Practices (ISMP) includes among its list of drugs which have a heightened risk of causing significant patient harm when used in error.

Synonyms 5-fluorouracil; 5-FU; FU

U.S. Brand Names Adrucil®

Therapeutic Category Antineoplastic Agent, Antimetabolite (Pyrimidine Analog)

Use Treatment of carcinomas of the breast, colon, rectum, pancreas, or stomach

General Dosage Range Dosage adjustment recommended in patients with hepatic or renal impairment

I.V.: *Adults:* Dosage varies greatly depending on indication

Dosage Forms

Injection, solution: 50 mg/mL (10 mL, 20 mL, 50 mL, 100 mL)

Adrucil®: 50 mg/mL (10 mL, 50 mL, 100 mL)

fluorouracil (topical) (flure oh YOOR a sil)

Medication Safety Issues

Sound-alike/look-alike issues:

Fluorouracil may be confused with flucytosine

High alert medication:

The Institute for Safe Medication Practices (ISMP) includes this medication among its list of drugs which have a heightened risk of causing significant patient harm when used in error.

Synonyms 5-fluorouracil; 5-FU; FU

U.S. Brand Names Carac®; Efudex®; Fluoroplex®

Canadian Brand Names Efudex®; Fluoroplex®

Therapeutic Category Antineoplastic Agent, Antimetabolite (Pyrimidine Analog)

Use Management of actinic or solar keratoses and superficial basal cell carcinomas

General Dosage Range **Topical:** *Adults:* Apply to lesions once (Carac™) or twice daily (Efudex®; Fluoroplex®)

Dosage Forms

Cream, topical: 5% (40 g)

Carac®: 0.5% (30 g)

Efudex®: 5% (40 g)

Fluoroplex®: 1% (30 g)

Solution, topical: 2% (10 mL); 5% (10 mL)

Efudex®: 5% (10 mL)

fluoxetine (floo OKS e teen)

Medication Safety Issues

Sound-alike/look-alike issues:

FLUoxetine may be confused with DULoxetine, famotidine, Feldene®, fluconazole, fluvastatin, fluvoxaMINE, fosinopril, furosemide, PARoxetine, thiothixene

PROzac® may be confused with Paxil®, Prelone®, PriLOSEC®, Prograf®, Proscar®, ProSom, Provera®

Sarafem® may be confused with Serophene®

BEERS Criteria medication:

This drug may be potentially inappropriate for use in geriatric patients (Quality of evidence - moderate; Strength of recommendation - strong).

International issues:

Reneuron [Spain] may be confused with Remeron brand name for mirtazapine [U.S., Canada, and multiple international markets]

Synonyms fluoxetine hydrochloride

Tall-Man **FLU**oxetine

U.S. Brand Names PROzac®; PROzac® Weekly™; Sarafem®

Canadian Brand Names Apo-Fluoxetine®; Ava-Fluoxetine; CO Fluoxetine; Dom-Fluoxetine; Fluoxetine Capsules BP; FXT 40; Gen-Fluoxetine; JAMP-Fluoxetine; Mint-Fluoxetine; Mylan-Fluoxetine; Novo-Fluoxetine; Nu-Fluoxetine; PHL-Fluoxetine; PMS-Fluoxetine; PRO-Fluoxetine; Prozac®; Q-Fluoxetine; ratio-Fluoxetine; Riva-Fluoxetine; Sandoz-Fluoxetine; Teva-Fluoxetine; ZYM-Fluoxetine

Therapeutic Category Antidepressant, Selective Serotonin Reuptake Inhibitor

Use Treatment of major depressive disorder (MDD); treatment of binge-eating and vomiting in patients with moderate-to-severe bulimia nervosa; obsessive-compulsive disorder (OCD); premenstrual dysphoric disorder (PMDD); panic disorder with or without agoraphobia; in combination with olanzapine for treatment-resistant or bipolar I depression

General Dosage Range Dosage adjustment recommended in patients with hepatic impairment

Oral:

Children 7-18 years: Initial: 10-20 mg once daily; Maintenance: 10-60 mg once daily

Adults: 10-80 mg once daily **or** 90 mg once weekly

Elderly: 10 mg/day

Dosage Forms

Capsule, oral: 10 mg, 20 mg, 40 mg

PROzac®: 10 mg, 20 mg, 40 mg

Capsule, delayed release, enteric coated pellets, oral: 90 mg

PROzac® Weekly™: 90 mg

Solution, oral: 20 mg/5 mL (5 mL, 120 mL)
Tablet, oral: 10 mg, 20 mg, 60 mg
Sarafem®: 10 mg, 15 mg, 20 mg

fluoxetine and olanzapine *see* olanzapine and fluoxetine *on page 661*
Fluoxetine Capsules BP (Can) *see* fluoxetine *on page 396*
fluoxetine hydrochloride *see* fluoxetine *on page 396*

fluoxymesterone (floo oks i MES te rone)

Medication Safety Issues
International issues:
Halotestin [Great Britain] may be confused with Haldol brand name for haloperidol [U.S. and multiple international markets]

U.S. Brand Names Androxy™

Therapeutic Category Androgen

Controlled Substance C-III

Use Replacement of endogenous testicular hormone; in females, palliative treatment of breast cancer

General Dosage Range Oral:
Adults (females): 10-40 mg/day in divided doses
Adults (males): 2.5-20 mg/day

Dosage Forms
Tablet, oral:
Androxy™: 10 mg

flupenthixol decanoate *see* flupentixol *(Canada only) on page 397*
flupenthixol dihydrochloride *see* flupentixol *(Canada only) on page 397*

flupentixol *(Canada only)* (floo pen TIKS ol)

Synonyms flupenthixol decanoate; flupenthixol dihydrochloride; flupentixol decanoate; flupentixol dihydrochloride

Canadian Brand Names Fluanxol®; Fluanxol® Depot

Therapeutic Category Antipsychotic Agent; Thioxanthene Derivative

Use Maintenance therapy of chronic schizophrenic patients whose main manifestations do **not** include excitement, agitation, or hyperactivity

General Dosage Range
I.M. (Depot): *Adults:* Initial test dose: 5-20 mg; Usual maintenance dose: 20-40 mg at 2- to 3-week intervals
Oral: *Adults:* Initial: 1 mg 3 times/day; Usual maintenance: 3-6 mg/day in divided doses

Product Availability Not available in U.S.

Dosage Forms - Canada
Injection, solution [depot]:
Fluanxol®: 20 mg/mL (1 mL); 100 mg/mL (1 mL)
Tablet, oral:
Fluanxol®: 0.5 mg, 3 mg, 5 mg

flupentixol decanoate *see* flupentixol *(Canada only) on page 397*
flupentixol dihydrochloride *see* flupentixol *(Canada only) on page 397*

fluphenazine (floo FEN a zeen)

Medication Safety Issues
Sound-alike/look-alike issues:
FluPHENAZine may be confused with fluvoxaMINE
BEERS Criteria medication:
This drug may be potentially inappropriate for use in geriatric patients (Quality of evidence - moderate; Strength of recommendation - strong).
International issues:
Prolixin [Turkey] may be confused with Prolixan brand name for azapropazone [Greece]

Synonyms fluphenazine decanoate; fluphenazine hydrochloride

Tall-Man flu**PHENAZ**ine

Canadian Brand Names Apo-Fluphenazine Decanoate®; Apo-Fluphenazine®; Modecate®; Modecate® Concentrate; PMS-Fluphenazine Decanoate

Therapeutic Category Phenothiazine Derivative

Use Management of manifestations of psychotic disorders and schizophrenia; depot formulation may offer improved outcome in individuals with psychosis who are nonadherent with oral antipsychotics

General Dosage Range

I.M. (hydrochloride): *Adults:* Initial: 1.25 mg as a single dose; Maintenance: 2.5-10 mg/day in divided doses every 6-8 hours

I.M., SubQ (Depot): *Adults:* Initial: 6.25-25 mg every 2-4 weeks (maximum: 100 mg)

Oral: *Adults:* 1-20 mg/day in divided doses every 6-8 hours (maximum: 40 mg/day)

Dosage Forms

Elixir, oral: 2.5 mg/5 mL (60 mL, 473 mL)

Injection, oil: 25 mg/mL (5 mL)

Injection, solution: 2.5 mg/mL (10 mL)

Solution, oral: 5 mg/mL (118 mL)

Tablet, oral: 1 mg, 2.5 mg, 5 mg, 10 mg

fluphenazine decanoate *see* fluphenazine *on page* 397

fluphenazine hydrochloride *see* fluphenazine *on page* 397

Flura-Drops® *see* fluoride *on page* 393

flurandrenolide (flure an DREN oh lide)

Medication Safety Issues

Sound-alike/look-alike issues:

Cordran® may be confused with Cardura®, codeine, Cordarone®

Synonyms flurandrenolone

U.S. Brand Names Cordran®; Cordran® SP

Canadian Brand Names Cordran®

Therapeutic Category Corticosteroid, Topical

Use Inflammation of corticosteroid-responsive dermatoses [medium potency topical corticosteroid]

General Dosage Range Topical:

Children: Apply 1-2 times/day

Adults: Apply 2-3 times/day

Dosage Forms

Cream, topical:

Cordran® SP: 0.05% (15 g, 30 g, 60 g)

Lotion, topical:

Cordran®: 0.05% (15 mL, 60 mL, 120 mL)

Tape, topical:

Cordran®: 4 mcg/cm^2 (24 inch, 80 inch)

flurandrenolone *see* flurandrenolide *on page* 398

flurazepam (flure AZ e pam)

Medication Safety Issues

Sound-alike/look-alike issues:

Flurazepam may be confused with temazepam

Dalmane® may be confused with Demulen®

BEERS Criteria medication:

This drug may be potentially inappropriate for use in geriatric patients (Quality of evidence - high; Strength of recommendation - strong).

Synonyms flurazepam hydrochloride

Canadian Brand Names Apo-Flurazepam®; Dalmane®; Som Pam

Therapeutic Category Benzodiazepine

Controlled Substance C-IV

Use Short-term treatment of insomnia

General Dosage Range Oral:

Children ≥15 years and Elderly: 15 mg at bedtime

Adults: 15-30 mg at bedtime

Dosage Forms

Capsule, oral: 15 mg, 30 mg

flurazepam hydrochloride *see* flurazepam *on page 398*

flurbiprofen (systemic) (flure BI proe fen)

Medication Safety Issues

Sound-alike/look-alike issues:

Flurbiprofen may be confused with fenoprofen

Ansaid® may be confused with Asacol®, Axid®

Synonyms flurbiprofen sodium

Canadian Brand Names Alti-Flurbiprofen; Ansaid®; Apo-Flurbiprofen®; Froben-SR®; Froben®; Novo-Flurprofen; Nu-Flurprofen

Therapeutic Category Nonsteroidal Antiinflammatory Drug (NSAID)

Use Treatment of rheumatoid arthritis and osteoarthritis

General Dosage Range Oral: *Adults:* 200-300 mg/day in 2-4 divided doses (maximum: 100 mg/dose; 300 mg/day)

Dosage Forms

Tablet, oral: 50 mg, 100 mg

flurbiprofen (ophthalmic) (flure BI proe fen)

Medication Safety Issues

Sound-alike/look-alike issues:

Flurbiprofen may be confused with fenoprofen

Ocufen® may be confused with Ocuflox®

International issues:

Ocufen [U.S., Canada, and multiple international markets] may be confused with Ocupres brand name for timolol [India]; Ocupress brand name for dorzolamide [Brazil]

Synonyms flurbiprofen sodium

U.S. Brand Names Ocufen®

Canadian Brand Names Ocufen®

Therapeutic Category Nonsteroidal Antiinflammatory Drug (NSAID), Ophthalmic

Use Inhibition of intraoperative miosis

General Dosage Range Ophthalmic: *Adults:* Instill 1 drop to each eye every 30 minutes (maximum: 4 doses)

Dosage Forms

Solution, ophthalmic: 0.03% (2.5 mL)

Ocufen®: 0.03% (2.5 mL)

flurbiprofen sodium *see* flurbiprofen (ophthalmic) *on page 399*

flurbiprofen sodium *see* flurbiprofen (systemic) *on page 399*

5-flurocytosine *see* flucytosine *on page 389*

flutamide (FLOO ta mide)

Medication Safety Issues

Sound-alike/look-alike issues:

Flutamide may be confused with Flumadine®, thalidomide

Eulexin® may be confused with Edecrin®, Eurax®

Synonyms 4′-nitro-3′-trifluoromethylisobutyrantide; Eulexin; Niftolid; NSC-147834; SCH 13521

Canadian Brand Names Apo-Flutamide®; Euflex®; Eulexin®; Novo-Flutamide; PMS-Flutamide; Teva-Flutamide

Therapeutic Category Antiandrogen

Use Treatment of metastatic prostatic carcinoma in combination therapy with LHRH agonist analogues

General Dosage Range Oral: *Adults:* 250 mg 3 times/day

Dosage Forms

Capsule, oral: 125 mg

fluticasone (oral inhalation) (floo TIK a sone)

Medication Safety Issues

Sound-alike/look-alike issues:

Flovent® may be confused with Flonase®

International issues:

Allegro: Brand name for fluticasone [Israel], but also the brand name for frovatriptan [Germany]

Allegro [Israel] may be confused with Allegra and Allegra-D brand names for fexofenadine and fexofenadine/pseudoephedrine, respectively, [U.S., Canada, and multiple international markets]

Flovent [U.S., Canada] may be confused with Flogen brand name for naproxen [Mexico]; Flogene brand name for piroxicam [Brazil]

Synonyms Flovent; fluticasone propionate

U.S. Brand Names Flovent® Diskus®; Flovent® HFA

Canadian Brand Names Flovent® Diskus®; Flovent® HFA

Therapeutic Category Corticosteroid, Inhalant (Oral)

Use Maintenance treatment of asthma as prophylactic therapy; also indicated for patients requiring oral corticosteroid therapy for asthma to assist in total discontinuation or reduction of total oral dose

General Dosage Range Inhalation:

Flovent® HFA:

Children 4-11 years: 88 mcg twice daily

Children ≥12 years and Adults: 88-880 mcg twice daily

Flovent® Diskus®:

Children 4-11 years: 50-100 mcg twice daily

Children ≥12 years and Adults: 100-1000 mcg twice daily

Dosage Forms

Aerosol, for oral inhalation:

Flovent® HFA: 44 mcg/inhalation (10.6 g); 110 mcg/inhalation (12 g); 220 mcg/inhalation (12 g)

Powder, for oral inhalation:

Flovent® Diskus®: 50 mcg (60s); 100 mcg (60s); 250 mcg (60s)

Dosage Forms - Canada

Aerosol, for oral inhalation:

Flovent® HFA: 50 mcg/inhalation (120 actuations); 125 mcg/inhalation (60 or 120 actuations); 250 mcg/inhalation (60 or 120 actuations)

Powder, for oral inhalation

Flovent® Diskus®: 50 mcg (60s); 100 mcg (60s); 250 mcg (60s); 500 mcg (60s)

fluticasone (nasal) (floo TIK a sone)

Medication Safety Issues

Sound-alike/look-alike issues:

Flonase® may be confused with Flovent®

International issues:

Allegro: Brand name for fluticasone [Israel], but also the brand name for frovatriptan [Germany]

Allegro [Israel] may be confused with Allegra and Allegra-D brand names for fexofenadine and fexofenadine/pseudoephedrine, respectively, [U.S., Canada, and multiple international markets]

Synonyms fluticasone furoate; fluticasone propionate

U.S. Brand Names Flonase®; Veramyst®

Canadian Brand Names Apo-Fluticasone®; Avamys®; Flonase®; ratio-Fluticasone

Therapeutic Category Corticosteroid, Nasal

Use

Flonase®: Management of seasonal and perennial allergic rhinitis and nonallergic rhinitis

Veramyst®, Avamys® [CAN]: Management of seasonal and perennial allergic rhinitis

General Dosage Range Intranasal:

Propionate (Flonase®):

Children ≥4 years: Initial: 1 spray (50 mcg/spray) per nostril once daily (100 mcg/day); Maintenance: 1-2 sprays per nostril once daily (100-200 mcg/day); (maximum: 2 sprays in each nostril [200 mcg]/day)

Adults: Initial: 2 sprays (50 mcg/spray) per nostril once daily (200 mcg/day); Maintenance: 1-2 sprays per nostril once daily (100-200 mcg/day)

Furoate (Veramyst®):

Children 2-11 years: Initial: 1 spray (27.5 mcg/spray) per nostril once daily (55 mcg/day); Maintenance 1-2 sprays per nostril once daily (55-110 mcg/day) (maximum: 2 sprays in each nostril [110 mcg]/day)

Children ≥12 years and Adults: Initial: 2 sprays (27.5 mcg/spray) per nostril once (110 mcg/day); Maintenance 1-2 sprays per nostril once daily (55-110 mcg/day) (maximum: 2 sprays in each nostril [110 mcg]/day)

Dosage Forms

Suspension, intranasal: 50 mcg/inhalation (16 g)

Flonase®: 50 mcg/inhalation (16 g)

Veramyst®: 27.5 mcg/inhalation (10 g)

Dosage Forms - Canada

Suspension, intranasal, as furoate [spray]:

Avamys®: 27.5 mcg/inhalation (4.5 g, 10 g)

fluticasone (topical) (floo TIK a sone)

Medication Safety Issues

Sound-alike/look-alike issues:

Cutivate® may be confused with Ultravate®

International issues:

Allegro: Brand name for fluticasone [Israel], but also the brand name for frovatriptan [Germany]

Allegro [Israel] may be confused with Allegra and Allegra-D brand names for fexofenadine and fexofenadine/pseudoephedrine, respectively [U.S., Canada, and multiple international markets]

Synonyms fluticasone propionate

U.S. Brand Names Cutivate®

Canadian Brand Names Cutivate™

Therapeutic Category Corticosteroid, Topical

Use Relief of inflammation and pruritus associated with corticosteroid-responsive dermatoses; atopic dermatitis

General Dosage Range Topical:

Cream: *Children ≥3 months and Adults:* Apply sparingly to affected area once or twice daily

Lotion:

Children ≥1 year: Apply sparingly to affected area once daily

Adults: Apply sparingly to affected area once or twice daily

Dosage Forms

Cream, topical: 0.05% (15 g, 30 g, 60 g)

Cutivate®: 0.05% (30 g, 60 g)

Lotion, topical: 0.05% (60 mL)

Cutivate®: 0.05% (120 mL)

Ointment, topical: 0.005% (15 g, 30 g, 60 g)

Cutivate®: 0.005% (30 g, 60 g)

fluticasone and salmeterol (floo TIK a sone & sal ME te role)

Medication Safety Issues

Sound-alike/look-alike issues:

Advair® may be confused with Adcirca®, Advicor®

Synonyms fluticasone propionate and salmeterol xinafoate; salmeterol and fluticasone

U.S. Brand Names Advair Diskus®; Advair® HFA

Canadian Brand Names Advair Diskus®; Advair®

Therapeutic Category $Beta_2$-Adrenergic Agonist, Long-Acting; Corticosteroid, Inhalant

Use Maintenance treatment of asthma; maintenance treatment of COPD

General Dosage Range Oral inhalation:

Children 4-11 years: Advair Diskus®: Fluticasone 100 mcg/salmeterol 50 mcg/inhalation: One inhalation twice daily (maximum dose)

Children ≥12 years:

Advair Diskus®: Fluticasone 100-500 mcg/salmeterol 50 mcg/inhalation: One inhalation twice daily. Maximum: Fluticasone 500 mcg/salmeterol 50 mcg/inhalation twice daily

Advair® HFA: Fluticasone 45-230 mcg/salmeterol 21 mcg/inhalation: Two inhalations twice daily

Adults:

Advair Diskus®: Initial, maximum: Fluticasone 250 mcg/salmeterol 50 mcg twice daily [COPD]; Maximum dose: Fluticasone 500 mcg/salmeterol 50 mcg/inhalation: One inhalation twice daily [Asthma]

Advair® HFA: Fluticasone 45-230 mcg/salmeterol 50 mcg/inhalation: Two inhalations twice daily

Dosage Forms

Aerosol, for oral inhalation:

Advair® HFA:

45/21: Fluticasone propionate 45 mcg and salmeterol 21 mcg (8 g, 12 g) [chlorofluorocarbon free]

115/21: Fluticasone propionate 115 mcg and salmeterol 21 mcg (8 g, 12 g) [chlorofluorocarbon free]

230/21: Fluticasone propionate 230 mcg and salmeterol 21 mcg (8 g, 12 g) [chlorofluorocarbon free]

Powder, for oral inhalation:

Advair Diskus®:

100/50: Fluticasone propionate 100 mcg and salmeterol 50 mcg (14s, 60s)

250/50: Fluticasone propionate 250 mcg and salmeterol 50 mcg (60s)

500/50: Fluticasone propionate 500 mcg and salmeterol 50 mcg (60s)

Dosage Forms - Canada

Aerosol, for oral inhalation:

Advair®: 125/25: Fluticasone propionate 125 mcg and salmeterol 25 mcg (12 g); 250/25: Fluticasone propionate 250 mcg and salmeterol 25 mcg (12 g)

fluticasone furoate *see* fluticasone (nasal) *on page 400*

fluticasone propionate *see* fluticasone (nasal) *on page 400*

fluticasone propionate *see* fluticasone (oral inhalation) *on page 400*

fluticasone propionate *see* fluticasone (topical) *on page 401*

fluticasone propionate and salmeterol xinafoate *see* fluticasone and salmeterol *on page 401*

fluticasone proprionate and azelastine hydrochloride *see* azelastine and fluticasone *on page 108*

fluvastatin (FLOO va sta tin)

Medication Safety Issues

Sound-alike/look-alike issues:

Fluvastatin may be confused with fluoxetine, nystatin, pitavastatin

U.S. Brand Names Lescol®; Lescol® XL

Canadian Brand Names Lescol®; Lescol® XL

Therapeutic Category HMG-CoA Reductase Inhibitor

Use To be used as a component of multiple risk factor intervention in patients at risk for atherosclerosis vascular disease due to hypercholesterolemia

Adjunct to dietary therapy to reduce elevated total cholesterol (total-C), LDL-C, triglyceride, and apolipoprotein B (apo-B) levels and to increase HDL-C in primary hypercholesterolemia and mixed dyslipidemia (Fredrickson types IIa and IIb); to slow the progression of coronary atherosclerosis in patients with coronary heart disease; reduce risk of coronary revascularization procedures in patients with coronary heart disease

General Dosage Range Oral:

Extended release: *Adolescents 10-16 years (females 1 year postmenarche) and Adults:* 80 mg once daily

Immediate release:

Adolescents 10-16 years (females 1 year postmenarche): Initial: 20 mg once daily; Maintenance: Up to 80 mg/day in 2 divided doses

Adults: Initial: 20-40 mg once daily; Maintenance: Up to 80 mg/day in 2 divided doses

Dosage Forms

Capsule, oral: 20 mg, 40 mg

Lescol®: 20 mg, 40 mg

Tablet, extended release, oral:

Lescol® XL: 80 mg

Fluviral® (Can) *see* influenza virus vaccine (inactivated) *on page 482*

Fluvirin® *see* influenza virus vaccine (inactivated) *on page 482*

fluvoxamine (floo VOKS a meen)

Medication Safety Issues

Sound-alike/look-alike issues:

FluvoxaMINE may be confused with flavoxATE, FLUoxetine, fluPHENAZine

Luvox may be confused with Lasix®, Levoxyl®, Lovenox®

BEERS Criteria medication:

This drug may be potentially inappropriate for use in geriatric patients (Quality of evidence - moderate; Strength of recommendation - strong).

Synonyms Luvox

Tall-Man fluvoxa**MINE**

U.S. Brand Names Luvox® CR

Canadian Brand Names Alti-Fluvoxamine; Apo-Fluvoxamine®; Luvox®; Novo-Fluvoxamine; Nu-Fluvoxamine; PMS-Fluvoxamine; Rhoxal-fluvoxamine; Riva-Fluvox; Sandoz-Fluvoxamine

Therapeutic Category Antidepressant, Selective Serotonin Reuptake Inhibitor

Use Treatment of obsessive-compulsive disorder (OCD)

General Dosage Range Dosage adjustment recommended in patients with hepatic impairment

Oral:

Children 8-11 years: Initial: 25 mg at bedtime; Maintenance: 50-200 mg/day (maximum: 200 mg/day)

Children 12-17 years: Initial: 25 mg at bedtime; Maintenance: 50-200 mg/day (maximum: 300 mg/day)

Adults: Initial: 50-100 mg at bedtime; Maintenance: 100-300 mg/day in 1-2 divided doses

Dosage Forms

Capsule, extended release, oral:

Luvox® CR: 100 mg, 150 mg

Tablet, oral: 25 mg, 50 mg, 100 mg

Fluzone® *see* influenza virus vaccine (inactivated) *on page 482*

Fluzone® High-Dose *see* influenza virus vaccine (inactivated) *on page 482*

Fluzone® Intradermal *see* influenza virus vaccine (inactivated) *on page 482*

FML® *see* fluorometholone *on page 395*

FML Forte® *see* fluorometholone *on page 395*

Focalin® *see* dexmethylphenidate *on page 269*

Focalin XR® *see* dexmethylphenidate *on page 269*

Foille® [OTC] *see* benzocaine *on page 121*

folacin *see* folic acid *on page 403*

Folacin-800 [OTC] *see* folic acid *on page 403*

folacin, vitamin B_{12}, and vitamin B_6 *see* folic acid, cyanocobalamin, and pyridoxine *on page 404*

Folastin *see* folic acid, cyanocobalamin, and pyridoxine *on page 404*

folate *see* folic acid *on page 403*

Folbee® *see* folic acid, cyanocobalamin, and pyridoxine *on page 404*

Folbic™ *see* folic acid, cyanocobalamin, and pyridoxine *on page 404*

Folcaps™ *see* folic acid, cyanocobalamin, and pyridoxine *on page 404*

Folcaps™ Care One *see* vitamins (multiple/prenatal) *on page 952*

Folgard® [OTC] *see* folic acid, cyanocobalamin, and pyridoxine *on page 404*

Folgard RX® *see* folic acid, cyanocobalamin, and pyridoxine *on page 404*

folic acid (FOE lik AS id)

Medication Safety Issues

Sound-alike/look-alike issues:

Folic acid may be confused with folinic acid

Synonyms folacin; folate; pteroylglutamic acid

U.S. Brand Names Folacin-800 [OTC]

Canadian Brand Names Apo-Folic®

Therapeutic Category Vitamin, Water Soluble

Use Treatment of megaloblastic and macrocytic anemias due to folate deficiency; dietary supplement to prevent neural tube defects

General Dosage Range

I.M., I.V., SubQ:

Infants: 0.1 mg/day

Children <4 years: Up to 0.3 mg/day

Children ≥4 years and Adults: 0.4 mg/day

Pregnant and lactating women: 0.8 mg/day (anemia)

Oral:

Infants: 0.1 mg/day

Children <4 years: Up to 0.3 mg/day

Children ≥4 years and Adults: 0.4 mg/day

Pregnant and lactating women: 0.8 mg/day (anemia) **or** 4 mg/day (prevention of neural tube defects)

Females of childbearing potential: Prevention of neural tube defects: 0.4-0.8 mg/day

Dosage Forms

Injection, solution: 5 mg/mL (10 mL)

Tablet, oral: 0.4 mg, 0.8 mg, 1 mg

Folacin-800 [OTC]: 0.8 mg

folic acid and polysaccharide-iron complex *see* polysaccharide-iron complex and folic acid *on page 740*

folic acid, cyanocobalamin, and pyridoxine

(FOE lik AS id, sye an oh koe BAL a min, & peer i DOKS een)

Synonyms cyanocobalamin, folic acid, and pyridoxine; folacin, vitamin B_{12}, and vitamin B_6; pyridoxine, folic acid, and cyanocobalamin

U.S. Brand Names FaBB; Folastin; Folbee®; Folbic™; Folcaps™; Folgard RX®; Folgard® [OTC]; Folplex 2.2; Foltabs™ 800 [OTC]; Foltx®; Homocysteine Guard [OTC]; Lev-Tov [OTC]; Tri-B® [OTC]; Tricardio B; Vita-Respa®

Therapeutic Category Vitamin

Use Nutritional supplement in end-stage renal failure, dialysis, hyperhomocysteinemia, homocystinuria, malabsorption syndromes, dietary deficiencies

General Dosage Range Oral: *Adults:* 1 tablet (folic acid 0.4-2.5 mg/cyanocobalamin 115-2000 mcg/ pyridoxine 10-25 mg) daily

Dosage Forms

Tablet: Folic acid 0.8 mg, cyanocobalamin 1000 mcg, and pyridoxine 50 mg

FaBB, Folgard RX®: Folic acid 2.2 mg, cyanocobalamin 1000 mcg, and pyridoxine 25 mg

Folbee®: Folic acid 2.5 mg, cyanocobalamin 1000 mcg, and pyridoxine 25 mg

Folastin, Folbic™, Foltx®: Folic acid 2.5 mg, cyanocobalamin 2000 mcg, and pyridoxine 25 mg

Folcaps™, Folplex 2.2: Folic acid 2.2 mg, cyanocobalamin 500 mcg, and pyridoxine 25 mg

Folgard® [OTC], Foltabs™ 800 [OTC]: Folic acid 0.8 mg, cyanocobalamin 115 mcg, and pyridoxine 10 mg

Homocysteine Guard [OTC], Tri-B® [OTC]: Folic acid 0.8 mg, cyanocobalamin 400 mcg, and pyridoxine 25 mg

Lev-Tov [OTC]: Folic acid 0.8 mg, cyanocobalamin 250 mcg, and pyridoxine 25 mg

Tricardio B: Folic acid 0.4 mg, cyanocobalamin 250 mcg, and pyridoxine 25 mg

Vita-Respa®: Folic acid 2.2 mg, cyanocobalamin 1300 mcg, and pyridoxine 25 mg

folic acid, magnesium carbonate, and calcium carbonate *see* magnesium carbonate, calcium carbonate, and folic acid *on page 557*

folinate calcium *see* leucovorin calcium *on page 527*

folinic acid (error prone synonym) *see* leucovorin calcium *on page 527*

follicle-stimulating hormone, human *see* urofollitropin *on page 931*

follicle stimulating hormone, recombinant *see* follitropin alfa *on page 404*

follicle stimulating hormone, recombinant *see* follitropin beta *on page 405*

Follistim® AQ *see* follitropin beta *on page 405*

Follistim® AQ Cartridge *see* follitropin beta *on page 405*

follitropin alfa (foe li TRO pin AL fa)

Synonyms follicle stimulating hormone, recombinant; FSH; rFSH-alpha; rhFSH-alpha

U.S. Brand Names Gonal-f®; Gonal-f® RFF; Gonal-f® RFF Pen

Canadian Brand Names Gonal-f®; Gonal-f® Pen

Therapeutic Category Ovulation Stimulator

Use

Gonal-f®: Induction of ovulation in anovulatory infertile patients in whom the cause of infertility is functional and not caused by primary ovarian failure; development of multiple follicles with Assisted Reproductive Technology (ART); induction of spermatogenesis in men with primary and secondary hypogonadotropic hypogonadism in whom the cause of infertility is not due to primary testicular failure.

Gonal-f® RFF: Induction of ovulation in oligo-anovulatory infertile patients in whom the cause of infertility is functional and not caused by primary ovarian failure; development of multiple follicles with ART

General Dosage Range SubQ:

Adults (females): Initial: 75-225 units/day; Maximum: Up to 300-450 units/day

Adults (males): Gonal-f®: Initial: 150 units 3 times/week; Maximum: Up to 300 units 3 times/week

Dosage Forms

Injection, powder for reconstitution:

Gonal-f®: 450 units, 1050 units

Gonal-f® RFF: 75 units

Injection, solution:

Gonal-f® RFF Pen: 300 units/0.5 mL (0.5 mL); 450 units/0.75 mL (0.75 mL); 900 units/1.5 mL (1.5 mL)

follitropin beta (foe li TRO pin BAY ta)

Synonyms follicle stimulating hormone, recombinant; FSH; rFSH-beta; rhFSH-beta

U.S. Brand Names Follistim® AQ; Follistim® AQ Cartridge

Canadian Brand Names Puregon®

Therapeutic Category Ovulation Stimulator

Use

Females: Induction of ovulation and pregnancy in anovulatory infertile patients in whom the cause of infertility is functional and not caused by primary ovarian failure; induction of pregnancy in normal ovulatory women undergoing Assisted Reproductive Technology (ART) (eg, *in vitro* fertilization [IVF], intracytoplasmic sperm injection [ICSI])

Males: Induction of spermatogenesis in men with primary and secondary hypogonadotropic hypogonadism in whom the cause of infertility is not due to primary testicular failure.

General Dosage Range

I.M., SubQ: *Adults (females):* Initial: 75-225 units/day; Maintenance: Up to 175-600 units/day

SubQ: *Adults (males):* 450 units/week

Dosage Forms

Injection, solution:

Follistim® AQ: 75 units/0.5 mL (0.5 mL); 150 units/0.5 mL (0.5 mL)

Follistim® AQ Cartridge: 350 units/0.42 mL (0.42 mL); 650 units/0.78 mL (0.78 mL); 975 units/1.17 mL (1.17 mL)

Folotyn® *see* pralatrexate *on page 748*
Folplex 2.2 *see* folic acid, cyanocobalamin, and pyridoxine *on page 404*
Foltabs™ 800 [OTC] *see* folic acid, cyanocobalamin, and pyridoxine *on page 404*
Foltabs™ Prenatal *see* vitamins (multiple/prenatal) *on page 952*
Foltabs™ Prenatal Plus DHA *see* vitamins (multiple/prenatal) *on page 952*
Foltrin® *see* vitamins (multiple/oral) *on page 951*
Foltx® *see* folic acid, cyanocobalamin, and pyridoxine *on page 404*

fomepizole (foe ME pi zole)

Medication Safety Issues

Sound-alike/look-alike issues:

Fomepizole may be confused with omeprazole

Synonyms 4-methylpyrazole; 4-MP

U.S. Brand Names Antizol®

Therapeutic Category Antidote

Use Treatment of methanol or ethylene glycol poisoning alone or in combination with hemodialysis

General Dosage Range Dosage adjustment recommended in patients with renal impairment

I.V.: *Adults:* Loading dose of 15 mg/kg, followed by 10 mg/kg every 12 hours for 4 doses, then 15 mg/kg every 12 hours

Dosage Forms

Injection, solution [preservative free]: 1 g/mL (1.5 mL)

Antizol®: 1 g/mL (1.5 mL)

fondaparinux (fon da PARE i nuks)

Medication Safety Issues

Sound-alike/look-alike issues:

Arixtra® may be confused with Arista® AH (hemostatic device)

High alert medication:

The Institute for Safe Medication Practices (ISMP) includes this medication among its list of drugs which have a heightened risk of causing significant patient harm when used in error.

Synonyms fondaparinux sodium

U.S. Brand Names Arixtra®

Canadian Brand Names Arixtra®

Therapeutic Category Factor Xa Inhibitor

Use Prophylaxis of deep vein thrombosis (DVT) in patients undergoing surgery for hip replacement, knee replacement, hip fracture (including extended prophylaxis following hip fracture surgery), or abdominal surgery (in patients at risk for thromboembolic complications); treatment of acute pulmonary embolism (PE); treatment of acute DVT without PE

Canadian labeling: Additional uses (not approved in U.S.): Unstable angina or non-ST segment elevation myocardial infarction (UA/NSTEMI) for the prevention of death and subsequent MI; ST segment elevation MI (STEMI) for the prevention of death and myocardial reinfarction

General Dosage Range SubQ:

Adults <50 kg: Treatment: 5 mg once daily

Adults 50-100 kg: Prophylaxis: 2.5 mg once daily; Treatment: 7.5 mg once daily

Adults >100 kg: Prophylaxis: 2.5 mg once daily; Treatment: 10 mg once daily

Dosage Forms

Injection, solution [preservative free]: 2.5 mg/0.5 mL (0.5 mL); 5 mg/0.4 mL (0.4 mL); 7.5 mg/0.6 mL (0.6 mL); 10 mg/0.8 mL (0.8 mL)

Arixtra®: 2.5 mg/0.5 mL (0.5 mL); 5 mg/0.4 mL (0.4 mL); 7.5 mg/0.6 mL (0.6 mL); 10 mg/0.8 mL (0.8 mL)

fondaparinux sodium *see* fondaparinux *on page 406*

Foradil® (Can) *see* formoterol *on page 406*

Foradil® Aerolizer® *see* formoterol *on page 406*

Forane® *see* isoflurane *on page 503*

formoterol (for MOH te rol)

Medication Safety Issues

Sound-alike/look-alike issues:

Foradil® may be confused with Toradol®

Administration issues:

Foradil® capsules for inhalation are for administration via Aerolizer™ inhaler and are **not** for oral use.

International issues:

Foradil [U.S., Canada, and multiple international markets] may be confused with Theradol brand name for tramadol [Netherlands]

Synonyms formoterol fumarate; formoterol fumarate dihydrate

U.S. Brand Names Foradil® Aerolizer®; Perforomist®

Canadian Brand Names Foradil®; Oxeze® Turbuhaler®

Therapeutic Category $Beta_2$-Adrenergic Agonist, Long-Acting

Use Maintenance treatment of asthma and prevention of bronchospasm (as concomitant therapy) in patients ≥5 years of age with reversible obstructive airway disease, including patients with symptoms of nocturnal asthma; maintenance treatment of bronchoconstriction in patients with COPD; prevention of exercise-induced bronchospasm in patients ≥5 years of age (monotherapy may be indicated in patients without persistent asthma)

Canadian labeling: Oxeze®: Also approved for acute relief of symptoms ("on demand" treatment) in patients ≥6 years of age

General Dosage Range Inhalation:

Foradil®: *Children ≥5 years and Adults:* 12 mcg capsule inhaled every 12 hours (maximum: 24 mcg/day) **or** 12 mcg capsule inhaled prior to exercise

Perforomist™: *Adults:* 20 mcg twice daily (maximum dose: 40 mcg/day)

Dosage Forms

Powder, for oral inhalation:

Foradil® Aerolizer®: 12 mcg/capsule (12s, 60s)

Solution, for nebulization:

Perforomist®: 20 mcg/2 mL (60s)

Dosage Forms - Canada

Powder for oral inhalation:

Oxeze® Turbuhaler®: 6 mcg/inhalation, 12 mcg/inhalation

formoterol and budesonide *see* budesonide and formoterol *on page 146*
formoterol and mometasone *see* mometasone and formoterol *on page 611*
formoterol and mometasone furoate *see* mometasone and formoterol *on page 611*
formoterol fumarate *see* formoterol *on page 406*
formoterol fumarate dihydrate *see* formoterol *on page 406*
formoterol fumarate dihydrate and budesonide *see* budesonide and formoterol *on page 146*
formoterol fumarate dihydrate and mometasone *see* mometasone and formoterol *on page 611*
Formula EM [OTC] *see* fructose, dextrose, and phosphoric acid *on page 411*
Formulation R™ [OTC] *see* phenylephrine (topical) *on page 717*
Formulex® (Can) *see* dicyclomine *on page 282*
5-formyl tetrahydrofolate *see* leucovorin calcium *on page 527*
Fortamet® *see* metformin *on page 579*
Fortaz® *see* ceftazidime *on page 185*
Forteo® *see* teriparatide *on page 880*
Fortesta™ *see* testosterone *on page 881*
Fortical® *see* calcitonin *on page 159*
Fosamax® *see* alendronate *on page 45*
Fosamax Plus D® *see* alendronate and cholecalciferol *on page 45*

fosamprenavir (FOS am pren a veer)

Medication Safety Issues

Sound-alike/look-alike issues:

Lexiva® may be confused with Levitra®

Synonyms fosamprenavir calcium; GW433908G

U.S. Brand Names Lexiva®

Canadian Brand Names Telzir®

Therapeutic Category Antiretroviral Agent, Protease Inhibitor

Use Treatment of HIV infections in combination with at least two other antiretroviral agents

General Dosage Range Dosage adjustment recommended in patients with hepatic impairment or on concomitant therapy

Oral:

Infants ≥4 weeks (PI-naive patients) or Infants ≥6 months (PI-experienced patients): Ritonavir-boosted regimen:

<11 kg: 45 mg/kg/dose twice daily (plus ritonavir); maximum: 700 mg/dose
11 to <15 kg: 30 mg/kg/dose twice daily (plus ritonavir); maximum: 700 mg/dose
15 to <20 kg: 23 mg/kg/dose twice daily (plus ritonavir); maximum: 700 mg/dose
≥20 kg: 18 mg/kg/dose twice daily (plus ritonavir); maximum: 700 mg/dose

Children ≥2 years (PI-naive patients): Unboosted regimen:

<47 kg: 30 mg/kg/dose twice daily; maximum: 1400 mg/dose
≥47 kg: 1400 mg twice daily

Adults:

Ritonavir-boosted regimen: 700 mg twice daily **or** 1400 mg once daily
Unboosted regimen: 1400 mg twice daily

Dosage Forms

Suspension, oral:

Lexiva®: 50 mg/mL (225 mL)

Tablet, oral:

Lexiva®: 700 mg

Dosage Forms - Canada

Tablet:

Telzir®: 700 mg

Suspension, oral:

Telzir®: 50 mg/mL

fosamprenavir calcium *see* fosamprenavir *on page 407*

fosaprepitant (fos a PRE pi tant)

Medication Safety Issues

Sound-alike/look-alike issues:

Fosaprepitant may be confused with aprepitant, fosamprenavir, fospropofol

Emend® for Injection (fosaprepitant) may be confused with Emend® (aprepitant) which is an oral capsule formulation.

Synonyms aprepitant injection; fosaprepitant dimeglumine; L-758,298; MK 0517

U.S. Brand Names Emend® for Injection

Canadian Brand Names Emend® IV

Therapeutic Category Antiemetic; Substance P/Neurokinin 1 Receptor Antagonist

Use Prevention of acute and delayed nausea and vomiting associated with moderately- and highly-emetogenic chemotherapy (in combination with other antiemetics)

General Dosage Range I.V.: *Adults:* 115 or 150 mg as a single dose

Dosage Forms

Injection, powder for reconstitution:

Emend® for Injection: 150 mg

fosaprepitant dimeglumine *see* fosaprepitant *on page 408*

Fosavance (Can) *see* alendronate and cholecalciferol *on page 45*

foscarnet (fos KAR net)

Synonyms PFA; phosphonoformate; phosphonoformic acid

U.S. Brand Names Foscavir®

Canadian Brand Names Foscavir®

Therapeutic Category Antiviral Agent

Use Treatment of acyclovir-resistant mucocutaneous herpes simplex virus (HSV) infections in immunocompromised persons (eg, with advanced AIDS); treatment of CMV retinitis in persons with HIV

General Dosage Range Dosage adjustment recommended in patients with renal impairment

I.V.: *Children >12 years and Adults:* Induction: CMV: 180 mg/kg/day in 2-3 evenly divided doses; HSV: 40 mg/kg/dose every 8-12 hours; Maintenance: CMV: 90-120 mg/kg once daily

Dosage Forms

Injection, solution [preservative free]: 24 mg/mL (250 mL, 500 mL)

Foscavir®: 24 mg/mL (250 mL)

Foscavir® *see* foscarnet *on page 408*

fosfomycin (fos foe MYE sin)

Medication Safety Issues

Sound-alike/look-alike issues:

Monurol® may be confused with Monopril®

Synonyms fosfomycin tromethamine

U.S. Brand Names Monurol®

Canadian Brand Names Monurol®

Therapeutic Category Antibiotic, Miscellaneous

Use Single oral dose in the treatment of uncomplicated urinary tract infections in women due to susceptible strains of *E. coli* and *Enterococcus faecalis*

General Dosage Range Oral: *Adults (females):* 3 g once

Dosage Forms

Powder for solution, oral:

Monurol®: 3 g/sachet (3s)

fosfomycin tromethamine *see* fosfomycin *on page 408*

fosinopril (foe SIN oh pril)

Medication Safety Issues

Sound-alike/look-alike issues:

Fosinopril may be confused with FLUoxetine, Fosamax®, furosemide, lisinopril

Monopril may be confused with Accupril®, minoxidil, moexipril, Monoket®, Monurol®, ramipril

Synonyms fosinopril sodium; Monopril

Canadian Brand Names Apo-Fosinopril®; Jamp-Fosinopril; Monopril®; Mylan-Fosinopril; PMS-Fosinopril; RAN™-Fosinopril; Riva-Fosinopril; Teva-Fosinopril

Therapeutic Category Angiotensin-Converting Enzyme (ACE) Inhibitor

Use Treatment of hypertension, either alone or in combination with other antihypertensive agents; treatment of heart failure (HF)

General Dosage Range Oral:

Children ≥6 years and >50 kg: Initial: 5-10 mg once daily (maximum: 40 mg/day)

Adults: Initial: 10 mg once daily; Maintenance: 10-40 mg/day in 1-2 divided doses (maximum: 80 mg/day)

Dosage Forms

Tablet, oral: 10 mg, 20 mg, 40 mg

fosinopril and hydrochlorothiazide (foe SIN oh pril & hye droe klor oh THYE a zide)

Medication Safety Issues

Sound-alike/look-alike issues:

Monopril® may be confused with Accupril®, minoxidil, moexipril, Monoket®, Monurol®, ramipril

Synonyms hydrochlorothiazide and fosinopril

U.S. Brand Names Monopril-HCT® [DSC]

Canadian Brand Names Monopril-HCT®

Therapeutic Category Angiotensin-Converting Enzyme (ACE) Inhibitor

Use Treatment of hypertension; not indicated for first-line treatment

General Dosage Range Oral: *Adults:* Fosinopril 10-80 mg and hydrochlorothiazide 12.5-50 mg once daily

Dosage Forms

Tablet:10/12.5: Fosinopril 10 mg and hydrochlorothiazide 12.5 mg; 20/12.5: Fosinopril 20 mg and hydrochlorothiazide 12.5 mg

fosinopril sodium *see* fosinopril *on page 409*

fosphenytoin (FOS fen i toyn)

Medication Safety Issues

Sound-alike/look-alike issues:

Cerebyx may be confused with CeleBREX®, CeleXA®, Cerezyme®, Cervarix®

Fosphenytoin may be confused with fospropofol

Administration issues:

Overdoses have occurred due to confusion between the **mg per mL concentration** of fosphenytoin (50 mg PE/mL) and **total drug content per vial** (either 100 mg PE/2 mL vial or 500 mg PE/10 mL vial). ISMP recommends that the total drug content per container is identified instead of the concentration in mg per mL to avoid confusion and potential overdosages. Additionally, since most errors have occurred with overdoses in children, they recommend that pediatric hospitals should consider stocking only the 2 mL vial.

Synonyms fosphenytoin sodium

Canadian Brand Names Cerebyx®

Therapeutic Category Hydantoin

Use Used for the control of generalized convulsive status epilepticus and prevention and treatment of seizures occurring during neurosurgery; indicated for short-term parenteral administration when other means of phenytoin administration are unavailable, inappropriate, or deemed less advantageous (the safety and effectiveness of fosphenytoin use for more than 5 days has not been systematically evaluated)

General Dosage Range

I.M.: *Adults:* Loading: 15-20 mg PE/kg; Maintenance: 4-6 mg PE/kg/day

I.V.: *Adults:* Loading: 10-20 mg PE/kg; Maintenance: 4-6 mg PE/kg/day

Dosage Forms

Injection, solution: 75 mg/mL (2 mL, 10 mL)

fosphenytoin sodium *see* fosphenytoin *on page* 409

fospropofol (fos PROE po fole)

Medication Safety Issues

Sound-alike/look-alike issues:

Fospropofol may be confused with fosaprepitant, fosphenytoin, propofol

High alert medication:

The Institute for Safe Medication Practices (ISMP) includes this medication among its list of drugs which have a heightened risk of causing significant patient harm when used in error.

Administration issues:

Onset of action: The onset of action will be delayed due to need for conversion to the active metabolite, propofol. If supplemental doses are administered before full effect occurs, the risk of dose-stacking may be elevated resulting in deeper sedation than intended.

Synonyms aquavan; fospropofol disodium; GPI 15715

U.S. Brand Names Lusedra™

Therapeutic Category Sedative

Controlled Substance C-IV

Use Monitored anesthesia care (MAC) sedation in patients undergoing diagnostic or therapeutic procedures

General Dosage Range I.V.:

Adults <65 years or with mild systemic disease (ASA-PS1 or -PS2): Initial: 6.5 mg/kg (maximum initial dose: 577.5 mg or 16.5 mL); Supplemental: 1.6 mg/kg (maximum supplemental dose: 140 mg or 4 mL) no more frequently than every 4 minutes as needed

Elderly ≥65 years or patients with severe systemic disease (ASA-PS3 or -PS4): Initial: 4.9 mg/kg (maximum initial dose: 437.5 mg or 12.5 mL); Supplemental 1.2 mg/kg (maximum supplemental dose: 105 mg or 3 mL) no more frequently than every 4 minutes as needed

Dosage Forms

Injection, solution [preservative free]:

Lusedra™: 35 mg/mL (30 mL)

fospropofol disodium *see* fospropofol *on page* 410

Fosrenol® *see* lanthanum *on page* 523

FR901228 *see* romidepsin *on page* 809

Fragmin® *see* dalteparin *on page* 252

Fraxiparine™ (Can) *see* nadroparin *(Canada only) on page* 624

Fraxiparine™ Forte (Can) *see* nadroparin *(Canada only) on page* 624

FreAmine® III *see* amino acid injection *on page* 61

FreAmine® HBC *see* amino acid injection *on page* 61

Freedavite [OTC] *see* vitamins (multiple/oral) *on page* 951

Freezone® [OTC] *see* salicylic acid *on page* 816

Frisium® (Can) *see* clobazam *on page* 220

Froben® (Can) *see* flurbiprofen (systemic) *on page* 399

Froben-SR® (Can) *see* flurbiprofen (systemic) *on page* 399

Frova® *see* frovatriptan *on page* 410

frovatriptan (froe va TRIP tan)

Medication Safety Issues

International issues:

Allegro: Brand name for frovatriptan [Germany], but also the brand name for fluticasone [Israel]

Allegro [Germany] may be confused with Allegra and Allegra-D brand names for fexofenadine and fexofenadine/pseudoehedrine, respectively, in the [U.S., Canada, and multiple international markets]

Synonyms frovatriptan succinate

U.S. Brand Names Frova®

Canadian Brand Names Frova®

Therapeutic Category Antimigraine Agent; Serotonin 5-$HT_{1B,\ 1D}$ Receptor Agonist

Use Acute treatment of migraine with or without aura

General Dosage Range Oral: *Adults:* 2.5 mg as a single dose, may repeat after 2 hours (maximum: 7.5 mg/day)

Dosage Forms

Tablet, oral:

Frova®: 2.5 mg

frovatriptan succinate *see* frovatriptan *on page* 410

fructose, dextrose, and phosphoric acid (FRUK tose, DEKS trose, & foss FOR ik AS id)

Synonyms dextrose, levulose and phosphoric acid; levulose, dextrose and phosphoric acid; phosphorated carbohydrate solution; phosphoric acid, levulose and dextrose

U.S. Brand Names Emetrol® [OTC]; Formula EM [OTC]; Kalmz [OTC]; Nausea Relief [OTC]; Nausetrol® [OTC]

Therapeutic Category Antiemetic

Use Relief of nausea associated with upset stomach that occurs with intestinal or stomach flu, and food indiscretions

General Dosage Range Oral:

Children ≥2-12 years: 5-10 mL every 15 minutes as needed; do not take for more than 1 hour (5 doses)

Children ≥12 years and Adults: 15-30 mL every 15 minutes as needed; do not take for more than 1 hour (5 doses)

Dosage Forms

Liquid, oral: Fructose 1.87 g, dextrose 1.87 g, and phosphoric acid 21.5 mg per 5 mL

Formula EM [OTC], Kalmz [OTC], Nausea Relief [OTC], Nausetrol® [OTC]: Fructose 1.87 g, dextrose 1.87 g, and phosphoric acid 21.5 mg per 5 mL

frusemide *see* furosemide *on page* 412

FS *see* fibrin sealant *on page* 383

FSH *see* follitropin alfa *on page* 404

FSH *see* follitropin beta *on page* 405

FSH *see* urofollitropin *on page* 931

FS VH S/D *see* fibrin sealant *on page* 383

FTC *see* emtricitabine *on page* 328

FTC/RPV/TDF *see* emtricitabine, rilpivirine, and tenofovir *on page* 329

FTC, TDF, and EFV *see* efavirenz, emtricitabine, and tenofovir *on page* 324

FTY720 *see* fingolimod *on page* 384

FU *see* fluorouracil (systemic) *on page* 395

FU *see* fluorouracil (topical) *on page* 396

5-FU *see* fluorouracil (systemic) *on page* 395

5-FU *see* fluorouracil (topical) *on page* 396

Fucidin® (Can) *see* fusidic acid *(Canada only) on page* 413

Fucidin H (Can) *see* fusidic acid and hydrocortisone *(Canada only) on page* 413

Fucithalmic® (Can) *see* fusidic acid *(Canada only) on page* 413

FUDR *see* floxuridine *on page* 388

FUDR® (Can) *see* floxuridine *on page* 388

Ful-Glo® *see* fluorescein *on page* 393

fulvestrant (fool VES trant)

Synonyms ICI-182,780; ZD9238

U.S. Brand Names Faslodex®

Canadian Brand Names Faslodex®

Therapeutic Category Antineoplastic Agent, Estrogen Receptor Antagonist

Use Treatment of hormone receptor-positive metastatic breast cancer in postmenopausal women with disease progression following antiestrogen therapy

General Dosage Range Dosage adjustment recommended in patients with hepatic impairment

I.M.: *Adults (postmenopausal women):* Initial: 500 mg on days 1, 15, and 29; Maintenance: 500 mg once monthly

Dosage Forms

Injection, solution:

Faslodex®: 50 mg/mL (5 mL)

Fungi-Nail® [OTC] *see* undecylenic acid and derivatives *on page 929*

Fungizone® (Can) *see* amphotericin B (conventional) *on page 71*

Fung-O® [OTC] *see* salicylic acid *on page 816*

Fungoid® [OTC] *see* miconazole (topical) *on page 599*

Furadantin® *see* nitrofurantoin *on page 644*

furazosin *see* prazosin *on page 753*

furosemide (fyoor OH se mide)

Medication Safety Issues

Sound-alike/look-alike issues:

Furosemide may be confused with famotidine, finasteride, fluconazole, FLUoxetine, fosinopril, loperamide, torsemide

Lasix® may be confused with Lanoxin®, Lidex®, Lomotil®, Lovenox®, Luvox®, Luxiq®

International issues:

Lasix [U.S., Canada, and multiple international markets] may be confused with Esidrex brand name for hydrochlorothiazide [multiple international markets]; Esidrix brand name for hydrochlorothiazide [Germany]

Urex [Australia, Hong Kong, Turkey] may be confused with Eurax brand name for crotamiton [U.S., Canada, and multiple international markets]

Synonyms frusemide

U.S. Brand Names Lasix®

Canadian Brand Names Apo-Furosemide®; Bio-Furosemide; Dom-Furosemide; Furosemide Injection, USP; Furosemide Special Injection; Lasix®; Lasix® Special; Novo-Semide; Nu-Furosemide; PMS-Furosemide

Therapeutic Category Diuretic, Loop

Use Management of edema associated with heart failure and hepatic or renal disease; acute pulmonary edema; treatment of hypertension (alone or in combination with other antihypertensives)

Canadian labeling: Additional use: Furosemide Special Injection and Lasix® Special (products not available in the U.S.): Adjunctive treatment of oliguria in patients with severe renal impairment

General Dosage Range

I.M.:

Children: Initial: 1 mg/kg/dose; Maintenance: Up to 6 mg/kg/dose every 6-12 hours

Adults: Initial: 20-40 mg/dose; Usual maintenance dose interval: 6-12 hours (maximum: 200 mg/dose)

Elderly: Initial: 20 mg/day

I.V.:

Children: Initial: 1 mg/kg/dose; Maintenance: Up to 6 mg/kg/dose every 6-12 hours

Adults: Initial: 20-40 mg/dose; Usual maintenance dose interval: 6-12 hours (maximum: 200 mg/dose) **or** 40 mg, followed by 80 mg within 1 hour if inadequate response **or** 20-40 mg bolus, followed by continuous I.V. infusion doses of 10-40 mg/hour, doubled as needed up to a maximum 160 mg/hour

Elderly: Initial: 20 mg/day

Oral:

Children: Initial: 2 mg/kg/dose every 6-8 hours (maximum: 6 mg/kg/dose)

Adults: Initial: 20-80 mg/dose every 6-8 hours; Usual maintenance dose interval: Once or twice daily (maximum: 600 mg/day)

Elderly: Initial: 20 mg/day

Dosage Forms

Injection, solution [preservative free]: 10 mg/mL (2 mL, 4 mL, 10 mL)

Solution, oral: 40 mg/5 mL (5 mL, 500 mL); 10 mg/mL (4 mL, 60 mL, 120 mL)

Tablet, oral: 20 mg, 40 mg, 80 mg

Lasix®: 20 mg, 40 mg, 80 mg

Dosage Forms - Canada

Injection, solution [preservative free]:

Furosemide Special Injection: 10 mg/mL (25 mL)

Tablet, oral:

Lasix® Special: 500 mg [scored]

Furosemide Injection, USP (Can) *see* furosemide *on page* 412

Furosemide Special Injection (Can) *see* furosemide *on page* 412

fusidic acid *(Canada only)* (fyoo SI dik AS id)

Synonyms sodium fusidate

Canadian Brand Names Fucidin®; Fucithalmic®

Therapeutic Category Antifungal Agent, Systemic

Use

Topical: Treatment of primary and secondary skin infections caused by susceptible organisms

Ophthalmic: Treatment of superficial infections of the eye and conjunctiva caused by susceptible organisms

General Dosage Range

Ophthalmic: *Children ≥2 years and Adults:* Instill 1 drop in each eye every 12 hours

Topical: *Children and Adults:* Apply to affected area 3-4 times/day or 1-2 times/day if gauze dressing used

Product Availability Not available in U.S.

Dosage Forms - Canada

Cream, topical:

Fucidin®: 2% (15 g, 30 g)

Ointment, topical:

Fucidin®: 2% (15 g, 30 g)

Suspension, ophthalmic:

Fucithalmic®: 10 mg/g [1%] (0.2 g) [unit-dose, without preservative]; (3 g, 5 g) [multidose, contains benzalkonium chloride]

fusidic acid and hydrocortisone *(Canada only)*

(fyoo SI dik AS id & hye droe KOR ti sone)

Synonyms hydrocortisone and fusidic acid

Canadian Brand Names Fucidin H

Therapeutic Category Antibiotic, Topical; Corticosteroid, Topical

Use Treatment of mild- to moderately-severe atopic dermatitis caused by susceptible organisms

General Dosage Range Topical: *Children ≥3 years and Adults:* Apply 3 times/day

Product Availability Not available in U.S.

Dosage Forms - Canada

Cream, topical:

Fusidin H: Fusidic acid 2% and hydrocortisone 1% (5 g, 15 g, 30 g)

Fusilev® *see* LEVOleucovorin *on page* 532

Fuzeon® *see* enfuvirtide *on page* 331

FVIII/vWF *see* antihemophilic factor/von Willebrand factor complex (human) *on page* 78

FXIII *see* factor XIII concentrate (human) *on page* 372

FXT 40 (Can) *see* fluoxetine *on page* 396

GAA *see* alglucosidase alfa *on page* 47

gabapentin (GA ba pen tin)

Medication Safety Issues

Sound-alike/look-alike issues:

Neurontin® may be confused with Motrin®, Neoral®, nitrofurantoin, Noroxin®, Zarontin®

U.S. Brand Names Gralise™; Neurontin®

Canadian Brand Names Apo-Gabapentin®; CO Gabapentin; Dom-Gabapentin; Mylan-Gabapentin; Neurontin®; PHL-Gabapentin; PMS-Gabapentin; PRO-Gabapentin; RAN™-Gabapentin; ratio-Gabapentin; Riva-Gabapentin; Teva-Gabapentin

Therapeutic Category Anticonvulsant

Use Adjunct for treatment of partial seizures with and without secondary generalized seizures in patients >12 years of age with epilepsy; adjunct for treatment of partial seizures in pediatric patients 3-12 years of age; management of postherpetic neuralgia (PHN) in adults

General Dosage Range Dosage adjustment recommended in patients with renal impairment

Oral:

Children 3-4 years: Initial: 10-15 mg/kg/day in 3 divided doses; Usual dose: 40 mg/kg/day in 3 divided doses (maximum: 50 mg/kg/day)

Children 5-12 years: Initial: 10-15 mg/kg/day in 3 divided doses; Usual dose: 25-35 mg/kg/day in 3 divided doses (maximum: 50 mg/kg/day)

Children >12 years: Initial: 300 mg 3 times/day; Usual dose: 900-1800 mg/day in 3 divided doses (maximum: 3600 mg/day [short-term])

Adults:

Immediate release: Initial: 300 mg 1-3 times/day; Maintenance: 900-3600 mg/day in 3 divided doses (maximum: 3600 mg/day [short-term])

Extended release: Initial: 300 mg; Maintenance: 1800 mg once daily

Dosage Forms

Capsule, oral: 100 mg, 300 mg, 400 mg

Neurontin®: 100 mg, 300 mg, 400 mg

Solution, oral: 250 mg/5 mL (470 mL)

Neurontin®: 250 mg/5 mL (470 mL)

Tablet, oral: 600 mg, 800 mg

Gralise™: 300 mg, 600 mg, 300 mg (9s) [white tablets; contains soybean lecithin] and 600 mg (69s) [beige tablets]

Neurontin®: 600 mg, 800 mg

gabapentin enacarbil (gab a PEN tin en a KAR bil)

Synonyms GSK 1838262; Solzira; XP13512

U.S. Brand Names Horizant™

Therapeutic Category Anticonvulsant, Miscellaneous

Use Treatment of moderate-to-severe restless leg syndrome (RLS); management of postherpetic neuralgia (PHN)

General Dosage Range Dosage adjustment recommended in patients with renal impairment.

Oral: *Adults:* 600 mg once daily (RLS) **or** 600 mg once daily for 3 days, then 600 mg twice daily (PHN)

Dosage Forms

Tablet, extended release, oral:

Horizant™: 600 mg

Gabitril® *see* tiagabine *on page 894*

Gablofen® *see* baclofen *on page 112*

^{67}Ga-citrate *see* gallium citrate Ga-67 *on page 418*

Gadavist™ *see* gadobutrol *on page 415*

gadobenate dimeglumine (gad oh BEN ate dye MEG loo meen)

Medication Safety Issues

High alert medication:

The Institute for Safe Medication Practices (ISMP) includes this medication among its list of drugs which have a heightened risk of causing significant patient harm when used in error.

Synonyms gadolinum-BOPTA; Gd-BOPTA

U.S. Brand Names Multihance®; Multihance® Multipack™

Therapeutic Category Diagnostic Agent; Radiological/Contrast Media, Nonionic

Use Contrast medium for magnetic resonance imaging (MRI) to visualize CNS lesions with abnormal vascularity in the brain, spine, and associated tissues

General Dosage Range I.V.: *Children ≥3 years and Adults:* 0.1 mmol/kg (0.2 mL/kg)

Dosage Forms

Injection, solution [preservative free]:

Multihance®: 529 mg/mL (5 mL, 10 mL, 15 mL, 20 mL)

Multihance® Multipack™: 529 mg/mL (50 mL, 100 mL)

gadobutrol (gad oh BYOO trol)

Medication Safety Issues

Sound-alike/look-alike issues:

Gadavist™ may be confused with Magnevist®

International issues:

Gadovist [Canada and multiple international markets] may be confused with Vasovist brand name for gadofosveset [Hungary, Turkey]

High alert medication:

The Institute for Safe Medication Practices (ISMP) includes this medication among its list of drug classes which have a heightened risk of causing significant patient harm when used in error.

Synonyms gadovist 1.0

U.S. Brand Names Gadavist™

Canadian Brand Names Gadovist™

Therapeutic Category Gadolinium-Containing Contrast Agent; Radiological/Contrast Media, Nonionic

Use

U.S. labeling: Contrast medium for magnetic resonance imaging (MRI) for the enhancement and detection of disruptions in the blood brain barrier and/or CNS vasculature

Canadian labeling: Contrast medium for magnetic resonance imaging (MRI) of CNS lesions (brain, spine, and associated tissues); perfusion studies to diagnose stroke, or to detect focal cerebral ischemia or tumor perfusion; contrast-enhanced magnetic resonance angiography (CE-MRA)

General Dosage Range Dosage adjustment recommended in patients with renal impairment

I.V.: *Children ≥2 years and Adults* 0.1 mmol/kg (0.1 mL/kg)

Dosage Forms

Injection, solution [preservative free]:

Gadavist™: 604.72 mg/mL (7.5 mL, 10 mL, 15 mL)

gadodiamide (gad oh DYE a mide)

Medication Safety Issues

High alert medication:

The Institute for Safe Medication Practices (ISMP) includes this medication among its list of drugs which have a heightened risk of causing significant patient harm when used in error.

Synonyms gadolinium-DTPA-BMA; Gd-DTPA-BMA

U.S. Brand Names Omniscan®

Canadian Brand Names Omniscan®

Therapeutic Category Radiological/Contrast Media, Nonionic

Use Contrast medium for magnetic resonance imaging (MRI) to visualize CNS lesions with abnormal vascularity in the brain, spine, and associated tissues, and to visualize body lesions with abnormal vascularity within the thoracic (noncardiac), abdominal, pelvic cavities, and retroperitoneal space

Canadian labeling: Additional indications (not in U.S. labeling): Contrast medium for MRI to visualize breast or musculoskeletal lesions with abnormal vascularity and for magnetic resonance angiography (MRA) to visualize and detect stenosis of the renal and aortoiliac arteries

General Dosage Range I.V.:

Children ≥2 years: 0.05-0.1 mmol/kg (0.1-0.2 mL/kg)

Adults: 0.05-0.1 mmol/kg (0.1-0.2 mL/kg); may repeat 0.2 mmol/kg (0.4 mL/kg) once if needed [CNS imaging]

Dosage Forms

Injection, solution [preservative free]:

Omniscan®: 287 mg/mL (5 mL, 10 mL, 15 mL, 20 mL, 50 mL, 100 mL)

gadofosveset (gad oh FOS ve set)

Medication Safety Issues

International issues:

Vasovist [Hungary, Turkey] may be confused with Gadavist brand name for gadobutrol [U.S.]; Gadovist brand name for gadobutrol [Canada and multiple international markets]; Magnevist brand name for gadopentetate dimeglumine [U.S., Canada, and multiple international markets]

High alert medication:

The Institute for Safe Medication Practices (ISMP) includes this medication among its list of drug classes which have a heightened risk of causing significant patient harm when used in error.

Synonyms gadofosveset trisodium

U.S. Brand Names Ablavar®

Therapeutic Category Gadolinium-Containing Contrast Agent; Radiological/Contrast Media, Paramagnetic Agent

Use Contrast medium used in magnetic resonance angiography (MRA) to evaluate or better define aortoiliac occlusive disease

General Dosage Range I.V.: *Adults:* 0.03 mmol/kg (0.12 mL/kg)

Dosage Forms

Injection, solution [preservative free]:

Ablavar®: 0.25 mmol/mL (10 mL, 15 mL)

Dosage Forms - Canada

Injection, solution [preservative free]:

Vasovist®: 0.25 mmoL/mL (10 mL, 15 mL, 20 mL)

gadofosveset trisodium *see* gadofosveset *on page 415*

gadolinium-DTPA *see* gadopentetate dimeglumine *on page 416*

gadolinium-DTPA-BMA *see* gadodiamide *on page 415*

gadolinium-DTPA-BMEA *see* gadoversetamide *on page 417*

gadolinium-HP-DO3A *see* gadoteridol *on page 416*

gadolinum-BOPTA *see* gadobenate dimeglumine *on page 414*

gadopentetate dimeglumine (gad oh PEN te tate dye MEG loo meen)

Medication Safety Issues

High alert medication:

The Institute for Safe Medication Practices (ISMP) includes this medication among its list of drugs which have a heightened risk of causing significant patient harm when used in error.

Synonyms gadolinium-DTPA; Gd-DTPA

U.S. Brand Names Magnevist®

Canadian Brand Names Magnevist®

Therapeutic Category Radiological/Contrast Media, Paramagnetic Agent

Use Contrast medium for magnetic resonance imaging (MRI) to visualize CNS lesions with abnormal vascularity in the brain, spine and associated tissues, extracranial/extraspinal lesions with abnormal vascularity in the head and neck, and body lesions with abnormal vascularity (excluding the heart)

General Dosage Range I.V.: *Children ≥2 years and Adults:* 0.1 mmol/kg (0.2 mL/kg)

Dosage Forms

Injection, solution [preservative free]:

Magnevist®: 469.01 mg/mL (5 mL, 10 mL, 15 mL, 20 mL, 50 mL, 100 mL)

gadoteridol (gad oh TER i dol)

Medication Safety Issues

High alert medication:

The Institute for Safe Medication Practices (ISMP) includes this medication among its list of drugs which have a heightened risk of causing significant patient harm when used in error.

Synonyms gadolinium-HP-DO3A; Gd-HP-DO3A

U.S. Brand Names ProHance®; ProHance® Multipack™

Therapeutic Category Radiological/Contrast Media, Nonionic

Use Contrast medium for magnetic resonance imaging (MRI) to visualize CNS lesions with abnormal vascularity in the brain, spine, and associated tissues and to visualize extracranial/extraspinal tissues in the head and neck

General Dosage Range I.V.:

Children ≥2 years: 0.1 mmol/kg (0.2 mL/kg)

Adults: 0.1 mmol/kg (0.2 mL/kg); may repeat 0.2 mmol/kg (0.4 mL/kg) once if needed [CNS imaging]

Dosage Forms

Injection, solution [preservative free]:

ProHance®: 279.3 mg/mL (5 mL, 10 mL, 15 mL, 17 mL, 20 mL)

ProHance® Multipack™: 279.3 mg/mL (50 mL)

gadoversetamide (gad oh ver SET a mide)

Medication Safety Issues

High alert medication:

The Institute for Safe Medication Practices (ISMP) includes this medication among its list of drugs which have a heightened risk of causing significant patient harm when used in error.

Synonyms gadolinium-DTPA-BMEA; Gd-DTPA-BMEA

U.S. Brand Names OptiMARK®

Therapeutic Category Radiological/Contrast Media, Nonionic

Use Contrast medium for magnetic resonance imaging (MRI) to visualize CNS lesions with abnormal vascularity in the brain, spine, and associated tissues and to visualize liver lesions with abnormal vascularity in patients highly suspect for liver structural abnormalities

General Dosage Range **I.V.:** *Adults:* 0.1 mmol/kg (0.2 mL/kg)

Dosage Forms

Injection, solution [preservative free]:

OptiMARK®: 330.9 mg/mL (5 mL, 10 mL, 15 mL, 20 mL, 30 mL, 50 mL)

Gadovist™ (Can) *see* gadobutrol *on page* 415
gadovist 1.0 *see* gadobutrol *on page* 415

gadoxetate (gad OX e tate)

Medication Safety Issues

Sound-alike/look-alike issues:

Eovist® may be confused with Evista®

High alert medication:

The Institute for Safe Medication Practices (ISMP) includes this medication among its list of drugs which have a heightened risk of causing significant patient harm when used in error.

Synonyms gadoxetate disodium; Gd-EOB-DTPA

U.S. Brand Names Eovist®

Canadian Brand Names Primovist

Therapeutic Category Gadolinium-Containing Contrast Agent; Radiological/Contrast Media, Ionic (Low Osmolality); Radiological/Contrast Media, Paramagnetic Agent

Use Contrast medium for magnetic resonance imaging (MRI) to detect and characterize lesions within focal liver disease

General Dosage Range **I.V.:** *Adults:* 0.025 mmol/kg (0.1 mL/kg)

Dosage Forms

Injection, solution [preservative free]:

Eovist®: 181.43 mg/mL (10 mL)

gadoxetate disodium *see* gadoxetate *on page* 417
^{67}Ga-gallium citrate *see* gallium citrate Ga-67 *on page* 418

galantamine (ga LAN ta meen)

Medication Safety Issues

Sound-alike/look-alike issues:

Razadyne® may be confused with Rozerem®

International issues:

Reminyl [Canada and multiple international markets] may be confused with Amarel brand name for glimepiride [France]; Amaryl brand name for glimepiride [U.S., Canada, and multiple international markets]; Robinul brand name for glycopyrrolate [U.S. and multiple international markets]

Synonyms galantamine hydrobromide

U.S. Brand Names Razadyne®; Razadyne® ER

Canadian Brand Names Mylan-Galantamine ER; PAT-Galantamine ER; Reminyl®; Reminyl® ER

Therapeutic Category Acetylcholinesterase Inhibitor (Central)

Use Treatment of mild-to-moderate dementia of Alzheimer disease

General Dosage Range Dosage adjustment recommended in patients with hepatic or renal impairment

Oral:

Extended-release: *Adults:* Initial: 8 mg once daily; Maintenance: 16-24 mg once daily
Immediate release: *Adults:* Initial: 4 mg twice daily; Maintenance: 16-24 mg/day in 2 divided doses

Dosage Forms

Capsule, extended release, oral: 8 mg, 16 mg, 24 mg
Razadyne® ER: 8 mg, 16 mg, 24 mg

Solution, oral: 4 mg/mL (100 mL)
Razadyne®: 4 mg/mL (100 mL)

Tablet, oral: 4 mg, 8 mg, 12 mg
Razadyne®: 4 mg, 8 mg, 12 mg

galantamine hydrobromide *see* galantamine *on page* 417

gallium citrate Ga-67 (GAL ee um SIT rate jee aye SIX tee SEV en)

Medication Safety Issues

Other safety concerns:

Radiopharmaceutical: Use appropriate precaution for handling, disposal, and minimizing exposure to patients and healthcare personnel. Use under supervision of experienced personnel. Should be stored in original lead container or adequate radiation shield.

Synonyms ^{67}Ga-citrate; ^{67}Ga-gallium citrate

Therapeutic Category Radiopharmaceutical

Use Diagnostic imaging of Hodgkin disease, lymphoma, bronchogenic carcinoma, and inflammatory lesions to identify fevers of unknown origin; nonbacterial infections

galsulfase (gal SUL fase)

Synonyms recombinant N-acetylgalactosamine 4-sulfatase; rhASB

U.S. Brand Names Naglazyme®

Therapeutic Category Enzyme

Use Replacement therapy in mucopolysaccharidosis VI (MPS VI; Maroteaux-Lamy Syndrome) for improvement of walking and stair-climbing capacity

General Dosage Range I.V.: *Children >5 years and Adults:* 1 mg/kg once weekly

Dosage Forms

Injection, solution [preservative free]:
Naglazyme®: 5 mg/5 mL (5 mL)

Galzin® *see* zinc acetate *on page* 962
GamaSTAN™ S/D *see* immune globulin *on page* 477
Gamastan S/D (Can) *see* immune globulin *on page* 477
Gamimune® N (Can) *see* immune globulin *on page* 477
gamma benzene hexachloride *see* lindane *on page* 541
Gamma E-Gems® [OTC] *see* vitamin E *on page* 950
Gamma-E PLUS [OTC] *see* vitamin E *on page* 950
Gammagard® Liquid *see* immune globulin *on page* 477
Gammagard Liquid (Can) *see* immune globulin *on page* 477
Gammagard S/D® *see* immune globulin *on page* 477
Gammagard S/D (Can) *see* immune globulin *on page* 477
gamma globulin *see* immune globulin *on page* 477
gamma hydroxybutyric acid *see* sodium oxybate *on page* 844
Gammaked™ *see* immune globulin *on page* 477
gammaphos *see* amifostine *on page* 59
Gammaplex® *see* immune globulin *on page* 477
Gamunex® [DSC] *see* immune globulin *on page* 477
Gamunex® (Can) *see* immune globulin *on page* 477
Gamunex®-C *see* immune globulin *on page* 477

ganciclovir (systemic) (gan SYE kloe veer)

Medication Safety Issues

Sound-alike/look-alike issues:

Cytovene® may be confused with Cytosar®, Cytosar-U
Ganciclovir may be confused with acyclovir

Synonyms DHPG sodium; GCV sodium; nordeoxyguanosine

U.S. Brand Names Cytovene®-IV

Canadian Brand Names Cytovene®

Therapeutic Category Antiviral Agent

Use Treatment of CMV retinitis in immunocompromised individuals, including patients with acquired immunodeficiency syndrome; prophylaxis of CMV infection in transplant patients

General Dosage Range Dosage adjustment recommended in patients with renal impairment

I.V.: *Children and Adults:* Induction: 30-35 mg/kg/week, given as once-daily dose for 5-7 days per week

Dosage Forms

Injection, powder for reconstitution: 500 mg

Cytovene®-IV: 500 mg

ganciclovir (ophthalmic) (gan SYE kloe veer)

Medication Safety Issues

Sound-alike/look-alike issues:

Ganciclovir may be confused with acyclovir

Synonyms nordeoxyguanosine

U.S. Brand Names Vitrasert®; Zirgan®

Therapeutic Category Antiviral Agent

Use

Intravitreal implant: Treatment of CMV retinitis in patients with acquired immunodeficiency syndrome

Ophthalmic gel: Treatment of acute herpetic keratitis (dendritic ulcers)

General Dosage Range

Ocular implant: *Children ≥9 years and Adults:* 1 implant for 5-8 month period

Ophthalmic gel: *Children ≥2 months and Adults:* 1 drop in affected eye 3-5 times/day

Dosage Forms

Gel, ophthalmic:

Zirgan®: 0.15% (5 g)

Implant, intravitreal:

Vitrasert®: 4.5 mg (1s)

ganirelix (ga ni REL ix)

Medication Safety Issues

International issues:

Antagon former U.S. brand name for ganirelix, but also the brand name for ranitidine in Brazil

Synonyms antagon; ganirelix acetate

Canadian Brand Names Orgalutran®

Therapeutic Category Antigonadotropic Agent

Use Inhibits premature luteinizing hormone (LH) surges in women undergoing controlled ovarian hyperstimulation

General Dosage Range SubQ: *Adults:* 250 mcg/day

Dosage Forms

Injection, solution: 250 mcg/0.5 mL (0.5 mL)

ganirelix acetate *see* ganirelix *on page 419*

GAR-936 *see* tigecycline *on page 896*

Garamycin® *see* gentamicin (ophthalmic) *on page 424*

Garasone (Can) *see* gentamicin (ophthalmic) *on page 424*

Gardasil® *see* papillomavirus (types 6, 11, 16, 18) vaccine (human, recombinant) *on page 690*

Gas-X® [OTC] *see* simethicone *on page 834*

Gas-X® Children's Tongue Twisters™ [OTC] *see* simethicone *on page 834*

Gas-X® Extra Strength [OTC] *see* simethicone *on page 834*

Gas-X® Maximum Strength [OTC] *see* simethicone *on page 834*

Gas-X® Thin Strips™ [OTC] *see* simethicone *on page 834*

Gas Ban™ [OTC] *see* calcium carbonate and simethicone *on page 163*

Gas Free Extra Strength [OTC] *see* simethicone *on page 834*

Gas Relief Ultra Strength [OTC] *see* simethicone *on page 834*

Gastrocrom® *see* cromolyn (systemic, oral inhalation) *on page 240*

Gastrografin® *see* diatrizoate meglumine and diatrizoate sodium *on page* 277
Gastroview *see* diatrizoate meglumine and diatrizoate sodium *on page* 277

gatifloxacin (gat i FLOKS a sin)

U.S. Brand Names Zymaxid™
Canadian Brand Names Zymar™
Therapeutic Category Antibiotic, Quinolone
Use Treatment of bacterial conjunctivitis
General Dosage Range Ophthalmic: *Children ≥1 year and Adults:* 1 drop into affected eye(s) every 2 hours while awake (maximum: 8 times/day) for 1 day; followed by 1 drop into affected eye(s) 2-4 times/day for 6 days
Dosage Forms
Solution, ophthalmic:
Zymaxid™: 0.5% (2.5 mL)
Dosage Forms - Canada
Solution, ophthalmic [drops]:
Zymar™: 0.3% (1 mL, 2.5 mL, 5 mL)

GaviLyte™-C *see* polyethylene glycol-electrolyte solution *on page* 738
GaviLyte™-G *see* polyethylene glycol-electrolyte solution *on page* 738
GaviLyte™-N *see* polyethylene glycol-electrolyte solution *on page* 738
Gaviscon® Extra Strength [OTC] *see* aluminum hydroxide and magnesium carbonate *on page* 55
Gaviscon® Liquid [OTC] *see* aluminum hydroxide and magnesium carbonate *on page* 55
Gaviscon® Tablet [OTC] *see* aluminum hydroxide and magnesium trisilicate *on page* 56
Gax-X® Infant [OTC] *see* simethicone *on page* 834
G-CSF *see* filgrastim *on page* 384
G-CSF (PEG conjugate) *see* pegfilgrastim *on page* 696
GCV sodium *see* ganciclovir (systemic) *on page* 418
GD-Amlodipine (Can) *see* amlodipine *on page* 65
GD-Atorvastatin (Can) *see* atorvastatin *on page* 100
GD-Azithromycin (Can) *see* azithromycin (systemic) *on page* 108
Gd-BOPTA *see* gadobenate dimeglumine *on page* 414
GDC-0449 *see* vismodegib *on page* 948
Gd-DTPA *see* gadopentetate dimeglumine *on page* 416
Gd-DTPA-BMA *see* gadodiamide *on page* 415
Gd-DTPA-BMEA *see* gadoversetamide *on page* 417
Gd-EOB-DTPA *see* gadoxetate *on page* 417
Gd-HP-DO3A *see* gadoteridol *on page* 416
GD-Latanoprost (Can) *see* latanoprost *on page* 524
GD-Mirtazapine (Can) *see* mirtazapine *on page* 606
GD-Sertraline (Can) *see* sertraline *on page* 831
GD-Terbinafine (Can) *see* terbinafine (systemic) *on page* 878
GD-Venlafaxine XR (Can) *see* venlafaxine *on page* 942
Gebauer's Ethyl Chloride® *see* ethyl chloride *on page* 364

gefitinib (ge FI tye nib)

Medication Safety Issues
Sound-alike/look-alike issues:
Gefitinib may be confused with axitinib, crizotinib, erlotinib, imatinib, SORAfenib, SUNItinib, vandetanib
High alert medication:
This medication is in a class the Institute for Safe Medication Practices (ISMP) includes among its list of drug classes which have a heightened risk of causing significant patient harm when used in error.
Synonyms ZD1839
U.S. Brand Names Iressa®
Canadian Brand Names IRESSA®
Therapeutic Category Antineoplastic Agent, Tyrosine Kinase Inhibitor

Use Treatment of locally advanced or metastatic nonsmall cell lung cancer (NSCLC) after failure of platinum-based and docetaxel therapies. Treatment is limited to patients who are benefiting or have benefited from treatment with gefitinib.

Note: Due to the lack of improved survival data from clinical trials of gefitinib, and in response to positive survival data with another EGFR inhibitor, according to the U.S. labeling, physicians are advised to use treatment options other than gefitinib in patients with advanced nonsmall cell lung cancer following one or two prior chemotherapy regimens when they are refractory/intolerant to their most recent regimen.

Canada labeling: First-line treatment of locally advanced or metastatic NSCLC with activating mutations of EGFR-TK

General Dosage Range Dosage adjustment recommended in patients on concomitant therapy or who develop toxicities.

Oral: *Adults:* 250 mg once daily

Dosage Forms

Tablet, oral:

Iressa®: 250 mg

gelatin (absorbable) (JEL a tin, ab SORB a ble)

Synonyms absorbable gelatin sponge

U.S. Brand Names Gelfilm®; Gelfoam®

Therapeutic Category Hemostatic Agent

Use Adjunct to provide hemostasis in surgical procedures; adjunct in neuro, thoracic, or ocular surgeries to promote tissue repair and/or prevent adhesions (Gelfilm®)

General Dosage Range Topical: *Children and Adults:* Dosage and administration vary by product formulation and/or surgical procedure.

Dosage Forms

Film, ophthalmic:

Gelfilm®: (6s)

Film, topical:

Gelfilm®: (1s)

Powder, topical:

Gelfoam®: (1 g)

Sponge, oral topical:

Gelfoam®: (12s)

Sponge, topical:

Gelfoam®: (4s, 6s, 12s)

gelatin, pectin, and methylcellulose (JEL a tin, PEK tin, & meth il SEL yoo lose)

Synonyms methylcellulose, gelatin, and pectin; pectin, gelatin, and methylcellulose

Therapeutic Category Protectant, Topical

Use Temporary relief from minor oral irritations

General Dosage Range Topical: *Children and Adults:* Press small dabs into place until the involved area is coated with a thin film as needed

Gelclair® *see* mucosal barrier gel, oral *on page* 618

Gelfilm® *see* gelatin (absorbable) *on page* 421

Gelfoam® *see* gelatin (absorbable) *on page* 421

Gel-Kam® [OTC] *see* fluoride *on page* 393

Gel-Kam® Rinse *see* fluoride *on page* 393

Gelnique® *see* oxybutynin *on page* 677

Gelnique 3%™ *see* oxybutynin *on page* 677

GelRite™ [OTC] *see* alcohol (ethyl) *on page* 43

Gel-Stat™ [OTC] *see* alcohol (ethyl) *on page* 43

Gelucast® *see* zinc gelatin *on page* 963

Gelusil® [OTC] *see* aluminum hydroxide, magnesium hydroxide, and simethicone *on page* 56

Gelusil® (Can) *see* aluminum hydroxide, magnesium hydroxide, and simethicone *on page* 56

Gelusil® Extra Strength (Can) *see* aluminum hydroxide and magnesium hydroxide *on page* 56

gemcitabine (jem SITE a been)

Medication Safety Issues

Sound-alike/look-alike issues:

Gemcitabine may be confused with gemtuzumab

Gemzar® may be confused with Zinecard®

High alert medication:

This medication is in a class the Institute for Safe Medication Practices (ISMP) includes among its list of drug classes which have a heightened risk of causing significant patient harm when used in error.

Synonyms dFdC; dFdCyd; difluorodeoxycytidine hydrochlorothiazide; gemcitabine hydrochloride; LY-188011

U.S. Brand Names Gemzar®

Canadian Brand Names Gemcitabine For Injection, USP; Gemzar®

Therapeutic Category Antineoplastic Agent

Use Treatment of metastatic breast cancer; inoperable locally-advanced or metastatic nonsmall cell lung cancer (NSCLC); locally advanced or metastatic pancreatic cancer; advanced, relapsed ovarian cancer

General Dosage Range Dosage adjustment recommended in patients with hepatic impairment or who develop toxicities

I.V.: *Adults:* Dosage varies greatly depending on indication

Dosage Forms

Injection, powder for reconstitution: 200 mg, 1 g, 2 g

Gemzar®: 200 mg, 1 g

Injection, solution: 38 mg/mL (5.26 mL, 26.3 mL, 52.6 mL)

Gemcitabine For Injection, USP (Can) *see* gemcitabine *on page* 422

gemcitabine hydrochloride *see* gemcitabine *on page* 422

gemfibrozil (jem FI broe zil)

Medication Safety Issues

Sound-alike/look-alike issues:

Lopid® may be confused with Levbid®, Lipitor®, Lodine

Synonyms CI-719

U.S. Brand Names Lopid®

Canadian Brand Names Apo-Gemfibrozil®; Gen-Gemfibrozil; GMD-Gemfibrozil; Lopid®; Mylan-Gemfibrozil; Novo-Gemfibrozil; Nu-Gemfibrozil; PMS-Gemfibrozil

Therapeutic Category Antihyperlipidemic Agent, Miscellaneous

Use Treatment of hypertriglyceridemia in Fredrickson types IV and V hyperlipidemia for patients who are at greater risk for pancreatitis and who have not responded to dietary intervention; to reduce the risk of CHD development in Fredrickson type IIb patients without a history or symptoms of existing CHD who have not responded to dietary and other interventions (including pharmacologic treatment) and who have decreased HDL, increased LDL, and increased triglycerides

General Dosage Range **Oral:** *Adults:* 600 mg twice daily

Dosage Forms

Tablet, oral: 600 mg

Lopid®: 600 mg

gemifloxacin (je mi FLOKS a sin)

Synonyms DW286; gemifloxacin mesylate; LA 20304a; SB-265805

U.S. Brand Names Factive®

Canadian Brand Names Factive®

Therapeutic Category Antibiotic, Quinolone

Use Treatment of acute exacerbation of chronic bronchitis; treatment of community-acquired pneumonia (CAP), including pneumonia caused by multidrug-resistant strains of *S. pneumoniae* (MDRSP)

General Dosage Range Dosage adjustment recommended in patients with renal impairment

Oral: *Adults:* 320 mg once daily

Dosage Forms

Tablet, oral:

Factive®: 320 mg

gemifloxacin mesylate *see* gemifloxacin *on page* 422

gemtuzumab ozogamicin (gem TOO zoo mab oh zog a MY sin)

Medication Safety Issues

Sound-alike/look-alike issues:

Gemtuzumab may be confused with gemcitabine

High alert medication:

This medication is in a class the Institute for Safe Medication Practices (ISMP) includes among its list of drug classes which have a heightened risk of causing significant patient harm when used in error.

Synonyms CMA-676; Mylotarg

Therapeutic Category Antineoplastic Agent, Natural Source (Plant) Derivative

Use Due to safety concerns, as well as lack of clinical benefit demonstrated in a post-approval clinical trial, gemtuzumab was withdrawn from the U.S. commercial market in 2010.

Product Availability No longer commercially available in the U.S. market for new patients. Available in Canada through a special access program.

Gemzar® *see* gemcitabine *on page 422*
Gen-Amilazide (Can) *see* amiloride and hydrochlorothiazide *on page 60*
Gen-Clozapine (Can) *see* clozapine *on page 228*
Gen-Combo Sterinebs (Can) *see* ipratropium and albuterol *on page 499*
Gen-Doxazosin (Can) *see* doxazosin *on page 311*
gene-activated human acid-beta-glucosidase *see* velaglucerase alfa *on page 941*
Generess™ Fe *see* ethinyl estradiol and norethindrone *on page 359*
Generlac *see* lactulose *on page 519*
Gen-Fluoxetine (Can) *see* fluoxetine *on page 396*
Gen-Gemfibrozil (Can) *see* gemfibrozil *on page 422*
Gengraf® *see* cyclosporine (systemic) *on page 245*
Gen-Hydroxychloroquine (Can) *see* hydroxychloroquine *on page 462*
Gen-Hydroxyurea (Can) *see* hydroxyurea *on page 464*
Gen-Ipratropium (Can) *see* ipratropium (oral inhalation) *on page 499*
Gen-Lovastatin (Can) *see* lovastatin *on page 553*
Gen-Medroxy (Can) *see* medroxyprogesterone *on page 567*
Gen-Nabumetone (Can) *see* nabumetone *on page 623*
Gen-Nizatidine (Can) *see* nizatidine *on page 647*
Genotropin® *see* somatropin *on page 849*
Genotropin Miniquick® *see* somatropin *on page 849*
Gen-Selegiline (Can) *see* selegiline *on page 828*
Gentak® *see* gentamicin (ophthalmic) *on page 424*

gentamicin (systemic) (jen ta MYE sin)

Medication Safety Issues

Sound-alike/look-alike issues:

Gentamicin may be confused with gentian violet, kanamycin, vancomycin

High alert medication:

The Institute for Safe Medication Practices (ISMP) includes this medication (intrathecal administration) among its list of drug classes which have a heightened risk of causing significant patient harm when used in error.

Synonyms gentamicin sulfate

Canadian Brand Names Gentamicin Injection, USP

Therapeutic Category Antibiotic, Aminoglycoside

Use Treatment of susceptible bacterial infections, normally gram-negative organisms, including *Pseudomonas*, *Proteus*, *Serratia*, and gram-positive *Staphylococcus*; treatment of bone infections, respiratory tract infections, skin and soft tissue infections, as well as abdominal and urinary tract infections, and septicemia; treatment of infective endocarditis

General Dosage Range Dosage adjustment recommended for the I.M. and I.V. routes in patients with renal impairment

I.M., I.V.:

Children <5 years: 2.5 mg/kg/dose every 8 hours
Children ≥5 years: 2-2.5 mg/kg/dose every 8 hours

Adults: 1-2.5 mg/kg/dose every 8-12 hours **or** 4-7 mg/kg once daily
Intrathecal: *Adults:* 4-8 mg/day

Dosage Forms
Infusion, premixed in NS: 60 mg (50 mL, 100 mL); 80 mg (50 mL, 100 mL); 100 mg (50 mL, 100 mL); 120 mg (50 mL, 100 mL)
Injection, solution: 40 mg/mL (2 mL, 20 mL, 50 mL)
Injection, solution [preservative free]: 10 mg/mL (2 mL)

gentamicin (ophthalmic) (jen ta MYE sin)

Medication Safety Issues
Sound-alike/look-alike issues:
Gentamicin may be confused with gentian violet, kanamycin, vancomycin

Synonyms gentamicin sulfate

U.S. Brand Names Garamycin®; Gentak®

Canadian Brand Names Diogent®; Garamycin®; Garasone; Gentak®; Gentocin; PMS-Gentamicin

Therapeutic Category Antibiotic, Aminoglycoside; Antibiotic, Ophthalmic

Use Treatment of ophthalmic infections caused by susceptible bacteria

General Dosage Range Ophthalmic: *Children and Adults:* Ointment: Instill 1/2" (1.25 cm) 2-3 times/day to every 3-4 hours; Solution: Instill 1-2 drops every 4 hours, up to 2 drops every hour for severe infections

Dosage Forms
Ointment, ophthalmic:
Gentak®: 0.3% (3.5 g)
Ointment, ophthalmic [preservative free]:
Garamycin®: 0.3% (3.5 g)
Solution, ophthalmic: 0.3% (5 mL, 15 mL)
Garamycin®: 0.3% (5 mL)
Gentak®: 0.3% (5 mL)

gentamicin (topical) (jen ta MYE sin)

Medication Safety Issues
Sound-alike/look-alike issues:
Gentamicin may be confused with gentian violet, kanamycin, vancomycin

Canadian Brand Names PMS-Gentamicin; ratio-Gentamicin

Therapeutic Category Antibiotic, Aminoglycoside; Antibiotic, Topical

Use Used topically to treat superficial infections of the skin

General Dosage Range Topical: *Children and Adults:* Apply 3-4 times/day to affected area

Dosage Forms
Cream, topical: 0.1% (15 g, 30 g)
Ointment, topical: 0.1% (15 g, 30 g)

gentamicin and prednisolone *see* prednisolone and gentamicin *on page* 755
Gentamicin Injection, USP (Can) *see* gentamicin (systemic) *on page* 423
gentamicin sulfate *see* gentamicin (ophthalmic) *on page* 424
gentamicin sulfate *see* gentamicin (systemic) *on page* 423
GenTeal® [OTC] *see* hydroxypropyl methylcellulose *on page* 463
Genteal® (Can) *see* hydroxypropyl methylcellulose *on page* 463
GenTeal® Mild [OTC] *see* hydroxypropyl methylcellulose *on page* 463
Gen-Temazepam (Can) *see* temazepam *on page* 875
Gen-Ticlopidine (Can) *see* ticlopidine *on page* 895
Gen-Tizanidine (Can) *see* tizanidine *on page* 900
Gentocin (Can) *see* gentamicin (ophthalmic) *on page* 424
Gen-Triazolam (Can) *see* triazolam *on page* 917
Geodon® *see* ziprasidone *on page* 964
Geriation [OTC] *see* vitamins (multiple/oral) *on page* 951
Geri-Dryl *see* diphenhydramine (systemic) *on page* 292
Geri-Freeda [OTC] *see* vitamins (multiple/oral) *on page* 951
Geri-Hydrolac™ [OTC] *see* lactic acid and ammonium hydroxide *on page* 517
Geri-Hydrolac™-12 [OTC] *see* lactic acid and ammonium hydroxide *on page* 517

Geri-kot [OTC] *see* senna *on page 829*
Geri-Stool [OTC] *see* docusate and senna *on page 305*
Geritol Complete® [OTC] *see* vitamins (multiple/oral) *on page 951*
Geritol Extend® [OTC] *see* vitamins (multiple/oral) *on page 951*
Geritol® Tonic [OTC] *see* vitamins (multiple/oral) *on page 951*
Geri-Tussin [OTC] *see* guaifenesin *on page 433*
Gesticare® DHA *see* vitamins (multiple/prenatal) *on page 952*
Gets-It® [OTC] *see* salicylic acid *on page 816*
GF196960 *see* tadalafil *on page 866*
GG *see* guaifenesin *on page 433*
GHB *see* sodium oxybate *on page 844*
GI87084B *see* remifentanil *on page 793*
Gianvi™ *see* ethinyl estradiol and drospirenone *on page 356*
Giazo™ *see* balsalazide *on page 114*
Gildess® FE 1.5/30 *see* ethinyl estradiol and norethindrone *on page 359*
Gildess® FE 1/20 *see* ethinyl estradiol and norethindrone *on page 359*
Gilenya® *see* fingolimod *on page 384*
glargine insulin *see* insulin glargine *on page 486*
Glassia™ *see* alpha$_1$-proteinase inhibitor *on page 51*

glatiramer acetate (gla TIR a mer AS e tate)

Medication Safety Issues

Sound-alike/look-alike issues:

Copaxone® may be confused with Compazine

Synonyms copolymer-1

U.S. Brand Names Copaxone®

Canadian Brand Names Copaxone®

Therapeutic Category Biological, Miscellaneous

Use Management of relapsing-remitting type multiple sclerosis, including patients with a first clinical episode with MRI features consistent with multiple sclerosis

General Dosage Range SubQ: *Adults:* 20 mg daily

Dosage Forms

Injection, solution [preservative free]:

Copaxone®: 20 mg/mL (1 mL)

glcCerase *see* velaglucerase alfa *on page 941*
Gleevec® *see* imatinib *on page 474*
Gliadel® *see* carmustine *on page 178*
Gliadel Wafer® (Can) *see* carmustine *on page 178*
glibenclamide *see* glyburide *on page 428*
Gliclazide-80 (Can) *see* gliclazide *(Canada only) on page 425*

gliclazide *(Canada only)* (GLYE kla zide)

Medication Safety Issues

High alert medication:

This medication is in a class the Institute for Safe Medication Practices (ISMP) includes among its list of drugs which have a heightened risk of causing significant patient harm when used in error.

Canadian Brand Names Apo-Gliclazide®; AVA-Gliclazide; Diamicron®; Diamicron® MR; Gliclazide MR; Gliclazide-80; Mylan-Gliclazide; Novo-Gliclazide; PMS-Gliclazide

Therapeutic Category Antidiabetic Agent, Oral; Hypoglycemic Agent, Oral; Sulfonylurea Agent

Use Management of type 2 diabetes mellitus (noninsulin-dependent, NIDDM)

General Dosage Range Oral:

Immediate release: *Adults:* Initial: 80 mg twice daily; Maintenance: 80-320 mg/day (maximum: 320 mg/day)

Modified release: *Adults:* 30-120 mg once daily (maximum: 120 mg/day)

Product Availability Not available in U.S.

Dosage Forms - Canada

Tablet, oral:

Diamicron®: 80 mg

Tablet, modified release, oral:

Diamicron® MR: 30 mg, 60 mg

Gliclazide MR (Can) *see* gliclazide *(Canada only) on page 425*

glimepiride (GLYE me pye ride)

Medication Safety Issues

Sound-alike/look-alike issues:

Glimepiride may be confused with glipiZIDE

Amaryl® may be confused with Altace®, Amerge®

High alert medication:

The Institute for Safe Medication Practices (ISMP) includes this medication among its list of drugs which have a heightened risk of causing significant patient harm when used in error.

International issues:

Amarel [France], Amaryl [U.S., Canada, and multiple international markets] may be confused with Reminyl brand name for galantamine [multiple international markets]

Amaryl [U.S., Canada, and multiple international markets] may be confused with Almarl brand name for arotinolol [Japan]

U.S. Brand Names Amaryl®

Canadian Brand Names Amaryl®; Apo-Glimepiride®; CO Glimepiride; Novo-Glimepiride; PMS-Glimepiride; ratio-Glimepiride; Rhoxal-glimepiride; Sandoz-Glimepiride

Therapeutic Category Antidiabetic Agent, Oral

Use Management of type 2 diabetes mellitus (noninsulin-dependent, NIDDM) as an adjunct to diet and exercise to lower blood glucose; may be used in combination with metformin or insulin in patients whose hyperglycemia cannot be controlled by diet and exercise in conjunction with a single oral hypoglycemic agent

General Dosage Range Dosage adjustment recommended in patients with renal impairment

Oral:

Adults: Initial: 1-2 mg once daily; Maintenance: 1-4 mg once daily (maximum: 8 mg/day)

Elderly: Initial: 1 mg/day

Dosage Forms

Tablet, oral: 1 mg, 2 mg, 4 mg

Amaryl®: 1 mg, 2 mg, 4 mg

glimepiride and pioglitazone *see* pioglitazone and glimepiride *on page 725*

glimepiride and pioglitazone hydrochloride *see* pioglitazone and glimepiride *on page 725*

glimepiride and rosiglitazone maleate *see* rosiglitazone and glimepiride *on page 811*

glipizide (GLIP i zide)

Medication Safety Issues

Sound-alike/look-alike issues:

GlipiZIDE may be confused with glimepiride, glyBURIDE

Glucotrol® may be confused with Glucophage®, Glucotrol® XL, glyBURIDE

High alert medication:

The Institute for Safe Medication Practices (ISMP) includes this medication among its list of drugs which have a heightened risk of causing significant patient harm when used in error.

Synonyms glydiazinamide

Tall-Man glipiZIDE

U.S. Brand Names Glucotrol XL®; Glucotrol®

Therapeutic Category Antidiabetic Agent, Oral

Use Management of type 2 diabetes mellitus (noninsulin-dependent, NIDDM)

General Dosage Range Dosage adjustment recommended in patients with hepatic impairment

Oral:

Immediate release:

Adults: Initial: 5 mg/day; Maintenance: Up to 40 mg/day

Elderly: Initial: 2.5 mg/day

Extended release: *Adults:* Initial: 5 mg/day; Maintenance: Up to 20 mg/day

Dosage Forms

Tablet, oral: 5 mg, 10 mg

Glucotrol®: 5 mg, 10 mg

Tablet, extended release, oral: 2.5 mg, 5 mg, 10 mg

Glucotrol XL®: 2.5 mg, 5 mg, 10 mg

glipizide and metformin (GLIP i zide & met FOR min)

Medication Safety Issues

High alert medication:

The Institute for Safe Medication Practices (ISMP) includes this medication among its list of drugs which have a heightened risk of causing significant patient harm when used in error.

Synonyms glipizide and metformin hydrochloride; metformin and glipizide

U.S. Brand Names Metaglip™

Therapeutic Category Antidiabetic Agent (Biguanide); Antidiabetic Agent (Sulfonylurea)

Use Indicated as an adjunct to diet and exercise to improve glycemic control in adults with type 2 diabetes mellitus (noninsulin-dependent, NIDDM)

General Dosage Range Oral: *Adults:* Initial: Glipizide 2.5 mg and metformin 250 mg once daily; Maintenance: Up to glipizide 20 mg/day and metformin 2000 mg/day in divided doses

Dosage Forms

Tablet, oral: 2.5/250: Glipizide 2.5 mg and metformin 250 mg; 2.5/500: Glipizide 2.5 mg and metformin 500 mg; 5/500: Glipizide 5 mg and metformin 500 mg

Metaglip™: 2.5/500: Glipizide 2.5 mg and metformin 500 mg; 5/500: Glipizide 5 mg and metformin 500 mg

glipizide and metformin hydrochloride *see* glipizide and metformin *on page 427*

Glivec *see* imatinib *on page 474*

GlucaGen® *see* glucagon *on page 427*

GlucaGen® Diagnostic Kit *see* glucagon *on page 427*

GlucaGen® HypoKit® *see* glucagon *on page 427*

glucagon (GLOO ka gon)

Synonyms glucagon hydrochloride

U.S. Brand Names GlucaGen®; GlucaGen® Diagnostic Kit; GlucaGen® HypoKit®; Glucagon Emergency Kit

Canadian Brand Names GlucaGen®; GlucaGen® HypoKit®

Therapeutic Category Antihypoglycemic Agent

Use Management of hypoglycemia; diagnostic aid in radiologic examinations to temporarily inhibit GI tract movement

General Dosage Range

I.M.:

Children <20 kg: 0.5 mg **or** 20-30 mcg/kg/dose, may repeat

Children ≥20 kg: 1 mg, may repeat

Adults: 1 mg, may repeat **or** 1-2 mg prior to gastrointestinal procedure

I.V.:

Children <20 kg: 0.5 mg or 20-30 mcg/kg/dose, may repeat

Children ≥20 kg: 1 mg, may repeat

Adults: 1 mg, may repeat in 20 minutes **or** 0.25-2 mg 10 minutes prior to gastrointestinal procedure

SubQ:

Children <20 kg: 0.5 mg **or** 20-30 mcg/kg/dose, may repeat

Children ≥20 kg and Adults: 1 mg, may repeat

Dosage Forms

Injection, powder for reconstitution:

GlucaGen®: 1 mg

GlucaGen® Diagnostic Kit: 1 mg

GlucaGen® HypoKit®: 1 mg

Glucagon Emergency Kit: 1 mg

Glucagon Emergency Kit *see* glucagon *on page 427*

glucagon hydrochloride *see* glucagon *on page 427*

Glucobay™ (Can) *see* acarbose *on page 19*

GlucoBurst® [OTC] *see* dextrose *on page 275*
GlucoNorm® (Can) *see* repaglinide *on page 794*
Glucophage® *see* metformin *on page 579*
Glucophage® XR *see* metformin *on page 579*
glucose *see* dextrose *on page 275*
glucose monohydrate *see* dextrose *on page 275*

glucose polymers (GLOO kose POL i merz)

U.S. Brand Names Polycose® [OTC]

Therapeutic Category Nutritional Supplement

Use Supplies calories for those persons not able to meet the caloric requirement with usual dietary intake

General Dosage Range Oral: *Adults:* Add to foods, beverages, or water as needed

Dosage Forms

Powder for suspension, oral:
Polycose® [OTC]: 349 g

Glucotrol® *see* glipizide *on page 426*
Glucotrol XL® *see* glipizide *on page 426*
Glucovance® *see* glyburide and metformin *on page 429*
glulisine insulin *see* insulin glulisine *on page 487*
Glumetza® *see* metformin *on page 579*
Glutofac®-MX *see* vitamins (multiple/oral) *on page 951*
Glutol™ [OTC] *see* dextrose *on page 275*
Glutose 15™ [OTC] *see* dextrose *on page 275*
Glutose 45™ [OTC] *see* dextrose *on page 275*
glybenclamide *see* glyburide *on page 428*
glybenzcyclamide *see* glyburide *on page 428*

glyburide (GLYE byoor ide)

Medication Safety Issues

Sound-alike/look-alike issues:
GlyBURIDE may be confused with glipiZIDE, Glucotrol®
Diaβeta® may be confused with Zebeta®
Micronase may be confused with microK®, miconazole, Micronor®, Microzide®

High alert medication:
The Institute for Safe Medication Practices (ISMP) includes this medication among its list of drugs which have a heightened risk of causing significant patient harm when used in error.

BEERS Criteria medication:
This drug may be potentially inappropriate for use in geriatric patients (Quality of evidence - high; Strength of recommendation - strong).

Synonyms glibenclamide; glybenclamide; glybenzcyclamide; Micronase

Tall-Man gly**BURIDE**

U.S. Brand Names DiaBeta®; Glynase® PresTab®

Canadian Brand Names Apo-Glyburide®; DiaBeta®; Dom-Glyburide; Euglucon®; Med-Glybe; Mylan-Glybe; Novo-Glyburide; Nu-Glyburide; PMS-Glyburide; PRO-Glyburide; ratio-Glyburide; Riva-Glyburide; Sandoz-Glyburide; Teva-Glyburide

Therapeutic Category Antidiabetic Agent, Oral

Use Adjunct to diet and exercise for the management of type 2 diabetes mellitus (noninsulin-dependent, NIDDM)

General Dosage Range Oral:
Regular tablets: *Adults:* Initial: 1.25-5 mg once daily; Maintenance: 1.25-20 mg/day as single or divided doses (maximum: 20 mg/day)
Micronized tablets: *Adults:* Initial: 0.75-3 mg once daily; Maintenance: 0.75-12 mg/day as single or divided doses (maximum: 12 mg/day)

Dosage Forms

Tablet, oral: 1.25 mg, 1.5 mg, 2.5 mg, 3 mg, 5 mg, 6 mg
DiaBeta®: 1.25 mg, 2.5 mg, 5 mg
Glynase® PresTab®: 1.5 mg, 3 mg, 6 mg

glyburide and metformin (GLYE byoor ide & met FOR min)

Medication Safety Issues

Sound-alike/look-alike issues:

Glucovance® may be confused with Vyvanse®

High alert medication:

The Institute for Safe Medication Practices (ISMP) includes this medication among its list of drugs which have a heightened risk of causing significant patient harm when used in error.

Synonyms glyburide and metformin hydrochloride; metformin and glyburide

U.S. Brand Names Glucovance®

Therapeutic Category Antidiabetic Agent (Sulfonylurea); Antidiabetic Agent, Oral

Use Adjunct to diet and exercise for the management of type 2 diabetes mellitus (noninsulin-dependent, NIDDM)

General Dosage Range Oral: *Adults:* Initial: Glyburide 1.25-5 mg and metformin 250-500 mg once or twice daily; Maintenance: Up to glyburide 20 mg/day and metformin 2000 mg/day

Dosage Forms

Tablet: Glyburide 1.25 mg and metformin 250 mg; glyburide 2.5 mg and metformin 500 mg; glyburide 5 mg and metformin 500 mg

Glucovance®: 2.5 mg/500 mg: Glyburide 2.5 mg and metformin 500 mg; 5 mg/500 mg: Glyburide 5 mg and metformin 500 mg

glyburide and metformin hydrochloride *see* glyburide and metformin *on page 429*

glycerin (GLIS er in)

Synonyms glycerol

U.S. Brand Names Fleet® Glycerin Suppositories [OTC]; Fleet® Liquid Glycerin [OTC]; Fleet® Pedia-Lax™ Glycerin Suppositories [OTC]; Fleet® Pedia-Lax™ Liquid Glycerin Suppositories [OTC]; Orajel® Dry Mouth [OTC]; Sani-Supp® [OTC]

Therapeutic Category Laxative; Ophthalmic Agent, Miscellaneous

Use Constipation; reduction of intraocular pressure; reduction of corneal edema; glycerin has been administered orally to reduce intracranial pressure

General Dosage Range

Ophthalmic: *Children and Adults:* Instill 1-2 drops in eye(s) once or every 3-4 hours

Oral: *Children and Adults:* 1.5 g/kg/day divided every 4 hours **or** 1 g/kg/dose every 6 hours **or** 1-1.8 g/kg once

Rectal:

Children <6 years: 1 infant suppository 1-2 times/day as needed **or** 2-5 mL as an enema

Children ≥6 years and Adults: 1 adult suppository 1-2 times/day as needed **or** 5-15 mL as an enema

Dosage Forms

Gel, oral:

Orajel® Dry Mouth [OTC]: 18% (42 g)

Liquid, for prescription compounding: USP: 100% (3840 mL)

Liquid, topical: USP: 100% (120 mL, 180 mL, 480 mL, 3840 mL)

Solution, rectal:

Fleet® Liquid Glycerin [OTC]: 5.6 g/5.5 mL (7.5 mL)

Fleet® Pedia-Lax™ Liquid Glycerin Suppositories [OTC]: 2.3 g/2.3 mL (4 mL)

Suppository, rectal: 82.5% (12s, 25s, 50s, 100s)

Fleet® Glycerin Suppositories [OTC]: 2 g (12s, 50s)

Fleet® Pedia-Lax™ Glycerin Suppositories [OTC]: 1 g (12s)

Sani-Supp® [OTC]: 82.5% (10s, 25s)

glycerol *see* glycerin *on page 429*

glycerol guaiacolate *see* guaifenesin *on page 433*

glyceryl trinitrate *see* nitroglycerin *on page 645*

Glycon (Can) *see* metformin *on page 579*

glycopyrrolate (glye koe PYE roe late)

Medication Safety Issues

International issues:

Robinul [U.S. and multiple international markets] may be confused with Reminyl brand name for galantamine [Canada and multiple international markets]

Synonyms glycopyrronium bromide

U.S. Brand Names Cuvposa™; Robinul®; Robinul® Forte

Canadian Brand Names Glycopyrrolate Injection, USP

Therapeutic Category Anticholinergic Agent

Use Inhibit salivation and excessive secretions of the respiratory tract preoperatively; control of upper airway secretions; intraoperatively to counteract drug-induced or vagal mediated bradyarrhythmias; adjunct in treatment of peptic ulcer (indication listed in product labeling but currently has no place in management of peptic ulcer disease)

Cuvposa™: Reduce chronic, severe drooling in those with neurologic conditions (eg, cerebral palsy) associated with drooling

General Dosage Range

I.M.:

Children <2 years: 4-9 mcg/kg once **or** 4-10 mcg/kg every 3-4 hours (maximum: 0.2 mg/dose; 0.8 mg/day)

Children ≥2 years: 4 mcg/kg once **or** 4-10 mcg/kg every 3-4 hours (maximum: 0.2 mg/dose; 0.8 mg/day)

Adults: 4 mcg/kg once **or** 0.1-0.2 mg 3-4 times/day

I.V.:

Children: 4-10 mcg/kg every 3-4 hours (maximum: 0.2 mg/dose; 0.8 mg/day) **or** 4 mcg/kg (maximum: 0.1 mg); repeat as needed

Adults: 0.1-0.2 mg 3-4 times/day **or** 0.1 mg repeated as needed

Oral: *Children 3-16 years:* 0.02-0.1 mg/kg/dose 3 times/day (maximum 3 mg/dose)

Dosage Forms

Injection, solution: 0.2 mg/mL (1 mL, 2 mL, 5 mL, 20 mL)

Robinul®: 0.2 mg/mL (1 mL, 2 mL, 5 mL, 20 mL)

Solution, oral:

Cuvposa™: 1 mg/5 mL (473 mL)

Tablet, oral: 1 mg, 2 mg

Robinul®: 1 mg

Robinul® Forte: 2 mg

Glycopyrrolate Injection, USP (Can) *see* glycopyrrolate *on page 429*

glycopyrronium bromide *see* glycopyrrolate *on page 429*

glycosum *see* dextrose *on page 275*

glydiazinamide *see* glipizide *on page 426*

Glynase® PresTab® *see* glyburide *on page 428*

Gly-Oxide® [OTC] *see* carbamide peroxide *on page 173*

Glyquin® XM (Can) *see* hydroquinone *on page 461*

Glyset® *see* miglitol *on page 602*

GM-CSF *see* sargramostim *on page 824*

GMD-Gemfibrozil (Can) *see* gemfibrozil *on page 422*

GnRH *see* gonadorelin *(Canada only) on page 431*

gold sodium thiomalate (gold SOW dee um thye oh MAL ate)

Synonyms sodium aurothiomalate

U.S. Brand Names Myochrysine® [DSC]

Canadian Brand Names Myochrysine®

Therapeutic Category Gold Compound

Use Adjunctive treatment of active rheumatoid arthritis

General Dosage Range Dosage adjustment recommended in patients with renal impairment or who develop toxicities

I.M.:

Children: Test dose (recommended): 10 mg first week; Initial dosing: 1 mg/kg/week (maximum: 50 mg/injection); Maintenance: 1 mg/kg/dose (maximum: 50 mg/injection)

Adults: Test dose: 10 mg first week; Initial dosing: 25 mg second week, then 25-50 mg/week until 1 g cumulative dose has been given; Maintenance: 25-50 mg every other week for 2-20 weeks, then every 3-4 weeks

golimumab (goe LIM ue mab)

Synonyms CNTO-148

U.S. Brand Names Simponi®

Canadian Brand Names Simponi®

Therapeutic Category Antipsoriatic Agent; Antirheumatic, Disease Modifying; Monoclonal Antibody; Tumor Necrosis Factor (TNF) Blocking Agent

Use Treatment of active rheumatoid arthritis (moderate-to-severe), active psoriatic arthritis, and active ankylosing spondylitis

General Dosage Range SubQ: *Adults:* 50 mg once per month

Dosage Forms

Injection, solution [preservative free]:
Simponi®: 50 mg/0.5 mL (0.5 mL)

GoLYTELY® *see* polyethylene glycol-electrolyte solution *on page 738*

gonadorelin acetate *see* gonadorelin *(Canada only) on page 431*

gonadorelin *(Canada only)* (goe nad oh RELL in)

Synonyms GnRH; gonadorelin acetate; gonadotropin releasing hormone; LHRH; LRH; luteinizing hormone releasing hormone

Canadian Brand Names Lutrepulse™

Therapeutic Category Gonadotropin

Use Induction of ovulation in females with hypothalamic amenorrhea

General Dosage Range I.V., SubQ: *Adults:* 1-20 mcg every 90 minutes

Product Availability Not available in U.S.

Dosage Forms - Canada

Injection, powder for reconstitution:
Lutrepulse®: 0.8 mg, 3.2 mg

gonadotropin releasing hormone *see* gonadorelin *(Canada only) on page 431*

Gonak™ *see* hydroxypropyl methylcellulose *on page 463*

Gonal-f® *see* follitropin alfa *on page 404*

Gonal-f® Pen (Can) *see* follitropin alfa *on page 404*

Gonal-f® RFF *see* follitropin alfa *on page 404*

Gonal-f® RFF Pen *see* follitropin alfa *on page 404*

gonioscopic ophthalmic solution *see* hydroxypropyl methylcellulose *on page 463*

Goniosoft™ [OTC] *see* hydroxypropyl methylcellulose *on page 463*

Goody's® Extra Strength Headache Powder [OTC] *see* acetaminophen, aspirin, and caffeine *on page 26*

Goody's® Extra Strength Pain Relief [OTC] *see* acetaminophen, aspirin, and caffeine *on page 26*

Goody's PM® [OTC] *see* acetaminophen and diphenhydramine *on page 23*

Gordofilm [OTC] *see* salicylic acid *on page 816*

Gordon Boro-Packs [OTC] *see* aluminum sulfate and calcium acetate *on page 57*

Gordon's® Urea [OTC] *see* urea *on page 930*

Gormel® [OTC] *see* urea *on page 930*

Gormel® Ten [OTC] *see* urea *on page 930*

goserelin (GOE se rel in)

Synonyms goserelin acetate; ICI-118630; ZDX

U.S. Brand Names Zoladex®

Canadian Brand Names Zoladex®; Zoladex® LA

Therapeutic Category Gonadotropin-Releasing Hormone Analog

Use Treatment of locally confined prostate cancer; palliative treatment of advanced prostate cancer; palliative treatment of advanced breast cancer in pre- and perimenopausal women; treatment of endometriosis, including pain relief and reduction of endometriotic lesions; endometrial thinning agent as part of treatment for dysfunctional uterine bleeding

General Dosage Range SubQ: *Adults:* 3.6 mg every 28 days **or** 10.8 mg every 12 weeks

Dosage Forms

Implant, subcutaneous:

Zoladex®: 3.6 mg (1s); 10.8 mg (1s)

goserelin acetate *see* goserelin *on page* 431

GP 47680 *see* oxcarbazepine *on page* 676

GPI 15715 *see* fospropofol *on page* 410

GR38032R *see* ondansetron *on page* 667

Gralise™ *see* gabapentin *on page* 413

gramicidin, neomycin, and polymyxin B *see* neomycin, polymyxin B, and gramicidin *on page* 634

granisetron (gra NI se tron)

Medication Safety Issues

Sound-alike/look-alike issues:

Granisetron may be confused with dolasetron, ondansetron, palonosetron

Synonyms BRL 43694; Kytril

U.S. Brand Names Granisol™; Sancuso®

Canadian Brand Names Granisetron Hydrochloride Injection; Kytril®

Therapeutic Category Selective 5-HT_3 Receptor Antagonist

Use Prophylaxis of nausea and vomiting associated with emetogenic chemotherapy and radiation therapy; prophylaxis and treatment of postoperative nausea and vomiting (PONV)

General Dosage Range

I.V.:

Children ≥2 years: 10 mcg/kg/dose (maximum: 1 mg/dose) as a single dose or every 12 hours

Adults: 10 mcg/kg/dose (maximum: 1 mg/dose) as a single dose or every 12 hours **or** 1 mg as a single dose

Oral: *Adults:* 2 mg/day in 1-2 divided dose

Transdermal: *Adults:* 1 patch prior to chemotherapy; Maximum duration: Patch may be worn up to 7 days

Dosage Forms

Injection, solution: 1 mg/mL (1 mL, 4 mL)

Injection, solution [preservative free]: 0.1 mg/mL (1 mL); 1 mg/mL (1 mL)

Patch, transdermal:

Sancuso®: 3.1 mg/24 hours (1s)

Solution, oral:

Granisol™: 2 mg/10 mL (30 mL)

Tablet, oral: 1 mg

Granisetron Hydrochloride Injection (Can) *see* granisetron *on page* 432

Granisol™ *see* granisetron *on page* 432

Granulex® *see* trypsin, balsam Peru, and castor oil *on page* 925

granulocyte colony stimulating factor *see* filgrastim *on page* 384

granulocyte colony stimulating factor (PEG conjugate) *see* pegfilgrastim *on page* 696

granulocyte-macrophage colony-stimulating factor *see* sargramostim *on page* 824

Gravol® [OTC] (Can) *see* dimenhydrinate *on page* 289

Gravol IM (Can) *see* dimenhydrinate *on page* 289

green tea extract *see* sinecatechins *on page* 836

Grifulvin V® *see* griseofulvin *on page* 432

griseofulvin (gri see oh FUL vin)

Synonyms griseofulvin microsize; griseofulvin ultramicrosize

U.S. Brand Names Grifulvin V®; Gris-PEG®

Therapeutic Category Antifungal Agent

Use Treatment of susceptible tinea infections of the skin, hair, and nails

General Dosage Range Oral:

Microsize:

Children >2 years: 10-20 mg/kg/day in single or divided doses

Adults: 500-1000 mg/day in single or divided doses

Ultramicrosize:
Children >2 years: 5-15 mg/kg/day in single dose or 2 divided doses (maximum: 750 mg/day)
Adults: 375-750 mg/day in single or divided doses

Dosage Forms

Suspension, oral: 125 mg/5 mL (118 mL, 120 mL)

Tablet, oral:
Grifulvin V®: 500 mg
Gris-PEG®: 125 mg, 250 mg

griseofulvin microsize *see* griseofulvin *on page* 432
griseofulvin ultramicrosize *see* griseofulvin *on page* 432
Gris-PEG® *see* griseofulvin *on page* 432
growth hormone, human *see* somatropin *on page* 849
GSK-580299 *see* papillomavirus (types 16, 18) vaccine (human, recombinant) *on page* 691
GSK 1838262 *see* gabapentin enacarbil *on page* 414
Guaiatussin AC *see* guaifenesin and codeine *on page* 434
Guaicon DMS [OTC] *see* guaifenesin and dextromethorphan *on page* 434

guaifenesin (gwye FEN e sin)

Medication Safety Issues

Sound-alike/look-alike issues:
GuaiFENesin may be confused with guanFACINE
Mucinex® may be confused with Mucomyst®

Synonyms cheratussin; GG; glycerol guaiacolate

Tall-Man guai**FEN**esin

U.S. Brand Names Allfen [OTC]; Bidex®-400 [OTC]; Diabetic Siltussin DAS-Na [OTC]; Diabetic Tussin® EX [OTC]; Fenesin IR [OTC]; Geri-Tussin [OTC]; Humibid® Maximum Strength [OTC]; Iophen NR [OTC]; Liquituss GG [OTC]; Mucinex® Kid's Mini-Melts™ [OTC]; Mucinex® Kid's [OTC]; Mucinex® Maximum Strength [OTC]; Mucinex® [OTC]; Mucus Relief [OTC] [DSC]; Organ-I NR [OTC]; Q-Tussin [OTC]; Refenesen™ 400 [OTC]; Refenesen™ [OTC]; Robafen [OTC]; Scot-Tussin® Expectorant [OTC]; Siltussin SA [OTC]; Vicks® Casero™ Chest Congestion Relief [OTC]; Vicks® DayQuil® Mucus Control [OTC]; Xpect™ [OTC]

Canadian Brand Names Balminil Expectorant; Benylin® E Extra Strength; Koffex Expectorant; Robitussin®

Therapeutic Category Expectorant

Use Help loosen phlegm and thin bronchial secretions to make coughs more productive

General Dosage Range Oral:

Extended release: *Children ≥12 years and Adults:* 600-1200 mg every 12 hours (maximum: 2.4 g/day)
Immediate release:
Children 6 months to 2 years: 25-50 mg every 4 hours (maximum: 300 mg/day)
Children 2-5 years: 50-100 mg every 4 hours (maximum: 600 mg/day)
Children 6-11 years: 100-200 mg every 4 hours (maximum: 1.2 g/day)
Children ≥12 years and Adults: 200-400 mg every 4 hours (maximum: 2.4 g/day)

Dosage Forms

Caplet, oral:
Fenesin IR [OTC]: 400 mg
Refenesen™ 400 [OTC]: 400 mg

Granules, oral:
Mucinex® Kid's Mini-Melts™ [OTC]: 50 mg/packet (12s); 100 mg/packet (12s)

Liquid, oral:
Diabetic Tussin® EX [OTC]: 100 mg/5 mL (118 mL)
Iophen NR [OTC]: 100 mg/5 mL (480 mL)
Liquituss GG [OTC]: 200 mg/5 mL (118 mL, 473 mL)
Mucinex® Kid's [OTC]: 100 mg/5 mL (118 mL)
Q-Tussin [OTC]: 100 mg/5 mL (118 mL, 237 mL, 473 mL)
Scot-Tussin® Expectorant [OTC]: 100 mg/5 mL (120 mL)
Vicks® Casero™ Chest Congestion Relief [OTC]: 100 mg/6.25 mL (120 mL, 240 mL)
Vicks® DayQuil® Mucus Control [OTC]: 200 mg/15 mL (295 mL)

Syrup, oral: 100 mg/5 mL (5 mL, 10 mL, 15 mL, 118 mL, 240 mL, 473 mL)
Diabetic Siltussin DAS-Na [OTC]: 100 mg/5 mL (118 mL)
Geri-Tussin [OTC]: 100 mg/5 mL (480 mL)
Robafen [OTC]: 100 mg/5 mL (120 mL, 240 mL, 480 mL)
Siltussin SA [OTC]: 100 mg/5 mL (120 mL, 240 mL, 480 mL)
Tablet, oral: 200 mg, 400 mg
Allfen [OTC]: 400 mg
Bidex®-400 [OTC]: 400 mg
Organ-I NR [OTC]: 200 mg
Refenesen™ [OTC]: 200 mg
Xpect™ [OTC]: 400 mg
Tablet, extended release, oral:
Humibid® Maximum Strength [OTC]: 1200 mg
Mucinex® [OTC]: 600 mg
Mucinex® Maximum Strength [OTC]: 1200 mg

guaifenesin and codeine (gwye FEN e sin & KOE deen)

Synonyms codeine and guaifenesin; Robitussin AC

U.S. Brand Names Allfen CD; Allfen CDX; Codar® GF; Dex-Tuss; Guaiatussin AC; Iophen C-NR; M-Clear; M-Clear WC; Mar-Cof® CG; Robafen AC

Therapeutic Category Antitussive/Expectorant

Controlled Substance Capsule: C-V; Liquid products: C-V; Tablet: C-III

Use Temporary control of cough due to minor throat and bronchial irritation

General Dosage Range Oral: *Children ≥6 years and Adults:* Dosage varies greatly depending on product

Dosage Forms

Capsule, oral:
M-Clear: Guaifenesin 200 mg and codeine 9 mg
Liquid, oral:
Codar® GF: Guaifenesin 200 mg and codeine 8 mg per 5 mL
Dex-Tuss: Guaifenesin 300 mg and codeine 10 mg per 5 mL
Iophen C-NR: Guaifenesin 100 mg and codeine 10 mg per 5 mL
M-Clear WC: Guaifenesin 100 mg and codeine 6.33 mg per 5 mL
Solution, oral: Guaifenesin 100 mg and codeine 10 mg per 5 mL
Mar-Cof® CG: Guaifenesin 225 mg and codeine 7.5 mg per 5 mL
Syrup, oral: Guaifenesin 100 mg and codeine 10 mg per 5 mL (473 mL)
Guaiatussin AC, Robafen AC: Guaifenesin 100 mg and codeine 10 mg per 5 mL
Tablet, oral:
Allfen CD: Guaifenesin 400 mg and codeine 10 mg
Allfen CDX: Guaifenesin 400 mg and codeine 20 mg

guaifenesin and dextromethorphan (gwye FEN e sin & deks troe meth OR fan)

Medication Safety Issues

Sound-alike/look-alike issues:
Benylin® may be confused with Benadryl®, Ventolin®

Synonyms dextromethorphan and guaifenesin

U.S. Brand Names Cheracol® D [OTC]; Cheracol® Plus [OTC]; Coricidin HBP® Chest Congestion and Cough [OTC]; Diabetic Siltussin-DM DAS-Na Maximum Strength [OTC]; Diabetic Siltussin-DM DAS-Na [OTC]; Diabetic Tussin® DM Maximum Strength [OTC]; Diabetic Tussin® DM [OTC]; Double Tussin DM [OTC]; Fenesin DM IR [OTC]; Guaicon DMS [OTC]; Iophen DM-NR [OTC]; Kolephrin® GG/DM [OTC]; Mucinex® DM Maximum Strength [OTC]; Mucinex® DM [OTC]; Mucinex® Kid's Cough Mini-Melts™ [OTC]; Mucinex® Kid's Cough [OTC]; Q-Tussin DM [OTC]; Refenesen™ DM [OTC]; Robafen DM Clear [OTC]; Robafen DM [OTC]; Robitussin® Peak Cold Cough + Chest Congestion DM [OTC]; Robitussin® Peak Cold Maximum Strength Cough + Chest Congestion DM [OTC]; Robitussin® Peak Cold Sugar-Free Cough + Chest Congestion DM [OTC]; Safe Tussin® DM [OTC]; Scot-Tussin® Senior [OTC]; Silexin [OTC]; Siltussin DM DAS [OTC]; Siltussin DM [OTC]; Vicks® 44E [OTC]; Vicks® DayQuil® Mucus Control DM [OTC]; Vicks® Nature Fusion™ Cough & Chest Congestion [OTC]; Vicks® Pediatric Formula 44E [OTC]

Canadian Brand Names Balminil DM E; Benylin® DM-E

Therapeutic Category Antitussive/Expectorant

Use Temporary control of cough due to minor throat and bronchial irritation

General Dosage Range Oral:

Children 2-6 years: Guaifenesin 50-100 mg and dextromethorphan 2.5-5 mg every 4 hours (maximum: Guaifenesin 600 mg/day; Dextromethorphan 30 mg/day)

Children 6-12 years: Guaifenesin 100-200 mg and dextromethorphan 5-10 mg every 4 hours (maximum: Guaifenesin 1200 mg/day; Dextromethorphan 60 mg/day)

Children ≥12 years and Adults: Guaifenesin 200-400 mg and dextromethorphan 10-20 mg every 4 hours (maximum: Guaifenesin 2400 mg/day; Dextromethorphan 120 mg/day)

Dosage Forms

Caplet, oral:

Fenesin DM IR [OTC]: Guaifenesin 400 mg and dextromethorphan 15 mg

Refenesen™ DM [OTC]: Guaifenesin 400 mg and dextromethorphan 20 mg

Capsule, softgel, oral:

Coricidin HBP® Chest Congestion and Cough [OTC]: Guaifenesin 200 mg and dextromethorphan 10 mg

Granules, oral:

Mucinex® Kid's Cough Mini-Melts™: Guaifenesin 100 mg and dextromethorphan 5 mg per packet (12s)

Liquid, oral: Guaifenesin 100 mg and dextromethorphan 10 mg per 5 mL

Diabetic Tussin® DM [OTC], Iophen DM-NR [OTC]: Guaifenesin 100 mg and dextromethorphan 10 mg per 5 mL

Iophen DM-NR: Guaifenesin 100 mg and dextromethorphan hydrobromide 10 mg per 5 mL (480 mL)

Diabetic Tussin® DM Maximum Strength [OTC]: Guaifenesin 200 mg and dextromethorphan 10 mg per 5 mL

Double Tussin DM [OTC]: Guaifenesin 300 mg and dextromethorphan 20 mg per 5 mL

Kolephrin® GG/DM [OTC]: Guaifenesin 150 mg and dextromethorphan 10 mg per 5 mL

Mucinex® Kid's Cough: Guaifenesin 100 mg and dextromethorphan 5 mg per 5 mL

Safe Tussin® DM [OTC]: Guaifenesin 100 mg and dextromethorphan 15 mg per 5 mL

Scot-Tussin® Senior [OTC]: Guaifenesin 200 mg and dextromethorphan 15 mg per 5 mL

Vicks® 44E [OTC]: Guaifenesin 200 mg and dextromethorphan 20 mg per 15 mL

Vicks® DayQuil® Mucus Control DM [OTC]: Guaifenesin 200 mg and dextromethorphan 10 mg per 15 mL

Vicks® Nature Fusion™ Cough & Chest Congestion [OTC]: Guaifenesin 200 mg and dextromethorphan 20 mg per 30 mL

Vicks® Pediatric Formula 44E [OTC]: Guaifenesin 100 mg and dextromethorphan 10 mg per 15 mL

Syrup, oral: Guaifenesin 100 mg and dextromethorphan 10 mg per 5 mL

Cheracol® D [OTC], Cheracol® Plus [OTC], Diabetic Siltussin-DM DAS-Na [OTC], Diabetic Siltussin-DM DAS-Na Maximum Strength [OTC], Guaicon DMS [OTC], Robafen DM [OTC], Robafen DM Clear [OTC], Robitussin® Peak Cold Cough + Chest Congestion DM [OTC], Robitussin® Peak Cold Sugar-Free Cough + Chest Congestion DM [OTC], Silexin [OTC], Siltussin DM [OTC], Siltussin DM DAS [OTC]: Guaifenesin 100 mg and dextromethorphan 10 mg per 5 mL

Q-Tussin DM [OTC]: Guaifenesin 100 mg and dextromethorphan 10 mg per 5 mL

Robitussin® Peak Cold Maximum Strength Cough + Chest Congestion DM [OTC]: Guaifenesin 200 mg and dextromethorphan 10 mg per 5 mL

Tablet, oral: Guaifenesin 1000 mg and dextromethorphan 60 mg; guaifenesin 1200 mg and dextromethorphan 60 mg

Silexin [OTC]: Guaifenesin 100 mg and dextromethorphan 10 mg

Tablet, extended release, oral:

Mucinex® DM [OTC]: Guaifenesin 600 mg and dextromethorphan 30 mg

Mucinex® DM Maximum Strength [OTC]: Guaifenesin 1200 mg and dextromethorphan 60 mg

Tablet, timed release, oral [scored]: Guaifenesin 1200 mg and dextromethorphan 60 mg

guaifenesin and dyphylline *see* dyphylline and guaifenesin *on page 321*

guaifenesin and phenylephrine (gwye FEN e sin & fen il EF rin)

Medication Safety Issues

Sound-alike/look-alike issues:

Entex® may be confused with Tenex®

Entex® LA brand name represents a different product in the U.S. than it does in Canada. Formerly available in the U.S., Entex® LA contains guaifenesin and phenylephrine, while in Canada the product bearing this brand name contains guaifenesin and pseudoephedrine.

Synonyms guaifenesin and phenylephrine tannate; phenylephrine hydrochloride and guaifenesin

U.S. Brand Names Ambi 10PEH/400GFN [OTC]; Crantex® [DSC]; Fenesin PE IR; J-Max [OTC]; Liquibid® D-R [OTC]; Liquibid® PD-R [OTC]; Medent®-PEI [OTC]; Mucinex® Cold [OTC]; Mucus Relief Sinus [OTC]; Nu-COPD [OTC]; OneTab™ Congestion & Cold [OTC]; Refenesen™ PE [OTC]; Rescon GG [OTC]; Sudafed PE® Non-Drying Sinus [OTC]; Triaminic® Children's Chest & Nasal Congestion [OTC]

Therapeutic Category Cold Preparation

Use Temporary relief of nasal congestion, sinusitis, rhinitis, and hay fever; temporary relief of cough associated with upper respiratory tract conditions, especially when associated with dry, nonproductive cough

General Dosage Range Oral: *Children >2 years and Adults:* Dosage varies greatly depending on product

Dosage Forms

Caplet, oral:

Fenesin PE IR, OneTab™ Congestion & Cold [OTC], Refenesen™ PE [OTC]: Guaifenesin 400 mg and phenylephrine 10 mg

Sudafed PE® Non-Drying Sinus [OTC]: Guaifenesin 200 mg and phenylephrine 5 mg

Liquid, oral:

Mucinex® Cold [OTC]: Guaifenesin 100 mg and phenylephrine 2.5 mg per 5 mL (480 mL)

Nu-COPD [OTC]: Guaifenesin 200 mg and phenylephrine 10 mg per 5 mL (480 mL)

Rescon GG [OTC]: Guaifenesin 100 mg and phenylephrine 5 mg per 5 mL (120 mL, 480 mL)

Syrup, oral:

J-Max [OTC]: Guaifenesin 200 mg and phenylephrine hydrochloride 5 mg per 5 mL (473 mL)

Triaminic® Children's Chest & Nasal Congestion [OTC]: Guaifenesin 50 mg and phenylephrine 2.5 mg per 5 mL (118 mL)

Tablet, oral:

Ambi 10PEH/400GFN [OTC], Liquibid® D-R [OTC], Medent®-PEI [OTC], Mucus Relief Sinus [OTC], Nu-COPD [OTC]: Guaifenesin 400 mg and phenylephrine 10 mg

Liquibid® PD-R [OTC]: Guaifenesin 200 mg and phenylephrine 5 mg

guaifenesin and phenylephrine tannate *see* guaifenesin and phenylephrine *on page* 435

guaifenesin and pseudoephedrine (gwye FEN e sin & soo doe e FED rin)

Medication Safety Issues

Sound-alike/look-alike issues:

Entex® may be confused with Tenex®

Entex® LA brand name represents a different product in the U.S. than it does in Canada. In the U.S., Entex® LA contains guaifenesin and phenylephrine, while in Canada the product bearing this brand name contains guaifenesin and pseudoephedrine.

Synonyms pseudoephedrine and guaifenesin

U.S. Brand Names Ambifed-G [OTC]; Congestac® [OTC]; ExeFen-IR; Maxifed [OTC]; Maxifed-G [OTC]; Mucinex® D Maximum Strength [OTC]; Mucinex® D [OTC]; Refenesen Plus [OTC]; SudaTex-G [OTC]

Canadian Brand Names Contac® Cold-Chest Congestion, Non Drowsy, Regular Strength; Entex® LA; Novahistex® Expectorant with Decongestant

Therapeutic Category Expectorant/Decongestant

Use Temporary relief of nasal congestion and to help loosen phlegm and thin bronchial secretions in the treatment of cough

General Dosage Range Oral: *Children >2 years and Adults:* Dosage varies greatly depending on product

Dosage Forms

Caplet, oral:

Congestac® [OTC], Refenesen Plus [OTC]: Guaifenesin 400 mg and pseudoephedrine 60 mg

Tablet, oral:

Ambifed-G [OTC]: Guaifenesin 400 mg and pseudoephedrine 20 mg

ExeFen-IR: Guaifenesin 400 mg and pseudoephedrine 30 mg

Maxifed [OTC]: Guaifenesin 400 mg and pseudoephedrine 60 mg

Maxifed-G [OTC], SudaTex-G [OTC]: Guaifenesin 400 mg and pseudoephedrine 40 mg

Tablet, extended release, oral:

Mucinex® D [OTC]: Guaifenesin 600 mg and pseudoephedrine 60 mg

Mucinex® D Maximum Strength [OTC]: Guaifenesin 1200 mg and pseudoephedrine 120 mg

guaifenesin, dextromethorphan, and phenylephrine

(gwye FEN e sin, deks troe meth OR fan, & fen il EF rin)

Synonyms dextromethorphan hydrobromide, guaifenesin, and phenylephrine hydrochloride; guaifenesin, dextromethorphan hydrobromide, and phenylephrine hydrochloride; phenylephrine hydrochloride, guaifenesin, and dextromethorphan hydrobromide

U.S. Brand Names Maxiphen DM; Maxiphen DMX; Mucinex® Children's Multi-Symptom Cold [OTC]; Robafen CF Cough & Cold [OTC]; Robitussin® Children's Cough & Cold CF [OTC]; Robitussin® Cough & Cold CF Max [OTC] [DSC]; Robitussin® Cough & Cold CF [OTC] [DSC]; Robitussin® Peak Cold Maximum Strength Multi-Symptom Cold [OTC]; Robitussin® Peak Cold Multi-Symptom Cold [OTC]; SINUtuss® DM [DSC]; Tusso™-DMR [DSC]

Therapeutic Category Antitussive; Decongestant

Use Symptomatic relief of dry nonproductive coughs and upper respiratory symptoms associated with hay fever, colds, or the flu

General Dosage Range Oral: *Children >4 years and Adults:* Dosage varies greatly depending on product

Dosage Forms

Liquid, oral:

Maxiphen DMX: Guaifenesin 200 mg, dextromethorphan 20 mg, and phenylephrine 10 mg per 5 mL

Mucinex® Children's Multi-Symptom Cold [OTC]: Guaifenesin 100 mg, dextromethorphan 5 mg, and phenylephrine 2.5 mg per 5 mL

Robitussin® Children's Cough & Cold CF [OTC]: Guaifenesin 50 mg, dextromethorphan 5 mg, and phenylephrine 2.5 mg per 5 mL

Robitussin® Peak Cold Maximum Strength Multi-Symptom Cold [OTC]: Guaifenesin 200 mg, dextromethorphan 10 mg, and phenylephrine 5 mg per 5 mL

Robitussin® Peak Cold Multi-Symptom Cold [OTC]: Guaifenesin 100 mg, dextromethorphan 10 mg, and phenylephrine 5 mg per 5 mL

Syrup, oral:

Robafen CF Cough & Cold [OTC]: Guaifenesin 100 mg, dextromethorphan 10 mg, and phenylephrine 5 mg per 5 mL

Tablet, oral [scored]:

Maxiphen DM: Guaifenesin 400 mg, dextromethorphan 20 mg, and phenylephrine 10 mg

guaifenesin, dextromethorphan hydrobromide, and phenylephrine hydrochloride *see* guaifenesin, dextromethorphan, and phenylephrine *on page 437*

guaifenesin, pseudoephedrine, and codeine

(gwye FEN e sin, soo doe e FED rin, & KOE deen)

Synonyms codeine, guaifenesin, and pseudoephedrine; pseudoephedrine, guaifenesin, and codeine

U.S. Brand Names Cheratussin® DAC; Mytussin® DAC; Tricode® GF

Canadian Brand Names Benylin® 3.3 mg-D-E; Calmylin with Codeine

Therapeutic Category Antitussive/Decongestant/Expectorant

Controlled Substance C-V

Use Temporarily relieves nasal congestion and controls cough associated with upper respiratory infections and related conditions (common cold, sinusitis, bronchitis, influenza)

General Dosage Range Oral:

Children 6-12 years: 5 mL every 4 hours (maximum: 20 mL/24 hours)

Children >12 years and Adults: 10 mL every 4 hours (maximum: 40 mL/24 hours)

Dosage Forms

Syrup, oral: Guaifenesin 100 mg, pseudoephedrine 30 mg, and codeine 10 mg per 5 mL (473 mL)

Cheratussin® DAC: Guaifenesin 100 mg, pseudoephedrine 30 mg and codeine 10 mg per 5 mL (473 mL)

Mytussin® DAC: Guaifenesin 100 mg, pseudoephedrine 30 mg, and codeine 10 mg per 5 mL (118 mL, 473 mL)

Tricode® GF: Guaifenesin 200 mg, pseudoephedrine 30 mg, and codeine 8 mg per 5 mL (473 mL)

guaifenesin, pseudoephedrine, and dextromethorphan

(gwye FEN e sin, soo doe e FED rin, & deks troe meth OR fan)

Synonyms dextromethorphan, guaifenesin, and pseudoephedrine; pseudoephedrine, dextromethorphan, and guaifenesin

U.S. Brand Names Ambifed DM; Ambifed-G DM; ExeFen-DMX; Maxifed DM; Maxifed DMX

Canadian Brand Names Balminil DM + Decongestant + Expectorant; Benylin® DM-D-E

Therapeutic Category Cold Preparation

Use Temporarily relieves nasal congestion and controls cough due to minor throat and bronchial irritation; helps loosen phlegm and thin bronchial secretions to make coughs more productive

General Dosage Range Oral: *Children ≥6 years and Adults:* Dosage varies greatly depending on product

Dosage Forms

Liquid, oral:

Maxifed DM: Guaifenesin 200 mg, pseudoephedrine 20 mg, and dextromethorphan 10 mg per 5 mL

Tablet, oral:

Ambifed DM: Guaifenesin 400 mg, pseudoephedrine 30 mg, and dextromethorphan 20 mg

Ambifed-G DM: Guaifenesin 400 mg, pseudoephedrine 20 mg, and dextromethorphan 20 mg

ExeFen-DMX, Maxifed DMX: Guaifenesin 400 mg, pseudoephedrine 60 mg, and dextromethorphan 20 mg

Maxifed DM: Guaifenesin 400 mg, pseudoephedrine 40 mg, and dextromethorphan 20 mg

guanfacine (GWAHN fa seen)

Medication Safety Issues

Sound-alike/look-alike issues:

GuanFACINE may be confused with guaiFENesin, guanabenz, guanidine

Tenex® may be confused with Entex®, Xanax®

BEERS Criteria medication:

This drug may be potentially inappropriate for use in geriatric patients (Quality of evidence - low; Strength of recommendation - strong).

International issues:

Tenex [U.S., Canada] may be confused with Kinex brand name for biperiden [Mexico]

Synonyms guanfacine hydrochloride

Tall-Man guan**FACINE**

U.S. Brand Names Intuniv®; Tenex®

Therapeutic Category Alpha-Adrenergic Agonist

Use

Tablet, immediate release: Management of hypertension

Tablet, extended release: Treatment of attention-deficit/hyperactivity disorder (ADHD) as monotherapy or adjunctive therapy to stimulants

General Dosage Range Oral:

Immediate release: *Children ≥12 years and Adults:* 0.5-2 mg once daily

Extended release: *Children ≥6 years and Adolescents:* 1-4 mg once daily

Dosage Forms

Tablet, oral: 1 mg, 2 mg

Tenex®: 1 mg, 2 mg

Tablet, extended release, oral:

Intuniv®: 1 mg, 2 mg, 3 mg, 4 mg

guanfacine hydrochloride *see* guanfacine *on page 438*

guanidine (GWAHN i deen)

Medication Safety Issues

Sound-alike/look-alike issues:

Guanidine may be confused with guanFACINE

Synonyms guanidine hydrochloride

Therapeutic Category Cholinergic Agent

Use Reduction of the symptoms of muscle weakness associated with the myasthenic syndrome of Eaton-Lambert, not for myasthenia gravis

General Dosage Range Oral: *Adults:* Initial: 10-15 mg/kg/day in 3-4 divided doses; Maintenance: Up to 35 mg/kg/day

Dosage Forms

Tablet, oral: 125 mg

guanidine hydrochloride *see* guanidine *on page 438*

gum benjamin *see* benzoin *on page 124*

GW506U78 *see* nelarabine *on page 632*

GW-1000-02 *see* tetrahydrocannabinol and cannabidiol *(Canada only) on page 884*

GW433908G *see* fosamprenavir *on page 407*
GW572016 *see* lapatinib *on page 523*
GW786034 *see* pazopanib *on page 694*
Gynazole-1® [DSC] *see* butoconazole *on page 155*
Gynazole-1® (Can) *see* butoconazole *on page 155*
Gyne-Lotrimin® 3 [OTC] *see* clotrimazole (topical) *on page 227*
Gyne-Lotrimin® 7 [OTC] *see* clotrimazole (topical) *on page 227*
Gynol II® [OTC] *see* nonoxynol 9 *on page 647*
Gynol II® Extra Strength [OTC] *see* nonoxynol 9 *on page 647*
Gynovite® Plus [OTC] *see* vitamins (multiple/oral) *on page 951*
H1N1 influenza vaccine *see* influenza virus vaccine (inactivated) *on page 482*
H1N1 influenza vaccine *see* influenza virus vaccine (live/attenuated) *on page 484*
h5G1.1 *see* eculizumab *on page 322*
H5N1 influenza vaccine *see* influenza virus vaccine (H5N1) *on page 482*
HA *see* typhoid and hepatitis A vaccine *(Canada only) on page 927*
Habitrol *see* nicotine *on page 640*
Habitrol® (Can) *see* nicotine *on page 640*

Haemophilus B conjugate and hepatitis B vaccine

(he MOF i lus bee KON joo gate & hep a TYE tis bee vak SEEN)

Medication Safety Issues

Sound-alike/look-alike issues:

Comvax® may be confused with Recombivax [Recombivax HB®]

Synonyms *Haemophilus* b (meningococcal protein conjugate) conjugate vaccine; hepatitis B vaccine (recombinant); hib conjugate vaccine; hib-hepB

U.S. Brand Names Comvax®

Therapeutic Category Vaccine, Inactivated Virus

Use

Immunization against invasive disease caused by *H. influenzae* type b and against infection caused by all known subtypes of hepatitis B virus in infants 6 weeks to 15 months of age born of hepatitis B surface antigen (HB_sAg)-negative mothers

Infants born of HB_sAg-positive mothers or mothers of unknown HB_sAg status should receive hepatitis B vaccine (recombinant) at birth and should complete the hepatitis B vaccination series given according to a particular schedule (refer to current ACIP recommendations).

General Dosage Range I.M.: *Infants ≥6 weeks:* 0.5 mL (series includes 3 doses)

Dosage Forms

Injection, suspension [preservative free]:

Comvax®: *Haemophilus* b capsular polysaccharide 7.5 mcg and hepatitis B surface antigen 5 mcg per 0.5 mL (0.5 mL)

***Haemophilus* B conjugate (Hib)** *see* diphtheria and tetanus toxoids, acellular pertussis, poliovirus and *Haemophilus* b conjugate vaccine *on page 298*

Haemophilus B conjugate vaccine (he MOF fi lus bee KON joo gate vak SEEN)

Synonyms *Haemophilus influenzae* type b; Hib; PRP-OMP; PRP-T

U.S. Brand Names ActHIB®; Hiberix®; PedvaxHIB®

Canadian Brand Names ActHIB®; PedvaxHIB®

Therapeutic Category Vaccine, Inactivated Bacteria

Use Routine immunization of children against invasive disease caused by *H. influenzae* type b

The Advisory Committee on Immunization Practices (ACIP) recommends routine vaccination of all children through age 59 months. Efficacy data are not available for use in older children and adults with chronic conditions associated with an increased risk of Hib disease. However, a single dose may also be considered for older children, adolescents, and adults who did not receive the childhood series and who have a chronic condition associated with an increased risk of Hib disease (eg, splenectomy, sickle cell disease, leukemia, HIV infection).

General Dosage Range I.M.: *Children:* 0.5 mL (number of doses determined by age at first dose)

Dosage Forms

Injection, powder for reconstitution [preservative free]:

ActHIB® *Haemophilus* b capsular polysaccharide 10 mcg per 0.5 mL

Hiberix®: *Haemophilus* b capsular polysaccharide 10 mcg per 0.5 mL

Injection, suspension:

PedvaxHIB®: *Haemophilus* b capsular polysaccharide 7.5 mcg

***Haemophilus* b (meningococcal protein conjugate) conjugate vaccine** *see* *Haemophilus* B conjugate and hepatitis B vaccine *on page 439*

***Haemophilus* B polysaccharide** *see* diphtheria and tetanus toxoids, acellular pertussis, poliovirus and *Haemophilus* b conjugate vaccine *on page 298*

***Haemophilus influenzae* b conjugate vaccine and diphtheria, tetanus toxoids, and acellular pertussis vaccine** *see* diphtheria and tetanus toxoids, acellular pertussis and *Haemophilus influenzae* b conjugate vaccine *on page 296*

***Haemophilus influenzae* type b** *see* *Haemophilus* B conjugate vaccine *on page 439*

HAL *see* hexaminolevulinate *on page 447*

Halaven™ *see* eribulin *on page 341*

halcinonide (hal SIN oh nide)

Medication Safety Issues

Sound-alike/look-alike issues:

Halcinonide may be confused with Halcion®

Halog® may be confused with Haldol®

U.S. Brand Names Halog®

Canadian Brand Names Halog®

Therapeutic Category Corticosteroid, Topical

Use Inflammation of corticosteroid-responsive dermatoses [high potency topical corticosteroid]

General Dosage Range Topical: *Children and Adults:* Apply sparingly 1-3 times/day

Dosage Forms

Cream, topical:

Halog®: 0.1% (30 g, 60 g, 216 g)

Ointment, topical:

Halog®: 0.1% (30 g, 60 g)

Halcion® *see* triazolam *on page 917*

Haldol® *see* haloperidol *on page 441*

Haldol® Decanoate *see* haloperidol *on page 441*

Haley's M-O *see* magnesium hydroxide and mineral oil *on page 559*

HalfLytely® and Bisacodyl *see* polyethylene glycol-electrolyte solution and bisacodyl *on page 739*

Halfprin® [OTC] *see* aspirin *on page 96*

halichondrin B analog *see* eribulin *on page 341*

halobetasol (hal oh BAY ta sol)

Medication Safety Issues

Sound-alike/look-alike issues:

Ultravate® may be confused with Cutivate®

Synonyms halobetasol propionate

U.S. Brand Names Halonate™; Ultravate®

Canadian Brand Names Ultravate®

Therapeutic Category Corticosteroid, Topical

Use Relief of inflammatory and pruritic manifestations of corticosteroid-response dermatoses [super high potency topical corticosteroid]

General Dosage Range Topical: *Children ≥12 years and Adults:* Apply sparingly to affected area of skin once or twice daily (maximum: 50 g/week; 2 consecutive weeks)

Dosage Forms

Cream, topical: 0.05% (15 g, 50 g)
Ultravate®: 0.05% (50 g)
Ointment, topical: 0.05% (15 g, 50 g)
Halonate™: 0.05% (50 g)
Ultravate®: 0.05% (50 g)

halobetasol propionate *see* halobetasol *on page 440*
Halog® *see* halcinonide *on page 440*
Halonate™ *see* halobetasol *on page 440*

haloperidol (ha loe PER i dole)

Medication Safety Issues

Sound-alike/look-alike issues:
Haldol® may be confused with Halcion®, Halog®, Stadol
BEERS Criteria medication:
This drug may be potentially inappropriate for use in geriatric patients (Quality of evidence - moderate; Strength of recommendation - strong).
International issues:
Haldol [U.S. and multiple international markets] may be confused with Halotestin brand name for fluoxymesterone [Great Britain]

Synonyms haloperidol decanoate; haloperidol lactate

U.S. Brand Names Haldol®; Haldol® Decanoate

Canadian Brand Names Apo-Haloperidol LA®; Apo-Haloperidol®; Haloperidol Injection, USP; Haloperidol Long Acting; Haloperidol-LA; Haloperidol-LA Omega; Novo-Peridol; PMS-Haloperidol; PMS-Haloperidol LA

Therapeutic Category Antipsychotic Agent, Butyrophenone

Use Management of schizophrenia; control of tics and vocal utterances of Tourette disorder in children and adults; severe behavioral problems in children

General Dosage Range

I.M.:
Decanoate: *Adults:* Initial: 10-20 times daily oral dose at 4-week intervals; Maintenance: 10-15 times initial oral dose
Lactate:
Children 6-12 years: 1-3 mg/dose every 4-8 hours (maximum: 0.15 mg/kg/day)
Adults: 2-5 mg every 4-8 hours as needed
Oral:
Children 3-12 years (15-40 kg): Initial: 0.5 mg/day in 2-3 divided doses; Maintenance: 0.05-0.15 mg/kg/day in 2-3 divided doses
Adults: Initial: 0.5-5 mg 2-3 times/day; Maintenance: Up to 30 mg/day in 2-3 divided doses

Dosage Forms

Injection, oil: 50 mg/mL (1 mL, 5 mL); 100 mg/mL (1 mL, 5 mL)
Haldol® Decanoate: 50 mg/mL (1 mL); 100 mg/mL (1 mL)
Injection, solution: 5 mg/mL (1 mL, 10 mL)
Haldol®: 5 mg/mL (1 mL)
Solution, oral: 2 mg/mL (5 mL, 15 mL, 120 mL)
Tablet, oral: 0.5 mg, 1 mg, 2 mg, 5 mg, 10 mg, 20 mg

haloperidol decanoate *see* haloperidol *on page 441*
Haloperidol Injection, USP (Can) *see* haloperidol *on page 441*
Haloperidol-LA (Can) *see* haloperidol *on page 441*
haloperidol lactate *see* haloperidol *on page 441*
Haloperidol-LA Omega (Can) *see* haloperidol *on page 441*
Haloperidol Long Acting (Can) *see* haloperidol *on page 441*
hamamelis water *see* witch hazel *on page 956*
harkoseride *see* lacosamide *on page 517*
Havrix® *see* hepatitis A vaccine *on page 444*
HAVRIX® (Can) *see* hepatitis A vaccine *on page 444*
Havrix® and Engerix-B® *see* hepatitis A and hepatitis B recombinant vaccine *on page 444*
HBIG *see* hepatitis B immune globulin (human) *on page 445*

hBNP *see* nesiritide *on page* 636
hCG *see* chorionic gonadotropin (human) *on page* 206
HCTZ (error-prone abbreviation) *see* hydrochlorothiazide *on page* 452
HDA® Toothache [OTC] *see* benzocaine *on page* 121
HDCV *see* rabies vaccine *on page* 784
Head & Shoulders® Citrus Breeze [OTC] *see* pyrithione zinc *on page* 779
Head & Shoulders® Citrus Breeze 2-in-1 [OTC] *see* pyrithione zinc *on page* 779
Head & Shoulders® Classic Clean [OTC] *see* pyrithione zinc *on page* 779
Head & Shoulders® Classic Clean 2-in-1 [OTC] *see* pyrithione zinc *on page* 779
Head & Shoulders® Clinical Strength [OTC] *see* selenium sulfide *on page* 828
Head & Shoulders® Dry Scalp [OTC] *see* pyrithione zinc *on page* 779
Head & Shoulders® Dry Scalp 2-in-1 [OTC] *see* pyrithione zinc *on page* 779
Head & Shoulders® Dry Scalp Care [OTC] *see* pyrithione zinc *on page* 779
Head & Shoulders® Dry Scalp Care 2-in-1 [OTC] *see* pyrithione zinc *on page* 779
Head & Shoulders® Extra Volume [OTC] *see* pyrithione zinc *on page* 779
Head & Shoulders® intensive solutions 2 in 1 [OTC] *see* pyrithione zinc *on page* 779
Head & Shoulders® intensive solutions for dry/damaged hair [OTC] *see* pyrithione zinc *on page* 779
Head & Shoulders® intensive solutions for fine/oily hair [OTC] *see* pyrithione zinc *on page* 779
Head & Shoulders® intensive solutions for normal hair [OTC] *see* pyrithione zinc *on page* 779
Head & Shoulders® Ocean Lift [OTC] *see* pyrithione zinc *on page* 779
Head & Shoulders® Ocean Lift 2-in-1 [OTC] *see* pyrithione zinc *on page* 779
Head & Shoulders® Refresh [OTC] *see* pyrithione zinc *on page* 779
Head & Shoulders® Refresh 2-in-1 [OTC] *see* pyrithione zinc *on page* 779
Head & Shoulders® Restoring Shine [OTC] *see* pyrithione zinc *on page* 779
Head & Shoulders® Restoring Shine 2 in 1 [OTC] *see* pyrithione zinc *on page* 779
Head & Shoulders® Sensitive Care [OTC] *see* pyrithione zinc *on page* 779
Head & Shoulders® Sensitive Care 2 in 1 [OTC] *see* pyrithione zinc *on page* 779
Head & Shoulders® Smooth & Silky [OTC] *see* pyrithione zinc *on page* 779
Head & Shoulders® Smooth & Silky 2-in-1 [OTC] *see* pyrithione zinc *on page* 779
Heartburn Relief [OTC] *see* famotidine *on page* 372
Heartburn Relief Maximum Strength [OTC] *see* famotidine *on page* 372
Heather *see* norethindrone *on page* 648
Hecoria™ *see* tacrolimus (systemic) *on page* 865
Hectorol® *see* doxercalciferol *on page* 313
hedgehog antagonist GDC-0449 *see* vismodegib *on page* 948
Helidac® *see* bismuth, metronidazole, and tetracycline *on page* 136
Helistat® *see* collagen hemostat *on page* 234
Helitene® *see* collagen hemostat *on page* 234
Helixate® FS *see* antihemophilic factor (recombinant) *on page* 78
Hemabate® *see* carboprost tromethamine *on page* 176
hematide *see* peginesatide *on page* 696
hematin *see* hemin *on page* 442
hemiacidrin *see* citric acid, magnesium carbonate, and glucono-delta-lactone *on page* 214

hemin (HEE min)

Synonyms hematin

U.S. Brand Names Panhematin®

Therapeutic Category Blood Modifiers

Use Treatment of recurrent attacks of acute intermittent porphyria (AIP)

General Dosage Range I.V.: *Children ≥16 years and Adults:* 1-4 mg/kg/day divided every 12 hours (maximum: 6 mg/kg/24 hours)

Dosage Forms

Injection, powder for reconstitution:
Panhematin®: 313 mg

Hemocyte® [OTC] *see* ferrous fumarate *on page 379*
Hemocyte Plus® *see* vitamins (multiple/oral) *on page 951*
Hemofil M *see* antihemophilic factor (human) *on page 78*
hemorrhoidal HC *see* hydrocortisone (topical) *on page 457*
Hemril®-30 *see* hydrocortisone (topical) *on page 457*
HepA *see* hepatitis A vaccine *on page 444*
HepaGam B® *see* hepatitis B immune globulin (human) *on page 445*
HepA-HepB *see* hepatitis A and hepatitis B recombinant vaccine *on page 444*
Hepalean® (Can) *see* heparin *on page 443*
Hepalean® Leo (Can) *see* heparin *on page 443*
Hepalean®-LOK (Can) *see* heparin *on page 443*

heparin (HEP a rin)

Medication Safety Issues

Sound-alike/look-alike issues:
Heparin may be confused with Hespan®

High alert medication:
The Institute for Safe Medication Practices (ISMP) includes this medication among its list of drugs which have a heightened risk of causing significant patient harm when used in error.

National Patient Safety Goals:
The Joint Commission (TJC) requires healthcare organizations that provide anticoagulant therapy to have a process in place to reduce the risk of anticoagulant-associated patient harm. Patients receiving anticoagulants should receive individualized care through a defined process that includes standardized ordering, dispensing, administration, monitoring and education. This does not apply to routine short-term use of anticoagulants for prevention of venous thromboembolism when the expectation is that the patient's laboratory values will remain within or close to normal values (NPSG.03.05.01).

Administration issues:
The 100 unit/mL concentration should not be used to flush heparin locks, I.V. lines, or intraarterial lines in neonates or infants <10 kg (systemic anticoagulation may occur). The 10 unit/mL flush concentration may inadvertently cause systemic anticoagulation in infants <1 kg who receive frequent flushes.

Other safety concerns:
Heparin sodium injection 10,000 units/mL and Hep-Lock U/P 10 units/mL have been confused with each other. Fatal medication errors have occurred between the two whose labels are both blue. **Never rely on color as a sole indicator to differentiate product identity.**

Heparin lock flush solution is intended only to maintain patency of I.V. devices and is **not** to be used for anticoagulant therapy.

Synonyms heparin calcium; heparin lock flush; heparin sodium

U.S. Brand Names Hep-Lock; HepFlush®-10

Canadian Brand Names Hepalean®; Hepalean® Leo; Hepalean®-LOK

Therapeutic Category Anticoagulant (Other)

Use Prophylaxis and treatment of thromboembolic disorders; as an anticoagulant for extracorporeal and dialysis procedures

Note: Heparin lock flush solution is intended only to maintain patency of I.V. devices and is **not** to be used for systemic anticoagulant therapy.

General Dosage Range

I.V.:

Children: Bolus: 50-100 units/kg; Initial infusion: 15-25 units/kg/hour; Maintenance: Increase dose by 2-4 units/kg/hour every 6-8 hours as needed **or** 50-100 units/kg every 4 hours intermittently

Adults: Bolus: 60-80 units/kg; Infusion: 10-30 units/kg/hour **or** 10,000 units (initially), then 50-70 units/kg (5000-10,000 units) every 4-6 hours intermittently

SubQ: *Adults:* Thromboprophylaxis: 5000 units every 8-12 hours; Treatment: 17,500 units every 12 hours

Dosage Forms

Infusion, premixed in 1/2 NS: 25,000 units (250 mL, 500 mL)

Infusion, premixed in D_5W: 10,000 units (100 mL, 250 mL); 12,500 units (250 mL); 20,000 units (500 mL); 25,000 units (250 mL, 500 mL)

Infusion, premixed in NS: 1000 units (500 mL); 2000 units (1000 mL)

Infusion, premixed in NS [preservative free]: 1000 units (500 mL); 2000 units (1000 mL)
Injection, solution: 10 units/mL (1 mL, 2 mL, 3 mL, 5 mL, 10 mL, 30 mL); 100 units/mL (1 mL, 2 mL, 3 mL, 5 mL, 10 mL, 30 mL); 1000 units/mL (1 mL, 10 mL, 30 mL); 5000 units/mL (1 mL, 10 mL); 10,000 units/mL (1 mL, 4 mL, 5 mL); 20,000 units/mL (1 mL)
Hep-Lock: 100 units/mL (1 mL)
Injection, solution [preservative free]: 1 units/mL (2 mL, 3 mL, 5 mL); 2 units/mL (3 mL); 10 units/mL (1 mL, 2 mL, 2.5 mL, 3 mL, 5 mL, 6 mL, 10 mL); 100 units/mL (1 mL, 2 mL, 2.5 mL, 3 mL, 5 mL, 10 mL); 1000 units/mL (2 mL); 5000 units/mL (0.5 mL); 10,000 units/mL (0.5 mL)
HepFlush®-10: 10 units/mL (10 mL)

heparin calcium *see* heparin *on page 443*

heparin lock flush *see* heparin *on page 443*

heparin sodium *see* heparin *on page 443*

HepatAmine® *see* amino acid injection *on page 61*

Hepatasol® *see* amino acid injection *on page 61*

hepatitis A and hepatitis B recombinant vaccine

(hep a TYE tis aye & hep a TYE tis bee ree KOM be nant vak SEEN)

Synonyms Engerix-B® and Havrix®; Havrix® and Engerix-B®; HepA-HepB; hepatitis B and hepatitis A vaccine

U.S. Brand Names Twinrix®

Canadian Brand Names Twinrix®; Twinrix® Junior

Therapeutic Category Vaccine

Use Active immunization against disease caused by hepatitis A virus and hepatitis B virus (all known subtypes) in populations desiring protection against or at high risk of exposure to these viruses.

Populations include travelers or people living in or relocating to areas of intermediate/high endemicity for **both** HAV and HBV and are at increased risk of HBV infection due to behavioral or occupational factors; patients with chronic liver disease; laboratory workers who handle live HAV and HBV; healthcare workers, police, and other personnel who render first-aid or medical assistance; workers who come in contact with sewage; employees of day care centers and correctional facilities; patients/staff of hemodialysis units; men who have sex with men; patients frequently receiving blood products; military personnel; users of injectable illicit drugs; close household contacts of patients with hepatitis A and hepatitis B infection; residents of drug and alcohol treatment centers

General Dosage Range I.M.: *Adults:* 3 doses (1 mL each) given on a 0-, 1-, and 6-month schedule

Dosage Forms

Injection, suspension [preservative free]:
Twinrix®: Hepatitis A virus antigen 720 ELISA units and hepatitis B surface antigen 20 mcg per mL (1 mL)

Dosage Forms - Canada

Injection, suspension [preservative free]:
Twinrix® Junior: Hepatitis A virus antigen 360 ELISA units and hepatitis B surface antigen 10 mcg per 0.5 mL (0.5 mL)

hepatitis A and typhoid vaccine *see* typhoid and hepatitis A vaccine *(Canada only) on page 927*

hepatitis A vaccine (hep a TYE tis aye vak SEEN)

Medication Safety Issues

International issues:
Avaxim [Canada and multiple international markets] may be confused with Avastin brand name for bevacizumab [U.S., Canada, and multiple international markets]

Synonyms HepA

U.S. Brand Names Havrix®; VAQTA®

Canadian Brand Names Avaxim®; Avaxim®-Pediatric; HAVRIX®; VAQTA®

Therapeutic Category Vaccine, Inactivated Virus

Use

Active immunization against disease caused by hepatitis A virus (HAV)

The Advisory Committee on Immunization Practices (ACIP) recommends routine vaccination for:

- All children ≥12 months of age
- All unvaccinated adults requesting protection from HAV infection
- All unvaccinated adults at risk for HAV infection, such as:
  Behavioral risks: Men who have sex with men; injection drug users
  Occupational risks: Persons who work with HAV-infected primates or with HAV in a research laboratory setting
  Medical risks: Persons with chronic liver disease; patients who receive clotting-factor concentrates
- Other risks: International travelers to regions with high or intermediate levels of endemic HAV infection (a list of countries is available at http://wwwn.cdc.gov/travel/contentdiseases.aspx)
- Unvaccinated persons who anticipate close personal contact with international adoptee from a country of intermediate to high endemicity of HAV, during their first 60 days of arrival into the United States (eg, household contacts, babysitters)

General Dosage Range I.M.:

Children 12 months to 18 years: 0.5 mL

Adults: 1 mL

Dosage Forms

Injection, suspension [preservative free]:

Havrix®: Hepatitis A virus antigen 720 ELISA units/0.5 mL (0.5 mL); Hepatitis A virus antigen 1440 ELISA units/mL (1 mL)

VAQTA®: Hepatitis A virus antigen 25 units/0.5 mL (0.5 mL); Hepatitis A virus antigen 50 units/mL (1 mL)

hepatitis B and hepatitis A vaccine *see* hepatitis A and hepatitis B recombinant vaccine *on page 444*

hepatitis B immune globulin (human) (hep a TYE tis bee i MYUN GLOB yoo lin YU man)

Medication Safety Issues

Sound-alike/look-alike issues:

HBIG may be confused with BabyBIG

Synonyms HBIG

U.S. Brand Names HepaGam B®; HyperHEP B™ S/D; Nabi-HB®

Canadian Brand Names HepaGam B®; HyperHEP B™ S/D

Therapeutic Category Immune Globulin

Use

Passive prophylactic immunity to hepatitis B following: Acute exposure to blood containing hepatitis B surface antigen (HB_sAg); perinatal exposure of infants born to HB_sAg-positive mothers; sexual exposure to HB_sAg-positive persons; household exposure to persons with acute HBV infection

Prevention of hepatitis B virus recurrence after liver transplantation in HB_sAg-positive transplant patients

Note: Hepatitis B immune globulin is not indicated for treatment of active hepatitis B infection and is ineffective in the treatment of chronic active hepatitis B infection.

General Dosage Range

I.M.:

Newborns and Infants <12 months: 0.5 mL/dose

Children ≥12 months and Adults: 0.06 mL/kg/dose

I.V.: *Adults:* 20,000 units/dose daily for 8 days, then every 2 weeks for 6 doses, then once monthly

Dosage Forms

Injection, solution [preservative free]:

HepaGam B®: Anti-HBs >312 units/mL (1 mL, 5 mL)

HyperHEP B™ S/D: Anti-HBs ≥220 units/mL (0.5 mL, 1 mL, 5 mL)

Nabi-HB®: Anti-HBs >312 units/mL (1 mL, 5 mL)

hepatitis B inactivated virus vaccine (recombinant DNA) *see* hepatitis B vaccine (recombinant) *on page 445*

hepatitis B vaccine (recombinant) (hep a TYE tis bee vak SEEN ree KOM be nant)

Medication Safety Issues

Sound-alike/look-alike issues:

Engerix-B® adult may be confused with Engerix-B® pediatric/adolescent

Recombivax HB® may be confused with Comvax®

Synonyms hepatitis B inactivated virus vaccine (recombinant DNA); HepB

U.S. Brand Names Engerix-B®; Recombivax HB®

Canadian Brand Names Engerix-B®; Recombivax HB®

Therapeutic Category Vaccine, Inactivated Virus

Use Immunization against infection caused by all known subtypes of hepatitis B virus (HBV)

The Advisory Committee on Immunization Practices (ACIP) recommends routine vaccination for the following (CDC, 2005; CDC, 2006; CDC, 2011):

- All infants at birth
- All infants and children (post-birth dose; refer to recommended vaccination schedule)
- All unvaccinated adults requesting protection from HBV infection
- All unvaccinated adults at risk for HBV infection such as those with:

Behavioral risks: Sexually-active persons with >1 partner in a 6-month period; persons seeking evaluation or treatment for a sexually-transmitted disease; men who have sex with men; injection drug users

Occupational risks: Healthcare and public safety workers with reasonably anticipated risk for exposure to blood or blood contaminated body fluids

Medical risks: Persons with end-stage renal disease (including predialysis, hemodialysis, peritoneal dialysis, and home dialysis); persons with HIV infection; persons with chronic liver disease. Adults (19 through 59 years of age) with diabetes mellitus type 1 or type 2 should be vaccinated as soon as possible following diagnosis. Adults ≥60 years with diabetes mellitus may also be vaccinated at the discretion of their treating clinician.

Other risks: Household contacts and sex partners of persons with chronic HBV infection; residents and staff of facilities for developmentally disabled persons; international travelers to regions with high or intermediate levels of endemic HBV infection

In addition, the ACIP recommends vaccination for any persons who are wounded in bombings or similar mass casualty events who have penetrating injuries or nonintact skin exposure, or who have contact with mucous membranes (exception - superficial contact with intact skin), and who cannot confirm receipt of a hepatitis B vaccination (CDC, 2008).

General Dosage Range Dosage adjustment recommended in patients with renal impairment.

I.M.:

Birth to 19 years: 0.5 mL

Adults ≥20 years: 1 mL

Dosage Forms

Injection, suspension [preservative free]:

Engerix-B®: Hepatitis B surface antigen 10 mcg/0.5 mL (0.5 mL); Hepatitis B surface antigen 20 mcg/mL (1 mL)

Recombivax HB®: Hepatitis B surface antigen 5 mcg/0.5 mL (0.5 mL); Hepatitis B surface antigen 10 mcg/mL (1 mL); Hepatitis B surface antigen 40 mcg/mL (1 mL)

hepatitis B vaccine (recombinant) *see Haemophilus* B conjugate and hepatitis B vaccine *on page 439*

HepB *see* hepatitis B vaccine (recombinant) *on page 445*

HepFlush®-10 *see* heparin *on page 443*

Hep-Lock *see* heparin *on page 443*

Hepsera® *see* adefovir *on page 37*

Hepsera™ (Can) *see* adefovir *on page 37*

Heptovir® (Can) *see* lamivudine *on page 520*

Herceptin® *see* trastuzumab *on page 911*

HES *see* hetastarch *on page 447*

HES *see* pentastarch *(Canada only) on page 704*

HES *see* tetrastarch *on page 885*

HES 130/0.4 *see* tetrastarch *on page 885*

HES 200/0.5 *see* pentastarch *(Canada only) on page 704*

HES 450/0.7 *see* hetastarch *on page 447*

Hespan® *see* hetastarch *on page 447*

hetastarch (HET a starch)

Medication Safety Issues

Sound-alike/look-alike issues:

Hespan® may be confused with heparin

Synonyms HES; HES 450/0.7; hydroxyethyl starch

U.S. Brand Names Hespan®; Hextend®

Canadian Brand Names Hextend®

Therapeutic Category Plasma Volume Expander

Use Blood volume expander used in treatment of hypovolemia; adjunct in leukapheresis to improve harvesting and increase the yield of granulocytes by centrifugation (Hespan®)

General Dosage Range Dosage adjustment recommended in patients with renal impairment

I.V.: *Adults:* 500-1500 mL/day **or** 20 mL/kg/day (up to 1500 mL/day)

Leukapheresis: *Adults:* 250-700 mL

Dosage Forms

Infusion, premixed in NS: 6% (500 mL)

Hespan®: 6% (500 mL)

Infusion, premixed in lactated electrolyte solution:

Hextend®: 6% (500 mL)

Hexabrix™ *see* ioxaglate meglumine and ioxaglate sodium *on page 498*

hexachlorocyclohexane *see* lindane *on page 541*

hexachlorophene (heks a KLOR oh feen)

Medication Safety Issues

Sound-alike/look-alike issues:

pHisoHex® may be confused with Fostex®, pHisoDerm®

U.S. Brand Names pHisoHex®

Canadian Brand Names pHisoHex®

Therapeutic Category Antibacterial, Topical

Use Surgical scrub and as a bacteriostatic skin cleanser; control an outbreak of gram-positive infection when other procedures have been unsuccessful

General Dosage Range Topical: *Children and Adults:* Apply 5 mL cleanser and water to area to be cleansed

Dosage Forms

Liquid, topical:

pHisoHex®: 3% (150 mL, 480 mL)

Hexalen® *see* altretamine *on page 54*

hexamethylenetetramine *see* methenamine *on page 582*

hexamethylmelamine *see* altretamine *on page 54*

hexamethylpropylene amine oxime *see* technetium Tc 99m exametazime *on page 871*

hexaminolevulinate (hex a mee noe LEV ue lin ate)

Synonyms HAL; hexaminolevulinate hydrochloride

U.S. Brand Names Cysview™

Therapeutic Category Contrast Agent

Use Detection of non-muscle invasive papillary cancer of the bladder; used in conjunction with the Karl Storz D-Light C Photodynamic Diagnostic (PDD) system

General Dosage Range Intravesical instillation: *Adults:* 50 mL instilled into empty bladder via urinary catheter

Dosage Forms

Powder for solution, intravesical:

Cysview™: 100 mg

hexaminolevulinate hydrochloride *see* hexaminolevulinate *on page 447*

Hexit™ (Can) *see* lindane *on page 541*

Hextend® *see* hetastarch *on page 447*

hexylresorcinol (heks il re ZOR si nole)

U.S. Brand Names Sucrets® Original [OTC]

Therapeutic Category Local Anesthetic

Use Minor antiseptic and local anesthetic for sore throat; topical antiseptic for minor cuts or abrasions

General Dosage Range Oral: *Children ≥6 years and Adults:* Up to 10 lozenges/day

Dosage Forms

Lozenge, oral:

Sucrets® Original [OTC]: 2.4 mg (18s)

hFSH *see* urofollitropin *on page 931*

hGH *see* somatropin *on page 849*

Hib *see Haemophilus* B conjugate vaccine *on page 439*

hib conjugate vaccine *see Haemophilus* B conjugate and hepatitis B vaccine *on page 439*

Hiberix® *see Haemophilus* B conjugate vaccine *on page 439*

hib-hepB *see Haemophilus* B conjugate and hepatitis B vaccine *on page 439*

Hibiclens® [OTC] *see* chlorhexidine gluconate *on page 196*

Hibidil® 1:2000 (Can) *see* chlorhexidine gluconate *on page 196*

Hibistat® [OTC] *see* chlorhexidine gluconate *on page 196*

High Gamma Vitamin E Complete™ [OTC] *see* vitamin E *on page 950*

high-molecular-weight iron dextran (DexFerrum®) *see* iron dextran complex *on page 501*

Hi-Kovite [OTC] *see* vitamins (multiple/oral) *on page 951*

Hiprex® *see* methenamine *on page 582*

hirulog *see* bivalirudin *on page 137*

Histantil (Can) *see* promethazine *on page 763*

Histaprin [OTC] *see* diphenhydramine (systemic) *on page 292*

Hizentra® *see* immune globulin *on page 477*

hMG *see* menotropins *on page 573*

HMM *see* altretamine *on page 54*

HMR 3647 *see* telithromycin *on page 874*

HN_2 *see* mechlorethamine *on page 566*

HOE 140 *see* icatibant *on page 471*

Hold® DM [OTC] *see* dextromethorphan *on page 272*

Homatropaire *see* homatropine *on page 448*

homatropine (hoe MA troe peen)

Medication Safety Issues

Sound-alike/look-alike issues:

Homatropine may be confused with Humatrope®, somatropin

Synonyms homatropine hydrobromide

U.S. Brand Names Homatropaire; Isopto® Homatropine

Therapeutic Category Anticholinergic Agent

Use Producing cycloplegia and mydriasis for refraction; treatment of acute inflammatory conditions of the uveal tract; optical aid in axial lens opacities

General Dosage Range Ophthalmic:

Children: Instill 1 drop (2% solution) 2-3 times/day **or** immediately prior to procedure, repeat every 10 minutes as needed

Adults: Instill 1-2 drops (2% or 5% solution) 2-3 times/day, up to every 3-4 hours as needed **or** 1-2 drops (2% solution) or 1 drop (5% solution) prior to procedure, repeat every 5-10 minutes as needed up to 3 doses

Dosage Forms

Solution, ophthalmic: 5% (5 mL)

Homatropaire: 5% (5 mL)

Isopto® Homatropine: 2% (5 mL); 5% (5 mL)

homatropine and hydrocodone *see* hydrocodone and homatropine *on page 455*

homatropine hydrobromide *see* homatropine *on page 448*

Homocysteine Guard [OTC] *see* folic acid, cyanocobalamin, and pyridoxine *on page 404*

Horizant™ *see* gabapentin enacarbil *on page 414*
horse antihuman thymocyte gamma globulin *see* antithymocyte globulin (equine) *on page 80*
12 Hour Nasal Relief [OTC] *see* oxymetazoline (nasal) *on page 681*
H.P. Acthar® *see* corticotropin *on page 237*
hpAT *see* antithrombin III *on page 80*
Hp-PAC® (Can) *see* lansoprazole, amoxicillin, and clarithromycin *on page 523*
HPV2 *see* papillomavirus (types 16, 18) vaccine (human, recombinant) *on page 691*
HPV4 *see* papillomavirus (types 6, 11, 16, 18) vaccine (human, recombinant) *on page 690*
HPV 16/18 L1 VLP/AS04 VAC *see* papillomavirus (types 16, 18) vaccine (human, recombinant) *on page 691*
HPV vaccine *see* papillomavirus (types 6, 11, 16, 18) vaccine (human, recombinant) *on page 690*
HPV vaccine *see* papillomavirus (types 16, 18) vaccine (human, recombinant) *on page 691*
HRIG *see* rabies immune globulin (human) *on page 784*
^{131}I-HSA *see* iodinated I 131 albumin *on page 493*
HTF919 *see* tegaserod *on page 873*
HumaLOG® *see* insulin lispro *on page 487*
Humalog® (Can) *see* insulin lispro *on page 487*
HumaLOG® KwikPen™ *see* insulin lispro *on page 487*
Humalog® Mix 25 (Can) *see* insulin lispro protamine and insulin lispro *on page 488*
HumaLOG® Mix 50/50™ *see* insulin lispro protamine and insulin lispro *on page 488*
HumaLOG® Mix 50/50™ KwikPen™ *see* insulin lispro protamine and insulin lispro *on page 488*
HumaLOG® Mix 75/25™ *see* insulin lispro protamine and insulin lispro *on page 488*
HumaLOG® Mix 75/25™ KwikPen™ *see* insulin lispro protamine and insulin lispro *on page 488*
Human Albumin Grifols® 25% *see* albumin *on page 41*
human antitumor necrosis factor alpha *see* adalimumab *on page 36*
human C1 inhibitor *see* C1 inhibitor (human) *on page 156*
human corticotrophin-releasing hormone, analogue *see* corticorelin *on page 237*
human diploid cell cultures rabies vaccine *see* rabies vaccine *on page 784*
human growth hormone *see* somatropin *on page 849*
humanized IgG1 anti-CD52 monoclonal antibody *see* alemtuzumab *on page 45*
human LFA-3/IgG(1) fusion protein *see* alefacept *on page 44*
human menopausal gonadotropin *see* menotropins *on page 573*
human papillomavirus vaccine *see* papillomavirus (types 6, 11, 16, 18) vaccine (human, recombinant) *on page 690*
human papillomavirus vaccine *see* papillomavirus (types 16, 18) vaccine (human, recombinant) *on page 691*
human rotavirus vaccine, attenuated (HRV) *see* rotavirus vaccine *on page 813*
human thyroid stimulating hormone *see* thyrotropin alpha *on page 894*
Humate-P® *see* antihemophilic factor/von Willebrand factor complex (human) *on page 78*
Humatin® (Can) *see* paromomycin *on page 693*
Humatrope® *see* somatropin *on page 849*
huMax-CD20 *see* ofatumumab *on page 659*
Humibid® Maximum Strength [OTC] *see* guaifenesin *on page 433*
Humira® *see* adalimumab *on page 36*
Humira® Pen *see* adalimumab *on page 36*
HuMist® [OTC] *see* sodium chloride *on page 840*
Humulin® 20/80 (Can) *see* insulin NPH and insulin regular *on page 489*
HumuLIN® 70/30 *see* insulin NPH and insulin regular *on page 489*
Humulin® 70/30 (Can) *see* insulin NPH and insulin regular *on page 489*
HumuLIN® N *see* insulin NPH *on page 488*
Humulin® N (Can) *see* insulin NPH *on page 488*
HumuLIN® R *see* insulin regular *on page 489*
Humulin® R (Can) *see* insulin regular *on page 489*
HumuLIN® R U-500 *see* insulin regular *on page 489*

Hurricaine® [OTC] *see* benzocaine *on page* 121
HurriCaine ONE™ *see* benzocaine *on page* 121
HXM *see* altretamine *on page* 54
Hyalgan® *see* hyaluronate and derivatives *on page* 450
hyaluronan *see* hyaluronate and derivatives *on page* 450

hyaluronate and derivatives (hye al yoor ON ate & dah RIV ah tives)

Medication Safety Issues

Sound-alike/look-alike issues:

Synvisc® may be confused with Synagis®

Synonyms hyaluronan; hyaluronic acid; hylan G-F 20; hylan polymers; sodium hyaluronate

U.S. Brand Names Amvisc®; Amvisc® Plus; Bionect®; Euflexxa®; Hyalgan®; Hylase® Wound; Juvéderm® Ultra; Juvéderm® Ultra Plus; Juvéderm® Ultra Plus XC; Juvéderm® Ultra XC; Orthovisc®; Perlane®; Provisc®; Restylane®; Supartz®; Synvisc-One®; Synvisc®

Canadian Brand Names Cystistat®; Durolane®; OrthoVisc®; Suplasyn®

Therapeutic Category Antirheumatic Miscellaneous; Ophthalmic Agent, Viscoelastic; Skin and Mucous Membrane Agent

Use

Intraarticular injection: Treatment of pain in osteoarthritis in knee in patients who have failed nonpharmacologic treatment and simple analgesics (Euflexxa®, Hyalgan®, OrthoVisc®, Supartz®, Synvisc®, Synvisc-One®)

Intradermal: Correction of moderate-to-severe facial wrinkles or folds (Juvederm® [all formulations], Perlane®, Restylane®)

Ophthalmic: Surgical aid in cataract extraction (Amvisc®, Amvisc® Plus, Provisc®); intraocular lens implantation (Amvisc®, Amvisc® Plus, Provisc®); corneal transplant (Amvisc®, Amvisc® Plus); glaucoma filtration (Amvisc®, Amvisc® Plus); and retinal attachment surgery (Amvisc®, Amvisc® Plus)

Submucosal: Lip augmentation (Restylane®)

Topical cream, gel: Management of skin ulcers and wounds (Bionect®, Hylase® Wound)

General Dosage Range

Intra-articular: *Adults:* 16-30 mg once weekly for 3-5 doses (total injections: 3-5) **or** 48 mg once

Intradermal: *Adults:* Inject as required for cosmetic effect (maximum: 20 mL/60 kg/year [Juvederm® all formulations] or maximum: 6 mL/treatment [Perlane®, Restylane®])

Ophthalmic: *Adults:* Depends upon procedure (slowly introduce a sufficient quantity into eye)

Submucosal: *Adults ≥21 years:* Maximum 1.5 mL per lip (upper or lower) per treatment session (Restylane®)

Topical: *Adults:* Apply to affected area 1-3 times daily

Dosage Forms

Cream, topical:

Bionect®: 0.2% (25 g)

Gel, topical:

Bionect®: 0.2% (30 g, 60 g)

Hylase® Wound: 2.5% (75 g)

Injection, gel, intradermal [hyaluronate acid]:

Juvéderm® Ultra: 24 mg/mL (0.4 mL, 0.8 mL)

Juvéderm® Ultra Plus: 24 mg/mL (0.4 mL, 0.8 mL)

Juvéderm® Ultra Plus XC: Hyaluronic acid 24 mg/mL and lidocaine 0.3% (0.4 mL, 0.8 mL)

Juvéderm® Ultra XC: Hyaluronic acid 24 mg/mL and lidocaine 0.3% (0.4 mL, 0.8 mL)

Injection, gel, intradermal [sodium hyaluronate]:

Perlane®: 20 mg/mL (1 mL)

Restylane®: 20 mg/mL (0.4 mL, 1 mL, 2 mL)

Injection, solution, intraarticular:

Euflexxa®: 10 mg/mL (2 mL)

Hyalgan®: 10 mg/mL (2 mL)

Orthovisc®: 15 mg/mL (2 mL)

Supartz®: 10 mg/mL (2.5 mL)

Synvisc-One®: 8 mg/mL (6 mL)

Synvisc®: 8 mg/mL (2 mL)

Injection, solution, intraocular:
Amvisc®: 12 mg/mL (0.5 mL, 0.8 mL)
Amvisc® Plus: 16 mg/mL (0.5 mL, 0.8 mL)
Provisc®: 10 mg/mL (0.4 mL, 0.55 mL, 0.85 mL)

hyaluronic acid *see* hyaluronate and derivatives *on page 450*

hyaluronidase (hye al yoor ON i dase)

U.S. Brand Names Amphadase™; Hylenex [DSC]; Vitrase®

Therapeutic Category Enzyme

Use Increase the dispersion and absorption of other injected drugs; increase rate of absorption of parenteral fluids given by subcutaneous administration (hypodermoclysis)

General Dosage Range

Intradermal: *Children and Adults:* 0.02 mL (3 units) of a 150 units/mL solution

SubQ:

Premature Infants: Volume of a single clysis/day should not exceed 25 mL/kg; rate of administration should not exceed 2 mL/minute

Children <3 years: Volume of a single clysis should not exceed 200 mL **or** 75 units over each scapula followed by injection of contrast medium at the same site

Children ≥3 years and Adults: Rate and volume of a single clysis should not exceed those used for infusion of I.V. fluids **or** 75 units over each scapula followed by injection of contrast medium at the same site

Dosage Forms

Injection, solution:
Amphadase™: 150 units/mL (1 mL)

Injection, solution [preservative free]:
Vitrase®: 200 units/mL (1.2 mL)

hycamptamine *see* topotecan *on page 906*
Hycamtin® *see* topotecan *on page 906*
hycet® *see* hydrocodone and acetaminophen *on page 454*
Hycodan *see* hydrocodone and homatropine *on page 455*
Hycort™ (Can) *see* hydrocortisone (topical) *on page 457*
Hydeltra T.B.A.® (Can) *see* prednisolone (systemic) *on page 754*
Hydergine [DSC] *see* ergoloid mesylates *on page 340*
Hydergine® (Can) *see* ergoloid mesylates *on page 340*
Hyderm (Can) *see* hydrocortisone (topical) *on page 457*

hydralazine (hye DRAL a zeen)

Medication Safety Issues

Sound-alike/look-alike issues:
HydrALAZINE may be confused with hydrOXYzine

Synonyms Apresoline [DSC]; hydralazine hydrochloride

Tall-Man hydr**ALAZINE**

Canadian Brand Names Apo-Hydralazine®; Apresoline®; Novo-Hylazin; Nu-Hydral

Therapeutic Category Vasodilator

Use Management of moderate-to-severe hypertension

General Dosage Range Dosage adjustment recommended in patients with renal impairment

I.M., I.V.:

Children: 0.1-0.2 mg/kg/dose (not to exceed 20 mg) every 4-6 hours as needed (maximum: 3.5 mg/kg/day in 4-6 divided doses)

Adults: Initial: 10-20 mg/dose every 4-6 hours as needed; Maintenance: Up to 40 mg/dose every 4-6 hours **or** Eclampsia/pre-eclampsia: 5 mg/dose then 5-10 mg every 20-30 minutes as needed

Oral:

Children: Initial: 0.75-1 mg/kg/day in 2-4 divided doses; Maintenance: Up to 7.5 mg/kg/day in 2-4 divided doses (maximum: 200 mg/day)

Adults: Initial: 10-25 mg 3-4 times/day; Maintenance: 25-300 mg/day (target dose: 225-300 mg/day for CHF) in 2-4 divided doses (maximum: 300 mg/day)

Elderly: Initial: 10 mg 2-3 times/day, increase by 10-25 mg/day every 2-5 days; Target dose: 225-300 mg/day for CHF

Dosage Forms

Injection, solution: 20 mg/mL (1 mL)

Tablet, oral: 10 mg, 25 mg, 50 mg, 100 mg

hydralazine and isosorbide dinitrate *see* isosorbide dinitrate and hydralazine *on page 505*
hydralazine hydrochloride *see* hydralazine *on page 451*
hydrated chloral *see* chloral hydrate *on page 194*
Hydrea® *see* hydroxyurea *on page 464*
Hydrisalic® [OTC] *see* salicylic acid *on page 816*
Hydro 35™ *see* urea *on page 930*
Hydro 40™ *see* urea *on page 930*

hydrochlorothiazide (hye droe klor oh THYE a zide)

Medication Safety Issues

Sound-alike/look-alike issues:

HCTZ is an error-prone abbreviation (mistaken as hydrocortisone)

Hydrochlorothiazide may be confused with hydrocortisone, Viskazide®

Microzide™ may be confused with Maxzide®, Micronase®

International issues:

Esidrex [multiple international markets] may be confused with Lasix brand name for furosemide [U.S., Canada, and multiple international markets]

Esidrix [Germany] may be confused with Lasix brand name for furosemide [U.S., Canada, and multiple international markets]

Synonyms HCTZ (error-prone abbreviation); Hydrodiuril

U.S. Brand Names Microzide®

Canadian Brand Names Apo-Hydro®; Bio-Hydrochlorothiazide; Dom-Hydrochlorothiazide; Novo-Hydrazide; Nu-Hydro; PMS-Hydrochlorothiazide

Therapeutic Category Diuretic, Thiazide

Use Management of mild-to-moderate hypertension; treatment of edema in heart failure and nephrotic syndrome

General Dosage Range Oral:

Children <6 months: 1-3 mg/kg/day in 2 divided doses

Children >6 months to 2 years: 1-3 mg/kg/day in 2 divided doses (maximum: 37.5 mg/day)

Children >2-17 years: Initial: 1 mg/kg/day (maximum: 3 mg/kg/day [50 mg/day])

Adults: 12.5-100 mg/day in 1-2 divided doses (maximum: 200 mg/day)

Elderly: 12.5-25 once daily

Dosage Forms

Capsule, oral: 12.5 mg

Microzide®: 12.5 mg

Tablet, oral: 12.5 mg, 25 mg, 50 mg

hydrochlorothiazide, aliskiren, and amlodipine *see* aliskiren, amlodipine, and hydrochlorothiazide *on page 48*
hydrochlorothiazide, amlodipine, and aliskiren *see* aliskiren, amlodipine, and hydrochlorothiazide *on page 48*
hydrochlorothiazide, amlodipine, and valsartan *see* amlodipine, valsartan, and hydrochlorothiazide *on page 68*
hydrochlorothiazide and aliskiren *see* aliskiren and hydrochlorothiazide *on page 48*
hydrochlorothiazide and amiloride *see* amiloride and hydrochlorothiazide *on page 60*
hydrochlorothiazide and benazepril *see* benazepril and hydrochlorothiazide *on page 119*
hydrochlorothiazide and bisoprolol *see* bisoprolol and hydrochlorothiazide *on page 137*
hydrochlorothiazide and candesartan *see* candesartan and hydrochlorothiazide *on page 168*
hydrochlorothiazide and captopril *see* captopril and hydrochlorothiazide *on page 171*
hydrochlorothiazide and cilazapril *see* cilazapril and hydrochlorothiazide *(Canada only) on page 209*
hydrochlorothiazide and enalapril *see* enalapril and hydrochlorothiazide *on page 330*
hydrochlorothiazide and eprosartan *see* eprosartan and hydrochlorothiazide *on page 338*
hydrochlorothiazide and fosinopril *see* fosinopril and hydrochlorothiazide *on page 409*
hydrochlorothiazide and irbesartan *see* irbesartan and hydrochlorothiazide *on page 501*

hydrochlorothiazide and lisinopril *see* lisinopril and hydrochlorothiazide *on page 544*
hydrochlorothiazide and losartan *see* losartan and hydrochlorothiazide *on page 551*
hydrochlorothiazide and methyldopa *see* methyldopa and hydrochlorothiazide *on page 588*
hydrochlorothiazide and metoprolol *see* metoprolol and hydrochlorothiazide *on page 595*
hydrochlorothiazide and metoprolol succinate *see* metoprolol and hydrochlorothiazide *on page 595*
hydrochlorothiazide and metoprolol tartrate *see* metoprolol and hydrochlorothiazide *on page 595*
hydrochlorothiazide and moexipril *see* moexipril and hydrochlorothiazide *on page 609*
hydrochlorothiazide and olmesartan medoxomil *see* olmesartan and hydrochlorothiazide *on page 663*
hydrochlorothiazide and pindolol *see* pindolol and hydrochlorothiazide *(Canada only) on page 724*
hydrochlorothiazide and propranolol *see* propranolol and hydrochlorothiazide *on page 768*
hydrochlorothiazide and quinapril *see* quinapril and hydrochlorothiazide *on page 782*
hydrochlorothiazide and ramipril *see* ramipril and hydrochlorothiazide *(Canada only) on page 787*

hydrochlorothiazide and spironolactone

(hye droe klor oh THYE a zide & speer on oh LAK tone)

Medication Safety Issues

Sound-alike/look-alike issues:

Aldactazide® may be confused with Aldactone®

Synonyms spironolactone and hydrochlorothiazide

U.S. Brand Names Aldactazide®

Canadian Brand Names Aldactazide 25®; Aldactazide 50®; Novo-Spirozine

Therapeutic Category Antihypertensive Agent, Combination

Use Management of mild-to-moderate hypertension; treatment of edema in congestive heart failure and nephrotic syndrome, and cirrhosis of the liver accompanied by edema and/or ascites

General Dosage Range Oral: *Adults:* 12.5-50 mg hydrochlorothiazide and 12.5-50 mg spironolactone/day in 1-2 divided doses

Dosage Forms

Tablet: Hydrochlorothiazide 25 mg and spironolactone 25 mg

Aldactazide®: 25/25: Hydrochlorothiazide 25 mg and spironolactone 25 mg; 50/50: Hydrochlorothiazide 50 mg and spironolactone 50 mg

hydrochlorothiazide and telmisartan *see* telmisartan and hydrochlorothiazide *on page 875*

hydrochlorothiazide and triamterene

(hye droe klor oh THYE a zide & trye AM ter een)

Medication Safety Issues

Sound-alike/look-alike issues:

Dyazide® may be confused with diazoxide, Dynacin®
Maxzide® may be confused with Maxidex®, Microzide®

Synonyms triamterene and hydrochlorothiazide

U.S. Brand Names Dyazide®; Maxzide®; Maxzide®-25

Canadian Brand Names Apo-Triazide®; Nu-Triazide; Pro-Triazide; Riva-Zide; Teva-Triamterene HCTZ

Therapeutic Category Antihypertensive Agent, Combination

Use Treatment of hypertension or edema (not recommended for initial treatment) when hypokalemia has developed on hydrochlorothiazide alone or when the development of hypokalemia must be avoided

General Dosage Range Oral: *Adults:* 25-50 mg hydrochlorothiazide and 37.5-75 mg triamterene once daily

Dosage Forms

Capsule: Hydrochlorothiazide 25 mg and triamterene 37.5 mg; hydrochlorothiazide 25 mg and triamterene 50 mg

Dyazide®: Hydrochlorothiazide 25 mg and triamterene 37.5 mg

Tablet: Hydrochlorothiazide 25 mg and triamterene 37.5 mg; hydrochlorothiazide 50 mg and triamterene 75 mg

Maxzide®: Hydrochlorothiazide 50 mg and triamterene 75 mg [scored]
Maxzide®-25: Hydrochlorothiazide 25 mg and triamterene 37.5 mg [scored]

hydrochlorothiazide and valsartan *see* valsartan and hydrochlorothiazide *on page 936*

hydrochlorothiazide, olmesartan, and amlodipine *see* olmesartan, amlodipine, and hydrochlorothiazide *on page 662*

Hydrocil® Instant [OTC] *see* psyllium *on page 774*

hydrocodone and acetaminophen (hye droe KOE done & a seet a MIN oh fen)

Medication Safety Issues

Sound-alike/look-alike issues:

Lorcet® may be confused with Fioricet®
Lortab® may be confused with Cortef®
Vicodin® may be confused with Hycodan, Indocin®
Zydone® may be confused with Vytone

High alert medication:

The Institute for Safe Medication Practices (ISMP) includes this medication among its list of drug classes which have a heightened risk of causing significant patient harm when used in error.

Other safety concerns:

Duplicate therapy issues: This product contains acetaminophen, which may be a component of other combination products. Do not exceed the maximum recommended daily dose of acetaminophen.

Synonyms acetaminophen and hydrocodone

U.S. Brand Names hycet®; Lorcet® 10/650; Lorcet® Plus; Lortab®; Margesic® H; Maxidone®; Norco®; Stagesic™; Vicodin®; Vicodin® ES; Vicodin® HP; Xodol® 10/300; Xodol® 5/300; Xodol® 7.5/300; Zamicet™; Zolvit®; Zydone®

Therapeutic Category Analgesic, Narcotic

Controlled Substance C-III

Use Relief of moderate-to-severe pain

General Dosage Range Oral:

Children 2-13 years or <50 kg: Hydrocodone 0.1-0.2 mg/kg/dose every 4-6 hours (maximum: 6 doses/day or maximum recommended dose of acetaminophen for age/weight)

Children ≥50 kg and Adults: Hydrocodone 2.5-10 mg every 4-6 hours (maximum: 4 g/day [acetaminophen])

Elderly: Hydrocodone 2.5-5 mg every 4-6 hours

Dosage Forms

Capsule, oral: Hydrocodone 5 mg and acetaminophen 500 mg

Margesic® H, Stagesic™: Hydrocodone 5 mg and acetaminophen 500 mg

Elixir, oral:

Lortab®: Hydrocodone 7.5 mg and acetaminophen 500 mg per 15 mL

Solution, oral: Hydrocodone 7.5 mg and acetaminophen 325 mg per 15 mL; hydrocodone 7.5 mg and acetaminophen 500 mg per 15 mL; hydrocodone 10 mg and acetaminophen 325 mg per 15 mL

hycet®: Hydrocodone 7.5 mg and acetaminophen 325 mg per 15 mL
Zamicet™: Hydrocodone 10 mg and acetaminophen 325 mg per 15 mL
Zolvit®: Hydrocodone 10 mg and acetaminophen 300 mg per 15 mL (480 mL)

Tablet, oral:

Generics:

Hydrocodone 2.5 mg and acetaminophen 500 mg
Hydrocodone 5 mg and acetaminophen 300 mg
Hydrocodone 5 mg and acetaminophen 325 mg
Hydrocodone 5 mg and acetaminophen 500 mg
Hydrocodone 7.5 mg and acetaminophen 300 mg
Hydrocodone 7.5 mg and acetaminophen 325 mg
Hydrocodone 7.5 mg and acetaminophen 500 mg
Hydrocodone 7.5 mg and acetaminophen 650 mg
Hydrocodone 7.5 mg and acetaminophen 750 mg
Hydrocodone 10 mg and acetaminophen 300 mg
Hydrocodone 10 mg and acetaminophen 325 mg
Hydrocodone 10 mg and acetaminophen 500 mg
Hydrocodone 10 mg and acetaminophen 650 mg
Hydrocodone 10 mg and acetaminophen 660 mg
Hydrocodone 10 mg and acetaminophen 750 mg

Brands:

Lorcet® 10/650: Hydrocodone 10 mg and acetaminophen 650 mg

Lorcet® Plus: Hydrocodone 7.5 mg and acetaminophen 650 mg

Lortab®: 5/500: Hydrocodone 5 mg and acetaminophen 500 mg; 7.5/500: Hydrocodone 7.5 mg and acetaminophen 500 mg; 10/500: Hydrocodone 10 mg and acetaminophen 500 mg

Maxidone®: Hydrocodone 10 mg and acetaminophen 750 mg

Norco®: Hydrocodone 5 mg and acetaminophen 325 mg; hydrocodone 7.5 mg and acetaminophen 325 mg; hydrocodone 10 mg and acetaminophen 325 mg

Vicodin®: Hydrocodone 5 mg and acetaminophen 500 mg

Vicodin® ES: Hydrocodone 7.5 mg and acetaminophen 750 mg

Vicodin® HP: Hydrocodone 10 mg and acetaminophen 660 mg

Xodol®: 5/300: Hydrocodone 5 mg and acetaminophen 300 mg; 7.5/300: Hydrocodone 7.5 mg and acetaminophen 300 mg; 10/300: Hydrocodone 10 mg and acetaminophen 300 mg

Zydone®: Hydrocodone 5 mg and acetaminophen 400 mg; hydrocodone 7.5 mg and acetaminophen 400 mg; hydrocodone 10 mg and acetaminophen 400 mg

hydrocodone and chlorpheniramine (hye droe KOE done & klor fen IR a meen)

Medication Safety Issues

Sound-alike/look-alike issues:

Tussionex® represents a different product in the U.S. than it does in Canada. In the U.S., Tussionex® contains hydrocodone and chlorpheniramine, while in Canada the product bearing this name contains hydrocodone and phenyltoloxamine.

High alert medication:

The Institute for Safe Medication Practices (ISMP) includes this medication among its list of drug classes which have a heightened risk of causing significant patient harm when used in error.

Synonyms chlorpheniramine maleate and hydrocodone bitartrate; hydrocodone polistirex and chlorpheniramine polistirex

U.S. Brand Names TussiCaps®; Tussionex®

Therapeutic Category Antihistamine/Antitussive

Controlled Substance C-III

Use Symptomatic relief of cough and upper respiratory symptoms associated with cold and allergy

General Dosage Range Oral:

Children 6-12 years: TussiCaps® 5 mg/4 mg: 1 capsule every 12 hours (maximum: 2 capsules/24 hours); Tussionex®: 2.5 mL every 12 hours (maximum: 5 mL/24 hours)

Children >12 years and Adults: TussiCaps® 10 mg/8 mg: 1 capsule every 12 hours (maximum: 2 capsules/24 hours); Tussionex®: 5 mL every 12 hours (maximum: 10 mL/24 hours)

Dosage Forms

Capsule, extended release:

TussiCaps® 5/4: Hydrocodone bitartrate 5 mg and chlorpheniramine maleate 4 mg

TussiCaps® 10/8: Hydrocodone bitartrate 10 mg and chlorpheniramine maleate 8 mg

Suspension, extended release: Hydrocodone bitartrate 10 mg and chlorpheniramine maleate 8 mg per 5 mL

Tussionex®: Hydrocodone bitartrate 10 mg and chlorpheniramine maleate 8 mg per 5 mL

hydrocodone and homatropine (hye droe KOE done & hoe MA troe peen)

Medication Safety Issues

Sound-alike/look-alike issues:

Hycodan may be confused with Vicodin®

High alert medication:

The Institute for Safe Medication Practices (ISMP) includes this medication among its list of drug classes which have a heightened risk of causing significant patient harm when used in error.

Synonyms homatropine and hydrocodone; Hycodan; hydrocodone bitartrate and homatropine methylbromide

U.S. Brand Names Hydromet®; Tussigon®

Therapeutic Category Antitussive

Controlled Substance C-III

Use Symptomatic relief of cough

General Dosage Range Oral:
Children 6-11 years: 1/2 tablet or 2.5 mL every 4-6 hours as needed (maximum: 3 tablets or 15 mL/24 hours)
Children ≥12 years and Adults: 1 tablet or 5 mL every 4-6 hours as needed (maximum: 6 tablets/24 hours or 30 mL/24 hours)

Dosage Forms
Syrup: Hydrocodone 5 mg and homatropine 1.5 mg per 5 mL
Hydromet®: Hydrocodone 5 mg and homatropine 1.5 mg per 5 mL
Tablet:
Tussigon®: Hydrocodone 5 mg and homatropine 1.5 mg

hydrocodone and ibuprofen (hye droe KOE done & eye byoo PROE fen)

Medication Safety Issues
Sound-alike/look-alike issues:
Reprexain™ may be confused with ZyPREXA®
High alert medication:
The Institute for Safe Medication Practices (ISMP) includes this medication among its list of drug classes which have a heightened risk of causing significant patient harm when used in error.

Synonyms hydrocodone bitartrate and ibuprofen; ibuprofen and hydrocodone

U.S. Brand Names Ibudone®; Reprexain™; Vicoprofen®

Canadian Brand Names Vicoprofen®

Therapeutic Category Analgesic, Narcotic

Controlled Substance C-III

Use Short-term (generally <10 days) management of moderate-to-severe acute pain; is not indicated for treatment of such conditions as osteoarthritis or rheumatoid arthritis

General Dosage Range Oral: *Adults:* 1 tablet every 4-6 hours (maximum: 5 tablets/day; <10 days total therapy)

Dosage Forms
Tablet: Hydrocodone 2.5 mg and ibuprofen 200 mg; hydrocodone 5 mg and ibuprofen 200 mg; hydrocodone 7.5 mg and ibuprofen 200 mg
Ibudone®: 5/200: Hydrocodone 5 mg and ibuprofen 200 mg; 10/200: Hydrocodone 10 mg and ibuprofen 200 mg
Reprexain™: 2.5/200: Hydrocodone 2.5 mg and ibuprofen 200 mg; 5/200: Hydrocodone 5 mg and ibuprofen 200 mg; 10/200: Hydrocodone 10 mg and ibuprofen 200 mg
Vicoprofen®: 7.5/200: Hydrocodone 7.5 mg and ibuprofen 200 mg

hydrocodone and pseudoephedrine (hye droe KOE done & soo doe e FED rin)

Medication Safety Issues
High alert medication:
The Institute for Safe Medication Practices (ISMP) includes this medication among its list of drug classes which have a heightened risk of causing significant patient harm when used in error.

Synonyms pseudoephedrine and hydrocodone; pseudoephedrine hydrochloride and hydrocodone bitartrate

U.S. Brand Names Rezira™

Therapeutic Category Antitussive/Decongestant

Controlled Substance C-III

Use Symptomatic relief of cough and nasal congestion associated with common cold

General Dosage Range Oral: *Adults:* 5 mL every 4-6 hours as needed (maximum: 20 mL/24 hours)

Dosage Forms
Solution, oral:
Rezira™: Hydrocodone 5 mg and pseudoephedrine 60 mg per 5 mL (480 mL)

hydrocodone bitartrate and homatropine methylbromide *see* hydrocodone and homatropine *on page 455*

hydrocodone bitartrate and ibuprofen *see* hydrocodone and ibuprofen *on page 456*

hydrocodone, chlorpheniramine, and pseudoephedrine

(hye droe KOE done, klor fen IR a meen, & soo doe e FED rin)

Medication Safety Issues

High alert medication:

The Institute for Safe Medication Practices (ISMP) includes this medication among its list of drug classes which have a heightened risk of causing significant patient harm when used in error.

Synonyms chlorpheniramine, pseudoephedrine, and hydrocodone; pseudoephedrine hydrochloride, hydrocodone bitartrate, and chlorpheniramine maleate; pseudoephedrine, hydrocodone, and chlorpheniramine

U.S. Brand Names Zutripro™

Therapeutic Category Alpha/Beta Agonist; Analgesic, Opioid; Antitussive; Decongestant; Histamine H_1 Antagonist; Histamine H_1 Antagonist, First Generation

Controlled Substance C-III

Use Temporary relief of cough and nasal congestion due to colds or upper respiratory allergies

General Dosage Range

Oral: *Adults:* 5 mL every 4-6 hours as needed (maximum: 4 doses/24 hours)

Dosage Forms

Solution, oral:

Zutripro™: Hydrocodone bitartrate 5 mg, chlorpheniramine maleate 4 mg, and pseudoephedrine hydrochloride 60 mg per 5 mL (480 mL) [contains propylene glycol; grape flavor]

hydrocodone polistirex and chlorpheniramine polistirex *see* hydrocodone and chlorpheniramine *on page 455*

hydrocortisone (systemic) (hye droe KOR ti sone)

Medication Safety Issues

Sound-alike/look-alike issues:

Hydrocortisone may be confused with hydrocodone, hydroxychloroquine, hydrochlorothiazide

Cortef® may be confused with Coreg®, Lortab®

HCT (occasional abbreviation for hydrocortisone) is an error-prone abbreviation (mistaken as hydrochlorothiazide)

Solu-CORTEF® may be confused with Solu-MEDROL®

Synonyms A-hydroCort; compound F; cortisol; hydrocortisone sodium succinate

U.S. Brand Names A-Hydrocort®; Cortef®; Solu-CORTEF®

Canadian Brand Names Cortef®; Solu-Cortef®

Therapeutic Category Corticosteroid, Systemic

Use Management of adrenocortical insufficiency; antiinflammatory or immunosuppressive

General Dosage Range

I.M., I.V.: *Children and Adults:* Dosage varies greatly depending on indication

Oral:

Children: 0.5-10 mg/kg/day **or** 10-300 mg/m²/day divided every 6-8 hours

Adolescents: 0.5-10 mg/kg/day **or** 10-300 mg/m²/day divided every 6-8 hours **or** 15-240 mg every 12 hours

Adults: 20-480 mg/day in divided doses every 8-12 hours **or** 10-20 mg/m²/day in 3 divided doses

Dosage Forms

Injection, powder for reconstitution:

A-Hydrocort®: 100 mg

Solu-CORTEF®: 100 mg

Injection, powder for reconstitution [preservative free]:

Solu-CORTEF®: 100 mg, 250 mg, 500 mg, 1000 mg

Tablet, oral: 5 mg, 10 mg, 20 mg

Cortef®: 5 mg, 10 mg, 20 mg

hydrocortisone (topical) (hye droe KOR ti sone)

Medication Safety Issues

Sound-alike/look-alike issues:

Hydrocortisone may be confused with hydrocodone, hydroxychloroquine, hydrochlorothiazide

Anusol® may be confused with Anusol-HC®, Aplisol®, Aquasol®

Cortizone® may be confused with cortisone

HCT (occasional abbreviation for hydrocortisone) is an error-prone abbreviation (mistaken as hydrochlorothiazide)

Hytone® may be confused with Vytone®

Proctocort® may be confused with ProctoCream®

International issues:

Nutracort [multiple international markets] may be confused with Nitrocor brand name of nitroglycerin [Italy, Russia, and Venezuela]

Synonyms A-hydroCort; compound F; cortisol; hemorrhoidal HC; hydrocortisone acetate; hydrocortisone butyrate; hydrocortisone probutate; hydrocortisone valerate; nutracort

U.S. Brand Names Ala-Cort; Ala-Scalp; Anu-med HC; Anucort-HC™; Anusol-HC®; Aquanil HC® [OTC]; Beta-HC® [OTC]; Caldecort® [OTC]; Colocort®; Cortaid® Advanced [OTC]; Cortaid® Intensive Therapy [OTC]; Cortaid® Maximum Strength [OTC]; Cortenema®; CortiCool® [OTC]; Cortifoam®; Cortizone-10® Hydratensive Healing [OTC]; Cortizone-10® Hydratensive Soothing [OTC]; Cortizone-10® Intensive Healing Eczema [OTC]; Cortizone-10® Maximum Strength Cooling Relief [OTC]; Cortizone-10® Maximum Strength Easy Relief [OTC]; Cortizone-10® Maximum Strength Intensive Healing Formula [OTC]; Cortizone-10® Maximum Strength [OTC]; Cortizone-10® Plus Maximum Strength [OTC]; Dermarest® Eczema Medicated [OTC]; Hemril®-30; Hydrocortisone Plus [OTC]; Hydroskin® [OTC]; Locoid Lipocream®; Locoid®; Pandel®; Pediaderm™ HC; Preparation H® Hydrocortisone [OTC]; Procto-Pak™; Proctocort®; ProctoCream®-HC; Proctosol-HC®; Proctozone-HC 2.5%™; Recort [OTC]; Scalpana [OTC]; Texacort™; U-Cort®; Westcort®

Canadian Brand Names Aquacort®; Cortamed®; Cortenema®; Cortifoam™; Emo-Cort®; Hycort™; Hyderm; HydroVal®; Locoid®; Prevex® HC; Sarna® HC; Westcort®

Therapeutic Category Corticosteroid, Rectal; Corticosteroid, Topical

Use Relief of inflammation of corticosteroid-responsive dermatoses (low and medium potency topical corticosteroid); adjunctive treatment of ulcerative colitis; mild-to-moderate atopic dermatitis; inflamed hemorrhoids, postirradiation (factitial) proctitis, and other inflammatory conditions of anorectum and pruritus ani

General Dosage Range

Rectal: *Adults:* Foam: One applicatorful 1-2 times/day; Suppository: 1-2 suppositories 2-3 times/day; Suspension: One enema at bedtime

Topical: *Children and Adults:* Apply thin film to affected area 2-4 times/day

Dosage Forms

Aerosol, foam, rectal:

Cortifoam®: 10% (15 g)

Cream, topical: 0.1% (15 g, 45 g); 0.2% (15 g, 45 g, 60 g); 0.5% (0.9 g, 15 g, 28.4 g, 30 g, 60 g); 1% (0.9 g, 1 g, 1.5 g, 15 g, 20 g, 28.35 g, 28.4 g, 30 g, 114 g, 120 g, 454 g); 2% (43 g); 2.5% (20 g, 28 g, 28.35 g, 30 g, 454 g)

Ala-Cort: 1% (28.4 g, 85.2 g)

Anusol-HC®: 2.5% (30 g)

Caldecort® [OTC]: 1% (28.4 g)

Cortaid® Advanced [OTC]: 1% (42 g)

Cortaid® Intensive Therapy [OTC]: 1% (37 g, 56 g)

Cortaid® Maximum Strength [OTC]: 1% (14 g, 28 g, 37 g, 56 g)

Cortizone-10® Maximum Strength [OTC]: 1% (15 g, 28 g, 56 g)

Cortizone-10® Maximum Strength Intensive Healing Formula [OTC]: 1% (28 g, 56 g)

Cortizone-10® Plus Maximum Strength [OTC]: 1% (28 g, 56 g)

Hydrocortisone Plus [OTC]: 1% (28.4 g)

Hydroskin® [OTC]: 1% (28 g)

Locoid Lipocream®: 0.1% (45 g, 60 g)

Locoid®: 0.1% (15 g, 45 g)

Pandel®: 0.1% (15 g, 45 g, 80 g)

Preparation H® Hydrocortisone [OTC]: 1% (26 g)

Procto-Pak™: 1% (28.4 g)

Proctocort®: 1% (28.35 g)

ProctoCream®-HC: 2.5% (30 g)

Proctosol-HC®: 2.5% (28.35 g)

Proctozone-HC 2.5%™: 2.5% (30 g)

Recort [OTC]: 1% (30 g)

U-Cort®: 1% (28 g)

Gel, topical:
CortiCool® [OTC]: 1% (0.9 g, 42.5 g)
Cortizone-10® Maximum Strength Cooling Relief [OTC]: 1% (28 g)

Liquid, topical:
Cortizone-10® Maximum Strength Easy Relief [OTC]: 1% (36 mL)
Scalpana [OTC]: 1% (85.5 mL)

Lotion, topical: 1% (114 g, 118 mL, 120 mL); 2.5% (59 mL, 60 mL, 118 mL)
Ala-Scalp: 2% (29.6 mL)
Aquanil HC® [OTC]: 1% (120 mL)
Beta-HC® [OTC]: 1% (60 mL)
Cortaid® Intensive Therapy [OTC]: 1% (98 g)
Cortizone-10® Hydratensive Healing [OTC]: 1% (113 g)
Cortizone-10® Hydratensive Soothing [OTC]: 1% (113 g)
Cortizone-10® Intensive Healing Eczema [OTC]: 1% (99 g)
Dermarest® Eczema Medicated [OTC]: 1% (118 mL)
Hydroskin® [OTC]: 1% (118 mL)
Locoid®: 0.1% (60 mL)
Pediaderm™ HC: 2% (29.6 mL)

Ointment, topical: 0.1% (15 g, 45 g); 0.2% (15 g, 45 g, 60 g); 0.5% (30 g); 1% (25 g, 28.4 g, 30 g, 110 g, 430 g, 454 g); 2.5% (20 g, 28.35 g, 30 g, 454 g)
Cortaid® Maximum Strength [OTC]: 1% (28 g, 37 g)
Cortizone-10® Maximum Strength [OTC]: 1% (28 g, 56 g)
Locoid®: 0.1% (15 g, 45 g)
Westcort®: 0.2% (45 g, 60 g)

Powder, for prescription compounding: USP: 100% (10 g, 25 g, 50 g, 100 g, 1000 g)

Solution, topical: 0.1% (20 mL, 60 mL)
Cortaid® Intensive Therapy [OTC]: 1% (59 mL)
Locoid®: 0.1% (20 mL, 60 mL)
Texacort™: 2.5% (30 mL)

Suppository, rectal: 25 mg (12s, 24s, 1000s); 30 mg (12s)
Anu-med HC: 25 mg (12s)
Anucort-HC™: 25 mg (12s, 24s, 100s)
Anusol-HC®: 25 mg (12s, 24s)
Hemril® -30: 30 mg (12s, 24s)
Proctocort®: 30 mg (12s, 24s)

Suspension, rectal: 100 mg/60 mL (60 mL)
Colocort®: 100 mg/60 mL (60 mL)
Cortenema®: 100 mg/60 mL (60 mL)

hydrocortisone acetate *see* hydrocortisone (topical) *on page 457*

hydrocortisone, acetic acid, and propylene glycol diacetate *see* acetic acid, propylene glycol diacetate, and hydrocortisone *on page 31*

hydrocortisone and acyclovir *see* acyclovir and hydrocortisone *on page 35*

hydrocortisone and benzoyl peroxide *see* benzoyl peroxide and hydrocortisone *on page 125*

hydrocortisone and ciprofloxacin *see* ciprofloxacin and hydrocortisone *on page 212*

hydrocortisone and fusidic acid *see* fusidic acid and hydrocortisone *(Canada only) on page 413*

hydrocortisone and iodoquinol *see* iodoquinol and hydrocortisone *on page 495*

hydrocortisone and lidocaine *see* lidocaine and hydrocortisone *on page 538*

hydrocortisone and pramoxine *see* pramoxine and hydrocortisone *on page 751*

hydrocortisone and urea *see* urea and hydrocortisone *on page 931*

hydrocortisone, bacitracin, neomycin, and polymyxin B *see* bacitracin, neomycin, polymyxin B, and hydrocortisone *on page 112*

hydrocortisone butyrate *see* hydrocortisone (topical) *on page 457*

hydrocortisone, neomycin, and polymyxin B *see* neomycin, polymyxin B, and hydrocortisone *on page 634*

hydrocortisone, neomycin, colistin, and thonzonium *see* neomycin, colistin, hydrocortisone, and thonzonium *on page 633*

Hydrocortisone Plus [OTC] *see* hydrocortisone (topical) *on page 457*

hydrocortisone probutate *see* hydrocortisone (topical) *on page 457*

hydrocortisone sodium succinate *see* hydrocortisone (systemic) *on page 457*

hydrocortisone valerate *see* hydrocortisone (topical) *on page* 457
Hydrodiuril *see* hydrochlorothiazide *on page* 452
Hydromet® *see* hydrocodone and homatropine *on page* 455
Hydromorph Contin® (Can) *see* hydromorphone *on page* 460
Hydromorph-IR® (Can) *see* hydromorphone *on page* 460

hydromorphone (hye droe MOR fone)

Medication Safety Issues

Sound-alike/look-alike issues:

Dilaudid® may be confused with Demerol®, Dilantin®

HYDROmorphone may be confused with morphine; significant overdoses have occurred when hydromorphone products have been inadvertently administered instead of morphine sulfate. Commercially available prefilled syringes of both products looks similar and are often stored in close proximity to each other. **Note:** Hydromorphone 1 mg oral is approximately equal to morphine 4 mg oral; hydromorphone 1 mg I.V. is approximately equal to morphine 5 mg I.V.

High alert medication:

The Institute for Safe Medication Practices (ISMP) includes this medication among its list of drug classes which have a heightened risk of causing significant patient harm when used in error.

Administration issues:

Dilaudid®, Dilaudid-HP®: Extreme caution should be taken to avoid confusing the highly-concentrated (Dilaudid-HP®) injection with the less-concentrated (Dilaudid®) injectable product.

Exalgo®: Extreme caution should be taken to avoid confusing the extended release Exalgo® 8 mg tablets with immediate release hydromorphone 8 mg tablets.

Significant differences exist between oral and I.V. dosing. Use caution when converting from one route of administration to another.

Synonyms dihydromorphinone; hydromorphone hydrochloride

Tall-Man **HYDRO**morphone

U.S. Brand Names Dilaudid-HP®; Dilaudid®; Exalgo®

Canadian Brand Names Dilaudid-HP-Plus®; Dilaudid-HP®; Dilaudid-XP®; Dilaudid®; Dilaudid® Sterile Powder; Hydromorph Contin®; Hydromorph-IR®; Hydromorphone HP; Hydromorphone HP® 10; Hydromorphone HP® 20; Hydromorphone HP® 50; Hydromorphone HP® Forte; Hydromorphone Hydrochloride Injection, USP; Jurnista™; PMS-Hydromorphone

Therapeutic Category Analgesic, Narcotic

Controlled Substance C-II

Use Management of moderate-to-severe pain

Exalgo®: Management of moderate-to-severe pain in opioid-tolerant patients (requiring around-the-clock analgesia for an extended period of time)

General Dosage Range Dosage adjustment recommended in patients with hepatic or renal impairment

I.M., SubQ: *Children >50 kg and Adults:* 0.8-2 mg every 4-6 hours

I.V.:

Children ≥6 months and <50 kg: 0.015 mg/kg/dose every 3-6 hours as needed

Children >50 kg and Adults: 0.2-0.6 mg every 2-3 hours as needed

Adults (mechanically ventilated): Infusion: 0.5-1 mg/**hour** (based on 70 kg patient) **or** 7-15 mcg/kg/**hour**

Epidural PCA: *Children >50 kg and Adults:* Bolus: 0.4-1 mg; Infusion: 0.03-0.3 mg/**hour**; Demand dose: 0.02-0.5 mg; Lockout interval: 10-15 minutes

Oral:

Children ≥6 months and <50 kg: 0.03-0.08 mg/kg/dose every 3-4 hours as needed

Children >50 kg: 2-8 mg every 3-4 hours as needed

Adults: 2-8 mg every 3-4 hours as needed; Extended release: 8-64 mg every 24 hours

Elderly: 1-2 mg every 3-6 hours

PCA:

Children <50 kg: Usual concentration: 0.2 mg/mL; Demand dose: 0.003-0.005 mg/kg/dose; Lockout interval: 6-10 minutes; Usual basal rate: 0-0.004 mg/kg/hour

Children >50 kg and Adults: Usual concentration: 0.2 mg/mL; Demand dose: 0.05-0.4 mg; Lockout interval: 5-10 minutes

Rectal: *Children >50 kg and Adults:* 3 mg every 6-8 hours as needed

Dosage Forms

Injection, powder for reconstitution:

Dilaudid-HP®: 250 mg

Injection, solution: 1 mg/mL (1 mL); 2 mg/mL (1 mL, 20 mL); 4 mg/mL (1 mL); 10 mg/mL (1 mL, 5 mL, 50 mL)
Dilaudid-HP®: 10 mg/mL (1 mL, 5 mL, 50 mL)
Dilaudid®: 1 mg/mL (1 mL); 2 mg/mL (1 mL); 4 mg/mL (1 mL)
Injection, solution [preservative free]: 10 mg/mL (1 mL, 5 mL, 50 mL)
Liquid, oral: 1 mg/mL (473 mL)
Dilaudid®: 1 mg/mL (473 mL)
Powder, for prescription compounding: USP: 100% (972 mg)
Suppository, rectal: 3 mg (6s)
Tablet, oral: 2 mg, 4 mg, 8 mg
Dilaudid®: 2 mg, 4 mg, 8 mg
Tablet, extended release, oral:
Exalgo®: 8 mg, 12 mg, 16 mg, 32 mg

Dosage Forms - Canada
Capsule, controlled release:
Hydromorph Contin®: 3 mg, 6 mg, 12 mg, 18 mg, 24 mg, 30 mg [not available in U.S.]

Hydromorphone HP (Can) *see* hydromorphone *on page 460*
Hydromorphone HP® 10 (Can) *see* hydromorphone *on page 460*
Hydromorphone HP® 20 (Can) *see* hydromorphone *on page 460*
Hydromorphone HP® 50 (Can) *see* hydromorphone *on page 460*
Hydromorphone HP® Forte (Can) *see* hydromorphone *on page 460*
hydromorphone hydrochloride *see* hydromorphone *on page 460*
Hydromorphone Hydrochloride Injection, USP (Can) *see* hydromorphone *on page 460*
hydroquinol *see* hydroquinone *on page 461*

hydroquinone (HYE droe kwin one)

Medication Safety Issues
Sound-alike/look-alike issues:
Eldopaque® may be confused with Eldoquin®
Eldopaque Forte® may be confused with Eldoquin Forte®

Synonyms hydroquinol; quinol

U.S. Brand Names Aclaro PD®; Aclaro®; Alphaquin HP®; Eldopaque Forte®; Eldopaque® [OTC]; Eldoquin Forte®; Eldoquin® [OTC]; EpiQuin® Micro; Esoterica® Daytime [OTC]; Esoterica® Nighttime [OTC]; Lustra-AF®; Lustra-Ultra™; Lustra®; Melpaque HP®; Melquin HP®; Melquin-3®; NeoStrata® HQ Skin Lightening [OTC]; Nuquin HP®; Palmer's® Skin Success® Eventone® Fade Cream [OTC]; Palmer's® Skin Success® Eventone® Fade Milk [OTC]; Palmer's® Skin Success® Eventone® Ultra Fade Serum [OTC]

Canadian Brand Names Eldopaque®; Eldoquin®; Glyquin® XM; Lustra®; NeoStrata® HQ; Solaquin Forte®; Solaquin®; Ultraquin™

Therapeutic Category Topical Skin Product

Use Gradual bleaching of hyperpigmented skin conditions

General Dosage Range Topical: *Children >12 years and Adults:* Apply thin layer and rub in twice daily

Dosage Forms
Cream, topical: 4% (28.35 g, 28.4 g, 30 g)
Alphaquin HP®: 4% (28.4 g, 56.7 g)
Eldopaque Forte®: 4% (28.35 g)
Eldopaque® [OTC]: 2% (28.35 g)
Eldoquin Forte®: 4% (28.4 g)
Eldoquin® [OTC]: 2% (28.35 g)
EpiQuin® Micro: 4% (40 g)
Esoterica® Daytime [OTC]: 2% (70 g, 85 g)
Esoterica® Nighttime [OTC]: 2% (85 g)
Lustra-AF®: 4% (56.8 g)
Lustra-Ultra™: 4% (56.8 g)
Lustra®: 4% (56.8 g)
Melpaque HP®: 4% (14.2 g, 28.4 g)
Melquin HP®: 4% (14.2 g, 28.4 g)
Nuquin HP®: 4% (14.2 g, 28.4 g, 56.7 g)
Palmer's® Skin Success® Eventone® Fade Cream [OTC]: 2% (75 g, 125 g)

Emulsion, topical:
Aclaro PD®: 4% (42.5 g)
Aclaro®: 4% (48.2 g)
Gel, topical: 4% (28.35 g, 30 g)
NeoStrata® HQ Skin Lightening [OTC]: 2% (30 g)
Nuquin HP®: 4% (14.2 g, 28.4 g)
Lotion, topical:
Palmer's® Skin Success® Eventone® Fade Milk [OTC]: 2% (250 mL)
Solution, topical:
Melquin-3®: 3% (29.57 mL)
Palmer's® Skin Success® Eventone® Ultra Fade Serum [OTC]: 2% (30 mL)

hydroquinone, fluocinolone acetonide, and tretinoin *see* fluocinolone, hydroquinone, and tretinoin *on page* *392*
Hydroskin® [OTC] *see* hydrocortisone (topical) *on page* *457*
HydroVal® (Can) *see* hydrocortisone (topical) *on page* *457*

hydroxyamphetamine and tropicamide (hye droks ee am FET a meen & troe PIK a mide)

Synonyms hydroxyamphetamine hydrobromide and tropicamide; tropicamide and hydroxyamphetamine
U.S. Brand Names Paremyd®
Therapeutic Category Adrenergic Agonist Agent, Ophthalmic
Use Short-term pupil dilation for diagnostic procedures and exams
General Dosage Range **Ophthalmic:** *Adults:* Instill 1-2 drops into conjunctival sac(s)
Dosage Forms
Solution, ophthalmic:
Paremyd®: Hydroxyamphetamine 1% and tropicamide 0.25% (15 mL)

hydroxyamphetamine hydrobromide and tropicamide *see* hydroxyamphetamine and tropicamide *on page* *462*
4-hydroxybutyrate *see* sodium oxybate *on page* *844*
hydroxycarbamide *see* hydroxyurea *on page* *464*

hydroxychloroquine (hye droks ee KLOR oh kwin)

Medication Safety Issues
Sound-alike/look-alike issues:
Hydroxychloroquine may be confused with hydrocortisone
Plaquenil® may be confused with Platinol
Synonyms hydroxychloroquine sulfate
U.S. Brand Names Plaquenil®
Canadian Brand Names Apo-Hydroxyquine®; Gen-Hydroxychloroquine; Mylan-Hydroxychloroquine; Plaquenil®; PRO-Hydroxyquine
Therapeutic Category Aminoquinoline (Antimalarial)
Use Suppression and treatment of acute attacks of malaria; treatment of systemic lupus erythematosus (SLE) and rheumatoid arthritis
General Dosage Range **Oral:**
Children: 13 mg/kg for 1-2 doses, followed by 6.5 mg/kg for 3 doses or once weekly
Adults: Initial: 400-800 mg/day divided 1-2 times/day; Maintenance: 200-400 mg/day **or** 800 mg for 1-2 doses, followed by 400 mg for 3 doses or once weekly
Dosage Forms
Tablet, oral: 200 mg
Plaquenil®: 200 mg

hydroxychloroquine sulfate *see* hydroxychloroquine *on page* *462*
1-α-hydroxycholecalciferol *see* alfacalcidol *(Canada only) on page* *46*
hydroxydaunomycin hydrochloride *see* doxorubicin *on page* *313*
hydroxyethylcellulose *see* artificial tears *on page* *93*
hydroxyethyl starch *see* hetastarch *on page* *447*
hydroxyethyl starch *see* pentastarch *(Canada only) on page* *704*
hydroxyethyl starch *see* tetrastarch *on page* *885*
hydroxyldaunorubicin hydrochloride *see* doxorubicin *on page* *313*

hydroxyprogesterone caproate (hye droks ee proe JES te rone CAP ro ate)

Medication Safety Issues

Sound-alike/look-alike issues:

Hydroxyprogesterone caproate may be confused with medroxyPROGESTERone

Synonyms 17OHPC

U.S. Brand Names Makena™

Therapeutic Category Progestin

Use To reduce the risk of preterm birth in women with singleton pregnancies who have a history of spontaneous preterm birth (delivery <37 weeks gestation) with previous singleton pregnancies

General Dosage Range I.M.: *Pregnant females:* 250 mg every 7 days

Dosage Forms

Injection, solution:

Makena™: 250 mg/mL (5 mL)

hydroxypropyl cellulose (hye droks ee PROE pil SEL yoo lose)

U.S. Brand Names Lacrisert®

Canadian Brand Names Lacrisert®

Therapeutic Category Ophthalmic Agent, Miscellaneous

Use Dry eyes (moderate-to-severe)

General Dosage Range Ophthalmic: *Adults:* Apply once daily

Dosage Forms

Insert, ophthalmic [preservative free]:

Lacrisert®: 5 mg (60s)

hydroxypropyl methylcellulose (hye droks ee PROE pil meth il SEL yoo lose)

Medication Safety Issues

Sound-alike/look-alike issues:

Isopto® Tears may be confused with Isoptin®

Synonyms gonioscopic ophthalmic solution; hypromellose

U.S. Brand Names Cellugel®; GenTeal® Mild [OTC]; GenTeal® [OTC]; Gonak™; Goniosoft™ [OTC]; Isopto® Tears [OTC]; Natural Balance Tears [OTC]; Nature's Tears [OTC]; Tears Again® MC Gel Drops™ [OTC]

Canadian Brand Names Genteal®; Isopto® Tears

Therapeutic Category Ophthalmic Agent, Miscellaneous

Use Relief of burning and minor irritation due to dry eyes; diagnostic agent in gonioscopic examination

General Dosage Range Ophthalmic: *Adults:* Instill 1-2 drops in affected eye(s) as needed

Dosage Forms

Gel, ophthalmic [preservative free]:

GenTeal® [OTC]: 0.3% (10 mL)

Injection, solution, ophthalmic:

Cellugel®: 2% (1 mL)

Solution, ophthalmic:

Gonak™: 2.5% (15 mL)

Goniosoft™ [OTC]: 2.5% (15 mL)

Isopto® Tears [OTC]: 0.5% (15 mL)

Natural Balance Tears [OTC]: 0.4% (15 mL)

Nature's Tears [OTC]: 0.4% (15 mL)

Tears Again® MC Gel Drops™ [OTC]: 0.3% (15 mL)

Solution, ophthalmic [preservative free]:

GenTeal® [OTC]: 0.3% (15 mL, 25 mL)

GenTeal® Mild [OTC]: 0.2% (15 mL, 25 mL)

9-hydroxy-risperidone *see* paliperidone *on page 685*

hydroxyurea (hye droks ee yoor EE a)

Medication Safety Issues

Sound-alike/look-alike issues:

Hydroxyurea may be confused with hydrOXYzine

High alert medication:

This medication is in a class the Institute for Safe Medication Practices (ISMP) includes among its list of drugs which have a heightened risk of causing significant patient harm when used in error.

International issues:

Hydrea [U.S., Canada, and multiple international markets] may be confused with Hydra brand name for isoniazid [Japan]

Synonyms hydroxycarbamide; hydurea

U.S. Brand Names Droxia®; Hydrea®

Canadian Brand Names Apo-Hydroxyurea®; Gen-Hydroxyurea; Hydrea®; Mylan-Hydroxyurea

Therapeutic Category Antineoplastic Agent

Use Treatment of melanoma, refractory chronic myelocytic leukemia (CML); recurrent, metastatic, or inoperable ovarian cancer; radiosensitizing agent in the treatment of squamous cell head and neck cancer (excluding lip cancer); adjunct in the management of sickle cell patients who have had at least three painful crises in the previous 12 months (to reduce frequency of these crises and the need for blood transfusions)

General Dosage Range Dosage adjustment recommended in patients with renal impairment

Oral: *Adults:* 15-35 mg/kg/day **or** 500-3000 mg/day as single or divided dose **or** 80 mg/kg as a single dose every third day

Dosage Forms

Capsule, oral: 500 mg

Droxia®: 200 mg, 300 mg, 400 mg

Hydrea®: 500 mg

1-α-hydroxyvitamin D_3 *see* alfacalcidol *(Canada only) on page 46*

hydroxyzine (hye DROKS i zeen)

Medication Safety Issues

Sound-alike/look-alike issues:

HydrOXYzine may be confused with hydrALAZINE, hydroxyurea

Atarax® may be confused with Ativan®

Vistaril® may be confused with Restoril™, Versed, Zestril®

BEERS Criteria medication:

This drug may be potentially inappropriate for use in geriatric patients (Quality of evidence - high; Strength of recommendation - strong).

International issues:

Vistaril [U.S. and Turkey] may be confused with Vastarel brand name for trimetazidine [multiple international markets]

Synonyms hydroxyzine hydrochloride; hydroxyzine pamoate

Tall-Man hydr**OXY**zine

U.S. Brand Names Vistaril®

Canadian Brand Names Apo-Hydroxyzine®; Atarax®; Hydroxyzine Hydrochloride Injection, USP; Novo-Hydroxyzin; Nu-Hydroxyzine; PMS-Hydroxyzine; Riva-Hydroxyzine

Therapeutic Category Antiemetic; Antihistamine

Use Treatment of anxiety/agitation (including adjunctive therapy in alcoholism); adjunct to pre- and postoperative analgesia and anesthesia; antipruritic; antiemetic

General Dosage Range Dosage adjustment recommended in patients with hepatic impairment

I.M.:

Children: 1.1 mg/kg/dose

Adults: 25-100 mg/dose

Oral:

Children: 0.6 mg/kg/dose (sedation)

Children <6 years: 50 mg/day in divided doses

Children ≥6 years: 50-100 mg/day in divided doses

Adults: 25-100 mg/dose

Dosage Forms

Capsule, oral: 25 mg, 50 mg, 100 mg
Vistaril®: 25 mg, 50 mg
Injection, solution: 25 mg/mL (1 mL); 50 mg/mL (1 mL, 2 mL, 10 mL)
Solution, oral: 10 mg/5 mL (473 mL)
Syrup, oral: 10 mg/5 mL (118 mL, 473 mL, 480 mL)
Tablet, oral: 10 mg, 25 mg, 50 mg

hydroxyzine hydrochloride *see* hydroxyzine *on page 464*
Hydroxyzine Hydrochloride Injection, USP (Can) *see* hydroxyzine *on page 464*
hydroxyzine pamoate *see* hydroxyzine *on page 464*
hydurea *see* hydroxyurea *on page 464*
Hygroton *see* chlorthalidone *on page 204*
hylan G-F 20 *see* hyaluronate and derivatives *on page 450*
hylan polymers *see* hyaluronate and derivatives *on page 450*
Hylase® Wound *see* hyaluronate and derivatives *on page 450*
Hylatopic™ *see* emollients *on page 328*
HylatopicPlus™ *see* emollients *on page 328*
HylatopicPlus™-Aurstat [DSC] *see* emollients *on page 328*
Hylenex [DSC] *see* hyaluronidase *on page 451*
HyoMax™-DT *see* hyoscyamine *on page 465*
HyoMax™-FT *see* hyoscyamine *on page 465*
HyoMax®-SL *see* hyoscyamine *on page 465*
HyoMax®-SR *see* hyoscyamine *on page 465*
Hyonatol *see* hyoscyamine, atropine, scopolamine, and phenobarbital *on page 467*
Hyophen™ *see* methenamine, phenyl salicylate, methylene blue, benzoic acid, and hyoscyamine *on page 583*
hyoscine butylbromide *see* scopolamine (systemic) *on page 826*
hyoscine hydrobromide *see* scopolamine (ophthalmic) *on page 826*

hyoscyamine (hye oh SYE a meen)

Medication Safety Issues

Sound-alike/look-alike issues:
Anaspaz® may be confused with Anaprox®, Antispas®
Levbid® may be confused with Enbrel®, Lithobid®, Lopid®, Lorabid®
Levsinex® may be confused with Lanoxin®
Levsin/SL® maybe confused with Levaquin®

BEERS Criteria medication:
This drug may be potentially inappropriate for use in geriatric patients (Quality of evidence - moderate; Strength of recommendation - strong).

Synonyms *l*-hyoscyamine sulfate; hyoscyamine sulfate

U.S. Brand Names Anaspaz®; ED-SPAZ; HyoMax® -SR; HyoMax®-SL; HyoMax™-DT; HyoMax™-FT; Hyosyne; Levbid®; Levsin®; Levsin®/SL; NuLev®; Oscimin; Symax® DuoTab; Symax® FasTab; Symax® SL; Symax® SR

Canadian Brand Names Levsin®

Therapeutic Category Anticholinergic Agent

Use

Oral: Adjunctive therapy for peptic ulcers, irritable bowel, neurogenic bladder/bowel; treatment of infant colic, GI tract disorders caused by spasm; to reduce rigidity, tremors, sialorrhea, and hyperhidrosis associated with parkinsonism; as a drying agent in acute rhinitis

Injection: Preoperative antimuscarinic to reduce secretions and block cardiac vagal inhibitory reflexes; to improve radiologic visibility of the kidneys; symptomatic relief of biliary and renal colic; reduce GI motility to facilitate diagnostic procedures (ie, endoscopy, hypotonic duodenography); reduce pain and hypersecretion in pancreatitis, certain cases of partial heart block associated with vagal activity; reversal of neuromuscular blockade

General Dosage Range

I.M., SubQ: *Adults:* 0.25-0.5 mg 4 times/day as needed

I.V.:

Children ≥2 years: 5 mcg/kg given 30-60 minutes prior to induction of anesthesia

Adults: 0.125-0.5 mg 4 times/day as needed **or** 0.25-0.5 mg or 5 mcg/kg as a single dose **or** 0.2 mg for every 1 mg neostigmine

Oral:

Regular release:

Children <2 years and 3.4 kg: 4 drops every 4 hours as needed (maximum: 24 drops/day)

Children <2 years and 5 kg: 5 drops every 4 hours as needed (maximum: 30 drops/day)

Children <2 years and 7 kg: 6 drops every 4 hours as needed (maximum: 36 drops/day)

Children <2 years and 10 kg: 8 drops every 4 hours as needed (maximum: 48 drops/day)

Children ≥2 years and 10 kg: 0.031-0.033 mg every 4 hours as needed (maximum: 0.75 mg/day)

Children ≥2 years and 20 kg: 0.0625 mg every 4 hours as needed (maximum: 0.75 mg/day)

Children ≥2 years and 40 kg: 0.0938 mg every 4 hours as needed (maximum: 0.75 mg/day)

Children ≥2 years and 50 kg: 0.125 mg every 4 hours as needed (maximum: 0.75 mg/day)

Adults: 0.125-0.25 mg every 4 hours or as needed (maximum: 1.5 mg/day)

Timed release: *Adults:* 0.375-0.75 mg every 12 hours (maximum: 1.5 mg/day)

S.L.:

Children ≥2 years and 10 kg: 0.031-0.033 mg every 4 hours as needed (maximum: 0.75 mg/day)

Children ≥2 years and 20 kg: 0.0625 mg every 4 hours as needed (maximum: 0.75 mg/day)

Children ≥2 years and 40 kg: 0.0938 mg every 4 hours as needed (maximum: 0.75 mg/day)

Children ≥2 years and 50 kg: 0.125 mg every 4 hours as needed (maximum: 0.75 mg/day)

Adults: 0.125-0.25 mg every 4 hours or as needed (maximum: 1.5 mg/day)

Dosage Forms

Elixir, oral: 0.125 mg/5 mL (473 mL, 480 mL)

Hyosyne: 0.125 mg/5 mL (473 mL)

Injection, solution:

Levsin®: 0.5 mg/mL (1 mL)

Solution, oral: 0.125 mg/mL (15 mL)

Hyosyne: 0.125 mg/mL (15 mL)

Tablet, oral: 0.125 mg

Levsin®: 0.125 mg

Tablet, sublingual: 0.125 mg

HyoMax®-SL: 0.125 mg

Levsin®/SL: 0.125 mg

Oscimin: 0.125 mg

Symax® SL: 0.125 mg

Tablet, chewable/disintegrating, oral:

HyoMax™-FT: 0.125 mg

NuLev®: 0.125 mg

Oscimin: 0.125 mg

Symax® FasTab: 0.125 mg

Tablet, dispersible, oral:

Oscimin: 0.125 mg

Tablet, extended release, oral: 0.375 mg

Levbid®: 0.375 mg

Oscimin: 0.375 mg

Tablet, orally disintegrating, oral: 0.125 mg

Anaspaz®: 0.125 mg

ED-SPAZ: 0.125 mg

Tablet, sustained release, oral: 0.375 mg

HyoMax® -SR: 0.375 mg

Symax® SR: 0.375 mg

Tablet, variable release, oral:

HyoMax™-DT: Hyoscyamine sulfate 0.125 mg [immediate release] and hyoscyamine sulfate 0.25 mg [sustained release]

Symax® DuoTab: Hyoscyamine sulfate 0.125 mg [immediate release] and hyoscyamine sulfate 0.25 mg [sustained release]

hyoscyamine, atropine, scopolamine, and phenobarbital

(hye oh SYE a meen, A troe peen, skoe POL a meen, & fee noe BAR bi tal)

Medication Safety Issues

Sound-alike/look-alike issues:

Donnatal® may be confused with Donnagel, Donnatal Extentabs®

BEERS Criteria medication:

This drug may be potentially inappropriate for use in geriatric patients (Quality of evidence - moderate; Strength of recommendation - strong).

Synonyms atropine, hyoscyamine, phenobarbital, and scopolamine; belladonna alkaloids with phenobarbital; phenobarbital, hyoscyamine, atropine, and scopolamine; scopolamine, hyoscyamine, atropine, and phenobarbital

U.S. Brand Names Donnatal Extentabs®; Donnatal®; Hyonatol

Therapeutic Category Anticholinergic Agent

Use Adjunct in treatment of irritable bowel syndrome, acute enterocolitis, duodenal ulcer

General Dosage Range Oral:

Extended release: *Adults:* 1 tablet every 8-12 hours

Immediate release:

Children ≥2 years:

9.1 kg: 1 mL every 4 hours **or** 1.5 mL every 6 hours

13.6 kg: 1.5 mL every 4 hours **or** 2 mL every 6 hours

22.7 kg: 2.5 mL every 4 hours **or** 3.75 mL every 6 hours

34 kg: 3.75 mL every 4 hours **or** 5 mL every 6 hours

45.4 kg: 5 mL every 4 hours **or** 7.5 mL every 6 hours

Adults: 1-2 tablets **or** 5-10 mL of elixir 3-4 times/day

Dosage Forms

Elixir: Hyoscyamine sulfate 0.1037 mg, atropine sulfate 0.0194 mg, scopolamine hydrobromide 0.0065 mg, and phenobarbital 16.2 mg per 5 mL

Donnatal®: Hyoscyamine 0.1037 mg, atropine 0.0194 mg, scopolamine 0.0065 mg, and phenobarbital 16.2 mg per 5 mL

Tablet: Hyoscyamine 0.1037 mg, atropine 0.0194 mg, scopolamine 0.0065 mg, and phenobarbital 16.2 mg

Donnatal®: Hyoscyamine 0.1037 mg, atropine 0.0194 mg, scopolamine 0.0065 mg, and phenobarbital 16.2 mg

Hyonatol: Hyoscyamine 0.1037 mg, atropine 0.0194 mg, scopolamine 0.0065 mg, and phenobarbital 16.2 mg

Tablet, extended release:

Donnatal Extentabs®: Hyoscyamine 0.3111 mg, atropine 0.0582 mg, scopolamine 0.0195 mg, and phenobarbital 48.6 mg

hyoscyamine, methenamine, benzoic acid, phenyl salicylate, and methylene blue *see* methenamine, phenyl salicylate, methylene blue, benzoic acid, and hyoscyamine *on page* 583

hyoscyamine sulfate *see* hyoscyamine *on page* 465

Hyosyne *see* hyoscyamine *on page* 465

Hyperal *see* total parenteral nutrition *on page* 908

hyperalimentation *see* total parenteral nutrition *on page* 908

Hypercare™ *see* aluminum chloride hexahydrate *on page* 55

HyperHEP B™ S/D *see* hepatitis B immune globulin (human) *on page* 445

HyperRAB® S/D *see* rabies immune globulin (human) *on page* 784

HyperRHO™ S/D Full Dose *see* Rh_o(D) immune globulin *on page* 797

HyperRHO™ S/D Mini-Dose *see* Rh_o(D) immune globulin *on page* 797

HyperSal® *see* sodium chloride *on page* 840

HyperTET™ S/D *see* tetanus immune globulin (human) *on page* 882

hypertonic saline *see* sodium chloride *on page* 840

HypoTears [OTC] *see* artificial tears *on page* 93

hypromellose *see* hydroxypropyl methylcellulose *on page* 463

Hytrin *see* terazosin *on page* 878

Hytrin® (Can) *see* terazosin *on page* 878

Hyzaar® *see* losartan and hydrochlorothiazide *on page* 551

Hyzaar® DS (Can) *see* losartan and hydrochlorothiazide *on page* 551

HZT-501 *see* ibuprofen and famotidine *on page* 470

I^{123} iobenguane *see* iobenguane I 123 *on page* 493

I-123 MIBG *see* iobenguane I 123 *on page* 493

ibandronate (eye BAN droh nate)

Synonyms ibandronate sodium; ibandronic acid

U.S. Brand Names Boniva®

Therapeutic Category Bisphosphonate Derivative

Use Treatment and prevention of osteoporosis in postmenopausal females

General Dosage Range

I.V.: *Adults:* 3 mg every 3 months

Oral: *Adults:* 150 mg once a month

Dosage Forms

Injection, solution:

Boniva®: 1 mg/mL (3 mL)

Tablet, oral: 150 mg

Boniva®: 150 mg

ibandronate sodium *see* ibandronate *on page* 468

ibandronic acid *see* ibandronate *on page* 468

Iberet®-500 [OTC] [DSC] *see* vitamins (multiple/oral) *on page* 951

ibidomide hydrochloride *see* labetalol *on page* 516

ibritumomab (ib ri TYOO mo mab)

Medication Safety Issues

High alert medication:

The Institute for Safe Medication Practices (ISMP) includes this medication among its list of drug classes which have a heightened risk of causing significant patient harm when used in error.

Administration issues:

Dosage maximum: Do not exceed the Y-90 Ibritumomab maximum allowable dose of 332 mCi (1184 MBq), regardless of the patient's body weight.

Synonyms ibritumomab tiuxetan; IDEC-Y2B8; Y-90 ibritumomab; Y-90 zevalin

U.S. Brand Names Zevalin®

Canadian Brand Names Zevalin®

Therapeutic Category Antineoplastic Agent, Monoclonal Antibody; Radiopharmaceutical

Use Treatment of relapsed or refractory low-grade or follicular B-cell non-Hodgkin lymphoma (NHL); treatment of follicular NHL in patients (previously untreated) who achieve a response (partial or complete) to first-line chemotherapy

General Dosage Range I.V.: *Adults:* Day 7, 8, or 9: 0.3-0.4 mCi/kg (11.1-14.8 MBq/kg) actual body weight (maximum: 32 mCi [1184 MBq])

Dosage Forms

Injection, solution [preservative free]:

Zevalin®: 1.6 mg/mL (2 mL)

ibritumomab tiuxetan *see* ibritumomab *on page* 468

Ibu® *see* ibuprofen *on page* 468

Ibu-200 [OTC] *see* ibuprofen *on page* 468

Ibudone® *see* hydrocodone and ibuprofen *on page* 456

ibuprofen (eye byoo PROE fen)

Medication Safety Issues

Sound-alike/look-alike issues:

Haltran® may be confused with Halfprin®

Motrin® may be confused with Neurontin®

BEERS Criteria medication:

This drug may be potentially inappropriate for use in geriatric patients (Quality of evidence - moderate; Strength of recommendation - strong).

Administration issues:

Injectable formulations: Both ibuprofen and ibuprofen lysine are available for parenteral use. Ibuprofen lysine is **only** indicated for closure of a clinically-significant patent ductus arteriosus.

Synonyms *p*-isobutylhydratropic acid; ibuprofen lysine

U.S. Brand Names Addaprin [OTC]; Advil® Children's [OTC]; Advil® Infants' [OTC]; Advil® Migraine [OTC]; Advil® [OTC]; Caldolor®; I-Prin [OTC]; Ibu-200 [OTC]; Ibu®; Midol® Cramps & Body Aches [OTC]; Motrin® Children's [OTC]; Motrin® IB [OTC]; Motrin® Infants' [OTC]; Motrin® Junior [OTC]; NeoProfen®; Proprinal® [OTC]; TopCare® Junior Strength [OTC]; Ultraprin [OTC]

Canadian Brand Names Advil®; Apo-Ibuprofen®; Motrin® (Children's); Motrin® IB; Novo-Profen; Nu-Ibuprofen

Therapeutic Category Analgesic, Nonnarcotic; Antipyretic; Nonsteroidal Antiinflammatory Drug (NSAID)

Use

Oral: Inflammatory diseases and rheumatoid disorders including juvenile idiopathic arthritis (JIA), mild-to-moderate pain, fever, dysmenorrhea, osteoarthritis

Ibuprofen injection (Caldolor®): Management of mild-to-moderate pain; management moderate-to-severe pain when used concurrently with an opioid analgesic; reduction of fever

Ibuprofen lysine injection (NeoProfen®): To induce closure of a clinically-significant patent ductus arteriosus (PDA) in premature infants weighing between 500-1500 g and who are ≤32 weeks gestational age (GA) when usual treatments are ineffective

General Dosage Range

I.V. (ibuprofen [Caldolor®]): *Adults:* 100-400 mg every 4-6 hours or 400-800 mg every 6 hours (maximum: 3.2 g/day)

I.V. (ibuprofen lysine [NeoProfen®]): *Infants between 500-1500 g and ≤32 weeks GA:* Initial: 10 mg/kg, followed by two doses of 5 mg/kg at 24 and 48 hours; **Note:** Dose should be based on birth weight.

Oral:

Analgesic/antipyretic:

Children 6-11 months and 12-17 lbs: 50 mg every 6-8 hours (maximum: 4 doses/day) **or** 4-10 mg/kg every 6-8 hours (maximum: 40 mg/kg/day)

Children 12-23 months and 18-23 lbs: 75 mg every 6-8 hours (maximum: 4 doses/day) **or** 4-10 mg/kg every 6-8 hours (maximum: 40 mg/kg/day)

Children 2-3 years and 24-35 lbs: 100 mg every 6-8 hours (maximum: 4 doses/day) **or** 4-10 mg/kg every 6-8 hours (maximum: 40 mg/kg/day)

Children 4-5 years and 36-47 lbs: 150 mg every 6-8 hours (maximum: 4 doses/day) **or** 4-10 mg/kg every 6-8 hours (maximum: 40 mg/kg/day)

Children 6-8 years and 48-59 lbs: 200 mg every 6-8 hours (maximum: 4 doses/day) **or** 4-10 mg/kg every 6-8 hours (maximum: 40 mg/kg/day)

Children 9-10 years and 60-71 lbs: 250 mg every 6-8 hours (maximum: 4 doses/day) **or** 4-10 mg/kg every 6-8 hours (maximum: 40 mg/kg/day)

Children 11-12 years and 72-95 lbs: 300 mg every 6-8 hours (maximum: 4 doses/day) **or** 4-10 mg/kg every 6-8 hours (maximum: 40 mg/kg/day)

Children >12 years: 200 mg every 4-6 hours as needed (maximum: 1200 mg/day) **or** 4-10 mg/kg every 6-8 hours (maximum: 40 mg/kg/day)

Adults: 200-400 mg every 4-6 hours

Inflammatory disease: *Adults:* 400-800 mg 3-4 times/day (maximum: 3200 mg/day)

JIA: *Children >6 months:* 30-50 mg/kg/day divided every 8 hours (maximum: 2.4 g/day)

Dosage Forms

Caplet, oral: 200 mg

Advil® [OTC]: 200 mg

Motrin® IB [OTC]: 200 mg

Motrin® Junior [OTC]: 100 mg

Capsule, liquid filled, oral: 200 mg

Advil® [OTC]: 200 mg

Advil® Migraine [OTC]: 200 mg

Gelcap, oral:

Advil® [OTC]: 200 mg

Injection, solution:

Caldolor®: 100 mg/mL (4 mL, 8 mL)

Injection, solution [preservative free]:
NeoProfen®: 17.1 mg/mL (2 mL)
Suspension, oral: 100 mg/5 mL (5 mL, 10 mL, 120 mL, 240 mL, 480 mL); 40 mg/mL (15 mL)
Advil® Children's [OTC]: 100 mg/5 mL (120 mL)
Advil® Infants' [OTC]: 40 mg/mL (15 mL)
Motrin® Children's [OTC]: 100 mg/5 mL (60 mL, 120 mL)
Motrin® Infants' [OTC]: 40 mg/mL (15 mL)
Tablet, oral: 200 mg, 400 mg, 600 mg, 800 mg
Addaprin [OTC]: 200 mg
Advil® [OTC]: 200 mg
I-Prin [OTC]: 200 mg
Ibu-200 [OTC]: 200 mg
Ibu®: 400 mg, 600 mg, 800 mg
Midol® Cramps & Body Aches [OTC]: 200 mg
Motrin® IB [OTC]: 200 mg
Proprinal® [OTC]: 200 mg
Ultraprin [OTC]: 200 mg
Tablet, chewable, oral:
Motrin® Junior [OTC]: 100 mg
TopCare® Junior Strength [OTC]: 100 mg

ibuprofen and famotidine (eye byoo PROE fen & fa MOE ti deen)

Synonyms famotidine and ibuprofen; HZT-501

U.S. Brand Names Duexis®

Therapeutic Category Histamine H_2 Antagonist; Nonsteroidal Antiinflammatory Drug (NSAID), Oral

Use Reduction of the risk of NSAID-associated gastric ulcers in patients who require an NSAID for the treatment of rheumatoid arthritis or osteoarthritis

General Dosage Range Oral: *Adults:* One tablet (800 mg ibuprofen/26.6 mg famotidine) 3 times daily

Dosage Forms

Tablet, oral:
Duexis®: Ibuprofen 800 mg and famotidine 26.6 mg

ibuprofen and hydrocodone *see* hydrocodone and ibuprofen *on page 456*

ibuprofen and oxycodone *see* oxycodone and ibuprofen *on page 680*

ibuprofen and pseudoephedrine *see* pseudoephedrine and ibuprofen *on page 773*

ibuprofen lysine *see* ibuprofen *on page 468*

ibuprofen, pseudoephedrine, and chlorpheniramine

(eye byoo PROE fen, soo doe e FED rin, & klor fen IR a meen)

Synonyms chlorpheniramine maleate, ibuprofen, and pseudoephedrine; ibuprofen, pseudoephedrine, and chlorpheniramine maleate; pseudoephedrine, chlorpheniramine, and ibuprofen

U.S. Brand Names Advil® Allergy Sinus; Advil® Multi-Symptom Cold

Canadian Brand Names Advil® Cold and Sinus Nighttime; Advil® Cold and Sinus Plus; Children's Advil® Cold and Flu Multi-Symptom

Therapeutic Category Antihistamine/Decongestant/Analgesic

Use Temporary relief of symptoms associated with the common cold, hay fever, or other respiratory allergies

General Dosage Range Oral: *Children ≥12 years and Adults:* 1 caplet every 4-6 hours (maximum: 6 caplets/day)

Dosage Forms

Caplet:
Advil® Allergy Sinus, Advil® Multi-Symptom Cold: Ibuprofen 200 mg, pseudoephedrine 30 mg, and chlorpheniramine 2 mg

ibuprofen, pseudoephedrine, and chlorpheniramine maleate *see* ibuprofen, pseudoephedrine, and chlorpheniramine *on page 470*

ibutilide (i BYOO ti lide)

Medication Safety Issues

High alert medication:

The Institute for Safe Medication Practices (ISMP) includes this medication among its list of drugs which have a heightened risk of causing significant patient harm when used in error.

BEERS Criteria medication:

This drug may be potentially inappropriate for use in geriatric patients (Quality of evidence - high; Strength of recommendation - strong).

Synonyms ibutilide fumarate

U.S. Brand Names Corvert®

Therapeutic Category Antiarrhythmic Agent, Class III

Use Acute termination of atrial fibrillation or flutter of recent onset; the effectiveness of ibutilide has not been determined in patients with arrhythmias >90 days in duration

General Dosage Range I.V.:

Adults <60 kg: 0.01 mg/kg; may repeat once

Adults ≥60 kg: 1 mg; may repeat once

Dosage Forms

Injection, solution: 0.1 mg/mL (10 mL)

Corvert®: 0.1 mg/mL (10 mL)

ibutilide fumarate *see* ibutilide *on page 471*

IC51 *see* Japanese encephalitis virus vaccine (inactivated) *on page 509*

icatibant (eye KAT i bant)

Synonyms HOE 140; icatibant acetate

U.S. Brand Names Firazyr®

Therapeutic Category Selective Bradykinin B2 Receptor Antagonist

Use Treatment of acute attacks of hereditary angioedema (HAE)

General Dosage Range SubQ: *Adults:* 30 mg/dose; maximum: 3 doses/24 hours

Dosage Forms

Injection, solution [preservative free]:

Firazyr®: 10 mg/mL (3 mL)

icatibant acetate *see* icatibant *on page 471*

IC-Green™ *see* indocyanine green *on page 480*

ICI-182,780 *see* fulvestrant *on page 411*

ICI-204,219 *see* zafirlukast *on page 958*

ICI-46474 *see* tamoxifen *on page 868*

ICI-118630 *see* goserelin *on page 431*

ICI-176334 *see* bicalutamide *on page 133*

ICI-D1033 *see* anastrozole *on page 75*

ICI-D1694 *see* raltitrexed *(Canada only) on page 786*

ICL670 *see* deferasirox *on page 258*

icodextrin (eye KOE dex trin)

Medication Safety Issues

High alert medication:

The Institute for Safe Medication Practices (ISMP) includes this medication among its list of drug classes which have a heightened risk of causing significant patient harm when used in error.

Other safety concerns:

Special care is warranted in patients with diabetes: Due to potential interference by maltose, careful attention must be given to glucose monitoring; only glucose monitors and test strips which employ the glucose-specific method should be used. Inaccurate methods (glucose dehydrogenase pyrroloquinolinequinone [GDH-PQQ] or glucose-dye-oxidoreductase methods [GDO]) can result in falsely-elevated readings. Inaccurate readings may mask recognition of true hypoglycemia, or may prompt the administration of insulin, potentially leading to life-threatening consequences.

U.S. Brand Names Extraneal

Therapeutic Category Adhesiolytic; Peritoneal Dialysate, Osmotic

Use

Adept®: Reduction of postsurgical adhesions in gynecologic laparoscopic procedures

Extraneal®: Daily exchange for the long dwell (8- to 16-hour) during continuous ambulatory peritoneal dialysis (CAPD) or automated peritoneal dialysis (APD) for the management of end-stage renal disease (ESRD); improvement of long-dwell ultrafiltration and clearance of creatinine and urea nitrogen (compared to 4.25% dextrose) in patients with high/average or greater transport characteristics as measured by peritoneal equilibration test (PET)

General Dosage Range Intraperitoneal: *Adults:*

CAPD or APD (Extraneal®): Given as a single daily exchange in CAPD or APD; dwell time of 8-16 hours is suggested

Laparoscopic gynecologic surgery (Adept®): Irrigate with at least 100 mL every 30 minutes during surgery; aspirate remaining fluid after surgery is completed, then instill 1 L into the cavity

Dosage Forms

Solution, intraperitoneal [preservative free]:

Extraneal: 7.5% (2 L, 2.5 L)

icosapent ethyl (eye KOE sa pent ETH il)

Synonyms AMR101; ethyl eicosapentaenoate; ethyl icosapentate; ethyl-eicosapentaenoic acid; ethyl-EPA; Vascepa™

Therapeutic Category Antilipemic Agent, Miscellaneous

Use Adjunct to dietary therapy in the treatment of hypertriglyceridemia (≥500 mg/dL)

Product Availability Vascepa™: FDA approved July 2012; availability anticipated in the first quarter 2013. Consult prescribing information for additional information.

ICRF-187 *see* dexrazoxane *on page* 269

Icy Hot® [OTC] *see* methyl salicylate and menthol *on page* 592

Idamycin® (Can) *see* idarubicin *on page* 472

Idamycin PFS® *see* idarubicin *on page* 472

idarubicin (eye da ROO bi sin)

Medication Safety Issues

Sound-alike/look-alike issues:

IDArubicin may be confused with DOXOrubicin, DAUNOrubicin, epirubicin

Idamycin PFS® may be confused with Adriamycin

High alert medication:

The Institute for Safe Medication Practices (ISMP) includes this medication among its list of drugs which have a heightened risk of causing significant patient harm when used in error.

Synonyms 4-demethoxydaunorubicin; 4-DMDR; idarubicin hydrochloride; IDR; IMI 30; SC 33428

Tall-Man IDArubicin

U.S. Brand Names Idamycin PFS®

Canadian Brand Names Idamycin®

Therapeutic Category Antineoplastic Agent

Use Treatment of acute myeloid leukemia (AML)

General Dosage Range Dosage adjustment recommended in patients with hepatic or renal impairment

I.V.: *Adults:* Induction: 12 mg/m^2/day for 3 days; Consolidation: 10-12 mg/m^2/day for 2 days

Dosage Forms

Injection, solution [preservative free]: 1 mg/mL (5 mL, 10 mL, 20 mL)

Idamycin PFS®: 1 mg/mL (5 mL, 10 mL, 20 mL)

idarubicin hydrochloride *see* idarubicin *on page* 472

IDEC-C2B8 *see* rituximab *on page* 805

IDEC-Y2B8 *see* ibritumomab *on page* 468

IDR *see* idarubicin *on page* 472

idursulfase (eye dur SUL fase)

Medication Safety Issues

Sound-alike/look-alike issues:

Elaprase® may be confused with Elspar®

U.S. Brand Names Elaprase®

Canadian Brand Names Elaprase®

Therapeutic Category Enzyme

Use Replacement therapy in mucopolysaccharidosis II (MPS II, Hunter syndrome) for improvement of walking capacity

General Dosage Range **I.V.**: *Children ≥5 years and Adults:* 0.5 mg/kg once weekly

Dosage Forms

Injection, solution [preservative free]:

Elaprase®: 2 mg/mL (5 mL)

IDV *see* indinavir *on page* *479*

Ifex *see* ifosfamide *on page* *473*

ifosfamide (eye FOSS fa mide)

Medication Safety Issues

Sound-alike/look-alike issues:

Ifosfamide may be confused with cyclophosphamide

High alert medication:

This medication is in a class the Institute for Safe Medication Practices (ISMP) includes its list of drug classes which have a heightened risk of causing significant patient harm when used in error.

Synonyms isophosphamide; Z4942

U.S. Brand Names Ifex

Canadian Brand Names Ifex

Therapeutic Category Antineoplastic Agent

Use

U.S. labeling: Treatment (third-line) of germ cell testicular cancer (in combination with other chemotherapy drugs and with concurrent mesna)

Canadian labeling (not approved indications in the U.S.): Treatment of soft tissue sarcoma, pancreatic cancer (relapsed or refractory), cervical cancer (advanced or recurrent; as monotherapy or in combination with cisplatin and bleomycin)

General Dosage Range Dosage adjustment recommended in patients with hepatic or renal impairment or who develop toxicities.

I.V.: *Adults:* 1200 mg/m^2/day for 5 days every 21 days

Dosage Forms

Injection, powder for reconstitution: 1 g, 3 g

Ifex: 1 g, 3 g

Injection, solution: 50 mg/mL (20 mL, 60 mL)

IG *see* immune globulin *on page* *477*

IgG4-kappa monoclonal antibody *see* natalizumab *on page* *630*

IGIM *see* immune globulin *on page* *477*

IGIV *see* immune globulin *on page* *477*

IGIVnex® (Can) *see* immune globulin *on page* *477*

123I-ioflupane *see* ioflupane I 123 *on page* *495*

IL-1Ra *see* anakinra *on page* *75*

IL-2 *see* aldesleukin *on page* *44*

IL-11 *see* oprelvekin *on page* *670*

Ilaris® *see* canakinumab *on page* *168*

Ilaris™ (Can) *see* canakinumab *on page* *168*

iloperidone (eye loe PER i done)

Medication Safety Issues

Sound-alike/look-alike issues:

Fanapt® may be confused with Xanax®

Iloperidone may be confused with domperidone

BEERS Criteria medication:

This drug may be potentially inappropriate for use in geriatric patients (Quality of evidence - moderate; Strength of recommendation - strong).

U.S. Brand Names Fanapt®

Therapeutic Category Antipsychotic Agent, Atypical

Use Acute treatment of schizophrenia

General Dosage Range **Oral:** *Adults:* Initial: 1 mg twice daily; Dosage range: 6-12 mg twice daily (maximum: 24 mg/day)

Dosage Forms

Tablet, oral:

Fanapt®: 1 mg, 2 mg, 4 mg, 6 mg, 8 mg, 10 mg, 12 mg, 1 mg (2s), 2 mg (2s), 4 mg (2s), and 6 mg (2s)

iloprost (EYE loe prost)

Synonyms iloprost tromethamine; prostacyclin PGI_2

U.S. Brand Names Ventavis®

Therapeutic Category Prostaglandin

Use Treatment of pulmonary arterial hypertension (PAH) (WHO Group I) in patients with NYHA Class III or IV symptoms to improve exercise tolerance, symptoms, and diminish clinical deterioration

General Dosage Range Dosage adjustment recommended in patients with hepatic impairment.

Inhalation: *Adults:* Initial: 2.5 mcg/dose; Maintenance: 2.5-5 mcg/dose 6-9 times/day (maximum: 45 mcg/day)

Dosage Forms

Solution, for oral inhalation [preservative free]:

Ventavis®: 10 mcg/mL (1 mL); 20 mcg/mL (1 mL)

iloprost tromethamine *see* iloprost *on page 474*

Ilotycin™ *see* erythromycin (ophthalmic) *on page 343*

imatinib (eye MAT eh nib)

Medication Safety Issues

Sound-alike/look-alike issues:

Imatinib may be confused with axitinib, dasatinib, erlotinib, gefitinib, nilotinib, SORAfenib, SUNItinib, vandetanib

High alert medication:

This medication is in a class the Institute for Safe Medication Practices (ISMP) includes among its list of drug classes which have a heightened risk of causing significant patient harm when used in error.

Synonyms CGP-57148B; Glivec; imatinib mesylate; STI-571

U.S. Brand Names Gleevec®

Canadian Brand Names Gleevec®

Therapeutic Category Antineoplastic Agent, Tyrosine Kinase Inhibitor

Use Treatment of:

Gastrointestinal stromal tumors (GIST) kit-positive (CD117), including unresectable and/or metastatic malignant and adjuvant treatment following complete resection

Philadelphia chromosome-positive (Ph+) chronic myeloid leukemia (CML) in chronic phase (newly-diagnosed)

Ph+ CML in blast crisis, accelerated phase, or chronic phase after failure of interferon therapy

Ph+ acute lymphoblastic leukemia (ALL) (relapsed or refractory)

Aggressive systemic mastocytosis (ASM) without D816V c-Kit mutation (or c-Kit mutation status unknown)

Dermatofibrosarcoma protuberans (DFSP) (unresectable, recurrent and/or metastatic)

Hypereosinophilic syndrome (HES) and/or chronic eosinophilic leukemia (CEL)

Myelodysplastic/myeloproliferative disease (MDS/MPD) associated with platelet-derived growth factor receptor (PDGFR) gene rearrangements

Canadian labeling (not an approved indication in the U.S.): Ph+ ALL induction therapy (newly diagnosed)

General Dosage Range Dosage adjustment recommended in patients with hepatic or renal impairment, on concomitant therapy, and/or who develop toxicities

Oral:

Children ≥2 years: 340 mg/m^2/day in 1-2 divided doses (maximum: 600 mg/day)

Adults: 100-800 mg/day in 1-2 divided doses

Dosage Forms

Tablet, oral:

Gleevec®: 100 mg, 400 mg

imatinib mesylate *see* imatinib *on page 474*

IMC-C225 *see* cetuximab *on page 192*

Imdur® *see* isosorbide mononitrate *on page 505*

123I-metaiodobenzylguanidine (MIBG) *see* iobenguane I 123 *on page 493*

imferon *see* iron dextran complex *on page 501*

IMI 30 *see* idarubicin *on page 472*

IMid-1 *see* lenalidomide *on page 525*

imidazole carboxamide *see* dacarbazine *on page 250*

imidazole carboxamide dimethyltriazene *see* dacarbazine *on page 250*

imiglucerase (i mi GLOO ser ace)

Medication Safety Issues

Sound-alike/look-alike issues:

Cerezyme® may be confused with Cerebyx®, Ceredase®

U.S. Brand Names Cerezyme®

Canadian Brand Names Cerezyme®

Therapeutic Category Enzyme

Use Long-term enzyme replacement therapy for patients with Type 1 Gaucher disease

General Dosage Range I.V.: *Children ≥2 years and Adults:* 2.5 units/kg 3 times weekly to 60 units/kg every 2 weeks.

Dosage Forms

Injection, powder for reconstitution:

Cerezyme®: 200 units, 400 units

imipemide *see* imipenem and cilastatin *on page 475*

imipenem and cilastatin (i mi PEN em & sye la STAT in)

Medication Safety Issues

Sound-alike/look-alike issues:

Imipenem may be confused with ertapenem, meropenem

Primaxin® may be confused with Premarin®, Primacor®

Synonyms imipemide; Primaxin® I.M. [DSC]

U.S. Brand Names Primaxin® I.V.

Canadian Brand Names Imipenem and Cilastatin for Injection; Primaxin® I.V. Infusion; RAN™-Imipenem-Cilastatin

Therapeutic Category Carbapenem (Antibiotic)

Use Treatment of lower respiratory tract, urinary tract, intraabdominal, gynecologic, bone and joint, skin and skin structure, endocarditis (caused by *Staphylococcus aureus*) and polymicrobic infections as well as bacterial septicemia. Antibacterial activity includes gram-positive bacteria (methicillin-sensitive *S. aureus* and *Streptococcus* spp), resistant gram-negative bacilli (including extended spectrum beta-lactamase-producing *Escherichia coli* and *Klebsiella* spp, *Enterobacter* spp, and *Pseudomonas aeruginosa*), and anaerobes.

General Dosage Range Dosage adjustment recommended in patients with renal impairment

I.V.:

Children >3 months: 15-25 mg/kg every 6 hours (maximum: 4 g/day)

Adults 30 to <70 kg: 125 mg every 12 hours up to 1000 mg every 8 hours

Adults ≥70 kg: 250-1000 mg every 6-8 hours (maximum: 50 mg/kg/day; 4 g/day)

Dosage Forms

Injection, powder for reconstitution: Imipenem 250 mg and cilastatin 250 mg; imipenem 500 mg and cilastatin 500 mg

Primaxin® I.V.: Imipenem 250 mg and cilastatin 250 mg; imipenem 500 mg and cilastatin 500 mg

Imipenem and Cilastatin for Injection (Can) *see* imipenem and cilastatin *on page 475*

imipramine (im IP ra meen)

Medication Safety Issues

Sound-alike/look-alike issues:

Imipramine may be confused with amitriptyline, desipramine, Norpramin®

BEERS Criteria medication:

This drug may be potentially inappropriate for use in geriatric patients (Quality of evidence - high [moderate for SIADH]; Strength of recommendation - strong).

Synonyms imipramine hydrochloride; imipramine pamoate

U.S. Brand Names Tofranil-PM®; Tofranil®

Canadian Brand Names Apo-Imipramine®; Novo-Pramine; Tofranil®

Therapeutic Category Antidepressant, Tricyclic (Tertiary Amine)

Use Treatment of depression; treatment of nocturnal enuresis in children

General Dosage Range Oral:

Children ≥6-12 years: Initial: 25 mg at bedtime, may increase to 50 mg at bedtime if no response (maximum: 2.5 mg/kg/day; 50 mg/day)

Children >12 years: Initial: 25 mg at bedtime, may increase to 75 mg at bedtime if not response (maximum: 75 mg/day) **or** 30-40 mg/day, increase gradually, to a maximum of 100 mg/day in single or divided doses

Adults: Initial: 75-150 mg/day, increase gradually to a maximum of 200 mg/day (outpatients) or 300 mg/day (inpatients) in divided doses or a single dose at bedtime

Elderly: Initial: 25-50 mg at bedtime (maximum: 100 mg/day)

Dosage Forms

Capsule, oral: 75 mg, 100 mg, 125 mg, 150 mg

Tofranil-PM®: 75 mg, 100 mg, 125 mg, 150 mg

Tablet, oral: 10 mg, 25 mg, 50 mg

Tofranil®: 10 mg, 25 mg, 50 mg

imipramine hydrochloride *see* imipramine *on page 476*
imipramine pamoate *see* imipramine *on page 476*

imiquimod (i mi KWI mod)

Medication Safety Issues

Sound-alike/look-alike issues:

Aldara® may be confused with Alora®, Lialda®

U.S. Brand Names Aldara®; Zyclara®

Canadian Brand Names Aldara®; Vyloma™; Zyclara®

Therapeutic Category Immune Response Modifier

Use Treatment of external genital and perianal warts/condyloma acuminata; nonhyperkeratotic actinic keratosis on face or scalp; superficial basal cell carcinoma (sBCC) with a maximum tumor diameter of 2 cm located on the trunk, neck, or extremities (excluding hands or feet)

General Dosage Range Topical:

Children ≥12 years: Apply a thin layer 3 times/week on alternate days, leave on for 6-10 hours

Adults:

Actinic keratosis: Apply twice weekly or once daily at bedtime for 2 treatment cycles (14 days each) separated by a 14-day rest period with no treatment; leave on for 8 hours

External genital and/or perianal warts/condyloma acuminata: Apply a thin layer 3 times/week on alternate days; leave on for 6-10 hours

Superficial basal cell carcinoma: Apply once daily at bedtime 5 days/week; leave on for 8 hours before washing

Dosage Forms

Cream, topical: 5% (24s)

Aldara®: 5% (12s)

Zyclara®: 3.75% (7.5 g, 28s)

Imitrex® *see* sumatriptan *on page 863*
Imitrex® DF (Can) *see* sumatriptan *on page 863*
Imitrex® Injection (Can) *see* sumatriptan *on page 863*
Imitrex® Nasal Spray (Can) *see* sumatriptan *on page 863*
ImmuCyst® (Can) *see* BCG *on page 116*

immune globulin (i MYUN GLOB yoo lin)

Medication Safety Issues

Sound-alike/look-alike issues:

Gamimune® N may be confused with CytoGam®

Immune globulin (intravenous) may be confused with hepatitis B immune globulin

Synonyms gamma globulin; IG; IGIM; IGIV; immune globulin subcutaneous (human); immune serum globulin; ISG; IV immune globulin; IVIG; panglobulin; SCIG

U.S. Brand Names Carimune® NF; Flebogamma® DIF; GamaSTAN™ S/D; Gammagard S/D®; Gammagard® Liquid; Gammaked™; Gammaplex®; Gamunex® [DSC]; Gamunex®-C; Hizentra®; Octagam®; Privigen®; Vivaglobin® [DSC]

Canadian Brand Names Gamastan S/D; Gamimune® N; Gammagard Liquid; Gammagard S/D; Gamunex®; Hizentra®; IGIVnex®; Privigen®; Vivaglobin®

Therapeutic Category Blood Product Derivative; Immune Globulin

Use

Treatment of primary humoral immunodeficiency syndromes (congenital agammaglobulinemia, severe combined immunodeficiency syndromes [SCIDS], common variable immunodeficiency, X-linked immunodeficiency, Wiskott-Aldrich syndrome) (Carimune® NF, Flebogamma® DIF, Gammagard® Liquid, Gammagard S/D®, Gammaked™, Gammaplex®, Gamunex®, Gamunex®-C, Hizentra®, Octagam®, Privigen®, Vivaglobin®)

Treatment of acute and chronic immune (idiopathic) thrombocytopenic purpura (ITP) (Carimune® NF, Gammagard S/D®, Gammaked™, Gamunex®, Gamunex®-C, Privigen® [chronic only])

Treatment of chronic inflammatory demyelinating polyneuropathy (CIDP) (Gammaked™, Gamunex®, Gamunex®-C)

Prevention of coronary artery aneurysms associated with Kawasaki syndrome (in combination with aspirin) (Gammagard S/D®)

Prevention of bacterial infection in patients with hypogammaglobulinemia and/or recurrent bacterial infections with B-cell chronic lymphocytic leukemia (CLL) (Gammagard S/D®)

Prevention of serious infection in immunoglobulin deficiency (select agammaglobulinemias) (GamaSTAN™ S/D)

Provision of passive immunity in the following susceptible individuals (GamaSTAN™ S/D):

Hepatitis A: Pre-exposure prophylaxis; postexposure: within 14 days and/or prior to manifestation of disease

Measles: For use within 6 days of exposure in an unvaccinated person, who has not previously had measles

Rubella: Postexposure prophylaxis (within 72 hours) to reduce the risk of infection and fetal damage in exposed pregnant women who will not consider therapeutic abortion

Varicella: For immunosuppressed patients when varicella zoster immune globulin is not available

General Dosage Range

I.M.: *Children and Adults:*

Hepatitis A:

Pre-exposure prophylaxis upon travel into endemic areas:

0.02 mL/kg for anticipated risk of exposure <3 months

0.06 mL/kg for anticipated risk of exposure ≥3 months

Postexposure prophylaxis: 0.02 mL/kg

Measles:

Postexposure, immunocompetent: 0.25 mL/kg

Postexposure, immunocompromised: 0.5 mL/kg (maximum dose: 15 mL)

Rubella: Prophylaxis during pregnancy: 0.55 mL/kg

Varicella: Prophylaxis: 0.6-1.2 mL/kg

Immune globulin deficiency: 0.66 mL/kg; administer a double dose at onset of therapy

I.V.: *Children and Adults:*

B-cell chronic lymphocytic leukemia (CLL): 400 mg/kg

Chronic inflammatory demyelinating polyneuropathy (CIDP): Loading dose: 2000 mg/kg; Maintenance: 500-1000 mg/kg

Immune (idiopathic) thrombocytopenic purpura (ITP): Dosage varies greatly depending on product

Kawasaki syndrome: 400-2000 mg/kg

Measles: >400 mg/kg

Primary humoral immunodeficiency disorders: 200-800 mg/kg

SubQ: *Children and Adults:*

Measles: ≥200 mg/kg

Primary humoral immunodeficiency disorders: Dosage varies greatly depending on product

Dosage Forms

Injection, powder for reconstitution [preservative free]:

Carimune® NF: 3 g, 6 g, 12 g

Gammagard S/D®: 2.5 g, 5 g, 10 g

Injection, solution [preservative free]:

Flebogamma® DIF: 5% [50 mg/mL] (10 mL, 50 mL, 100 mL, 200 mL, 400 mL); 10% [100 mg/mL] (100 mL, 200 mL)

GamaSTAN™ S/D: 15% to 18% [150 to 180 mg/mL] (2 mL, 10 mL)

Gammagard® Liquid: 10% [100 mg/mL] (10 mL, 25 mL, 50 mL, 100 mL, 200 mL)

Gammaked™: 10% [100 mg/mL] (10 mL, 25 mL, 50 mL, 100 mL, 200 mL)

Gammaplex®: 5% [50 mg/mL] (50 mL, 100 mL, 200 mL)

Gamunex®-C: 10% [100 mg/mL] (10 mL, 25 mL, 50 mL, 100 mL, 200 mL)

Hizentra®: 200 mg/mL (5 mL, 10 mL, 20 mL)

Octagam®: 5% [50 mg/mL] (20 mL, 50 mL, 100 mL, 200 mL)

Privigen®: 10% [100 mg/mL] (50 mL, 100 mL, 200 mL)

immune globulin subcutaneous (human) *see* immune globulin *on page 477*
immune serum globulin *see* immune globulin *on page 477*
Immunine® VH (Can) *see* factor IX *on page 371*
Imodium® (Can) *see* loperamide *on page 547*
Imodium® A-D [OTC] *see* loperamide *on page 547*
Imodium® A-D EZ Chews [OTC] *see* loperamide *on page 547*
Imodium® A-D for children [OTC] *see* loperamide *on page 547*
Imodium® Advanced Multi-Symptom (Can) *see* loperamide and simethicone *on page 548*
Imodium® Multi-Symptom Relief [OTC] *see* loperamide and simethicone *on page 548*
Imogam® Rabies-HT *see* rabies immune globulin (human) *on page 784*
Imogam® Rabies Pasteurized (Can) *see* rabies immune globulin (human) *on page 784*
Imovane® (Can) *see* zopiclone *(Canada only) on page 967*
Imovax® Polio (Can) *see* poliovirus vaccine (inactivated) *on page 736*
Imovax® Rabies *see* rabies vaccine *on page 784*
Implanon® *see* etonogestrel *on page 366*
Imuran® *see* azathioprine *on page 106*
INCB424 *see* ruxolitinib *on page 815*
INCB 18424 *see* ruxolitinib *on page 815*
Incivek™ *see* telaprevir *on page 873*

incobotulinumtoxinA (in kuh BOT yoo lin num TOKS in aye)

Medication Safety Issues

Other safety concerns:

Botulinum products are not interchangeable; potency differences may exist between the products.

Synonyms botulinum toxin type A

U.S. Brand Names Xeomin®

Canadian Brand Names Xeomin®

Therapeutic Category Neuromuscular Blocker Agent, Toxin; Ophthalmic Agent, Toxin

Use Treatment of blepharospasm in patients previously treated with onabotulinumtoxinA (Botox®); treatment of cervical dystonia in botulinum toxin-naïve and previously treated patients; temporary improvement in the appearance of moderate-to-severe glabellar lines associated with corrugator and/or procerus muscle activity

Canadian labeling: Treatment of hypertonicity disorders of the seventh nerve (eg, blepharospasm, hemifacial spasm); treatment of poststroke spasticity of upper limb(s); treatment of cervical dystonia (spasmodic torticollis)

General Dosage Range I.M.: *Adults:*

Blepharospasm: Initial: Total dose should be the same as previously administered onabotulinumtoxinA dose or 1.25-2.5 units/injection site (maximum dose: 35 units/eye or 70 units/both eyes/every 3 months)

Cervical dystonia: Initial total dose: 120 units

Reduction of glabellar lines: 4 units/injection site into each of the 5 sites (maximum dose: 20 units/treatment session every 3 months)

Dosage Forms

Injection, powder for reconstitution:

Xeomin®: 50 units, 100 units

Increlex® *see* mecasermin *on page 565*

indacaterol (in da KA ter ol)

Synonyms indacaterol maleate; QAB149

U.S. Brand Names Arcapta™ Neohaler™

Canadian Brand Names Onbrez® Breezhaler®

Therapeutic Category $Beta_2$-Adrenergic Agonist; $Beta_2$-Adrenergic Agonist, Long-Acting

Use Long-term maintenance treatment of airflow obstruction in chronic obstructive pulmonary disease (COPD) including chronic bronchitis and/or emphysema

General Dosage Range Inhalation: *Adults:* One inhalation once daily

Dosage Forms

Powder, for oral inhalation:

Arcapta™ Neohaler™: 75 mcg/capsule (30s)

indacaterol maleate *see* indacaterol *on page 479*

indapamide (in DAP a mide)

Medication Safety Issues

Sound-alike/look-alike issues:

Indapamide may be confused with Iopidine®

International issues:

Pretanix [Hungary] may be confused with Protonix brand name for pantoprazole [U.S., Canada]

Canadian Brand Names Apo-Indapamide®; Dom-Indapamide; Indapamide Hemihydrate; JAMP-Indapamide; Lozide®; Mylan-Indapamide; Novo-Indapamide; Nu-Indapamide; PHL-Indapamide; PMS-Indapamide; PRO-Indapamide; Riva-Indapamide

Therapeutic Category Diuretic, Miscellaneous

Use Management of mild-to-moderate hypertension; treatment of edema in heart failure

General Dosage Range Oral: *Adults:* 1.25-5 mg once daily

Dosage Forms

Tablet, oral: 1.25 mg, 2.5 mg

indapamide and perindopril erbumine *see* perindopril erbumine and indapamide *(Canada only) on page 709*

Indapamide Hemihydrate (Can) *see* indapamide *on page 479*

Inderal® (Can) *see* propranolol *on page 767*

Inderal® LA *see* propranolol *on page 767*

Inderide *see* propranolol and hydrochlorothiazide *on page 768*

indigo carmine *see* indigotindisulfonate sodium *on page 479*

indigotindisulfonate sodium (in di goe tin dye SUL foe nate SOW dee um)

Synonyms indigo carmine

Therapeutic Category Diagnostic Agent, Kidney Function

Use Localizing ureteral orifices during cystoscopy and ureteral catheterization

General Dosage Range I.M., I.V.:

Infants and Children: <5 mL

Adults: 5 mL

Dosage Forms

Injection, solution: 8 mg/mL (5 mL)

indinavir (in DIN a veer)

Medication Safety Issues

Sound-alike/look-alike issues:

Indinavir may be confused with Denavir®

Synonyms IDV; indinavir sulfate

U.S. Brand Names Crixivan®

Canadian Brand Names Crixivan®

Therapeutic Category Antiviral Agent

Use Treatment of HIV infection; should always be used as part of a multidrug regimen (at least three antiretroviral agents)

General Dosage Range Dosage adjustment recommended in patients with hepatic impairment or on concomitant therapy

Oral: *Adults:* 800 mg every 8 hours; Boosted regimen: 800 mg every 12 hours

Dosage Forms

Capsule, oral:

Crixivan®: 100 mg, 200 mg, 400 mg

indinavir sulfate *see* indinavir *on page 479*

Indium DTPA In 111 *see* pentetate indium disodium in 111 *on page 706*

indium IN-111 pentetate disodium *see* pentetate indium disodium in 111 *on page 706*

indium in-111 pentetreotide kit *see* indium in-111 pentetreotide *on page 480*

indium in-111 pentetreotide (IN dee um eye en won e LEV en pen te TREE oh tide)

Medication Safety Issues

Other safety concerns:

Radiopharmaceutical: Use appropriate precaution for handling, disposal, and minimizing exposure to patients and healthcare personnel. Use under supervision of experienced personnel. Should be stored in original lead container or adequate radiation shield.

Synonyms ^{111}in-pentetreotide; indium in-111 pentetreotide kit; OctreoScan® (Prep Kit)

U.S. Brand Names OctreoScan®

Therapeutic Category Radiopharmaceutical

Use Scintigraphic localization of primary and metastatic neuroendocrine tumors with somatostatin receptors

Dosage Forms

Kit, [preservative free]:

OctreoScan®:

Injection, powder for reconstitution: Pentetreotide 10 mcg

Injection, solution: Indium In-111 chloride 111 MBq (3.0 mCi) per 1 mL (1.1 mL)

Indocid® P.D.A. (Can) *see* indomethacin *on page 480*

Indocin® *see* indomethacin *on page 480*

Indocin® I.V. *see* indomethacin *on page 480*

indocyanine green (in doe SYE a neen green)

U.S. Brand Names IC-Green™

Therapeutic Category Diagnostic Agent

Use Determining hepatic function, cardiac output, and liver blood flow; ophthalmic angiography

General Dosage Range

Cardiac catheter:

Infants: 1.25 mg (maximum total dose: 2 mg/kg)

Children: 2.5 mg (maximum total dose: 2 mg/kg)

Adults: 5 mg (maximum total dose: 2 mg/kg)

I.V.: *Adults:* Hepatic function: 0.5 mg/kg; Ophthalmic angiography: ≤40 mg bolus

Dosage Forms

Injection, powder for reconstitution: 25 mg

IC-Green™: 25 mg

indometacin *see* indomethacin *on page 480*

indomethacin (in doe METH a sin)

Medication Safety Issues

Sound-alike/look-alike issues:

Indocin® may be confused with Imodium®, Lincocin®, Minocin®, Vicodin®

BEERS Criteria medication:

This drug may be potentially inappropriate for use in geriatric patients (Quality of evidence - moderate; Strength of recommendation - strong).

Synonyms indometacin; indomethacin sodium trihydrate

U.S. Brand Names Indocin®; Indocin® I.V.

Canadian Brand Names Apo-Indomethacin®; Indocid® P.D.A.; Novo-Methacin; Nu-Indo; Pro-Indo; ratio-Indomethacin; Sandoz-Indomethacin

Therapeutic Category Analgesic, Nonnarcotic; Nonsteroidal Antiinflammatory Drug (NSAID)

Use Acute gouty arthritis, acute bursitis/tendonitis, moderate-to-severe osteoarthritis, rheumatoid arthritis, ankylosing spondylitis; I.V. form used as alternative to surgery for closure of patent ductus arteriosus in neonates

General Dosage Range

I.V.:

Neonates <48 hours old at time of first dose: Initial: 0.2 mg/kg, followed by 2 doses of 0.1 mg/kg at 12- to 24-hour intervals

Neonates 2-7 days old at time of first dose: Initial: 0.2 mg/kg, followed by 2 doses of 0.2 mg/kg at 12- to 24-hour intervals

Neonates >7 days old at time of first dose: Initial: 0.2 mg/kg, followed by 2 doses of 0.25 mg/kg at 12- to 24-hour intervals

Oral:

Extended release: *Children >14 years and Adults:* 75-150 mg/day in 1-2 divided doses (maximum: 150 mg/day)

Immediate release:

Children ≥2 years: 1-2 mg/kg/day in 2-4 divided doses (maximum: 4 mg/kg/day; 200 mg/day)

Adults: 50-150 mg/day in 2-4 divided doses (maximum: 200 mg/day)

Rectal: *Children >14 years and Adults:* 50-150 mg/day in 2-4 divided doses (maximum: 200 mg/day)

Dosage Forms

Capsule, oral: 25 mg, 50 mg

Capsule, extended release, oral: 75 mg

Injection, powder for reconstitution: 1 mg

Indocin® I.V.: 1 mg

Suppository, rectal:

Indocin®: 50 mg (30s)

Suspension, oral:

Indocin®: 25 mg/5 mL (237 mL)

indomethacin sodium trihydrate *see* indomethacin *on page 480*

^{111}in-DTPA *see* pentetate indium disodium in 111 *on page 706*

INF-alpha 2 *see* interferon alfa-2b *on page 490*

Infanrix® *see* diphtheria and tetanus toxoids, and acellular pertussis vaccine *on page 298*

Infanrix Hexa™ (Can) *see* diphtheria and tetanus toxoids, acellular pertussis, hepatitis B (recombinant), poliovirus (inactivated), and *Haemophilus influenzae* B conjugate (adsorbed) vaccine *on page 297*

Infantaire [OTC] *see* acetaminophen *on page 20*

Infantaire Gas [OTC] *see* simethicone *on page 834*

Infants Gas Relief Drops [OTC] [DSC] *see* simethicone *on page 834*

Infasurf® *see* calfactant *on page 167*

INFeD® *see* iron dextran complex *on page 501*

Infergen® *see* interferon alfacon-1 *on page 491*

infliximab (in FLIKS e mab)

Medication Safety Issues

Sound-alike/look-alike issues:

InFLIXimab may be confused with riTUXimab

Remicade® may be confused with Renacidin®, Rituxan®

Synonyms avakine; infliximab, recombinant

Tall-Man in**FLIX**imab

U.S. Brand Names Remicade®

Canadian Brand Names Remicade®

Therapeutic Category Monoclonal Antibody

Use

Treatment of moderately- to severely-active rheumatoid arthritis (with methotrexate)

Treatment of moderately- to severely-active Crohn disease with inadequate response to conventional therapy (to reduce signs/symptoms and induce and maintain clinical remission) or to reduce the number of draining enterocutaneous and rectovaginal fistulas and maintain fistula closure

Treatment of psoriatic arthritis (to reduce signs/symptoms of active arthritis and inhibit progression of structural damage and improve physical function)

Treatment of chronic severe plaque psoriasis

Treatment of active ankylosing spondylitis (reduce signs/symptoms)

Treatment of moderately- to severely-active ulcerative colitis with inadequate response to conventional therapy (reduce signs/symptoms and induce and maintain clinical remission, mucosal healing and eliminate corticosteroid use)

General Dosage Range Dosage adjustment is required in heart failure patients.

I.V.:

Children ≥6 years: Initial: 5 mg/kg at 0, 2, and 6 weeks; Maintenance: 5 mg/kg every 8 weeks

Adults: Initial: 3-10 mg/kg at 0, 2, and 6 weeks; Maintenance: 3-10 mg/kg every 8 weeks **or** 5 mg/kg every 6 weeks

Dosage Forms

Injection, powder for reconstitution:

Remicade®: 100 mg

infliximab, recombinant *see* infliximab *on page 481*

influenza vaccine *see* influenza virus vaccine (inactivated) *on page 482*

influenza vaccine *see* influenza virus vaccine (live/attenuated) *on page 484*

influenza virus vaccine (H5N1) (in floo EN za VYE rus vak SEEN H5N1)

Medication Safety Issues

Sound-alike/look-alike issues:

Influenza virus vaccine (H5N1) may be confused with the nonavian strain of influenza virus vaccine

Synonyms avian influenza virus vaccine; bird flu vaccine; H5N1 influenza vaccine; influenza virus vaccine (monovalent)

Therapeutic Category Vaccine

Use Active immunization of adults at increased risk of exposure to the H5N1 viral subtype of influenza

General Dosage Range I.M.: *Adults 18-64 years:* 1 mL, followed by second 1 mL dose given 28 days later

Dosage Forms

Injection, suspension: Hemagglutinin (H5N1strain) 90 mcg/mL (5 mL)

influenza virus vaccine (inactivated) (in floo EN za VYE rus vak SEEN, in ak ti VAY ted)

Medication Safety Issues

Sound-alike/look-alike issues:

Fluarix® may be confused with Flarex®

Influenza virus vaccine may be confused with flumazenil

Influenza virus vaccine may be confused with tetanus toxoid and tuberculin products. Medication errors have occurred when tuberculin skin tests (PPD) have been inadvertently administered instead of tetanus toxoid products and influenza virus vaccine. These products are refrigerated and often stored in close proximity to each other.

International issues:

Fluarix [U.S., Canada, and multiple international markets] may be confused with Flarex brand name for fluorometholone [U.S. and multiple international markets] and Fluorex brand name for fluoride [France]

Synonyms H1N1 influenza vaccine; influenza vaccine; influenza virus vaccine (purified surface antigen); influenza virus vaccine (split-virus); TIV; trivalent inactivated influenza vaccine

U.S. Brand Names Afluria®; Fluarix®; FluLaval®; Fluvirin®; Fluzone®; Fluzone® High-Dose; Fluzone® Intradermal

Canadian Brand Names Agriflu™; Fluad™; Fluviral®; Influvac®; Intanza®; Vaxigrip®

Therapeutic Category Vaccine, Inactivated (Viral)

Use Provide active immunity to influenza virus strains contained in the vaccine

The Advisory Committee on Immunization Practices (ACIP) recommends annual vaccination with the seasonal trivalent inactivated influenza vaccine (TIV) (injection) for all persons ≥6 months of age.

When vaccine supply is limited, target groups for vaccination (those at higher risk of complications from influenza infection and their close contacts) include the following:

- Persons ≥50 years of age
- Residents of nursing homes and other chronic-care facilities that house persons of any age with chronic medical conditions
- Adults and children with chronic disorders of the pulmonary or cardiovascular systems (except hypertension), including asthma
- Adults and children who have chronic metabolic diseases (including diabetes mellitus), hepatic disease, renal dysfunction, hematologic disorders, or immunosuppression (including immunosuppression caused by medications or HIV)
- Adults and children with cognitive or neurologic/neuromuscular conditions (including conditions such as spinal cord injuries or seizure disorders) which may compromise respiratory function, the handling of respiratory secretions, or that can increase the risk of aspiration
- Children and adolescents (6 months to 18 years of age) who are receiving long-term aspirin therapy, and therefore, may be at risk for developing Reye syndrome after influenza
- Women who are or will be pregnant during the influenza season
- Children 6-59 months of age
- Healthcare personnel
- Household contacts and caregivers of children <5 years (particularly children <6 months) and adults ≥50 years
- Household contacts and caregivers of persons with medical conditions which put them at high risk of complications from influenza infection
- American Indians/Alaska Natives
- Morbidly obese (BMI ≥40)

The Advisory Committee on Immunization Practices (ACIP) states that healthy, nonpregnant persons aged 2-49 years may receive vaccination with either the seasonal live, attenuated influenza vaccine (LAIV) (nasal spray) or the seasonal trivalent inactivated influenza vaccine (TIV) (injection).

General Dosage Range

I.M.:

Children 6-35 months: 0.25 mL/dose (1 or 2 doses per season)

Children 3-9 years: 0.5 mL/dose (1 or 2 doses per season)

Children ≥9 years and Adults: 0.5 mL/dose (1 dose per season)

Intradermal: *Adults:* 18-64 years: 0.1 mL/dose (1 dose per season)

Dosage Forms

Injection, suspension:

Afluria®: Hemagglutinin 45 mcg/0.5 mL (5 mL)

FluLaval®: Hemagglutinin 45 mcg/0.5 mL (5 mL)

Fluvirin®: Hemagglutinin 45 mcg/0.5 mL (5 mL)

Fluzone®: Hemagglutinin 45 mcg/0.5 mL (5 mL)

Injection, suspension [preservative free]:

Afluria®: Hemagglutinin 45 mcg/0.5 mL (0.5 mL)

Fluarix®: Hemagglutinin 45 mcg/0.5 mL (0.5 mL)

Fluvirin®: Hemagglutinin 45 mcg/0.5 mL (0.5 mL)

Fluzone®: Hemagglutinin 22.5 mcg/0.25 mL (0.25 mL); Hemagglutinin 45 mcg/0.5 mL (0.5 mL)

Fluzone® High-Dose: Hemagglutinin 180 mcg/0.5 mL (0.5 mL)

Fluzone® Intradermal: Hemagglutinin 27 mcg/0.1 mL (0.1 mL)

Dosage Forms - Canada

Injection, suspension:

Fluviral®: Hemagglutinin 45 mcg/0.5 mL (5 mL)

Vaxigrip®: Hemagglutinin 45 mcg/0.5 mL (5 mL)

Injection, suspension [preservative free]:

Agriflu™: Hemagglutinin 45 mcg/0.5 mL (0.5 mL)

Fluad™: Hemagglutinin 45 mcg/0.5 mL (0.5 mL)

Influvac®: Hemagglutinin 45 mcg/0.5 mL (0.5 mL)

Intanza®: Hemagglutinin 27 mcg/0.1 mL (0.1 mL); Hemagglutinin 45 mcg/0.1 mL (0.1 mL)

Vaxigrip®: Hemagglutinin 45 mcg/0.5 mL (0.25 mL, 0.5 mL)

influenza virus vaccine (live/attenuated)

(in floo EN za VYE rus vak SEEN live ah TEN yoo aye ted)

Medication Safety Issues

Sound-alike/look-alike issues:

Influenza virus vaccine may be confused with flumazenil

Synonyms H1N1 influenza vaccine; influenza vaccine; influenza virus vaccine (trivalent, live); LAIV; live attenuated influenza vaccine

U.S. Brand Names FluMist®

Canadian Brand Names FluMist®

Therapeutic Category Vaccine, Live (Viral)

Use Provide active immunity to influenza virus strains contained in the vaccine

The Advisory Committee on Immunization Practices (ACIP) states that healthy, nonpregnant persons aged 2-49 years may receive vaccination with either the seasonal live, attenuated influenza vaccine (LAIV) (nasal spray) or the seasonal trivalent inactivated influenza vaccine (TIV) (injection).

General Dosage Range Intranasal:

Children 2-8 years: 0.2 mL/dose (1 or 2 doses per season)

Children ≥9 years and Adults ≤49 years: 0.2 mL/dose (1 dose per season)

Product Availability FluMist® Quadrivalent Vaccine: FDA approved February 2012; availability anticipated for the 2013-2014 flu season. Consult prescribing information for additional information.

Dosage Forms

Solution, intranasal [preservative free]:

FluMist®: (0.2 mL)

influenza virus vaccine (monovalent) *see* influenza virus vaccine (H5N1) *on page 482*

influenza virus vaccine (purified surface antigen) *see* influenza virus vaccine (inactivated) *on page 482*

influenza virus vaccine (split-virus) *see* influenza virus vaccine (inactivated) *on page 482*

influenza virus vaccine (trivalent, live) *see* influenza virus vaccine (live/attenuated) *on page 484*

Influvac® (Can) *see* influenza virus vaccine (inactivated) *on page 482*

Infufer® (Can) *see* iron dextran complex *on page 501*

Infumorph 200 *see* morphine (systemic) *on page 612*

Infumorph 500 *see* morphine (systemic) *on page 612*

Infuvite® Adult *see* vitamins (multiple/injectable) *on page 951*

Infuvite® Pediatric *see* vitamins (multiple/injectable) *on page 951*

ingenol mebutate (IN je nol MEB u tate)

Synonyms *Euphorbia peplus* derivative; PEP005

U.S. Brand Names Picato®

Therapeutic Category Skin and Mucous Membrane Agent, Miscellaneous; Topical Skin Product

Use Topical treatment of actinic keratosis

General Dosage Range Topical: *Adults:* Apply once daily for 2 days (0.05%) or 3 days (0.015%)

Dosage Forms

Gel, topical:

Picato®: 0.015% (3s); 0.05% (2s)

INH *see* isoniazid *on page 503*

Inhibace® (Can) *see* cilazapril *(Canada only) on page 208*

Inhibace® Plus (Can) *see* cilazapril and hydrochlorothiazide *(Canada only) on page 209*

Inlyta® *see* axitinib *on page 105*

Innohep® (Can) *see* tinzaparin *on page 898*

InnoPran XL® *see* propranolol *on page 767*

INOmax® *see* nitric oxide *on page 644*

Inova® *see* benzoyl peroxide *on page 124*

^{111}in-pentetate *see* pentetate indium disodium in 111 *on page 706*

^{111}in-pentetreotide *see* indium in-111 pentetreotide *on page 480*

insect sting kit *see* epinephrine and chlorpheniramine *on page 335*

insoluble prussian blue *see* ferric hexacyanoferrate *on page 379*

Inspra™ *see* eplerenone *on page 337*

Insta-Glucose® [OTC] *see* dextrose *on page 275*

Instat™ MCH *see* collagen hemostat *on page 234*

Instillagel® (Can) *see* lidocaine and chlorhexidine *(Canada only) on page 537*

insulin aspart (IN soo lin AS part)

Medication Safety Issues

Sound-alike/look-alike issues:

NovoLOG® may be confused with HumaLOG®, HumuLIN® R, NovoLIN® N, NovoLIN® R, NovoLOG® Mix 70/30

High alert medication:

The Institute for Safe Medication Practices (ISMP) includes this medication among its list of drugs which have a heightened risk of causing significant patient harm when used in error. ***Due to the number of insulin preparations, it is essential to identify/clarify the type of insulin to be used.***

Other safety concerns:

Cross-contamination may occur if insulin pens are shared among multiple patients. Steps should be taken to prohibit sharing of insulin pens.

Synonyms aspart insulin

U.S. Brand Names NovoLOG®; NovoLOG® FlexPen®; NovoLOG® Penfill®

Canadian Brand Names NovoRapid®

Therapeutic Category Antidiabetic Agent, Insulin

Use Treatment of type 1 diabetes mellitus (insulin-dependent, IDDM) and type 2 diabetes mellitus (noninsulin-dependent, NIDDM) to improve glycemic control

General Dosage Range SubQ: *Children ≥2 years, Adolescents, and Adults:* Daily doses are expressed as the **total units/kg/day of all insulin formulations combined.** Diabetes mellitus, type 1: Initial: 0.2-0.6 units/kg/day in divided doses; usual maintenance: 0.5-1 units/kg/day in divided doses.

Dosage Forms

Injection, solution:

NovoLOG®: 100 units/mL (10 mL)

NovoLOG® FlexPen®: 100 units/mL (3 mL)

NovoLOG® Penfill®: 100 units/mL (3 mL)

insulin aspart and insulin aspart protamine *see* insulin aspart protamine and insulin aspart *on page 485*

insulin aspart protamine and insulin aspart

(IN soo lin AS part PROE ta meen & IN soo lin AS part)

Medication Safety Issues

Sound-alike/look-alike issues:

NovoLOG® Mix 70/30 may be confused with HumaLOG® Mix 75/25™, HumuLIN® 70/30, NovoLIN® 70/30, NovoLOG®

High alert medication:

The Institute for Safe Medication Practices (ISMP) includes this medication among its list of drugs which have a heightened risk of causing significant patient harm when used in error. ***Due to the number of insulin preparations, it is essential to identify/clarify the type of insulin to be used.***

Other safety concerns:

Cross-contamination may occur if insulin pens are shared among multiple patients. Steps should be taken to prohibit sharing of insulin pens.

Synonyms insulin aspart and insulin aspart protamine; NovoLog 70/30

U.S. Brand Names NovoLOG® Mix 70/30; NovoLOG® Mix 70/30 FlexPen®

Canadian Brand Names NovoMix® 30

Therapeutic Category Antidiabetic Agent, Insulin

Use Treatment of type 1 diabetes mellitus (insulin-dependent, IDDM) and type 2 diabetes mellitus (noninsulin-dependent, NIDDM) to improve glycemic control

General Dosage Range SubQ: *Adults:* Diabetes mellitus, type 1 or 2: **Not** intended for initial therapy; basal insulin requirements should be established **first** to direct dosing of combination insulin products.

Dosage Forms

Injection, suspension:

NovoLOG® Mix 70/30: Insulin aspart protamine suspension 70% [intermediate acting] and insulin aspart solution 30% [rapid acting]: 100 units/mL (10 mL)

NovoLOG® Mix 70/30 FlexPen®: Insulin aspart protamine suspension 70% [intermediate acting] and insulin aspart solution 30% [rapid acting]: 100 units/mL (3 mL)

insulin detemir (IN soo lin DE te mir)

Medication Safety Issues

High alert medication:

The Institute for Safe Medication Practices (ISMP) includes this medication among its list of drugs which have a heightened risk of causing significant patient harm when used in error. ***Due to the number of insulin preparations, it is essential to identify/clarify the type of insulin to be used.***

Administration issues:

Insulin detemir is a clear solution, but it is NOT intended for I.V. or I.M. administration.

Other safety concerns:

Cross-contamination may occur if insulin pens are shared among multiple patients. Steps should be taken to prohibit sharing of insulin pens.

Synonyms detemir insulin

U.S. Brand Names Levemir®; Levemir® FlexPen®

Canadian Brand Names Levemir®

Therapeutic Category Antidiabetic Agent, Insulin

Use Treatment of type 1 diabetes mellitus (insulin-dependent, IDDM) and type 2 diabetes mellitus (noninsulin-dependent, NIDDM) to improve glycemic control

General Dosage Range SubQ:

Children ≥2 years, Adolescents, and Adults: Diabetes mellitus, type 1: Initial dose: Approximately one-third of the total daily insulin requirement administered in 1-2 divided doses.

Adults: Diabetes mellitus, type 2: Initial: 10 units **or** 0.1-0.2 units/kg in 1-2 divided doses

Dosage Forms

Injection, solution:

Levemir®: 100 units/mL (10 mL)

Levemir® FlexPen®: 100 units/mL (3 mL)

insulin glargine (IN soo lin GLAR jeen)

Medication Safety Issues

Sound-alike/look-alike issues:

Insulin glargine may be confused with insulin glulisine

Lantus® may be confused with latanoprost, Latuda®, Xalatan®

High alert medication:

The Institute for Safe Medication Practices (ISMP) includes this medication among its list of drugs which have a heightened risk of causing significant patient harm when used in error. ***Due to the number of insulin preparations, it is essential to identify/clarify the type of insulin to be used.***

Administration issues:

Insulin glargine is a clear solution, but it is NOT intended for I.V. or I.M. administration.

Other safety concerns:

Cross-contamination may occur if insulin pens are shared among multiple patients. Steps should be taken to prohibit sharing of insulin pens.

International issues:

Lantus [U.S., Canada, and multiple international markets] may be confused with Lanvis brand name for thioguanine [Canada and multiple international markets]

Synonyms glargine insulin

U.S. Brand Names Lantus®; Lantus® Solostar®

Canadian Brand Names Lantus®; Lantus® OptiSet®

Therapeutic Category Antidiabetic Agent, Insulin

Use Treatment of type 1 diabetes mellitus (insulin-dependent, IDDM) and type 2 diabetes mellitus (noninsulin-dependent, NIDDM) to improve glycemic control

General Dosage Range SubQ:

Children ≥6 years, Adolescents, and Adults: Diabetes mellitus, type 1: Initial dose: Approximately one-third of the total daily insulin requirement administered once daily

Adults: Diabetes mellitus, type 2: Initial: 10 units or 0.2 units/kg once daily

Dosage Forms

Injection, solution:

Lantus®: 100 units/mL (3 mL, 10 mL)

Lantus® Solostar®: 100 units/mL (3 mL)

insulin glulisine (IN soo lin gloo LIS een)

Medication Safety Issues

Sound-alike/look-alike issues:

Insulin glulisine may be confused with insulin glargine

High alert medication:

The Institute for Safe Medication Practices (ISMP) includes this medication among its list of drugs which have a heightened risk of causing significant patient harm when used in error. ***Due to the number of insulin preparations, it is essential to identify/clarify the type of insulin to be used.***

Other safety concerns:

Cross-contamination may occur if insulin pens are shared among multiple patients. Steps should be taken to prohibit sharing of insulin pens.

Synonyms glulisine insulin

U.S. Brand Names Apidra®; Apidra® SoloStar®

Canadian Brand Names Apidra®

Therapeutic Category Antidiabetic Agent, Insulin

Use Treatment of type 1 diabetes mellitus (insulin-dependent, IDDM) and type 2 diabetes mellitus (noninsulin-dependent, NIDDM) to improve glycemic control

General Dosage Range SubQ: *Children ≥4 years, Adolescents and Adults:* Diabetes mellitus, type 1: **Note:** Multiple daily doses or continuous subcutaneous infusions guided by blood glucose monitoring are the standard of diabetes care. Combinations of insulin formulations are commonly used. The daily doses presented below are expressed as the **total units/kg/day of all insulin formulations combined.** Initial: 0.2-0.6 units/kg/day in divided doses; usual maintenance: 0.5-1 units/kg/day in divided doses.

Dosage Forms

Injection, solution:

Apidra®: 100 units/mL (3 mL, 10 mL)

Apidra® SoloStar®: 100 units/mL (3 mL)

insulin lispro (IN soo lin LYE sproe)

Medication Safety Issues

Sound-alike/look-alike issues:

HumaLOG® may be confused with HumaLOG® Mix 50/50, Humira®, HumuLIN® N, HumuLIN® R, NovoLOG®

High alert medication:

The Institute for Safe Medication Practices (ISMP) includes this medication among its list of drugs which have a heightened risk of causing significant patient harm when used in error. ***Due to the number of insulin preparations, it is essential to identify/clarify the type of insulin to be used.***

Other safety concerns:

Cross-contamination may occur if insulin pens are shared among multiple patients. Steps should be taken to prohibit sharing of insulin pens.

Synonyms lispro insulin

U.S. Brand Names HumaLOG®; HumaLOG® KwikPen™

Canadian Brand Names Humalog®

Therapeutic Category Antidiabetic Agent, Insulin

Use Treatment of type 1 diabetes mellitus (insulin-dependent, IDDM) and type 2 diabetes mellitus (noninsulin-dependent, NIDDM) to improve glycemic control

General Dosage Range SubQ: *Children ≥3 years, Adolescents and Adults:* Daily doses are expressed as the **total units/kg/day of all insulin formulations combined.** Diabetes mellitus, type 1: Initial: 0.2-0.6 units/kg/day in divided doses; usual maintenance: 0.5-1 units/kg/day in divided doses.

Dosage Forms

Injection, solution:

HumaLOG®: 100 units/mL (3 mL, 10 mL)

HumaLOG® KwikPen™: 100 units/mL (3 mL)

insulin lispro and insulin lispro protamine *see* insulin lispro protamine and insulin lispro *on page 488*

insulin lispro protamine and insulin lispro

(IN soo lin LYE sproe PROE ta meen & IN soo lin LYE sproe)

Medication Safety Issues

Sound-alike/look-alike issues:

HumaLOG® Mix 50/50™ may be confused with HumaLOG®

HumaLOG® Mix 75/25™ may be confused with HumuLIN® 70/30, NovoLIN® 70/30, and NovoLOG® Mix 70/30

High alert medication:

The Institute for Safe Medication Practices (ISMP) includes this medication among its list of drugs which have a heightened risk of causing significant patient harm when used in error. ***Due to the number of insulin preparations, it is essential to identify/clarify the type of insulin to be used.***

Other safety concerns:

Cross-contamination may occur if insulin pens are shared among multiple patients. Steps should be taken to prohibit sharing of insulin pens.

Synonyms insulin lispro and insulin lispro protamine

U.S. Brand Names HumaLOG® Mix 50/50™; HumaLOG® Mix 50/50™ KwikPen™; HumaLOG® Mix 75/25™; HumaLOG® Mix 75/25™ KwikPen™

Canadian Brand Names Humalog® Mix 25

Therapeutic Category Antidiabetic Agent, Insulin

Use Treatment of type 1 diabetes mellitus (insulin-dependent, IDDM) and type 2 diabetes mellitus (noninsulin-dependent, NIDDM) to improve glycemic control

General Dosage Range SubQ: *Adults:* Diabetes mellitus, type 1 or 2: **Not** intended for initial therapy; basal insulin requirements should be established **first** to direct dosing of combination insulin products.

Dosage Forms

Injection, suspension:

HumaLOG® Mix 50/50™: Insulin lispro protamine suspension 50% [intermediate acting] and insulin lispro solution 50% [rapid acting]: 100 units/mL (10 mL)

HumaLOG® Mix 50/50™ KwikPen™: Insulin lispro protamine suspension 50% [intermediate acting] and insulin lispro solution 50% [rapid acting]: 100 units/mL (3 mL)

HumaLOG® Mix 75/25™: Insulin lispro protamine suspension 75% [intermediate acting] and insulin lispro solution 25% [rapid acting]: 100 units/mL (10 mL)

HumaLOG® Mix 75/25™ KwikPen™: Insulin lispro protamine suspension 75% [intermediate acting] and insulin lispro solution 25% [rapid acting]: 100 units/mL (3 mL)

insulin NPH (IN soo lin N P H)

Medication Safety Issues

Sound-alike/look-alike issues:

HumuLIN® N may be confused with HumuLIN® R, HumaLOG®, Humira®

NovoLIN® N may be confused with NovoLIN® R, NovoLOG®

High alert medication:

The Institute for Safe Medication Practices (ISMP) includes this medication among its list of drugs which have a heightened risk of causing significant patient harm when used in error. ***Due to the number of insulin preparations, it is essential to identify/clarify the type of insulin to be used.***

Other safety concerns:

Cross-contamination may occur if insulin pens are shared among multiple patients. Steps should be taken to prohibit sharing of insulin pens.

Synonyms isophane insulin; NPH insulin

U.S. Brand Names HumuLIN® N; NovoLIN® N

Canadian Brand Names Humulin® N; Novolin® ge NPH

Therapeutic Category Antidiabetic Agent, Insulin

Use Treatment of type 1 diabetes mellitus (insulin-dependent, IDDM) and type 2 diabetes mellitus (noninsulin-dependent, NIDDM) to improve glycemic control

General Dosage Range SubQ:

Children ≥2 years, Adolescents, and Adults: Daily doses are expressed as the **total units/kg/day of all insulin formulations combined.** Diabetes mellitus, type 1: Initial: 0.2-0.6 units/kg/day in divided doses; usual maintenance: 0.5-1 units/kg/day in divided doses.

Adults: Diabetes mellitus, type 2: Initial: 0.2 units/kg/day or 10 units/day in divided doses before meals.

Dosage Forms

Injection, suspension:

HumuLIN® N: 100 units/mL (3 mL, 10 mL)

NovoLIN® N: 100 units/mL (10 mL)

Dosage Forms - Canada

Injection, suspension:

Novolin® ge NPH: 100 units/mL (3 mL, 10 mL)

insulin NPH and insulin regular (IN soo lin N P H & IN soo lin REG yoo ler)

Medication Safety Issues

Sound-alike/look-alike issues:

HumuLIN® 70/30 may be confused with HumaLOG® Mix 75/25, HumuLIN® R, NovoLIN® 70/30, NovoLOG® Mix 70/30

NovoLIN® 70/30 may be confused with HumaLOG® Mix 75/25, HumuLIN® 70/30, HumuLIN® R, NovoLIN® R, and NovoLOG® Mix 70/30

High alert medication:

The Institute for Safe Medication Practices (ISMP) includes this medication among its list of drugs which have a heightened risk of causing significant patient harm when used in error. ***Due to the number of insulin preparations, it is essential to identify/clarify the type of insulin to be used.***

Other safety concerns:

Cross-contamination may occur if insulin pens are shared among multiple patients. Steps should be taken to prohibit sharing of insulin pens.

Synonyms insulin regular and insulin NPH; isophane insulin and regular insulin; NPH insulin and regular insulin

U.S. Brand Names HumuLIN® 70/30; NovoLIN® 70/30

Canadian Brand Names Humulin® 20/80; Humulin® 70/30; Novolin® ge 30/70; Novolin® ge 40/60; Novolin® ge 50/50

Therapeutic Category Antidiabetic Agent, Insulin

Use Treatment of type 1 diabetes mellitus (insulin-dependent, IDDM) and type 2 diabetes mellitus (noninsulin-dependent, NIDDM) to improve glycemic control

General Dosage Range SubQ:

Children, Adolescents, and Adults: Daily doses are expressed as the **total units/kg/day of all insulin formulations combined.** Diabetes mellitus, type 1: Initial: 0.2-0.6 units/kg/day in divided doses; usual maintenance: 0.5-1 units/kg/day in divided doses.

Adults: Diabetes mellitus, type 2: **Not** intended for initial therapy; basal insulin requirements should be established **first** to direct dosing of combination insulin products.

Dosage Forms

Injection, suspension:

HumuLIN® 70/30: Insulin NPH suspension 70% [intermediate acting] and insulin regular solution 30% [short acting]: 100 units/mL (3 mL, 10 mL)

NovoLIN® 70/30: Insulin NPH suspension 70% [intermediate acting] and insulin regular solution 30% [short acting]: 100 units/mL (10 mL)

Dosage Forms - Canada

Injection, suspension:

Humulin® 20/80: Insulin regular solution 20% [short acting] and insulin NPH suspension 80% [intermediate acting]: 100 units/mL (3 mL)

Novolin® ge 30/70: Insulin regular solution 30% [short acting] and insulin NPH suspension 70% [intermediate acting]: 100 units/mL (3 mL)

Novolin® ge 40/60: Insulin regular solution 40% [short acting] and insulin NPH suspension 60% [intermediate acting]: 100 units/mL (3 mL)

Novolin® ge 50/50: Insulin regular solution 50% [short acting] and insulin NPH suspension 50% [intermediate acting]: 100 units/mL (3 mL)

insulin regular (IN soo lin REG yoo ler)

Medication Safety Issues

Sound-alike/look-alike issues:

HumuLIN® R may be confused with HumaLOG®, Humira®, HumuLIN® 70/30, HumuLIN® N, NovoLIN® 70/30, NovoLIN® R, NovoLOG®

NovoLIN® R may be confused with HumuLIN® R, NovoLIN® 70/30, NovoLIN® N, NovoLOG®

High alert medication:

The Institute for Safe Medication Practices (ISMP) includes this medication among its list of drugs which have a heightened risk of causing significant patient harm when used in error. ***Due to the number of insulin preparations, it is essential to identify/clarify the type of insulin to be used.***

BEERS Criteria medication:

This drug may be potentially inappropriate for use in geriatric patients (Quality of evidence - moderate; Strength of recommendation - strong).

Administration issues:

Concentrated solutions (eg, U-500) should not be available in patient care areas. U-500 regular insulin should be stored, dispensed, and administered separately from U-100 regular insulin. For patients who receive U-500 insulin in the hospital setting, highlighting the strength prominently on the patient's medical chart and medication record may help to reduce dispensing errors.

Other safety concerns:

Cross-contamination may occur if insulin pens are shared among multiple patients. Steps should be taken to prohibit sharing of insulin pens.

Synonyms regular insulin

U.S. Brand Names HumuLIN® R; HumuLIN® R U-500; NovoLIN® R

Canadian Brand Names Humulin® R; Novolin® ge Toronto

Therapeutic Category Antidiabetic Agent, Insulin; Antidote

Use Treatment of type 1 diabetes mellitus (insulin-dependent, IDDM) and type 2 diabetes mellitus (noninsulin-dependent, NIDDM) to improve glycemic control

General Dosage Range Dosage adjustment recommended in patients with renal impairment

I.V., SubQ: *Children and Adults:*

Diabetes mellitus, type 1: Initial: 0.5-1 unit/kg/day in divided doses; Usual maintenance: 0.5-1.2 units/kg/day in divided doses. **Note:** Generally, 50% to 75% of the total daily dose (TDD) is given as an intermediate- or long-acting form of insulin (1-2 daily injections) and the remaining portion is then divided and administered before or at mealtime (depending on the formulation) as a rapid-acting or short-acting form of insulin.

Diabetes mellitus, type 2: Initial basal insulin dose: 0.2 units/kg or 10 units/day given as an intermediate- or long-acting insulin at bedtime or long-acting insulin given in the morning

Dosage Forms

Injection, solution:

HumuLIN® R: 100 units/mL (3 mL, 10 mL)
HumuLIN® R U-500: 500 units/mL (20 mL)
NovoLIN® R: 100 units/mL (10 mL)

insulin regular and insulin NPH *see* insulin NPH and insulin regular *on page 489*
Intanza® (Can) *see* influenza virus vaccine (inactivated) *on page 482*
Integrilin® *see* eptifibatide *on page 339*
Intelence® *see* etravirine *on page 367*
α-2-interferon *see* interferon alfa-2b *on page 490*
interferon alfa-2a (PEG conjugate) *see* peginterferon alfa-2a *on page 697*
interferon alfa-2b (PEG conjugate) *see* peginterferon alfa-2b *on page 698*

interferon alfa-2b (in ter FEER on AL fa too bee)

Medication Safety Issues

Sound-alike/look-alike issues:

Interferon alfa-2b may be confused with interferon alfa-2a, interferon alfa-n3, pegylated interferon alfa-2b

Intron® A may be confused with PEG-Intron

International issues:

Interferon alfa-2b may be confused with interferon alpha multi-subtype which is available in international markets

Synonyms INF-alpha 2; interferon alpha-2b; rLFN-α2; α-2-interferon

U.S. Brand Names Intron® A

Canadian Brand Names Intron® A

Therapeutic Category Biological Response Modulator

Use

Patients ≥1 year of age: Chronic hepatitis B

Patients ≥3 years of age: Chronic hepatitis C (in combination with ribavirin)

Patients ≥18 years of age: Condyloma acuminata, chronic hepatitis B, chronic hepatitis C, hairy cell leukemia, malignant melanoma, AIDS-related Kaposi sarcoma, follicular non-Hodgkin lymphoma

General Dosage Range Dosage adjustment is recommended in patients who develop toxicities

I.M.:

Children 1-17 years: 3-5 million units/m^2 3 times weekly (maximum: 3 million units per dose)

Adults: Dosage varies greatly depending on indication

I.V.: *Adults:* 20 million units/m^2 for 5 consecutive days per week

Intralesional: *Adults:* 1 million units/lesion 3 times weekly, on alternate days (maximum: 5 lesions per treatment)

SubQ:

Children 1-17 years: Initial: 3 million units/m^2 3 times weekly for 1 week; Maintenance: 6 million units/m^2 3 times weekly (maximum: 10 million units 3 times weekly) **or** 3-5 million units/m^2 3 times weekly (maximum: 3 million units per dose)

Adults: Dosage varies greatly depending on indication

Dosage Forms

Injection, powder for reconstitution [preservative free]:

Intron® A: 10 million units, 18 million units, 50 million units

Injection, solution:

Intron® A: 6 million units/mL (3 mL); 10 million units/mL (2.5 mL); 3 million units/0.2 mL (1.2 mL); 5 million units/0.2 mL (1.2 mL); 10 million units/0.2 mL (1.2 mL)

interferon alfacon-1 (in ter FEER on AL fa con one)

Medication Safety Issues

Sound-alike/look-alike issues:

Interferon alfacon-1 may be confused with interferon alfa-2a, interferon alfa-2b, interferon alfa-n3, peginterferon alfa-2b

International issues:

Interferon alfacon-1 may be confused with interferon alpha multi-subtype which is available in international markets

U.S. Brand Names Infergen®

Therapeutic Category Interferon

Use Treatment of chronic hepatitis C virus (HCV) infection in patients ≥18 years of age with compensated liver disease and anti-HCV serum antibodies or HCV RNA; concurrent use with ribavirin in HCV-infected patients who have failed treatment with pegylated interferon/ribavirin (Bacon, 2009)

General Dosage Range Dosage adjustment recommended in patients who develop toxicities

SubQ: *Adults:* 9-15 mcg 3 times/week; may increase to 15 mcg 3 times/week

Dosage Forms

Injection, solution [preservative free]:

Infergen®: 30 mcg/mL (0.3 mL, 0.5 mL)

interferon alfa-n3 (in ter FEER on AL fa en three)

Medication Safety Issues

Sound-alike/look-alike issues:

Alferon® may be confused with Alkeran®

U.S. Brand Names Alferon® N

Canadian Brand Names Alferon® N

Therapeutic Category Biological Response Modulator

Use Patients ≥18 years of age: Intralesional treatment of refractory or recurring genital or venereal warts (condylomata acuminata)

General Dosage Range Intralesional: *Adults:* Inject 250,000 units (0.05 mL) in each wart twice weekly (maximum: 8 weeks)

Dosage Forms

Injection, solution:

Alferon® N: 5 million units (1 mL)

interferon alpha-2b *see* interferon alfa-2b *on page 490*

interferon beta-1a (in ter FEER on BAY ta won aye)

Medication Safety Issues

Sound-alike/look-alike issues:

Avonex® may be confused with Avelox®

Synonyms rIFN beta-1a

U.S. Brand Names Avonex®; Avonex® Pen™; Rebif®

Canadian Brand Names Avonex®; Rebif®

Therapeutic Category Biological Response Modulator

Use Treatment of relapsing forms of multiple sclerosis (MS)

Canadian labeling: Additional uses (not in U.S. labeling): Avonex®: To decrease the number and volume of active brain lesions, decrease overall disease burden, and delay onset of clinically definite MS in patients who have experienced a single demyelinating event.

General Dosage Range Dosage adjustment recommended in patients who develop toxicities

I.M.: *Adults:* Initial: 30 mcg once weekly **or** 7.5 mcg (week 1) then titrate in increments of 7.5 mcg once weekly (weeks 2-4) to 30 mcg once weekly

SubQ: *Adults:* Initial: 4.4 or 8.8 mcg 3 times/week for 2 weeks; Titration: 11 or 22 mcg 3 times/week for 2 weeks; Maintenance: 22 or 44 mcg 3 times/week

Dosage Forms

Injection, powder for reconstitution [preservative free]:

Avonex®: 33 mcg [contains albumin (human); provides 30 mcg/mL following reconstitution; supplied with diluent]

Injection, solution:

Avonex®, Avonex® Pen™: 30 mcg/0.5 mL (0.5 mL)

Injection, solution [preservative free]:

Rebif®: 22 mcg/0.5 mL (0.5 mL), 44 mcg/0.5 mL (0.5 mL)

Injection, solution [preservative free, combination package]:

Rebif®: Titration Pack: 22 mcg/0.5 mL (6s) and 8.8 mcg/0.2 mL (6s)

interferon beta-1b (in ter FEER on BAY ta won bee)

Synonyms rIFN beta-1b

U.S. Brand Names Betaseron®; Extavia®

Canadian Brand Names Betaseron®; Extavia®

Therapeutic Category Biological Response Modulator

Use Treatment of relapsing forms of multiple sclerosis (MS); treatment of first clinical episode with MRI features consistent with MS

Canadian labeling: Additional use (not in U.S. labeling): Treatment of secondary-progressive MS

General Dosage Range SubQ: *Adults:* 0.0625-0.25 mg (2-8 million units) every other day

Dosage Forms

Injection, powder for reconstitution [preservative free]:

Betaseron®: 0.3 mg [~9.6 million units]

Extavia®: 0.3 mg [~9.6 million units]

interferon gamma-1b (in ter FEER on GAM ah won bee)

U.S. Brand Names Actimmune®

Canadian Brand Names Actimmune®

Therapeutic Category Biological Response Modulator

Use Reduce frequency and severity of serious infections associated with chronic granulomatous disease; delay time to disease progression in patients with severe, malignant osteopetrosis

General Dosage Range Dosage adjustment recommended in patients who develop toxicities

SubQ: *Children and Adults:*

BSA ≤0.5 m^2: 1.5 mcg/kg/dose 3 times/week

BSA >0.5 m^2: 50 mcg/m^2 (1 million units/m^2) 3 times/week

Dosage Forms

Injection, solution [preservative free]:

Actimmune®: 100 mcg (0.5 mL)

interleukin-1 receptor antagonist *see* anakinra *on page* 75

interleukin 2 *see* aldesleukin *on page* 44

interleukin-11 *see* oprelvekin *on page 670*
Intermezzo® *see* zolpidem *on page 966*
Intralipid® *see* fat emulsion *on page 373*
intrapleural talc *see* talc (sterile) *on page 867*
intravenous fat emulsion *see* fat emulsion *on page 373*
intrifiban *see* eptifibatide *on page 339*
Intron® A *see* interferon alfa-2b *on page 490*
Intropin *see* dopamine *on page 309*
Introvale™ *see* ethinyl estradiol and levonorgestrel *on page 357*
Intuniv® *see* guanfacine *on page 438*
INVanz® *see* ertapenem *on page 342*
Invanz® (Can) *see* ertapenem *on page 342*
Invega® *see* paliperidone *on page 685*
Invega® Sustenna® *see* paliperidone *on page 685*
Invirase® *see* saquinavir *on page 824*

iobenguane I 123 (eye oh BEN gwane eye one TWEN tee three)

Synonyms 123 meta-iodobenzlyguanidine sulfate; 123I-metaiodobenzylguanidine (MIBG); I-123 MIBG; I^{123} iobenguane; iobenguane sulfate I 123

U.S. Brand Names AdreView™

Therapeutic Category Radiopharmaceutical

Use As an adjunct to other diagnostic tests, in the detection of primary or metastatic pheochromocytoma or neuroblastoma

Dosage Forms

Injection, solution:

AdreView™: Iobenguane sulfate 0.08 mg and I 123 74 MBq (2 mCi) per mL (5 mL)

iobenguane sulfate I 123 *see* iobenguane I 123 *on page 493*
Iodex® [OTC] *see* iodine *on page 493*

iodinated I 131 albumin (EYE oh di nay ted eye won thur tee won al BYOO min)

Medication Safety Issues

Other safety concerns:

Radiopharmaceutical: Use appropriate precaution for handling, disposal, and minimizing exposure to patients and healthcare personnel. Use under supervision of experienced personnel. Should be stored in original lead container or adequate radiation shield.

Synonyms ^{131}I-albumin; ^{131}I-HSA

U.S. Brand Names Megatope; Volumex HSA I-131

Therapeutic Category Radiopharmaceutical

Use For the determination of total blood and plasma volumes, cardiac output, cardiac and pulmonary blood volumes and circulation times; and in protein turnover studies, heart and great vessel delineation, localization of the placenta, and localization of cerebral neoplasms

iodine (EYE oh dyne)

Medication Safety Issues

Sound-alike/look-alike issues:

Iodine may be confused with codeine, Iopidine®, Lodine

U.S. Brand Names Iodex® [OTC]; Iodoflex™ [OTC]; Iodosorb® [OTC]

Therapeutic Category Topical Skin Product

Use Used topically as an antiseptic in the management of minor, superficial skin wounds and has been used to disinfect the skin preoperatively

General Dosage Range Topical: *Adults:* Antiseptic: Apply to affected area 1-3 times/day; Ulcer/wound cleansing: Apply to clean wound 3 times/week (maximum: 50 g/application; 150 g/week)

Dosage Forms

Dressing, topical:

Iodoflex™ [OTC]: 0.9% (3s, 5s)

Gel, topical:

Iodosorb® [OTC]: 0.9% (40 g)

Ointment, topical:
Iodex® [OTC]: 4.7% (30 g, 720 g)
Tincture, topical: 2% (30 mL, 59 mL, 473 mL); 7% (30 mL, 473 mL)
Tincture, swabstick, topical: 2% (50s)

iodine I 131 tositumomab and tositumomab *see* tositumomab and iodine I 131 tositumomab *on page* 907

iodipamide meglumine (eye oh DI pa mide MEG loo meen)

Medication Safety Issues
High alert medication:
The Institute for Safe Medication Practices (ISMP) includes this medication among its list of drugs which have a heightened risk of causing significant patient harm when used in error.

U.S. Brand Names Cholografin® Meglumine

Therapeutic Category Iodinated Contrast Media; Radiological/Contrast Media, Ionic

Use Contrast medium for intravenous cholangiography and cholecystography

General Dosage Range I.V.:
Infants and Children: 0.3-0.6 mL/kg (maximum: 20 mL)
Adults: 20 mL

Dosage Forms
Injection, solution:
Cholografin® Meglumine: 520 mg/mL (20 mL)

iodipamide meglumine and diatrizoate meglumine *see* diatrizoate meglumine and iodipamide meglumine *on page* 277

iodixanol (EYE oh dix an ole)

Medication Safety Issues
High alert medication:
The Institute for Safe Medication Practices (ISMP) includes this medication among its list of drugs which have a heightened risk of causing significant patient harm when used in error.
Administration issues:
Not for intrathecal use.

U.S. Brand Names Visipaque™

Canadian Brand Names Visipaque™

Therapeutic Category Iodinated Contrast Media; Radiological/Contrast Media, Nonionic

Use
Intraarterial: Digital subtraction angiography, angiocardiography, peripheral arteriography, visceral arteriography, cerebral arteriography
Intravenous: Contrast enhanced computed tomography imaging, excretory urography, and peripheral venography

General Dosage Range
I.V.:
Children >1-12 years: Iodixanol 270 mg iodine/mL: 1-2 mL/kg (maximum: 2 mL/kg)
Children >12 years and Adults: Iodixanol 270 mg and 320 mg iodine/mL: Concentration and dose vary based on study type; refer to product labeling (maximum total dose: 80 g iodine)
Intraarterial:
Children >1-12 years: Iodixanol 320 mg iodine/mL: 1-2 mL/kg (maximum: 4 mL/kg)
Children >12 years and Adults: Iodixanol 320 mg iodine/mL: Dose individualized based on injection site and study type; refer to product labeling (maximum total dose: 80 g iodine)

Dosage Forms
Injection, solution [preservative free]:
Visipaque™: 270: 550 mg/mL (50 mL, 100 mL, 150 mL, 200 mL); 320: 652 mg/mL (50 mL, 100 mL, 150 mL, 200 mL, 500 mL)

iodochlorhydroxyquin and flumethasone *see* clioquinol and flumethasone *(Canada only) on page* 220

Iodoflex™ [OTC] *see* iodine *on page* 493

iodoquinol (eye oh doe KWIN ole)

Synonyms diiodohydroxyquin

U.S. Brand Names Yodoxin®

Canadian Brand Names Diodoquin®

Therapeutic Category Amebicide

Use Treatment of acute and chronic intestinal amebiasis; asymptomatic cyst passers; *Blastocystis hominis* infections; ineffective for amebic hepatitis or hepatic abscess

General Dosage Range Oral:

Children: 30-40 mg/kg/day in 3 divided doses (maximum: 1.95 g/day)

Adults: 650 mg 3 times/day (maximum: 2 g/day)

Dosage Forms

Tablet, oral:

Yodoxin®: 210 mg, 650 mg

iodoquinol and hydrocortisone (eye oh doe KWIN ole & hye droe KOR ti sone)

Medication Safety Issues

Sound-alike/look-alike issues:

Vytone may be confused with Hytone®, Zydone®

Synonyms hydrocortisone and iodoquinol; Vytone

U.S. Brand Names Alcortin® A; Dermazene®

Therapeutic Category Antifungal/Corticosteroid

Use Treatment of eczema (including impetiginized, nuchal, and nummular); acne urticaria; anogenital pruritus, atopic dermatitis, chronic infectious dermatitis; chronic eczematoid otitis externa; folliculitis, intertrigo; lichen simplex chronicus; moniliasis; mycotic dermatoses; neurodermatitis (localized or systemic); pyoderma, stasis dermatitis

General Dosage Range Topical: *Children ≥12 years and Adults:* Apply 3-4 times/day

Dosage Forms

Cream, topical: Iodoquinol 1% and hydrocortisone 1% (30 g)

Dermazene®: Iodoquinol 1% and hydrocortisone 1% (30 g)

Gel, topical:

Alcortin® A: Iodoquinol 1% and hydrocortisone 2% (2 g)

Iodosorb® [OTC] *see* iodine *on page 493*

ioflupane *see* ioflupane I 123 *on page 495*

ioflupane-123 I *see* ioflupane I 123 *on page 495*

ioflupane I 123 (eye oh FLOO pane eye one TWEN tee three)

Synonyms 123I-ioflupane; DaTSCAN; ioflupane; ioflupane-123 I

U.S. Brand Names DaTscan™

Therapeutic Category Radiopharmaceutical

Controlled Substance C-II

Use Striatal dopamine transporter (DaT) visualization using single photon emission computed tomography (SPECT) brain imaging as an adjunct to other diagnostic tests to assist in the evaluation of patients with suspected Parkinsonian syndromes (PS); specifically, to differentiate essential tremor (ET) from tremor due to PS (idiopathic Parkinson disease, multiple system atrophy, and progressive supranuclear palsy)

Dosage Forms

Injection, solution [preservative free]:

DaTscan™: Ioflupane 0.07-0.13 mcg and I 123 74 MBq (2 mCi) per 1 mL (2.5 mL)

iohexol (eye oh HEX ole)

Medication Safety Issues

High alert medication:

The Institute for Safe Medication Practices (ISMP) includes this medication among its list of drugs which have a heightened risk of causing significant patient harm when used in error.

U.S. Brand Names Omnipaque™ 140 [DSC]; Omnipaque™ 180; Omnipaque™ 240; Omnipaque™ 300; Omnipaque™ 350

Canadian Brand Names Omnipaque™

Therapeutic Category Polypeptide Hormone; Radiological/Contrast Media, Nonionic

Use

Intrathecal: Myelography; contrast enhancement for computerized tomography

Intravascular: Angiocardiography, aortography, digital subtraction angiography, peripheral arteriography, excretory urography; contrast enhancement for computed tomographic imaging

Oral/body cavity: Arthrography, GI tract examination, hysterosalpingography, pancreatography, cholangiopancreatography, herniography, cystourethrography; enhanced computed tomography of the abdomen

Dosage Forms

Injection, solution [preservative free]:

Omnipaque™ 180: 388 mg/mL (10 mL, 20 mL)

Omnipaque™ 240: 518 mg/mL (10 mL, 20 mL, 50 mL, 100 mL, 150 mL, 200 mL)

Omnipaque™ 300: 647 mg/mL (10 mL, 30 mL, 50 mL, 75 mL, 100 mL, 125 mL, 150 mL, 200 mL, 500 mL)

Omnipaque™ 350: 755 mg/mL (50 mL, 75 mL, 100 mL, 125 mL, 150 mL, 200 mL, 500 mL)

Ionil® [OTC] *see* salicylic acid *on page 816*

Ionil Plus® [OTC] *see* salicylic acid *on page 816*

ionil-T® [OTC] *see* coal tar *on page 228*

ionil-T® Plus [OTC] *see* coal tar *on page 228*

iopamidol (eye oh PA mi dole)

Medication Safety Issues

High alert medication:

The Institute for Safe Medication Practices (ISMP) includes this medication among its list of drugs which have a heightened risk of causing significant patient harm when used in error.

U.S. Brand Names Isovue Multipack®; Isovue-M®; Isovue® 200; Isovue® 250; Isovue® 300; Isovue® 370

Therapeutic Category Iodinated Contrast Media; Radiological/Contrast Media, Nonionic

Use

Intrathecal (Isovue-M®): Myelography contrast enhancement of computed tomographic cisternography and ventriculography; thoracolumbar myelography

Intravascular (Isovue®, Isovue Multipack®): Angiography (eg, coronary, cerebral, peripheral arteriogram), pediatric angiocardiography, excretory urography; contrast enhancement of computed tomographic imaging (in adults and children); evaluation of certain malignancies; image enhancement of non-neoplastic lesions

Dosage Forms

Injection, solution:

Isovue Multipack®: 51% (200 mL); 61% (200 mL, 500 mL); 76% (200 mL, 500 mL)

Isovue® 200: 41% (50 mL, 200 mL)

Isovue® 250: 51% (50 mL, 100 mL, 150 mL)

Isovue® 300: 61% (30 mL, 50 mL, 75 mL, 100 mL, 150 mL)

Isovue® 370: 76% (50 mL, 75 mL, 100 mL, 125 mL, 150 mL)

Injection, solution, intrathecal:

Isovue-M®: 41% (10 mL, 20 mL); 61% (15 mL)

Iophen C-NR *see* guaifenesin and codeine *on page 434*

Iophen DM-NR [OTC] *see* guaifenesin and dextromethorphan *on page 434*

Iophen NR [OTC] *see* guaifenesin *on page 433*

Iopidine® *see* apraclonidine *on page 88*

iopromide (eye oh PROE mide)

Medication Safety Issues

High alert medication:

The Institute for Safe Medication Practices (ISMP) includes this medication among its list of drugs which have a heightened risk of causing significant patient harm when used in error.

U.S. Brand Names Ultravist®

Canadian Brand Names Ultravist®

Therapeutic Category Radiological/Contrast Media, Nonionic

Use Enhance imaging in cerebral arteriography and peripheral arteriography; coronary arteriography and left ventriculography, visceral angiography and aortography; contrast-enhanced computed tomographic imaging of the head and body, excretory urography, intraarterial digital subtraction angiography, peripheral venography

Dosage Forms

Injection, solution:

Ultravist®: Iodine 240 mg/mL (100 mL, 200 mL); Iodine 300 mg/mL (50 mL, 100 mL, 125 mL, 150 mL, 200 mL, 500 mL); Iodine 370 mg/mL (50 mL, 100 mL, 150 mL, 200 mL, 250 mL, 500 mL)

iOSAT™ [OTC] *see* potassium iodide *on page 746*

iothalamate meglumine (eye oh thal A mate MEG loo meen)

Medication Safety Issues

High alert medication:

The Institute for Safe Medication Practices (ISMP) includes this medication among its list of drugs which have a heightened risk of causing significant patient harm when used in error.

U.S. Brand Names Conray®; Conray® 30; Conray® 43; Cysto-Conray™ II

Therapeutic Category Iodinated Contrast Media; Radiological/Contrast Media, Ionic

Use

Solution for injection: Arthrography, cerebral angiography, cranial computerized angiotomography, digital subtraction angiography, direct cholangiography, endoscopic retrograde cholangiopancreatography, excretory urography, peripheral arteriography, urography, venography; contrast enhancement of computed tomographic images

Solution for instillation: Retrograde cystography and cystourethrography

Dosage Forms

Injection, solution:

Conray® 30: 30% (150 mL)

Conray® 43: 43% (50 mL, 250 mL)

Conray®: 60% (30 mL, 50 mL, 100 mL, 150 mL)

Injection, solution for instillation:

Cysto-Conray™ II: 17.2% (250 mL)

iotrolan *(Canada only)* (eye OH troe lan)

Medication Safety Issues

Sound-alike/look-alike issues:

Osmovist® may be confused with Gadavist™, Gadovist™, Magnevist®

High alert medication:

The Institute for Safe Medication Practices (ISMP) includes this medication among its list of drug classes which have a heightened risk of causing significant patient harm when used in error.

International issues:

Osmovist [Canada] may be confused with Vasovist brand name for gadofosveset [Hungary, Turkey]

Canadian Brand Names Osmovist®

Therapeutic Category Iodinated Contrast Media; Radiological/Contrast Media, Nonionic (Iso-Osmolality)

Use Myelography (lumbar, cervical, total columnar); computerized tomography (CT) of spinal and subarachnoid spaces

Product Availability Not available in U.S.

Dosage Forms - Canada

Injection, solution, intrathecal [preservative free]:

Osmovist®:

240 [contains iotrolan 513 mg equivalent to iodine 240 mg/mL] (10 mL)

300 [contains iotrolan 641 mg equivalent to iodine 300 mg /mL] (10 mL)

ioversol (EYE oh ver sole)

Medication Safety Issues

High alert medication:

The Institute for Safe Medication Practices (ISMP) includes this medication among its list of drugs which have a heightened risk of causing significant patient harm when used in error.

U.S. Brand Names Optiray® 240; Optiray® 300; Optiray® 320; Optiray® 350

Therapeutic Category Iodinated Contrast Media; Radiological/Contrast Media, Nonionic

Use Arteriography, angiography, angiocardiography, ventriculography, excretory urography, and venography procedures; contrast enhanced tomographic imaging

General Dosage Range Dosage varies greatly depending on product.

Dosage Forms

Injection, solution [preservative free]:

Optiray® 240: 51% (50 mL, 100 mL, 125 mL, 150 mL, 200 mL)
Optiray® 300: 64% (50 mL, 100 mL, 150 mL, 200 mL, 500 mL)
Optiray® 320: 68% (20 mL, 30 mL, 50 mL, 75 mL, 100 mL, 125 mL, 150 mL, 200 mL)
Optiray® 350: 74% (50 mL, 75 mL, 100 mL, 125 mL, 150 mL, 200 mL, 250 mL, 500 mL)

ioxaglate meglumine and ioxaglate sodium

(eye ox AG late MEG loo meen & eye ox AG late SOW dee um)

Medication Safety Issues

High alert medication:

The Institute for Safe Medication Practices (ISMP) includes this medication among its list of drugs which have a heightened risk of causing significant patient harm when used in error.

Synonyms ioxaglate sodium and ioxaglate meglumine

U.S. Brand Names Hexabrix™

Therapeutic Category Iodinated Contrast Media; Radiological/Contrast Media, Ionic

Use Angiocardiography, arteriography, aortography, arthrography, angiography, hysterosalpingography, venography, and urography procedures; contrast enhancement of computed tomographic imaging

Dosage Forms

Injection, solution:

Hexabrix™: Ioxaglate meglumine 39.3% and ioxaglate sodium 19.6% (20 mL, 50 mL, 100 mL, 150 mL, 200 mL)

ioxaglate sodium and ioxaglate meglumine *see* ioxaglate meglumine and ioxaglate sodium *on page 498*

ioxilan (eye OKS ee lan)

Medication Safety Issues

High alert medication:

The Institute for Safe Medication Practices (ISMP) includes this medication among its list of drugs which have a heightened risk of causing significant patient harm when used in error.

U.S. Brand Names Oxilan® 300; Oxilan® 350

Canadian Brand Names Oxilan® 300; Oxilan® 350

Therapeutic Category Iodinated Contrast Media; Radiological/Contrast Media, Nonionic

Use

Intraarterial: Ioxilan 300 mgI/mL is indicated for cerebral arteriography. Ioxilan 350 mgI/mL is indicated for coronary arteriography and left ventriculography, visceral angiography, aortography, and peripheral arteriography

Intravenous: Both products are indicated for excretory urography and contrast-enhanced computed tomographic (CECT) imaging of the head and body

Dosage Forms

Injection, solution [preservative free]:

Oxilan® 300: 62% (50 mL, 100 mL, 150 mL, 200 mL, 500 mL)
Oxilan® 350: 73% (50 mL, 100 mL, 150 mL, 200 mL, 500 mL)

ipilimumab (ip i LIM u mab)

Medication Safety Issues

High alert medication:

This medication is in a class the Institute for Safe Medication Practices (ISMP) includes among its list of drug classes which have a heightened risk of causing significant patient harm when used in error.

Synonyms MDX-010; MDX-CTLA-4; MOAB-CTLA-4

U.S. Brand Names Yervoy™

Canadian Brand Names Yervoy™

Therapeutic Category Antineoplastic Agent, Monoclonal Antibody; Monoclonal Antibody

Use Treatment of unresectable or metastatic melanoma

General Dosage Range Dosage adjustment recommended in patients who develop toxicities.
I.V.: *Adults:* 3 mg/kg every 3 weeks

Dosage Forms
Injection, solution [preservative free]:
Yervoy™: 5 mg/mL (10 mL, 40 mL)

Iplex *see* mecasermin *on page* 565
IPOL® *see* poliovirus vaccine (inactivated) *on page* 736

ipratropium (oral inhalation) (i pra TROE pee um)

Medication Safety Issues
Sound-alike/look-alike issues:
Atrovent® may be confused with Alupent, Serevent®
Ipratropium may be confused with tiotropium

Synonyms ipratropium bromide
U.S. Brand Names Atrovent® HFA
Canadian Brand Names Atrovent® HFA; Gen-Ipratropium; Mylan-Ipratropium Sterinebs; Novo-Ipramide; Nu-Ipratropium; PMS-Ipratropium
Therapeutic Category Anticholinergic Agent
Use Anticholinergic bronchodilator used in bronchospasm associated with COPD, bronchitis, and emphysema

General Dosage Range
Inhalation: *Children >12 years and Adults:* 2 inhalations 4 times/day (maximum: 12 inhalations/day)
Nebulization: *Children >12 years and Adults:* 500 mcg every 6-8 hours

Dosage Forms
Aerosol, for oral inhalation:
Atrovent® HFA: 17 mcg/actuation (12.9 g)
Solution, for nebulization: 0.02% [500 mcg/2.5 mL] (25s, 30s, 60s)
Solution, for nebulization [preservative free]: 0.02% [500 mcg/2.5 mL] (25s, 30s, 60s)

ipratropium (nasal) (i pra TROE pee um)

Medication Safety Issues
Sound-alike/look-alike issues:
Atrovent® may be confused with Alupent, Serevent®
Ipratropium may be confused with tiotropium

Synonyms ipratropium bromide
U.S. Brand Names Atrovent®
Canadian Brand Names Alti-Ipratropium; Apo-Ipravent®; Atrovent®; Mylan-Ipratropium Solution
Therapeutic Category Anticholinergic Agent
Use Symptomatic relief of rhinorrhea associated with the common cold and allergic and nonallergic rhinitis

General Dosage Range **Intranasal:**
0.03% solution: *Children ≥6 years and Adults:* 2 sprays in each nostril 2-3 times/day
0.06% solution: *Children ≥5 years and Adults:* 2 sprays in each nostril 3-4 times/day

Dosage Forms
Solution, intranasal: 0.03% (30 mL); 0.06% (15 mL)
Atrovent®: 0.03% (30 mL); 0.06% (15 mL)

ipratropium and albuterol (i pra TROE pee um & al BYOO ter ole)

Medication Safety Issues
Sound-alike/look-alike issues:
Combivent® may be confused with Combivir®, Serevent®
DuoNeb® may be confused with DuoTrav™, Duovent® UDV

Synonyms albuterol and ipratropium; salbutamol and ipratropium
U.S. Brand Names Combivent®; Combivent® Respimat®; DuoNeb®
Canadian Brand Names CO Ipra-Sal; Combivent UDV; Gen-Combo Sterinebs; ratio-Ipra Sal UDV
Therapeutic Category Bronchodilator
Use Treatment of COPD in those patients who are currently on a regular bronchodilator who continue to have bronchospasms and require a second bronchodilator

General Dosage Range

Inhalation: *Adults:* 1 inhalation (Combivent® Respimat®) or 2 inhalations (Combivent®) 4 times daily (maximum: Combivent® Respimat®: 6 inhalations/24 hours; Combivent®: 12 inhalations/24 hours)

Nebulization: *Adults:* 3 mL every 6 hours (maximum: 3 mL every 4 hours)

Dosage Forms

Aerosol, for oral inhalation:

Combivent®: Ipratropium bromide 18 mcg and albuterol (base) 90 mcg per inhalation (14.7 g) [200 metered actuations]

Solution, for nebulization: Ipratropium 0.5 mg and albuterol (base) 2.5 mg per 3 mL (30s, 60s)

DuoNeb®: Ipratropium 0.5 mg and albuterol (base) 2.5 mg per 3 mL (30s, 60s)

Solution, for oral inhalation [spray]:

Combivent® Respimat®: Ipratropium bromide 20 mcg and albuterol (base) 100 mcg per inhalation (4 g) [120 metered actuations]

ipratropium and fenoterol *(Canada only)* (i pra TROE pee um & fen oh TER ole)

Medication Safety Issues

Sound-alike/look-alike issues:

Duovent® UDV may be confused with Combivent® UDV, DuoNeb®

Synonyms fenoterol and ipratropium; fenoterol hydrobromide and ipratropium bromide; ipratropium bromide and fenoterol hydrobromide

Canadian Brand Names Duovent® UDV

Therapeutic Category Anticholinergic Agent; Beta$_2$-Adrenergic Agonist

Use Treatment of bronchospasm associated with acute severe exacerbation of COPD or bronchial asthma

General Dosage Range Nebulization: *Children ≥12 years and Adults:* Usual dose: 4 mL; may repeat every 6 hours as needed

Product Availability Not available in U.S.

Dosage Forms - Canada

Solution for nebulization:

Duovent® UDV: Ipratropium bromide 0.5 mg and fenoterol 1.25 mg per 4 mL (20s)

ipratropium bromide *see* ipratropium (nasal) *on page 499*

ipratropium bromide *see* ipratropium (oral inhalation) *on page 499*

ipratropium bromide and fenoterol hydrobromide *see* ipratropium and fenoterol *(Canada only) on page 500*

I-Prin [OTC] *see* ibuprofen *on page 468*

Iprivask® *see* desirudin *on page 263*

iproveratril hydrochloride *see* verapamil *on page 942*

IPV *see* poliovirus vaccine (inactivated) *on page 736*

Iquix® *see* levofloxacin (ophthalmic) *on page 532*

irbesartan (ir be SAR tan)

Medication Safety Issues

Sound-alike/look-alike issues:

Avapro® may be confused with Anaprox®

U.S. Brand Names Avapro®

Canadian Brand Names Avapro®; CO Irbesartan; PMS-Irbesartan; ratio-Irbesartan; Sandoz-Irbesartan; Teva-Irbesartan

Therapeutic Category Angiotensin II Receptor Antagonist

Use Treatment of hypertension alone or in combination with other antihypertensives; treatment of diabetic nephropathy in patients with type 2 diabetes mellitus (noninsulin-dependent, NIDDM) and hypertension

General Dosage Range Oral:

Children 6-12 years: Initial: 75 mg once daily; Maintenance: 75-150 mg once daily

Children ≥13 years and Adults: Initial: 75-150 mg once daily; Maintenance: 75-300 mg once daily

Dosage Forms

Tablet, oral: 75 mg, 150 mg, 300 mg

Avapro®: 75 mg, 150 mg, 300 mg

irbesartan and hydrochlorothiazide (ir be SAR tan & hye droe klor oh THYE a zide)

Medication Safety Issues

Sound-alike/look-alike issues:

Avalide® may be confused with Avandia®

Synonyms Avapro® HCT; hydrochlorothiazide and irbesartan

U.S. Brand Names Avalide®

Canadian Brand Names Avalide®; CO Irbesartan HCT; Irbesartan-HCTZ; PMS-Irbesartan HCTZ; Ran™-Irbesartan HCTZ; ratio-Irbesartan HCTZ; Sandoz-Irbesartan HCT; Teva-Irbesartan HCTZ

Therapeutic Category Antihypertensive Agent, Combination

Use Combination therapy for the management of hypertension; may be used as initial therapy in patients likely to need multiple drugs to achieve blood pressure goals

General Dosage Range Oral: *Adults:* Irbesartan 150-300 mg and hydrochlorothiazide 12.5-25 mg once daily

Dosage Forms

Tablet: 150/12.5: Irbesartan 150 mg and hydrochlorothiazide 12.5 mg; 300/12.5: Irbesartan 300 mg and hydrochlorothiazide 12.5 mg

Avalide®: Irbesartan 150 mg and hydrochlorothiazide 12.5 mg; irbesartan 300 mg and hydrochlorothiazide 12.5 mg

Irbesartan-HCTZ (Can) *see* irbesartan and hydrochlorothiazide *on page* 501

Ircon® [OTC] *see* ferrous fumarate *on page* 379

Iressa® *see* gefitinib *on page* 420

IRESSA® (Can) *see* gefitinib *on page* 420

irinotecan (eye rye no TEE kan)

Medication Safety Issues

Sound-alike/look-alike issues:

Irinotecan may be confused with topotecan

High alert medication:

This medication is in a class the Institute for Safe Medication Practices (ISMP) includes among its list of drug classes which have a heightened risk of causing significant patient harm when used in error.

Synonyms camptothecin-11; CPT-11; irinotecan HCl; irinotecan hydrochloride

U.S. Brand Names Camptosar®

Canadian Brand Names Camptosar®; Irinotecan Hydrochloride Trihydrate

Therapeutic Category Antineoplastic Agent

Use Treatment of metastatic carcinoma of the colon or rectum

General Dosage Range Dosage adjustment recommended in patients with hepatic impairment or who develop toxicities

I.V.: *Adults:* Dosage varies greatly depending on indication

Dosage Forms

Injection, solution: 20 mg/mL (2 mL, 5 mL, 25 mL)

Injection, solution [preservative free]: 20 mg/mL (2 mL, 5 mL)

Camptosar®: 20 mg/mL (2 mL, 5 mL, 15 mL)

irinotecan HCl *see* irinotecan *on page* 501

irinotecan hydrochloride *see* irinotecan *on page* 501

Irinotecan Hydrochloride Trihydrate (Can) *see* irinotecan *on page* 501

iron dextran *see* iron dextran complex *on page* 501

iron dextran complex (EYE ern DEKS tran KOM pleks)

Medication Safety Issues

Sound-alike/look-alike issues:

Dexferrum® may be confused with Desferal®

Iron dextran complex may be confused with ferumoxytol

Synonyms high-molecular-weight iron dextran (DexFerrum®); imferon; iron dextran; low-Molecular-weight iron dextran (INFeD®)

U.S. Brand Names Dexferrum®; INFeD®

Canadian Brand Names Dexiron™; Infufer®

Therapeutic Category Electrolyte Supplement, Oral

Use Treatment of iron deficiency in patients in whom oral administration is infeasible or ineffective

General Dosage Range Note: A 0.5 mL test dose (0.25 mL in infants) should be given prior to starting iron dextran therapy.

I.M., I.V.:

Children <5 kg and >4 months: Replacement iron (mg) = blood loss (mL) x Hct; **Note:** Total dose should be divided daily at not more than 25 mg/day

Children 5-15 kg and >4 months: Total Dose (mL) = 0.0442 (desired Hgb [usually 12 g/dL] - observed Hgb) x W (in kg) + (0.26 x W [in kg]) **or** replacement iron (mg) = blood loss (mL) x hematocrit; **Note:** Total dose should be divided daily at not more than 50 mg/day (5-10 kg) or 100 mg/day (10-15 kg)

Children >15 kg: Total Dose (mL) = 0.0442 (desired Hgb [usually 14.8 g/dL] - observed Hgb) x LBW + (0.26 x LBW) **or** replacement iron (mg) = blood loss (mL) x Hct; **Note:** Total dose should be divided daily at not more than 100 mg/day

Adults: Total Dose (mL) = 0.0442 (desired Hgb [usually 14.8 g/dL] - observed Hgb) x LBW + (0.26 x LBW) **or** replacement iron (mg) = blood loss (mL) x Hct; **Note:** Total dose should be divided daily at not more than 100 mg/day

Dosage Forms

Injection, solution:

Dexferrum®: Elemental iron 50 mg/mL (1 mL, 2 mL)

INFeD®: Elemental iron 50 mg/mL (2 mL)

iron fumarate *see* ferrous fumarate *on page 379*

iron gluconate *see* ferrous gluconate *on page 380*

iron-polysaccharide complex *see* polysaccharide-iron complex *on page 740*

iron-polysaccharide complex and folic acid *see* polysaccharide-iron complex and folic acid *on page 740*

iron-polysaccharide complex, vitamin B12, and folic acid *see* polysaccharide-iron complex, vitamin B12, and folic acid *on page 741*

iron sucrose (EYE ern SOO krose)

Medication Safety Issues

Sound-alike/look-alike issues:

Iron sucrose may be confused with ferumoxytol

U.S. Brand Names Venofer®

Canadian Brand Names Venofer®

Therapeutic Category Iron Salt

Use Treatment of iron-deficiency anemia in chronic renal failure, including nondialysis-dependent patients (with or without erythropoietin therapy) and dialysis-dependent patients receiving erythropoietin therapy

General Dosage Range I.V.: *Adults:* 100 mg (5 mL) 1-3 times/week during dialysis **or** 200 mg on 5 different occasions within a 14-day period **or** two 300 mg infusion 14 days apart, followed by a single 400 mg infusion 14 days later (maximum: 1000 mg cumulative total)

Dosage Forms

Injection, solution [preservative free]:

Venofer®: Elemental iron 20 mg/mL (2.5 mL, 5 mL, 10 mL)

iron sulfate *see* ferrous sulfate *on page 380*

Isagel® [OTC] *see* alcohol (ethyl) *on page 43*

ISD *see* isosorbide dinitrate *on page 504*

ISDN *see* isosorbide dinitrate *on page 504*

Isentress® *see* raltegravir *on page 785*

ISG *see* immune globulin *on page 477*

ISMN *see* isosorbide mononitrate *on page 505*

isoamyl nitrite *see* amyl nitrite *on page 74*

isobamate *see* carisoprodol *on page 177*

isocarboxazid (eye soe kar BOKS a zid)

U.S. Brand Names Marplan®

Therapeutic Category Antidepressant, Monoamine Oxidase Inhibitor

Use Treatment of depression

General Dosage Range Oral: *Adults:* Initial: 10 mg 2-4 times/day; may increase to a maximum of 60 mg/day divided in 2-4 doses

Dosage Forms

Tablet, oral:

Marplan®: 10 mg

isoflurane (eye soe FLURE ane)

Medication Safety Issues

Sound-alike/look-alike issues:

Isoflurane may be confused with enflurane

High alert medication:

The Institute for Safe Medication Practices (ISMP) includes this medication among its list of drug classes which have a heightened risk of causing significant patient harm when used in error.

U.S. Brand Names Forane®; Terrell™

Canadian Brand Names Forane®

Therapeutic Category General Anesthetic

Use Maintenance of general anesthesia

Note: Use of isoflurane for induction of general anesthesia is an FDA-labeled indication; however, it is not recommended clinically due to its irritant properties and unpleasant odor, which causes breath-holding or coughing.

General Dosage Range Inhalation: *Adults:* Maintenance: With nitrous oxide: 1% to 2.5%; without nitrous oxide: 1.5% to 3.5%

Dosage Forms

Liquid, for inhalation: USP: ≥99.9 mL/100 mL (100 mL, 250 mL)

Forane®: USP: ≥99.9 mL/100 mL (100 mL, 250 mL)

Terrell™: USP: ≥99.9 mL/100 mL (100 mL, 250 mL)

isometheptene, acetaminophen, and dichloralphenazone *see* acetaminophen, isometheptene, and dichloralphenazone *on page 30*

isometheptene, dichloralphenazone, and acetaminophen *see* acetaminophen, isometheptene, and dichloralphenazone *on page 30*

IsonaRif™ *see* rifampin and isoniazid *on page 800*

isoniazid (eye soe NYE a zid)

Medication Safety Issues

International issues:

Hydra [Japan] may be confused with Hydrea brand name for hydroxyurea [U.S., Canada, and multiple international markets]

Synonyms INH; isonicotinic acid hydrazide

Canadian Brand Names Isotamine®; PMS-Isoniazid

Therapeutic Category Antitubercular Agent

Use Treatment of susceptible tuberculosis infections; treatment of latent tuberculosis infection (LTBI)

General Dosage Range Oral, I.M.:

Children: 10-20 mg/kg/day once daily (maximum: 300 mg/day) **or** 20-40 mg/kg 2-3 times/week (maximum: 900 mg/dose)

Adults: 300 mg (5 mg/kg) once daily **or** 900 mg (15 mg/kg) 2-3 times/week

Dosage Forms

Injection, solution: 100 mg/mL (10 mL)

Solution, oral: 50 mg/5 mL (473 mL)

Tablet, oral: 100 mg, 300 mg

isoniazid and rifampin *see* rifampin and isoniazid *on page 800*

isoniazid, pyrazinamide, and rifampin *see* rifampin, isoniazid, and pyrazinamide *on page 800*

isonicotinic acid hydrazide *see* isoniazid *on page 503*

isonipecaine hydrochloride *see* meperidine *on page 574*

isophane insulin *see* insulin NPH *on page 488*

isophane insulin and regular insulin *see* insulin NPH and insulin regular *on page 489*

isophosphamide *see* ifosfamide *on page 473*

isoproterenol (eye soe proe TER e nole)

Medication Safety Issues

Sound-alike/look-alike issues:

Isuprel® may be confused with Disophrol®, Isordil®

Synonyms isoproterenol hydrochloride

U.S. Brand Names Isuprel®

Therapeutic Category Adrenergic Agonist Agent

Use Manufacturer's labeled indications (see **"Note"**): Mild or transient episodes of heart block that do not require electric shock or pacemaker therapy; serious episodes of heart block and Adams-Stokes attacks (except when caused by ventricular tachycardia or fibrillation); cardiac arrest until electric shock or pacemaker therapy is available; bronchospasm during anesthesia; adjunct to fluid and electrolyte replacement therapy and other drugs and procedures in the treatment of hypovolemic or septic shock and low cardiac output states (eg, decompensated heart failure, cardiogenic shock)

Note: The use of isoproterenol in advanced cardiac life support (ACLS) has largely been supplanted by the use of other adrenergic agents (eg, epinephrine and dopamine). The use of isoproterenol for bronchospasm during anesthesia and cardiogenic, hypovolemic, or septic shock is no longer recommended.

General Dosage Range Continuous I.V. infusion:

Children: 0.05-2 mcg/**kg**/minute; titrate to patient response

Adults: 2-10 mcg/minute; titrate to patient response

Dosage Forms

Injection, solution:

Isuprel®: 0.2 mg/mL (1 mL, 5 mL)

isoproterenol hydrochloride *see* isoproterenol *on page 504*
Isoptin® SR *see* verapamil *on page 942*
Isopto® Atropine *see* atropine *on page 102*
Isopto® Carbachol *see* carbachol *on page 172*
Isopto® Carpine *see* pilocarpine (ophthalmic) *on page 723*
Isopto® Homatropine *see* homatropine *on page 448*
Isopto® Hyoscine *see* scopolamine (ophthalmic) *on page 826*
Isopto® Tears [OTC] *see* hydroxypropyl methylcellulose *on page 463*
Isopto® Tears (Can) *see* hydroxypropyl methylcellulose *on page 463*
Isordil® Titradose™ *see* isosorbide dinitrate *on page 504*
Isosorbide (Can) *see* isosorbide dinitrate *on page 504*

isosorbide dinitrate (eye soe SOR bide dye NYE trate)

Medication Safety Issues

Sound-alike/look-alike issues:

Isordil® may be confused with Inderal®, Isuprel®, Plendil®

Synonyms ISD; ISDN

U.S. Brand Names Dilatrate®-SR; Isordil® Titradose™

Canadian Brand Names ISDN; Isosorbide; Novo-Sorbide; PMS-Isosorbide

Therapeutic Category Vasodilator

Use Prevention and treatment of angina pectoris

Note: Due to slower onset of action, not the drug of choice to abort an acute anginal episode.

General Dosage Range

Oral:

Immediate release: *Adults:* 5-40 mg 2-3 times/day

Sustained release: *Adults:* 40-160 mg/day in divided doses

Sublingual: *Adults:* 2.5-5 mg every 5-10 minutes for maximum of 3 doses in 15-30 minutes **or** 2.5-5 mg 15 minutes prior to activities which may provoke an anginal episode

Dosage Forms

Capsule, sustained release, oral:

Dilatrate®-SR: 40 mg

Tablet, oral: 5 mg, 10 mg, 20 mg, 30 mg
Isordil® Titradose™: 5 mg, 40 mg
Tablet, sublingual: 2.5 mg, 5 mg
Tablet, extended release, oral: 40 mg

isosorbide dinitrate and hydralazine

(eye soe SOR bide dye NYE trate & hye DRAL a zeen)

Synonyms hydralazine and isosorbide dinitrate
U.S. Brand Names BiDil®
Therapeutic Category Vasodilator
Use Treatment of heart failure, adjunct to standard therapy, in self-identified African-Americans
General Dosage Range Dosage adjustment recommended in patients who develop toxicities.
Oral: *Adults:* 1-2 tablets 3 times/day
Dosage Forms
Tablet:
BiDil®: Isosorbide dinitrate 20 mg and hydralazine 37.5 mg

isosorbide mononitrate (eye soe SOR bide mon oh NYE trate)

Medication Safety Issues
Sound-alike/look-alike issues:
Imdur® may be confused with Imuran®, Inderal® LA, K-Dur®
Monoket® may be confused with Monopril®
Synonyms ISMN
U.S. Brand Names Imdur®; Monoket® [DSC]
Canadian Brand Names Apo-ISMN®; Imdur®; PMS-ISMN; PRO-ISMN
Therapeutic Category Vasodilator
Use Prevention of angina pectoris
General Dosage Range Oral:
Extended release: *Adults:* Initial: 30-60 mg once daily; Maintenance: 30-240 mg once daily (maximum: 240 mg/day)
Regular release: *Adults:* 5-20 mg twice daily
Dosage Forms
Tablet, oral: 10 mg, 20 mg
Tablet, extended release, oral: 30 mg, 60 mg, 120 mg
Imdur®: 30 mg, 60 mg, 120 mg

isosulfan blue (eye soe SUL fan bloo)

U.S. Brand Names Lymphazurin™
Therapeutic Category Contrast Agent
Use Adjunct to lymphography for visualization of the lymphatic system; sentinel node identification
General Dosage Range SubQ: *Adults:* Inject 0.5 mL into 3 interdigital spaces of each extremity per study (maximum: 3 mL [30 mg])
Dosage Forms
Injection, solution [preservative free]: 1% (5 mL)
Lymphazurin™: 1% (5 mL)

Isotamine® (Can) *see* isoniazid *on page* 503

isotretinoin (eye soe TRET i noyn)

Medication Safety Issues
Sound-alike/look-alike issues:
Accutane® may be confused with Accolate®, Accupril®
Claravis™ may be confused with Cleviprex®
ISOtretinoin may be confused with tretinoin
Synonyms 13-*cis*-retinoic acid; 13-*cis*-vitamin A acid; 13-CRA; *Cis*-retinoic acid; absorica; Accutane; isotretinoinum
Tall-Man **ISO**tretinoin
U.S. Brand Names Amnesteem®; Claravis™; Myorisan™; Sotret®
Canadian Brand Names Accutane®; Clarus™

Therapeutic Category Retinoic Acid Derivative

Use Treatment of severe recalcitrant nodular acne unresponsive to conventional therapy

General Dosage Range Dosage adjustments recommended in patients with hepatic impairment

Oral:

Children 12-17 years: 0.5-1 mg/kg/day in 2 divided doses

Adults: 0.5-2 mg/kg/day in 2 divided doses

Product Availability

Absorica™: FDA approved May 2012; availability expected in the fourth quarter of 2012. Consult prescribing information for additional information.

Dosage Forms

Capsule, oral:

Claravis™: 10 mg, 20 mg, 30 mg, 40 mg

Myorisan™: 10 mg, 20 mg, 40 mg

Capsule, softgel, oral:

Amnesteem®: 10 mg, 20 mg, 40 mg

Sotret®: 10 mg, 20 mg, 30 mg, 40 mg

isotretinoinum *see* isotretinoin *on page* 505

Isovue® 200 *see* iopamidol *on page* 496

Isovue® 250 *see* iopamidol *on page* 496

Isovue® 300 *see* iopamidol *on page* 496

Isovue® 370 *see* iopamidol *on page* 496

Isovue-M® *see* iopamidol *on page* 496

Isovue Multipack® *see* iopamidol *on page* 496

isoxsuprine (eye SOKS syoo preen)

Medication Safety Issues

Sound-alike/look-alike issues:

Vasodilan may be confused with Vasocidin®

BEERS Criteria medication:

This drug may be potentially inappropriate for use in geriatric patients (Quality of evidence - high; Strength of recommendation - strong).

Synonyms isoxsuprine hydrochloride; Vasodilan

Therapeutic Category Vasodilator

Use Treatment of peripheral vascular diseases, such as arteriosclerosis obliterans, thromboangiitis obliterans (Buerger disease), and Raynaud disease; relief of symptoms associated with cerebrovascular insufficiency

Note: More appropriate therapies (medical or surgical) should be considered; efficacy of isoxsuprine in the treatment of these conditions has not been well established.

General Dosage Range Oral:

Adults: 10-20 mg 3-4 times/day

Elderly: Start with lower dose due to potential hypotension.

Dosage Forms

Tablet, oral: 10 mg, 20 mg

isoxsuprine hydrochloride *see* isoxsuprine *on page* 506

isradipine (iz RA di peen)

Medication Safety Issues

Sound-alike/look-alike issues:

DynaCirc® may be confused with Dynacin®

U.S. Brand Names DynaCirc CR® [DSC]

Therapeutic Category Calcium Channel Blocker

Use Treatment of hypertension

General Dosage Range Dosage adjustment recommended in patients with hepatic or renal impairment

Oral: *Adults:*

Capsule: Initial: 2.5 mg twice daily; Usual range: 2.5-10 mg/day

Controlled release tablet: Initial: 5 mg once daily; Maintenance: 5-20 mg once daily (maximum: 20 mg/day)

Dosage Forms

Capsule, oral: 2.5 mg, 5 mg

Istalol® *see* timolol (ophthalmic) *on page 897*

Istodax® *see* romidepsin *on page 809*

Isuprel® *see* isoproterenol *on page 504*

Itch-X® [OTC] *see* pramoxine *on page 750*

itraconazole (i tra KOE na zole)

Medication Safety Issues

Sound-alike/look-alike issues:

Itraconazole may be confused with fluconazole

Sporanox® may be confused with Suprax®, Topamax®

U.S. Brand Names Sporanox®

Canadian Brand Names Sporanox®

Therapeutic Category Antifungal Agent

Use

Oral capsules: Treatment of susceptible fungal infections in immunocompromised and immunocompetent patients including blastomycosis and histoplasmosis; indicated for aspergillosis (in patients intolerant/refractory to amphotericin B), and onychomycosis of the toenail and fingernail (in nonimmunocompromised patients)

Oral solution: Treatment of oral and esophageal candidiasis

General Dosage Range Dosage adjustment recommended in patients with renal impairment

Oral: *Adults:* 100-600 mg/day; doses >200 mg/day are given in 2-3 divided doses

Dosage Forms

Capsule, oral: 100 mg

Sporanox®: 100 mg

Solution, oral:

Sporanox®: 10 mg/mL (150 mL)

ivacaftor (eye va KAF tor)

Synonyms VX-770

U.S. Brand Names Kalydeco™

Therapeutic Category Cystic Fibrosis Transmembrane Conductance Regulator Potentiator

Use Treatment of cystic fibrosis (CF) in patients who have a G551D mutation in the cystic fibrosis transmembrane conductance regulator (CFTR) gene

Note: Not effective in patients with CF who are homozygous for the F508del mutation in the CTFR gene

General Dosage Range Dosage adjustment recommended in patients with hepatic impairment or on concomitant therapy.

Oral: *Children ≥6 years and Adults:* 150 mg every 12 hours

Dosage Forms

Tablet, oral:

Kalydeco™: 150 mg

ivermectin (systemic) (eye ver MEK tin)

U.S. Brand Names Stromectol®

Therapeutic Category Anthelmintic

Use Treatment of the following infections: Strongyloidiasis of the intestinal tract due to the nematode parasite *Strongyloides stercoralis*. Onchocerciasis due to the immature form of the nematode parasite *Onchocerca volvulus*

General Dosage Range Oral: *Children ≥15 kg and Adults:* 150-200 mcg/kg as a single dose

Dosage Forms

Tablet, oral:

Stromectol®: 3 mg

ivermectin (topical) (eye ver MEK tin)

U.S. Brand Names Sklice™

Therapeutic Category Antiparasitic Agent, Topical; Pediculocide

Use Topical treatment of head lice (*Pediculus capitis*) infestation

General Dosage Range Topical: *Children ≥6 months and Adults:* Apply sufficient amount (up to 1 tube) to completely cover dry scalp and hair; for single-dose use only

Dosage Forms

Lotion, topical:

Sklice™: 0.5% (117 g)

IVIG *see* immune globulin *on page* 477

IV immune globulin *see* immune globulin *on page* 477

Ivy Block® [OTC] *see* bentoquatam *on page* 120

Ivy-Rid® [OTC] *see* benzocaine *on page* 121

ixabepilone (ix ab EP i lone)

Medication Safety Issues

High alert medication:

This medication is in a class the Institute for Safe Medication Practices (ISMP) includes among its list of drug classes which have a heightened risk of causing significant patient harm when used in error.

Synonyms azaepothilone B; BMS-247550; epothilone B lactam

U.S. Brand Names Ixempra®

Therapeutic Category Antineoplastic Agent, Antimicrotubular; Antineoplastic Agent, Epothilone B Analog

Use Treatment of metastatic or locally-advanced breast cancer (refractory or resistant)

General Dosage Range Dosage adjustment recommended in patients with hepatic impairment or who develop toxicities

I.V.: *Adults:* 40 mg/m^2 every 3 weeks (maximum dose: 88 mg)

Dosage Forms

Injection, powder for reconstitution:

Ixempra®: 15 mg, 45 mg

Ixempra® *see* ixabepilone *on page* 508

Ixiaro® *see* Japanese encephalitis virus vaccine (inactivated) *on page* 509

JAA-Aminophylline (Can) *see* aminophylline *on page* 62

Jakafi™ *see* ruxolitinib *on page* 815

Jakavi™ (Can) *see* ruxolitinib *on page* 815

Jalyn™ *see* dutasteride and tamsulosin *on page* 320

JAMP-Alendronate (Can) *see* alendronate *on page* 45

JAMP-Amlodipine (Can) *see* amlodipine *on page* 65

JAMP-Atenolol (Can) *see* atenolol *on page* 99

JAMP-Bicalutamide (Can) *see* bicalutamide *on page* 133

JAMP-Candesartan (Can) *see* candesartan *on page* 168

JAMP-Carvedilol (Can) *see* carvedilol *on page* 179

JAMP-Ciprofloxacin (Can) *see* ciprofloxacin (systemic) *on page* 210

JAMP-Citalopram (Can) *see* citalopram *on page* 213

Jamp-Colchicine (Can) *see* colchicine *on page* 231

JAMP-Cyclobenzaprine (Can) *see* cyclobenzaprine *on page* 243

Jamp-Dicyclomine (Can) *see* dicyclomine *on page* 282

Jamp-Dimenhydrinate [OTC] (Can) *see* dimenhydrinate *on page* 289

JAMP-Finasteride (Can) *see* finasteride *on page* 384

JAMP-Fluoxetine (Can) *see* fluoxetine *on page* 396

Jamp-Fosinopril (Can) *see* fosinopril *on page* 409

JAMP-Indapamide (Can) *see* indapamide *on page* 479

JAMP-Letrozole (Can) *see* letrozole *on page* 526

JAMP-Lisinopril (Can) *see* lisinopril *on page* 544

JAMP-Metformin (Can) *see* metformin *on page* 579

JAMP-Metformin Blackberry (Can) *see* metformin *on page* 579

JAMP-Metoprolol-L (Can) *see* metoprolol *on page* 595

Jamp-Mirtazapine (Can) *see* mirtazapine *on page* 606

JAMP-Mycophenolate (Can) *see* mycophenolate *on page 619*
JAMP-Ondansetron (Can) *see* ondansetron *on page 667*
JAMP-Pioglitazone (Can) *see* pioglitazone *on page 725*
JAMP-Pravastatin (Can) *see* pravastatin *on page 752*
JAMP-Quetiapine (Can) *see* quetiapine *on page 781*
JAMP-Ramipril (Can) *see* ramipril *on page 786*
JAMP-Risperidone (Can) *see* risperidone *on page 803*
JAMP-Rizatriptan (Can) *see* rizatriptan *on page 807*
JAMP-Ropinirole (Can) *see* ropinirole *on page 810*
JAMP-Simvastatin (Can) *see* simvastatin *on page 835*
JAMP-Tamsulosin (Can) *see* tamsulosin *on page 868*
JAMP-Terbinafine (Can) *see* terbinafine (systemic) *on page 878*
Jantoven® *see* warfarin *on page 954*
Janumet® *see* sitagliptin and metformin *on page 837*
Janumet® XR *see* sitagliptin and metformin *on page 837*
Januvia® *see* sitagliptin *on page 837*

Japanese encephalitis virus vaccine (inactivated)

(jap a NEESE en sef a LYE tis VYE rus vak SEEN, in ak ti VAY ted)

Synonyms IC51; JE-VC (Ixiaro®)

U.S. Brand Names Ixiaro®

Canadian Brand Names Ixiaro®

Therapeutic Category Vaccine, Inactivated Virus

Use Active immunization against Japanese encephalitis

Japanese encephalitis vaccine is not recommended for all persons traveling to or residing in Asia. The Advisory Committee on Immunization Practices (ACIP) recommends vaccination for:

- Persons spending ≥1 month in endemic areas during transmission season
- Research laboratory workers who may be exposed to the Japanese encephalitis virus

Vaccination may also be considered for the following:

- Travelers to areas with an ongoing outbreak
- Travelers spending <30 days in endemic areas during the transmission season and planning to go outside of urban areas and have an increased risk of exposure. For example, high-risk activities include extensive outdoor activity in rural areas especially at night; extensive outdoor activities such as camping, hiking, etc; staying in accommodations without air conditioning, screens or bed nets.
- Travelers to endemic areas who are unsure of specific destination, activities, or duration of travel

General Dosage Range

I.M.: *Adults ≥17 years:* 0.5 mL/dose on days 0 and 28

Dosage Forms

Injection, suspension:

Ixiaro®: Inactivated JEV proteins 6 mcg/0.5 mL (0.5 mL)

Jentadueto™ *see* linagliptin and metformin *on page 540*
Jevantique™ [DSC] *see* ethinyl estradiol and norethindrone *on page 359*
JE-VC (Ixiaro®) *see* Japanese encephalitis virus vaccine (inactivated) *on page 509*
Jevtana® *see* cabazitaxel *on page 157*
Jinteli™ *see* ethinyl estradiol and norethindrone *on page 359*
J-Max [OTC] *see* guaifenesin and phenylephrine *on page 435*
Jolessa™ *see* ethinyl estradiol and levonorgestrel *on page 357*
Jolivette® *see* norethindrone *on page 648*
J-Tan D PD [OTC] *see* brompheniramine and pseudoephedrine *on page 144*
J-Tan PD [OTC] *see* brompheniramine *on page 143*
Junel® 1.5/30 *see* ethinyl estradiol and norethindrone *on page 359*
Junel® 1/20 *see* ethinyl estradiol and norethindrone *on page 359*
Junel® Fe 1.5/30 *see* ethinyl estradiol and norethindrone *on page 359*
Junel® Fe 1/20 *see* ethinyl estradiol and norethindrone *on page 359*
Jurnista™ (Can) *see* hydromorphone *on page 460*
Just For Kids™ [OTC] *see* fluoride *on page 393*

kanamycin (kan a MYE sin)

Medication Safety Issues

Sound-alike/look-alike issues:

Kanamycin may be confused with Garamycin®, gentamicin

Synonyms kanamycin sulfate

Therapeutic Category Aminoglycoside (Antibiotic)

Use Treatment of serious infections caused by susceptible strains of *E. coli*, *Proteus* species, *Enterobacter aerogenes*, *Klebsiella pneumoniae*, *Serratia marcescens*, and *Acinetobacter* species; second-line treatment of *Mycobacterium tuberculosis*

General Dosage Range Dosage adjustment of I.M. and I.V. route recommended in patients with renal impairment

I.M., I.V.:

Children: 15 mg/kg/day divided every 8-12 hours
Adults: 5-7.5 mg/kg every 8-12 hours
Elderly: 5-7.5 mg/kg every 12-24 hours

Inhalation, aerosol: *Adults:* 250 mg 2-4 times/day
Intraperitoneal: *Adults:* 500 mg
Irrigation: *Adults:* 0.25% (maximum: 1.5 g/day)

Dosage Forms

Injection, solution: 1 g/3 mL (3 mL)

ketamine (KEET a meen)

Medication Safety Issues

Sound-alike/look-alike issues:

Ketalar® may be confused with Kenalog®, ketorolac

High alert medication:

The Institute for Safe Medication Practices (ISMP) includes this medication among its list of drugs which have a heightened risk of causing significant patient harm when used in error.

Synonyms ketamine hydrochloride

U.S. Brand Names Ketalar®

Canadian Brand Names Ketalar®; Ketamine Hydrochloride Injection, USP

Therapeutic Category General Anesthetic

Controlled Substance C-III

Use Induction and maintenance of general anesthesia

General Dosage Range

I.M.: *Children ≥16 years and Adults:* 2-6 mg/kg

I.V.: *Children ≥16 years and Adults:* 0.2-2 mg/kg **or** 0.1-0.5 mg/minute as a continuous infusion

Dosage Forms

Injection, solution: 10 mg/mL (20 mL); 50 mg/mL (10 mL); 100 mg/mL (5 mL, 10 mL)

Ketalar®: 10 mg/mL (20 mL); 50 mg/mL (10 mL); 100 mg/mL (5 mL)

ketoconazole (systemic) (kee toe KOE na zole)

Medication Safety Issues

Sound-alike/look-alike issues:

Nizoral® may be confused with Nasarel, Neoral®, Nitrol®

Canadian Brand Names Apo-Ketoconazole®; Novo-Ketoconazole

Therapeutic Category Antifungal Agent, Oral

Use Treatment of susceptible fungal infections, including candidiasis, oral thrush, blastomycosis, histoplasmosis, paracoccidioidomycosis, coccidioidomycosis, chromomycosis, candiduria, chronic mucocutaneous candidiasis, as well as certain recalcitrant cutaneous dermatophytoses

General Dosage Range Oral:

Children ≥2 years: 3.3-6.6 mg/kg once daily

Adults: 200-400 mg once daily

Dosage Forms

Tablet, oral: 200 mg

ketoconazole (topical) (kee toe KOE na zole)

Medication Safety Issues

Sound-alike/look-alike issues:

Nizoral® may be confused with Nasarel, Neoral®, Nitrol®

U.S. Brand Names Extina®; Nizoral®; Nizoral® A-D [OTC]; Xolegel®

Canadian Brand Names Ketoderm®; Xolegel®

Therapeutic Category Antifungal Agent, Topical

Use

Cream: Treatment of tinea corporis, tinea cruris, tinea versicolor, cutaneous candidiasis, seborrheic dermatitis

Foam, gel: Treatment of seborrheic dermatitis

Shampoo: Treatment of dandruff, seborrheic dermatitis, tinea versicolor

General Dosage Range Topical:

Cream: *Children ≥12 years and Adults:* Rub gently into the affected area 1-2 times daily

Foam: *Children ≥12 years and Adults:* Apply to affected area twice daily

Gel: *Children ≥12 years and Adults:* Apply gently to affected area once daily

Shampoo: *Children ≥12 years and Adults:* Apply up to twice weekly

Dosage Forms

Aerosol, foam, topical: 2% (50 g, 100 g)

Extina®: 2% (50 g, 100 g)

Cream, topical: 2% (15 g, 30 g, 60 g)

Gel, topical:

Xolegel®: 2% (45 g)

Shampoo, topical: 2% (120 mL)

Nizoral®: 2% (120 mL)

Nizoral® A-D [OTC]: 1% (120 mL, 210 mL)

Ketoderm® (Can) *see* ketoconazole (topical) *on page 512*

3-keto-desogestrel *see* etonogestrel *on page 366*

ketoprofen (kee toe PROE fen)

Medication Safety Issues

Sound-alike/look-alike issues:

Ketoprofen may be confused with ketotifen

BEERS Criteria medication:

This drug may be potentially inappropriate for use in geriatric patients (Quality of evidence - moderate; Strength of recommendation - strong).

Canadian Brand Names Apo-Keto SR®; Apo-Keto-E®; Apo-Keto®; Ketoprofen SR; Ketoprofen-E; Nu-Ketoprofen; Nu-Ketoprofen-E; PMS-Ketoprofen; PMS-Ketoprofen-E

Therapeutic Category Analgesic, Nonnarcotic; Nonsteroidal Antiinflammatory Drug (NSAID)

Use Acute and long-term treatment of rheumatoid arthritis and osteoarthritis; primary dysmenorrhea; mild-to-moderate pain

General Dosage Range Dosage adjustment recommended in patients with hepatic and renal impairment

Oral:

Extended release: *Adults:* 200 mg once daily

Regular release: *Adults:* 25-50 mg 4 times/day or 75 mg 3 times/day (maximum: 300 mg/day)

Dosage Forms

Capsule, oral: 50 mg, 75 mg

Capsule, extended release, oral: 200 mg

Ketoprofen-E (Can) *see* ketoprofen *on page 512*

Ketoprofen SR (Can) *see* ketoprofen *on page 512*

ketorolac (systemic) (KEE toe role ak)

Medication Safety Issues

Sound-alike/look-alike issues:

Ketorolac may be confused with Ketalar®

Toradol® may be confused with Foradil®, Inderal®, TEGretol®, traMADol, tromethamine

BEERS Criteria medication:

This drug may be potentially inappropriate for use in geriatric patients (Quality of evidence - high; Strength of recommendation - strong).

International issues:

Toradol [Canada and multiple international markets] may be confused with Theradol brand name for tramadol [Netherlands]

Synonyms ketorolac tromethamine; Toradol

Canadian Brand Names Apo-Ketorolac Injectable®; Apo-Ketorolac®; Ketorolac Tromethamine Injection, USP; Novo-Ketorolac; Nu-Ketorolac; Toradol®; Toradol® IM

Therapeutic Category Nonsteroidal Antiinflammatory Drug (NSAID), Oral; Nonsteroidal Antiinflammatory Drug (NSAID), Parenteral

Use Short-term (≤5 days) management of moderate-to-severe acute pain requiring analgesia at the opioid level

General Dosage Range Dosage adjustment recommended in patients with renal impairment

I.M.:

Children ≥16 years and Adults <50 kg and Elderly ≥65 years: 30 mg as a single dose **or** 15 mg every 6 hours (maximum: 60 mg/day)

Children ≥16 years and Adults ≥50 kg: 60 mg as a single dose **or** 30 mg every 6 hours (maximum: 120 mg/day)

I.V.:

Children ≥16 years and Adults <50 kg and Elderly ≥65 years: 15 mg as a single dose **or** 15 mg every 6 hours (maximum: 60 mg/day)

Children ≥16 years and Adults ≥50 kg: 30 mg as a single dose **or** 30 mg every 6 hours (maximum: 120 mg/day)

Oral:

Children ≥17 years and Adults <50 kg and Elderly ≥65 years: 10 mg every 4-6 hours (maximum: 40 mg/day)

Children ≥17 years and Adults ≥50 kg: 20 mg, followed by 10 mg every 4-6 hours (maximum: 40 mg/day)

Dosage Forms

Injection, solution: 15 mg/mL (1 mL, 2 mL); 30 mg/mL (1 mL, 2 mL, 10 mL)

Tablet, oral: 10 mg

ketorolac (nasal) (KEE toe role ak)

Medication Safety Issues

Sound-alike/look-alike issues:

Ketorolac may be confused with Ketalar®

BEERS Criteria medication:

This drug may be potentially inappropriate for use in geriatric patients (Quality of evidence - high; Strength of recommendation - strong).

Synonyms ketorolac tromethamine

U.S. Brand Names Sprix®

Therapeutic Category Nonsteroidal Antiinflammatory Drug (NSAID), Nasal

Use Short-term (≤5 days) management of moderate-to-moderately-severe acute pain requiring analgesia at the opioid level

General Dosage Range Dosage adjustment recommended in patients with renal impairment.

Intranasal:

Adults <65 years and ≥50 kg: one spray (15.75 mg) in each nostril (total dose: 31.5 mg) every 6-8 hours; maximum dose: 4 doses (126 mg)/day

Adults <50 kg and/or Elderly ≥65 years: One spray (15.75 mg) in 1 nostril (total dose: 15.75 mg) every 6-8 hours; maximum dose: 4 doses (63 mg)/day

Dosage Forms

Solution, intranasal [preservative free]:

Sprix®: 15.75 mg/spray (1.7 g)

ketorolac (ophthalmic) (KEE toe role ak)

Medication Safety Issues

Sound-alike/look-alike issues:

Acular® may be confused with Acthar®, Ocular

Ketorolac may be confused with Ketalar®

Synonyms ketorolac tromethamine

U.S. Brand Names Acular LS®; Acular®; Acuvail®

Canadian Brand Names Acular LS®; Acular®; ratio-Ketorolac

Therapeutic Category Nonsteroidal Antiinflammatory Drug (NSAID), Ophthalmic

Use Temporary relief of ocular itching due to seasonal allergic conjunctivitis; postoperative inflammation following cataract extraction; reduction of ocular pain and photophobia following incisional refractive surgery; reduction of ocular pain, burning, and stinging following corneal refractive surgery

General Dosage Range Ophthalmic: *Children ≥3 years and Adults:* Instill 1 drop (0.25 mg) 4 times/day to eye(s)

Dosage Forms

Solution, ophthalmic: 0.4% (5 mL); 0.5% (3 mL, 5 mL, 10 mL)

Acular LS®: 0.4% (5 mL)

Acular®: 0.5% (5 mL)

Solution, ophthalmic [preservative free]:

Acuvail®: 0.45% (0.4 mL)

ketorolac tromethamine *see* ketorolac (nasal) *on page* 513

ketorolac tromethamine *see* ketorolac (ophthalmic) *on page* 513

ketorolac tromethamine *see* ketorolac (systemic) *on page* 512

Ketorolac Tromethamine Injection, USP (Can) *see* ketorolac (systemic) *on page* 512

ketotifen (systemic) *(Canada only)* (kee toe TYE fen)

Medication Safety Issues

Sound-alike/look-alike issues:

Ketotifen may be confused with ketoprofen

Zaditen® may be confused with Zaditor®

Synonyms ketotifen fumarate

Canadian Brand Names APO-Ketotifen®; Novo-Ketotifen; Nu-Ketotifen®; PMS-Ketotifen; Zaditen®

Therapeutic Category Histamine H_1 Antagonist; Histamine H_1 Antagonist, Second Generation; Mast Cell Stabilizer; Piperidine Derivative

Use Adjunctive therapy in the chronic treatment of pediatric patients ≥6 months of age with mild, atopic asthma

General Dosage Range Oral:

Children 6 months to 3 years: Initial: 0.05 mg/kg once daily or in 2 divided doses for 5 days; Maintenance: 0.05 mg/kg twice daily (maximum dose: 1 mg twice daily)

Children >3 years: Initial: 1 mg once daily or in 2 divided doses for 5 days; Maintenance: 1 mg twice daily

Product Availability Not available in the U.S.

Dosage Forms - Canada

Syrup, oral:

Zaditen®: 1 mg/5 mL (250 mL)

Tablet, oral:

Zaditen®: 1 mg

ketotifen (ophthalmic) (kee toe TYE fen)

Medication Safety Issues

Sound-alike/look-alike issues:

Claritin™ Eye (ketotifen) may be confused with Claritin® (loratadine)

Ketotifen may be confused with ketoprofen

ZyrTEC® Itchy Eye (ketotifen) may be confused with ZyrTEC® (cetirizine)

Synonyms ketotifen fumarate

U.S. Brand Names Alaway™ [OTC]; Claritin™ Eye [OTC]; Zaditor® [OTC]; ZyrTEC® Itchy Eye [OTC]

Canadian Brand Names Zaditor®

Therapeutic Category Antihistamine, H_1 Blocker, Ophthalmic

Use Temporary relief of eye itching due to allergic conjunctivitis

General Dosage Range Ophthalmic: *Children ≥3 years and Adults:* Instill 1 drop into the affected eye(s) twice daily, every 8-12 hours

Dosage Forms

Solution, ophthalmic: 0.025% (5 mL)
Alaway™ [OTC]: 0.025% (10 mL)
Claritin™ Eye [OTC]: 0.025% (5 mL)
Zaditor® [OTC]: 0.025% (5 mL)
ZyrTEC® Itchy Eye [OTC]: 0.025% (5 mL)

Dosage Forms - Canada

Solution, ophthalmic [drops]:
Zaditor®: 0.025% (5 mL)
Solution, ophthalmic [drops], preservative free:
Zaditor®: 0.025% (0.4 mL) (30s)

K-Phos® MF *see* potassium phosphate and sodium phosphate *on page 747*
K-Phos® Neutral *see* potassium phosphate and sodium phosphate *on page 747*
K-Phos® No. 2 *see* potassium phosphate and sodium phosphate *on page 747*
K-Phos® Original *see* potassium acid phosphate *on page 743*
KPN Prenatal [OTC] *see* vitamins (multiple/prenatal) *on page 952*
Kristalose® *see* lactulose *on page 519*
Krystexxa™ *see* pegloticase *on page 699*
K-Tab® *see* potassium chloride *on page 744*
kunecatechins *see* sinecatechins *on page 836*
Kuvan™ *see* sapropterin *on page 823*
Kwellada-P™ (Can) *see* permethrin *on page 709*
Kyprolis™ *see* carfilzomib *on page 177*
Kytril *see* granisetron *on page 432*
Kytril® (Can) *see* granisetron *on page 432*
L-749,345 *see* ertapenem *on page 342*
L-758,298 *see* fosaprepitant *on page 408*
L-M-X® 4 [OTC] *see* lidocaine (topical) *on page 535*
L-M-X® 5 [OTC] *see* lidocaine (topical) *on page 535*
L 754030 *see* aprepitant *on page 88*
LA 20304a *see* gemifloxacin *on page 422*

labetalol (la BET a lole)

Medication Safety Issues

Sound-alike/look-alike issues:

Labetalol may be confused with betaxolol, lamoTRIgine, Lipitor®
Normodyne® may be confused with Norpramin®
Trandate® may be confused with traMADol, TRENtal®

High alert medication:

The Institute for Safe Medication Practices (ISMP) includes this medication among its list of drugs which have a heightened risk of causing significant patient harm when used in error.

Administration issues:

Significant differences exist between oral and I.V. dosing. Use caution when converting from one route of administration to another.

Synonyms ibidomide hydrochloride; labetalol hydrochloride

U.S. Brand Names Trandate®

Canadian Brand Names Apo-Labetalol®; Labetalol Hydrochloride Injection, USP; Normodyne®; Trandate®

Therapeutic Category Alpha-/Beta- Adrenergic Blocker

Use Treatment of mild-to-severe hypertension; I.V. for severe hypertension (eg, hypertensive emergencies)

General Dosage Range

I.V.:

Children: 0.3-1 mg/kg/dose intermittently **or** 0.4-1 mg/kg/hour infusion (maximum: 3 mg/kg/hour)
Adults: Bolus: 20 mg, may give 40-80 mg at 10-minute intervals; Infusion: 2 mg/minute (maximum: 300 mg total cumulative dose)

Oral: *Adults:* Initial: 100 mg twice daily; Maintenance: 200-800 mg/day in 2 divided doses (maximum: 2.4 g/day)

Dosage Forms

Injection, solution: 5 mg/mL (4 mL, 8 mL, 20 mL, 40 mL)
Trandate®: 5 mg/mL (20 mL, 40 mL)
Tablet, oral: 100 mg, 200 mg, 300 mg
Trandate®: 100 mg, 200 mg, 300 mg

labetalol hydrochloride *see* labetalol *on page 516*
Labetalol Hydrochloride Injection, USP (Can) *see* labetalol *on page 516*
Lac-Dose® [OTC] *see* lactase *on page 517*
Lac-Hydrin® *see* lactic acid and ammonium hydroxide *on page 517*
Lac-Hydrin® Five [OTC] *see* lactic acid and ammonium hydroxide *on page 517*

LAClotion™ *see* lactic acid and ammonium hydroxide *on page 517*

lacosamide (la KOE sa mide)

Medication Safety Issues

Sound-alike/look-alike issues:

Lacosamide may be confused with zonisamide

Vimpat® may be confused with Vimovo™

Synonyms ADD 234037; harkoseride; LCM; SPM 927

U.S. Brand Names Vimpat®

Canadian Brand Names Vimpat®

Therapeutic Category Anticonvulsant, Miscellaneous

Controlled Substance C-V

Use Adjunctive therapy in the treatment of partial-onset seizures

General Dosage Range Dosage adjustment recommended in patients with hepatic or renal impairment

Oral: *Adolescents ≥17 years and Adults:* Initial: 50 mg twice daily; Maintenance dose: 200-400 mg/day

Dosage Forms

Injection, solution:

Vimpat®: 10 mg/mL (20 mL)

Solution, oral:

Vimpat®: 10 mg/mL (465 mL)

Tablet, oral:

Vimpat®: 50 mg, 100 mg, 150 mg, 200 mg

Lacrisert® *see* hydroxypropyl cellulose *on page 463*

LaCrosse Complete [OTC] *see* sodium phosphates *on page 845*

Lactaid® Fast Act [OTC] *see* lactase *on page 517*

Lactaid® Original [OTC] *see* lactase *on page 517*

lactase (LAK tase)

U.S. Brand Names Lac-Dose® [OTC]; Lactaid® Fast Act [OTC]; Lactaid® Original [OTC]; Lactose Intolerance [OTC]; Lactrase® [OTC]

Canadian Brand Names Dairyaid®

Therapeutic Category Nutritional Supplement

Use Help digest lactose in milk for patients with lactose intolerance

General Dosage Range Oral: *Adults:* 1-2 capsules with meals **or** 5-15 drops or 1-2 capsules/quart of milk **or** 1-3 tablets with meals

Dosage Forms

Caplet, oral: 3000 FCC lactase units

Lactaid® Fast Act [OTC]: 9000 FCC lactase units

Lactaid® Original [OTC]: 3000 FCC lactase units

Capsule, oral:

Lactrase® [OTC]: 250 mg standardized enzyme lactase

Capsule, softgel, oral:

Lactose Intolerance [OTC]: 250 mg standardized enzyme lactase

Tablet, oral: 9000 units

Lac-Dose® [OTC]: 3000 FCC lactase units

Tablet, chewable, oral:

Lactaid® Fast Act [OTC]: 9000 FCC lactase units

lactic acid (LAK tik AS id)

Synonyms sodium-PCA and lactic acid

Therapeutic Category Topical Skin Product

Use Lubricate and moisturize the skin counteracting dryness and itching

General Dosage Range Topical: *Adults:* Apply twice daily

lactic acid and ammonium hydroxide (LAK tik AS id & a MOE nee um hye DROKS ide)

Synonyms ammonium hydroxide and lactic acid; ammonium lactate

U.S. Brand Names AmLactin® [OTC]; Geri-Hydrolac™ [OTC]; Geri-Hydrolac™-12 [OTC]; Lac-Hydrin®; Lac-Hydrin® Five [OTC]; LAClotion™

Therapeutic Category Topical Skin Product

Use Treatment of moderate-to-severe xerosis and ichthyosis vulgaris

General Dosage Range Topical:

Cream: *Children ≥2 years and Adults:* Apply twice daily to affected area

Lotion: *Children and Adults:* Apply twice daily to affected area

Dosage Forms

Cream, topical: Lactic acid 12% with ammonium hydroxide (140 g, 280 g, 385 g)

AmLactin® [OTC]: Lactic acid 12% with ammonium hydroxide (140 g)

Lac-Hydrin®: Lactic acid 12% with ammonium hydroxide (280 g, 385 g)

Lotion, topical: Lactic acid 12% with ammonium hydroxide (225 g, 400 g)

AmLactin® [OTC], Lac-Hydrin®, LAClotion™: Lactic acid 12% with ammonium hydroxide (225 g, 400 g)

Geri-Hydrolac™ [OTC], Lac-Hydrin® Five: Lactic acid 5% with ammonium hydroxide (120 mL, 240 mL)

Geri-Hydrolac™-12 [OTC]: Lactic acid 12% with ammonium hydroxide (120 mL, 240 mL)

Lactinex™ [OTC] *see* Lactobacillus *on page 518*

Lactobacillus (lak toe ba SIL us)

Synonyms *Lactobacillus acidophilus*; *Lactobacillus bifidus*; *Lactobacillus bulgaricus*; *Lactobacillus casei*; *Lactobacillus paracasei*; *Lactobacillus plantarum*; *Lactobacillus reuteri*; *Lactobacillus rhamnosus* GG

U.S. Brand Names Bacid® [OTC]; Culturelle® [OTC]; Dofus [OTC]; Flora-Q™ [OTC]; Floranex™ [OTC]; Kala® [OTC]; Lactinex™ [OTC]; Lacto-Bifidus [OTC]; Lacto-Key [OTC]; Lacto-Pectin [OTC]; Lacto-TriBlend [OTC]; Megadophilus® [OTC]; MoreDophilus® [OTC]; RisaQuad®-2 [OTC]; RisaQuad™ [OTC]; Superdophilus® [OTC]; VSL #3® [OTC]; VSL #3®-DS

Canadian Brand Names Bacid®; Fermalac

Therapeutic Category Gastrointestinal Agent, Miscellaneous

Use Promote normal bacterial flora of the intestinal tract

General Dosage Range Oral: *Children and Adults:* Dosage varies greatly depending on product

Dosage Forms

Capsule:

Culturelle® [OTC]: *L. rhamnosus* GG 10 billion colony-forming units

Dofus [OTC]: *L. acidophilus* and *L. bifidus* 10:1 ratio

Flora-Q™ [OTC]: *L. acidophilus* and *L. paracasei* ≥8 billion colony-forming units

Lacto-Key [OTC]:

100: *L. acidophilus* 1 billion colony-forming units

600: *L. acidophilus* 6 billion colony-forming units

Lacto-Bifidus [OTC]:

100: *L. bifidus* 1 billion colony-forming units

600: *L. bifidus* 6 billion colony-forming units

Lacto-Pectin [OTC]: *L. acidophilus* and *L. casei* ≥5 billion colony-forming units

Lacto-TriBlend [OTC]:

100: *L. acidophilus, L. bifidus,* and *L. bulgaricus* 1 billion colony-forming units

600: *L. acidophilus, L. bifidus,* and *L. bulgaricus* 6 billion colony-forming units

Megadophilus® [OTC], Superdophilus® [OTC]: *L. acidophilus* 2 billion units

RisaQuad™ [OTC]: *L. acidophilus* and *L. paracasei* 8 billion colony-forming units

VSL #3® [OTC]: *L. acidophilus, L. plantarum, L. paracasei, L. bulgaricus* 112 billion live cells

Capsule, double strength:

RisaQuad®-2 [OTC]: *L. acidophilus* and *L. paracasei* 16 billion colony-forming units

Capsule, softgel: *L. acidophilus* 100 active units

Caplet:

Bacid® [OTC]: *L. acidophilus 80%* and *L. bulgaricus* 10%

Granules:

Floranex™ [OTC], Lactinex™ [OTC]: *L. acidophilus* and *L. bulgaricus* 100 million live cells per 1 g packet (12s)

Powder:

Lacto-TriBlend [OTC]: *L. acidophilus, L. bifidus,* and *L. bulgaricus* 10 billion colony-forming units per ¼ teaspoon

Megadophilus® [OTC], Superdophilus® [OTC]: *L. acidophilus* 2 billion units per half-teaspoon

MoreDophilus® [OTC]: *L. acidophilus* 12.4 billion units per teaspoon

VSL #3® [OTC]: *L. acidophilus, L. plantarum, L. paracasei, L. bulgaricus* 450 billion live cells

VSL #3®-DS: *L. acidophilus, L. plantarum, L. paracasei, L. bulgaricus* 900 billion live cells

Tablet:
Kala® [OTC]: *L. acidophilus* 200 million units
Tablet, chewable: *L. reuteri* 100 million organisms
Floranex™ [OTC]: *L. acidophilus* and *L. bulgaricus* 1 million colony-forming units
Lactinex™ [OTC]: *L. acidophilus* and *L. bulgaricus* 1 million live cells
Wafer: *L. acidophilus* 90 mg and *L. bifidus* 25 mg (100s)

Lactobacillus acidophilus *see* Lactobacillus *on page 518*
Lactobacillus bifidus *see* Lactobacillus *on page 518*
Lactobacillus bulgaricus *see* Lactobacillus *on page 518*
Lactobacillus casei *see* Lactobacillus *on page 518*
Lactobacillus paracasei *see* Lactobacillus *on page 518*
Lactobacillus plantarum *see* Lactobacillus *on page 518*
Lactobacillus reuteri *see* Lactobacillus *on page 518*
***Lactobacillus rhamnosus* GG** *see* Lactobacillus *on page 518*
Lacto-Bifidus [OTC] *see* Lactobacillus *on page 518*
lactoflavin *see* riboflavin *on page 799*
Lacto-Key [OTC] *see* Lactobacillus *on page 518*
Lacto-Pectin [OTC] *see* Lactobacillus *on page 518*
Lactose Intolerance [OTC] *see* lactase *on page 517*
Lacto-TriBlend [OTC] *see* Lactobacillus *on page 518*
Lactrase® [OTC] *see* lactase *on page 517*

lactulose (LAK tyoo lose)

Medication Safety Issues

Sound-alike/look-alike issues:
Lactulose may be confused with lactose

U.S. Brand Names Constulose; Enulose; Generlac; Kristalose®

Canadian Brand Names Acilac; Apo-Lactulose®; Laxilose; PMS-Lactulose

Therapeutic Category Ammonium Detoxicant; Laxative

Use Prevention and treatment of portal-systemic encephalopathy (including hepatic precoma and coma); treatment of constipation

General Dosage Range

Oral:
Infants: 1.7-6.7 g/day (2.5-10 mL/day) in divided doses
Older Children and Adolescents: 26.7-60 g/day (40-90 mL/day) in divided doses
Adults: PSE: 20-30 g (30-45 mL) every hour initially, then 3-4 times/day; Constipation: 10-40 g (15-60 mL) daily

Rectal: *Adults:* Constipation: 200 g (300 mL); may repeat every 4-6 hours

Dosage Forms

Crystals for solution, oral:
Kristalose®: 10 g/packet (30s); 20 g/packet (30s)
Solution, oral: 10 g/15 mL (15 mL, 30 mL, 237 mL, 240 mL, 473 mL, 480 mL, 500 mL, 946 mL, 960 mL, 1000 mL, 1890 mL, 1892 mL, 1920 mL)
Constulose: 10 g/15 mL (946 mL)
Enulose: 10 g/15 mL (473 mL)
Solution, oral/rectal: 10 g/15 mL (237 mL, 473 mL, 946 mL, 1920 mL)
Generlac: 10 g/15 mL (473 mL, 1892 mL)

ladakamycin *see* azacitidine *on page 106*
LAIV *see* influenza virus vaccine (live/attenuated) *on page 484*
L-AmB *see* amphotericin B liposomal *on page 72*
LaMICtal® *see* lamotrigine *on page 521*
Lamictal® (Can) *see* lamotrigine *on page 521*
LaMICtal® ODT™ *see* lamotrigine *on page 521*
LaMICtal® XR™ *see* lamotrigine *on page 521*
LamISIL® *see* terbinafine (systemic) *on page 878*
Lamisil® (Can) *see* terbinafine (systemic) *on page 878*

Lamisil® (Can) *see* terbinafine (topical) *on page 879*
LamISIL AT® [OTC] *see* terbinafine (topical) *on page 879*

lamivudine (la MI vyoo deen)

Medication Safety Issues
Sound-alike/look-alike issues:
LamiVUDine may be confused with lamoTRIgine
Epivir® may be confused with Combivir®

Synonyms 3TC

Tall-Man lamiVUDine

U.S. Brand Names Epivir-HBV®; Epivir®

Canadian Brand Names 3TC®; Apo-Lamivudine®; Heptovir®

Therapeutic Category Antiviral Agent

Use
Epivir®: Treatment of HIV infection when antiretroviral therapy is warranted; should always be used as part of a multidrug regimen (at least three antiretroviral agents)
Epivir-HBV®: Treatment of chronic hepatitis B associated with evidence of hepatitis B viral replication and active liver inflammation. Resistance develops rapidly in hepatitis B; consider use only if other anti-HBV antiviral agents with more favorable resistance patterns cannot be used.

General Dosage Range Dosage adjustment recommended in patients with renal impairment
Oral:
Infants 1-3 months: HIV (DHHS [pediatric], 2010): 4 mg/kg/dose twice daily
Children 3 months to 2 years: HIV: 4 mg/kg/dose twice daily (maximum: 150 mg/dose twice daily)
Children 2-16 years and >16 years and <50 kg: Hepatitis B: 3 mg/kg/dose once daily (maximum: 100 mg/day); HIV: 4 mg/kg/dose twice daily (maximum: 150 mg/dose twice daily)
Children >16 years and ≥50 kg: Hepatitis B: 3 mg/kg/dose once daily (maximum: 100 mg/day); HIV: 150 mg twice daily **or** 300 mg once daily
Adults <50 kg: Hepatitis B: 100 mg/day; HIV (DHHS [pediatric], 2010): 4 mg/kg/dose twice daily (maximum: 150 mg/dose twice daily)
Adults ≥50 kg: Hepatitis B: 100 mg/day; HIV: 150 mg twice daily **or** 300 mg once daily

Dosage Forms
Solution, oral:
Epivir-HBV®: 5 mg/mL
Epivir®: 10 mg/mL
Tablet, oral: 150 mg, 300 mg
Epivir-HBV®: 100 mg
Epivir®: 150 mg, 300 mg

lamivudine, abacavir, and zidovudine *see* abacavir, lamivudine, and zidovudine *on page 16*
lamivudine and abacavir *see* abacavir and lamivudine *on page 16*

lamivudine and zidovudine (la MI vyoo deen & zye DOE vyoo deen)

Medication Safety Issues
Sound-alike/look-alike issues:
Combivir® may be confused with Combivent®, Epivir®
Other safety concerns:
AZT is an error-prone abbreviation (mistaken as azaTHIOprine, aztreonam)

Synonyms AZT + 3TC (error-prone abbreviation); zidovudine and lamivudine

U.S. Brand Names Combivir®

Canadian Brand Names Combivir®; Teva-Lamivudine/Zidovudine

Therapeutic Category Antiviral Agent

Use Treatment of HIV infection when therapy is warranted based on clinical and/or immunological evidence of disease progression

General Dosage Range Oral: *Adolescents ≥30 kg and Adults:* 1 tablet (lamivudine 150 mg/zidovudine 300 mg) twice daily

Dosage Forms
Tablet, oral: Lamivudine 150 mg and zidovudine 300 mg
Combivir®: Lamivudine 150 mg and zidovudine 300 mg [scored]

lamotrigine (la MOE tri jeen)

Medication Safety Issues

Sound-alike/look-alike issues:

LamoTRIgine may be confused with labetalol, LamISIL®, lamiVUDine, levothyroxine, Lomotil®

LaMICtal® may be confused with LamISIL®, Lomotil®

Administration issues:

Potential exists for medication errors to occur among different formulations of LaMICtal® (tablets, extended release tablets, orally disintegrating tablets, and chewable/dispersible tablets). Patients should be instructed to visually inspect tablets dispensed to verify receiving the correct medication and formulation. The medication guide includes illustrations to aid in tablet verification.

International issues:

Lamictal [U.S., Canada, and multiple international markets] may be confused with Ludiomil brand name for maprotiline [multiple international markets]

Lamotrigine [U.S., Canada, and multiple international markets] may be confused with Ludiomil brand name for maprotiline [multiple international markets]

Synonyms BW-430C; LTG

Tall-Man lamo**TRI**gine

U.S. Brand Names LaMICtal®; LaMICtal® ODT™; LaMICtal® XR™

Canadian Brand Names Apo-Lamotrigine®; Lamictal®; Mylan-Lamotrigine; Novo-Lamotrigine; PMS-Lamotrigine; ratio-Lamotrigine; Teva-Lamotrigine

Therapeutic Category Anticonvulsant

Use Adjunctive therapy in the treatment of generalized seizures of Lennox-Gastaut syndrome, primary generalized tonic-clonic seizures, and partial seizures; conversion to monotherapy in patients with partial seizures who are receiving treatment with valproic acid or a single enzyme-inducing antiepileptic drug (specifically carbamazepine, phenytoin, phenobarbital or primidone); maintenance treatment of bipolar I disorder

General Dosage Range Dosage adjustment recommended in patients with hepatic or renal impairment or on concomitant therapy

Oral:

Immediate release formulation:

Children 2-12 years: Dosage varies greatly depending on indication

Children ≥13 years and Adults: Dosage varies greatly depending on indication

Extended release formulation: *Children ≥13 years and Adults:* Dosage varies greatly depending on indication

Dosage Forms

Tablet, oral: 25 mg, 100 mg, 150 mg, 200 mg

LaMICtal®: 25 mg, 100 mg, 150 mg, 200 mg, 25 mg (42s) [white tablets] and 100 mg (7s) [peach tablets], 25 mg (84s) [white tablets] and 100 mg (14s) [peach tablets]

Tablet, chewable/dispersible, oral: 5 mg, 25 mg

LaMICtal®: 2 mg, 5 mg, 25 mg

Tablet, extended release, oral:

LaMICtal® XR™: 25 mg, 50 mg, 100 mg, 200 mg, 250 mg, 300 mg, 25 mg (21s) [yellow/white tablets] and 50 mg (7s) [green/white tablets], 50 mg (14s) [green/white tablets], 100 mg (14s) [orange/white tablets], and 200 mg (7s) [blue/white tablets], 25 mg (14s) [yellow/white tablets], 50 mg (14s) [green/white tablets], and 100 mg (7s) [orange/white tablets]

Tablet, orally disintegrating, oral:

LaMICtal® ODT™: 25 mg, 50 mg, 100 mg, 200 mg, 25 mg (21s) and 50 mg (7s), 50 mg (42s) and 100 mg (14s), 25 mg (14s), 50 mg (14s), and 100 mg (7s)

Lanacane® [OTC] *see* benzocaine *on page 121*

Lanacane® Maximum Strength [OTC] *see* benzocaine *on page 121*

Lanaphilic® with Urea [OTC] *see* urea *on page 930*

lanolin, cetyl alcohol, glycerin, petrolatum, and mineral oil

(LAN oh lin, SEE til AL koe hol, GLIS er in, pe troe LAY tum, & MIN er al oyl)

Synonyms cetyl alcohol, glycerin, lanolin, mineral oil, and petrolatum; mineral oil, petrolatum, lanolin, cetyl alcohol, and glycerin

U.S. Brand Names Lubriderm® Fragrance Free [OTC]; Lubriderm® [OTC]

Therapeutic Category Topical Skin Product

Use Treatment of dry skin

General Dosage Range Topical: *Adults:* Apply to skin as necessary

Dosage Forms

Lotion, topical [bottle]: 180 mL, 300 mL, 480 mL

Lubriderm® Fragrance Free [OTC], Lubriderm® [OTC]: 180 mL, 300 mL, 480 mL

Lotion, topical [tube]: 100 mL

Lubriderm® Fragrance Free [OTC], Lubriderm® [OTC]: 100 mL

Lanoxin® *see* digoxin *on page* 285

lanreotide (lan REE oh tide)

Medication Safety Issues

Sound-alike/look-alike issues:

Somatuline® may be confused with Soma, somatropin, SUMAtriptan

Synonyms lanreotide acetate

U.S. Brand Names Somatuline® Depot

Canadian Brand Names Somatuline® Autogel®

Therapeutic Category Somatostatin Analog

Use Long-term treatment of acromegaly in patients who are not candidates for or are unresponsive to surgery and/or radiotherapy

General Dosage Range Dosage adjustment recommended in patients with hepatic or renal impairment

SubQ: *Adults:* Initial: 90 mg once every 4 weeks for 3 months; Maintenance: 60-120 mg every 4 weeks **or** 120 mg every 6-8 weeks

Dosage Forms

Injection, solution:

Somatuline® Depot: 60 mg/0.4 mL (0.4 mL); 90 mg/0.4 mL (0.4 mL); 120 mg/0.5 mL (0.5 mL)

Dosage Forms - Canada

Injection, solution:

Somatuline® Autogel®: 60 mg/~0.3 mL (~0.3 mL); 90 mg/~0.4 mL (~0.4 mL); 120 mg/~0.5 mL (~0.5 mL)

lanreotide acetate *see* lanreotide *on page* 522

lansoprazole (lan SOE pra zole)

Medication Safety Issues

Sound-alike/look-alike issues:

Lansoprazole may be confused with aripiprazole, dexlansoprazole

Prevacid® may be confused with Pravachol®, Prevpac®, PriLOSEC®, Prinivil®

U.S. Brand Names First®-Lansoprazole; Prevacid®; Prevacid® 24 HR [OTC]; Prevacid® SoluTab™

Canadian Brand Names Apo-Lansoprazole®; Mylan-Lansoprazole; Prevacid®; Prevacid® FasTab; Teva-Lansoprazole

Therapeutic Category Gastric Acid Secretion Inhibitor; Proton Pump Inhibitor

Use Short-term treatment of active duodenal ulcers; maintenance treatment of healed duodenal ulcers; as part of a multidrug regimen for *H. pylori* eradication to reduce the risk of duodenal ulcer recurrence; short-term treatment of active benign gastric ulcer; treatment of NSAID-associated gastric ulcer; to reduce the risk of NSAID-associated gastric ulcer in patients with a history of gastric ulcer who require an NSAID; short-term treatment of symptomatic GERD; short-term treatment for all grades of erosive esophagitis; to maintain healing of erosive esophagitis; long-term treatment of pathological hypersecretory conditions, including Zollinger-Ellison syndrome

OTC labeling: Relief of frequent heartburn (≥2 days/week)

General Dosage Range Oral:

Children 1-11 years and ≤30 kg: 15 mg once daily (maximum: 30 mg twice daily)

Children 1-11 years and >30 kg: 30 mg once daily (maximum: 30 mg twice daily)

Children 12-17 years: 15-30 mg once daily

Adults: 15-180 mg/day in 1-2 divided doses

Dosage Forms

Capsule, delayed release, oral: 15 mg, 30 mg

Prevacid®: 15 mg, 30 mg

Prevacid® 24 HR [OTC]: 15 mg

Powder for suspension, oral:
First®-Lansoprazole: 3 mg/mL (90 mL, 150 mL, 300 mL)
Tablet, delayed release, orally disintegrating, oral:
Prevacid® SoluTab™: 15 mg, 30 mg

lansoprazole, amoxicillin, and clarithromycin
(lan SOE pra zole, a moks i SIL in, & kla RITH roe mye sin)

Medication Safety Issues
Sound-alike/look-alike issues:
Prevpac® may be confused with Prevacid®

Synonyms amoxicillin, clarithromycin, and lansoprazole; clarithromycin, lansoprazole, and amoxicillin; lansoprazole, amoxicillin, and clarithromycin

U.S. Brand Names Prevpac®

Canadian Brand Names Hp-PAC®

Therapeutic Category Antibiotic, Macrolide Combination; Antibiotic, Penicillin; Gastrointestinal Agent, Miscellaneous

Use Eradication of *H. pylori* to reduce the risk of recurrent duodenal ulcer

General Dosage Range Oral: *Adults:* Lansoprazole 30 mg, amoxicillin 1 g, and clarithromycin 500 mg taken together twice daily

Dosage Forms
Combination package [each administration card contains]:
Prevpac®:
Capsule: Amoxicillin 500 mg (4 capsules/day)
Capsule, delayed release (Prevacid®): Lansoprazole 30 mg (2 capsules/day)
Tablet (Biaxin®): Clarithromycin 500 mg (2 tablets/day)

lansoprazole, amoxicillin, and clarithromycin *see* lansoprazole, amoxicillin, and clarithromycin *on page 523*

lanthanum (LAN tha num)

Medication Safety Issues
Sound-alike/look-alike issues:
Lanthanum may be confused with lithium

Synonyms lanthanum carbonate

U.S. Brand Names Fosrenol®

Canadian Brand Names Fosrenol®

Therapeutic Category Phosphate Binder

Use Reduction of serum phosphate in patients with stage 5 chronic kidney disease (end-stage renal disease [ESRD]; kidney failure: GFR <15 mL/minute/1.73 m^2 or dialysis)

General Dosage Range Oral: *Adults:* Initial: 1500 mg/day in divided doses; Usual range: 1500-3000 mg/day

Dosage Forms
Tablet, chewable, oral:
Fosrenol®: 500 mg, 750 mg, 1000 mg

lanthanum carbonate *see* lanthanum *on page 523*
Lantus® *see* insulin glargine *on page 486*
Lantus® OptiSet® (Can) *see* insulin glargine *on page 486*
Lantus® Solostar® *see* insulin glargine *on page 486*
Lanvis® (Can) *see* thioguanine *on page 890*

lapatinib (la PA ti nib)

Medication Safety Issues
Sound-alike/look-alike issues:
Lapatinib may be confused with dasatinib, erlotinib, imatinib, SUNItinib, vandetanib
High alert medication:
This medication is in a class the Institute for Safe Medication Practices (ISMP) includes among its list of drug classes which have a heightened risk of causing significant patient harm when used in error.

Synonyms GW572016; lapatinib ditosylate

U.S. Brand Names Tykerb®

Canadian Brand Names Tykerb®

Therapeutic Category Antineoplastic Agent, Tyrosine Kinase Inhibitor; Epidermal Growth Factor Receptor (EGFR) Inhibitor

Use Treatment of HER2 overexpressing advanced or metastatic breast cancer (in combination with capecitabine) in patients who have received prior therapy (with an anthracycline, a taxane, and trastuzumab) and HER2 overexpressing hormone receptor positive metastatic breast cancer in postmenopausal women where hormone therapy is indicated (in combination with letrozole)

General Dosage Range Dosage adjustment recommended in patients with hepatic impairment, on concomitant therapy, or who develop toxicities

Oral: *Adults:* 1250-1500 mg once daily

Dosage Forms

Tablet, oral:

Tykerb®: 250 mg

lapatinib ditosylate *see* lapatinib *on page 523*

L-arginine *see* arginine *on page 90*

L-arginine hydrochloride *see* arginine *on page 90*

Lariam® (Can) *see* mefloquine *on page 568*

laronidase (lair OH ni days)

Synonyms recombinant α-L-iduronidase (glycosaminoglycan α-L-iduronohydrolase)

U.S. Brand Names Aldurazyme®

Canadian Brand Names Aldurazyme®

Therapeutic Category Enzyme

Use Treatment of Hurler and Hurler-Scheie forms of mucopolysaccharidosis I (MPS I); treatment of Scheie form of MPS I in patients with moderate-to-severe symptoms

General Dosage Range I.V.: *Children ≥6 months and Adults:* 0.58 mg/kg once weekly

Dosage Forms

Injection, solution [preservative free]:

Aldurazyme®: 2.9 mg/5 mL (5 mL)

Lasix® *see* furosemide *on page 412*

Lasix® Special (Can) *see* furosemide *on page 412*

L-asparaginase (*E. coli*) *see* asparaginase (*E. coli*) *on page 95*

L-asparaginase (*Erwinia*) *see* asparaginase (*Erwinia*) *on page 96*

L-asparaginase with polyethylene glycol *see* pegaspargase *on page 696*

lassar's zinc paste *see* zinc oxide *on page 963*

Lastacaft™ *see* alcaftadine *on page 42*

latanoprost (la TA noe prost)

Medication Safety Issues

Sound-alike/look-alike issues:

Latanoprost may be confused with Lantus®

Xalatan® may be confused with Lantus®, Travatan®, Xalacom™, Zarontin®

U.S. Brand Names Xalatan®

Canadian Brand Names Apo-Latanoprost®; CO Latanoprost; GD-Latanoprost; Xalatan®

Therapeutic Category Prostaglandin

Use Reduction of elevated intraocular pressure in patients with open-angle glaucoma or ocular hypertension

General Dosage Range Ophthalmic: *Adults:* 1 drop (1.5 mcg) in the affected eye(s) once daily

Dosage Forms

Solution, ophthalmic: 0.005% (2.5 mL)

Xalatan®: 0.005% (2.5 mL)

latanoprost and timolol *(Canada only)* (la TA noe prost & TIM oh lol)

Medication Safety Issues

Sound-alike/look-alike issues:

Xalacom™ may be confused with Xalatan®

Synonyms timolol maleate and latanoprost

Canadian Brand Names Xalacom™

Therapeutic Category Beta-Blocker, Nonselective; Ophthalmic Agent, Antiglaucoma; Prostaglandin, Ophthalmic

Use Reduction of intraocular pressure (IOP) in patients with open-angle glaucoma or ocular hypertension who are insufficiently responsive to topical beta-blockers, prostaglandin analogues, or other IOP-reducing agents and in whom combination therapy is appropriate

General Dosage Range Ophthalmic: *Adults:* Instill 1 drop once daily

Product Availability Not available in U.S.

Dosage Forms - Canada

Solution, ophthalmic:

Xalacom™: Latanoprost (0.005%) and timolol 0.5% (as base) (2.5 mL)

Latisse® *see* bimatoprost *on page 133*

***Latrodectus* antivenin** *see* antivenin *(Latrodectus mactans) on page 81*

***Latrodectus* antivenom** *see* antivenin *(Latrodectus mactans) on page 81*

***Latrodectus mactans* antivenin** *see* antivenin *(Latrodectus mactans) on page 81*

***Latrodectus mactans* antivenom** *see* antivenin *(Latrodectus mactans) on page 81*

Latuda® *see* lurasidone *on page 555*

Lavacol® [OTC] *see* alcohol (ethyl) *on page 43*

Laxilose (Can) *see* lactulose *on page 519*

Lazanda® *see* fentanyl *on page 377*

***l*-bunolol hydrochloride** *see* levobunolol *on page 529*

L-carnitine *see* levocarnitine *on page 530*

L-Carnitine [OTC] *see* levocarnitine *on page 530*

LCD *see* coal tar *on page 228*

LCM *see* lacosamide *on page 517*

L-deoxythymidine *see* telbivudine *on page 874*

L-deprenyl *see* selegiline *on page 828*

LDP-341 *see* bortezomib *on page 139*

LdT *see* telbivudine *on page 874*

LEA29Y *see* belatacept *on page 118*

Lectopam® (Can) *see* bromazepam *(Canada only) on page 142*

Lederle Leucovorin (Can) *see* leucovorin calcium *on page 527*

Leena® *see* ethinyl estradiol and norethindrone *on page 359*

leflunomide (le FLOO noh mide)

U.S. Brand Names Arava®

Canadian Brand Names Apo-Leflunomide®; Arava®; Mylan-Leflunomide; Novo-Leflunomide; PHL-Leflunomide; PMS-Leflunomide; Sandoz-Leflunomide

Therapeutic Category Antiinflammatory Agent

Use Treatment of active rheumatoid arthritis; indicated to reduce signs and symptoms, and to inhibit structural damage and improve physical function

General Dosage Range Dosage adjustment recommended in patients who develop toxicities

Oral: *Adults:* Initial: 100 mg/day for 3 days; Maintenance range: 10-20 mg/day

Dosage Forms

Tablet, oral: 10 mg, 20 mg

Arava®: 10 mg, 20 mg

Legatrin PM® [OTC] *see* acetaminophen and diphenhydramine *on page 23*

lenalidomide (le na LID oh mide)

Medication Safety Issues

Sound-alike/look-alike issues:

Lenalidomide may be confused with thalidomide

High alert medication:

This medication is in a class the Institute for Safe Medication Practices (ISMP) includes among its list of drug classes which have a heightened risk of causing significant patient harm when used in error.

Synonyms CC-5013; IMid-1
U.S. Brand Names Revlimid®
Canadian Brand Names Revlimid®
Therapeutic Category Angiogenesis Inhibitor; Immunosuppressant Agent; Tumor Necrosis Factor (TNF) Blocking Agent
Use Treatment of low- or intermediate-1-risk myelodysplastic syndrome (MDS) in patients with deletion 5q (del 5q) cytogenetic abnormality with transfusion-dependent anemia (with or without other cytogenetic abnormalities); treatment of multiple myeloma (in combination with dexamethasone) in patients who have received at least one prior therapy
General Dosage Range Dosage adjustment recommended in patients with renal impairment or who develop toxicities
Oral: *Adults:* 10 once daily **or** 25 mg once daily for 21 of 28 days
Dosage Forms
Capsule, oral:
Revlimid®: 2.5 mg, 5 mg, 10 mg, 15 mg, 25 mg

lepargylic acid *see* azelaic acid *on page* 107

lepirudin (leh puh ROO din)

Medication Safety Issues
High alert medication:
The Institute for Safe Medication Practices (ISMP) includes this medication among its list of drugs which have a heightened risk of causing significant patient harm when used in error.
Synonyms lepirudin (rDNA); recombinant hirudin
U.S. Brand Names Refludan® [DSC]
Canadian Brand Names Refludan®
Therapeutic Category Anticoagulant (Other)
Use Indicated for anticoagulation in patients with heparin-induced thrombocytopenia (HIT) and associated thromboembolic disease in order to prevent further thromboembolic complications
General Dosage Range Dosage adjustment recommended in patients with renal impairment
I.V.: *Adults:* Bolus: 0.2-0.4 mg/kg; Infusion: 0.1-0.15 mg/kg/hour (maximum: 0.21 mg/kg/hour)

lepirudin (rDNA) *see* lepirudin *on page* 526
Lescol® *see* fluvastatin *on page* 402
Lescol® XL *see* fluvastatin *on page* 402
Lessina® *see* ethinyl estradiol and levonorgestrel *on page* 357
Letairis® *see* ambrisentan *on page* 58

letrozole (LET roe zole)

Medication Safety Issues
Sound-alike/look-alike issues:
Femara® may be confused with Famvir®, femhrt®, Provera®
Letrozole may be confused with anastrozole
Synonyms CGS-20267
U.S. Brand Names Femara®
Canadian Brand Names Femara®; JAMP-Letrozole; Letrozole Tablets, USP; MED-Letrozole; Myl-Letrozole; PMS-Letrozole; Sandoz-Letrozole
Therapeutic Category Antineoplastic Agent, Hormone (Antiestrogen)
Use For use in postmenopausal women in the adjuvant treatment of hormone receptor-positive early breast cancer, extended adjuvant treatment of early breast cancer after 5 years of tamoxifen, advanced breast cancer with disease progression following antiestrogen therapy, hormone receptor-positive or hormone receptor-unknown, locally-advanced, or first-line (or second-line) treatment of advanced or metastatic breast cancer
General Dosage Range Dosage adjustment recommended in patients with hepatic impairment
Oral: *Adults (postmenopausal females):* 2.5 mg once daily
Dosage Forms
Tablet, oral: 2.5 mg
Femara®: 2.5 mg

Letrozole Tablets, USP (Can) *see* letrozole *on page* 526

leucovorin *see* leucovorin calcium *on page 527*

leucovorin calcium (loo koe VOR in KAL see um)

Medication Safety Issues

Sound-alike/look-alike issues:

Leucovorin may be confused with Leukeran®, Leukine®, LEVOleucovorin

Folinic acid may be confused with folic acid

Folinic acid is an error prone synonym and should not be used

Synonyms 5-formyl tetrahydrofolate; calcium folinate; calcium leucovorin; citrovorum factor; folinate calcium; folinic acid (error prone synonym); leucovorin

Canadian Brand Names Lederle Leucovorin

Therapeutic Category Folic Acid Derivative

Use Antidote for folic acid antagonists (methotrexate, trimethoprim, pyrimethamine) and rescue therapy following high-dose methotrexate; in combination with fluorouracil in the treatment of colon cancer; treatment of megaloblastic anemias when folate is deficient as in infancy, sprue, pregnancy, and nutritional deficiency when oral folate therapy is not possible

General Dosage Range

I.M.: *Children and Adults:* ≤1 mg/day [folate deficient megaloblastic anemia] **or** 15 mg (~10 mg/m^2) every 6 hours for 10 doses [methotrexate rescue dose]

I.V.:

Children: 15 mg (~10 mg/m^2) every 6 hours for 10 doses

Adults: Initial: 15 mg (~10 mg/m^2) every 6 hours for 10 doses [methotrexate rescue dose] **or** 200 mg/m^2 **or** 20 mg/m^2 as a single dose [colorectal cancer]

Oral: *Children and Adults:* 5-15 mg/day [weak folic acid antagonist overdose] **or** 15 mg (~10 mg/m^2) every 6 hours for 10 doses [methotrexate rescue dose]

Dosage Forms

Injection, powder for reconstitution: 50 mg, 100 mg, 200 mg, 350 mg, 500 mg

Injection, solution [preservative free]: 10 mg/mL (50 mL)

Tablet, oral: 5 mg, 10 mg, 15 mg, 25 mg

Leukeran® *see* chlorambucil *on page 195*

Leukine® *see* sargramostim *on page 824*

leuprolide (loo PROE lide)

Medication Safety Issues

Sound-alike/look-alike issues:

Lupron Depot® (1-month or 3-month formulation) may be confused with Lupron Depot-Ped® (1-month or 3-month formulation)

Lupron Depot-Ped® is available in two formulations, a 1-month formulation and a 3-month formulation. Both formulations offer an 11.25 mg strength which may further add confusion.

Synonyms abbott-43818; leuprolide acetate; leuprorelin acetate; TAP-144

U.S. Brand Names Eligard®; Lupron Depot-Ped®; Lupron Depot®

Canadian Brand Names Eligard®; Lupron®; Lupron® Depot®

Therapeutic Category Antineoplastic Agent; Luteinizing Hormone-Releasing Hormone Analog

Use Palliative treatment of advanced prostate cancer; management of endometriosis; treatment of anemia caused by uterine leiomyomata (fibroids); central precocious puberty

General Dosage Range I.M., SubQ: *Children and Adults:* Dosage varies greatly depending on indication

Dosage Forms

Injection, powder for reconstitution [preservative free]:

Eligard®: 7.5 mg (monthly), 22.5 mg (3 month), 30 mg (4 month), 45 mg (6 month)

Lupron Depot-Ped®: 7.5 mg (monthly), 11.25 mg (3 month), 11.25 mg (monthly), 15 mg (monthly), 30 mg (3 month)

Lupron Depot®: 3.75 mg (monthly), 7.5 mg (monthly), 11.25 mg (3 month), 22.5 mg (3 month), 30 mg (4 month), 45 mg (6 month)

Injection, solution: 5 mg/mL (2.8 mL)

leuprolide acetate *see* leuprolide *on page 527*

leuprorelin acetate *see* leuprolide *on page 527*

leurocristine sulfate *see* vincristine *on page 946*

Leustatin® [DSC] *see* cladribine *on page 215*

levalbuterol (leve al BYOO ter ole)

Medication Safety Issues

Sound-alike/look-alike issues:

Xopenex® may be confused with Xanax®

Synonyms levalbuterol hydrochloride; levalbuterol tartrate; R-albuterol

U.S. Brand Names Xopenex HFA™; Xopenex®

Canadian Brand Names Xopenex®

Therapeutic Category Adrenergic Agonist Agent; $Beta_2$-Adrenergic Agonist Agent; Bronchodilator

Use Treatment or prevention of bronchospasm in children and adults with reversible obstructive airway disease

General Dosage Range

Inhalation (metered-dose inhaler): *Children ≥4 years and Adults:* 1-2 puffs every 4-6 hours

Nebulization (solution):

Children ≤4 years: 0.31-1.25 mg every 4-6 hours as needed

Children 5-11 years: 0.31-0.63 mg 3 times/day

Children ≥12 years and Adults: 0.63-1.25 mg every 8 hours as needed

Elderly: Initial: 0.63 mg

Dosage Forms

Aerosol, for oral inhalation:

Xopenex HFA™: 45 mcg/actuation (15 g)

Solution, for nebulization [preservative free]: 0.31 mg/3 mL (3 mL); 0.63 mg/3 mL (3 mL); 1.25 mg/3 mL (3 mL); 1.25 mg/0.5 mL (30s)

Xopenex®: 0.31 mg/3 mL (24s); 0.63 mg/3 mL (24s); 1.25 mg/3 mL (24s)

levalbuterol hydrochloride *see* levalbuterol *on page 528*
levalbuterol tartrate *see* levalbuterol *on page 528*
Levaquin® *see* levofloxacin (systemic) *on page 531*
levarterenol bitartrate *see* norepinephrine *on page 648*
Levate® (Can) *see* amitriptyline *on page 64*
Levatol® *see* penbutolol *on page 701*
Levbid® *see* hyoscyamine *on page 465*
Levemir® *see* insulin detemir *on page 486*
Levemir® FlexPen® *see* insulin detemir *on page 486*

levetiracetam (lee va tye RA se tam)

Medication Safety Issues

Sound-alike/look-alike issues:

Keppra® may be confused with Keflex®, Keppra XR®

LevETIRAcetam may be confused with levOCARNitine, levofloxacin

Potential for dispensing errors between Keppra® and Kaletra® (lopinavir/ritonavir)

Tall-Man lev**ETIRA**cetam

U.S. Brand Names Keppra XR®; Keppra®

Canadian Brand Names Apo-Levetiracetam®; Ava-Levetiracetam; CO Levetiracetam; Dom-Levetiracetam; Keppra®; PHL-Levetiracetam; PMS-Levetiracetam; PRO-Levetiracetam

Therapeutic Category Anticonvulsant

Use Adjunctive therapy in the treatment of partial-onset, myoclonic, and/or primary generalized tonic-clonic seizures

General Dosage Range Dosage adjustment recommended in patients with renal impairment

Oral:

Immediate release:

Children 1 to <6 months: Initial: 7 mg/kg twice daily; Maintenance: 7-21 mg/kg/dose twice daily (maximum: 42 mg/kg/day)

Children 6 months to <4 years: Initial: 10 mg/kg twice daily; Maintenance: 10-25 mg/kg twice daily (maximum: 50 mg/kg/day)

Children 4 to <16 years: Initial: 10 mg/kg twice daily; Maintenance: 10-30 mg/kg twice daily (maximum: 60 mg/kg/day or 3000 mg/day)

Children ≥12 years: Initial: 500 mg twice daily; Maintenance: 500-1500 mg twice daily (maximum: 3000 mg/day)

Adults: Initial: 500 mg twice daily; Maintenance: 500-1500 mg twice daily (maximum: 3000 mg/day)

Extended release: *Children ≥16 years and Adults:* Initial: 1000 mg once daily; Maintenance: 1000-3000 mg once daily (maximum: 3000 mg/day)

I.V.: *Children ≥16 years and Adults:* Initial: 500 mg twice daily; Maintenance: 500-1500 mg twice daily (maximum: 3000 mg/day)

Dosage Forms

Infusion, premixed in sodium chloride 0.54%: 1500 mg (100 mL)
Infusion, premixed in sodium chloride 0.75%: 1000 mg (100 mL)
Infusion, premixed in sodium chloride 0.82%: 500 mg (100 mL)
Injection, solution: 100 mg/mL (5 mL)
Keppra®: 100 mg/mL (5 mL)
Solution, oral: 100 mg/mL (5 mL, 118 mL, 472 mL, 473 mL, 480 mL, 500 mL)
Keppra®: 100 mg/mL (480 mL)
Tablet, oral: 250 mg, 500 mg, 750 mg, 1000 mg
Keppra®: 250 mg, 500 mg, 750 mg, 1000 mg
Tablet, extended release, oral: 500 mg, 750 mg
Keppra XR®: 500 mg, 750 mg

Levitra® *see* vardenafil *on page 938*

levobunolol (lee voe BYOO noe lole)

Medication Safety Issues

Sound-alike/look-alike issues:
Levobunolol may be confused with levocabastine
Betagan® may be confused with Betadine®, Betoptic® S

Synonyms *l*-bunolol hydrochloride; levobunolol hydrochloride

U.S. Brand Names Betagan®

Canadian Brand Names Apo-Levobunolol®; Betagan®; Novo-Levobunolol; Optho-Bunolol®; PMS-Levobunolol; Sandoz-Levobunolol

Therapeutic Category Beta-Adrenergic Blocker

Use To lower intraocular pressure in chronic open-angle glaucoma or ocular hypertension

General Dosage Range Ophthalmic: *Adults:* Instill 1 drop in the affected eye(s) 1-2 times/day

Dosage Forms

Solution, ophthalmic: 0.25% (5 mL, 10 mL); 0.5% (5 mL, 10 mL, 15 mL)
Betagan®: 0.5% (5 mL, 10 mL, 15 mL)

levobunolol hydrochloride *see* levobunolol *on page 529*
levocabastine hydrochloride *see* levocabastine (nasal) *(Canada only) on page 529*
levocabastine hydrochloride *see* levocabastine (ophthalmic) *(Canada only) on page 530*

levocabastine (nasal) *(Canada only)* (LEE voe kab as teen)

Medication Safety Issues

Sound-alike/look-alike issues:
Levocabastine may be confused with levobunolol, levOCARNitine
Livostin® may be confused with lovastatin

International issues:
Livostin [Canada and multiple international markets] may be confused with Limoxin brand name for ambroxol [Indonesia] and amoxicillin [Mexico]; Lovastin brand name for lovastatin [Malaysia, Poland, Singapore]

Synonyms levocabastine hydrochloride

Canadian Brand Names Livostin®

Therapeutic Category Histamine H_1 Antagonist; Histamine H_1 Antagonist, Second Generation; Piperidine Derivative

Use Symptomatic treatment of allergic rhinitis

General Dosage Range Intranasal: *Children ≥12 years and Adults ≤65 years:* 2 sprays in each nostril 2-4 times/day

Product Availability Not available in U.S.

Dosage Forms - Canada

Microsuspension, intranasal, as hydrochloride [spray]:
Livostin®: 0.05% [50 mcg/spray] (15 mL) [contains benzalkonium chloride]

levocabastine (ophthalmic) *(Canada only)* (LEE voe kab as teen)

Medication Safety Issues

Sound-alike/look-alike issues:

Levocabastine may be confused with levobunolol, levOCARNitine

Livostin® may be confused with lovastatin

International issues:

Livostin [Canada and multiple international markets] may be confused with Limoxin brand name for ambroxol [Indonesia] and amoxicillin [Mexico]; Lovastin brand name for lovastatin [Malaysia, Poland, Singapore]

Synonyms levocabastine hydrochloride

Canadian Brand Names Livostin® Eye Drops

Therapeutic Category Histamine H_1 Antagonist; Histamine H_1 Antagonist, Second Generation; Piperidine Derivative

Use Treatment of seasonal allergic conjunctivitis

General Dosage Range **Ophthalmic:** *Children ≥12 years and Adults ≤65 years:* Instill 1 drop in affected eye(s) 2-4 times/day

Product Availability Not available in U.S.

Dosage Forms - Canada

Suspension, ophthalmic:

Livostin®: 0.05% (5 mL, 10 mL)

Levocarb CR (Can) *see* carbidopa and levodopa *on page 174*

levocarnitine (lee voe KAR ni teen)

Medication Safety Issues

Sound-alike/look-alike issues:

LevOCARNitine may be confused with levETIRAcetam, levocabastine

Synonyms carnitine; L-carnitine

Tall-Man lev**OCARN**itine

U.S. Brand Names Carnitine-300 [OTC]; Carnitor®; Carnitor® SF; L-Carnitine [OTC]

Canadian Brand Names Carnitor®

Therapeutic Category Dietary Supplement

Use

Oral: Primary systemic carnitine deficiency; acute and chronic treatment of patients with an inborn error of metabolism which results in secondary carnitine deficiency

I.V.: Acute and chronic treatment of patients with an inborn error of metabolism which results in secondary carnitine deficiency; prevention and treatment of carnitine deficiency in patients with end-stage renal disease (ESRD) who are undergoing hemodialysis.

General Dosage Range

I.V.:

Children: 50 mg/kg/day in divided doses (maximum: 300 mg/kg/day)

Adults: 50 mg/kg/day in divided doses (maximum: 300 mg/kg/day) **or** 20 mg/kg after each hemodialysis session

Oral:

Infants and Children: Initial: 50 mg/kg/day in divided doses; Maintenance: 50-100 mg/kg/day in divided doses (maximum: 3000 mg daily)

Adults: 990 mg (tablet) 2-3 times daily **or** 1000-3000 g daily (oral solution) in divided doses

Dosage Forms

Capsule, oral:

Carnitine-300 [OTC]: 300 mg

L-Carnitine [OTC]: 250 mg

Injection, solution [preservative free]: 200 mg/mL (5 mL, 12.5 mL)

Carnitor®: 200 mg/mL (5 mL)

Solution, oral: 100 mg/mL (118 mL)

Carnitor®: 100 mg/mL (118 mL)

Carnitor® SF: 100 mg/mL (118 mL)

Tablet, oral: 330 mg

Carnitor®: 330 mg

L-Carnitine [OTC]: 500 mg

levocetirizine (LEE vo se TI ra zeen)

Medication Safety Issues

Sound-alike/look-alike issues:

Levocetirizine may be confused with cetirizine

Synonyms levocetirizine dihydrochloride

U.S. Brand Names Xyzal®

Therapeutic Category Antihistamine

Use Relief of symptoms of perennial and seasonal allergic rhinitis; treatment of skin manifestations (uncomplicated) of chronic idiopathic urticaria

General Dosage Range Dosage adjustment recommended in patients with renal impairment

Oral:

Children 6 months to 5 years: 1.25 mg once daily

Children 6-11 years: 2.5 mg once daily

Children ≥12 years and Adults: 2.5-5 mg once daily

Dosage Forms

Solution, oral: 0.5 mg/mL (150 mL)

Xyzal®: 0.5 mg/mL (150 mL)

Tablet, oral: 5 mg

Xyzal®: 5 mg

levocetirizine dihydrochloride *see* levocetirizine *on page 531*

levodopa and benserazide *see* benserazide and levodopa *(Canada only) on page 120*

levodopa and carbidopa *see* carbidopa and levodopa *on page 174*

levodopa, carbidopa, and entacapone (lee voe DOE pa, kar bi DOE pa, & en TA ka pone)

Medication Safety Issues

Administration issues:

Strengths listed in Stalevo® brand names correspond to the **levodopa** component of the formulation only. All strengths of Stalevo® contain a levodopa/carbidopa ratio of 4:1 plus entacapone 200 mg.

Synonyms carbidopa, entacapone, and levodopa; carbidopa, levodopa, and entacapone; entacapone, carbidopa, and levodopa

U.S. Brand Names Stalevo®

Canadian Brand Names Stalevo®

Therapeutic Category Anti-Parkinson Agent (Dopamine Agonist); Anti-Parkinson Agent, COMT Inhibitor

Use Treatment of idiopathic Parkinson disease

General Dosage Range Oral: *Adults:* 1 tablet (50-200 mg levodopa/12.5-50 mg carbidopa/200 mg entacapone) at each dosing interval (maximum: 1600 mg/day entacapone or 300 mg/day carbidopa)

Dosage Forms

Tablet:

Stalevo®: 50: Levodopa 50 mg, carbidopa 12.5 mg, and entacapone 200 mg; 75: Levodopa 75 mg, carbidopa 18.75 mg, and entacapone 200 mg; 100: Levodopa 100 mg, carbidopa 25 mg, and entacapone 200 mg; 125: Levodopa 125 mg, carbidopa 31.25 mg, and entacapone 200 mg; 150: Levodopa 150 mg, carbidopa 37.5 mg, and entacapone 200 mg; 200: Levodopa 200 mg, carbidopa 50 mg, and entacapone 200 mg

Levo-Dromoran *see* levorphanol *on page 533*

levofloxacin (systemic) (lee voe FLOKS a sin)

Medication Safety Issues

Sound-alike/look-alike issues:

Levaquin® may be confused with Levoxyl®, Levsin/SL®, Lovenox®

Levofloxacin may be confused with levETIRAcetam, levodopa, Levophed®, levothyroxine

U.S. Brand Names Levaquin®

Canadian Brand Names Levaquin®; Novo-Levofloxacin; PMS-Levofloxacin

Therapeutic Category Antibiotic, Quinolone; Respiratory Fluoroquinolone

Use Treatment of community-acquired pneumonia, including multidrug resistant strains of *S. pneumoniae* (MDRSP); nosocomial pneumonia; chronic bronchitis (acute bacterial exacerbation); acute bacterial rhinosinusitis (ABRS); prostatitis, urinary tract infection (uncomplicated or complicated); acute pyelonephritis; skin or skin structure infections (uncomplicated or complicated); reduce incidence or disease progression of inhalational anthrax (postexposure); prophylaxis and treatment of plague (pneumonic and septicemic) due to *Y. pestis*

General Dosage Range Dosage adjustment recommended in patients with renal impairment

Oral, I.V.:

Infants ≥6 months and Children ≤50 kg: 8 mg/kg every 12 hours (maximum: 250 mg/dose)
Children >50 kg: 500 mg once daily
Adults: 250-750 mg once daily

Dosage Forms

Infusion, premixed in D_5W [preservative free]: 250 mg (50 mL); 500 mg (100 mL); 750 mg (150 mL)
Levaquin®: 250 mg (50 mL); 500 mg (100 mL); 750 mg (150 mL)
Injection, solution [preservative free]: 25 mg/mL (20 mL, 30 mL)
Solution, oral: 25 mg/mL (100 mL, 200 mL, 480 mL)
Levaquin®: 25 mg/mL (480 mL)
Tablet, oral: 250 mg, 500 mg, 750 mg
Levaquin®: 250 mg, 500 mg, 750 mg

levofloxacin (ophthalmic) (lee voe FLOKS a sin)

Medication Safety Issues

Sound-alike/look-alike issues:
Levofloxacin may be confused with levETIRAcetam, levodopa, levothyroxine

U.S. Brand Names Iquix®; Quixin®

Therapeutic Category Antibiotic, Ophthalmic; Antibiotic, Quinolone

Use Treatment of bacterial conjunctivitis caused by susceptible organisms (Quixin® 0.5% ophthalmic solution); treatment of corneal ulcer caused by susceptible organisms (Iquix® 1.5% ophthalmic solution)

General Dosage Range Ophthalmic: *Children ≥1 year and Adults:* 1-2 drops every 30 minutes to 6 hours

Dosage Forms

Solution, ophthalmic: 0.5% (5 mL)
Iquix®: 1.5% (5 mL)
Quixin®: 0.5% (5 mL)

levo-folinic acid *see* LEVOleucovorin *on page* 532

LEVOleucovorin (lee voe loo koe VOR in)

Medication Safety Issues

Sound-alike/look-alike issues:
LEVOleucovorin may be confused with leucovorin calcium, Leukeran®, Leukine®

Synonyms 6S-leucovorin; calcium levoleucovorin; L-leucovorin; levo-folinic acid; levo-leucovorin; levoleucovorin calcium pentahydrate; S-leucovorin

U.S. Brand Names Fusilev®

Therapeutic Category Antidote; Rescue Agent (Chemotherapy)

Use Treatment of advanced, metastatic colorectal cancer (palliative) in combination with fluorouracil; rescue agent after high-dose methotrexate therapy in osteosarcoma; antidote for impaired methotrexate elimination and for inadvertent overdosage of folic acid antagonists

General Dosage Range I.V.: *Children and Adults:* Dosing varies greatly depending on indication

Product Availability

Fusilev® solution for injection: FDA approved April 2011; availability expected in the third quarter of 2011
Fusilev® solution for injection is a ready-to-use formulation and will be available in 175 mg/17.5 mL and 250 mg/25 mL presentations.

Dosage Forms

Injection, powder for reconstitution:
Fusilev®: 50 mg

levo-leucovorin *see* LEVOleucovorin *on page* 532
levoleucovorin calcium pentahydrate *see* LEVOleucovorin *on page* 532
levomefolate calcium, drospirenone, and ethinyl estradiol *see* ethinyl estradiol, drospirenone, and levomefolate *on page* 363
levomefolate, drospirenone, and ethinyl estradiol *see* ethinyl estradiol, drospirenone, and levomefolate *on page* 363
levomepromazine *see* methotrimeprazine *(Canada only) on page* 585
levonordefrin and mepivacaine hydrochloride *see* mepivacaine and levonordefrin *on page* 576

levonorgestrel (LEE voe nor jes trel)

Synonyms LNg 20; Plan B

U.S. Brand Names Mirena®; Next Choice®; Next Choice™ One Dose; Plan B® One Step

Canadian Brand Names Mirena®; Norlevo; Plan B®

Therapeutic Category Contraceptive, Implant (Progestin); Contraceptive, Progestin Only

Use

Intrauterine device (IUD): Prevention of pregnancy; treatment of heavy menstrual bleeding in women who also choose to use an IUD for contraception

Oral: Emergency contraception following unprotected intercourse or possible contraceptive failure

Plan B® One-Step is approved for OTC use by women ≥17 years of age and available by prescription only for women <17 years of age. Next Choice™ (generic of the original Plan-B® 2-dose regimen) is also approved for OTC use by women ≥17 years of age and by prescription only for women <17 years of age.

General Dosage Range

Intrauterine: *Adults:* Insert into uterine cavity, releases 20 mcg/day over 5 years

Oral: *Adults:* 0.75 mg every 12 hours for 2 doses **or** 1.5 mg as a single dose

Dosage Forms

Intrauterine device, intrauterine:

Mirena®: 52 mg/device

Tablet, oral: 0.75 mg

Next Choice®: 0.75 mg

Next Choice™ One Dose: 1.5 mg

Plan B® One Step: 1.5 mg

levonorgestrel and estradiol *see* estradiol and levonorgestrel *on page 349*

levonorgestrel and ethinyl estradiol *see* ethinyl estradiol and levonorgestrel *on page 357*

Levophed® *see* norepinephrine *on page 648*

Levora® *see* ethinyl estradiol and levonorgestrel *on page 357*

levorphanol (lee VOR fa nole)

Medication Safety Issues

High alert medication:

The Institute for Safe Medication Practices (ISMP) includes this medication among its list of drug classes which have a heightened risk of causing significant patient harm when used in error.

Synonyms Levo-Dromoran; levorphan tartrate; levorphanol tartrate

Therapeutic Category Analgesic, Narcotic

Controlled Substance C-II

Use Relief of moderate-to-severe pain; preoperative sedation/analgesia; management of chronic pain (eg, cancer) requiring opioid therapy

General Dosage Range Dosage adjustment recommended in patients with hepatic impairment

Oral: *Adults:* 2-4 mg every 6-8 hours as needed

Dosage Forms

Tablet, oral: 2 mg,

levorphanol tartrate *see* levorphanol *on page 533*

levorphan tartrate *see* levorphanol *on page 533*

Levothroid® *see* levothyroxine *on page 533*

levothyroxine (lee voe thye ROKS een)

Medication Safety Issues

Sound-alike/look-alike issues:

Levothyroxine may be confused with lamoTRIgine, Lanoxin®, levofloxacin, liothyronine

Levoxyl® may be confused with Lanoxin®, Levaquin®, Luvox®

Synthroid® may be confused with Symmetrel®

Administration issues:

Significant differences exist between oral and I.V. dosing. Use caution when converting from one route of administration to another.

Other safety concerns:

To avoid errors due to misinterpretation of a decimal point, always express dosage in mcg (**not** mg).

Synonyms *L*-thyroxine sodium; levothyroxine sodium; T_4
U.S. Brand Names Levothroid®; Levoxyl®; Synthroid®; Tirosint®; Unithroid®
Canadian Brand Names Eltroxin®; Euthyrox; Levothyroxine Sodium; Synthroid®
Therapeutic Category Thyroid Product
Use Replacement or supplemental therapy in hypothyroidism; pituitary TSH suppression
General Dosage Range

I.M.: *Children and Adults:* 50% of oral dose
I.V.:
Children: 50% of oral dose
Adults: 50% of oral dose or 200-500 mcg, then 100-300 mcg the next day if needed
Oral:
Children 1-3 months: 10-15 mcg/kg/day
Children 3-6 months: 8-10 mcg/kg/day
Children 6-12 months: 6-8 mcg/kg/day
Children 1-5 years: 5-6 mcg/kg/day
Children 6-12 years: 4-5 mcg/kg/day
Children >12 years: 2-3 mcg/kg/day
Adults: Initial: 12.5-25 mcg/day **or** 1.7 mcg/kg/day (usual doses are ≤200 mcg/day)
Elderly >50 years without cardiac disease ***or*** *<50 years with cardiac disease:* Initial: 25-50 mcg/day
Elderly >50 years with cardiac disease: Initial: 12.5-25 mcg/day

Dosage Forms

Capsule, soft gelatin, oral:
Tirosint®: 13 mcg, 25 mcg, 50 mcg, 75 mcg, 88 mcg, 100 mcg, 112 mcg, 125 mcg, 137 mcg, 150 mcg
Injection, powder for reconstitution: 100 mcg, 500 mcg
Tablet, oral: 25 mcg, 50 mcg, 75 mcg, 88 mcg, 100 mcg, 112 mcg, 125 mcg, 137 mcg, 150 mcg, 175 mcg, 200 mcg, 300 mcg
Levothroid®: 25 mcg, 50 mcg, 75 mcg, 88 mcg, 100 mcg, 112 mcg, 125 mcg, 137 mcg, 150 mcg, 175 mcg, 200 mcg, 300 mcg
Levoxyl®: 25 mcg, 50 mcg, 75 mcg, 88 mcg, 100 mcg, 112 mcg, 125 mcg, 137 mcg, 150 mcg, 175 mcg, 200 mcg
Synthroid®: 25 mcg, 50 mcg, 75 mcg, 88 mcg, 100 mcg, 112 mcg, 125 mcg, 137 mcg, 150 mcg, 175 mcg, 200 mcg, 300 mcg
Unithroid®: 25 mcg, 50 mcg, 75 mcg, 88 mcg, 100 mcg, 112 mcg, 125 mcg, 150 mcg, 175 mcg, 200 mcg, 300 mcg

levothyroxine and liothyronine *see* liotrix *on page 542*
levothyroxine and liothyronine *see* thyroid, desiccated *on page 893*
levothyroxine sodium *see* levothyroxine *on page 533*
Levothyroxine Sodium (Can) *see* levothyroxine *on page 533*
Levoxyl® *see* levothyroxine *on page 533*
Levsin® *see* hyoscyamine *on page 465*
Levsin®/SL *see* hyoscyamine *on page 465*
Lev-Tov [OTC] *see* folic acid, cyanocobalamin, and pyridoxine *on page 404*
Levulan® Kerastick® *see* aminolevulinic acid *on page 62*
levulose, dextrose and phosphoric acid *see* fructose, dextrose, and phosphoric acid *on page 411*
Lexapro® *see* escitalopram *on page 345*
Lexiscan® *see* regadenoson *on page 792*
Lexiva® *see* fosamprenavir *on page 407*
LFA-3/IgG(1) fusion protein, human *see* alefacept *on page 44*
LHRH *see* gonadorelin *(Canada only) on page 431*
***l*-hyoscyamine sulfate** *see* hyoscyamine *on page 465*
Lialda® *see* mesalamine *on page 577*
Librax® *see* clidinium and chlordiazepoxide *on page 218*
Librium *see* chlordiazepoxide *on page 196*
Licide® [OTC] *see* pyrethrins and piperonyl butoxide *on page 776*
LidaMantle® *see* lidocaine (topical) *on page 535*
LidaMantle HC® *see* lidocaine and hydrocortisone *on page 538*
LidaMantle HC® Relief Pad™ *see* lidocaine and hydrocortisone *on page 538*

Lidemol® (Can) *see* fluocinonide *on page* 392
Lidex *see* fluocinonide *on page* 392
Lidex® (Can) *see* fluocinonide *on page* 392

lidocaine (systemic) (LYE doe kane)

Medication Safety Issues

High alert medication:

The Institute for Safe Medication Practices (ISMP) includes this medication (epidural administration; I.V. formulation) among its list of drugs which have a heightened risk of causing significant patient harm when used in error.

International issues:

Lidosen [Italy] may be confused with Lincocin brand name for lincomycin [U.S., Canada, and multiple international markets]; Lodosyn brand name for carbidopa [U.S.]

Synonyms lidocaine hydrochloride; lignocaine hydrochloride

U.S. Brand Names Xylocaine®; Xylocaine® Dental; Xylocaine® MPF

Canadian Brand Names Xylocard®

Therapeutic Category Antiarrhythmic Agent, Class I-B; Local Anesthetic

Use Local and regional anesthesia by infiltration, nerve block, epidural, or spinal techniques; acute treatment of ventricular arrhythmias from myocardial infarction or cardiac manipulation

General Dosage Range Dosage adjustment recommended in patients with hepatic impairment.

I.V.:

Children: Loading dose: 1 mg/kg, may repeat 0.5-1 mg/kg; Infusion: 20-50 mcg/kg/minute

Adults: Bolus: 1-1.5 mg/kg, may repeat 0.5-0.75 mg/kg up to a total of 3 mg/kg; Infusion: 1-4 mg/minute

Local injection: *Children and Adults:* Maximum: 4.5 mg/kg/dose; do not repeat within 2 hours

Dosage Forms

Infusion, premixed in D_5W: 0.4% [4 mg/mL] (250 mL, 500 mL); 0.8% [8 mg/mL] (250 mL, 500 mL)

Injection, solution: 1% [10 mg/mL] (2 mL, 10 mL, 20 mL, 30 mL, 50 mL); 2% [20 mg/mL] (2 mL, 5 mL, 20 mL, 50 mL)

Xylocaine®: 0.5% [5 mg/mL] (50 mL); 1% [10 mg/mL] (10 mL, 20 mL, 50 mL); 2% [20 mg/mL] (10 mL, 20 mL, 50 mL)

Xylocaine® Dental: 2% [20 mg/mL] (1.8 mL)

Injection, solution [preservative free]: 0.5% [5 mg/mL] (50 mL); 1% [10 mg/mL] (2 mL, 5 mL, 30 mL); 1.5% [15 mg/mL] (20 mL); 2% [20 mg/mL] (2 mL, 5 mL, 10 mL); 4% [40 mg/mL] (5 mL)

Xylocaine®: 2% [20 mg/mL] (5 mL)

Xylocaine® MPF: 0.5% [5 mg/mL] (50 mL); 1% [10 mg/mL] (2 mL, 5 mL, 10 mL, 30 mL); 1.5% [15 mg/mL] (10 mL, 20 mL); 2% [20 mg/mL] (2 mL, 5 mL, 10 mL); 4% [40 mg/mL] (5 mL)

Injection, solution, premixed in $D_{7.5}W$ [preservative free]: 5% [50 mg/mL] (2 mL)

lidocaine (ophthalmic) (LYE doe kane)

Synonyms lidocaine hydrochloride; lignocaine hydrochloride

U.S. Brand Names Akten™

Therapeutic Category Local Anesthetic; Local Anesthetic, Ophthalmic

Use To provide local anesthesia to ocular surface during ophthalmologic procedures

General Dosage Range **Ophthalmic:** *Children and Adults:* 2 drops to ocular surface; may repeat to maintain effect

Dosage Forms

Gel, ophthalmic [preservative free]:

Akten™: 3.5% (5 mL)

lidocaine (topical) (LYE doe kane)

Synonyms lidocaine hydrochloride; lidocaine patch; lignocaine hydrochloride; Viscous Lidocaine; Xylocaine Viscous

U.S. Brand Names AneCream™ [OTC]; Anestafoam™ [OTC]; Band-Aid® Hurt Free™ Antiseptic Wash [OTC]; Burn Jel Plus [OTC]; Burn Jel® [OTC]; L-M-X® 4 [OTC]; L-M-X® 5 [OTC]; LidaMantle®; Lidoderm®; LidoPatch™ [OTC]; LTA® 360; Premjact®; RectiCare™ [OTC]; Regenecare®; Regenecare® HA [OTC]; Solarcaine® cool aloe Burn Relief [OTC]; Topicaine® [OTC]; Unburn® [OTC]; Xylocaine®

Canadian Brand Names Betacaine®; Lidodan™; Lidoderm®; Maxilene®; Xylocaine®

Therapeutic Category Analgesic, Topical; Local Anesthetic

Use

Rectal: Temporary relief of pain and itching due to anorectal disorders

Topical: Local anesthetic for oral mucous membrane; use in laser/cosmetic surgeries; minor burns, cuts, and abrasions of the skin

Oral topical solution (viscous): Topical anesthesia of irritated oral mucous membranes and pharyngeal tissue

Patch (Lidoderm®): Relief of allodynia (painful hypersensitivity) and chronic pain in postherpetic neuralgia

Patch (LidoPatch™): Temporary relief of localized pain

General Dosage Range Topical:

Cream: *Children and Adults:* Dosage varies greatly depending on product

Gel, ointment, solution: *Adults:* Apply to affected area ≤4 times/day as needed (maximum: 4.5 mg/kg/dose; 300 mg/dose)

Jelly:

Children: Maximum: 4.5 mg/kg/dose

Adults: 3-30 mL (maximum: 30 mL [600 mg]/12-hour period)

Oral topical solution (viscous):

Infants and Children <3 years: 1.25 mL applied no more frequently than every 3 hours (maximum: 4 doses per 12-hour period)

Children ≥3 years: Should not exceed 4.5 mg/kg/dose (or 300 mg/dose); swished in the mouth and spit out no more frequently than every 3 hours

Adults: 15 mL swished in the mouth and spit out or gargled no more frequently than every 3 hours (maximum: 8 doses per 24-hour period)

Patch: *Adults:*

Lidoderm®: Apply up to 3 patches in a single application for up to 12 hours in any 24-hour period

LidoPatch™: Apply 1 patch in a single application for up to 12 hours in any 24-hour period

Dosage Forms

Aerosol, foam, topical:

Anestafoam™ [OTC]: 4% (30 g)

Aerosol, spray, topical:

Solarcaine® cool aloe Burn Relief [OTC]: 0.5% (127 g)

Cream, rectal:

L-M-X® 5 [OTC]: 5% (15 g, 30 g)

Cream, topical: 0.5% (0.9 g)

AneCream™ [OTC]: 4% (5 g, 15 g, 30 g)

L-M-X® 4 [OTC]: 4% (5 g, 15 g, 30 g)

LidaMantle®: 3% (85 g)

RectiCare™ [OTC]: 5% (30 g)

Gel, topical:

Burn Jel Plus [OTC]: 2.5% (118 mL)

Burn Jel® [OTC]: 2% (59 mL, 118 mL); 2% (3.5 g)

Regenecare®: 2% (14 g, 85 g)

Regenecare® HA [OTC]: 2% (85 g)

Solarcaine® cool aloe Burn Relief [OTC]: 0.5% (113 g, 226 g)

Topicaine® [OTC]: 4% (10 g, 30 g, 113 g); 5% (10 g, 30 g, 113 g)

Unburn® [OTC]: 2.5% (59 mL)

Jelly, topical: 2% (5 mL, 30 mL)

Jelly, topical [preservative free]: 2% (5 mL, 10 mL, 20 mL)

Lotion, topical:

LidaMantle®: 3% (177 mL)

Ointment, topical: 5% (30 g, 35.4 g, 50 g)

Patch, topical:

Lidoderm®: 5% (30s)

LidoPatch™ [OTC]: 3.99% (3s)

Solution, topical: 4% [40 mg/mL] (50 mL)

Band-Aid® Hurt Free™ Antiseptic Wash [OTC]: 2% [20 mg/mL] (177 mL)

LTA® 360: 4% [40 mg/mL] (4 mL)

Premjact®: 9.6% (13 mL)

Xylocaine®: 4% [40 mg/mL] (50 mL)

Solution, topical [preservative free]: 4% [40 mg/mL] (4 mL)

Solution, viscous, oral topical: 2% [20 mg/mL] (20 mL, 100 mL, 500 mL)

lidocaine and chlorhexidine *(Canada only)* (LYE doe kane & klor HEKS i deen)

Synonyms chlorhexidine and lidocaine; lidocaine hydrochloride and chlorhexidine gluconate

Canadian Brand Names Instillagel®

Therapeutic Category Analgesic, Topical; Antibiotic, Topical; Local Anesthetic

Use To provide local anesthesia, lubrication, and antisepsis during urologic procedures including catheterization, cystoscopy, ultrasound or other intraurethral procedures

General Dosage Range Intraurethral:

Children <12 years: Maximum lidocaine dose: 6 mg/kg or 3 mL per 10 kg; maximum of 4 doses per 24-hour period

Children ≥12 years: Dose should correspond with the patient's weight and physical condition; maximum of 4 doses per 24-hour period

Adults: Instill 6 mL (females) or 6-39 mL (males) in 3-4 portions; maximum of 4 doses per 24-hour period

Product Availability Not available in the U.S.

Dosage Forms - Canada

Gel, topical:

Instillagel®: Lidocaine 2% and chlorhexidine 0.05% (6 mL, 11 mL)

lidocaine and epinephrine (LYE doe kane & ep i NEF rin)

Synonyms epinephrine and lidocaine

U.S. Brand Names Lignospan® Forte; Lignospan® Standard; Xylocaine® MPF With Epinephrine; Xylocaine® With Epinephrine

Canadian Brand Names Xylocaine® With Epinephrine

Therapeutic Category Local Anesthetic

Use Local infiltration anesthesia; AVS for nerve block

General Dosage Range Conduction block or infiltration (dental):

Children <12 years: 20-30 mg (1-1.5 mL) of 2% lidocaine with epinephrine 1:100,000 (maximum: 4.5 mg/kg of lidocaine or 100-150 mg as a single dose)

Children ≥12 years and Adults: Do not exceed 7 mg/kg body weight up to a maximum range of 300 mg (usual dental practice) to 500 mg (approved product labeling) of lidocaine hydrochloride and 3 mcg (0.003 mg) of epinephrine/kg of body weight **or** 0.2 mg epinephrine per dental appointment.

Dosage Forms

Injection, solution:

Generics:

0.5% / 1:200,000: Lidocaine hydrochloride 0.5% [5 mg/mL] and epinephrine 1:200,000 (50 mL)

1% / 1:100,000: Lidocaine hydrochloride 1% [10 mg/mL] and epinephrine 1:100,000 (20 mL, 30 mL, 50 mL)

2% / 1:100,000: Lidocaine hydrochloride 2% [20 mg/mL] and epinephrine 1:100,000 (30 mL, 50 mL)

Brands:

Xylocaine® with Epinephrine:

0.5% / 1:200,000: Lidocaine hydrochloride 0.5% [5 mg/mL] and epinephrine 1:200,000 (50 mL)

1% / 1:100,000: Lidocaine hydrochloride 1% [10 mg/mL] and epinephrine 1:100,000 (10 mL, 20 mL, 50 mL)

2% / 1:100,000: Lidocaine hydrochloride 2% [20 mg/mL] and epinephrine 1:100,000 (10 mL, 20 mL, 50 mL)

Injection, solution [preservative free]:

Generics:

1.5% / 1:200,000: Lidocaine hydrochloride 1.5% [15 mg/mL] and epinephrine 1:200,000 (5 mL, 30 mL)

2% / 1:200,000: Lidocaine hydrochloride 2% [20 mg/mL] and epinephrine 1:200,000 (20 mL)

Brands:

Xylocaine®-MPF with Epinephrine:

1% / 1:200,000: Lidocaine hydrochloride 1% [10 mg/mL] and epinephrine 1:200,000 (5 mL, 10 mL, 30 mL)

1.5% / 1:200,000: Lidocaine hydrochloride 1.5% [15 mg/mL] and epinephrine 1:200,000 (5 mL, 10 mL, 30 mL)

2% / 1:200,000: Lidocaine hydrochloride 2% [20 mg/mL] and epinephrine 1:200,000 (5 mL, 10 mL, 20 mL)

Injection, solution [for dental use]:

Generics:

2% / 1:50,000: Lidocaine hydrochloride 2% [20 mg/mL] and epinephrine 1:50,000 (1.7 mL, 1.8 mL)

2% / 1:100,000: Lidocaine hydrochloride 2% [20 mg/mL] and epinephrine 1:100,000 (1.7 mL, 1.8 mL)

Brands:

Lignospan® Forte: 2% / 1:50,000: Lidocaine hydrochloride 2% [20 mg/mL] and epinephrine 1:50,000 (1.7 mL)

Lignospan® Standard: 2% / 1:100,000: Lidocaine hydrochloride 2% [20 mg/mL] and epinephrine 1:100,000 (1.7 mL)

lidocaine and hydrocortisone (LYE doe kane & hye droe KOR ti sone)

Synonyms hydrocortisone and lidocaine

U.S. Brand Names AnaMantle HC® Cream; AnaMantle HC® Forte; AnaMantle HC® Gel; LidaMantle HC®; LidaMantle HC® Relief Pad™; LidoCort™; Peranex™ HC; Peranex™ HC Medi-Pad; RectaGel™ HC

Therapeutic Category Anesthetic/Corticosteroid

Use Topical antiinflammatory and anesthetic for skin disorders; rectal for the treatment of hemorrhoids, anal fissures, pruritus ani, or similar conditions

General Dosage Range

Rectal: *Adults:* 1 applicatorful twice daily

Topical: *Adults:* Apply 2-3 times/day

Dosage Forms

Cream, rectal: Lidocaine 3% and hydrocortisone 0.5% (7 g); lidocaine 3% and hydrocortisone 1% (7 g)

AnaMantle HC® Forte: Lidocaine 3% and hydrocortisone 1% (7 g)

AnaMantle HC®: Lidocaine 3% and hydrocortisone 0.5% (7 g)

Peranex™ HC: Lidocaine 2% and hydrocortisone 2% (7 g)

Cream, topical:

LidaMantle HC®: Lidocaine 3% and hydrocortisone 0.5% (85 g)

Gel, rectal: Lidocaine 3% and hydrocortisone 2.5% (7 g)

AnaMantle HC®, LidoCort™: Lidocaine 3% and hydrocortisone 2.5% (7 g)

RectaGel™ HC: Lidocaine 2.8% and hydrocortisone 0.55% (20 g)

Lotion, topical:

LidaMantle HC®: Lidocaine 3% and hydrocortisone 0.5% (177 mL)

Pad, topical:

LidaMantel HC® Relief Pad™: Lidocaine 2% and hydrocortisone 2% (60s)

Peranex™ HC Medi-Pad: Lidocaine 3% and hydrocortisone 1% (60s)

lidocaine and prilocaine (LYE doe kane & PRIL oh kane)

Synonyms prilocaine and lidocaine

U.S. Brand Names EMLA®; Oraqix®

Canadian Brand Names EMLA®

Therapeutic Category Analgesic, Topical

Use

Topical anesthetic for use on normal intact skin to provide local analgesia for minor procedures such as I.V. cannulation or venipuncture; has also been used for painful procedures such as lumbar puncture and skin graft harvesting; for superficial minor surgery of genital mucous membranes and as an adjunct for local infiltration anesthesia in genital mucous membranes.

Periodontal gel: Topical anesthetic for use in periodontal pockets during scaling or root planning procedures

General Dosage Range

Periodontal: *Adults:* Maximum recommended dose: 1 treatment session: 5 cartridges (8.5 g)

Topical, cream:

Children 0-3 months or <5 kg: Apply up to 1 g over no more than 10 cm^2 of skin for no longer than 1 hour

Children 3-12 months and >5 kg: Apply up to 2 g total over no more than 20 cm^2 of skin for no longer than 4 hours

Children 1-6 years and >10 kg: Apply up to 10 g total over no more than 100 cm^2 of skin for no longer than 4 hours

Children 7-12 years and >20 kg: Apply up to 20 g total over no more than 200 cm^2 of skin for no longer than 4 hours
Adults: Apply 2-2.5 g per 10-25 cm^2 of skin for at least 1-2 hours **or** 5-10 g for 5-10 minutes
Adults (males): Apply 1 g/10 cm^2 for 15 minutes

Dosage Forms
Cream, topical: Lidocaine 2.5% and prilocaine 2.5% (5 g, 30 g)
EMLA®: Lidocaine 2.5% and prilocaine 2.5% (5 g, 30 g)
Gel, periodontal:
Oraqix®: Lidocaine 2.5% and prilocaine 2.5% (1.7 g)

Dosage Forms - Canada
Patch, transdermal:
EMLA® Patch: Lidocaine 2.5% and prilocaine 2.5% per patch (2s, 20s)

lidocaine and tetracaine (LYE doe kane & TET ra kane)

Medication Safety Issues
Other safety concerns:
Transdermal patch may contain conducting metal (eg, aluminum); remove patch prior to MRI.

Synonyms eutectic mixture of lidocaine and tetracaine; tetracaine and lidocaine

U.S. Brand Names Synera®

Therapeutic Category Analgesic, Topical; Local Anesthetic

Use Topical anesthetic for use on normal intact skin for minor procedures (eg, I.V. cannulation or venipuncture) and superficial dermatologic procedures

General Dosage Range Topical: *Children ≥3 years and Adults:* Apply patch to intact skin for 20-30 minutes, prior to procedure

Dosage Forms
Patch, transdermal:
Synera®: Lidocaine 70 mg and tetracaine 70 mg (10s)

lidocaine hydrochloride *see* lidocaine (ophthalmic) *on page* 535
lidocaine hydrochloride *see* lidocaine (systemic) *on page* 535
lidocaine hydrochloride *see* lidocaine (topical) *on page* 535
lidocaine hydrochloride and chlorhexidine gluconate *see* lidocaine and chlorhexidine *(Canada only) on page* 537
lidocaine patch *see* lidocaine (topical) *on page* 535
LidoCort™ *see* lidocaine and hydrocortisone *on page* 538
Lidodan™ (Can) *see* lidocaine (topical) *on page* 535
Lidoderm® *see* lidocaine (topical) *on page* 535
LidoPatch™ [OTC] *see* lidocaine (topical) *on page* 535
LID-Pack® (Can) *see* bacitracin and polymyxin B *on page* 111
lignocaine hydrochloride *see* lidocaine (ophthalmic) *on page* 535
lignocaine hydrochloride *see* lidocaine (systemic) *on page* 535
lignocaine hydrochloride *see* lidocaine (topical) *on page* 535
Lignospan® Forte *see* lidocaine and epinephrine *on page* 537
Lignospan® Standard *see* lidocaine and epinephrine *on page* 537
Limbitrol *see* amitriptyline and chlordiazepoxide *on page* 64
Limbrel™ [DSC] *see* flavocoxid *on page* 385
Limbrel 250™ *see* flavocoxid *on page* 385
Limbrel 500™ *see* flavocoxid *on page* 385

linagliptin (lin a GLIP tin)

Medication Safety Issues
High alert medication:
The Institute for Safe Medication Practices (ISMP) includes this medication among its list of drug classes which have a heightened risk of causing significant patient harm when used in error.

Synonyms BI-1356

U.S. Brand Names Tradjenta™

Canadian Brand Names Trajenta™

Therapeutic Category Antidiabetic Agent, Dipeptidyl Peptidase IV (DPP-IV) Inhibitor

Use Management of type 2 diabetes mellitus (noninsulin dependent, NIDDM) as an adjunct to diet and exercise as monotherapy or in combination with other antidiabetic agents

General Dosage Range Oral: *Adults:* 5 mg once daily

Concomitant use with insulin and/or insulin secretagogues (eg, sulfonylureas): Reduced dose of insulin and/or insulin secretagogues may be needed.

Dosage Forms

Tablet, oral:

Tradjenta™: 5 mg

linagliptin and metformin (lin a GLIP tin & met FOR min)

Medication Safety Issues

Sound-alike/look-alike issues:

Linagliptin and Metformin may be confused with Sitagliptin and Metformin

High alert medication:

The Institute for Safe Medication Practices (ISMP) includes this medication among its list of drug classes which have a heightened risk of causing significant patient harm when used in error.

Synonyms linagliptin and metformin hydrochloride; metformin and linagliptin; metformin hydrochloride and linagliptin

U.S. Brand Names Jentadueto™

Therapeutic Category Antidiabetic Agent, Biguanide; Antidiabetic Agent, Dipeptidyl Peptidase IV (DPP-IV) Inhibitor

Use Management of type 2 diabetes mellitus (noninsulin dependent, NIDDM) as an adjunct to diet and exercise in patients not adequately controlled on metformin or linagliptin monotherapy

General Dosage Range Oral: *Adults:* Linagliptin 2.5 mg and metformin 500-1000 mg twice daily (maximum: 5 mg/day [linagliptin], 2000 mg/day [metformin])

Dosage Forms

Tablet, oral:

Jentadueto™ 2.5/500: Linagliptin 2.5 mg and metformin 500 mg
Jentadueto™ 2.5/850: Linagliptin 2.5 mg and metformin 850 mg
Jentadueto™ 2.5/1000: Linagliptin 2.5 mg and metformin 1000 mg

linagliptin and metformin hydrochloride *see* linagliptin and metformin *on page* 540
Lincocin® *see* lincomycin *on page* 540

lincomycin (lin koe MYE sin)

Medication Safety Issues

Sound-alike/look-alike issues:

Lincocin® may be confused with Cleocin®, Indocin®, Minocin®

International issues:

Lincocin [U.S., Canada, and multiple international markets] may be confused with Lidosen brand name for lidocaine [Italy] and Limoxin brand name for ambroxol [Indonesia]; amoxicillin [Mexico]

Synonyms lincomycin hydrochloride

U.S. Brand Names Lincocin®

Canadian Brand Names Lincocin®

Therapeutic Category Antibiotic, Lincosamide

Use Treatment of serious susceptible bacterial infections, mainly those caused by streptococci, pneumococci, and staphylococci resistant to other agents

General Dosage Range Dosage adjustment recommended in patients with renal impairment

I.M.:

Children >1 month: 10 mg/kg every 12-24 hours
Adults: 600 mg every 12-24 hours

I.V.:

Children >1 month: 10-20 mg/kg/day divided every 8-12 hours
Adults: 600 mg to 1 g every 8-12 hours (maximum: 8 g/day)

Subconjunctival injection: *Adults:* 75 mg

Dosage Forms

Injection, solution:

Lincocin®: 300 mg/mL (2 mL, 10 mL)

lincomycin hydrochloride *see* lincomycin *on page* 540

lindane (LIN dane)

Synonyms benzene hexachloride; gamma benzene hexachloride; hexachlorocyclohexane

Canadian Brand Names Hexit™; PMS-Lindane

Therapeutic Category Scabicides/Pediculicides

Use Treatment of *Sarcoptes scabiei* (scabies), *Pediculus capitis* (head lice), and *Phthirus pubis* (crab lice); FDA recommends reserving lindane as a second-line agent or with inadequate response to other therapies

General Dosage Range Topical:

Lotion: *Children and Adults:* Apply a thin layer; bathe and remove drug after 8-12 hours
Shampoo: *Children and Adults:* Apply to dry hair (maximum: 60 mL)

Dosage Forms

Lotion, topical: 1% (60 mL)
Shampoo, topical: 1% (60 mL)

Linessa® (Can) *see* ethinyl estradiol and desogestrel *on page* 356

linezolid (li NE zoh lid)

Medication Safety Issues

Sound-alike/look-alike issues:

Zyvox® may be confused with Zosyn®, Zovirax®

U.S. Brand Names Zyvox®

Canadian Brand Names Zyvoxam®

Therapeutic Category Antibiotic, Oxazolidinone

Use Treatment of vancomycin-resistant *Enterococcus faecium* (VRE) infections, nosocomial pneumonia caused by *Staphylococcus aureus* (including MRSA) or *Streptococcus pneumoniae* (including multidrug-resistant strains [MDRSP]), complicated and uncomplicated skin and skin structure infections (including diabetic foot infections without concomitant osteomyelitis), and community-acquired pneumonia caused by susceptible gram-positive organisms

General Dosage Range

I.V.:

Children ≤11 years: 10 mg/kg (maximum dose: 600 mg) every 8 hours
Children ≥12 years and Adults: 600 mg every 12 hours

Oral:

Children <5 years: 10 mg/kg every 8 hours (maximum: 600 mg/dose)
Children 5-11 years: 10 mg/kg every 8-12 hours (maximum: 600 mg/dose)
Children ≥12 years and Adults: 400-600 mg every 12 hours

Dosage Forms

Infusion, premixed:
Zyvox®: 200 mg (100 mL); 600 mg (300 mL)

Powder for suspension, oral:
Zyvox®: 100 mg/5 mL (150 mL)

Tablet, oral:
Zyvox®: 600 mg

Lioresal® *see* baclofen *on page* 112

Lioresal® D.S. (Can) *see* baclofen *on page* 112

Lioresal® Intrathecal (Can) *see* baclofen *on page* 112

liothyronine (lye oh THYE roe neen)

Medication Safety Issues

Sound-alike/look-alike issues:

Liothyronine may be confused with levothyroxine

Other safety concerns:

T3 is an error-prone abbreviation (mistaken as acetaminophen and codeine [ie, Tylenol® #3])

Synonyms liothyronine sodium; sodium *L*-triiodothyronine; T_3 sodium (error-prone abbreviation)

U.S. Brand Names Cytomel®; Triostat®

Canadian Brand Names Cytomel®

Therapeutic Category Thyroid Product

Use

Oral: Replacement or supplemental therapy in hypothyroidism; management of nontoxic goiter; a diagnostic aid

I.V.: Treatment of myxedema coma/precoma

General Dosage Range

I.V.: *Adults:* 10-50 mcg/dose

Oral:

Infants: Initial: 5 mcg/day; Usual maintenance dose: 20 mcg/day

Children 1-3 years: Initial: 5 mcg/day; Usual maintenance dose: 50 mcg/day

Children >3 years: Initial: 5 mcg/day; Maintenance: Up to 100 mcg/day

Adults: Initial 5-25 mcg/day; Maintenance range 5-100 mcg/day

Elderly: Initial: 5 mcg/day

Dosage Forms

Injection, solution: 10 mcg/mL (1 mL)

Triostat®: 10 mcg/mL (1 mL)

Tablet, oral: 5 mcg, 25 mcg, 50 mcg

Cytomel®: 5 mcg, 25 mcg, 50 mcg

liothyronine and levothyroxine *see* liotrix *on page* *542*

liothyronine sodium *see* liothyronine *on page* *541*

liotrix (LYE oh triks)

Medication Safety Issues

Sound-alike/look-alike issues:

Liotrix may be confused with Klotrix®

Thyrolar® may be confused with Thyrogen®

Synonyms levothyroxine and liothyronine; liothyronine and levothyroxine; T_3/T_4 liotrix

U.S. Brand Names Thyrolar®

Canadian Brand Names Thyrolar®

Therapeutic Category Thyroid Product

Use

Replacement or supplemental therapy in hypothyroidism (uniform mixture of T_4:T_3 in 4:1 ratio by weight)

Thyroid-stimulating hormone (TSH) suppressant therapy used in the management of thyroid cancer (levothyroxine is generally recommended for this indication); prevention or treatment of euthyroid goiters (eg, thyroid nodules, subacute or chronic lymphocytic thyroiditis [Hashimoto], multinodular goiters)

Diagnostic agent in suppression tests to diagnose suspected mild hyperthyroidism or to demonstrate thyroid gland autonomy

General Dosage Range Oral:

Children 0-6 months: Levothyroxine 12.5-25 mcg/Liothyronine 3.1-6.25 mcg once daily

Children 6-12 months: Levothyroxine 25-37.5 mcg/Liothyronine 6.25-9.35 mcg once daily

Children 1-5 years: Levothyroxine 37.5-50 mcg/Liothyronine 9.35-12.5 mcg once daily

Children 6-12 years: Levothyroxine 50-75 mcg/Liothyronine 12.5-18.75 mcg once daily

Children >12 years: Levothyroxine 75 mcg/Liothyronine 18.75 mcg once daily

Adults: Initial: Levothyroxine 25 mcg/Liothyronine 6.25 mcg once daily; Usual maintenance: Levothyroxine 50-100 mcg/Liothyronine 12.5-25 mcg once daily

Elderly: Initial: Levothyroxine 12.5-25 mcg/Liothyronine 3.1-6.25 mcg once daily

Dosage Forms

Tablet, oral:

Thyrolar®:

1/4 [levothyroxine 12.5 mcg and liothyronine 3.1 mcg]

1/2 [levothyroxine 25 mcg and liothyronine 6.25 mcg]

1 [levothyroxine 50 mcg and liothyronine 12.5 mcg]

2 [levothyroxine 100 mcg and liothyronine 25 mcg]

3 [levothyroxine 150 mcg and liothyronine 37.5 mcg]

lipancreatin *see* pancrelipase *on page* *687*

lipase, protease, and amylase *see* pancrelipase *on page* *687*

lipiarrmycin *see* fidaxomicin *on page* *383*

Lipidil EZ® (Can) *see* fenofibrate *on page* *375*

Lipidil Micro® (Can) *see* fenofibrate *on page* *375*

Lipidil Supra® (Can) *see* fenofibrate *on page* 375
Lipitor® *see* atorvastatin *on page* 100
Lipodox *see* doxorubicin (liposomal) *on page* 314
Lipofen® *see* fenofibrate *on page* 375
liposomal bupivacaine *see* bupivacaine (liposomal) *on page* 149
liposomal cytarabine *see* cytarabine (liposomal) *on page* 248
liposomal DAUNOrubicin *see* daunorubicin (liposomal) *on page* 257
liposomal DOXOrubicin *see* doxorubicin (liposomal) *on page* 314
liposome vincristine *see* vincristine (liposomal) *on page* 947
Liposyn® II (Can) *see* fat emulsion *on page* 373
Liposyn® III *see* fat emulsion *on page* 373
Liqua-Cal [OTC] *see* calcium and vitamin D *on page* 161
Liquibid® D-R [OTC] *see* guaifenesin and phenylephrine *on page* 435
Liquibid® PD-R [OTC] *see* guaifenesin and phenylephrine *on page* 435
liquid antidote *see* charcoal, activated *on page* 193
Liquid Entero Vu™ *see* barium *on page* 114
Liquid Polibar® *see* barium *on page* 114
Liquid Polibar Plus® *see* barium *on page* 114
Liquituss GG [OTC] *see* guaifenesin *on page* 433

liraglutide (lir a GLOO tide)

Medication Safety Issues

Other safety concerns:

Cross-contamination may occur if pens are shared among multiple patients. Steps should be taken to prohibit sharing of pens.

Synonyms NN2211

U.S. Brand Names Victoza®

Canadian Brand Names Victoza®

Therapeutic Category Antidiabetic Agent, Glucagon-Like Peptide-1 (GLP-1) Receptor Agonist

Use Treatment of type 2 diabetes mellitus (noninsulin-dependent, NIDDM) to improve glycemic control

General Dosage Range SubQ: *Adults:* Initial: 0.6 mg once daily; maintenance: 1.2-1.8 mg/day

Dosage Forms

Injection, solution:

Victoza®: 6 mg/mL (3 mL)

lisdexamfetamine (lis dex am FET a meen)

Medication Safety Issues

Sound-alike/look-alike issues:

Vyvanse® may be confused with Visanne®, ViVAXIM®, Vytorin®, Glucovance®, Vivactil®

Synonyms lisdexamfetamine dimesylate; lisdexamphetamine; NRP104

U.S. Brand Names Vyvanse®

Canadian Brand Names Vyvanse®

Therapeutic Category Stimulant

Controlled Substance C-II

Use Treatment of attention-deficit/hyperactivity disorder (ADHD)

General Dosage Range Oral: *Children ≥6 years and Adults:* Initial: 30 mg once daily; Maintenance: Up to 70 mg once daily

Dosage Forms

Capsule, oral:

Vyvanse®: 20 mg, 30 mg, 40 mg, 50 mg, 60 mg, 70 mg

lisdexamfetamine dimesylate *see* lisdexamfetamine *on page* 543
lisdexamphetamine *see* lisdexamfetamine *on page* 543

lisinopril (lyse IN oh pril)

Medication Safety Issues

Sound-alike/look-alike issues:

Lisinopril may be confused with fosinopril, Lioresal®, Lipitor®, RisperDAL®

Prinivil® may be confused with Plendil®, Pravachol®, Prevacid®, PriLOSEC®, Proventil®

Zestril® may be confused with Desyrel, Restoril™, Vistaril®, Zegerid®, Zerit®, Zetia®, Zostrix®, ZyPREXA®

International issues:

Acepril [Malaysia] may be confused with Accupril which is a brand name for quinapril [U.S.]

Acepril: Brand name for lisinopril [Malaysia], but also the brand name for captopril [Great Britain]; enalapril [Hungary, Switzerland]

U.S. Brand Names Prinivil®; Zestril®

Canadian Brand Names Apo-Lisinopril®; CO Lisinopril; Dom-Lisinopril; JAMP-Lisinopril; Mint-Lisinopril; Mylan-Lisinopril; PMS-Lisinopril; Prinivil®; PRO-Lisinopril; RAN™-Lisinopril; ratio-Lisinopril; ratio-Lisinopril P; ratio-Lisinopril Z; Riva-Lisinopril; Sandoz-Lisinopril; Teva-Lisinopril (Type P); Teva-Lisinopril (Type Z); Zestril®

Therapeutic Category Angiotensin-Converting Enzyme (ACE) Inhibitor

Use Treatment of hypertension, either alone or in combination with other antihypertensive agents; adjunctive therapy in treatment of heart failure (afterload reduction); treatment of acute myocardial infarction within 24 hours in hemodynamically-stable patients to improve survival; treatment of left ventricular dysfunction after myocardial infarction

General Dosage Range Dosage adjustment recommended in patients with renal impairment

Oral:

Children ≥6 years: Initial: 0.07 mg/kg once daily (up to 5 mg); Maintenance: Maximum: Doses >0.61 mg/kg or >40 mg have not been evaluated

Adults: Initial: 2.5-10 mg/day; Maintenance: 10-80 mg/day

Elderly: Initial: 2.5-5 mg/day (maximum: 40 mg/day)

Dosage Forms

Tablet, oral: 2.5 mg, 5 mg, 10 mg, 20 mg, 30 mg, 40 mg

Prinivil®: 5 mg, 10 mg, 20 mg

Zestril®: 2.5 mg, 5 mg, 10 mg, 20 mg, 30 mg, 40 mg

lisinopril and hydrochlorothiazide (lyse IN oh pril & hye droe klor oh THYE a zide)

Synonyms hydrochlorothiazide and lisinopril

U.S. Brand Names Prinzide®; Zestoretic®

Canadian Brand Names Apo-Lisinopril®/Hctz; Mylan-Lisinopril/Hctz; Novo-Lisinopril/Hctz; Prinzide®; Sandoz-Lisinopril/Hctz; Teva-Lisinopril/Hctz (Type P); Teva-Lisinopril/Hctz (Type Z); Zestoretic®

Therapeutic Category Antihypertensive Agent, Combination

Use Treatment of hypertension

General Dosage Range Oral: *Adults:* Lisinopril 10-80 mg and hydrochlorothiazide 12.5-50 mg once daily

Dosage Forms

Tablet, oral: 10/12.5: Lisinopril 10 mg and hydrochlorothiazide 12.5 mg; 20/12.5: Lisinopril 20 mg and hydrochlorothiazide 12.5 mg; 20/25: Lisinopril 20 mg and hydrochlorothiazide 25 mg

Prinzide®:

10/12.5: Lisinopril 10 mg and hydrochlorothiazide 12.5 mg

20/12.5: Lisinopril 20 mg and hydrochlorothiazide 12.5 mg

Zestoretic®:

10/12.5: Lisinopril 10 mg and hydrochlorothiazide 12.5 mg

20/12.5: Lisinopril 20 mg and hydrochlorothiazide 12.5 mg

20/25: Lisinopril 20 mg and hydrochlorothiazide 25 mg

lispro insulin *see* insulin lispro *on page 487*

Lithane™ (Can) *see* lithium *on page 544*

lithium (LITH ee um)

Medication Safety Issues

Sound-alike/look-alike issues:

Eskalith may be confused with Estratest

Lithium may be confused with lanthanum

Lithobid® may be confused with Levbid®, Lithostat®

Other safety concerns:

Do not confuse **mEq** (milliequivalent) with **mg** (milligram). **Note:** 300 mg lithium carbonate or citrate contain 8 mEq lithium. Dosage should be written in **mg** (milligrams) to avoid confusion.

Check prescriptions for unusually high volumes of the syrup for dosing errors.

Synonyms Eskalith; lithium carbonate; lithium citrate

U.S. Brand Names Lithobid®

Canadian Brand Names Apo-Lithium® Carbonate; Apo-Lithium® Carbonate SR; Carbolith™; Duralith®; Euro-Lithium; Lithane™; Lithmax; PHL-Lithium Carbonate; PMS-Lithium Carbonate; PMS-Lithium Citrate

Therapeutic Category Antimanic Agent

Use Management of bipolar disorders; treatment of mania in individuals with bipolar disorder (maintenance treatment prevents or diminishes intensity of subsequent episodes)

General Dosage Range Dosage adjustment recommended in patients with renal impairment

Oral:

Immediate release:

Adults: 900-2400 mg/day in 3-4 divided doses

Elderly: Initial: 300 mg twice daily (maximum: >900-1200 mg/day)

Extended release: *Adults:* 900-1800 mg/day in 2 divided doses

Dosage Forms

Capsule, oral: 150 mg, 300 mg, 600 mg

Solution, oral: 300 mg/5 mL (500 mL)

Tablet, oral: 300 mg, 600 mg

Tablet, extended release, oral: 300 mg, 450 mg

Lithobid®: 300 mg

lithium carbonate *see* lithium *on page 544*

lithium citrate *see* lithium *on page 544*

Lithmax (Can) *see* lithium *on page 544*

Lithobid® *see* lithium *on page 544*

Lithostat® *see* acetohydroxamic acid *on page 31*

Little Fevers™ [OTC] *see* acetaminophen *on page 20*

Little Noses® Decongestant [OTC] *see* phenylephrine (nasal) *on page 716*

Little Noses® Saline [OTC] *see* sodium chloride *on page 840*

Little Noses® Sterile Saline Nasal Mist [OTC] *see* sodium chloride *on page 840*

Little Noses® Stuffy Nose Kit [OTC] *see* sodium chloride *on page 840*

Little Phillips'® Milk of Magnesia [OTC] *see* magnesium hydroxide *on page 558*

Little Teethers® [OTC] *see* benzocaine *on page 121*

Little Tummys® Gas Relief [OTC] *see* simethicone *on page 834*

Little Tummys® Laxative [OTC] *see* senna *on page 829*

Livalo® *see* pitavastatin *on page 728*

live attenuated influenza vaccine *see* influenza virus vaccine (live/attenuated) *on page 484*

live smallpox vaccine *see* smallpox vaccine *on page 839*

Livostin® (Can) *see* levocabastine (nasal) *(Canada only) on page 529*

Livostin® Eye Drops (Can) *see* levocabastine (ophthalmic) *(Canada only) on page 530*

L-leucovorin *see* LEVOleucovorin *on page 532*

l-lysine (el LYE seen)

Synonyms l-lysine hydrochloride

U.S. Brand Names Lysinyl [OTC]

Therapeutic Category Dietary Supplement

Use Improves utilization of vegetable proteins; prevention of recurrent herpes simplex infection

General Dosage Range Oral: *Adults:* 334-1500 mg/day

Dosage Forms

Capsule, oral: 500 mg

Lysinyl [OTC]: 500 mg

Powder, oral: (100 g)

Lysinyl [OTC]: (150 g)

Tablet, oral: 500 mg, 1000 mg

l-lysine hydrochloride *see* l-lysine *on page 545*
LM3100 *see* plerixafor *on page 729*
LMD® *see* dextran *on page 270*
10% LMD *see* dextran *on page 270*
L-methylfolate *see* methylfolate *on page 589*
L-methylfolate, methylcobalamin, and N-acetylcysteine *see* methylfolate, methylcobalamin, and acetylcysteine *on page 590*
LNg 20 *see* levonorgestrel *on page 533*
Locacorten® Vioform® (Can) *see* clioquinol and flumethasone *(Canada only) on page 220*
Locoid® *see* hydrocortisone (topical) *on page 457*
Locoid Lipocream® *see* hydrocortisone (topical) *on page 457*
Lodine *see* etodolac *on page 365*
Lodosyn® *see* carbidopa *on page 174*

lodoxamide (loe DOKS a mide)

Medication Safety Issues

International issues:

Thilomide [Greece, Turkey] may be confused with Thalomid brand name for thalidomide [U.S., Canada]

Synonyms lodoxamide tromethamine

U.S. Brand Names Alomide®

Canadian Brand Names Alomide®

Therapeutic Category Mast Cell Stabilizer

Use Treatment of vernal keratoconjunctivitis, vernal conjunctivitis, and vernal keratitis

General Dosage Range Ophthalmic: *Children >2 years and Adults:* Instill 1-2 drops in eye(s) 4 times/day

Dosage Forms

Solution, ophthalmic:

Alomide®: 0.1% (10 mL)

lodoxamide tromethamine *see* lodoxamide *on page 546*
Lodrane® D [OTC] *see* brompheniramine and pseudoephedrine *on page 144*
Loestrin™ 1.5/30 (Can) *see* ethinyl estradiol and norethindrone *on page 359*
Loestrin® 21 1.5/30 *see* ethinyl estradiol and norethindrone *on page 359*
Loestrin® 21 1/20 *see* ethinyl estradiol and norethindrone *on page 359*
Loestrin® 24 Fe *see* ethinyl estradiol and norethindrone *on page 359*
Loestrin® Fe 1.5/30 *see* ethinyl estradiol and norethindrone *on page 359*
Loestrin® Fe 1/20 *see* ethinyl estradiol and norethindrone *on page 359*
Lo-Femenal 21 (Can) *see* ethinyl estradiol and norgestrel *on page 362*
Lofibra® *see* fenofibrate *on page 375*
LoHist [OTC] *see* chlorpheniramine and phenylephrine *on page 200*
LoHist-12 [DSC] *see* brompheniramine *on page 143*
LoHist-D [OTC] *see* chlorpheniramine and pseudoephedrine *on page 200*
LoHist PEB [OTC] *see* brompheniramine and phenylephrine *on page 144*
LoHist PSB [OTC] *see* brompheniramine and pseudoephedrine *on page 144*
LoHist PSB DM [OTC] *see* brompheniramine, pseudoephedrine, and dextromethorphan *on page 144*
L-OHP *see* oxaliplatin *on page 674*
LoKara™ *see* desonide *on page 265*
Lo Loestrin™ Fe *see* ethinyl estradiol and norethindrone *on page 359*
Lomotil® *see* diphenoxylate and atropine *on page 295*

lomustine (loe MUS teen)

Medication Safety Issues

Sound-alike/look-alike issues:

Lomustine may be confused with bendamustine, carmustine

High alert medication:

This medication is in a class the Institute for Safe Medication Practices (ISMP) includes among its list of drug classes which have a heightened risk of causing significant patient harm when used in error.

Administration issues:

Lomustine should only be administered as a single dose once every 6 weeks; serious errors have occurred when lomustine was inadvertently administered daily.

Synonyms CCNU; lomustinum

U.S. Brand Names CeeNU®

Canadian Brand Names CeeNU®

Therapeutic Category Antineoplastic Agent

Use Treatment of primary and metastatic brain tumors (after surgery and/or radiation therapy); treatment of relapsed or refractory Hodgkin disease (as part of a combination chemotherapy regimen)

General Dosage Range Dosage adjustment recommended in patients with renal impairment or who develop toxicities

Oral: *Children and Adults:* 100-130 mg/m^2 as a single dose once every 6 weeks

Dosage Forms

Capsule, oral:

CeeNU®: 10 mg, 40 mg, 100 mg

lomustinum *see* lomustine *on page* 547

longastatin *see* octreotide *on page* 658

Loniten® (Can) *see* minoxidil (systemic) *on page* 605

Lo Ovral *see* ethinyl estradiol and norgestrel *on page* 362

Lo/Ovral®-28 *see* ethinyl estradiol and norgestrel *on page* 362

Loperacap (Can) *see* loperamide *on page* 547

loperamide (loe PER a mide)

Medication Safety Issues

Sound-alike/look-alike issues:

Imodium® A-D may be confused with Indocin®

Loperamide may be confused with furosemide, Lomotil®

International issues:

Indiaral [France] may be confused with Inderal and Inderal LA brand names for propranolol [U.S., Canada, and multiple international markets]

Lomotil: Brand name for loperamide [Mexico, Philippines], but also the brand name for diphenoxylate [U.S., Canada, and multiple international markets]

Lomotil [Mexico, Phillipines] may be confused with Ludiomil brand name for maprotiline [multiple international markets]

Synonyms loperamide hydrochloride

U.S. Brand Names Anti-Diarrheal [OTC]; Diamode [OTC]; Imodium® A-D EZ Chews [OTC]; Imodium® A-D for children [OTC]; Imodium® A-D [OTC]

Canadian Brand Names Apo-Loperamide®; Diarr-Eze; Dom-Loperamide; Imodium®; Loperacap; Novo-Loperamide; PMS-Loperamine; Rhoxal-loperamide; Rho®-Loperamine; Riva-Loperamide; Sandoz-Loperamide

Therapeutic Category Antidiarrheal

Use Control and symptomatic relief of chronic diarrhea associated with inflammatory bowel disease and of acute nonspecific diarrhea; to reduce volume of ileostomy discharge

OTC labeling: Control of symptoms of diarrhea, including Traveler's diarrhea

General Dosage Range Oral:

Children 2-5 years (13-20 kg): Initial: 1 mg 3 times/day for first 24 hours; Maintenance: 0.1 mg/kg after each loose stool

Children 6-8 years (20-30 kg): Initial: 2 mg twice daily for first 24 hours; Maintenance: 0.1 mg/kg after each loose stool **or** 2 mg after first loose stool, followed by 1 mg after each subsequent stool (maximum: 4 mg/day)

Children 8-12 years (>30 kg): Initial: 2 mg 3 times/day for first 24 hours; Maintenance: 0.1 mg/kg after each loose stool

Children 9-11 years: 2 mg after first loose stool, followed by 1 mg after each subsequent stool (maximum: 6 mg/day)

Children ≥12 years: Initial: 4 mg after first loose stool, followed by 2 mg after each subsequent stool (maximum: 8 mg/day)

Adults: Initial: 4 mg followed by 2 mg after each loose stool (maximum: 8-16 mg/day) **or** 4-8 mg/day in divided doses

Dosage Forms

Caplet, oral: 2 mg
- Anti-Diarrheal [OTC]: 2 mg
- Diamode [OTC]: 2 mg
- Imodium® A-D [OTC]: 2 mg

Capsule, oral: 2 mg

Liquid, oral: 1 mg/7.5 mL (120 mL)
- Imodium® A-D [OTC]: 1 mg/7.5 mL (120 mL, 240 mL)
- Imodium® A-D for children [OTC]: 1 mg/7.5 mL (120 mL)

Solution, oral: 1 mg/5 mL (5 mL, 10 mL, 118 mL, 120 mL)
- Anti-Diarrheal [OTC]: 1 mg/5 mL (120 mL)

Tablet, chewable, oral:
- Imodium® A-D EZ Chews [OTC]: 2 mg

loperamide and simethicone (loe PER a mide & sye METH i kone)

Synonyms simethicone and loperamide hydrochloride

U.S. Brand Names Imodium® Multi-Symptom Relief [OTC]

Canadian Brand Names Imodium® Advanced Multi-Symptom

Therapeutic Category Antidiarrheal; Antiflatulent

Use Control of symptoms of diarrhea and gas (bloating, pressure, and cramps)

General Dosage Range Oral:

Children 6-8 years (48-59 lbs): 1 caplet/tablet after first loose stool, followed by 1/2 caplet/tablet with each subsequent loose stool (maximum: 2 caplets or tablets/24 hours)

Children 9-11 years (60-95 lbs): 1 caplet/tablet after first loose stool, followed by 1/2 caplet/tablet with each subsequent loose stool (maximum: 3 caplets or tablets/24 hours)

Children ≥12 years and Adults: 1 caplet/tablet after each loose stool (maximum: 4 caplets or tablets/24 hours)

Dosage Forms

Caplet:
- Imodium® Multi-Symptom Relief: Loperamide hydrochloride 2 mg and simethicone 125 mg

Tablet, chewable:
- Imodium® Muliti-Symptom Relief: Loperamide hydrochloride 2 mg and simethicone 125 mg

loperamide hydrochloride *see* loperamide *on page* 547

Lopid® *see* gemfibrozil *on page* 422

lopinavir and ritonavir (loe PIN a veer & rit ON uh veer)

Medication Safety Issues

Sound-alike/look-alike issues:

Potential for dispensing errors between Kaletra® and Keppra® (levETIRAcetam)

Administration issues:

Children's doses are based on weight and calculated by milligrams of lopinavir. Care should be taken to accurately calculate the dose. The oral solution contains lopinavir 80 mg and ritonavir 20 mg per one mL. Children <12 years of age (and ≤40 kg) who are not taking certain concomitant antiretroviral medications will receive <5 mL of solution per dose.

Synonyms ritonavir and lopinavir

U.S. Brand Names Kaletra®

Canadian Brand Names Kaletra®

Therapeutic Category Antiretroviral Agent, Nonnucleoside Reverse Transcriptase Inhibitor (NNRTI)

Use Treatment of HIV infection in combination with other antiretroviral agents

General Dosage Range Dosage adjustment recommended in patients on concomitant therapy

Oral:

Children 14 days to 6 months: Lopinavir 16 mg/kg or 300 mg/m^2 twice daily

Children 6 months to 18 years and <15 kg: 12 mg lopinavir/kg twice daily (maximum dose: Lopinavir 400 mg/ritonavir 100 mg)

Children 6 months to 18 years and 15-40 kg: 10 mg lopinavir/kg twice daily (maximum dose: Lopinavir 400 mg/ritonavir 100 mg)

Children 6 months to 18 years and >40 kg: Lopinavir 400 mg/ritonavir 100 mg twice daily

Adults: Lopinavir 400 mg/ritonavir 100 mg twice daily **or** lopinavir 800 mg/ritonavir 200 mg once daily

Dosage Forms

Solution, oral:

Kaletra®: Lopinavir 80 mg and ritonavir 20 mg per mL

Tablet:

Kaletra®:

Lopinavir 100 mg and ritonavir 25 mg

Lopinavir 200 mg and ritonavir 50 mg

Lopresor® (Can) *see* metoprolol *on page* 595

Lopresor SR® (Can) *see* metoprolol *on page* 595

Lopressor® *see* metoprolol *on page* 595

Lopressor HCT® *see* metoprolol and hydrochlorothiazide *on page* 595

Loprox® *see* ciclopirox *on page* 207

Loradamed [OTC] *see* loratadine *on page* 549

loratadine (lor AT a deen)

Medication Safety Issues

Sound-alike/look-alike issues:

Claritin® may be confused with clarithromycin

Claritin® (loratadine) may be confused with Claritin™ Eye (ketotifen)

BEERS Criteria medication:

This drug may be potentially inappropriate for use in geriatric patients (Quality of evidence - varies based on comorbidity; Strength of recommendation - varies based on comorbidity)

Synonyms Tavist ND

U.S. Brand Names Alavert® Allergy 24 Hour [OTC]; Alavert® Children's Allergy [OTC]; Claritin® 24 Hour Allergy [OTC]; Claritin® Children's Allergy [OTC]; Claritin® Liqui-Gels® 24 Hour Allergy [OTC]; Claritin® RediTabs® 24 Hour Allergy [OTC]; Loradamed [OTC]

Canadian Brand Names Apo-Loratadine®; Claritin®; Claritin® Kids

Therapeutic Category Antihistamine

Use Relief of nasal and nonnasal symptoms of seasonal allergic rhinitis; treatment of chronic idiopathic urticaria

General Dosage Range Dosage adjustment recommended in patients with hepatic or renal impairment

Oral:

Children 2-5 years: 5 mg once daily

Children ≥6 years and Adults: 10 mg once daily

Dosage Forms

Capsule, liquid gel, oral:

Claritin® Liqui-Gels® 24 Hour Allergy [OTC]: 10 mg

Solution, oral: 5 mg/5 mL (120 mL)

Syrup, oral: 5 mg/5 mL (120 mL, 240 mL)

Claritin® Children's Allergy [OTC]: 5 mg/5 mL (60 mL, 120 mL)

Tablet, oral: 10 mg

Alavert® Allergy 24 Hour [OTC]: 10 mg

Claritin® 24 Hour Allergy [OTC]: 10 mg

Loradamed [OTC]: 10 mg

Tablet, chewable, oral:

Claritin® Children's Allergy [OTC]: 5 mg

Tablet, orally disintegrating, oral: 10 mg

Alavert® Allergy 24 Hour [OTC]: 10 mg

Alavert® Children's Allergy [OTC]: 10 mg

Claritin® RediTabs® 24 Hour Allergy [OTC]: 10 mg

Loratadine-D 12 Hour [OTC] *see* loratadine and pseudoephedrine *on page* 550

loratadine and pseudoephedrine (lor AT a deen & soo doe e FED rin)

Medication Safety Issues

Sound-alike/look-alike issues:

Claritin-D® may be confused with Claritin-D® 24

Claritin-D® 24 may be confused with Claritin-D®

Synonyms pseudoephedrine and loratadine

U.S. Brand Names Alavert™ Allergy and Sinus [OTC]; Claritin-D® 12 Hour Allergy & Congestion [OTC]; Claritin-D® 24 Hour Allergy & Congestion [OTC]; Loratadine-D 12 Hour [OTC]

Canadian Brand Names Chlor-Tripolon ND®; Claritin® Extra; Claritin® Liberator

Therapeutic Category Antihistamine/Decongestant Combination

Use Temporary relief of symptoms of seasonal allergic rhinitis, other upper respiratory allergies, or the common cold

General Dosage Range Dosage adjustment recommended in patients with renal impairment

Oral: *Children ≥12 years and Adults:* Alavert™ Allergy and Sinus, Claritin-D® 24-Hour: 1 tablet every 24 hours; Claritin-D® 12-Hour: 1 tablet every 12 hours

Dosage Forms

Tablet, extended release: Loratadine 10 mg and pseudoephedrine 240 mg

Alavert™ Allergy and Sinus [OTC]: Loratadine 5 mg and pseudoephedrine 120 mg

Claritin-D® 12 Hour Allergy & Congestion [OTC]: Loratadine 5 mg and pseudoephedrine 120 mg

Claritin-D® 24 Hour Allergy & Congestion [OTC]: Loratadine 10 mg and pseudoephedrine 240 mg

Loratadine-D 12 Hour [OTC]: Loratadine 5 mg and pseudoephedrine sulfate 120 mg

lorazepam (lor A ze pam)

Medication Safety Issues

Sound-alike/look-alike issues:

LORazepam may be confused with ALPRAZolam, clonazePAM, diazepam, KlonoPIN®, Lovaza®, temazepam, zolpidem

Ativan® may be confused with Ambien®, Atarax®, Atgam®, Avitene®

BEERS Criteria medication:

This drug may be potentially inappropriate for use in geriatric patients (Quality of evidence - high; Strength of recommendation - strong).

Administration issues:

Injection dosage form contains propylene glycol. Monitor for toxicity when administering continuous lorazepam infusions.

Tall-Man LORazepam

U.S. Brand Names Ativan®; Lorazepam Intensol™

Canadian Brand Names Apo-Lorazepam®; Ativan®; Dom-Lorazepam; Lorazepam Injection, USP; Novo-Lorazem; Nu-Loraz; PHL-Lorazepam; PMS-Lorazepam; PRO-Lorazepam

Therapeutic Category Benzodiazepine

Controlled Substance C-IV

Use

Oral: Management of anxiety disorders or short-term (≤4 months) relief of the symptoms of anxiety, anxiety associated with depressive symptoms, or insomnia due to anxiety or transient stress

I.V.: Status epilepticus, amnesia, sedation

General Dosage Range

I.M.:

Children: 0.02-0.09 mg/kg as a single dose

Adults: 0.5-1 mg every 30-60 minutes as needed **or** 0.05 mg/kg as a single dose (maximum: 4 mg/dose)

I.V.: *Children and Adults:* Dosage varies greatly depending on indication

Oral:

Children: 0.02-0.09 mg/kg every 4-8 hours or as a single dose

Adults: Dosage varies greatly depending on indication

Dosage Forms

Injection, solution: 2 mg/mL (1 mL, 10 mL); 4 mg/mL (1 mL, 10 mL)

Solution, oral: 2 mg/mL (30 mL)

Lorazepam Intensol™: 2 mg/mL (30 mL)

Tablet, oral: 0.5 mg, 1 mg, 2 mg
Ativan®: 0.5 mg, 1 mg, 2 mg

Lorazepam Injection, USP (Can) *see* lorazepam *on page 550*
Lorazepam Intensol™ *see* lorazepam *on page 550*

lorcaserin (lor KA ser in)

Synonyms Belviq®; lorcaserin hydrochloride

Use Chronic weight management, as an adjunct to a reduced-calorie diet and increased physical activity, in patients with either an initial body mass index (BMI) of ≥30 kg/m^2 **or** an initial BMI of ≥27 kg/m^2 and at least one weight-related comorbid condition (eg, hypertension, dyslipidemia, type 2 diabetes)

Product Availability Belviq®: FDA approved June 2012; expected availability is currently undetermined

lorcaserin hydrochloride *see* lorcaserin *on page 551*
Lorcet® 10/650 *see* hydrocodone and acetaminophen *on page 454*
Lorcet® Plus *see* hydrocodone and acetaminophen *on page 454*
Lortab® *see* hydrocodone and acetaminophen *on page 454*
Loryna™ *see* ethinyl estradiol and drospirenone *on page 356*
Lorzone™ *see* chlorzoxazone *on page 204*

losartan (loe SAR tan)

Medication Safety Issues

Sound-alike/look-alike issues:

Cozaar® may be confused with Colace®, Coreg®, Hyzaar®, Zocor®
Losartan may be confused with valsartan

Synonyms DuP 753; losartan potassium; MK594

U.S. Brand Names Cozaar®

Canadian Brand Names Apo-Losartan; CO Losartan; Cozaar®; Mylan-Losartan; PMS-Losartan; Teva-Losartan

Therapeutic Category Angiotensin II Receptor Antagonist

Use Treatment of hypertension (HTN); treatment of diabetic nephropathy in patients with type 2 diabetes mellitus (noninsulin-dependent, NIDDM) and a history of hypertension; stroke risk reduction in patients with HTN and left ventricular hypertrophy (LVH)

General Dosage Range Dosage adjustment recommended in patients with hepatic impairment

Oral:

Children 6-16 years: Initial: 0.7 mg/kg once daily (maximum: 50 mg/day); Maintenance: Maximum: ≤1.4 mg/kg; 100 mg

Adults: Initial: 25-50 mg once daily; Maintenance: 25-100 mg/day in 1-2 divided doses (maximum: 100 mg/day)

Dosage Forms

Tablet, oral: 25 mg, 50 mg, 100 mg
Cozaar®: 25 mg, 50 mg, 100 mg

losartan and hydrochlorothiazide (loe SAR tan & hye droe klor oh THYE a zide)

Medication Safety Issues

Sound-alike/look-alike issues:

Hyzaar® may be confused with Cozaar®

Synonyms hydrochlorothiazide and losartan

U.S. Brand Names Hyzaar®

Canadian Brand Names Apo-Losartan/HCTZ; Hyzaar®; Hyzaar® DS; Mylan-Losartan/HCTZ; Teva-Losartan/HCTZ

Therapeutic Category Antihypertensive Agent, Combination

Use Treatment of hypertension; stroke risk reduction in patients with HTN and left ventricular hypertrophy (LVH)

General Dosage Range Oral: *Adults:* Losartan 50-100 mg and hydrochlorothiazide 12.5-50 mg once daily

Dosage Forms

Tablet: 50/12.5: Losartan 50 mg and hydrochlorothiazide 12.5 mg; 100/12.5: Losartan 100 mg and hydrochlorothiazide 12.5 mg; 100/25: Losartan 100 mg and hydrochlorothiazide 25 mg

Hyzaar®: 50/12.5: Losartan 50 mg and hydrochlorothiazide 12.5 mg; 100/12.5: Losartan 100 mg and hydrochlorothiazide 12.5 mg; 100/25: Losartan 100 mg and hydrochlorothiazide 25 mg

losartan potassium *see* losartan *on page 551*

LoSeasonique® *see* ethinyl estradiol and levonorgestrel *on page 357*

Losec® (Can) *see* omeprazole *on page 665*

Lotemax® *see* loteprednol *on page 552*

Lotensin® *see* benazepril *on page 119*

Lotensin HCT® *see* benazepril and hydrochlorothiazide *on page 119*

loteprednol (loe te PRED nol)

Synonyms loteprednol etabonate

U.S. Brand Names Alrex®; Lotemax®

Canadian Brand Names Alrex®; Lotemax®

Therapeutic Category Corticosteroid, Ophthalmic

Use

Ointment, 0.5% (Lotemax®): Treatment of postoperative inflammation and pain following ocular surgery

Suspension, 0.2% (Alrex®): Temporary relief of signs and symptoms of seasonal allergic conjunctivitis

Suspension, 0.5% (Lotemax®): Inflammatory conditions (treatment of steroid-responsive inflammatory conditions of the palpebral and bulbar conjunctiva, cornea, and anterior segment of the globe such as allergic conjunctivitis, acne rosacea, superficial punctate keratitis, herpes zoster keratitis, iritis, cyclitis, selected infective conjunctivitis, when the inherent hazard of steroid use is accepted to obtain an advisable diminution in edema and inflammation) and treatment of postoperative inflammation following ocular surgery

General Dosage Range Ophthalmic: *Adults:* Ointment: Apply ~1/2 inch ribbon into affected eye(s) 4 times/day; Solution: Instill 1-2 drops into affected eye(s) 4 times/day

Product Availability

Lotemax® 0.5% ointment: FDA approved April 2011; expected availability undetermined

Lotemax® 0.5% ointment is a topical corticosteroid approved for the treatment of postoperative inflammation and pain following ocular surgery.

Dosage Forms

Ointment, ophthalmic:

Lotemax®: 0.5% (3.5 g)

Suspension, ophthalmic:

Alrex®: 0.2% (5 mL, 10 mL)

Lotemax®: 0.5% (5 mL, 10 mL, 15 mL)

loteprednol and tobramycin (loe te PRED nol & toe bra MYE sin)

Synonyms loteprednol etabonate and tobramycin; tobramycin and loteprednol etabonate

U.S. Brand Names Zylet®

Therapeutic Category Antibiotic/Corticosteroid, Ophthalmic

Use Treatment of steroid-responsive ocular inflammatory conditions where either a superficial bacterial ocular infection or the risk of a superficial bacterial ocular infection exists

General Dosage Range Ophthalmic: *Children and Adults:* Instill 1-2 drops into the affected eye(s) every 4-6 hours

Dosage Forms

Suspension, ophthalmic [drops]:

Zylet®: Loteprednol 0.5% and tobramycin 0.3% (2.5 mL, 5 mL, 10 mL)

loteprednol etabonate *see* loteprednol *on page 552*

loteprednol etabonate and tobramycin *see* loteprednol and tobramycin *on page 552*

Lotrel® *see* amlodipine and benazepril *on page 66*

Lotriderm® (Can) *see* betamethasone and clotrimazole *on page 130*

Lotrimin AF® [OTC] *see* miconazole (topical) *on page 599*

Lotrimin® AF Athlete's Foot [OTC] *see* clotrimazole (topical) *on page 227*

Lotrimin® AF for Her [OTC] *see* clotrimazole (topical) *on page 227*

Lotrimin® AF Jock Itch [OTC] *see* clotrimazole (topical) *on page* 227

Lotrimin® ultra™ [OTC] *see* butenafine *on page* 155

Lotrisone® *see* betamethasone and clotrimazole *on page* 130

Lotronex® *see* alosetron *on page* 51

lovastatin (LOE va sta tin)

Medication Safety Issues

Sound-alike/look-alike issues:

Lovastatin may be confused with atorvaSTATin, Leustatin®, Livostin®, Lotensin®, nystatin, pitavastatin

Mevacor® may be confused with Benicar®, Lipitor®

International issues:

Lovacol [Chile and Finland] may be confused with Levatol brand name for penbutolol [U.S.]

Lovastin [Malaysia, Poland, and Singapore] may be confused with Livostin brand name for levocabastine [multiple international markets]

Mevacor [U.S., Canada, and multiple international markets} may be confused with Mivacron brand name for mivacurium [multiple international markets]

Synonyms mevinolin; monacolin K

U.S. Brand Names Altoprev®; Mevacor®

Canadian Brand Names Apo-Lovastatin®; CO Lovastatin; Dom-Lovastatin; Gen-Lovastatin; Mevacor®; Mylan-Lovastatin; Novo-Lovastatin; Nu-Lovastatin; PHL-Lovastatin; PMS-Lovastatin; PRO-Lovastatin; RAN™-Lovastatin; ratio-Lovastatin; Riva-Lovastatin; Sandoz-Lovastatin

Therapeutic Category HMG-CoA Reductase Inhibitor

Use

Adjunct to dietary therapy to decrease elevated serum total and LDL-cholesterol concentrations in primary hypercholesterolemia

Primary prevention of coronary artery disease (patients without symptomatic disease with average to moderately elevated total and LDL-cholesterol and below average HDL-cholesterol); slow progression of coronary atherosclerosis in patients with coronary heart disease and reduce the risk of myocardial infarction, unstable angina, and coronary revascularization procedures.

Adjunct to dietary therapy in adolescent patients (10-17 years of age, females >1 year postmenarche) with heterozygous familial hypercholesterolemia having LDL >189 mg/dL, **or** LDL >160 mg/dL with positive family history of premature cardiovascular disease (CVD), **or** LDL >160 mg/dL with the presence of at least two other CVD risk factors

General Dosage Range Dosage adjustment recommended in patients with renal impairment or on concomitant therapy

Oral:

Extended release: *Adults:* 20-60 mg once daily (maximum: 60 mg daily)

Immediate release:

Children 10-17 years: Initial: 10-20 mg once daily; Maintenance: 10-40 mg once daily (maximum: 40 mg daily)

Adults: Initial: 20 mg once daily; Maintenance: 20-80 mg once daily (maximum: 80 mg daily)

Dosage Forms

Tablet, oral: 10 mg, 20 mg, 40 mg

Mevacor®: 20 mg, 40 mg

Tablet, extended release, oral:

Altoprev®: 20 mg, 40 mg, 60 mg

lovastatin and niacin *see* niacin and lovastatin *on page* 639

Lovaza® *see* omega-3-acid ethyl esters *on page* 665

Lovenox® *see* enoxaparin *on page* 332

Lovenox® HP (Can) *see* enoxaparin *on page* 332

low-Molecular-weight iron dextran (INFeD®) *see* iron dextran complex *on page* 501

Low-Ogestrel® *see* ethinyl estradiol and norgestrel *on page* 362

Loxapac (Can) *see* loxapine *on page* 554

loxapine (LOKS a peen)

Medication Safety Issues

Sound-alike/look-alike issues:

Loxitane® may be confused with Lexapro®, Soriatane®

BEERS Criteria medication:

This drug may be potentially inappropriate for use in geriatric patients (Quality of evidence - moderate; Strength of recommendation - strong).

International issues:

Loxitane [U.S.] may be confused with Lexotan which is a brand name for bromazepam [multiple international markets]

Synonyms loxapine succinate; oxilapine succinate

U.S. Brand Names Loxitane®

Canadian Brand Names Apo-Loxapine®; Dom-Loxapine; Loxapac; Nu-Loxapine; PHL-Loxapine; Xylac™

Therapeutic Category Antipsychotic Agent, Dibenzoxazepine

Use Management of psychotic disorders

General Dosage Range Oral:

Adults: Initial: 10 mg twice daily (up to 50 mg/day); Usual maintenance: 20-100 mg/day in 2-4 divided doses (maximum: 250 mg/day)

Dosage Forms

Capsule, oral: 5 mg, 10 mg, 25 mg, 50 mg

Loxitane®: 5 mg, 10 mg, 25 mg, 50 mg

Dosage Forms - Canada

Injection, solution:

Loxapac: 50 mg/mL (1 mL)

Solution, oral [concentrate]:

Xylac™: 25 mg/mL (100 mL)

Tablet, oral:

Xylac™: 2.5 mg, 5 mg, 10 mg, 25 mg, 50 mg

loxapine succinate *see* loxapine *on page* 554

Loxitane® *see* loxapine *on page* 554

Lozide® (Can) *see* indapamide *on page* 479

Lozi-Flur™ *see* fluoride *on page* 393

L-PAM *see* melphalan *on page* 570

L-phenylalanine mustard *see* melphalan *on page* 570

LRH *see* gonadorelin *(Canada only) on page* 431

L-sarcolysin *see* melphalan *on page* 570

LTA® 360 *see* lidocaine (topical) *on page* 535

LTG *see* lamotrigine *on page* 521

***L*-thyroxine sodium** *see* levothyroxine *on page* 533

Lu-26-054 *see* escitalopram *on page* 345

lubiprostone (loo bi PROS tone)

Synonyms RU 0211; SPI 0211

U.S. Brand Names Amitiza®

Therapeutic Category Gastrointestinal Agent, Miscellaneous

Use Treatment of chronic idiopathic constipation; treatment of irritable bowel syndrome with constipation in adult women

General Dosage Range Dosage adjustment recommended in hepatic impairment and in patients who develop toxicities

Oral:

Adults (females): 8 mcg twice daily **or** 24 mcg twice daily

Adults (males): 24 mcg twice daily

Dosage Forms

Capsule, softgel, oral:

Amitiza®: 8 mcg, 24 mcg

Lubriderm® [OTC] *see* lanolin, cetyl alcohol, glycerin, petrolatum, and mineral oil *on page* 521

Lubriderm® Fragrance Free [OTC] *see* lanolin, cetyl alcohol, glycerin, petrolatum, and mineral oil *on page 521*

Lucentis® *see* ranibizumab *on page 787*

lucinactant (loo sin AK tant)

Synonyms Surfaxin®

Therapeutic Category Lung Surfactant

Use Prevention of respiratory distress syndrome (RDS) in premature infants at high risk for RDS

General Dosage Range Endotracheal: *Premature infants:* 5.8 mL/kg birth weight; up to 3 subsequent doses (total of 4 doses) may be administered at ≥6-hour intervals within the first 48 hours of life

Product Availability Surfaxin®: FDA approved March 2012; availability anticipated late 2012. Consult prescribing information for additional information.

Ludiomil *see* maprotiline *on page 562*

Lufyllin® *see* dyphylline *on page 321*

lumefantrine and artemether *see* artemether and lumefantrine *on page 92*

Lumigan® *see* bimatoprost *on page 133*

Lumigan® RC (Can) *see* bimatoprost *on page 133*

luminal sodium *see* phenobarbital *on page 712*

Lumitene™ [OTC] *see* beta-carotene *on page 128*

Lumizyme® *see* alglucosidase alfa *on page 47*

Lunesta® *see* eszopiclone *on page 354*

LupiCare® Dandruff [OTC] *see* salicylic acid *on page 816*

LupiCare® Psoriasis [OTC] *see* salicylic acid *on page 816*

Lupron® (Can) *see* leuprolide *on page 527*

Lupron Depot® *see* leuprolide *on page 527*

Lupron® Depot® (Can) *see* leuprolide *on page 527*

Lupron Depot-Ped® *see* leuprolide *on page 527*

lurasidone (loo RAS i done)

Medication Safety Issues

Sound-alike/look-alike issues:

Latuda® may be confused with Lantus®

BEERS Criteria medication:

This drug may be potentially inappropriate for use in geriatric patients (Quality of evidence - moderate; Strength of recommendation - strong).

Synonyms lurasidone hydrochloride; SM-13496

U.S. Brand Names Latuda®

Therapeutic Category Antipsychotic Agent, Atypical

Use Treatment of schizophrenia

General Dosage Range Dosage adjustment recommended in patients with hepatic or renal impairment or on concomitant therapy.

Oral: *Adults:* Initial: 40 mg once daily (maximum: 160 mg/day)

Dosage Forms

Tablet, oral:

Latuda®: 20 mg, 40 mg, 80 mg

lurasidone hydrochloride *see* lurasidone *on page 555*

Lusedra™ *see* fospropofol *on page 410*

Lustra® *see* hydroquinone *on page 461*

Lustra-AF® *see* hydroquinone *on page 461*

Lustra-Ultra™ *see* hydroquinone *on page 461*

luteinizing hormone releasing hormone *see* gonadorelin *(Canada only) on page 431*

Lutera® *see* ethinyl estradiol and levonorgestrel *on page 357*

Lutrepulse™ (Can) *see* gonadorelin *(Canada only) on page 431*

lutropin alfa (LOO troe pin AL fa)

Synonyms r-hLH; recombinant human luteinizing hormone

U.S. Brand Names Luveris® [DSC]

Therapeutic Category Gonadotropin; Ovulation Stimulator

Use Stimulation of follicular development in infertile hypogonadotropic hypogonadal (HH) women with profound luteinizing hormone (LH) deficiency (<1.2 units/L); to be used in combination with follitropin alfa

General Dosage Range SubQ: *Adults (females):* 75 units daily

Luveris® [DSC] *see* lutropin alfa *on page 556*
Luvox *see* fluvoxamine *on page 403*
Luvox® (Can) *see* fluvoxamine *on page 403*
Luvox® CR *see* fluvoxamine *on page 403*
Luxiq® *see* betamethasone *on page 129*
LY139603 *see* atomoxetine *on page 99*
LY146032 *see* daptomycin *on page 254*
LY170053 *see* olanzapine *on page 660*
LY-188011 *see* gemcitabine *on page 422*
LY231514 *see* pemetrexed *on page 700*
LY246736 *see* alvimopan *on page 57*
LY248686 *see* duloxetine *on page 319*
LY303366 *see* anidulafungin *on page 76*
LY570310 *see* telaprevir *on page 873*
LY-640315 *see* prasugrel *on page 752*
LY2148568 *see* exenatide *on page 369*
Lybrel® *see* ethinyl estradiol and levonorgestrel *on page 357*
Lyderm® (Can) *see* fluocinonide *on page 392*
Lymphazurin™ *see* isosulfan blue *on page 505*
lymphocyte immune globulin *see* antithymocyte globulin (equine) *on page 80*
lymphocyte mitogenic factor *see* aldesleukin *on page 44*
Lyrica® *see* pregabalin *on page 756*
Lysinyl [OTC] *see* l-lysine *on page 545*
Lysodren® *see* mitotane *on page 607*
Lysteda™ *see* tranexamic acid *on page 910*
Maalox® Advanced Maximum Strength [OTC] *see* aluminum hydroxide, magnesium hydroxide, and simethicone *on page 56*
Maalox® Advanced Maximum Strength [OTC] *see* calcium carbonate and simethicone *on page 163*
Maalox® Advanced Regular Strength [OTC] *see* aluminum hydroxide, magnesium hydroxide, and simethicone *on page 56*
Maalox® Children's [OTC] *see* calcium carbonate *on page 161*
Maalox® Junior Plus Antigas [OTC] *see* calcium carbonate and simethicone *on page 163*
Maalox® Regular Strength [OTC] *see* calcium carbonate *on page 161*
MabCampath® (Can) *see* alemtuzumab *on page 45*
Macrobid® *see* nitrofurantoin *on page 644*
Macrodantin® *see* nitrofurantoin *on page 644*
Macugen® *see* pegaptanib *on page 695*

mafenide (MA fe nide)

Synonyms mafenide acetate

U.S. Brand Names Sulfamylon®

Therapeutic Category Antibacterial, Topical

Use

Cream: Adjunctive antibacterial agent in the treatment of second- and third-degree burns

Solution: Adjunctive antibacterial agent for use under moist dressings over meshed autografts on excised burn wounds

General Dosage Range Topical: *Children and Adults:* Apply to a thickness of approximately 1/16" once or twice daily

Dosage Forms

Cream, topical:

Sulfamylon®: 85 mg/g (56.7 g, 113.4 g, 453.6 g)

Powder for solution, topical:

Sulfamylon®: 50 g/packet (5s)

mafenide acetate *see* mafenide *on page* 556

Mag 64® [OTC] *see* magnesium chloride *on page* 557

Mag-Al [OTC] *see* aluminum hydroxide and magnesium hydroxide *on page* 56

magaldrate and simethicone (MAG al drate & sye METH i kone)

Medication Safety Issues

Sound-alike/look-alike issues:

Riopan Plus® may be confused with Repan®

Synonyms Riopan Plus; simethicone and magaldrate

Therapeutic Category Antacid; Antiflatulent

Use Relief of hyperacidity associated with peptic ulcer, gastritis, peptic esophagitis, and hiatal hernia which are accompanied by symptoms of gas

General Dosage Range Oral: *Adults:* 5-10 mL (540-1080 mg magaldrate) between meals and at bedtime

Dosage Forms

Suspension, oral: Magaldrate 540 mg and simethicone 20 mg per 5 mL

Mag-Al Ultimate [OTC] *see* aluminum hydroxide and magnesium hydroxide *on page* 56

mag citrate *see* magnesium citrate *on page* 558

Mag Delay™ [OTC] *see* magnesium chloride *on page* 557

Mag®-G [OTC] *see* magnesium gluconate *on page* 558

Maginex™ [OTC] *see* magnesium L-aspartate hydrochloride *on page* 559

Maginex™ DS [OTC] *see* magnesium L-aspartate hydrochloride *on page* 559

MagneBind® 400 Rx *see* magnesium carbonate, calcium carbonate, and folic acid *on page* 557

magnesia magma *see* magnesium hydroxide *on page* 558

magnesium carbonate and aluminum hydroxide *see* aluminum hydroxide and magnesium carbonate *on page* 55

magnesium carbonate, calcium carbonate, and folic acid

(mag NEE zhum KAR bun ate, KAL see um KAR bun ate, & FOE lik AS id)

Synonyms calcium carbonate, folic acid, and magnesium carbonate; folic acid, magnesium carbonate, and calcium carbonate

U.S. Brand Names MagneBind® 400 Rx

Therapeutic Category Calcium Salt; Electrolyte Supplement, Oral; Magnesium Salt; Vitamin; Vitamin, Water Soluble

Use Prevention or treatment of nutritional deficiencies

General Dosage Range Oral: *Adults:* 1-3 tablets 3 times/day

Dosage Forms

Tablet, oral:

MagneBind® 400 Rx: Magnesium carbonate 400 mg, calcium carbonate 200 mg, and folic acid 1 mg

magnesium chloride (mag NEE zhum KLOR ide)

U.S. Brand Names Chloromag®; Mag 64® [OTC]; Mag Delay™ [OTC]; Slow-Mag® [OTC]

Therapeutic Category Electrolyte Supplement, Oral

Use Correction or prevention of hypomagnesemia; dietary supplement

General Dosage Range

I.V.:

Children <50 kg: 0.3-0.5 mEq/kg/day
Children >50 kg: 10-30 mEq/day
Adults: 8-24 mEq/day added to TPN

Oral: RDA (elemental magnesium):
Children: 80-240 mg/day
Adults: 360-410 mg/day

Dosage Forms
Injection, solution: 200 mg/mL (50 mL)
Chloromag®: 200 mg/mL (50 mL)
Tablet, delayed release, enteric coated, oral:
Mag 64® [OTC]: Elemental magnesium 64 mg
Mag Delay™ [OTC]: Elemental magnesium 64 mg
Tablet, enteric coated, oral:
Slow-Mag® [OTC]: Elemental magnesium 71.5 mg

magnesium citrate (mag NEE zhum SIT rate)

Synonyms citrate of magnesia; mag citrate
U.S. Brand Names Citroma® [OTC]
Canadian Brand Names Citro-Mag®
Therapeutic Category Laxative
Use Evacuation of bowel prior to certain surgical and diagnostic procedures or overdose situations; relieves occasional constipation
General Dosage Range Oral:
Children <6 years: 2-4 mL/kg given once or in divided doses
Children 6-12 years: 100-150 mL given once or in divided doses
Children >12 years and Adults: 150-300 mL given once or in divided doses

Dosage Forms
Solution, oral: 290 mg/5 mL (296 mL, 300 mL)
Citroma® [OTC]: 290 mg/5 mL (296 mL, 340 mL)
Tablet, oral: Elemental magnesium 100 mg

magnesium gluceptate *see* magnesium glucoheptonate *(Canada only) on page* 558
Magnesium Glucoheptonate (Can) *see* magnesium glucoheptonate *(Canada only) on page* 558

magnesium glucoheptonate *(Canada only)* (mag NEE zhum gloo koh HEP toh nate)

Synonyms magnesium gluceptate
Canadian Brand Names Magnesium Glucoheptonate
Therapeutic Category Electrolyte Supplement, Parenteral; Magnesium Salt
Use Dietary supplement
General Dosage Range Oral: *Adults:* 1500-3000 mg (75-150 mg elemental magnesium) 1-3 times/day
Product Availability Not available in U.S.

Dosage Forms - Canada
Solution, oral: 100 mg/mL

magnesium gluconate (mag NEE zhum GLOO koe nate)

U.S. Brand Names Magonate® [OTC]; Magtrate® [OTC]; Mag®-G [OTC]
Therapeutic Category Electrolyte Supplement, Oral
Use Dietary supplement
General Dosage Range Oral: RDA (elemental magnesium):
Children 1-13 years: 80-240 mg/day
Children ≥14 years and Adults: 310-420 mg/day

Dosage Forms
Liquid, oral:
Magonate® [OTC]: 1000 mg/5 mL (355 mL)
Tablet, oral: 500 mg, 550 mg
Magonate® [OTC]: 500 mg
Magtrate® [OTC]: 500 mg
Mag®-G [OTC]: 500 mg

magnesium hydroxide (mag NEE zhum hye DROKS ide)

Synonyms magnesia magma; MOM

U.S. Brand Names Fleet® Pedia-Lax™ Chewable Tablet [OTC]; Little Phillips'® Milk of Magnesia [OTC]; Milk of Magnesia [OTC]; Milk of Magnesium [OTC]; Phillips'® Milk of Magnesia [OTC]

Therapeutic Category Antacid; Electrolyte Supplement, Oral; Laxative

Use Short-term treatment of occasional constipation and symptoms of hyperacidity, laxative

General Dosage Range Oral:

Children 2-5 years: OTC laxative: Magnesium hydroxide 400 mg/5 mL: 5-15 mL/day
Children 6-11 years: OTC laxative: Magnesium hydroxide 400 mg/5 mL: 15-30 mL/day
Children ≥12 years and Adults: OTC laxative: Magnesium hydroxide 400 mg/5 mL: 30-60 mL/day

Dosage Forms

Suspension, oral: 400 mg/5 mL (30 mL, 473 mL, 3840 mL); 2400 mg/10 mL (10 mL)
Little Phillips'® Milk of Magnesia [OTC]: 800 mg/5 mL (120 mL)
Milk of Magnesia [OTC]: 400 mg/5 mL (360 mL, 480 mL); 800 mg/5 mL (100 mL, 400 mL)
Milk of Magnesium [OTC]: 400 mg/5 mL (3.78 L, 473 mL)
Phillips'® Milk of Magnesia [OTC]: 400 mg/5 mL (120 mL, 240 mL, 360 mL, 780 mL); 800 mg/5 mL (240 mL)

Tablet, chewable, oral:
Fleet® Pedia-Lax™ Chewable Tablet [OTC]: 400 mg
Phillips'® Milk of Magnesia [OTC]: 311 mg

magnesium hydroxide, aluminum hydroxide, and simethicone *see* aluminum hydroxide, magnesium hydroxide, and simethicone *on page 56*

magnesium hydroxide and aluminum hydroxide *see* aluminum hydroxide and magnesium hydroxide *on page 56*

magnesium hydroxide and calcium carbonate *see* calcium carbonate and magnesium hydroxide *on page 163*

magnesium hydroxide and mineral oil (mag NEE zhum hye DROKS ide & MIN er al oyl)

Synonyms Haley's M-O; MOM/mineral oil emulsion

U.S. Brand Names Phillips'® M-O [OTC]

Therapeutic Category Laxative

Use Short-term treatment of occasional constipation

General Dosage Range Oral:

Children 6-11 years: 20-30 mL at bedtime
Children ≥12 years and Adults: 45-60 mL at bedtime

Dosage Forms

Suspension, oral:
Phillips'® M-O [OTC]: Magnesium hydroxide 300 mg and mineral oil 1.25 mL per 5 mL

magnesium hydroxide, famotidine, and calcium carbonate *see* famotidine, calcium carbonate, and magnesium hydroxide *on page 373*

magnesium L-aspartate hydrochloride

(mag NEE zhum el as PAR tate hye droe KLOR ide)

Synonyms MAH

U.S. Brand Names Maginex™ DS [OTC]; Maginex™ [OTC]

Therapeutic Category Electrolyte Supplement, Oral

Use Dietary supplement

General Dosage Range Oral: RDA (elemental magnesium):

Children 1-13 years: 80-240 mg/day
Children ≥14 years and Adults: 310-420 mg/day

Dosage Forms

Granules for solution, oral [preservative free]:
Maginex™ DS [OTC]: 1230 mg/packet (30s)

Tablet, enteric coated, oral [preservative free]:
Maginex™ [OTC]: 615 mg

magnesium oxide (mag NEE zhum OKS ide)

Synonyms mag oxide

U.S. Brand Names Mag-Ox® 400 [OTC]; MAGnesium-Oxide™ [OTC]; Phillips'® Laxative Dietary Supplement Cramp-Free [OTC]; Uro-Mag® [OTC]

Therapeutic Category Antacid; Electrolyte Supplement, Oral; Laxative

Use Electrolyte replacement

General Dosage Range Oral: RDA (elemental magnesium):

Children 1-13 years: 80-240 mg/day

Children ≥14 years and Adults: 310-420 mg/day

Dosage Forms

Caplet, oral: Elemental magnesium 250 mg

Phillips'® Laxative Dietary Supplement Cramp-Free [OTC]: Elemental magnesium 500 mg

Capsule, oral:

Uro-Mag® [OTC]: 140 mg

Tablet, oral: 400 mg, 420 mg, 500 mg

Mag-Ox® 400 [OTC]: 400 mg

MAGnesium-Oxide™ [OTC]: 400 mg

MAGnesium-Oxide™ [OTC] *see* magnesium oxide *on page* 559

magnesium oxide, sodium picosulfate, and citric acid *see* sodium picosulfate, magnesium oxide, and citric acid *on page* 846

magnesium salicylate (mag NEE zhum sa LIS i late)

U.S. Brand Names Doan's® Extra Strength [OTC]; Keygesic [OTC]; Momentum® [OTC]; MST 600 [DSC]

Therapeutic Category Nonsteroidal Antiinflammatory Drug (NSAID)

Use Mild-to-moderate pain, fever, various inflammatory conditions; relief of pain and inflammation of rheumatoid arthritis and osteoarthritis

General Dosage Range Oral: *Children ≥12 years and Adults:*

Doan's® Extra Strength, Momentum®: 2 caplets every 6 hours as needed (maximum: 8 caplets/day)

Keygesic: 1 tablet every 4 hours as needed (maximum: 4 tablets/day)

Dosage Forms

Caplet, oral:

Doan's® Extra Strength [OTC]: 580 mg

Momentum® [OTC]: 580 mg

Tablet, oral:

Keygesic [OTC]: 650 mg

magnesium sulfate (mag NEE zhum SUL fate)

Medication Safety Issues

Sound-alike/look-alike issues:

Magnesium sulfate may be confused with manganese sulfate, morphine sulfate

$MgSO_4$ is an error-prone abbreviation (mistaken as morphine sulfate)

High alert medication:

The Institute for Safe Medication Practices (ISMP) includes this medication (I.V. formulation) among its list of drugs which have a heightened risk of causing significant patient harm when used in error.

Synonyms epsom salts; $MgSO_4$ (error-prone abbreviation)

Therapeutic Category Anticonvulsant; Electrolyte Supplement, Oral; Laxative

Use Treatment and prevention of hypomagnesemia; prevention and treatment of seizures in severe preeclampsia or eclampsia, pediatric acute nephritis; torsade de pointes; treatment of cardiac arrhythmias (VT/VF) caused by hypomagnesemia; soaking aid

General Dosage Range

I.V.: *Children and Adults:* Dosage varies greatly depending on indication

Oral: RDA (elemental magnesium):

Children 1-13 years: 80-240 mg/day

Children ≥14 years and Adults: 310-420 mg/day

I.M.: *Adults:* Hypomagnesemia: 1-4 g/day in divided doses

Topical: *Adults:* Soaking aid: Dissolve 2 cupfuls of powder per gallon of warm water

Dosage Forms

Infusion, premixed in D_5W: 10 mg/mL (100 mL)

Infusion, premixed in water for injection: 40 mg/mL (50 mL, 100 mL, 500 mL, 1000 mL); 80 mg/mL (50 mL)

Injection, solution: 500 mg/mL (5 mL, 10 mL, 20 mL, 25 mL, 50 mL)

Injection, solution [preservative free]: 500 mg/mL (2 mL, 5 mL, 10 mL, 20 mL, 50 mL)

Powder, oral/topical: USP: 100% (227 g, 454 g, 1810 g, 2720 g)

magnesium sulfate, potassium sulfate, and sodium sulfate *see* sodium sulfate, potassium sulfate, and magnesium sulfate *on page* 847
magnesium sulfate, sodium sulfate, and potassium sulfate *see* sodium sulfate, potassium sulfate, and magnesium sulfate *on page* 847
magnesium trisilicate and aluminum hydroxide *see* aluminum hydroxide and magnesium trisilicate *on page* 56
Magnevist® *see* gadopentetate dimeglumine *on page* 416
Magonate® [OTC] *see* magnesium gluconate *on page* 558
Mag-Ox® 400 [OTC] *see* magnesium oxide *on page* 559
mag oxide *see* magnesium oxide *on page* 559
Magtrate® [OTC] *see* magnesium gluconate *on page* 558
MAH *see* magnesium L-aspartate hydrochloride *on page* 559
Makena™ *see* hydroxyprogesterone caproate *on page* 463
Malarone® *see* atovaquone and proguanil *on page* 101
Malarone® Pediatric (Can) *see* atovaquone and proguanil *on page* 101

malathion (mal a THYE on)

U.S. Brand Names Ovide®

Therapeutic Category Scabicides/Pediculicides

Use Topical treatment of *Pediculus capitis* (head lice and their ova)

General Dosage Range Topical: *Children ≥6 years and Adults:* Apply sufficient amount to cover and thoroughly moisten dry hair and scalp; shampoo after 8-12 hours; may repeat in 7-9 days

Dosage Forms

Lotion, topical: 0.5% (59 mL)
Ovide®: 0.5% (59 mL)

maltodextrin (mal toe DEK strin)

U.S. Brand Names Carrington® Oral Wound Rinse [OTC]; Multidex® [OTC]

Therapeutic Category Skin and Mucous Membrane Agent

Use Topical: Treatment of infected or noninfected wounds

General Dosage Range

Oral: *Adults:* 1 packet or 15 mL 3-4 times/day or more if needed
Topical: *Adults:* Apply to wounds with dressing changes

Dosage Forms

Gel, topical [preservative free]:
Multidex® [OTC]: 7.1 mL (7.1 mL); 14.2 mL (14.2 mL); 85.2 mL (85.2 mL)
Powder, topical [preservative free]:
Multidex® [OTC]: 6 g (6 g); 12 g (12 g); 25 g (25 g); 45 g (45 g)
Powder for suspension, oral:
Carrington® Oral Wound Rinse [OTC]: 23 g
Solution, topical [preservative free]:
Multidex® [OTC]: 45 mL (45 mL)

Manda-Amlodipine (Can) *see* amlodipine *on page* 65
Manda-Citalopram (Can) *see* citalopram *on page* 213
Mandelamine® (Can) *see* methenamine *on page* 582
mandrake *see* podophyllum resin *on page* 736
Manerix® (Can) *see* moclobemide *(Canada only) on page* 609
manganese *see* trace elements *on page* 908

mannitol (MAN i tole)

Medication Safety Issues

Sound-alike/look-alike issues:
Osmitrol® may be confused with esmolol

Synonyms *D*-mannitol

U.S. Brand Names Aridol™; Osmitrol

Canadian Brand Names Osmitrol®

Therapeutic Category Diuretic, Osmotic

Use

Injection: Reduction of increased intracranial pressure associated with cerebral edema; reduction of increased intraocular pressure; promoting urinary excretion of toxic substances; genitourinary irrigant in transurethral prostatic resection or other transurethral surgical procedures

Note: Although FDA-labeled indications, the use of mannitol for the prevention of acute renal failure and/or promotion of diuresis is not routinely recommended (Kellum, 2008).

Genitourinary irrigation solution: Irrigation in transurethral prostatic resection or other transurethral surgical procedures

Powder for inhalation: Assessment of bronchial hyperresponsiveness

General Dosage Range

Inhalation: *Children ≥6 years and Adults:* 0-635 mg administered in a stepwise fashion until a positive response or the full dose has been administered (whichever comes first)

I.V.: *Adults:* Reduction of intraocular pressure: 1.5-2 g/kg

Transurethral: *Adults:* Use 5% urogenital solution as required for irrigation

Dosage Forms

Injection, solution: 20% [200 mg/mL] (250 mL, 500 mL); 25% [250 mg/mL] (50 mL)

Osmitrol: 5% [50 mg/mL] (1000 mL); 10% [100 mg/mL] (500 mL); 15% [150 mg/mL] (500 mL); 20% [200 mg/mL] (250 mL, 500 mL)

Injection, solution [preservative free]: 25% [250 mg/mL] (50 mL)

Powder, for oral inhalation:

Aridol™: 0 mg (1s) [empty], 5 mg (1s), 10 mg (1s), 20 mg (1s), 40 mg (15s) (19s)

Solution, genitourinary irrigation: 5% [50 mg/mL] (2000 mL)

Mantoux *see* tuberculin tests *on page 925*

Mapap® [OTC] *see* acetaminophen *on page 20*

Mapap® Arthritis Pain [OTC] *see* acetaminophen *on page 20*

Mapap® Children's [OTC] *see* acetaminophen *on page 20*

Mapap® Extra Strength [OTC] *see* acetaminophen *on page 20*

Mapap® Infant's [OTC] *see* acetaminophen *on page 20*

Mapap® Junior Rapid Tabs [OTC] *see* acetaminophen *on page 20*

Mapap® Multi-Symptom Cold [OTC] *see* acetaminophen, dextromethorphan, and phenylephrine *on page 28*

Mapap PM [OTC] *see* acetaminophen and diphenhydramine *on page 23*

Mapap® Sinus PE [OTC] *see* acetaminophen and phenylephrine *on page 24*

Mapezine® (Can) *see* carbamazepine *on page 172*

maprotiline (ma PROE ti leen)

Medication Safety Issues

International issues

Ludiomil [multiple international markets] may be confused with Lamictal brand name for lamotrigine [U.S., Canada, and multiple international markets]; lamotrigine [U.S., Canada, and multiple international markets]; Lomotil brand name for diphenoxylate [U.S, Canada, and multiple international markets] and brand name for loperamide [Mexico, Philippines]

Synonyms Ludiomil; maprotiline hydrochloride

Canadian Brand Names Novo-Maprotiline; Teva-Maprotiline

Therapeutic Category Antidepressant, Tetracyclic

Use Treatment of major depressive disorder (MDD) or of anxiety associated with depression

General Dosage Range Oral:

Adults: Initial: 75-150 mg once daily; Maintenance: 75-225 mg/day as a single dose or in divided doses

Elderly: Initial: 25 mg/day; Maintenance: 50-75 mg/day

Dosage Forms

Tablet, oral: 25 mg, 50 mg, 75 mg

maprotiline hydrochloride *see* maprotiline *on page 562*

maraviroc (mah RAV er rock)

Synonyms UK-427,857

U.S. Brand Names Selzentry®

Canadian Brand Names Celsentri™

Therapeutic Category Antiretroviral Agent, CCR5 Antagonist

Use Treatment of CCR5-tropic HIV-1 infection, in combination with other antiretroviral agents

General Dosage Range Dosage adjustment recommended in patients with renal impairment or on concomitant therapy

Oral: *Children ≥16 years and Adults:* 300 mg twice daily

Dosage Forms

Tablet, oral:

Selzentry®: 150 mg, 300 mg

M-Clear *see* guaifenesin and codeine *on page 434*

M-Clear WC *see* guaifenesin and codeine *on page 434*

m-cresyl acetate (em-KREE sil AS e tate)

U.S. Brand Names Cresylate™

Therapeutic Category Otic Agent, Antiinfective

Use Treatment of external otitis infections caused by susceptible bacteria or fungus

General Dosage Range Dose reduction may be necessary in children.

Otic: *Children and Adults:* Instill 3-5 drops into the affected ear(s) 3 times daily

Dosage Forms

Solution, otic:

Cresylate™: 25% (15 mL)

MCT *see* medium chain triglycerides *on page 567*

MCT Oil® [OTC] *see* medium chain triglycerides *on page 567*

MCT Oil® (Can) *see* medium chain triglycerides *on page 567*

MCV *see* meningococcal (groups A / C / Y and W-135) diphtheria conjugate vaccine *on page 571*

MCV4 *see* meningococcal (groups A / C / Y and W-135) diphtheria conjugate vaccine *on page 571*

MD-76®R *see* diatrizoate meglumine and diatrizoate sodium *on page 277*

MD-Gastroview® *see* diatrizoate meglumine and diatrizoate sodium *on page 277*

MDL 73,147EF *see* dolasetron *on page 306*

MDP Multidose *see* technetium Tc 99m medronate *on page 872*

MDX-010 *see* ipilimumab *on page 498*

MDX-CTLA-4 *see* ipilimumab *on page 498*

ME-609 *see* acyclovir and hydrocortisone *on page 35*

measles, mumps, and rubella virus vaccine

(MEE zels, mumpz & roo BEL a VYE rus vak SEEN)

Medication Safety Issues

Sound-alike/look-alike issues:

MMR (measles, mumps and rubella virus vaccine) may be confused with MMRV (measles, mumps, rubella, and varicella) vaccine

Synonyms MMR; mumps, measles and rubella vaccines; rubella, measles and mumps vaccines

U.S. Brand Names M-M-R® II

Canadian Brand Names M-M-R® II; Priorix™

Therapeutic Category Vaccine, Live Virus

Use Measles, mumps, and rubella prophylaxis

The Advisory Committee on Immunization Practices (ACIP) recommends routine vaccination for the following:

- All children (first dose given at 12-15 months of age)
- Adults born 1957 or later (without evidence of immunity or documentation of vaccination).
- Adults at higher risk for exposure to and transmission of measles mumps and rubella should receive special consideration for vaccination, unless an acceptable evidence of immunity exists. This includes international travelers, persons attending colleges and other post-high school education, persons working in healthcare facilities.

General Dosage Range SubQ:

Children ≥12 months: 0.5 mL

Adults: Born ≥1957 without evidence of immunity: 0.5 mL for 1 or 2 doses

Dosage Forms

Injection, powder for reconstitution [preservative free]:

M-M-R® II: Measles virus ≥1000 $TCID_{50}$, mumps virus ≥20,000 $TCID_{50}$, and rubella virus ≥1000 $TCID_{50}$

measles, mumps, rubella, and varicella virus vaccine

(MEE zels, mumpz, roo BEL a, & var i SEL a VYE rus vak SEEN)

Synonyms MMR-V; MMRV; mumps, rubella, varicella, and measles vaccine; rubella, varicella, measles, and mumps vaccine; varicella, measles, mumps, and rubella vaccine

U.S. Brand Names ProQuad®

Canadian Brand Names Priorix-Tetra™

Therapeutic Category Vaccine, Live Virus

Use To provide simultaneous active immunization against measles, mumps, rubella, and varicella

The Advisory Committee on Immunization Practices (ACIP) recommends routine vaccination against measles, mumps, rubella, and varicella in healthy children 12 months to 12 years of age. For children receiving their first dose at 12-47 months of age, either the MMRV combination vaccine or separate MMR and varicella vaccines can be used. (The ACIP prefers administration of separate MMR and varicella vaccines as the first dose in this age group unless the parent or caregiver expresses preference for the MMRV combination.) For children receiving the first dose at ≥48 months or their second dose at any age, use of MMRV is preferred.

Canadian labeling (not in U.S. labeling): MMRV combination vaccine is approved for use in healthy children 9 months to 6 years; may consider use in healthy children ≤12 years of age based upon prior experience with the separate component (live-attenuated MMR or live-attenuated varicella [OKA-strain]) vaccines.

General Dosage Range SubQ: *Children 12 months to 12 years:* 1 dose (0.5 mL)

Dosage Forms

Injection, powder for reconstitution [preservative free]:

ProQuad®: Measles virus ≥3.00 log_{10} $TCID_{50}$, mumps virus ≥4.30 log_{10} $TCID_{50}$, rubella virus ≥3.00 log_{10} $TCID_{50}$, and varicella virus ≥3.99 log_{10} PFU

Dosage Forms - Canada

Injection, powder for reconstitution [preservative free]:

Priorix-Tetra™ (CAN): Measles virus ≥3.00 log_{10} $CCID_{50}$, mumps virus ≥4.4 log_{10} $CCID_{50}$, rubella virus ≥3.00 log_{10} $CCID_{50}$, and varicella virus ≥3.3 log_{10} PFU

mebendazole (me BEN da zole)

Medication Safety Issues

Sound-alike/look-alike issues:

Mebendazole may be confused with metroNIDAZOLE

Synonyms Vermox

Canadian Brand Names Vermox®

Therapeutic Category Anthelmintic

Use Treatment of *Ancylostoma duodenale* or *Necator amiericanus* (hookworms), *Ascaris lumbricoides* (roundworms), *Enterobius vermicularis* (pinworms), *Strongyloides stercoralis* (roundworm), *Taenia solium* (tapeworms), *Trichuris trichiura* (whipworms),

General Dosage Range Oral: *Children ≥2 years and Adults:* 100 mg as a single dose **or** twice daily

Dosage Forms - Canada

Tablet, oral:

Vermox® 100 mg

mecasermin (mek a SER min)

Synonyms Iplex; mecasermin (rDNA origin); mecasermin rinfabate; recombinant human insulin-like growth factor-1; rhIGF-1 (mecasermin [Increlex®]); rhIGF-1/rhIGFBP-3 (mecasermin rinfabate [Iplex™])

U.S. Brand Names Increlex®

Therapeutic Category Growth Hormone

Use Treatment of growth failure in children with severe primary insulin-like growth factor-1 deficiency (IGF-1 deficiency; primary IGFD), or with growth hormone (GH) gene deletions who have developed neutralizing antibodies to GH

General Dosage Range SubQ:

Children ≥2 years: Increlex®: Initial: 0.04-0.08 mg/kg twice daily; Maintenance: 0.04-0.12 mg/kg twice daily

Children ≥3 years: Iplex™: Initial: 0.5 mg/kg once daily; Maintenance: 0.5-2 mg/kg once daily

Dosage Forms

Injection, solution:

Increlex®: 10 mg/mL (4 mL)

mecasermin (rDNA origin) *see* mecasermin *on page 565*

mecasermin rinfabate *see* mecasermin *on page 565*

mechlorethamine (me klor ETH a meen)

Medication Safety Issues

High alert medication:

The Institute for Safe Medication Practices (ISMP) includes this medication among its list of drugs which have a heightened risk of causing significant patient harm when used in error.

Synonyms chlorethazine; chlorethazine mustard; HN_2; mechlorethamine hydrochloride; mustine; nitrogen mustard

U.S. Brand Names Mustargen®

Therapeutic Category Antineoplastic Agent

Use Hodgkin disease; non-Hodgkin lymphoma; intracavitary injection for treatment of metastatic tumors; pleural and other malignant effusions

General Dosage Range

I.V.: *Adults:* 0.4 mg/kg as a single dose **or** in divided doses of 0.1 mg/kg/day (for 4 days) or 0.2 mg/kg/day (for 2 days) per treatment course

Intracavitary: *Adults:* 0.4 mg/kg as a single dose, although 0.2 mg/kg (10-20 mg) as a single dose has been used by the *intrapericardial* route

Dosage Forms

Injection, powder for reconstitution:

Mustargen®: 10 mg

mechlorethamine hydrochloride *see* mechlorethamine *on page 566*

meclizine (MEK li zeen)

Medication Safety Issues

Sound-alike/look-alike issues:

Antivert® may be confused with Anzemet®, Axert®

BEERS Criteria medication:

This drug may be potentially inappropriate for use in geriatric patients (Quality of evidence - varies based on comorbidity; Strength of recommendation - varies based on comorbidity)

Synonyms meclizine hydrochloride; meclozine hydrochloride

U.S. Brand Names Antivert®; Bonine® [OTC] [DSC]; Dramamine® Less Drowsy Formula [OTC]; Medi-Meclizine [OTC]; Trav-L-Tabs® [OTC]; VertiCalm™ [OTC]

Therapeutic Category Antihistamine

Use Prevention and treatment of symptoms of motion sickness; management of vertigo with diseases affecting the vestibular system

General Dosage Range Oral: *Children ≥12 years and Adults:* 25-50 mg 1 hour before travel, may repeat every 24 hours if needed **or** 25-100 mg/day in divided doses

Dosage Forms

Caplet, oral: 12.5 mg

Tablet, oral: 12.5 mg, 25 mg

Antivert®: 12.5 mg, 25 mg, 50 mg

Dramamine® Less Drowsy Formula [OTC]: 25 mg

Medi-Meclizine [OTC]: 25 mg

Trav-L-Tabs® [OTC]: 25 mg

VertiCalm™ [OTC]: 25 mg

Tablet, chewable, oral: 25 mg

meclizine hydrochloride *see* meclizine *on page 566*

meclofenamate (me kloe fen AM ate)

Medication Safety Issues

BEERS Criteria medication:

This drug may be potentially inappropriate for use in geriatric patients (Quality of evidence - moderate; Strength of recommendation - strong).

Synonyms meclofenamate sodium

Canadian Brand Names Meclomen®

Therapeutic Category Analgesic, Nonnarcotic; Nonsteroidal Antiinflammatory Drug (NSAID)

Use Treatment of inflammatory disorders, arthritis, mild-to-moderate pain, dysmenorrhea

General Dosage Range Oral: *Children >14 years and Adults:* 50-100 mg every 4-6 hours (maximum: 400 mg/day)

Dosage Forms

Capsule, oral: 50 mg, 100 mg

meclofenamate sodium *see* meclofenamate *on page 566*

Meclomen® (Can) *see* meclofenamate *on page 566*

meclozine hydrochloride *see* meclizine *on page 566*

Med-Baclofen (Can) *see* baclofen *on page 112*

Medent®-PEI [OTC] *see* guaifenesin and phenylephrine *on page 435*

Med-Glybe (Can) *see* glyburide *on page 428*

medicinal carbon *see* charcoal, activated *on page 193*

medicinal charcoal *see* charcoal, activated *on page 193*

Medicone® Hemorrhoidal [OTC] *see* benzocaine *on page 121*

Medicone® Suppositories [OTC] *see* phenylephrine (topical) *on page 717*

Medi-First® Sinus Decongestant [OTC] *see* phenylephrine (systemic) *on page 715*

Medi-Meclizine [OTC] *see* meclizine *on page 566*

Medi Pads [OTC] *see* witch hazel *on page 956*

Medi-Phenyl [OTC] *see* phenylephrine (systemic) *on page 715*

Mediproxen [OTC] *see* naproxen *on page 628*

medium chain triglycerides (mee DEE um chane trye GLIS er ides)

Synonyms MCT; triglycerides, medium chain

U.S. Brand Names MCT Oil® [OTC]

Canadian Brand Names MCT Oil®

Therapeutic Category Nutritional Supplement

Use Dietary supplement for those who cannot digest long-chain fats; malabsorption associated with disorders such as pancreatic insufficiency, bile salt deficiency, short bowel syndrome, and bacterial overgrowth of the small bowel; induce ketosis as a prevention for seizures

General Dosage Range Oral:

Infants: Initial: 0.5 mL every other feeding, then advance to every feeding, then increase in increments of 0.25-0.5 mL/feeding at intervals of 2-3 days as tolerated

Children: 45 mL/day in divided doses **or** ~39 mL with each meal **or** 50% to 70% (800-1120 kcal) of total calories (1600 kcal)

Adults: 45 mL/day in divided doses **or** 15 mL 3-4 times/day

Dosage Forms

Oil, oral:

MCT Oil® [OTC]: 14 g/15 mL (960 mL)

MED-Letrozole (Can) *see* letrozole *on page 526*

Med-Metformin (Can) *see* metformin *on page 579*

Medrol® *see* methylprednisolone *on page 591*

Medrol Dose Pack *see* methylprednisolone *on page 591*

Medrol® Dosepak™ *see* methylprednisolone *on page 591*

Medroxy (Can) *see* medroxyprogesterone *on page 567*

medroxyprogesterone (me DROKS ee proe JES te rone)

Medication Safety Issues

Sound-alike/look-alike issues:

Depo-Provera® may be confused with depo-subQ provera 104™

MedroxyPROGESTERone may be confused with hydroxyprogesterone caproate, methylPREDNISolone, methylTESTOSTERone

Provera® may be confused with Covera®, Femara®, Parlodel®, Premarin®, Proscar®, PROzac®

Administration issues:

The injectable dosage form is available in different formulations. Carefully review prescriptions to assure the correct formulation and route of administration.

Synonyms acetoxymethylprogesterone; medroxyprogesterone acetate; methylacetoxyprogesterone; MPA

Tall-Man medroxyPROGESTERone

U.S. Brand Names Depo-Provera®; Depo-Provera® Contraceptive; depo-subQ provera 104®; Provera®

Canadian Brand Names Alti-MPA; Apo-Medroxy®; Depo-Prevera®; Depo-Provera®; Dom-Medroxyprogesterone; Gen-Medroxy; Medroxy; Medroxyprogesterone Acetate Injectable Suspension USP; Novo-Medrone; PMS-Medroxyprogesterone; Provera-Pak; Provera®; Teva-Medroxyprogesterone

Therapeutic Category Contraceptive, Progestin Only; Progestin

Use Secondary amenorrhea or abnormal uterine bleeding due to hormonal imbalance; reduction of endometrial hyperplasia in nonhysterectomized postmenopausal women receiving conjugated estrogens; prevention of pregnancy; management of endometriosis-associated pain; adjunctive therapy and palliative treatment of recurrent and metastatic endometrial carcinoma

General Dosage Range Dosage adjustment recommended in patients with hepatic impairment.

I.M.:

Adolescents and Adults: Contraception: 150 mg every 3 months

Adults: Endometrial cancer: 400-1000 mg/week

Oral: *Adolescents and Adults:* 5-10 mg once daily

SubQ: *Adolescents and Adults:* 104 mg every 3 months (every 12-14 weeks)

Dosage Forms

Injection, suspension: 150 mg/mL (1 mL)

Depo-Provera®: 400 mg/mL (2.5 mL)

Depo-Provera® Contraceptive: 150 mg/mL (1 mL)

depo-subQ provera 104®: 104 mg/0.65 mL (0.65 mL)

Tablet, oral: 2.5 mg, 5 mg, 10 mg

Provera®: 2.5 mg, 5 mg, 10 mg

medroxyprogesterone acetate *see* medroxyprogesterone *on page 567*

Medroxyprogesterone Acetate Injectable Suspension USP (Can) *see* medroxyprogesterone *on page 567*

medroxyprogesterone and estrogens (conjugated) *see* estrogens (conjugated/equine) and medroxyprogesterone *on page 352*

Med-Sotalol (Can) *see* sotalol *on page 851*

Mefenamic-250 (Can) *see* mefenamic acid *on page 568*

mefenamic acid (me fe NAM ik AS id)

Medication Safety Issues

Sound-alike/look-alike issues:

Ponstel® may be confused with Pronestyl

BEERS Criteria medication:

This drug may be potentially inappropriate for use in geriatric patients (Quality of evidence - moderate; Strength of recommendation - strong).

U.S. Brand Names Ponstel®

Canadian Brand Names Apo-Mefenamic®; Dom-Mefenamic Acid; Mefenamic-250; Nu-Mefenamic; PMS-Mefenamic Acid; Ponstan®

Therapeutic Category Analgesic, Nonnarcotic; Nonsteroidal Antiinflammatory Drug (NSAID)

Use Short-term relief of mild-to-moderate pain including primary dysmenorrhea

General Dosage Range Oral: *Children >14 years and Adults:* Initial: 500 mg, then 250 mg every 6 hours as needed (maximum therapy: 1 week)

Dosage Forms

Capsule, oral: 250 mg

Ponstel®: 250 mg

mefloquine (ME floe kwin)

Synonyms mefloquine hydrochloride

Canadian Brand Names Apo-Mefloquine®; Lariam®

Therapeutic Category Antimalarial Agent

Use Treatment of mild-to-moderate acute malarial infections (including treatment of chloroquine-resistant malaria) and prevention of malaria caused by *Plasmodium falciparum* or *P. vivax*

Note: Due to geographical resistance and cross-resistance, consult current CDC guidelines.

General Dosage Range Oral:

Children ≥6 months: Prophylaxis: 5 mg/kg/once weekly (maximum: 250 mg/dose); Treatment: 20-25 mg/kg/day in 2 divided doses (maximum: 1250 mg)

Adults: Prophylaxis: 250 mg once weekly; Treatment: 1250 mg (5 tablets) as a single dose

Dosage Forms

Tablet, oral: 250 mg

mefloquine hydrochloride *see* mefloquine *on page 568*

Mefoxin® *see* cefoxitin *on page 184*

Megace® *see* megestrol *on page 569*

Megace® ES *see* megestrol *on page 569*

Megace® OS (Can) *see* megestrol *on page 569*

Megadophilus® [OTC] *see* Lactobacillus *on page 518*

Megatope *see* iodinated I 131 albumin *on page 493*

megestrol (me JES trole)

Medication Safety Issues

Sound-alike/look-alike issues:

Megace® may be confused with Reglan®

Megestrol may be confused with mesalamine

BEERS Criteria medication:

This drug may be potentially inappropriate for use in geriatric patients (Quality of evidence - moderate; Strength of recommendation - strong).

Synonyms 5071-1DL(6); megestrol acetate; NSC-71423

U.S. Brand Names Megace®; Megace® ES

Canadian Brand Names Apo-Megestrol®; Megace®; Megace® OS; Nu-Megestrol

Therapeutic Category Antineoplastic Agent; Progestin

Use Palliative treatment of breast and endometrial carcinoma; treatment of anorexia, cachexia, or unexplained significant weight loss in patients with AIDS

General Dosage Range Oral:

Adults (females): Tablet: 40-320 mg/day in divided doses

Adults (males/females): Suspension: 400-800 mg/day [Megace®] **or** 625 mg/day [Megace® ES]

Dosage Forms

Suspension, oral: 40 mg/mL (10 mL, 20 mL, 237 mL, 240 mL, 473 mL, 480 mL)

Megace®: 40 mg/mL (240 mL)

Megace® ES: 125 mg/mL (150 mL)

Tablet, oral: 20 mg, 40 mg

megestrol acetate *see* megestrol *on page 569*

Mellaril *see* thioridazine *on page 891*

meloxicam (mel OKS i kam)

Medication Safety Issues

BEERS Criteria medication:

This drug may be potentially inappropriate for use in geriatric patients (Quality of evidence - moderate; Strength of recommendation - strong).

U.S. Brand Names Mobic®

Canadian Brand Names Apo-Meloxicam®; CO Meloxicam; Dom-Meloxicam; Mobicox®; Mobic®; Mylan-Meloxicam; Novo-Meloxicam; PHL-Meloxicam; PMS-Meloxicam; ratio-Meloxicam; Teva-Meloxicam

Therapeutic Category Nonsteroidal Antiinflammatory Drug (NSAID)

Use Relief of signs and symptoms of osteoarthritis, rheumatoid arthritis, and juvenile idiopathic arthritis (JIA)

General Dosage Range Oral:

Children ≥2 years: 0.125 mg/kg/day (maximum: 7.5 mg/day)

Adults: Initial: 7.5 mg once daily; Maintenance: 7.5-15 mg once daily (maximum: 15 mg/day)

Dosage Forms

Suspension, oral: 7.5 mg/5 mL (100 mL)

Mobic®: 7.5 mg/5 mL (100 mL)

Tablet, oral: 7.5 mg, 15 mg

Mobic®: 7.5 mg, 15 mg

Melpaque HP® *see* hydroquinone *on page 461*

melphalan (MEL fa lan)

Medication Safety Issues

Sound-alike/look-alike issues:

Melphalan may be confused with Mephyton®, Myleran®

Alkeran® may be confused with Alferon®, Leukeran®, Myleran®

High alert medication:

This medication is in a class the Institute for Safe Medication Practices (ISMP) includes among its list of drug classes which have a heightened risk of causing significant patient harm when used in error.

Synonyms L-PAM; L-phenylalanine mustard; L-sarcolysin; phenylalanine mustard

U.S. Brand Names Alkeran®

Canadian Brand Names Alkeran®

Therapeutic Category Antineoplastic Agent

Use Palliative treatment of multiple myeloma and nonresectable epithelial ovarian carcinoma

General Dosage Range Dosage adjustment recommended in patients with renal impairment or who develop toxicities

I.V.: *Adults:* 16 mg/m^2 administered at 2-week intervals for 4 doses, then repeat at 4-week intervals

Oral: *Adults:* Dosage varies greatly depending on indication

Dosage Forms

Injection, powder for reconstitution: 50 mg

Alkeran®: 50 mg

Tablet, oral:

Alkeran®: 2 mg

Melquin-3® *see* hydroquinone *on page 461*

Melquin HP® *see* hydroquinone *on page 461*

memantine (me MAN teen)

Medication Safety Issues

Sound-alike/look-alike issues:

Memantine may be confused with mesalamine

Synonyms memantine hydrochloride; Namenda XR

U.S. Brand Names Namenda®

Canadian Brand Names Apo-Memantine; CO Memantine; Ebixa®; PMS-Memantine; ratio-Memantine; Riva-Memantine; Sandoz-Memantine

Therapeutic Category N-Methyl-D-Aspartate Receptor Antagonist

Use Treatment of moderate-to-severe dementia of the Alzheimer type

General Dosage Range Dosage adjustment recommended in patients with renal impairment

Oral: *Adults:* Initial: 5 mg once daily; Target: 20 mg daily in 2 divided doses

Product Availability

Namenda XR™: FDA approved in June 2010; anticipated availability is currently undetermined

Namenda XR™ is an extended release capsule (once-daily administration) approved for the treatment of moderate-to-severe dementia associated with Alzheimer disease

Dosage Forms

Combination package, oral:

Namenda®: Tablet: 5 mg (28s) and Tablet: 10 mg (21s)

Solution, oral:

Namenda®: 2 mg/mL (360 mL)

Tablet, oral:

Namenda®: 5 mg, 10 mg

memantine hydrochloride *see* memantine *on page 570*

Menactra® *see* meningococcal (groups A / C / Y and W-135) diphtheria conjugate vaccine *on page 571*

meningococcal group C-CRM197 conjugate vaccine *(Canada only)*

(me NIN joe kok al groop see see ahr em wuhn nahyn tee sev uhn KON joo gate vak SEEN)

Synonyms menC-CRM197; menCC

Canadian Brand Names Menjugate®

Therapeutic Category Vaccine

Use To provide active immunization against invasive meningococcal disease caused by *N. meningitidis* serogroup C, in children ≥2 months and adults

The National Advisory Committee on Immunization (NACI) recommendations for persons considered at an increased risk for meningococcal disease:

Chemoprophylaxis and immunoprophylaxis: Selection of meningococcal vaccination to be based upon serogroup(s):

Individuals living in the same household or with close contact (eg, kissing, shared cigarettes, shared eating or drinking utensils) of infected patient

Employees and children of nursery schools or day care

Immunoprophylaxis: Selection of meningococcal vaccination to be based upon serogroup(s):

Adolescents and young adults

Laboratory workers routinely exposed to isolates of *N. meningitidis*

Military recruits

Persons traveling to or who reside in countries where *N. meningitidis* is hyperendemic or epidemic, particularly if contact with local population will be prolonged

Persons with terminal complement component deficiencies

Persons with anatomic or functional asplenia

Note: Use is also recommended during meningococcal outbreaks caused by serogroup C.

Chemoprophylaxis:

Healthcare workers with intensive unprotected contact with infected patients

Airline passengers sitting directly next to an infected patient for duration of at least 8 hours

See NACI guidelines for specific drug treatment at http://www.phac-aspc.gc.ca/naci-ccni

General Dosage Range I.M.:

Infants ≥2-12 months: 0.5 mL as a single dose for a total of 3 doses

Infants ≥4-11 months without prior vaccination: 0.5 mL as a single dose for a total of 2 doses

Children ≥1 year and Adults: 0.5 mL as a single dose

Product Availability Not available in U.S.

Dosage Forms - Canada

Injection, powder for reconstitution:

Menjugate®: 10 mcg of oligosaccharide antigen group C

meningococcal (groups A / C / Y and W-135) diphtheria conjugate vaccine

(me NIN joe kok al groops aye, see, why & dubl yoo won thur tee fyve dif THEER ee a KON joo gate vak SEEN)

Medication Safety Issues

Administration issue:

Menactra® (MCV4) should be administered by intramuscular (I.M.) injection only. Inadvertent subcutaneous (SubQ) administration has been reported; possibly due to confusion of this product with Menomune® (MPSV4), also a meningococcal polysaccharide vaccine, which is administered by the SubQ route.

Synonyms MCV; MCV4; menACWY-CRM (Menveo®); menACWY-D (Menactra®); meningococcal conjugate vaccine

U.S. Brand Names Menactra®; Menveo®

Canadian Brand Names Menactra®; Menveo®

Therapeutic Category Vaccine

Use Provide active immunization of children and adults against invasive meningococcal disease caused by *N. meningitidis* serogroups A, C, Y, and W-135.

The Advisory Committee on Immunization Practices (ACIP) recommends routine vaccination of all persons at age 11 or 12 years of age, followed by a booster at age 16 years of age (CDC, 60[3], 2011).

The ACIP also recommends vaccination for:

Children 9 through 23 months of age at increased risk for meningococcal disease (CDC, 60[40], 2011). Children at increased risk include:

- Children traveling to or who reside in countries where *N. meningitidis* is hyperendemic or epidemic
- Children with persistent complement component deficiencies (eg, C5-C9, properdin, factor H, or factor D)

Persons 2 through 55 years of age at increased risk for meningococcal disease (CDC, 60[3], 2011). Meningococcal conjugate vaccine (MCV4) is preferred for persons aged 2-55 years; meningococcal polysaccharide vaccine (MPSV4) is preferred in adults ≥56 years of age (CDC, 2005). Persons at increased risk include:

- Previously unvaccinated college freshmen living in dormitories
- Microbiologists routinely exposed to isolates of *N. meningitidis*
- Military recruits
- Persons traveling to or who reside in countries where *N. meningitidis* is hyperendemic or epidemic, particularly if contact with local population will be prolonged
- Persons with persistent complement component deficiencies (eg, C5-C9, properdin, factor H, or factor D)
- Persons with anatomic or functional asplenia

Use is also recommended during meningococcal outbreaks caused by vaccine preventable serogroups (all recommended age groups) (CDC, 2005; CDC, 60[40], 2011).

General Dosage Range I.M.:

Children 9-23 months (Menactra®):0.5 mL/dose given as a 2-dose series, 3 months apart

Children ≥2 years and Adults ≤55 years: 0.5 mL as a single dose

Dosage Forms

Injection, solution [preservative free]:

Menactra®: 4 mcg each of polysaccharide antigen groups A, C, Y, and W-135 [bound to diphtheria toxoid 48 mcg] per 0.5 mL

Menveo®: MenA oligosaccharide 10 mcg, MenC oligosaccharide 5 mcg, MenY oligosaccharide 5 mcg, and MenW-135 oligosaccharide 5 mcg [bound to CRM_{197} protein 32.7-64.1 mcg] per 0.5 mL

meningococcal polysaccharide (groups C and Y) and *Haemophilus* b tetanus toxoid conjugate vaccine

(me NIN joe kok al pol i SAK a ride groops see & why & he MOF i lus bee TET a nus TOKS oyd KON joo gate vak SEEN)

Medication Safety Issues

Sound-alike/look-alike issues:

MenHibrix® (Meningococcal Polysaccharide (Groups C and Y) and *Haemophilus* b Tetanus Toxoid Conjugate Vaccine) may be confused with Hiberix® (*Haemophilus* b Conjugate Vaccine)

Synonyms Menhibrix

Therapeutic Category Vaccine, Inactivated (Bacterial)

Use To provide active immunity to prevent invasive disease caused by meningococcal serogroups C and Y and *Haemophilus influenzae* type b

General Dosage Range

I.M.: *Children 6 weeks to 18 months:* 0.5 mL/dose given as a four-dose series at 2, 4, 6, and 12-15 months of age

Product Availability MenHibrix®: FDA approved June 2012; availability expected October 2012. Consult prescribing information for additional information.

meningococcal polysaccharide vaccine *see* meningococcal polysaccharide vaccine (groups A / C / Y and W-135) *on page 573*

meningococcal polysaccharide vaccine (groups A / C / Y and W-135)

(me NIN joe kok al pol i SAK a ride vak SEEN groops aye, see, why & dubl yoo won thur tee fyve)

Medication Safety Issues

Administration issue:

Menomune® (MPSV4) should be administered by subcutaneous (SubQ) injection. Menactra® (MCV4), also a meningococcal polysaccharide vaccine, is to be administered by intramuscular (I.M.) injection only.

Synonyms meningococcal polysaccharide vaccine; MPSV; MPSV4

U.S. Brand Names Menomune®-A/C/Y/W-135

Canadian Brand Names Menomune®-A/C/Y/W-135

Therapeutic Category Vaccine, Live Bacteria

Use Provide active immunity to meningococcal serogroups contained in the vaccine

The Advisory Committee on Immunization Practices (ACIP) recommends routine vaccination for persons at increased risk for meningococcal disease. Meningococcal conjugate vaccine (MCV4) is preferred for persons aged 2-55 years; meningococcal polysaccharide vaccine (MPSV4) is preferred in adults ≥56 years of age (CDC, 2005).

Persons at increased risk include:

- Previously unvaccinated college freshmen living in dormitories
- Microbiologists routinely exposed to isolates of *N. meningitidis*
- Military recruits
- Persons traveling to or who reside in countries where *N. meningitidis* is hyperendemic or epidemic, particularly if contact with local population will be prolonged
- Persons with persistent complement component deficiencies (eg, C5-C9, properidin, factor H, or factor D)
- Persons with anatomic or functional asplenia
- Persons with HIV infection

Use is also recommended during meningococcal outbreaks caused by vaccine preventable serogroups.

General Dosage Range SubQ: *Children ≥2 years and Adults:* 0.5 mL as a single dose

Dosage Forms

Injection, powder for reconstitution [MPSV4]:

Menomune®-A/C/Y/W-135: 50 mcg each of polysaccharide antigen groups A, C, Y, and W-135 per 0.5 mL dose

Menjugate® (Can) *see* meningococcal group C-CRM197 conjugate vaccine *(Canada only) on page 571*

Menomune®-A/C/Y/W-135 *see* meningococcal polysaccharide vaccine (groups A / C / Y and W-135) *on page 573*

Menopur® *see* menotropins *on page 573*

Menostar® *see* estradiol (systemic) *on page 347*

menotropins (men oh TROE pins)

Medication Safety Issues

Sound-alike/look-alike issues:

Repronex® may be confused with Regranex®

Synonyms hMG; human menopausal gonadotropin

U.S. Brand Names Menopur®; Repronex®

Canadian Brand Names Menopur®; Repronex®

Therapeutic Category Gonadotropin

Use Female:

In conjunction with hCG to induce ovulation and pregnancy in infertile females experiencing oligoanovulation or anovulation when the cause of anovulation is functional and not caused by primary ovarian failure (Repronex®)

Stimulation of multiple follicle development in ovulatory patients as part of an assisted reproductive technology (ART) (Menopur®, Repronex®)

General Dosage Range

I.M.: *Adults:* Repronex®: Initial: 150 units **or** 225 units daily (maximum: 450 units/day; 12 days of therapy)

SubQ: *Adults:* Menopur®: Initial: 225 units daily (maximum: 450 units/day; 20 days of therapy); Repronex®: Initial: 150 units **or** 225 units daily (maximum: 450 units/day; 12 days of therapy)

Dosage Forms

Injection, powder for reconstitution:

Menopur®, Repronex®: Follicle stimulating hormone activity 75 units and luteinizing hormone activity 75 units

Mentax® *see* butenafine *on page 155*

menthol and methyl salicylate *see* methyl salicylate and menthol *on page 592*

menthol and zinc oxide (topical) (MEN thole & zink OKS ide)

U.S. Brand Names Calmoseptine® [OTC]; Risamine™ [OTC]

Therapeutic Category Protectant, Topical; Topical Skin Product

Use Provides a barrier to protect intact and/or injured skin from moisture, wound or fistula drainage, urine, or feces; diaper rash

General Dosage Range Topical: *Children and Adults:* Apply thin layer 2-4 times/day or after each incontinent episode/diaper change

Dosage Forms

Ointment, topical:

Calmoseptine®: Menthol 0.44% and zinc oxide 20.625% (3.5 g/packet, 75 g, 120 g)

Risamine™: Menthol 0.44% and zinc oxide 20.625% (113 g)

Menveo® *see* meningococcal (groups A / C / Y and W-135) diphtheria conjugate vaccine *on page 571*

mepenzolate (me PEN zoe late)

Medication Safety Issues

Sound-alike/look-alike issues:

Cantil® may be confused with Bentyl®

Synonyms mepenzolate bromide

U.S. Brand Names Cantil®

Canadian Brand Names Cantil®

Therapeutic Category Anticholinergic Agent

Use Adjunctive treatment of peptic ulcer disease; has not been shown to be effective in contributing to the healing of peptic ulcer, preventing complications, or decreasing the rate of recurrence

General Dosage Range Oral: *Adults:* 25-50 mg 4 times/day

Dosage Forms

Tablet, oral:

Cantil®: 25 mg

mepenzolate bromide *see* mepenzolate *on page 574*

meperidine (me PER i deen)

Medication Safety Issues

Sound-alike/look-alike issues:

Meperidine may be confused with meprobamate

Demerol® may be confused with Demulen®, Desyrel, Dilaudid®, Pamelor™

High alert medication:

The Institute for Safe Medication Practices (ISMP) includes this medication among its list of drug classes which have a heightened risk of causing significant patient harm when used in error.

BEERS Criteria medication:

This drug may be potentially inappropriate for use in geriatric patients (Quality of evidence - high; Strength of recommendation - strong).

Other safety concerns:

Avoid the use of meperidine for pain control, especially in elderly and renally-compromised patients because of the risk of neurotoxicity (American Pain Society, 2008; Institute for Safe Medication Practices [ISMP], 2007)

Synonyms isonipecaine hydrochloride; meperidine hydrochloride; pethidine hydrochloride

U.S. Brand Names Demerol®

Canadian Brand Names Demerol®

Therapeutic Category Analgesic, Narcotic

Controlled Substance C-II

Use Management of moderate-to-severe pain; adjunct to anesthesia and preoperative sedation

General Dosage Range Dosage adjustment recommended in patients with hepatic impairment

I.M., SubQ:

Children: 1.1-1.8 mg/kg/dose every 3-4 hours as needed (maximum: 50-150 mg/dose) **or** 1.1-2.2 mg/kg given 30-90 minutes before the beginning of anesthesia (maximum: 50-150 mg/dose)

Adults: 50-150 mg every 3-4 hours as needed **or** 50-150 mg given 30-90 minutes before the beginning of anesthesia **or** 50-100 mg when pain becomes regular; may repeat at every 1-3 hours

Elderly: Avoid use

Oral:

Children: 1.1-1.8 mg/kg/dose every 3-4 hours as needed (maximum: 50-150 mg/dose)

Adults: Initial: 50-150 mg every 3-4 hours as needed

Elderly: Avoid use

Dosage Forms

Injection, solution: 10 mg/mL (30 mL); 25 mg/mL (1 mL)

Demerol®: 25 mg/mL (1 mL); 25 mg/0.5 mL (0.5 mL); 50 mg/mL (1 mL, 1.5 mL, 2 mL, 30 mL); 75 mg/mL (1 mL); 100 mg/mL (1 mL, 20 mL)

Solution, oral: 50 mg/5 mL (500 mL)

Tablet, oral: 50 mg, 100 mg

Demerol®: 50 mg, 100 mg

meperidine hydrochloride *see* meperidine *on page 574*

Mephyton® *see* phytonadione *on page 722*

mepivacaine (me PIV a kane)

Medication Safety Issues

Sound-alike/look-alike issues:

Mepivacaine may be confused with bupivacaine

Polocaine® may be confused with prilocaine

High alert medication:

The Institute for Safe Medication Practices (ISMP) includes this medication (epidural administration) among its list of drug classes which have a heightened risk of causing significant patient harm when used in error.

Synonyms mepivacaine hydrochloride

U.S. Brand Names Carbocaine®; Polocaine®; Polocaine® MPF

Canadian Brand Names Carbocaine®; Polocaine®

Therapeutic Category Local Anesthetic

Use Local or regional analgesia; anesthesia by local infiltration, peripheral and central neural techniques (epidural and caudal); **not** for use in spinal anesthesia

General Dosage Range

Brachial, cervical, intercostal, pudendal nerve block: *Adults:* 5-40 mL of 1% solution **or** 5-20 mL of 2% solution (maximum: 400 mg)

Caudal and epidural block (preservative free solutions only): *Adults:* 15-30 mL of 1% solution (maximum: 300 mg) **or** 10-25 mL of 1.5% solution (maximum: 375 mg) **or** 10-20 mL of a 2% solution (maximum: 400 mg)

Infiltration: *Adults:* Up to 40 mL of 1% solution (maximum: 400 mg)

Local injection:

Children <3 years or <14 kg: Dose varies; only concentrations less than 2% should be used (maximum: 5-6 mg/kg)

Children ≥3 years or ≥14 kg: Dose varies (maximum: 5-6 mg/kg)

Adults: Dose varies (maximum: 400 mg/dose; 1000 mg/day)

Paracervical block: *Adults:* Up to 20 mL (total for both sides) of 1% solution (maximum: 200 mg)

Therapeutic block: *Adults:* 1-5 mL of 1% solution (maximum: 50 mg) or 1-5 mL of 2% solution (maximum: 100 mg)

Transvaginal block: *Adults:* Up to 30 mL (total for both sides) of a 1% solution (maximum: 300 mg)

Dosage Forms

Injection, solution: 3% [30 mg/mL] (1.8 mL)

Carbocaine®: 1% [10 mg/mL] (50 mL); 2% [20 mg/mL] (50 mL); 3% [30 mg/mL] (1.7 mL)

Polocaine®: 1% [10 mg/mL] (50 mL); 2% [20 mg/mL] (50 mL)

Injection, solution [preservative free]:

Carbocaine®: 1% [10 mg/mL] (30 mL); 1.5% [15 mg/mL] (30 mL); 2% [20 mg/mL] (20 mL)

Polocaine® MPF: 1% [10 mg/mL] (30 mL); 1.5% [15 mg/mL] (30 mL); 2% [20 mg/mL] (20 mL)

mepivacaine and levonordefrin (me PIV a kane & lee voe nor DEF rin)

Synonyms levonordefrin and mepivacaine hydrochloride

U.S. Brand Names Carbocaine® 2% with Neo-Cobefrin®; Polocaine® Dental with Levonordefrin; Scandonest® 2% L

Canadian Brand Names Polocaine® 2% and Levonordefrin 1:20,000

Therapeutic Category Local Anesthetic

General Dosage Range

Infiltration and nerve block (single site): *Children >10 years and Adults:* 36 mg (1.8 mL) of mepivacaine hydrochloride as a 2% solution with levonordefrin 1:20,000

Infiltration and nerve block (entire cavity):

Children ≤10 years: Carefully calculate on basis of patient's weight (maximum: 6.6 mg/kg; 180 mg of mepivacaine as 2% solution with levonordefrin 1:20,000)

Children >10 years and Adults: 180 mg (9 mL) of mepivacaine hydrochloride as 2% solution with levonordefrin 1:20,000 (maximum: 6.6 mg/kg; 400 mg of mepivacaine hydrochloride per appointment)

Dosage Forms

Injection, solution [for dental use]:

Carbocaine® 2% with Neo-Cobefrin®: Mepivacaine 2% and levonordefrin 1:20,000 (1.7 mL)

Polocaine® Dental with Levonordefrin: Mepivacaine 2% and levonordefrin 1:20,000 (1.7 mL)

Scandonest® 2% L: Mepivacaine 2% and levonordefrin 1:20,000 (1.7 mL)

mepivacaine hydrochloride *see* mepivacaine *on page* 575

meprobamate (me proe BA mate)

Medication Safety Issues

Sound-alike/look-alike issues:

Meprobamate may be confused with meperidine

Equanil may be confused with Elavil®

BEERS Criteria medication:

This drug may be potentially inappropriate for use in geriatric patients (Quality of evidence - moderate; Strength of recommendation - strong).

Synonyms Equanil

Canadian Brand Names Novo-Mepro

Therapeutic Category Antianxiety Agent

Controlled Substance C-IV

Use Management of anxiety disorders

General Dosage Range

Oral:

Children 6-12 years: 200-600 mg/day in 2-3 divided doses

Adults: 1200-1600 mg/day in 3-4 divided doses, up to 2400 mg/day

Dosage Forms

Tablet, oral: 200 mg, 400 mg

Mepron® *see* atovaquone *on page* 101

mercaptoethane sulfonate *see* mesna *on page* 578

mercaptopurine (mer kap toe PYOOR een)

Medication Safety Issues

Sound-alike/look-alike issues:

Mercaptopurine may be confused with methotrexate

Purinethol® may be confused with propylthiouracil

High alert medication:

This medication is in a class the Institute for Safe Medication Practices (ISMP) includes among its list of drug classes which have a heightened risk of causing significant patient harm when used in error.

Other safety concerns:

To avoid potentially serious dosage errors, the terms "6-mercaptopurine" or "6-MP" should be avoided; use of these terms has been associated with sixfold overdosages.

Azathioprine is metabolized to mercaptopurine; concurrent use of these commercially-available products has resulted in profound myelosuppression.

Synonyms 6-mercaptopurine (error-prone abbreviation); 6-MP (error-prone abbreviation)

U.S. Brand Names Purinethol®

Canadian Brand Names Purinethol®

Therapeutic Category Antineoplastic Agent

Use Maintenance treatment component of acute lymphoblastic leukemia (ALL)

General Dosage Range Dosage adjustment recommended in patients with hepatic or renal impairment or on concomitant therapy

Oral: *Children and Adults:* Maintenance: 1.5-2.5 mg/kg/day

Dosage Forms

Tablet, oral: 50 mg

Purinethol®: 50 mg

6-mercaptopurine (error-prone abbreviation) *see* mercaptopurine *on page* 576

mercapturic acid *see* acetylcysteine *on page* 32

meropenem (mer oh PEN em)

Medication Safety Issues

Sound-alike/look-alike issues:

Meropenem may be confused with ertapenem, imipenem, metroNIDAZOLE

U.S. Brand Names Merrem® I.V.

Canadian Brand Names Merrem®

Therapeutic Category Carbapenem (Antibiotic)

Use

Treatment of intraabdominal infections (complicated appendicitis and peritonitis); treatment of bacterial meningitis in pediatric patients ≥3 months of age caused by *S. pneumoniae*, *H. influenzae*, and *N. meningitidis*; treatment of complicated skin and skin structure infections caused by susceptible organisms

Canadian labeling: Additional indications (not in U.S. labeling): Treatment of lower respiratory tract infections (community-acquired and nosocomial pneumonias), complicated urinary tract infections, gynecologic infections (excluding chlamydia), and septicemia; treatment of bacterial meningitis in adults caused by *S. pneumoniae*, *H. influenzae*, and *N. meningitidis* (use in adult meningitis based on pediatric data)

General Dosage Range Dosage adjustment recommended in patients with renal impairment

I.V.:

Children ≥3 months and <50 kg: 10-40 mg/kg every 8 hours (maximum: 2 g every 8 hours)

Children ≥50 kg and Adults: 500 mg to 2 g every 8 hours

Dosage Forms

Injection, powder for reconstitution: 500 mg, 1 g

Merrem® I.V.: 500 mg, 1 g

Merrem® (Can) *see* meropenem *on page* 577

Merrem® I.V. *see* meropenem *on page* 577

Mersyndol® With Codeine (Can) *see* acetaminophen, codeine, and doxylamine *(Canada only) on page* 27

mesalamine (me SAL a meen)

Medication Safety Issues

Sound-alike/look-alike issues:

Mesalamine may be confused with mecamylamine, megestrol, memantine, metaxalone, methenamine

Apriso™ may be confused with Apri®

Asacol® may be confused with Ansaid®, Os-Cal®, Visicol®

Lialda® may be confused with Aldara®

Pentasa® may be confused with Pancrease®, Pangestyme®

Synonyms 5-aminosalicylic acid; 5-ASA; fisalamine; mesalazine

U.S. Brand Names Apriso™; Asacol®; Asacol® HD; Canasa®; Lialda®; Pentasa®; Rowasa®; sfRowasa™

Canadian Brand Names 5-ASA; Asacol®; Asacol® 800; Mesasal®; Mezavant®; Novo-5 ASA; Novo-5 ASA-ECT; Pentasa®; Salofalk®; Salofalk® 5-ASA

Therapeutic Category 5-Aminosalicylic Acid Derivative

Use

Oral:

Asacol®, Lialda®, Mezavant®, Pentasa®: Treatment and maintenance of remission of mildly- to moderately-active ulcerative colitis

Apriso™: Maintenance of remission of ulcerative colitis

Asacol® HD: Treatment of moderately-active ulcerative colitis

Rectal: Treatment of active mild-to-moderate distal ulcerative colitis, proctosigmoiditis, or proctitis

General Dosage Range

Oral: *Adults:*

Capsule: Apriso™: 1.5 g once daily; Pentasa®: 1 g 4 times/day

Tablet: Asacol®: 800 mg 3 times/day or 1.6 g/day in divided doses; Asacol® HD: 1.6 g 3 times/day; Lialda®, Mezavant®: 2.4-4.8 g once daily

Rectal: *Adults:* Retention enema: 60 mL (4 g) at bedtime, retained overnight (~8 hours); Suppository: Insert 1000 mg at bedtime

Dosage Forms

Capsule, controlled release, oral:

Pentasa®: 250 mg, 500 mg

Capsule, delayed and extended release, oral:

Apriso™: 0.375 g

Suppository, rectal:

Canasa®: 1000 mg (30s, 42s)

Suspension, rectal: 4 g/60 mL (7s, 28s)

Rowasa®: 4 g/60 mL (7s, 28s)

sfRowasa™: 4 g/60 mL (7s, 28s)

Tablet, delayed release, enteric coated, oral:

Asacol®: 400 mg

Asacol® HD: 800 mg

Lialda®: 1.2 g

Dosage Forms - Canada

Tablet, delayed and extended release:

Mezavant®: 1.2 g

mesalazine *see* mesalamine *on page 577*

Mesasal® (Can) *see* mesalamine *on page 577*

M-Eslon® (Can) *see* morphine (systemic) *on page 612*

mesna (MES na)

Synonyms mercaptoethane sulfonate; sodium 2-mercaptoethane sulfonate

U.S. Brand Names Mesnex®

Canadian Brand Names Mesna for injection; Uromitexan

Therapeutic Category Antidote

Use Preventative agent to reduce the incidence of ifosfamide-induced hemorrhagic cystitis

General Dosage Range

I.V.: *Children and Adults:* 60% of the ifosfamide dose given in 3 divided doses

I.V., Oral: *Children and Adults:* 100% of the ifosfamide dose, given as 20% I.V., followed by 2 (40% each) doses orally

Dosage Forms

Injection, solution: 100 mg/mL (10 mL)

Mesnex®: 100 mg/mL (10 mL)

Tablet, oral:

Mesnex®: 400 mg

Dosage Forms - Canada

Injection, solution:

Mesna for injection: 100 mg/mL (10 mL)

Mesna for injection (Can) *see* mesna *on page 578*

Mesnex® *see* mesna *on page 578*

Mestinon® *see* pyridostigmine *on page 777*

Mestinon®-SR (Can) *see* pyridostigmine *on page 777*

Mestinon® Timespan® *see* pyridostigmine *on page 777*

mestranol and norethindrone *see* norethindrone and mestranol *on page 649*

Metadate CD® *see* methylphenidate *on page 590*

Metadate® ER *see* methylphenidate *on page 590*

Metadol™ (Can) *see* methadone *on page 581*

Metadol-D™ (Can) *see* methadone *on page 581*

Metaglip™ *see* glipizide and metformin *on page 427*

123 meta-iodobenzlyguanidine sulfate *see* iobenguane I 123 *on page 493*

Metamucil® [OTC] *see* psyllium *on page 774*

Metamucil® (Can) *see* psyllium *on page 774*

Metamucil® Plus Calcium [OTC] *see* psyllium *on page 774*

Metamucil® Smooth Texture [OTC] *see* psyllium *on page 774*

metaproterenol (met a proe TER e nol)

Medication Safety Issues

Sound-alike/look-alike issues:

Metaproterenol may be confused with metipranolol, metoprolol

Alupent may be confused with Atrovent®

Synonyms Alupent; metaproterenol sulfate; orciprenaline sulfate

Canadian Brand Names Apo-Orciprenaline®; ratio-Orciprenaline®; Tanta-Orciprenaline®

Therapeutic Category Adrenergic Agonist Agent

Use Bronchodilator in reversible airway obstruction due to asthma or COPD

General Dosage Range Oral:

Children <6 years: 1.3-2.6 mg/kg/day divided every 6-8 hours

Children 6-9 years (or <27 kg): 10 mg/dose 3-4 times/day

Children >9 years (or ≥27 kg) and Adults: 20 mg 3-4 times/day

Dosage Forms

Syrup, oral: 10 mg/5 mL (473 mL)

Tablet, oral: 10 mg, 20 mg

metaproterenol sulfate *see* metaproterenol *on page 579*

Metastron® *see* strontium-89 *on page 854*

metaxalone (me TAKS a lone)

Medication Safety Issues

Sound-alike/look-alike issues:

Metaxalone may be confused with mesalamine, metolazone

Skelaxin® may be confused with Robaxin®

BEERS Criteria medication:

This drug may be potentially inappropriate for use in geriatric patients (Quality of evidence - moderate; Strength of recommendation - strong).

U.S. Brand Names Skelaxin®

Canadian Brand Names Skelaxin®

Therapeutic Category Skeletal Muscle Relaxant

Use Relief of discomfort associated with acute, painful musculoskeletal conditions

General Dosage Range Oral: *Children >12 years and Adults:* 800 mg 3-4 times/day

Dosage Forms

Tablet, oral: 800 mg

Skelaxin®: 800 mg

metformin (met FOR min)

Medication Safety Issues

Sound-alike/look-alike issues:

MetFORMIN may be confused with metroNIDAZOLE

Glucophage® may be confused with Glucotrol®, Glutofac®

High alert medication:

The Institute for Safe Medication Practices (ISMP) includes this medication among its list of drug classes which have a heightened risk of causing significant patient harm when used in error.

International issues:

Dianben [Spain] may be confused with Diovan brand name for valsartan [U.S., Canada, and multiple international markets]

Synonyms metformin hydrochloride

Tall-Man met**FORMIN**

U.S. Brand Names Fortamet®; Glucophage®; Glucophage® XR; Glumetza®; Riomet®

Canadian Brand Names Apo-Metformin®; Ava-Metformin; CO Metformin; Dom-Metformin; Glucophage®; Glumetza®; Glycon; JAMP-Metformin; JAMP-Metformin Blackberry; Med-Metformin; Mylan-Metformin; Novo-Metformin; Nu-Metformin; PHL-Metformin; PMS-Metformin; PRO-Metformin; Q-Metformin; RAN™-Metformin; ratio-Metformin; Riva-Metformin; Sandoz-Metformin FC

Therapeutic Category Antidiabetic Agent, Oral

Use Management of type 2 diabetes mellitus (noninsulin-dependent, NIDDM) when hyperglycemia cannot be managed with diet and exercise alone.

General Dosage Range Oral:

Extended release: *Adults:* Initial: 500 mg once daily; Maintenance: Up to 2000-2500 mg/day (varies by product) in 1-2 divided doses

Immediate release:

Children 10-16 years: Initial: 500 mg twice daily; Maintenance: Up to 2000 mg/day in divided doses

Children >16 years and Adults: Initial: 500 mg twice daily **or** 850 mg once daily; Maintenance: Up to 2000 mg/day in 2 divided doses **or** 2550 mg/day in 3 divided doses

Dosage Forms

Solution, oral:

Riomet®: 100 mg/mL (118 mL, 473 mL)

Tablet, oral: 500 mg, 850 mg, 1000 mg

Glucophage®: 500 mg, 850 mg, 1000 mg

Tablet, extended release, oral: 500 mg, 750 mg, 1000 mg

Fortamet®: 500 mg, 1000 mg

Glucophage® XR: 500 mg, 750 mg

Glumetza®: 500 mg, 1000 mg

metformin and glipizide *see* glipizide and metformin *on page* 427

metformin and glyburide *see* glyburide and metformin *on page* 429

metformin and linagliptin *see* linagliptin and metformin *on page* 540

metformin and repaglinide *see* repaglinide and metformin *on page* 794

metformin and rosiglitazone *see* rosiglitazone and metformin *on page* 812

metformin and saxagliptin *see* saxagliptin and metformin *on page* 825

metformin and sitagliptin *see* sitagliptin and metformin *on page* 837

metformin hydrochloride *see* metformin *on page* 579

metformin hydrochloride and linagliptin *see* linagliptin and metformin *on page* 540

metformin hydrochloride and pioglitazone hydrochloride *see* pioglitazone and metformin *on page* 725

metformin hydrochloride and rosiglitazone maleate *see* rosiglitazone and metformin *on page* 812

metformin hydrochloride and saxagliptin *see* saxagliptin and metformin *on page* 825

methacholine (meth a KOLE leen)

Synonyms methacholine chloride

U.S. Brand Names Provocholine®

Canadian Brand Names Methacholine Omega; Provocholine®

Therapeutic Category Diagnostic Agent

Use Diagnosis of bronchial airway hyperactivity

General Dosage Range Inhalation: *Children ≥5 years and Adults:* 5 breaths of each of the following concentrations: 0.025 mg/mL, 0.25 mg/mL, 2.5 mg/mL, 10 mg/mL, and 25 mg/mL

Dosage Forms

Powder for reconstitution, for oral inhalation:
Provocholine®: 100 mg

methacholine chloride *see* methacholine *on page 580*

Methacholine Omega (Can) *see* methacholine *on page 580*

methadone (METH a done)

Medication Safety Issues

Sound-alike/look-alike issues:
Methadone may be confused with dexmethylphenidate, Mephyton®, methylphenidate, Metadate CD®, Metadate® ER, morphine

High alert medication:
The Institute for Safe Medication Practices (ISMP) includes this medication among its list of drug classes which have a heightened risk of causing significant patient harm when used in error.

Synonyms methadone hydrochloride

U.S. Brand Names Dolophine®; Methadone Diskets®; Methadone Intensol™; Methadose®

Canadian Brand Names Metadol-D™; Metadol™

Therapeutic Category Analgesic, Narcotic

Controlled Substance C-II

Use Management of moderate-to-severe pain; detoxification and maintenance treatment of opioid addiction as part of an FDA-approved program

General Dosage Range Dosage adjustment recommended in patients with renal impairment or who develop toxicities

I.M.:
Adults: Initial: 2.5 mg every 8-12 hours
Elderly: 2.5 mg every 8-12 hours

I.V., SubQ: *Adults:* Initial: 2.5 mg every 8-12 hours

Oral:
Adults: Detoxification: Initial: Up to 40 mg/day; Maintenance: 80-120 mg/day; Pain: 2.5-10 mg every 4-12 hours as needed
Elderly: 2.5 mg every 8-12 hours

Dosage Forms

Injection, solution: 10 mg/mL (20 mL)

Solution, oral: 5 mg/5 mL (500 mL); 10 mg/5 mL (500 mL); 10 mg/mL (946 mL, 960 mL, 1000 mL, 1000s)
Methadone Intensol™: 10 mg/mL (30 mL)
Methadose®: 10 mg/mL (1000 mL)

Tablet, oral: 5 mg, 10 mg
Dolophine®: 5 mg, 10 mg

Tablet, dispersible, oral: 40 mg
Methadone Diskets®: 40 mg
Methadose®: 40 mg

Methadone Diskets® *see* methadone *on page 581*

methadone hydrochloride *see* methadone *on page 581*

Methadone Intensol™ *see* methadone *on page 581*

Methadose® *see* methadone *on page 581*

methaminodiazepoxide hydrochloride *see* chlordiazepoxide *on page 196*

methamphetamine (meth am FET a meen)

Medication Safety Issues

Sound-alike/look-alike issues:
Desoxyn® may be confused with digoxin

Synonyms desoxyephedrine hydrochloride; methamphetamine hydrochloride

U.S. Brand Names Desoxyn®

Canadian Brand Names Desoxyn®

Therapeutic Category Amphetamine

Controlled Substance C-II

Use Treatment of attention-deficit/hyperactivity disorder (ADHD); short-term (few weeks) adjunct to caloric restriction in exogenous obesity

Pharmacotherapy for weight loss is recommended only for obese patients with a body mass index ≥30 kg/m^2, or ≥27 kg/m^2 in the presence of other risk factors such as hypertension, diabetes, and/or dyslipidemia or a high waist circumference; therapy should be used in conjunction with a comprehensive weight management program.

General Dosage Range Oral:

Children ≥6 years: ADHD: Initial: 5 mg 1-2 times daily; Usual maintenance: 20-25 mg daily
Children ≥12 years and Adults: Exogenous obesity: 5 mg before each meal

Dosage Forms

Tablet, oral: 5 mg
Desoxyn®: 5 mg

methamphetamine hydrochloride *see* methamphetamine *on page* 581

methazolamide (meth a ZOE la mide)

Medication Safety Issues

Sound-alike/look-alike issues:

Methazolamide may be confused with methenamine, metolazone
Neptazane™ may be confused with Nesacaine®

U.S. Brand Names Neptazane™

Canadian Brand Names Apo-Methazolamide®

Therapeutic Category Carbonic Anhydrase Inhibitor

Use Treatment of chronic open-angle or secondary glaucoma; short-term therapy of acute angle-closure glaucoma prior to surgery

General Dosage Range Oral: *Adults:* 50-100 mg 2-3 times/day

Dosage Forms

Tablet, oral: 25 mg, 50 mg
Neptazane™: 25 mg, 50 mg

methenamine (meth EN a meen)

Medication Safety Issues

Sound-alike/look-alike issues:

Hiprex® may be confused with Mirapex®
Methenamine may be confused with mesalamine, methazolamide, methionine
Urex may be confused with Eurax®, Serax

International issues:

Urex: Brand name for methenamine [U.S. (discontinued)], but also the brand name for furosemide [Australia, China, Turkey]
Urex [U.S. (discontinued)] may be confused with Eurax brand name for crotamitin [U.S., Canada, and multiple international markets]

Synonyms hexamethylenetetramine; methenamine hippurate; methenamine mandelate; Urex

U.S. Brand Names Hiprex®

Canadian Brand Names Dehydral®; Hiprex®; Mandelamine®; Urasal®

Therapeutic Category Antibiotic, Miscellaneous

Use Prophylaxis or suppression of recurrent urinary tract infections; urinary tract discomfort secondary to hypermotility

General Dosage Range Oral:

Hippurate:
Children ≥6 years: 0.5-1 g twice daily
Adults: 1 g twice daily

Mandelate:
Children >2-6 years: 50-75 mg/kg/day in 3-4 divided doses **or** 0.25 g/30 lb 4 times/day
Children 6-12 years: 50-75 mg/kg/day in 3-4 divided doses **or** 0.5 g 4 times/day
Children >12 years and Adults: 1 g 4 times/day

Dosage Forms

Tablet, oral: 500 mg, 1 g
Hiprex®: 1 g

methenamine hippurate *see* methenamine *on page* 582

methenamine mandelate *see* methenamine *on page* 582

methenamine, phenyl salicylate, methylene blue, benzoic acid, and hyoscyamine

(meth EN a meen, fen nil sa LIS i late, METH i leen bloo, ben ZOE ik AS id & hye oh SYE a meen)

Medication Safety Issues

BEERS Criteria medication:

This drug may be potentially inappropriate for use in geriatric patients (Quality of evidence - moderate; Strength of recommendation - strong).

Synonyms benzoic acid, hyoscyamine, methenamine, methylene blue, and phenyl salicylate; benzoic acid, methenamine, methylene blue, phenyl salicylate, and hyoscyamine; hyoscyamine, methenamine, benzoic acid, phenyl salicylate, and methylene blue; methylene blue, methenamine, benzoic acid, phenyl salicylate, and hyoscyamine; phenyl salicylate, methenamine, methylene blue, benzoic acid, and hyoscyamine

U.S. Brand Names Hyophen™; Prosed®/DS

Therapeutic Category Antibiotic, Miscellaneous

Use Urinary tract discomfort secondary to hypermotility resulting from infection or diagnostic procedures

General Dosage Range Oral: *Adults:* 1 tablet 4 times/day

Dosage Forms

Tablet, oral:

Hyophen™, Prosed®/DS: Methenamine 81.6 mg, phenyl salicylate 36.2 mg, methylene blue 10.8 mg, benzoic acid 9 mg, hyoscyamine sulfate 0.12 mg

Methergine® [DSC] *see* methylergonovine *on page* 589

Methergine® (Can) *see* methylergonovine *on page* 589

methimazole (meth IM a zole)

Medication Safety Issues

Sound-alike/look-alike issues:

Methimazole may be confused with metolazone

Synonyms thiamazole

U.S. Brand Names Tapazole®

Canadian Brand Names Dom-Methimazole; PHL-Methimazole; Tapazole®

Therapeutic Category Antithyroid Agent

Use Treatment of hyperthyroidism; improve hyperthyroidism prior to thyroidectomy or radioactive iodine therapy

General Dosage Range Oral:

Children: Initial: 0.4 mg/kg/day in 3 divided doses; Maintenance: 0.2 mg/kg/day in 3 divided doses

Adults: Initial: 15-60 mg/day in 3 divided doses; Maintenance: 5-15 mg/day in 1-3 divided doses

Dosage Forms

Tablet, oral: 5 mg, 10 mg

Tapazole®: 5 mg, 10 mg

Methitest™ *see* methyltestosterone *on page* 593

methocarbamol (meth oh KAR ba mole)

Medication Safety Issues

Sound-alike/look-alike issues:

Methocarbamol may be confused with mephobarbital

Robaxin® may be confused with ribavirin, Skelaxin®

BEERS Criteria medication:

This drug may be potentially inappropriate for use in geriatric patients (Quality of evidence - moderate; Strength of recommendation - strong).

International issues:

Robaxin [U.S., Canada, Great Britain, Greece, Spain] may be confused with Rubex brand name for ascorbic acid [Ireland]; doxorubicin [Brazil]

U.S. Brand Names Robaxin®; Robaxin®-750

Canadian Brand Names Robaxin®

Therapeutic Category Skeletal Muscle Relaxant

Use Adjunctive treatment of muscle spasm associated with acute painful musculoskeletal conditions (eg, tetanus)

General Dosage Range

I.M.: *Adults:* 1 g every 8 hours (maximum dose: 3 g/day for 3 consecutive days)

I.V.:

Children: 15 mg/kg/dose **or** 500 mg/m²/dose every 6 hours as needed (maximum dose: 1.8 g/m²/day for 3 consecutive days)

Adults: 1-3 g every 6 hours **or** 1 g every 8 hours (maximum dose: 3 g/day for 3 consecutive days)

Oral: *Children ≥16 years and Adults:* Initial: 1.5 g 4 times/day for 2-3 days (maximum: 8 g/day); Maintenance: 4-4.5 g/day in 3-6 divided doses

Dosage Forms

Injection, solution:

Robaxin®: 100 mg/mL (10 mL)

Tablet, oral: 500 mg, 750 mg

Robaxin®: 500 mg

Robaxin®-750: 750 mg

methohexital (meth oh HEKS i tal)

Medication Safety Issues

Sound-alike/look-alike issues:

Brevital® may be confused with Brevibloc®

High alert medication:

The Institute for Safe Medication Practices (ISMP) includes this medication among its list of drugs which have a heightened risk of causing significant patient harm when used in error.

Synonyms methohexital sodium

U.S. Brand Names Brevital® Sodium

Canadian Brand Names Brevital®

Therapeutic Category Barbiturate

Controlled Substance C-IV

Use Induction of anesthesia; procedural sedation

General Dosage Range Dosage adjustment recommended in patients with hepatic impairment

I.M.: *Infants ≥1 month and Children:* Induction: 6.6-10 mg/kg of a 5% solution

I.V.: *Adults:* Induction: 1-1.5 mg/kg

Rectal: *Infants ≥1 month and Children:* Induction: 25 mg/kg of a 1% solution **or** 25 mg/kg of a 10% (100 mg/mL) solution; maximum dose: 500 mg

Dosage Forms

Injection, powder for reconstitution:

Brevital® Sodium: 500 mg, 2.5 g

methohexital sodium *see* methohexital *on page* 584

methotrexate (meth oh TREKS ate)

Medication Safety Issues

Sound-alike/look-alike issues:

Methotrexate may be confused with mercaptopurine, methylPREDNISolone sodium succinate, metolazone, metroNIDAZOLE, mitoXANtrone, PRALAtrexate

High alert medication:

The Institute for Safe Medication Practices (ISMP) includes this medication among its list of drugs which have a heightened risk of causing significant patient harm when used in error.

Administration issues:

Errors have occurred (resulting in death) when methotrexate was administered as "daily" dose instead of the recommended "weekly" dose.

Intrathecal medication safety: The American Society of Clinical Oncology (ASCO)/Oncology Nursing Society (ONS) chemotherapy administration safety standards (Jacobson, 2009) encourage the following safety measures for intrathecal chemotherapy:

- Intrathecal medication should not be prepared during the preparation of any other agents
- After preparation, store in an isolated location or container clearly marked with a label identifying as "intrathecal" use only
- Delivery to the patient should only be with other medications intended for administration into the central nervous system

Other safety concerns:

MTX is an error-prone abbreviation (mistaken as mitoxantrone)

International issues:

Trexall [U.S.] may be confused with Trexol brand name for tamadol [Mexico]; Truxal brand name for chlorprothixene [multiple international markets]

Synonyms amethopterin; methotrexate sodium; methotrexatum; MTX (error-prone abbreviation)

U.S. Brand Names Rheumatrex®; Trexall™

Canadian Brand Names Apo-Methotrexate®; ratio-Methotrexate

Therapeutic Category Antineoplastic Agent

Use

Oncology-related uses: Treatment of trophoblastic neoplasms (gestational choriocarcinoma, chorioadenoma destruens and hydatidiform mole), acute lymphocytic leukemia (ALL), meningeal leukemia, breast cancer, head and neck cancer (epidermoid), cutaneous T-Cell lymphoma (advanced mycosis fungoides), lung cancer (squamous cell and small cell), advanced non-Hodgkin lymphomas (NHL), osteosarcoma

Nononcology uses: Treatment of psoriasis (severe, recalcitrant, disabling) and severe rheumatoid arthritis (RA), including polyarticular-course juvenile idiopathic arthritis (JIA)

General Dosage Range Dosage adjustment recommended in patients with hepatic or renal impairment

I.M., oral:

Children: 5-30 mg/m^2 once weekly or every 2 weeks

Adults: Dosage varies greatly depending on indication

I.V.:

Children: 10-18,000 mg/m^2 bolus dosing or continuous infusion over 6-42 hours

Adults: Dosage varies greatly depending on indication

Intrathecal:

Children <1 year: 6 mg/dose

Children 1 year: 8 mg/dose

Children 2 years: 10 mg/dose

Children ≥3 years and Adults: 12 mg/dose

Dosage Forms

Injection, powder for reconstitution: 1 g

Injection, solution: 25 mg/mL (2 mL, 10 mL)

Injection, solution [preservative free]: 25 mg/mL (2 mL, 4 mL, 8 mL, 10 mL, 20 mL, 40 mL)

Tablet, oral: 2.5 mg

Rheumatrex®: 2.5 mg

Trexall™: 5 mg, 7.5 mg, 10 mg, 15 mg

methotrexate sodium *see* methotrexate *on page* 584

methotrexatum *see* methotrexate *on page* 584

methotrimeprazine *(Canada only)* (meth oh trye MEP ra zeen)

Synonyms levomepromazine; methotrimeprazine hydrochloride

Canadian Brand Names Apo-Methoprazine®; Novo-Meprazine; Nozinan®; PMS-Methotrimeprazine

Therapeutic Category Neuroleptic Agent

Use Treatment of schizophrenia; psychosis; manic-depressive syndromes; anxiety or tension disorders; management of pain, including pain caused by neuralgia or cancer; adjunct to general anesthesia; management of nausea and vomiting; sedation

General Dosage Range

I.M.:

Children: 0.063-0.125 mg/kg/day in 1-3 divided doses

Adults: 10-25 mg every 8 hours **or** 75-100 mg as a single dose

I.V.:
Children: 0.063 mg/kg in 250 mL D_5W infused at a rate of 20-40 drops/minute
Adults: 10-25 mg in 500 mL D_5W infused at a rate of 20-40 drops/minute
Oral:
Children: 0.25 mg/kg/day in 2-3 divided doses (maximum: 40 mg/day [children <12 years])
Adults: 6-75 mg/day in 2-3 divided doses (maximum: doses up to 1000 mg/day have been used) **or** 10-25 mg at bedtime

Product Availability Not available in U.S.

Dosage Forms - Canada
Injection, solution:
Nozinan®: 25 mg/mL (1 mL)
Tablet, oral: 2 mg, 5 mg, 25 mg, 50 mg

methotrimeprazine hydrochloride *see* methotrimeprazine *(Canada only) on page* 585

methoxsalen (systemic) (meth OKS a len)

Medication Safety Issues
Sound-alike/look-alike issues:
Methoxsalen soft gelatin capsules (Oxsoralen-Ultra®) may be confused with methoxsalen hard gelatin capsules (8-MOP®); bioavailability and photosensitization onset differ between the two products.

Synonyms 8-methoxypsoralen; methoxypsoralen

U.S. Brand Names 8-MOP®; Oxsoralen-Ultra®; Uvadex®

Canadian Brand Names Oxsoralen-Ultra®; Oxsoralen® Capsule; Ultramop™

Therapeutic Category Psoralen

Use
Oral: Symptomatic control of severe, recalcitrant disabling psoriasis; repigmentation of idiopathic vitiligo; palliative treatment of skin manifestations of cutaneous T-cell lymphoma (CTCL)
Extracorporeal: Palliative treatment of skin manifestations of CTCL

General Dosage Range
Extracorporeal: *Adults:* Amount of Uvadex® needed for each treatment may be calculated using the following equation: Treatment volume x 0.017 = mL of Uvadex® needed. Inject this amount into photoactivation bag and administer treatment for 2 consecutive days every 4 weeks for a minimum of 7 treatment cycles; may increase to every 2 weeks (maximum: 20 accelerated therapy cycles)
Oral: *Adults:* Psoriasis: Initial: 10-70 mg; may repeat 2-3 times/week (48 hours between doses); Maintenance: 1 treatment every 1-3 weeks; Vitiligo: 20 mg

Dosage Forms
Capsule, oral:
8-MOP®: 10 mg
Oxsoralen-Ultra®: 10 mg
Solution, for extracorporeal administration:
Uvadex®: 20 mcg/mL (10 mL)

methoxsalen (topical) (meth OKS a len)

Synonyms methoxypsoralen

U.S. Brand Names Oxsoralen®

Canadian Brand Names Oxsoralen® Lotion

Therapeutic Category Psoralen

Use Repigmentation of idiopathic vitiligo

General Dosage Range Topical: *Children ≥12 years and Adults:* Lotion is applied by healthcare provider prior to UVA light exposure, usually no more than once weekly

Dosage Forms
Lotion, topical:
Oxsoralen®: 1% (29.57 mL)

methoxypsoralen *see* methoxsalen (systemic) *on page* 586

methoxypsoralen *see* methoxsalen (topical) *on page* 586

8-methoxypsoralen *see* methoxsalen (systemic) *on page* 586

methscopolamine (meth skoe POL a meen)

Medication Safety Issues

International issues:

Pamine [U.S., Canada] may be confused with Pemine brand name for penicillamine [Italy]

Synonyms methscopolamine bromide

U.S. Brand Names Pamine®; Pamine® Forte

Canadian Brand Names Pamine®

Therapeutic Category Anticholinergic Agent

Use Adjunctive therapy in the treatment of peptic ulcer

General Dosage Range Oral: *Adults:* 2.5-5 mg twice daily

Dosage Forms

Tablet, oral: 2.5 mg, 5 mg

Pamine®: 2.5 mg

Pamine® Forte: 5 mg

methscopolamine bromide *see* methscopolamine *on page* 587

methsuximide (meth SUKS i mide)

Medication Safety Issues

Sound-alike/look-alike issues:

Methsuximide may be confused with ethosuximide

U.S. Brand Names Celontin®

Canadian Brand Names Celontin®

Therapeutic Category Anticonvulsant

Use Control of absence (petit mal) seizures that are refractory to other drugs

General Dosage Range Oral: *Adults:* Initial: 300 mg/day for 1 week; Maintenance: Up to 1.2 g/day in 2-4 divided doses

Dosage Forms

Capsule, oral:

Celontin®: 150 mg, 300 mg

methyclothiazide (meth i kloe THYE a zide)

Medication Safety Issues

Sound-alike/look-alike issues:

Enduron may be confused with Empirin, Imuran®, Inderal®

Synonyms Enduron

Therapeutic Category Diuretic, Thiazide

Use Management of hypertension; adjunctive therapy of edema

General Dosage Range Oral: *Adults:* 2.5-10 mg once daily

Dosage Forms

Tablet, oral: 5 mg

methylacetoxyprogesterone *see* medroxyprogesterone *on page* 567

methyl aminolevulinate (METH il a mee noe LEV ue lin ate)

Medication Safety Issues

Sound-alike/look-alike issues:

Methyl aminolevulinate may be confused with aminolevulinic acid

Synonyms methyl aminolevulinate hydrochloride; P-1202

U.S. Brand Names Metvixia™

Canadian Brand Names Metvix®

Therapeutic Category Photosensitizing Agent, Topical; Topical Skin Product

Use Treatment of thin and moderately thick, nonhyperkeratotic, nonpigmented actinic keratoses of the face and scalp; to be used in conjunction with red light illumination

General Dosage Range Topical: *Adults:* Apply up to 1 g once; repeat in 1 week

Dosage Forms

Cream, topical:

Metvixia™: 16.8% (2 g)

methyl aminolevulinate hydrochloride *see* methyl aminolevulinate *on page 587*

methylcellulose (meth il SEL yoo lose)

Medication Safety Issues

Sound-alike/look-alike issues:

Citrucel® may be confused with Citracal®

U.S. Brand Names Citrucel® [OTC]; Soluble Fiber Therapy [OTC]

Therapeutic Category Laxative

Use Adjunct in treatment of constipation

General Dosage Range Oral:

Caplet:

Children 6-11 years: 1 caplet up to 6 times/day (maximum: 6 caplets/day)

Children ≥12 years and Adults: 2 caplets up to 6 times/day (maximum: 12 caplets/day)

Powder:

Children 6-11 years: 1 g (2-2.5 level teaspoons) up to 3 times/day

Children ≥12 years and Adults: 2 g (1 rounded or heaping tablespoon) up to 3 times/day

Dosage Forms

Caplet, oral:

Citrucel® [OTC]: 500 mg

Powder, oral:

Citrucel® [OTC]: 2 g/scoop (454 g, 479 g, 850 g, 907 g, 1190 g, 1843 g)

Soluble Fiber Therapy [OTC]: 2 g/scoop (454 g)

methylcellulose, gelatin, and pectin *see* gelatin, pectin, and methylcellulose *on page 421*

methylcobalamin, acetylcysteine, and methylfolate *see* methylfolate, methylcobalamin, and acetylcysteine *on page 590*

methyldopa (meth il DOE pa)

Medication Safety Issues

Sound-alike/look-alike issues:

Methyldopa may be confused with L-dopa, levodopa

BEERS Criteria medication:

This drug may be potentially inappropriate for use in geriatric patients (Quality of evidence - low; Strength of recommendation - strong).

Synonyms Aldomet; methyldopate hydrochloride

Canadian Brand Names Apo-Methyldopa®; Nu-Medopa

Therapeutic Category Alpha-Adrenergic Blocking Agent

Use Management of moderate-to-severe hypertension

General Dosage Range Dosage adjustment recommended in patients with renal impairment

I.V.:

Children: 5-10 mg/kg/dose every 6-8 hours (maximum: 65 mg/kg/day; 3 g/day)

Adults: 250-500 mg every 6-8 hours (maximum: 1 g every 6 hours)

Oral:

Children: Initial: 10 mg/kg/day in 2-4 divided doses; Maintenance: Up to 65 mg/kg/day (maximum: 3 g/day)

Adults: Initial: 250 mg 2-3 times/day; Maintenance: 250-1000 mg/day in 2 divided doses (maximum: 3 g/day)

Dosage Forms

Injection, solution: 50 mg/mL (5 mL)

Tablet, oral: 250 mg, 500 mg

methyldopa and hydrochlorothiazide (meth il DOE pa & hye droe klor oh THYE a zide)

Medication Safety Issues

Sound-alike/look-alike issues:

Aldoril may be confused with Aldomet, Elavil®

BEERS Criteria medication:

This drug may be potentially inappropriate for use in geriatric patients (Quality of evidence - low; Strength of recommendation - strong).

Synonyms Aldoril; hydrochlorothiazide and methyldopa

Canadian Brand Names Apo-Methazide®

Therapeutic Category Antihypertensive Agent, Combination

Use Management of moderate-to-severe hypertension

General Dosage Range Oral: *Adults:* Methyldopa 250 mg and hydrochlorothiazide 15-25 mg twice daily **or** methyldopa 250 mg and hydrochlorothiazide 15 mg 3 times daily **or** methyldopa 500 mg and hydrochlorothiazide 30-50 mg once daily. Maximum daily dose, based on the hydrochlorothiazide content: Oral: 50 mg/day

Dosage Forms

Tablet: Methyldopa 250 mg and hydrochlorothiazide 15 mg; methyldopa 250 mg and hydrochlorothiazide 25 mg

methyldopate hydrochloride *see* methyldopa *on page* 588

methylene blue (METH i leen bloo)

Medication Safety Issues

Other safety concerns:

Due to the potential for dosing errors between mg and mL of methylene blue, prescribing and dosing should only be expressed in terms of mg of methylene blue (and not as mL)

Due to potential toxicity (hemolytic anemia), do not use methylene blue to color enteral feedings to detect aspiration.

Synonyms methylthionine chloride

Therapeutic Category Antidote

Use Antidote for cyanide poisoning and drug-induced methemoglobinemia, indicator dye

General Dosage Range I.V.: *Children and Adults:* 1-2 mg/kg **or** 25-50 mg/m^2 as a single dose; may repeat

Dosage Forms

Injection, solution: 10 mg/mL (1 mL, 10 mL)

methylene blue, methenamine, benzoic acid, phenyl salicylate, and hyoscyamine *see* methenamine, phenyl salicylate, methylene blue, benzoic acid, and hyoscyamine *on page* 583

methylergometrine maleate *see* methylergonovine *on page* 589

methylergonovine (meth il er goe NOE veen)

Medication Safety Issues

Sound-alike/look-alike issues:

Methergine® may be confused with Brethine

Methylergonovine and terbutaline parenteral dosage forms look similar. Due to their contrasting indications, use care when administering these agents.

Synonyms methylergometrine maleate; methylergonovine maleate

U.S. Brand Names Methergine® [DSC]

Canadian Brand Names Methergine®

Therapeutic Category Ergot Alkaloid and Derivative

Use Prevention and treatment of postpartum and postabortion hemorrhage caused by uterine atony or subinvolution

General Dosage Range

I.M., I.V.: *Adults:* 0.2 mg after delivery; may repeat every 2-4 hours

Oral: *Adults:* 0.2 mg 3-4 times/day in the puerperium

Dosage Forms

Injection, solution: 0.2 mg/mL (1 mL)

Tablet, oral: 0.2 mg

methylergonovine maleate *see* methylergonovine *on page* 589

methylfolate (meth il FO late)

Synonyms 6(S)-5-methyltetrahydrofolate; 6(S)-5-MTHF; L-methylfolate

U.S. Brand Names Deplin®

Therapeutic Category Dietary Supplement

Use Medicinal food for management of patients with low plasma and/or low red blood cell folate

General Dosage Range Oral: *Adults:* 7.5 mg daily

Dosage Forms

Tablet, oral: L-methylfolate 7.5 mg

Deplin™: L-methylfolate 7.5 mg

methylfolate, methylcobalamin, and acetylcysteine

(meth il FO late meth il koe BAL a min & a se teel SIS teen)

Synonyms acetylcysteine, methylcobalamin, and methylfolate; acetylcysteine, methylfolate, and methylcobalamin; L-methylfolate, methylcobalamin, and N-acetylcysteine; methylcobalamin, acetylcysteine, and methylfolate

U.S. Brand Names Cerefolin® NAC

Therapeutic Category Dietary Supplement

Use Medicinal food for use in patients with neurovascular oxidative stress and/or hyperhomocysteinemia

General Dosage Range Oral: *Children ≥12 years and Adults:* 1 caplet daily

Dosage Forms

Caplet, oral:

Cerefolin® NAC: L-methylfolate 5.6 mg, methylcobalamin 2 mg, and N-acetylcysteine 600 mg [gluten free, sugar free]

Methylin® *see* methylphenidate *on page 590*

methylmorphine *see* codeine *on page 230*

methylnaltrexone (meth il nal TREKS one)

Medication Safety Issues

Sound-alike/look-alike issues:

Methylnaltrexone may be confused with naltrexone

Synonyms methylnaltrexone bromide; N-methylnaltrexone bromide

U.S. Brand Names Relistor®

Canadian Brand Names Relistor®

Therapeutic Category Gastrointestinal Agent, Miscellaneous; Opioid Antagonist, Peripherally-Acting

Use Treatment of opioid-induced constipation in patients with advanced illness receiving palliative care with inadequate response to conventional laxative regimens

General Dosage Range Dosage adjustment recommended in patients with renal impairment

SubQ:

Adults <38 kg and >114 kg: 0.15 mg/kg (round dose up to nearest 0.1 mL of volume) every other day as needed (maximum: 1 dose/24 hours)

Adults 38 to <62 kg: 8 mg every other day as needed (maximum: 1 dose/24 hours)

Adults 62-114 kg: 12 mg every other day as needed (maximum: 1 dose/24 hours)

Dosage Forms

Injection, solution:

Relistor®: 8 mg/0.4 mL (0.4 mL); 12 mg/0.6 mL (0.6 mL)

methylnaltrexone bromide *see* methylnaltrexone *on page 590*

methylphenidate (meth il FEN i date)

Medication Safety Issues

Sound-alike/look-alike issues:

Metadate CD® may be confused with Metadate® ER

Metadate® ER may be confused with methadone

Methylphenidate may be confused with methadone

Ritalin® may be confused with Rifadin®, ritodrine

Ritalin LA® may be confused with Ritalin-SR®

Synonyms methylphenidate hydrochloride

U.S. Brand Names Concerta®; Daytrana®; Metadate CD®; Metadate® ER; Methylin®; Ritalin LA®; Ritalin-SR®; Ritalin®

Canadian Brand Names Apo-Methylphenidate®; Apo-Methylphenidate® SR; Biphentin®; Concerta®; PHL-Methylphenidate; PMS-Methylphenidate; ratio-Methylphenidate; Ritalin®; Ritalin® SR; Sandoz-Methylphenidate SR; Teva-Methylphenidate ER-C

Therapeutic Category Central Nervous System Stimulant, Nonamphetamine

Controlled Substance C-II

Use Treatment of attention-deficit/hyperactivity disorder (ADHD); symptomatic management of narcolepsy

General Dosage Range

Oral:

Immediate release:

Children ≥6 years: Initial: 5 mg twice daily; Maintenance: Increase by 5-10 mg/day at weekly intervals (maximum: 60 mg/day)

Adults: ADHD: Initial: 5 mg twice daily; Maintenance: Increase by 5-10 mg/day at weekly intervals (maximum: 60 mg/day); Narcolepsy: 10 mg 2-3 times/day (maximum: 60 mg/day)

Extended release:

Children 6-12 years: Concerta®: 18-54 mg once every morning (maximum: 54 mg/day); Metadate® ER, Ritalin® SR: Maximum: 60 mg/day; Metadate CD®, Ritalin LA®: Initial: 20 mg once daily (maximum: 60 mg/day)

Children 13-17 years and Adults: Concerta®: 18-72 mg once every morning (maximum: 72 mg/day); Metadate CD®, Ritalin LA®: Initial: 20 mg once daily (maximum: 60 mg/day)

Transdermal: *Children 6-17 years:* Initial: 10 mg patch once daily

Dosage Forms

Capsule, extended release, oral: 20 mg, 30 mg, 40 mg

Metadate CD®: 10 mg, 20 mg, 30 mg, 40 mg, 50 mg, 60 mg

Ritalin LA®: 10 mg, 20 mg, 30 mg, 40 mg

Patch, transdermal:

Daytrana®: 10 mg/9 hours (30s); 15 mg/9 hours (30s); 20 mg/9 hours (30s); 30 mg/9 hours (30s)

Solution, oral: 5 mg/5 mL (500 mL); 10 mg/mL (500 mL)

Methylin®: 5 mg/5 mL (500 mL); 10 mg/5 mL (500 mL)

Tablet, oral: 5 mg, 10 mg, 20 mg

Ritalin®: 5 mg, 10 mg, 20 mg

Tablet, chewable, oral:

Methylin®: 2.5 mg, 5 mg, 10 mg

Tablet, extended release, oral: 10 mg, 18 mg, 20 mg, 27 mg, 36 mg, 54 mg

Concerta®: 18 mg, 27 mg, 36 mg, 54 mg

Metadate® ER: 20 mg

Tablet, sustained release, oral: 20 mg

Ritalin-SR®: 20 mg

methylphenidate hydrochloride *see* methylphenidate *on page 590*

methylphenoxy-benzene propanamine *see* atomoxetine *on page 99*

methylphenyl isoxazolyl penicillin *see* oxacillin *on page 674*

methylphytyl napthoquinone *see* phytonadione *on page 722*

methylprednisolone (meth il pred NIS oh lone)

Medication Safety Issues

Sound-alike/look-alike issues:

MethylPREDNISolone may be confused with medroxyPROGESTERone, methotrexate, methylTESTOSTERone, predniSONE

Depo-Medrol® may be confused with Solu-Medrol®

Medrol® may be confused with Mebaral®

Solu-MEDROL® may be confused with salmeterol, Solu-CORTEF®

International issues:

Medrol [U.S., Canada, and multiple international markets] may be confused with Medral brand name for omeprazole [Mexico]

Synonyms 6-α-methylprednisolone; Medrol Dose Pack; methylprednisolone acetate; methylprednisolone sodium succinate; Solumedrol

Tall-Man methyl**PREDNIS**olone

U.S. Brand Names A-Methapred®; Depo-Medrol®; Medrol®; Medrol® Dosepak™; Solu-MEDROL®

Canadian Brand Names Depo-Medrol®; Medrol®; Methylprednisolone Acetate; Solu-Medrol®

Therapeutic Category Adrenal Corticosteroid

Use Primarily as an antiinflammatory or immunosuppressant agent in the treatment of a variety of diseases including those of hematologic, allergic, inflammatory, neoplastic, and autoimmune origin. Prevention and treatment of graft-versus-host disease following allogeneic bone marrow transplantation.

General Dosage Range

I.M.:

Acetate: *Adults:* 10-120 mg every 1-2 weeks

Sodium succinate:

Children: 0.5-1.7 mg/kg/day **or** 5-25 mg/m^2/day divided every 6-12 hours; "Pulse" therapy: 15-30 mg/kg/dose given once daily for 3 days

Adults: 10-80 mg once daily

I.V. (sodium succinate): *Children and Adults:* Dosage varies greatly by indication

Intraarticular (acetate): *Adults:* Administer every 1-5 weeks

Large joints (eg, knee, ankle): 20-80 mg

Medium joints (eg, elbow, wrist): 10-40 mg

Small joints: 4-10 mg

Intralesional (acetate): *Adults:* 20-60 mg every 1-5 weeks

Oral:

Children: 0.5-1.7 mg/kg/day **or** 5-25 mg/m^2/day divided every 6-12 hours; "Pulse" therapy: 15-30 mg/kg/dose once daily for 3 days

Adults: 2-60 mg/day in 1-4 divided doses

Dosage Forms

Injection, powder for reconstitution: 40 mg, 125 mg, 500 mg, 1 g

A-Methapred®: 40 mg, 125 mg

Solu-MEDROL®: 500 mg, 1 g, 2 g

Injection, powder for reconstitution [preservative free]:

Solu-MEDROL®: 40 mg, 125 mg, 500 mg, 1 g

Injection, suspension: 40 mg/mL (1 mL, 5 mL, 10 mL); 80 mg/mL (1 mL, 5 mL)

Depo-Medrol®: 20 mg/mL (5 mL); 40 mg/mL (1 mL, 5 mL, 10 mL); 80 mg/mL (5 mL)

Injection, suspension [preservative free]:

Depo-Medrol®: 80 mg/mL (1 mL)

Tablet, oral: 4 mg, 8 mg, 16 mg, 32 mg

Medrol®: 2 mg, 4 mg, 8 mg, 16 mg, 32 mg

Medrol® Dosepak™: 4 mg

6-α-methylprednisolone *see* methylprednisolone *on page 591*

methylprednisolone acetate *see* methylprednisolone *on page 591*

Methylprednisolone Acetate (Can) *see* methylprednisolone *on page 591*

methylprednisolone sodium succinate *see* methylprednisolone *on page 591*

4-methylpyrazole *see* fomepizole *on page 405*

methyl salicylate and menthol (METH il sa LIS i late & MEN thol)

Medication Safety Issues

Other safety concerns:

Transdermal patch may contain conducting metal (eg, aluminum); remove patch prior to MRI.

Synonyms menthol and methyl salicylate

U.S. Brand Names BenGay® [OTC]; Icy Hot® [OTC]; Precise® [OTC]; Salonpas® Arthritis Pain® [OTC]; Salonpas® Jet Spray [OTC]; Salonpas® Massage Foam [OTC]; Salonpas® Pain Relief Patch® [OTC]; Salonpas® [OTC]; Thera-Gesic® Plus [OTC]; Thera-Gesic® [OTC]

Therapeutic Category Analgesic, Topical; Salicylate; Topical Skin Product

Use Temporary relief of minor aches and pains of muscle and joints associated with arthritis, bruises, simple backache, sprains, and strains

General Dosage Range Topical:

Balm, cream, foam, patch (methyl salicylate 10%/menthol 1.5%), spray, stick: *Children ≥12 years and Adults:* Apply up to 3-4 times/day

Gel: *Children ≥2 years and Adults:* Apply up to 3-4 times/day

Patch (methyl salicylate 10%/menthol 3%): *Adults:* Apply 1 patch for up to 8-12 hours (maximum: 1 patch/application; 2 patches/24 hours; 3 days of consecutive use)

Dosage Forms

Aerosol, foam, topical:

Salonpas® Massage Foam [OTC]: Methyl salicylate 10% and menthol 3% (118 mL)

Aerosol, spray, topical:

Salonpas® Jet Spray [OTC]: Methyl salicylate 10% and menthol 3% (118 mL)

Balm, topical:

Icy Hot® Balm [OTC]: Methyl salicylate 29% and menthol 7.6% (99.2 g)

Cream, topical:

BenGay® Arthritis Formula [OTC]: Methyl salicylate 30% and menthol 8% (57 g, 113 g)
BenGay® Greaseless [OTC]: Methyl salicylate 15% and menthol 10% (57 g, 113 g)
Icy Hot® [OTC]: Methyl salicylate 30% and menthol 10% (35.4 g, 85 g)
Precise® [OTC]: Methyl salicylate 30% and menthol 10% (75 g)
Thera-Gesic® [OTC]: Methyl salicylate 15% and menthol 1% (85 g, 142 g)
Thera-Gesic® Plus [OTC]: Methyl salicylate 15% and menthol 4% (85 g) [contains aloe]

Patch, topical:

Salonpas® Arthritis Pain® [OTC]: Methyl salicylate 10% and menthol 3% (5s)
Salonpas® Pain Relief Patch®: Methyl salicylate 10% and menthol 1.5% (3s)
Salonpas® Pain Relief Patch®: Methyl salicylate 10% and menthol 3% (5s)

Stick, topical:

Icy Hot® [OTC]: Methyl salicylate 30% and menthol 10% (49 g)

methyltestosterone (meth il tes TOS te rone)

Medication Safety Issues

Sound-alike/look-alike issues:

MethylTESTOSTERone may be confused with medroxyPROGESTERone, methylPREDNISolone

BEERS Criteria medication:

This drug may be potentially inappropriate for use in geriatric patients (Quality of evidence - moderate; Strength of recommendation - weak).

Tall-Man methyl**TESTOSTER**one

U.S. Brand Names Android®; Methitest™; Testred®

Therapeutic Category Androgen

Controlled Substance C-III

Use

Male: Hypogonadism; delayed puberty; impotence and climacteric symptoms
Female: Palliative treatment of metastatic breast cancer

General Dosage Range

Oral:

Adults (females): 50-200 mg/day
Adults (males): 10-50 mg/day

Dosage Forms

Capsule, oral:

Android®: 10 mg
Testred®: 10 mg

Tablet, oral:

Methitest™: 10 mg

methyltestosterone and esterified estrogen *see* estrogens (esterified) and methyltestosterone *on page 353*

methylthionine chloride *see* methylene blue *on page 589*

metipranolol (met i PRAN oh lol)

Medication Safety Issues

Sound-alike/look-alike issues:

Metipranolol may be confused with metaproterenol

International issues:

Betanol [Monaco] may be confused with Beta-Val brand name for betamethasone [U.S.]; Betimol brand name for timolol [U.S.]; Patanol brand name for olopatadine [U.S., Canada, and multiple international markets]

Synonyms metipranolol hydrochloride

U.S. Brand Names OptiPranolol®

Canadian Brand Names OptiPranolol®

Therapeutic Category Beta-Adrenergic Blocker

Use Treatment of chronic open-angle glaucoma or ocular hypertension

General Dosage Range Ophthalmic: *Adults:* Instill 1 drop into affected eye(s) twice daily

Dosage Forms

Solution, ophthalmic: 0.3% (5 mL, 10 mL)

OptiPranolol®: 0.3% (5 mL, 10 mL)

metipranolol hydrochloride *see* metipranolol *on page* 593

metoclopramide (met oh KLOE pra mide)

Medication Safety Issues

Sound-alike/look-alike issues:

Metoclopramide may be confused with metolazone, metoprolol, metroNIDAZOLE

Reglan® may be confused with Megace®, Regonol®, Renagel®

BEERS Criteria medication:

This drug may be potentially inappropriate for use in geriatric patients (Quality of evidence - moderate; Strength of recommendation - strong).

U.S. Brand Names Metozolv™ ODT; Reglan®

Canadian Brand Names Apo-Metoclop®; Metoclopramide Hydrochloride Injection; Metoclopramide Omega; Nu-Metoclopramide; PMS-Metoclopramide

Therapeutic Category Gastrointestinal Agent, Prokinetic

Use

Oral: Symptomatic treatment of diabetic gastroparesis; gastroesophageal reflux

I.V., I.M.: Symptomatic treatment of diabetic gastroparesis; postpyloric placement of enteral feeding tubes; prevention and/or treatment of nausea and vomiting associated with chemotherapy, or postsurgery; to stimulate gastric emptying and intestinal transit of barium during radiological examination of the stomach/small intestine

General Dosage Range Dosage adjustment recommended in patients with renal impairment

I.M.: *Adults:* 10-20 mg as a single dose **or** 10 mg before each meal and at bedtime

I.V.:

Children <6 years: 0.1 mg/kg as a single dose

Children 6-14 years: 2.5-5 mg as a single dose

Children >14 years: 10 mg as a single dose

Adults: 10 mg before each meal and at bedtime **or** 1-2 mg/kg every 2-3 hours (maximum: 5 doses/day) **or** 10 mg as a single dose

Oral: *Adults:* 10-15 mg up to 4 times/day

Dosage Forms

Injection, solution [preservative free]: 5 mg/mL (2 mL, 10 mL, 20 mL, 30 mL)

Solution, oral: 5 mg/5 mL (0.9 mL, 10 mL, 473 mL, 480 mL)

Tablet, oral: 5 mg, 10 mg

Reglan®: 5 mg, 10 mg

Tablet, orally disintegrating, oral:

Metozolv™ ODT: 5 mg, 10 mg

Metoclopramide Hydrochloride Injection (Can) *see* metoclopramide *on page* 594

Metoclopramide Omega (Can) *see* metoclopramide *on page* 594

metolazone (me TOLE a zone)

Medication Safety Issues

Sound-alike/look-alike issues:

Metolazone may be confused with metaxalone, methazolamide, methimazole, methotrexate, metoclopramide, metoprolol, minoxidil

Zaroxolyn® may be confused with Zarontin®

U.S. Brand Names Zaroxolyn®

Canadian Brand Names Zaroxolyn®

Therapeutic Category Diuretic, Miscellaneous

Use Management of mild-to-moderate hypertension; treatment of edema in heart failure and nephrotic syndrome, impaired renal function

General Dosage Range Oral: *Adults:* 2.5-20 mg every 24 hours

Dosage Forms

Tablet, oral: 2.5 mg, 5 mg, 10 mg

Zaroxolyn®: 2.5 mg, 5 mg

Metopirone® *see* metyrapone *on page* 597

metoprolol (me toe PROE lole)

Medication Safety Issues

Sound-alike/look-alike issues:

Lopressor® may be confused with Lyrica®

Metoprolol may be confused with metaproterenol, metoclopramide, metolazone, misoprostol

Metoprolol succinate may be confused with metoprolol tartrate

Toprol-XL® may be confused with TEGretol®, TEGretol®-XR, Topamax®

High alert medication:

The Institute for Safe Medication Practices (ISMP) includes this medication among its list of drugs which have a heightened risk of causing significant patient harm when used in error.

Administration issues:

Significant differences exist between oral and I.V. dosing. Use caution when converting from one route of administration to another.

Synonyms metoprolol succinate; metoprolol tartrate

U.S. Brand Names Lopressor®; Toprol-XL®

Canadian Brand Names Apo-Metoprolol (Type L®); Apo-Metoprolol SR®; Apo-Metoprolol®; Ava-Metoprolol; Ava-Metoprolol (Type L); Betaloc®; Dom-Metoprolol-B; Dom-Metoprolol-L; JAMP-Metoprolol-L; Lopresor SR®; Lopresor®; Metoprolol Tartrate Injection, USP; Metoprolol-25; Metoprolol-L; Mylan-Metoprolol (Type L); Nu-Metop; PMS-Metoprolol-B; PMS-Metoprolol-L; Riva-Metoprolol-L; Sandoz-Metoprolol (Type L); Sandoz-Metoprolol SR; Teva-Metoprolol

Therapeutic Category Beta-Adrenergic Blocker

Use Treatment of angina pectoris, hypertension, or hemodynamically-stable acute myocardial infarction

Extended release: Treatment of angina pectoris or hypertension; to reduce mortality/hospitalization in patients with heart failure (stable NYHA Class II or III) already receiving ACE inhibitors, diuretics, and/or digoxin

General Dosage Range

I.V.: *Adults:* 1.25-5 mg every 6-12 hours (maximum: 15 mg every 3 hours) **or** 5 mg every 2 minutes for 3 doses (acute MI)

Oral:

Extended release:

Children ≥6 years: 1-2 mg/kg once daily (maximum: 2 mg/kg/day or 200 mg/day)

Adults: 12.5-200 mg/day (maximum: 400 mg/day)

Immediate release:

Children >1 year: 1-6 mg/kg/day divided twice daily (maximum: 200 mg/day)

Adults: 50-450 mg/day in 2-3 divided doses

Dosage Forms

Injection, solution: 1 mg/mL (5 mL)

Lopressor®: 1 mg/mL (5 mL)

Injection, solution [preservative free]: 1 mg/mL (5 mL)

Tablet, oral: 25 mg, 50 mg, 100 mg

Lopressor®: 50 mg, 100 mg

Tablet, extended release, oral: 25 mg, 50 mg, 100 mg, 200 mg

Toprol-XL®: 25 mg, 50 mg, 100 mg, 200 mg

Metoprolol-25 (Can) *see* metoprolol *on page* 595

Metoprolol-L (Can) *see* metoprolol *on page* 595

metoprolol and hydrochlorothiazide (me toe PROE lole & hye droe klor oh THYE a zide)

Synonyms hydrochlorothiazide and metoprolol; hydrochlorothiazide and metoprolol succinate; hydrochlorothiazide and metoprolol tartrate; metoprolol succinate and hydrochlorothiazide; metoprolol tartrate and hydrochlorothiazide

U.S. Brand Names Dutoprol™; Lopressor HCT®

Therapeutic Category Beta-Blocker, Beta-1 Selective; Diuretic, Thiazide

Use Treatment of hypertension (not recommended for initial treatment)

General Dosage Range Oral: *Adults:*

Metoprolol **tartrate** (immediate release) 50-200 mg and hydrochlorothiazide 12.5-50 mg administered daily as single or 2 divided doses (maximum: 200 mg/day [metoprolol tartrate] and 50 mg/day [hydrochlorothiazide])

Metoprolol **succinate** (extended release) 25-200 mg and hydrochlorothiazide 12.5-25 mg once daily (maximum: 200 mg [metoprolol succinate] and 25 mg/day [hydrochlorothiazide])

Dosage Forms

Tablet, oral: 50/25: Metoprolol 50 mg and hydrochlorothiazide 25 mg; 100/25: Metoprolol 100 mg and hydrochlorothiazide 25 mg; 100/50: Metoprolol 100 mg and hydrochlorothiazide 50 mg

Lopressor HCT®: 50/25: Metoprolol 50 mg and hydrochlorothiazide 25 mg; 100/25: Metoprolol 100 mg and hydrochlorothiazide 25 mg

Tablet, extended release, oral:

Dutoprol™: 25/12.5: Metoprolol succinate 25 mg and hydrochlorothiazide 12.5 mg

Dutoprol™: 50/12.5: Metoprolol succinate 50 mg and hydrochlorothiazide 12.5 mg

Dutoprol™: 100/12.5: Metoprolol succinate 100 mg and hydrochlorothiazide 12.5 mg [scored]

metoprolol succinate *see* metoprolol *on page 595*

metoprolol succinate and hydrochlorothiazide *see* metoprolol and hydrochlorothiazide *on page 595*

metoprolol tartrate *see* metoprolol *on page 595*

metoprolol tartrate and hydrochlorothiazide *see* metoprolol and hydrochlorothiazide *on page 595*

Metoprolol Tartrate Injection, USP (Can) *see* metoprolol *on page 595*

Metozolv™ ODT *see* metoclopramide *on page 594*

MetroCream® *see* metronidazole (topical) *on page 597*

MetroGel® *see* metronidazole (topical) *on page 597*

Metrogel® (Can) *see* metronidazole (topical) *on page 597*

MetroGel® 1% Kit [DSC] *see* metronidazole (topical) *on page 597*

MetroGel-Vaginal® *see* metronidazole (topical) *on page 597*

MetroLotion® *see* metronidazole (topical) *on page 597*

metronidazole (systemic) (met roe NYE da zole)

Medication Safety Issues

Sound-alike/look-alike issues:

MetroNIDAZOLE may be confused with mebendazole, meropenem, metFORMIN, methotrexate, metoclopramide, miconazole

Synonyms metronidazole hydrochloride

Tall-Man metro**NIDAZOLE**

U.S. Brand Names Flagyl®; Flagyl® 375; Flagyl® ER

Canadian Brand Names Apo-Metronidazole®; Flagyl®; Florazole® ER

Therapeutic Category Amebicide; Antibiotic, Miscellaneous; Antiprotozoal, Nitroimidazole

Use Treatment of susceptible anaerobic bacterial and protozoal infections in the following conditions: Amebiasis, symptomatic and asymptomatic trichomoniasis; skin and skin structure infections, bone and joint infections, CNS infections, endocarditis, gynecologic infections, intraabdominal infections (as part of combination regimen), respiratory tract infections (lower), systemic anaerobic infections; treatment of antibiotic-associated pseudomembranous colitis (AAPC); as part of a multidrug regimen for *H. pylori* eradication to reduce the risk of duodenal ulcer recurrence; surgical prophylaxis (colorectal); useful as single agent or in combination with amoxicillin, amoxicillin/clavulanic acid, or ciprofloxacin in the treatment of periodontitis associated with the presence of *Actinobacillus actinomycetemcomitans* (AA).

General Dosage Range Dosage adjustment recommended in patients with hepatic or renal impairment

I.V.: *Adults:* 500 mg every 6-8 hours (maximum: 4 g/day)

Oral:

Extended release: *Adults:* 750 mg once daily

Regular release:

Infants and Children: 35-50 mg/kg/day divided every 8 hours

Adults: 250-750 mg every 6-12 hours (maximum: 4 g/day) **or** 2 g as a single dose

Dosage Forms

Capsule, oral: 375 mg

Flagyl® 375: 375 mg

Infusion, premixed iso-osmotic sodium chloride solution: 500 mg (100 mL)

Tablet, oral: 250 mg, 500 mg

Flagyl®: 250 mg, 500 mg

Tablet, extended release, oral:

Flagyl® ER: 750 mg

metronidazole (topical) (met roe NYE da zole)

Synonyms metronidazole hydrochloride

Tall-Man metro**NIDAZOLE**

U.S. Brand Names MetroCream®; MetroGel-Vaginal®; MetroGel®; MetroGel® 1% Kit [DSC]; MetroLotion®; Noritate®; Rosadan™; Vandazole®

Canadian Brand Names MetroCream®; Metrogel®; MetroLotion®; Nidagel™; Noritate®; Rosasol®

Therapeutic Category Antibiotic, Topical

Use

Topical: Treatment of inflammatory lesions and erythema of rosacea

Vaginal gel: Bacterial vaginosis

General Dosage Range

Intravaginal: *Adults:* 1 applicatorful (~37.5 mg metronidazole) intravaginally once or twice daily

Topical: *Adults:* Apply a thin film to affected area once (1%) or twice (0.75%) daily

Dosage Forms

Cream, topical: 0.75% (45 g)

MetroCream®: 0.75% (45 g)

Noritate®: 1% (60 g)

Rosadan™: 0.75% (45 g)

Gel, topical: 0.75% (45 g)

MetroGel®: 1% (55 g, 60 g)

Gel, vaginal: 0.75% (70 g)

MetroGel-Vaginal®: 0.75% (70 g)

Vandazole®: 0.75% (70 g)

Lotion, topical: 0.75% (59 mL, 60 mL)

MetroLotion®: 0.75% (59 mL)

metronidazole and nystatin *(Canada only)* (met roe NYE da zole & nye STAT in)

Synonyms nystatin and metronidazole

Canadian Brand Names Flagystatin®

Therapeutic Category Antifungal Agent, Vaginal; Antiprotozoal, Nitroimidazole

Use Treatment of mixed vaginal infection due to *T. vaginalis* and *C. albicans*

General Dosage Range Intravaginal: *Adults:* Insert 1 applicatorful or tablet daily

Product Availability Not available in U.S.

Dosage Forms - Canada

Cream, vaginal:

Flagystatin®: Metronidazole 500 mg and nystatin 100,000 units per applicatorful (55 g)

Tablet, vaginal:

Flagystatin® Ovule: Metronidazole 500 mg and nystatin 100,000 units (10s)

metronidazole, bismuth subcitrate potassium, and tetracycline *see* bismuth, metronidazole, and tetracycline *on page* 136

metronidazole, bismuth subsalicylate, and tetracycline *see* bismuth, metronidazole, and tetracycline *on page* 136

metronidazole hydrochloride *see* metronidazole (systemic) *on page* 596

metronidazole hydrochloride *see* metronidazole (topical) *on page* 597

MET tyrosine kinase inhibitor PF-02341066 *see* crizotinib *on page* 240

Metvix® (Can) *see* methyl aminolevulinate *on page* 587

Metvixia™ *see* methyl aminolevulinate *on page* 587

metyrapone (me TEER a pone)

Medication Safety Issues

Sound-alike/look-alike issues:

Metyrapone may be confused with metyrosine

U.S. Brand Names Metopirone®

Therapeutic Category Diagnostic Agent

Use Diagnostic test for hypothalamic-pituitary ACTH function

General Dosage Range Oral:
Children: 15 mg/kg (minimum: 250 mg; maximum: 750 mg) every 4 hours for 6 doses **or** 30 mg/kg (maximum: 3 g) as a single dose
Adults: 750 mg every 4 hours for 6 doses **or** 30 mg/kg (maximum: 3 g) as a single dose

Dosage Forms
Capsule, oral:
Metopirone®: 250 mg

metyrosine (me TYE roe seen)

Medication Safety Issues
Sound-alike/look-alike issues:
Metyrosine may be confused with metyrapone

Synonyms AMPT; OGMT
U.S. Brand Names Demser®
Therapeutic Category Tyrosine Hydroxylase Inhibitor
Use Short-term management of pheochromocytoma before surgery, long-term management when surgery is contraindicated or when chronic malignant pheochromocytoma exists
General Dosage Range Oral: *Children ≥12 years and Adults:* Initial: 250 mg 4 times/day; Usual maintenance: 2-3 g/day in 4 divided doses (maximum: 4 g/day)

Dosage Forms
Capsule, oral:
Demser®: 250 mg

Mevacor® *see* lovastatin *on page 553*
mevinolin *see* lovastatin *on page 553*

mexiletine (meks IL e teen)

Canadian Brand Names Novo-Mexiletine
Therapeutic Category Antiarrhythmic Agent, Class I-B
Use Management of serious ventricular arrhythmias; suppression of PVCs
General Dosage Range Dosage adjustment recommended in patients with hepatic impairment
Oral: *Adults:* Initial: 200 mg every 8 hours; Maintenance: 200-300 mg every 8 hours (maximum: 1.2 g/day)

Dosage Forms
Capsule, oral: 150 mg, 200 mg, 250 mg

Mezavant® (Can) *see* mesalamine *on page 577*
MG217® Medicated Tar [OTC] *see* coal tar *on page 228*
MG217® Medicated Tar Extra Strength [OTC] *see* coal tar *on page 228*
MG217® Medicated Tar Intensive Strength [OTC] *see* coal tar *on page 228*
MG217® Sal-Acid [OTC] *see* salicylic acid *on page 816*
$MgSO_4$ (error-prone abbreviation) *see* magnesium sulfate *on page 560*
Miacalcin® *see* calcitonin *on page 159*
Miacalcin® NS (Can) *see* calcitonin *on page 159*
Mi-Acid [OTC] *see* aluminum hydroxide, magnesium hydroxide, and simethicone *on page 56*
Mi-Acid™ Double Strength [OTC] *see* calcium carbonate and magnesium hydroxide *on page 163*
Mi-Acid Gas Relief [OTC] *see* simethicone *on page 834*
Mi-Acid Maximum Strength [OTC] [DSC] *see* aluminum hydroxide, magnesium hydroxide, and simethicone *on page 56*
Micaderm® [OTC] *see* miconazole (topical) *on page 599*

micafungin (mi ka FUN gin)

Synonyms micafungin sodium
U.S. Brand Names Mycamine®
Canadian Brand Names Mycamine®
Therapeutic Category Antifungal Agent, Parenteral; Drug-induced Neuritis, Treatment Agent

Use Treatment of esophageal candidiasis; *Candida* prophylaxis in patients undergoing hematopoietic stem cell transplant (HSCT); treatment of candidemia, acute disseminated candidiasis, and other *Candida* infections (peritonitis and abscesses)

General Dosage Range I.V.: *Adults:* Prophylaxis: 50 mg daily; Treatment: 100-150 mg daily

Dosage Forms

Injection, powder for reconstitution:

Mycamine®: 50 mg, 100 mg

micafungin sodium *see* micafungin *on page 598*

Micanol® (Can) *see* anthralin *on page 76*

Micardis® *see* telmisartan *on page 874*

Micardis® HCT *see* telmisartan and hydrochlorothiazide *on page 875*

Micardis® Plus (Can) *see* telmisartan and hydrochlorothiazide *on page 875*

Micatin® [OTC] *see* miconazole (topical) *on page 599*

Micatin® (Can) *see* miconazole (topical) *on page 599*

miconazole (oral) (mi KON a zole)

Medication Safety Issues

Sound-alike/look-alike issues:

Miconazole may be confused with metroNIDAZOLE, Micronase, Micronor®

Synonyms miconazole nitrate

U.S. Brand Names Oravig® [DSC]

Therapeutic Category Antifungal Agent, Oral Nonabsorbed

Use Treatment of oropharyngeal candidiasis

General Dosage Range Buccal: *Children ≥16 years and Adults:* 50 mg (1 tablet) once daily

Dosage Forms

Tablet, for buccal application:

Oravig®: 50 mg

miconazole (topical) (mi KON a zole)

Medication Safety Issues

Sound-alike/look-alike issues:

Miconazole may be confused with metroNIDAZOLE, Micronase, Micronor®

Lotrimin® may be confused with Lotrisone®, Otrivin®

Micatin® may be confused with Miacalcin®

Synonyms miconazole nitrate

U.S. Brand Names 3M™ Cavilon™ Antifungal [OTC]; Aloe Vesta® Antifungal [OTC]; Baza® Antifungal [OTC]; Carrington® Antifungal [OTC]; Critic-Aid® Clear AF [OTC]; DermaFungal [OTC]; Dermagran® AF [OTC]; DiabetAid® Antifungal Foot Bath [OTC]; Fungoid® [OTC]; Lotrimin AF® [OTC]; Micaderm® [OTC]; Micatin® [OTC]; Micro-Guard® [OTC]; Miranel AF™ [OTC]; Mitrazol® [OTC]; Monistat® 1 Day or Night [OTC]; Monistat® 1 [OTC]; Monistat® 3 [OTC]; Monistat® 7 [OTC]; Neosporin® AF [OTC]; Podactin Cream [OTC]; Secura® Antifungal Extra Thick [OTC]; Secura® Antifungal Greaseless [OTC]; Ting® Spray Powder [OTC]; Zeasorb®-AF [OTC]

Canadian Brand Names Dermazole; Micatin®; Micozole; Monistat®; Monistat® 3

Therapeutic Category Antifungal Agent

Use Treatment of vulvovaginal candidiasis and a variety of skin and mucous membrane fungal infections

General Dosage Range

Intravaginal: *Children ≥12 years and Adults:* Insert 1 applicatorful or suppository (100 mg or 200 mg) once daily at bedtime **or** insert 1 suppository (1200 mg) as a single dose.

Topical: *Children and Adults:* Apply twice daily **or** dissolve 1 effervescent tablet in ~1 gallon of water and soak feet for 15-30 minutes

Dosage Forms

Aerosol, powder, topical:

Lotrimin AF® [OTC]: 2% (133 g)

Micatin® [OTC]: 2% (90 g)

Neosporin® AF [OTC]: 2% (85 g)

Ting® Spray Powder [OTC]: 2% (128 g)

Aerosol, spray, topical:
Micatin® [OTC]: 2% (90 g, 105 mL)
Neosporin® AF [OTC]: 2% (105 mL)
Combination package, topical/vaginal: Cream, topical: 2% (9 g) and Suppository, vaginal: 200 mg (3s)
Monistat® 1 [OTC]: Cream, topical: 2% (9 g) and Insert, vaginal: 1200 mg (1)
Monistat® 3 [OTC]: Cream, topical: 2% (9 g) and Cream, vaginal: 4% (25 g), Cream, topical: 2% (9 g) and Cream, vaginal: 4% (3 x 5 g), Cream, topical: 2% (9 g) and Insert, vaginal: 200 mg (3s)
Monistat® 7 [OTC]: Cream, topical: 2% (9 g) and Cream, vaginal: 2% (45 g), Cream, topical: 2% (9 g) and Cream, vaginal: 2% (7 x 5 g), Cream, topical: 2% (9 g) and Suppository, vaginal: 100 mg (7s)
Monistat® 1 Day or Night [OTC]: Cream, topical: 2% (9 g) and Insert, vaginal: 1200 mg (1)
Cream, topical: 2% (15 g, 30 g, 45 g)
Baza® Antifungal [OTC]: 2% (4 g, 57 g, 142 g)
Carrington® Antifungal [OTC]: 2% (150 g)
Micaderm® [OTC]: 2% (30 g)
Micatin® [OTC]: 2% (14 g)
Miranel AF™ [OTC]: 2% (28 g)
3M™ Cavilon™ Antifungal [OTC]: 2% (56 g, 141 g)
Neosporin® AF [OTC]: 2% (14 g, 15 g)
Podactin Cream [OTC]: 2% (30 g)
Secura® Antifungal Extra Thick [OTC]: 2% (97.5 g)
Secura® Antifungal Greaseless [OTC]: 2% (60 g)
Cream, vaginal: 2% (45 g)
Monistat® 7 [OTC]: 2% (45 g)
Monistat® 3 [OTC]: 4% (15 g, 25 g)
Liquid, topical:
Lotrimin AF® [OTC]: 2% (150 g)
Ointment, topical:
Aloe Vesta® Antifungal [OTC]: 2% (60 g, 150 g)
Critic-Aid® Clear AF [OTC]: 2% (57 g, 142 g, 300s)
DermaFungal [OTC]: 2% (120 g)
Dermagran® AF [OTC]: 2% (120 g)
Powder, topical:
Lotrimin AF® [OTC]: 2% (90 g)
Micro-Guard® [OTC]: 2% (90 g)
Mitrazol® [OTC]: 2% (30 g)
Zeasorb®-AF [OTC]: 2% (70 g)
Suppository, vaginal: 100 mg (7s); 200 mg (3s)
Tablet for solution, topical:
DiabetAid® Antifungal Foot Bath [OTC]: 2% (10s)
Tincture, topical:
Fungoid® [OTC]: 2% (7.39 mL, 30 mL)

miconazole and zinc oxide (mi KON a zole & zink OKS ide)

Synonyms zinc oxide and miconazole nitrate

U.S. Brand Names Vusion®

Therapeutic Category Antifungal Agent, Topical

Use Adjunctive treatment of diaper dermatitis complicated by *Candida albicans* infection

General Dosage Range Topical: *Children ≥4 weeks:* Apply to affected area with each diaper change (maximum therapy: 7 days)

Dosage Forms
Ointment, topical:
Vusion®: Miconazole 0.25% and zinc oxide 15% (50 g)

miconazole nitrate *see* miconazole (oral) *on page* 599
miconazole nitrate *see* miconazole (topical) *on page* 599
Micozole (Can) *see* miconazole (topical) *on page* 599
MICRhoGAM® UF Plus *see* Rh_o(D) immune globulin *on page* 797
microfibrillar collagen hemostat *see* collagen hemostat *on page* 234
Microgestin® 1.5/30 *see* ethinyl estradiol and norethindrone *on page* 359
Microgestin® 1/20 *see* ethinyl estradiol and norethindrone *on page* 359
Microgestin® Fe 1.5/30 *see* ethinyl estradiol and norethindrone *on page* 359

Microgestin® Fe 1/20 *see* ethinyl estradiol and norethindrone *on page 359*
Micro-Guard® [OTC] *see* miconazole (topical) *on page 599*
microK® *see* potassium chloride *on page 744*
microK® 10 *see* potassium chloride *on page 744*
Micro-K Extencaps® (Can) *see* potassium chloride *on page 744*
Micronase *see* glyburide *on page 428*
Micronor® (Can) *see* norethindrone *on page 648*
Microzide® *see* hydrochlorothiazide *on page 452*
***Micrurus fulvius* antivenin** *see* antivenin *(Micrurus fulvius) on page 81*
***Micrurus fulvius* antivenom** *see* antivenin *(Micrurus fulvius) on page 81*
Midamor (Can) *see* amiloride *on page 60*

midazolam (MID aye zoe lam)

Medication Safety Issues

Sound-alike/look-alike issues:

Versed may be confused with VePesid, Vistaril®

High alert medication:

The Institute for Safe Medication Practices (ISMP) includes this medication among its list of drugs which have a heightened risk of causing significant patient harm when used in error.

Synonyms midazolam hydrochloride; Versed

Canadian Brand Names Apo-Midazolam®; Midazolam Injection

Therapeutic Category Benzodiazepine

Controlled Substance C-IV

Use Preoperative sedation; moderate sedation prior to diagnostic or radiographic procedures; ICU sedation (continuous infusion); induction and maintenance of general anesthesia

General Dosage Range

I.M.:

Children: 0.1-0.15 mg/kg 30-60 minutes prior to surgery/procedure (maximum: 10 mg total)

Adults: 0.07-0.08 mg/kg 30-60 minutes prior to surgery/procedure; Usual dose: 5 mg

I.V.:

Infants <6 months: 0.05-0.2 mg/kg loading dose followed by 0.4-6 mcg/kg/minute infusion

Infants 6 months to Children 5 years: Initial: 0.05-0.1 mg/kg once (maximum: 6 mg or 0.6 mg/kg total) **or** 0.05-0.2 mg/kg loading dose followed by 0.4-6 mcg/kg/minute infusion

Children 6-12 years: 0.025-0.05 mg/kg once (maximum: 10 mg or 0.4 mg/kg total) **or** 0.05-0.2 mg/kg loading dose followed by 0.4-6 mcg/kg/minute infusion

Children ≥12 years and Adults: Dosage varies greatly depending on indication

Oral:

Children <6 years: 0.25-0.5 mg/kg as single dose; may require as much as 1 mg/kg (maximum: 20 mg total)

Children 6-16 years: 0.25-0.5 mg/kg as a single dose (maximum: 20 mg total)

Dosage Forms

Injection, solution: 1 mg/mL (2 mL, 5 mL, 10 mL); 5 mg/mL (1 mL, 2 mL, 5 mL, 10 mL)

Injection, solution [preservative free]: 1 mg/mL (2 mL, 5 mL); 5 mg/mL (1 mL, 2 mL)

Syrup, oral: 2 mg/mL (2.5 mL, 118 mL)

midazolam hydrochloride *see* midazolam *on page 601*
Midazolam Injection (Can) *see* midazolam *on page 601*

midodrine (MI doe dreen)

Medication Safety Issues

Sound-alike/look-alike issues:

Midodrine may be confused with Midrin®, minoxidil

ProAmatine may be confused with protamine

Synonyms midodrine hydrochloride; ProAmatine

Canadian Brand Names Amatine®; Apo-Midodrine®

Therapeutic Category Alpha-Adrenergic Agonist

Use **Orphan drug:** Treatment of symptomatic orthostatic hypotension

General Dosage Range Dosage adjustment recommended in patients with renal impairment

Oral: *Adults:* 10 mg 3 times/day (maximum: 40 mg/day)

Dosage Forms

Tablet, oral: 2.5 mg, 5 mg, 10 mg

midodrine hydrochloride *see* midodrine *on page 601*

Midol® Cramps & Body Aches [OTC] *see* ibuprofen *on page 468*

Midol® Extended Relief [OTC] *see* naproxen *on page 628*

Midol® Teen Formula [OTC] *see* acetaminophen and pamabrom *on page 24*

Midrin *see* acetaminophen, isometheptene, and dichloralphenazone *on page 30*

Mifeprex® *see* mifepristone *on page 602*

mifepristone (mi FE pris tone)

Medication Safety Issues

Sound-alike/look-alike issues:

Mifeprex® may be confused with Mirapex®

Mifepristone may be confused with misoprostol

High alert medication:

The Institute for Safe Medication Practices (ISMP) includes this medication among its list of drug classes which have a heightened risk of causing significant patient harm when used in error.

Synonyms RU-38486; RU-486

U.S. Brand Names Korlym™; Mifeprex®

Therapeutic Category Abortifacient; Antineoplastic Agent, Hormone Antagonist; Antiprogestin

Use

Korlym™: To control hyperglycemia occurring secondary to hypercortisolism in patients with endogenous Cushing syndrome who have type 2 diabetes mellitus or glucose intolerance and who failed surgery or who are not surgical candidates

Mifeprex®: Medical termination of intrauterine pregnancy, through day 49 of pregnancy. Patients may need treatment with misoprostol and possibly surgery to complete therapy.

General Dosage Range Dosage adjustment recommended in patients with hepatic or renal impairment or on concomitant therapy when treating hyperglycemia in patients with Cushing syndrome.

Oral: *Adults:* Hyperglycemia in patients with Cushing syndrome: 300-1200 mg once daily (maximum: 1200 mg once daily, not to exceed 20 mg/kg/day); Termination of pregnancy: Day 1: 600 mg (three 200 mg tablets) as a single dose

Dosage Forms

Tablet, oral:

Korlym™: 300 mg

Mifeprex®: 200 mg

Migergot® *see* ergotamine and caffeine *on page 340*

miglitol (MIG li tol)

Medication Safety Issues

Sound-alike/look-alike issues:

Glyset® may be confused with Cycloset®

U.S. Brand Names Glyset®

Therapeutic Category Antidiabetic Agent, Oral

Use Type 2 diabetes mellitus (noninsulin-dependent, NIDDM):

Monotherapy as an adjunct to diet to improve glycemic control in patients with type 2 diabetes mellitus (noninsulin-dependent, NIDDM) whose hyperglycemia cannot be managed with diet alone

Combination therapy with a sulfonylurea when diet plus either miglitol or a sulfonylurea alone do not result in adequate glycemic control. The effect of miglitol to enhance glycemic control is additive to that of sulfonylureas when used in combination.

General Dosage Range Oral: *Adults:* Initial: 25 mg 3 times/day; Maintenance: 25-100 mg 3 times/day (maximum: 300 mg/day)

Dosage Forms

Tablet, oral:

Glyset®: 25 mg, 50 mg, 100 mg

miglustat (MIG loo stat)

Medication Safety Issues

International issues:

Zavesca: Brand name for miglustat [U.S., Canada, and multiple international markets], but also brand name for escitalopram [in multiple international markets; ISMP April 21, 2010]

Synonyms OGT-918

U.S. Brand Names Zavesca®

Canadian Brand Names Zavesca®

Therapeutic Category Enzyme Inhibitor

Use Treatment of mild-to-moderate type 1 Gaucher disease when enzyme replacement therapy is not a therapeutic option

Canadian labeling: Additional use (not in U.S. labeling): Treatment to delay the progression of neurological manifestations in Niemann-Pick Type C disease

General Dosage Range Dosage adjustment recommended in patients with renal impairment

Oral: *Adults:* 100 mg 1-3 times/day

Dosage Forms

Capsule, oral:

Zavesca®: 100 mg

Migranal® *see* dihydroergotamine *on page 287*

Mild-C® [OTC] *see* ascorbic acid *on page 94*

Milk of Magnesia [OTC] *see* magnesium hydroxide *on page 558*

Milk of Magnesium [OTC] *see* magnesium hydroxide *on page 558*

Millipred™ *see* prednisolone (systemic) *on page 754*

Millipred™ DP *see* prednisolone (systemic) *on page 754*

milnacipran (mil NAY ci pran)

Medication Safety Issues

Sound-alike/look-alike issues:

Savella® may be confused with cevimeline, sevelamer

U.S. Brand Names Savella®

Therapeutic Category Antidepressant, Serotonin/Norepinephrine Reuptake Inhibitor

Use Management of fibromyalgia

General Dosage Range Dosage adjustment recommended in patients with renal impairment

Oral: *Adults:* 50 mg twice daily (maximum dose: 200 mg/day)

Dosage Forms

Combination package, oral:

Savella®: Tablet: 12.5 mg (5s), Tablet: 25 mg (8s), and Tablet: 50 mg (42s)

Tablet, oral:

Savella®: 12.5 mg, 25 mg, 50 mg, 100 mg

milrinone (MIL ri none)

Medication Safety Issues

Sound-alike/look-alike issues:

Primacor® may be confused with Primaxin®

High alert medication:

The Institute for Safe Medication Practices (ISMP) includes this medication among its list of drugs which have a heightened risk of causing significant patient harm when used in error.

Synonyms milrinone lactate

Canadian Brand Names Milrinone Lactate Injection; Primacor®

Therapeutic Category Cardiovascular Agent, Other

Use Short-term I.V. therapy of acutely-decompensated heart failure

General Dosage Range Dosage adjustment recommended in patients with renal impairment

I.V.: *Adults:* Loading dose (optional): 50 mcg/kg; Maintenance: 0.375-0.75 mcg/kg/minute

Dosage Forms

Infusion, premixed in D_5W: 200 mcg/mL (100 mL, 200 mL)
Injection, solution: 1 mg/mL (10 mL, 20 mL, 50 mL)
Injection, solution [preservative free]: 1 mg/mL (10 mL, 20 mL)

milrinone lactate *see* milrinone *on page 603*
Milrinone Lactate Injection (Can) *see* milrinone *on page 603*
Mimvey™ *see* estradiol and norethindrone *on page 349*
Mimyx® *see* emollients *on page 328*
mineral oil, petrolatum, lanolin, cetyl alcohol, and glycerin *see* lanolin, cetyl alcohol, glycerin, petrolatum, and mineral oil *on page 521*
Minestrin™ 1/20 (Can) *see* ethinyl estradiol and norethindrone *on page 359*
Minims Cyclopentolate (Can) *see* cyclopentolate *on page 244*
Mini-Prenatal [OTC] *see* vitamins (multiple/prenatal) *on page 952*
Minipress® *see* prazosin *on page 753*
Minirin® (Can) *see* desmopressin *on page 264*
Minitran™ *see* nitroglycerin *on page 645*
Minocin® *see* minocycline *on page 604*
Minocin® PAC *see* minocycline *on page 604*

minocycline (mi noe SYE kleen)

Medication Safety Issues

Sound-alike/look-alike issues:
Dynacin® may be confused with Dyazide®, DynaCirc®, Dynapen
Minocin® may be confused with Indocin®, Lincocin®, Minizide®, niacin

Synonyms minocycline hydrochloride

U.S. Brand Names Dynacin®; Minocin®; Minocin® PAC; Solodyn®

Canadian Brand Names Apo-Minocycline®; Arestin Microspheres; Dom-Minocycline; Minocin®; Mylan-Minocycline; Novo-Minocycline; PHL-Minocycline; PMS-Minocycline; ratio-Minocycline; Riva-Minocycline; Sandoz-Minocycline

Therapeutic Category Tetracycline Derivative

Use Treatment of susceptible bacterial infections of both gram-negative and gram-positive organisms; treatment of anthrax (inhalational, cutaneous, and gastrointestinal); moderate-to-severe acne; meningococcal (asymptomatic) carrier state; Rickettsial diseases (including Rocky Mountain spotted fever, Q fever); nongonococcal urethritis, gonorrhea; acute intestinal amebiasis; respiratory tract infection; skin/soft tissue infections; chlamydial infections

Extended release (Solodyn®): Only indicated for treatment of inflammatory lesions of non-nodular moderate-to-severe acne

General Dosage Range Dosage adjustment recommended in patients with renal impairment

I.V.:
Children >8 years: 4 mg/kg initially, followed by 2 mg/kg/dose every 12 hours (maximum: 400 mg daily)
Adults: 200 mg initially, followed by 100 mg every 12 hours (maximum: 400 mg daily)

Oral:
Children >8 years: 4 mg/kg initially, followed by 2 mg/kg/dose every 12 hours
Children ≥12 years: Solodyn®: 45-135 mg once daily (weight-based)
Adults: 200 mg initially, followed by 100 mg every 12 hours **or** 50-100 mg twice daily (acne); Solodyn®: 45-135 mg once daily (weight-based)

Dosage Forms

Capsule, oral: 50 mg, 75 mg, 100 mg
Capsule, pellet filled, oral:
Minocin®: 50 mg, 100 mg
Minocin® PAC: 50 mg, 100 mg
Injection, powder for reconstitution:
Minocin®: 100 mg
Tablet, oral: 50 mg, 75 mg, 100 mg
Dynacin®: 50 mg, 75 mg, 100 mg
Tablet, extended release, oral: 45 mg, 90 mg, 135 mg
Solodyn®: 45 mg, 65 mg, 90 mg, 115 mg, 135 mg

minocycline hydrochloride *see* minocycline *on page 604*

Min-Ovral® (Can) *see* ethinyl estradiol and levonorgestrel *on page* 357

minoxidil (systemic) (mi NOKS i dil)

Medication Safety Issues

Sound-alike/look-alike issues:

Loniten® may be confused with Lipitor®

Minoxidil may be confused with metolazone, midodrine, Minipress®, Minocin®, Monopril®, Noxafil®

International issues:

Noxidil [Thailand] may be confused with Noxafil brand name for posaconazole [U.S. and multiple international markets]

Canadian Brand Names Loniten®

Therapeutic Category Vasodilator, Direct-Acting

Use Management of severe hypertension (usually in combination with a diuretic and beta-blocker)

General Dosage Range Oral:

Children <12 years: Initial: 0.1-0.2 mg/kg once daily (maximum: 5 mg/day); Usual dosage range: 0.25-1 mg/kg/day in 1-2 divided doses (maximum: 50 mg/day)

Children ≥12 years and Adults: Initial: 5 mg once daily; Usual dosage range: 2.5-80 mg/day in 1-2 divided doses (maximum: 100 mg/day)

Elderly: Initial: 2.5 mg once daily

Dosage Forms

Tablet, oral: 2.5 mg, 10 mg

minoxidil (topical) (mi NOKS i dil)

U.S. Brand Names Rogaine® Extra Strength for Men [OTC]; Rogaine® for Men [OTC]; Rogaine® for Women [OTC]

Canadian Brand Names Apo-Gain®; Rogaine®

Therapeutic Category Topical Skin Product

Use Treatment of alopecia androgenetica in males and females

General Dosage Range Topical: *Adults:* Apply twice daily

Dosage Forms

Aerosol, foam, topical:

Rogaine® for Men [OTC]: 5% (60 g)

Solution, topical: 2% (60 mL); 5% (60 mL)

Rogaine® Extra Strength for Men [OTC]: 5% (60 mL)

Rogaine® for Women [OTC]: 2% (60 mL)

Mint-Amlodipine (Can) *see* amlodipine *on page* 65

Mint-Atenolol (Can) *see* atenolol *on page* 99

Mint-Ciprofloxacin (Can) *see* ciprofloxacin (systemic) *on page* 210

Mint-Citalopram (Can) *see* citalopram *on page* 213

Mint-Fluoxetine (Can) *see* fluoxetine *on page* 396

Mint-Lisinopril (Can) *see* lisinopril *on page* 544

Mint-Ondansetron (Can) *see* ondansetron *on page* 667

Mintox Plus [OTC] *see* aluminum hydroxide, magnesium hydroxide, and simethicone *on page* 56

Mint-Pioglitazone (Can) *see* pioglitazone *on page* 725

Mint-Pravastatin (Can) *see* pravastatin *on page* 752

Mint-Risperidon (Can) *see* risperidone *on page* 803

Mint-Simvastatin (Can) *see* simvastatin *on page* 835

Mint-Topiramate (Can) *see* topiramate *on page* 906

Miochol®-E *see* acetylcholine *on page* 32

Miostat® *see* carbachol *on page* 172

MiraLAX® [OTC] *see* polyethylene glycol 3350 *on page* 737

Miranel AF™ [OTC] *see* miconazole (topical) *on page* 599

Mirapex® *see* pramipexole *on page* 749

Mirapex® ER® *see* pramipexole *on page* 749

Mircette® *see* ethinyl estradiol and desogestrel *on page* 356

Mirena® *see* levonorgestrel *on page* 533

mirtazapine (mir TAZ a peen)

Medication Safety Issues

Sound-alike/look-alike issues:

Remeron® may be confused with Premarin®, ramelteon, Rozerem®, Zemuron®

BEERS Criteria medication:

This drug may be potentially inappropriate for use in geriatric patients (SIADH: Quality of evidence - moderate; Strength of recommendation - strong).

International issues:

Avanza [Australia] may be confused with Albenza brand name for albendazole [U.S.]; Avandia brand name for rosiglitazone [U.S., Canada, and multiple international markets]

Remeron [U.S., Canada, and multiple international markets] may be confused with Reneuron which is a brand name for fluoxetine [Spain]

U.S. Brand Names Remeron SolTab®; Remeron®

Canadian Brand Names Apo-Mirtazapine®; Auro-Mirtazapine; Ava-Mirtazapine; CO Mirtazapine; Dom-Mirtazapine; GD-Mirtazapine; Jamp-Mirtazapine; Mylan-Mirtazapine; Novo-Mirtazapine; PMS-Mirtazapine; PRO-Mirtazapine; ratio-Mirtazapine; Remeron®; Remeron® RD; Riva-Mirtazapine; Sandoz-Mirtazapine; Sandoz-Mirtazapine FC; ZYM-Mirtazapine

Therapeutic Category Antidepressant, Alpha-2 Antagonist

Use Treatment of depression

General Dosage Range Oral: *Adults:* Initial: 15 mg nightly; Maintenance: 15-45 mg nightly

Dosage Forms

Tablet, oral: 7.5 mg, 15 mg, 30 mg, 45 mg

Remeron®: 15 mg, 30 mg, 45 mg

Tablet, orally disintegrating, oral: 15 mg, 30 mg, 45 mg

Remeron SolTab®: 15 mg, 30 mg, 45 mg

misoprostol (mye soe PROST ole)

Medication Safety Issues

Sound-alike/look-alike issues:

Cytotec® may be confused with Cytoxan

Misoprostol may be confused with metoprolol, mifepristone

U.S. Brand Names Cytotec®

Canadian Brand Names Apo-Misoprostol®; Novo-Misoprostol; PMS-Misoprostol

Therapeutic Category Prostaglandin

Use Prevention of NSAID-induced gastric ulcers; medical termination of pregnancy of ≤49 days (in conjunction with mifepristone)

General Dosage Range Oral:

Adults: 100-200 mcg 4 times/day

Elderly: Initial: 100 mcg/day

Dosage Forms

Tablet, oral: 100 mcg, 200 mcg

Cytotec®: 100 mcg, 200 mcg

misoprostol and diclofenac *see* diclofenac and misoprostol *on page* 281

MITC *see* mitomycin (systemic) *on page* 606

MITO *see* mitomycin (systemic) *on page* 606

MITO-C *see* mitomycin (systemic) *on page* 606

mitomycin-X *see* mitomycin (systemic) *on page* 606

mitomycin-C *see* mitomycin (ophthalmic) *on page* 607

mitomycin-C *see* mitomycin (systemic) *on page* 606

mitomycin (systemic) (mye toe MYE sin)

Medication Safety Issues

Sound-alike/look-alike issues:

MitoMYcin (Systemic) may be confused with MitoMYcin (Ophthalmic), mitotane, mitoXANtrone

High alert medication:

This medication is in a class the Institute for Safe Medication Practices (ISMP) includes among its list of drug classes which have a heightened risk of causing significant patient harm when used in error.

Synonyms MITC; MITO; MITO-C; mitomycin-C; mitomycin-X; MMC; MTC; Mutamycin

Tall-Man mitoMYcin

Canadian Brand Names Mutamycin®

Therapeutic Category Antineoplastic Agent, Antibiotic

Use Treatment of adenocarcinoma of stomach or pancreas

General Dosage Range Dosage adjustment recommended in patients with renal impairment or who develop toxicities.

I.V.: *Adults:* 20 mg/m^2 every 6-8 weeks

Dosage Forms

Injection, powder for reconstitution: 5 mg, 20 mg, 40 mg

mitomycin (ophthalmic) (mye toe MYE sin)

Medication Safety Issues

Sound-alike/look-alike issues:

MitoMYcin (Ophthalmic) may be confused with MitoMYcin (Systemic), mitotane, mitoXANtrone

High alert medication:

This medication is in a class the Institute for Safe Medication Practices (ISMP) includes among its list of drug classes which have a heightened risk of causing significant patient harm when used in error.

Administration issues:

Mitosol® is not intended for intraocular administration; intraocular administration may result in cell death and lead to corneal and retinal infarction, and ciliary body atrophy.

Mitosol® is only intended for topical application to the surgical site of glaucoma filtration surgery.

Synonyms mitomycin-C; MMC

Tall-Man mitoMYcin

U.S. Brand Names Mitosol®

Therapeutic Category Antineoplastic Agent, Antibiotic; Ophthalmic Agent, Miscellaneous

Use Adjunct to *ab externo* glaucoma surgery

General Dosage Range Topical ophthalmic: *Adults:* 0.2 mg solution is aseptically applied via saturated sponges to surgical site of glaucoma filtration surgery for 2 minutes

Dosage Forms

Powder for solution, ophthalmic [kit]:

Mitosol®: 0.2 mg [supplied with diluent]

Mitosol® *see* mitomycin (ophthalmic) *on page* 607

mitotane (MYE toe tane)

Medication Safety Issues

Sound-alike/look-alike issues:

Mitotane may be confused with mitoMYcin, mitoXANtrone

High alert medication:

The Institute for Safe Medication Practices (ISMP) includes this medication among its list of drug classes which have a heightened risk of causing significant patient harm when used in error.

Synonyms chloditan; chlodithane; khloditan; mytotan; o,p'-DDD; ortho,para-DDD

U.S. Brand Names Lysodren®

Canadian Brand Names Lysodren®

Therapeutic Category Antineoplastic Agent

Use Treatment of inoperable adrenocortical carcinoma

General Dosage Range Dosage adjustment recommended in patients who develop toxicities

Oral: *Adults:* Initial: 2-6 g/day in divided doses; Maintenance: 9-10 g/day in 3-4 divided doses (maximum: 18 g/day)

Dosage Forms

Tablet, oral:

Lysodren®: 500 mg

mitoxantrone (mye toe ZAN trone)

Medication Safety Issues

Sound-alike/look-alike issues:

MitoXANtrone may be confused with methotrexate, mitoMYcin, mitotane, Mutamycin®

High alert medication:

This medication is in a class the Institute for Safe Medication Practices (ISMP) includes among its list of drug classes which have a heightened risk of causing significant patient harm when used in error.

Synonyms CL-232315; DHAD; DHAQ; dihydroxyanthracenedione; dihydroxyanthracenedione dihydrochloride; mitoxantrone dihydrochloride; mitoxantrone HCl; mitoxantrone hydrochloride; Mitozantrone; Novantrone

Tall-Man mitoXANtrone

Canadian Brand Names Mitoxantrone Injection®

Therapeutic Category Antineoplastic Agent

Use Treatment of acute nonlymphocytic leukemias (ANLL [includes myelogenous, promyelocytic, monocytic and erythroid leukemias]); advanced hormone-refractory prostate cancer; secondary progressive or relapsing-remitting multiple sclerosis (MS)

General Dosage Range I.V.: *Adults:* 12 mg/m^2/day once daily for 2-3 days **or** 12-14 mg/m^2 every 3 weeks **or** 12 mg/m^2 every 3 months (multiple sclerosis; maximum lifetime cumulative dose: 140 mg/m^2)

Dosage Forms

Injection, solution [concentrate, preservative free]: 2 mg/mL (10 mL, 12.5 mL, 15 mL)

mitoxantrone dihydrochloride *see* mitoxantrone *on page 608*

mitoxantrone HCl *see* mitoxantrone *on page 608*

mitoxantrone hydrochloride *see* mitoxantrone *on page 608*

Mitoxantrone Injection® (Can) *see* mitoxantrone *on page 608*

Mitozantrone *see* mitoxantrone *on page 608*

Mitrazol® [OTC] *see* miconazole (topical) *on page 599*

MK-217 *see* alendronate *on page 45*

MK383 *see* tirofiban *on page 900*

MK-0431 *see* sitagliptin *on page 837*

MK462 *see* rizatriptan *on page 807*

MK 0517 *see* fosaprepitant *on page 408*

MK-0518 *see* raltegravir *on page 785*

MK594 *see* losartan *on page 551*

MK0826 *see* ertapenem *on page 342*

MK 869 *see* aprepitant *on page 88*

MLN341 *see* bortezomib *on page 139*

MMC *see* mitomycin (ophthalmic) *on page 607*

MMC *see* mitomycin (systemic) *on page 606*

MMF *see* mycophenolate *on page 619*

MMR *see* measles, mumps, and rubella virus vaccine *on page 564*

M-M-R® II *see* measles, mumps, and rubella virus vaccine *on page 564*

MMR-V *see* measles, mumps, rubella, and varicella virus vaccine *on page 564*

MMRV *see* measles, mumps, rubella, and varicella virus vaccine *on page 564*

MOAB 2C4 *see* pertuzumab *on page 710*

MOAB ABX-EGF *see* panitumumab *on page 688*

MOAB C225 *see* cetuximab *on page 192*

MoAb CD52 *see* alemtuzumab *on page 45*

MOAB-CTLA-4 *see* ipilimumab *on page 498*

MOAB HER2 *see* trastuzumab *on page 911*

Mobic® *see* meloxicam *on page 569*

Mobicox® (Can) *see* meloxicam *on page 569*

Mobisyl® [OTC] *see* trolamine *on page 923*

moclobemide *(Canada only)* (moe KLOE be mide)

Canadian Brand Names Apo-Moclobemide®; Dom-Moclobemide; Manerix®; Novo-Moclobemide; Nu-Moclobemide; PMS-Moclobemide; Teva-Moclobemide

Therapeutic Category Antidepressant, Monoamine Oxidase Inhibitor

Use Symptomatic relief of depressive illness

General Dosage Range Dosage adjustment recommended in patients with hepatic impairment or on concomitant therapy

Oral: *Adults:* Initial: 300 mg/day in 2 divided doses; Maintenance: Up to 600 mg/day

Product Availability Not available in U.S.

Dosage Forms - Canada

Tablet, oral:

Apo-Moclobemide®, Dom-Moclobemide, Manerix®, Novo-Moclobemide, Nu-Moclobemide, PMS-Moclobemide: 100 mg, 150 mg, 300 mg

modafinil (moe DAF i nil)

U.S. Brand Names Provigil®

Canadian Brand Names Alertec®; Apo-Modafinil®

Therapeutic Category Central Nervous System Stimulant, Nonamphetamine

Controlled Substance C-IV

Use Improve wakefulness in patients with excessive daytime sleepiness associated with narcolepsy and shift work sleep disorder (SWSD); adjunctive therapy for obstructive sleep apnea/hypopnea syndrome (OSAHS)

General Dosage Range Dosage adjustment recommended in patients with hepatic impairment.

Oral: *Adults:* 200 mg once daily (maximum: 400 mg/day)

Dosage Forms

Tablet, oral: 100 mg, 200 mg

Provigil®: 100 mg, 200 mg

Modecate® (Can) *see* fluphenazine *on page 397*

Modecate® Concentrate (Can) *see* fluphenazine *on page 397*

Modicon® *see* ethinyl estradiol and norethindrone *on page 359*

modified Dakin's solution *see* sodium hypochlorite solution *on page 842*

Modulon® (Can) *see* trimebutine *(Canada only) on page 920*

Moduret (Can) *see* amiloride and hydrochlorothiazide *on page 60*

moexipril (mo EKS i pril)

Medication Safety Issues

Sound-alike/look-alike issues:

Moexipril may be confused with Monopril®

Synonyms moexipril hydrochloride

U.S. Brand Names Univasc®

Therapeutic Category Angiotensin-Converting Enzyme (ACE) Inhibitor

Use Treatment of hypertension, alone or in combination with thiazide diuretics

General Dosage Range Dosage adjustment recommended in patients with renal impairment

Oral: *Adults:* Initial: 3.75-7.5 mg once daily; Maintenance: 7.5-30 mg/day in 1 or 2 divided doses

Dosage Forms

Tablet, oral: 7.5 mg, 15 mg

Univasc®: 7.5 mg, 15 mg

moexipril and hydrochlorothiazide (mo EKS i pril & hye droe klor oh THYE a zide)

Synonyms hydrochlorothiazide and moexipril

U.S. Brand Names Uniretic®

Canadian Brand Names Uniretic®

Therapeutic Category Angiotensin-Converting Enzyme (ACE) Inhibitor; Diuretic, Thiazide

Use Treatment of hypertension; not indicated for initial treatment of hypertension

General Dosage Range Oral: *Adults:* 7.5-30 mg of moexipril/day and ≤50 mg hydrochlorothiazide/day in a single or divided dose

Dosage Forms

Tablet, oral: 7.5/12.5: Moexipril 7.5 mg and hydrochlorothiazide 12.5; 15/12.5: Moexipril 15 mg and hydrochlorothiazide 12.5; 15/25: Moexipril 15 mg and hydrochlorothiazide 25

Uniretic®: 7.5/12.5: Moexipril 7.5 mg and hydrochlorothiazide 12.5 mg [scored]; 15/12.5: Moexipril 15 mg and hydrochlorothiazide 12.5 mg [scored]; 15/25: Moexipril 15 mg and hydrochlorothiazide 25 mg [scored]

moexipril hydrochloride *see* moexipril *on page 609*

Mogadon (Can) *see* nitrazepam *(Canada only) on page 644*

Moi-Stir® [OTC] *see* saliva substitute *on page 819*

MOM *see* magnesium hydroxide *on page 558*

Momentum® [OTC] *see* magnesium salicylate *on page 560*

mometasone (oral inhalation) (moe MET a sone)

Synonyms mometasone furoate

U.S. Brand Names Asmanex® Twisthaler®

Canadian Brand Names Asmanex® Twisthaler®

Therapeutic Category Corticosteroid, Inhalant (Oral)

Use Maintenance treatment of asthma as prophylactic therapy

General Dosage Range Inhalation:

Children 4-11 years: 110 mcg once daily (maximum: 110 mcg/day)

Children ≥12 years and Adults: 1-4 inhalations (220-880 mcg) in 1-2 divided doses (maximum: 880 mcg/day)

Dosage Forms

Powder, for oral inhalation:

Asmanex® Twisthaler®: 110 mcg (7 units, 30 units); 220 mcg (14 units, 30 units, 60 units, 120 units)

Dosage Forms - Canada

Powder, for oral inhalation:

Asmanex® Twisthaler®: 200 mcg (30 doses, 60 doses); 400 mcg (30 doses, 60 doses)

mometasone (nasal) (moe MET a sone)

Synonyms mometasone furoate

U.S. Brand Names Nasonex®

Canadian Brand Names Nasonex®

Therapeutic Category Corticosteroid, Nasal

Use Treatment of nasal symptoms of seasonal and perennial allergic rhinitis; prevention of nasal symptoms associated with seasonal allergic rhinitis; treatment of nasal polyps in adults

Canadian labeling: Additional use (not in U.S. labeling): Treatment of mild-to-moderate uncomplicated rhinosinusitis or as adjunctive treatment (with antimicrobials) in acute rhinosinusitis

General Dosage Range Intranasal:

Children 2-11 years: 1 spray (50 mcg) in each nostril once daily

Children ≥12 years and Adults: 2 sprays (100 mcg) in each nostril once or twice daily

Dosage Forms

Suspension, intranasal:

Nasonex®: 50 mcg/spray (17 g)

Dosage Forms - Canada Excipient information presented when available (limited, particularly for generics); consult specific product labeling.

Suspension, intranasal:

Nasonex®: 50 mcg/spray [delivers 140 sprays]

mometasone (topical) (moe MET a sone)

Medication Safety Issues

Sound-alike/look-alike issues:

Elocon® lotion may be confused with ophthalmic solutions. Manufacturer's labeling emphasizes the product is **NOT** for use in the eyes.

Synonyms mometasone furoate

U.S. Brand Names Elocon®

Canadian Brand Names Elocom®; PMS-Mometasone; ratio-Mometasone; Taro-Mometasone

Therapeutic Category Corticosteroid, Topical

Use Relief of the inflammatory and pruritic manifestations of corticosteroid-responsive dermatoses (medium potency topical corticosteroid)

General Dosage Range Topical:
Cream, ointment: *Children ≥2 years and Adults:* Apply a thin film to affected area once daily
Lotion: *Children ≥12 years and Adults:* Apply a few drops to affected area once daily

Dosage Forms
Cream, topical: 0.1% (15 g, 45 g)
Elocon®: 0.1% (15 g, 45 g)
Lotion, topical: 0.1% (30 mL, 60 mL)
Elocon®: 0.1% (30 mL, 60 mL)
Ointment, topical: 0.1% (15 g, 45 g)
Elocon®: 0.1% (15 g, 45 g)

mometasone and formoterol (moe MET a sone & for MOH te rol)

Synonyms formoterol and mometasone; formoterol and mometasone furoate; formoterol fumarate dihydrate and mometasone

U.S. Brand Names Dulera®

Canadian Brand Names Zenhale™

Therapeutic Category $Beta_2$-Adrenergic Agonist Agent; $Beta_2$-Adrenergic Agonist, Long-Acting; Corticosteroid, Inhalant (Oral)

Use Maintenance treatment of asthma where combination therapy is indicated

General Dosage Range Inhalation: *Children ≥12 years and Adults:* 2 inhalations twice daily (maximum: 4 inhalations/day)

Dosage Forms
Aerosol, for oral inhalation:
Dulera®: Mometasone 100 mcg and formoterol 5 mcg per inhalation (13 g) [120 metered actuations]
Dulera®: Mometasone 200 mcg and formoterol 5 mcg per inhalation (13 g) [120 metered actuations]

Dosage Forms - Canada
Aerosol, for oral inhalation:
Zenhale™: Mometasone furoate 50 mcg and formoterol fumarate dihydrate 5 mcg per inhalation [120 metered actuations]

mometasone furoate *see* mometasone (nasal) *on page 610*
mometasone furoate *see* mometasone (oral inhalation) *on page 610*
mometasone furoate *see* mometasone (topical) *on page 610*
MOM/mineral oil emulsion *see* magnesium hydroxide and mineral oil *on page 559*
monacolin K *see* lovastatin *on page 553*
Monicure (Can) *see* fluconazole *on page 388*
***Monilia* skin test** *see Candida albicans (Monilia) on page 169*
Monistat® (Can) *see* miconazole (topical) *on page 599*
Monistat® 1 [OTC] *see* miconazole (topical) *on page 599*
Monistat® 1 Day or Night [OTC] *see* miconazole (topical) *on page 599*
Monistat® 3 [OTC] *see* miconazole (topical) *on page 599*
Monistat® 3 (Can) *see* miconazole (topical) *on page 599*
Monistat® 7 [OTC] *see* miconazole (topical) *on page 599*

monobenzone (mon oh BEN zone)

Therapeutic Category Topical Skin Product

Use Final depigmentation in extensive vitiligo

General Dosage Range Topical: *Children ≥12 years and Adults:* Initial: Apply 2-3 times/day; once depigmentation obtained apply as needed (usually 2 times/week)

Monocaps [OTC] *see* vitamins (multiple/oral) *on page 951*
Monoclate-P® *see* antihemophilic factor (human) *on page 78*
monoclonal antibody 2C4 *see* pertuzumab *on page 710*
monoclonal antibody 5G1.1 *see* eculizumab *on page 322*
monoclonal antibody ABX-EGF *see* panitumumab *on page 688*

monoclonal antibody anti-C5 *see* eculizumab *on page* 322
monoclonal antibody campath-1H *see* alemtuzumab *on page* 45
monoclonal antibody CD52 *see* alemtuzumab *on page* 45
Monodox® *see* doxycycline *on page* 314
monoethanolamine *see* ethanolamine oleate *on page* 355
Monoket® [DSC] *see* isosorbide mononitrate *on page* 505
MonoNessa® *see* ethinyl estradiol and norgestimate *on page* 361
Mononine® *see* factor IX *on page* 371
Monopril *see* fosinopril *on page* 409
Monopril® (Can) *see* fosinopril *on page* 409
Monopril-HCT® [DSC] *see* fosinopril and hydrochlorothiazide *on page* 409
Monopril-HCT® (Can) *see* fosinopril and hydrochlorothiazide *on page* 409
monsel's solution *see* ferric subsulfate *on page* 379

montelukast (mon te LOO kast)

Medication Safety Issues

Sound-alike/look-alike issues:

Singulair® may be confused with SINEquan®

Synonyms montelukast sodium

U.S. Brand Names Singulair®

Canadian Brand Names Apo-Montelukast; Montelukast Sodium Tablets; Mylan-Montelukast; PMS-Montelukast; PMS-Montelukast FC; Sandoz-Montelukast; Sandoz-Montelukast Granules; Singulair®; Teva-Montelukast

Therapeutic Category Leukotriene Receptor Antagonist

Use Prophylaxis and chronic treatment of asthma; relief of symptoms of seasonal allergic rhinitis and perennial allergic rhinitis; prevention of exercise-induced bronchoconstriction

General Dosage Range Oral:

Children 6 months-5 years: 4 mg once daily
Children 6-14 years: 5 mg once daily **or** 5 mg 2 hours prior to exercise
Children ≥15 years and Adults: 10 mg once daily **or** 10 mg 2 hours prior to exercise

Dosage Forms

Granules, oral:
Singulair®: 4 mg/packet (30s)
Tablet, oral: 10 mg
Singulair®: 10 mg
Tablet, chewable, oral: 4 mg, 5 mg
Singulair®: 4 mg, 5 mg

montelukast sodium *see* montelukast *on page* 612
Montelukast Sodium Tablets (Can) *see* montelukast *on page* 612
Monurol® *see* fosfomycin *on page* 408
8-MOP® *see* methoxsalen (systemic) *on page* 586
MoreDophilus® [OTC] *see* Lactobacillus *on page* 518
morning after pill *see* ethinyl estradiol and norgestrel *on page* 362

morphine (systemic) (MOR feen)

Medication Safety Issues

Sound-alike/look-alike issues:

Morphine may be confused with HYDROmorphone, methadone
Morphine sulfate may be confused with magnesium sulfate
Kadian® may be confused with Kapidex [DSC]
MS Contin® may be confused with OxyCONTIN®
MSO_4 and MS are error-prone abbreviations (mistaken as magnesium sulfate)
AVINza® may be confused with Evista®, INVanz®

Roxanol may be confused with OxyFast®, Roxicet™, Roxicodone®

High alert medication:

The Institute for Safe Medication Practices (ISMP) includes this medication (I.V. formulation) among its list of drug classes which have a heightened risk of causing significant patient harm when used in error.

Other safety concerns:

Use care when prescribing and/or administering morphine solutions. These products are available in different concentrations. Always prescribe dosage in mg; **not** by volume (mL).

Use caution when selecting a morphine formulation for use in neurologic infusion pumps (eg, Medtronic delivery systems). The product should be appropriately labeled as "preservative-free" and suitable for intraspinal use via continuous infusion. In addition, the product should be formulated in a pH range that is compatible with the device operation specifications.

Significant differences exist between oral and I.V. dosing. Use caution when converting from one route of administration to another.

Synonyms MS (error-prone abbreviation and should not be used); MSO_4 (error-prone abbreviation and should not be used); Roxanol

U.S. Brand Names Astramorph®/PF; AVINza®; Duramorph; Infumorph 200; Infumorph 500; Kadian®; MS Contin®; Oramorph® SR

Canadian Brand Names Doloral; Kadian®; M-Eslon®; M.O.S.-SR®; M.O.S.-Sulfate®; M.O.S.® 10; M.O.S.® 20; M.O.S.® 30; Morphine Extra Forte Injection; Morphine Forte Injection; Morphine HP®; Morphine LP® Epidural; Morphine SR; Morphine-EPD; MS Contin SRT; MS Contin®; MS-IR®; Novo-Morphine SR; PMS-Morphine Sulfate SR; ratio-Morphine; ratio-Morphine SR; Sandoz-Morphine SR; Statex®; Teva-Morphine SR

Therapeutic Category Analgesic, Opioid

Controlled Substance C-II

Use Relief of moderate-to-severe acute and chronic pain; relief of pain of myocardial infarction; relief of dyspnea of acute left ventricular failure and pulmonary edema; preanesthetic medication

Infumorph®: Used in continuous microinfusion devices for intrathecal or epidural administration in treatment of intractable chronic pain

Controlled-, extended-, or sustained-release products: Only intended/indicated for use when repeated doses for an extended period of time are required. The 100 mg and 200 mg tablets or capsules of Kadian®, MS Contin®, and morphine sulfate controlled-release tablets and the 60 mg, 90 mg, and 120 mg capsules of Avinza® should only be used in opioid-tolerant patients.

General Dosage Range Dosage adjustment recommended in patients with renal impairment

Epidural: *Adults:* 5 mg (Astromorph/PF™, Duramorph®) as a single dose **or** 1-6 mg bolus followed by 0.1-0.2 mg/hour (maximum: 10 mg/day) **or** continuous microinfusion (Infumorph®): Opioid-naive patients: 3.5-7.5 mg/day; Opioid-tolerant patients: 4.5-30 mg/day

I.M.:

Children >6 months and <50 kg: 0.1-0.2 mg/kg every 3-4 hours as needed

Adults: 5-20 mg every 4 hours as needed

I.T. (I.T. dose is usually 1/10 that of epidural dose): *Adults:* Opioid-naive: 0.2-1 mg/dose as single dose or once daily; Opioid-tolerant: 1-10 mg/day

I.V.:

Children >6 months and <50 kg: 0.1-0.2 mg/kg every 3-4 hours as needed **or** 10-60 mcg/kg/**hour** as a continuous infusion

Adults: 2.5-5 mg every 3-4 hours **or** 0.8-10 mg/hour; Usual range: Up to 80 mg/hour

Adults (mechanically-ventilated): 0.7-10 mg every 1-2 hours as needed **or** 5-35 mg/hour infusion

Oral:

Controlled, extended or sustained release: *Adults:*

Capsules: Established daily dose on prompt-release formulations administered in 1-2 divided doses (every 12 hours)

Tablets: Established daily dose on prompt-release formulations administered in divided doses every 8-12 hours

Immediate release:

Children >6 months and <50 kg: 0.15-0.3 mg/kg every 3-4 hours as needed

Adults: 10-30 mg every 4 hours as needed; **Note:** Much higher doses may be necessary for chronic pain

PCA: *Adults:* Concentration: 1 mg/mL; Demand dose: 0.5-2.5 mg; Lockout interval: 5-10 minutes

Rectal: *Adults:* 10-20 mg every 3-4 hours

SubQ:

Adults: 5-20 mg every 3-4 hours as needed **or** 0.8-10 mg/hour (up to 80 mg/hour) as continuous infusion

Adults (mechanically-ventilated): 0.7-10 mg every 1-2 hours as needed **or** 5-35 mg/hour infusion

Dosage Forms

Capsule, extended release, oral: 10 mg, 20 mg, 30 mg, 50 mg, 60 mg, 80 mg, 100 mg, 200 mg

AVINza®: 30 mg, 45 mg, 60 mg, 75 mg, 90 mg, 120 mg

Kadian®: 10 mg, 20 mg, 30 mg, 40 mg, 50 mg, 60 mg, 70 mg, 80 mg, 100 mg, 130 mg, 150 mg, 200 mg

Injection, solution: 1 mg/mL (10 mL, 30 mL, 50 mL); 2 mg/mL (1 mL); 4 mg/mL (1 mL); 5 mg/mL (1 mL, 30 mL, 50 mL); 8 mg/mL (1 mL); 10 mg/mL (1 mL, 10 mL); 10 mg/0.7 mL (0.7 mL); 15 mg/mL (1 mL, 20 mL); 25 mg/mL (4 mL, 10 mL, 20 mL); 50 mg/mL (20 mL, 40 mL, 50 mL)

Injection, solution [preservative free]: 0.5 mg/mL (10 mL, 30 mL); 1 mg/mL (10 mL, 30 mL); 5 mg/mL (30 mL); 25 mg/mL (4 mL, 10 mL, 20 mL)

Astramorph®/PF: 0.5 mg/mL (2 mL, 10 mL); 1 mg/mL (2 mL, 10 mL)

Duramorph: 0.5 mg/mL (10 mL); 1 mg/mL (10 mL)

Infumorph 200: 10 mg/mL (20 mL)

Infumorph 500: 25 mg/mL (20 mL)

Solution, oral: 10 mg/5 mL (5 mL, 100 mL, 500 mL); 20 mg/5 mL (100 mL, 500 mL); 100 mg/5 mL (15 mL, 30 mL, 120 mL, 240 mL)

Suppository, rectal: 5 mg (12s); 10 mg (12s); 20 mg (12s); 30 mg (12s)

Tablet, oral: 15 mg, 30 mg

Tablet, controlled release, oral:

MS Contin®: 15 mg, 30 mg, 60 mg, 100 mg, 200 mg

Tablet, extended release, oral: 15 mg, 30 mg, 60 mg, 100 mg, 200 mg

Tablet, sustained release, oral:

Oramorph® SR: 15 mg, 30 mg, 60 mg, 100 mg

Dosage Forms - Canada

Solution, oral:

Doloral: 1 mg/mL; 5 mg/mL [not available in U.S.]

morphine (liposomal) (MOR feen)

Medication Safety Issues

Sound-alike/look-alike issues:

Morphine may be confused with HYDROmorphone

Morphine sulfate may be confused with magnesium sulfate

MSO_4 and MS are error-prone abbreviations (mistaken as magnesium sulfate)

High alert medication:

The Institute for Safe Medication Practices (ISMP) includes this medication among its list of drug classes which have a heightened risk of causing significant patient harm when used in error.

Synonyms extended release epidural morphine; MS (error-prone abbreviation and should not be used); MSO_4 (error-prone abbreviation and should not be used)

U.S. Brand Names DepoDur®

Therapeutic Category Analgesic, Opioid

Controlled Substance C-II

Use Epidural (lumbar) single-dose management of surgical pain

General Dosage Range Epidural: *Adults:* 10-15 mg as a single dose

Dosage Forms

Injection, extended release liposomal suspension [preservative free]:

DepoDur®: 10 mg/mL (1 mL, 1.5 mL)

morphine and naltrexone (MOR feen & nal TREKS one)

Medication Safety Issues

Sound-alike/look-alike issues:

Morphine may be confused with HYDROmorphone

Morphine sulfate may be confused with magnesium sulfate

Naltrexone may be confused with methylnaltrexone, naloxone

MSO_4 and MS are error-prone abbreviations (mistaken as magnesium sulfate)

High alert medication:

The Institute for Safe Medication Practices (ISMP) includes this medication among its list of drug classes which have a heightened risk of causing significant patient harm when used in error.

Synonyms morphine sulfate and naltrexone hydrochloride; MS (error-prone abbreviation and should not be used); MSO_4 (error-prone abbreviation and should not be used); naltrexone and morphine

U.S. Brand Names Embeda™

Therapeutic Category Analgesic, Opioid; Opioid Antagonist

Controlled Substance C-II

Use Relief of moderate-to-severe pain when continual, around-the-clock therapy is needed for an extended period of time

General Dosage Range Oral: *Adults:* Initial: 20 mg/0.8 mg once or twice daily; Maintenance: Adjust based on individual patient requirement

Dosage Forms

Capsule, extended release, oral:

Embeda™ 20/0.8: Morphine 20 mg and naltrexone 0.8 mg
Embeda™ 30/1.2: Morphine 30 mg and naltrexone 1.2 mg
Embeda™ 50/2: Morphine 50 mg and naltrexone 2 mg
Embeda™ 80/3.2: Morphine 80 mg and naltrexone 3.2 mg
Embeda™ 100/4: Morphine 100 mg and naltrexone 4 mg

Morphine-EPD (Can) *see* morphine (systemic) *on page 612*
Morphine Extra Forte Injection (Can) *see* morphine (systemic) *on page 612*
Morphine Forte Injection (Can) *see* morphine (systemic) *on page 612*
Morphine HP® (Can) *see* morphine (systemic) *on page 612*
Morphine LP® Epidural (Can) *see* morphine (systemic) *on page 612*
Morphine SR (Can) *see* morphine (systemic) *on page 612*
morphine sulfate and naltrexone hydrochloride *see* morphine and naltrexone *on page 614*

morrhuate sodium (MOR yoo ate SOW dee um)

Therapeutic Category Sclerosing Agent

Use Treatment of small, uncomplicated varicose veins of the lower extremities

General Dosage Range I.V.: *Adults:* 50-250 mg

Dosage Forms

Injection, solution: 50 mg/mL (30 mL)

M.O.S.® 10 (Can) *see* morphine (systemic) *on page 612*
M.O.S.® 20 (Can) *see* morphine (systemic) *on page 612*
M.O.S.® 30 (Can) *see* morphine (systemic) *on page 612*
Mosco® Callus & Corn Remover [OTC] *see* salicylic acid *on page 816*
Mosco® One Step Corn Remover [OTC] *see* salicylic acid *on page 816*
M.O.S.-SR® (Can) *see* morphine (systemic) *on page 612*
M.O.S.-Sulfate® (Can) *see* morphine (systemic) *on page 612*
Motofen® *see* difenoxin and atropine *on page 284*
Motrin® Children's [OTC] *see* ibuprofen *on page 468*
Motrin® (Children's) (Can) *see* ibuprofen *on page 468*
Motrin® IB [OTC] *see* ibuprofen *on page 468*
Motrin® IB (Can) *see* ibuprofen *on page 468*
Motrin® Infants' [OTC] *see* ibuprofen *on page 468*
Motrin® Junior [OTC] *see* ibuprofen *on page 468*
Mouth Kote® [OTC] *see* saliva substitute *on page 819*
MoviPrep® *see* polyethylene glycol-electrolyte solution *on page 738*
Moxatag™ *see* amoxicillin *on page 69*
Moxeza™ *see* moxifloxacin (ophthalmic) *on page 616*

moxifloxacin (systemic) (moxs i FLOKS a sin)

Medication Safety Issues

Sound-alike/look-alike issues:

Avelox® may be confused with Avonex®

Synonyms moxifloxacin hydrochloride

U.S. Brand Names Avelox®; Avelox® ABC Pack; Avelox® I.V.

Canadian Brand Names Avelox®; Avelox® I.V.

Therapeutic Category Antibiotic, Quinolone; Respiratory Fluoroquinolone

Use Treatment of mild-to-moderate community-acquired pneumonia, including multidrug-resistant *Streptococcus pneumoniae* (MDRSP); acute bacterial exacerbation of chronic bronchitis; acute bacterial rhinosinusitis (ABRS); complicated and uncomplicated skin and skin structure infections; complicated intraabdominal infections

General Dosage Range I.V., oral: *Adults:* 400 mg every 24 hours

Dosage Forms

Infusion, premixed in sodium chloride 0.8% [preservative free]:

Avelox® I.V.: 400 mg (250 mL)

Tablet, oral:

Avelox®: 400 mg

Avelox® ABC Pack: 400 mg

moxifloxacin (ophthalmic) (moxs i FLOKS a sin)

Medication Safety Issues

International issues:

Vigamox [U.S., Canada, and multiple international markets] may be confused with Fisamox brand name for amoxicillin [Australia]

Synonyms moxifloxacin hydrochloride

U.S. Brand Names Moxeza™; Vigamox®

Canadian Brand Names Vigamox®

Therapeutic Category Antibiotic, Ophthalmic; Antibiotic, Quinolone

Use Treatment of bacterial conjunctivitis caused by susceptible organisms

General Dosage Range Ophthalmic:

Children ≥4 months and Adults: Moxeza™: Instill 1 drop into affected eye(s) 2 times/day

Children ≥1 year and Adults: Vigamox®: Instill 1 drop into affected eye(s) 3 times/day

Dosage Forms

Solution, ophthalmic:

Moxeza™: 0.5% (3 mL)

Vigamox®: 0.5% (3 mL)

moxifloxacin hydrochloride *see* moxifloxacin (ophthalmic) *on page* 616

moxifloxacin hydrochloride *see* moxifloxacin (systemic) *on page* 616

Mozobil™ *see* plerixafor *on page* 729

4-MP *see* fomepizole *on page* 405

MP-424 *see* telaprevir *on page* 873

MPA *see* medroxyprogesterone *on page* 567

MPA *see* mycophenolate *on page* 619

MPA and estrogens (conjugated) *see* estrogens (conjugated/equine) and medroxyprogesterone *on page* 352

6-MP (error-prone abbreviation) *see* mercaptopurine *on page* 576

MPSV *see* meningococcal polysaccharide vaccine (groups A / C / Y and W-135) *on page* 573

MPSV4 *see* meningococcal polysaccharide vaccine (groups A / C / Y and W-135) *on page* 573

MRA *see* tocilizumab *on page* 902

MS Contin® *see* morphine (systemic) *on page* 612

MS Contin SRT (Can) *see* morphine (systemic) *on page* 612

MS (error-prone abbreviation and should not be used) *see* morphine and naltrexone *on page* 614

MS (error-prone abbreviation and should not be used) *see* morphine (liposomal) *on page* 614

MS (error-prone abbreviation and should not be used) *see* morphine (systemic) *on page* 612

mucosal barrier gel, oral (myoo KOH sul BAR ee er GEL, OR al)

Synonyms mucosal bioadherent gel

U.S. Brand Names Gelclair®

Therapeutic Category Gastrointestinal Agent, Miscellaneous

Use Management of oral mucosal pain caused by oral mucositis/stomatitis (resulting from chemotherapy or radiation therapy), irritation due to oral surgery, traumatic ulcers caused by braces/ill-fitting dentures or disease, diffuse aphthous ulcers (canker sores)

General Dosage Range Oral: *Adults:* Gargle and spit the mixture of 1 single-use packet (15 mL) and water 3 times/day, or as needed.

Dosage Forms

Gel, oral:

Gelclair®: 15 mL/packet (15s)

mucosal bioadherent gel *see* mucosal barrier gel, oral *on page* 618

Mucus Relief [OTC] [DSC] *see* guaifenesin *on page* 433

Mucus Relief Sinus [OTC] *see* guaifenesin and phenylephrine *on page* 435

Multaq® *see* dronedarone *on page* 317

Multidex® [OTC] *see* maltodextrin *on page* 561

Multihance® *see* gadobenate dimeglumine *on page* 414

Multihance® Multipack™ *see* gadobenate dimeglumine *on page* 414

Multi-Nate 30 *see* vitamins (multiple/prenatal) *on page* 952

multiple vitamins *see* vitamins (multiple/oral) *on page* 951

Multitrace®-4 *see* trace elements *on page* 908

Multitrace®-4 Concentrate *see* trace elements *on page* 908

Multitrace®-4 Neonatal *see* trace elements *on page* 908

Multitrace®-4 Pediatric *see* trace elements *on page* 908

Multitrace®-5 *see* trace elements *on page* 908

Multitrace®-5 Concentrate *see* trace elements *on page* 908

multivitamins/fluoride *see* vitamins (multiple/pediatric) *on page* 952

mumps, measles and rubella vaccines *see* measles, mumps, and rubella virus vaccine *on page* 564

mumps, rubella, varicella, and measles vaccine *see* measles, mumps, rubella, and varicella virus vaccine *on page* 564

mupirocin (myoo PEER oh sin)

Medication Safety Issues

Sound-alike/look-alike issues:

Bactroban® may be confused with bacitracin, baclofen, Bactrim™

Synonyms mupirocin calcium; pseudomonic acid A

U.S. Brand Names Bactroban Cream®; Bactroban Nasal®; Bactroban®; Centany®; Centany® AT

Canadian Brand Names Bactroban®

Therapeutic Category Antibiotic, Topical

Use

Intranasal: Eradication of nasal colonization with MRSA in adult patients and healthcare workers

Topical: Treatment of impetigo or secondary infected traumatic skin lesions due to *S. aureus* and *S. pyogenes*

General Dosage Range

Intranasal: *Children ≥12 years and Adults:* Approximately one-half of the ointment from the single-use tube should be applied into one nostril and the other half into the other nostril twice daily

Topical: *Children ≥2 months and Adults:* Apply to affected area 3 times/day

Dosage Forms

Cream, topical:

Bactroban Cream®: 2% (15 g, 30 g)

Ointment, intranasal:
Bactroban Nasal®: 2% (1 g)
Ointment, topical: 2% (0.9 g, 15 g, 22 g, 30 g)
Bactroban®: 2% (22 g)
Centany®: 2% (30 g)
Centany® AT: 2% (1s)

mycophenolate (mye koe FEN oh late)

Synonyms MMF; MPA; mycophenolate mofetil; mycophenolate sodium; mycophenolic acid

U.S. Brand Names CellCept®; Myfortic®

Canadian Brand Names Apo-Mycophenolate; CellCept®; CO Mycophenolate; JAMP-Mycophenolate; Myfortic®; Mylan-Mycophenolate; Novo-Mycophenolate; Sandoz-Mycophenolate; Sandoz-Mycophenolate Mofetil

Therapeutic Category Immunosuppressant Agent

Use Prophylaxis of organ rejection concomitantly with cyclosporine and corticosteroids in patients receiving allogeneic renal (CellCept®, Myfortic®), cardiac (CellCept®), or hepatic (CellCept®) transplants

General Dosage Range Dosage adjustment recommended in patient with renal impairment and who develop toxicities

I.V.: *Adults:* 1-1.5 g twice daily
Oral:
Cellcept®:
Children (suspension): 600 mg/m^2/dose twice daily (maximum: 1 g twice daily)
Children with BSA 1.25-1.5 m^2: 750 mg capsule twice daily
Children with BSA >1.5 m^2: 1 g capsule or tablet twice daily
Adults: 1-1.5 g twice daily
Myfortic®:
Children with BSA 1.19-1.58 m^2: 540 mg twice daily (maximum: 1080 mg/day)
Children with BSA >1.58 m^2 and Adults: 720 mg twice daily (maximum: 1440 mg/day)

Dosage Forms
Capsule, oral: 250 mg
CellCept®: 250 mg
Injection, powder for reconstitution:
CellCept®: 500 mg
Powder for suspension, oral:
CellCept®: 200 mg/mL (175 mL)

Tablet, oral: 500 mg
CellCept®: 500 mg
Tablet, delayed release, oral:
Myfortic®: 180 mg, 360 mg

Myoflex® (Can) *see* trolamine *on page 923*
Myorisan™ *see* isotretinoin *on page 505*
Myozyme® *see* alglucosidase alfa *on page 47*
Myphetane DX [DSC] *see* brompheniramine, pseudoephedrine, and dextromethorphan *on page 144*
Mysoline® *see* primidone *on page 758*
Mytab Gas [OTC] *see* simethicone *on page 834*
Mytab Gas Maximum [OTC] *see* simethicone *on page 834*
Mytelase® [DSC] *see* ambenonium *on page 58*
mytotan *see* mitotane *on page 607*
Mytussin® DAC *see* guaifenesin, pseudoephedrine, and codeine *on page 437*
Myzilra™ *see* ethinyl estradiol and levonorgestrel *on page 357*
N-9 *see* nonoxynol 9 *on page 647*
N-0923 *see* rotigotine *on page 813*
NAAK *see* atropine and pralidoxime *on page 103*
Nabi-HB® *see* hepatitis B immune globulin (human) *on page 445*
nab-paclitaxel *see* paclitaxel (protein bound) *on page 684*

nabumetone (na BYOO me tone)

Medication Safety Issues

BEERS Criteria medication:

This drug may be potentially inappropriate for use in geriatric patients (Quality of evidence - moderate; Strength of recommendation - strong).

Synonyms Relafen

Canadian Brand Names Apo-Nabumetone®; Gen-Nabumetone; Mylan-Nabumetone; Novo-Nabumetone; Relafen®; Rhoxal-nabumetone; Sandoz-Nabumetone

Therapeutic Category Analgesic, Nonnarcotic; Nonsteroidal Antiinflammatory Drug (NSAID)

Use Management of osteoarthritis and rheumatoid arthritis

General Dosage Range Dosage adjustment recommended in patients with renal impairment

Oral: *Adults:* 1000 mg/day in 1-2 divided doses (maximum: 2000 mg/day)

Dosage Forms

Tablet, oral: 500 mg, 750 mg

NAC *see* acetylcysteine *on page 32*
***N*-acetyl-L-cysteine** *see* acetylcysteine *on page 32*
***N* acetylcysteine** *see* acetylcysteine *on page 32*
n-acetyl-p-aminophenol *see* acetaminophen *on page 20*
NaCl *see* sodium chloride *on page 840*
NACSA *see* antivenin *(Micrurus fulvius) on page 81*

nadolol (NAY doe lol)

Medication Safety Issues

Sound-alike/look-alike issues:

Corgard® may be confused with Cognex®, Coreg®

International issues:

Nadolol may be confused with Mandol brand name for cefamandole [Belgium, Netherlands, New Zealand, Russia]

U.S. Brand Names Corgard®

Canadian Brand Names Alti-Nadolol; Apo-Nadol®; Corgard®; Novo-Nadolol; Teva-Nadolol

Therapeutic Category Beta-Adrenergic Blocker

Use Treatment of hypertension and angina pectoris; prophylaxis of migraine headaches

General Dosage Range Dosage adjustment recommended in patients with renal impairment

Oral:

Adults: Initial: 40 mg once daily; Maintenance: 40-320 mg once daily
Elderly: Initial: 20 mg once daily; Maintenance: 20-240 mg once daily

Dosage Forms

Tablet, oral: 20 mg, 40 mg, 80 mg
Corgard®: 20 mg, 40 mg, 80 mg

nadolol and bendroflumethiazide (NAY doe lol & ben droe floo meth EYE a zide)

Synonyms bendroflumethiazide and nadolol

U.S. Brand Names Corzide®

Therapeutic Category Antihypertensive Agent, Combination; Beta-Adrenergic Blocker, Nonselective; Diuretic, Thiazide

Use Treatment of hypertension; combination product should not be used for initial therapy

General Dosage Range Dosage adjustment recommended in patients with renal impairment

Oral: *Adults:* Initial: Nadolol 40 mg and bendroflumethiazide 5 mg once daily; Maintenance: Nadolol 40-80 mg and bendroflumethiazide 5 mg once daily

Dosage Forms

Tablet: Nadolol 40 mg and bendroflumethiazide 5 mg; nadolol 80 mg and bendroflumethiazide 5 mg
Corzide® 40/5: Nadolol 40 mg and bendroflumethiazide 5 mg [scored]
Corzide® 80/5: Nadolol 80 mg and bendroflumethiazide 5 mg [scored]

nadroparin calcium *see* nadroparin *(Canada only) on page* 624

nadroparin *(Canada only)* (nad roe PA rin)

Medication Safety Issues

High alert medication:
This medication is in a class the Institute for Safe Medication Practices (ISMP) includes among its list of drug classes which have a heightened risk of causing significant patient harm when used in error.

Synonyms nadroparin calcium

Canadian Brand Names Fraxiparine™; Fraxiparine™ Forte

Therapeutic Category Low Molecular Weight Heparin

Use Prophylaxis of thromboembolic disorders (particularly deep venous thrombosis and pulmonary embolism) in general and orthopedic surgery; treatment of deep venous thrombosis; prevention of clotting during hemodialysis; treatment of unstable angina and non-Q-wave myocardial infarction

General Dosage Range Dosage varies greatly depending on indication.

Product Availability Not available in U.S.

Dosage Forms - Canada

Injection, solution:
Fraxiparine™: 9500 anti-Xa units/mL (0.2 mL, 0.3 mL, 0.4 mL, 0.6 mL, 0.8 mL, 1 mL)
Fraxiparine™ Forte: 19,000 anti-Xa units/mL (0.6 mL, 0.8 mL, 1 mL)

nafarelin (naf a REL in)

Medication Safety Issues

Sound-alike/look-alike issues:
Nafarelin may be confused with Anafranil®, enalapril

Synonyms nafarelin acetate

U.S. Brand Names Synarel®

Canadian Brand Names Synarel®

Therapeutic Category Hormone, Posterior Pituitary

Use Treatment of endometriosis, including pain and reduction of lesions; treatment of central precocious puberty (CPP; gonadotropin-dependent precocious puberty) in children of both sexes

General Dosage Range Nasal:
Children: 2 sprays (400 mcg) into each nostril twice daily; may increase to 3 sprays (600 mcg) into alternating nostrils 3 times/day
Adults: 1 spray (200 mcg) in 1-2 nostrils twice daily

Dosage Forms

Solution, intranasal:
Synarel®: 2 mg/mL (8 mL)

nafarelin acetate *see* nafarelin *on page* 624

nafcillin (naf SIL in)

Synonyms ethoxynaphthamido penicillin sodium; nafcillin sodium; Nallpen; sodium nafcillin

Canadian Brand Names Nallpen®; Unipen®

Therapeutic Category Penicillin

Use Treatment of infections such as osteomyelitis, septicemia, endocarditis, and CNS infections caused by susceptible strains of staphylococci species

General Dosage Range

I.M.:

Children: 25 mg/kg twice daily

Adults: 500 mg every 4-6 hours

I.V.:

Children: 50-200 mg/kg/day in divided every 4-6 hours (maximum: 12 g/day)

Adults: 500-2000 mg every 4-6 hours

Dosage Forms

Infusion, premixed iso-osmotic dextrose solution: 1 g (50 mL); 2 g (100 mL)

Injection, powder for reconstitution: 1 g, 2 g, 10 g

nafcillin sodium *see* nafcillin *on page 624*

naftifine (NAF ti feen)

Synonyms naftifine hydrochloride

U.S. Brand Names Naftin®

Therapeutic Category Antifungal Agent

Use Topical treatment of tinea cruris (jock itch), tinea corporis (ringworm), and tinea pedis (athlete's foot)

General Dosage Range Topical: *Adults:* Cream: Apply once daily; Gel: Apply twice daily

Dosage Forms

Cream, topical:

Naftin®: 1% (30 g, 60 g, 90 g); 2% (45 g)

Gel, topical:

Naftin®: 1% (40 g, 60 g, 90 g)

naftifine hydrochloride *see* naftifine *on page 625*

Naftin® *see* naftifine *on page 625*

Naglazyme® *see* galsulfase *on page 418*

$NaHCO_3$ *see* sodium bicarbonate *on page 840*

NaI I-123 *see* sodium iodide I^{123} *on page 843*

nalbuphine (NAL byoo feen)

Medication Safety Issues

Sound-alike/look-alike issues:

Nubain may be confused with Navane®, Nebcin

High alert medication:

The Institute for Safe Medication Practices (ISMP) includes this medication among its list of drug classes which have a heightened risk of causing significant patient harm when used in error.

Synonyms nalbuphine hydrochloride; Nubain

Therapeutic Category Analgesic, Narcotic

Use Relief of moderate-to-severe pain; preoperative analgesia, postoperative and surgical anesthesia, and obstetrical analgesia during labor and delivery

General Dosage Range

I.M., SubQ: *Adults:* 10 mg/70 kg every 3-6 hours (maximum: 20 mg/dose; 160 mg/day)

I.V.: *Adults:* 10 mg/70 kg every 3-6 hours (maximum: 20 mg/dose; 160 mg/day) **or** 0.3-3 mg/kg over 10-15 minutes, then 0.25-0.5 mg/kg as required for anesthesia **or** 2.5-5 mg (1-2 doses)

Dosage Forms

Injection, solution: 10 mg/mL (10 mL); 20 mg/mL (10 mL)

Injection, solution [preservative free]: 10 mg/mL (1 mL); 20 mg/mL (1 mL)

nalbuphine hydrochloride *see* nalbuphine *on page 625*

Nalcrom® (Can) *see* cromolyn (systemic, oral inhalation) *on page 240*

Nalfon® *see* fenoprofen *on page 376*

Nallpen *see* nafcillin *on page 624*

Nallpen® (Can) *see* nafcillin *on page 624*

***N*-allylnoroxymorphine hydrochloride** *see* naloxone *on page 626*

naloxone (nal OKS one)

Medication Safety Issues

Sound-alike/look-alike issues:

Naloxone may be confused with Lanoxin®, naltrexone

Narcan may be confused with Marcaine®, Norcuron®

International issues:

Narcan [multiple international markets] may be confused with Marcen brand name for ketazolam [Spain]

Synonyms *N*-allylnoroxymorphine hydrochloride; naloxone hydrochloride; Narcan

Canadian Brand Names Naloxone Hydrochloride Injection®; Naloxone Hydrochloride Injection® USP

Therapeutic Category Antidote

Use Complete or partial reversal of opioid drug effects, including respiratory depression; management of known or suspected opioid overdose; diagnosis of suspected opioid dependence or acute opioid overdose

General Dosage Range I.M., I.V., SubQ: *Adults:* 0.1-2 mg every 2-3 minutes as needed (maximum: 10 mg)

Dosage Forms

Injection, solution: 0.4 mg/mL (1 mL, 10 mL)

Injection, solution [preservative free]: 0.4 mg/mL (1 mL)

naloxone and buprenorphine *see* buprenorphine and naloxone *on page 150*

naloxone hydrochloride *see* naloxone *on page 626*

naloxone hydrochloride and pentazocine *see* pentazocine and naloxone *on page 705*

naloxone hydrochloride dihydrate and buprenorphine hydrochloride *see* buprenorphine and naloxone *on page 150*

Naloxone Hydrochloride Injection® (Can) *see* naloxone *on page 626*

Naloxone Hydrochloride Injection® USP (Can) *see* naloxone *on page 626*

naltrexone (nal TREKS one)

Medication Safety Issues

Sound-alike/look-alike issues:

Naltrexone may be confused with methylnaltrexone, naloxone

ReVia® may be confused with Revatio®, Revex®

Administration issues:

Vivitrol®: For intramuscular (I.M.) gluteal injection only

Synonyms naltrexone hydrochloride

U.S. Brand Names ReVia®; Vivitrol®

Canadian Brand Names ReVia®

Therapeutic Category Antidote

Use Treatment of ethanol dependence; prevention of relapse in opioid dependent patients, following opioid detoxification

General Dosage Range

I.M.: *Adults:* 380 mg once every 4 weeks

Oral: *Adults:* 25-50 mg once daily

Dosage Forms

Injection, microspheres for suspension, extended release:

Vivitrol®: 380 mg

Tablet, oral: 50 mg

ReVia®: 50 mg

naltrexone and morphine *see* morphine and naltrexone *on page 614*

naltrexone hydrochloride *see* naltrexone *on page 626*

Namenda® *see* memantine *on page 570*

Namenda XR *see* memantine *on page 570*

nanoparticle albumin-bound paclitaxel *see* paclitaxel (protein bound) *on page 684*

NAPA and NABZ *see* sodium phenylacetate and sodium benzoate *on page 844*

naphazoline (nasal) (naf AZ oh leen)

Synonyms naphazoline hydrochloride

U.S. Brand Names Privine® [OTC]

Therapeutic Category $Alpha_1$ Agonist

Use Temporary relief of nasal congestion associated with the common cold, upper respiratory allergies, or sinusitis

General Dosage Range Intranasal: *Children ≥12 years and Adults:* Instill 1-2 drops or sprays every 6 hours if needed

Dosage Forms

Solution, intranasal:

Privine® [OTC]: 0.05% (20 mL, 25 mL)

naphazoline (ophthalmic) (naf AZ oh leen)

Synonyms naphazoline hydrochloride

U.S. Brand Names AK-Con™; Clear eyes® for Dry Eyes Plus ACR Relief [OTC]; Clear eyes® for Dry Eyes plus Redness Relief [OTC]; Clear eyes® Redness Relief [OTC]; Clear eyes® Seasonal Relief [OTC]

Canadian Brand Names Naphcon Forte®; Vasocon®

Therapeutic Category $Alpha_1$ Agonist; Ophthalmic Agent, Vasoconstrictor

Use Topical ocular vasoconstrictor; relief of redness of the eye due to minor irritation

General Dosage Range Ophthalmic: *Adults:*

0.1% solution (prescription): 1-2 drops into conjunctival sac every 3-4 hours as needed

0.012% or 0.025% solution (OTC): 1-2 drops into affected eye(s) up to 4 times/day

Dosage Forms

Solution, ophthalmic:

AK-Con™: 0.1% (15 mL)

Clear eyes® for Dry Eyes Plus ACR Relief [OTC]: 0.025% (15 mL)

Clear eyes® for Dry Eyes plus Redness Relief [OTC]: 0.012% (15 mL)

Clear eyes® Redness Relief [OTC]: 0.012% (6 mL, 15 mL, 30 mL)

Clear eyes® Seasonal Relief [OTC]: 0.012% (15 mL, 30 mL)

naphazoline and pheniramine (naf AZ oh leen & fen NIR a meen)

Medication Safety Issues

Sound-alike/look-alike issues:

Visine® may be confused with Visken®

Synonyms pheniramine and naphazoline

U.S. Brand Names Naphcon-A® [OTC]; Opcon-A® [OTC]; Visine-A® [OTC]

Canadian Brand Names Naphcon-A®; Visine® Advanced Allergy

Therapeutic Category Antihistamine/Decongestant Combination

Use Treatment of ocular congestion, irritation, and itching

General Dosage Range Ophthalmic: *Children ≥6 years and Adults:* 1-2 drops into the affected eye(s) up to 4 times/day

Dosage Forms

Solution, ophthalmic:

Naphcon-A® [OTC]: Naphazoline 0.025% and pheniramine 0.3%

Opcon-A® [OTC]: Naphazoline 0.027% and pheniramine 0.3%

Visine-A® [OTC]: Naphazoline 0.025% and pheniramine 0.3%

naphazoline hydrochloride *see* naphazoline (nasal) *on page* 626

naphazoline hydrochloride *see* naphazoline (ophthalmic) *on page* 627

Naphcon-A® [OTC] *see* naphazoline and pheniramine *on page* 627

Naphcon-A® (Can) *see* naphazoline and pheniramine *on page* 627

Naphcon Forte® (Can) *see* naphazoline (ophthalmic) *on page* 627

Naprelan® *see* naproxen *on page* 628

Naprelan™ (Can) *see* naproxen *on page* 628

Naprosyn® *see* naproxen *on page* 628

Naprosyn® E (Can) *see* naproxen *on page* 628

Naprosyn® SR (Can) *see* naproxen *on page* 628

naproxen (na PROKS en)

Medication Safety Issues

Sound-alike/look-alike issues:

Naproxen may be confused with Natacyn®, Nebcin
Anaprox® may be confused with Anaspaz®, Avapro®
Naprelan® may be confused with Naprosyn®
Naprosyn® may be confused with Natacyn®, Nebcin

BEERS Criteria medication:

This drug may be potentially inappropriate for use in geriatric patients (Quality of evidence - moderate; Strength of recommendation - strong).

International issues:

Flogen [Mexico] may be confused with Flovent brand name for fluticasone [U.S., Canada]
Flogen [Mexico] may be confused with Floxin brand name for flunarizine [Thailand], norfloxacin [South Africa], ofloxacin [U.S., Canada], and perfloxacin [Philippines]

Synonyms naproxen sodium

U.S. Brand Names Aleve® [OTC]; All Day Relief [OTC]; Anaprox®; Anaprox® DS; EC-Naprosyn®; Mediproxen [OTC]; Midol® Extended Relief [OTC]; Naprelan®; Naprosyn®; Pamprin® Maximum Strength All Day Relief [OTC]

Canadian Brand Names Anaprox®; Anaprox® DS; Apo-Napro-Na DS®; Apo-Napro-Na®; Apo-Naproxen EC®; Apo-Naproxen SR®; Apo-Naproxen®; Mylan-Naproxen EC; Naprelan™; Naprosyn®; Naprosyn® E; Naprosyn® SR; Naproxen Sodium DS; Naproxen-NA; Naproxen-NA DF; PMS-Naproxen; PMS-Naproxen EC; PRO-Naproxen EC; Riva-Naproxen; Riva-Naproxen Sodium; Riva-Naproxen Sodium DS; Teva-Naproxen; Teva-Naproxen EC; Teva-Naproxen Sodium; Teva-Naproxen Sodium DS; Teva-Naproxen SR

Therapeutic Category Analgesic, Nonnarcotic; Antipyretic; Nonsteroidal Antiinflammatory Drug (NSAID)

Use Management of ankylosing spondylitis, osteoarthritis, and rheumatoid disorders (including juvenile idiopathic arthritis [JIA]); acute gout; mild-to-moderate pain; tendonitis, bursitis; dysmenorrhea; fever

General Dosage Range Oral:

Children >2-11 years: 10 mg/kg/day in 2 divided doses (maximum: 10 mg/kg/day)
Children ≥12 years: 10 mg/kg/day in 2 divided doses (maximum: 10 mg/kg/day) **or** 200 mg every 8-12 hours (maximum: 600 mg/day)
Adults: Initial: 200-750 mg as a single dose; Maintenance: 200-500 mg every 6-12 hours (maximum: 1500 mg/day)

Dosage Forms

Caplet, oral: 220 mg
Aleve® [OTC]: 220 mg
All Day Relief [OTC]: 220 mg
Midol® Extended Relief [OTC]: 220 mg
Pamprin® Maximum Strength All Day Relief [OTC]: 220 mg

Capsule, liquid gel, oral:
Aleve® [OTC]: 220 mg

Combination package, oral:
Naprelan®: Day 1-3: Tablet, controlled release: 825 mg [equivalent to naproxen base 750 mg] (6s) [contains sodium 75 mg] and Day 4-10: Tablet, controlled release: 550 mg [equivalent to naproxen base 500 mg] (14s) [contains sodium 50 mg]

Gelcap, oral:
Aleve® [OTC]: 220 mg

Suspension, oral: 125 mg/5 mL (500 mL)
Naprosyn®: 125 mg/5 mL (473 mL)

Tablet, oral: 220 mg, 250 mg, 275 mg, 375 mg, 500 mg, 550 mg
Aleve® [OTC]: 220 mg
Anaprox®: 275 mg
Anaprox® DS: 550 mg
Mediproxen [OTC]: 220 mg
Naprosyn®: 250 mg, 375 mg, 500 mg

Tablet, controlled release, oral:
Naprelan®: 412.5 mg, 550 mg, 825 mg

Tablet, delayed release, enteric coated, oral: 375 mg, 500 mg
EC-Naprosyn®: 375 mg, 500 mg

naproxen and esomeprazole (na PROKS en & es oh ME pray zol)

Medication Safety Issues

Sound-alike/look-alike issues:

Vimovo™ may be confused with Vimpat®

Synonyms esomeprazole and naproxen

U.S. Brand Names Vimovo™

Canadian Brand Names Vimovo™

Therapeutic Category Nonsteroidal Antiinflammatory Drug (NSAID); Proton Pump Inhibitor

Use Reduction of the risk of NSAID-associated gastric ulcers in patients at risk of developing gastric ulcers who require an NSAID for the treatment of rheumatoid arthritis, osteoarthritis, and ankylosing spondylitis

General Dosage Range Oral: *Adults:* 1 tablet (naproxen 375-500 mg/esomeprazole 20 mg) twice daily; Maximum daily dose of esomeprazole: 40 mg/day

Dosage Forms

Tablet, variable release, oral:

Vimovo™: Naproxen [delayed release] 375 mg and esomeprazole [immediate release] 20 mg, Naproxen [delayed release] 500 mg and esomeprazole [immediate release] 20 mg

naproxen and pseudoephedrine (na PROKS en & soo doe e FED rin)

Synonyms naproxen sodium and pseudoephedrine; pseudoephedrine and naproxen

U.S. Brand Names Aleve®-D Sinus & Cold [OTC]; Aleve®-D Sinus & Headache [OTC]; Sudafed® 12 Hour Pressure + Pain [OTC]

Therapeutic Category Decongestant/Analgesic

Use Temporary relief of cold, sinus, and flu symptoms (including nasal congestion, sinus congestion/pressure, headache, minor body aches and pains, and fever)

General Dosage Range Oral: *Children ≥12 years and Adults:* 1 caplet (naproxen sodium 220 mg/pseudoephedrine 120 mg) every 12 hours (maximum: 2 caplets/day)

Dosage Forms

Caplet, extended release:

Aleve®-D Sinus & Cold [OTC], Aleve®-D Sinus & Headache [OTC], Sudafed® 12 Hour Pressure + Pain [OTC]: Naproxen sodium 220 mg [equivalent to naproxen 200 mg and sodium 20 mg] and pseudoephedrine hydrochloride 120 mg

naproxen and sumatriptan *see* sumatriptan and naproxen *on page* 863
Naproxen-NA (Can) *see* naproxen *on page* 628
Naproxen-NA DF (Can) *see* naproxen *on page* 628
naproxen sodium *see* naproxen *on page* 628
naproxen sodium and pseudoephedrine *see* naproxen and pseudoephedrine *on page* 629
naproxen sodium and sumatriptan *see* sumatriptan and naproxen *on page* 863
naproxen sodium and sumatriptan succinate *see* sumatriptan and naproxen *on page* 863
Naproxen Sodium DS (Can) *see* naproxen *on page* 628

naratriptan (NAR a trip tan)

Medication Safety Issues

Sound-alike/look-alike issues:

Amerge® may be confused with Altace®, Amaryl®

Synonyms naratriptan hydrochloride

U.S. Brand Names Amerge®

Canadian Brand Names Amerge®; Sandoz-Naratriptan; Teva-Naratriptan

Therapeutic Category Antimigraine Agent; Serotonin Agonist

Use Treatment of acute migraine headache with or without aura

General Dosage Range Dosage adjustment recommended in patients with hepatic or renal impairment

Oral: *Adults:* 1-2.5 mg, may repeat after 4 hours (maximum: 5 mg/day)

Dosage Forms

Tablet, oral: 1 mg, 2.5 mg

Amerge®: 1 mg, 2.5 mg

naratriptan hydrochloride *see* naratriptan *on page* 629
Narcan *see* naloxone *on page* 626

Nardil® *see* phenelzine *on page 712*
Naropin® *see* ropivacaine *on page 810*
Nasacort® AQ *see* triamcinolone (nasal) *on page 915*
NasalCrom® [OTC] *see* cromolyn (nasal) *on page 241*
Nasalide® (Can) *see* flunisolide (nasal) *on page 391*
Nascobal® *see* cyanocobalamin *on page 242*
nasohist™ [OTC] *see* chlorpheniramine and phenylephrine *on page 200*
nasohist™ DM pediatric [OTC] *see* chlorpheniramine, phenylephrine, and dextromethorphan *on page 201*
Nasonex® *see* mometasone (nasal) *on page 610*
Natacyn® *see* natamycin *on page 630*
NataFort® [OTC] *see* vitamins (multiple/prenatal) *on page 952*

natalizumab (na ta LIZ u mab)

Synonyms AN100226; anti-4 alpha integrin; IgG4-kappa monoclonal antibody
U.S. Brand Names Tysabri®
Canadian Brand Names Tysabri®
Therapeutic Category Monoclonal Antibody, Selective Adhesion-Molecule Inhibitor
Use Monotherapy for the treatment of relapsing forms of multiple sclerosis; treatment of moderately- to severely-active Crohn disease

Canada labeling: Treatment of relapsing forms of multiple sclerosis

General Dosage Range I.V.: *Adults:* 300 mg every 4 weeks
Dosage Forms
Injection, solution [preservative free]:
Tysabri®: 300 mg/15 mL (15 mL)

natamycin (na ta MYE sin)

Medication Safety Issues
Sound-alike/look-alike issues:
Natacyn® may be confused with Naprosyn®
Synonyms pimaricin
U.S. Brand Names Natacyn®
Canadian Brand Names Natacyn®
Therapeutic Category Antifungal Agent
Use Treatment of blepharitis, conjunctivitis, and keratitis caused by susceptible fungi (*Aspergillus*, *Candida*, *Cephalosporium*, *Fusarium*, and *Penicillium*)
General Dosage Range Ophthalmic: *Adults:* Initial: Instill 1 drop in conjunctival sac every 1-2 hours for 3-4 days; Maintenance: 1 drop 4-8 times/day
Dosage Forms
Suspension, ophthalmic:
Natacyn®: 5% (15 mL)

Natazia® *see* estradiol and dienogest *on page 349*

nateglinide (na te GLYE nide)

Medication Safety Issues
High alert medication:
The Institute for Safe Medication Practices (ISMP) includes this medication among its list of drug classes which have a heightened risk of causing significant patient harm when used in error.
U.S. Brand Names Starlix®
Canadian Brand Names Starlix®
Therapeutic Category Antidiabetic Agent, Oral
Use Management of type 2 diabetes mellitus (noninsulin-dependent, NIDDM) as monotherapy when hyperglycemia cannot be managed by diet and exercise alone; in combination with metformin or a thiazolidinedione to lower blood glucose in patients whose hyperglycemia cannot be controlled by exercise, diet, or a single agent alone
General Dosage Range Oral: *Adults:* 60-120 mg 3 times/day

Dosage Forms

Tablet, oral: 60 mg, 120 mg

Starlix®: 60 mg, 120 mg

Natrecor® *see* nesiritide *on page* 636
natriuretic peptide *see* nesiritide *on page* 636
Natroba™ *see* spinosad *on page* 852
NatrOVA *see* spinosad *on page* 852
Natulan® (Can) *see* procarbazine *on page* 760
Natural Balance Tears [OTC] *see* hydroxypropyl methylcellulose *on page* 463
Natural Fiber Therapy [OTC] *see* psyllium *on page* 774
Natural Fiber Therapy Smooth Texture [OTC] *see* psyllium *on page* 774
natural lung surfactant *see* beractant *on page* 128
Nature's Tears [OTC] *see* hydroxypropyl methylcellulose *on page* 463
Nature-Throid™ *see* thyroid, desiccated *on page* 893
Nausea Relief [OTC] *see* fructose, dextrose, and phosphoric acid *on page* 411
Nauseatol [OTC] (Can) *see* dimenhydrinate *on page* 289
Nausetrol® [OTC] *see* fructose, dextrose, and phosphoric acid *on page* 411
Navane® [DSC] *see* thiothixene *on page* 892
Navane® (Can) *see* thiothixene *on page* 892
Navelbine® *see* vinorelbine *on page* 947
Na-Zone® [OTC] *see* sodium chloride *on page* 840
N-carbamoyl-L-glutamic acid *see* carglumic acid *on page* 177
N-carbamylglutamate *see* carglumic acid *on page* 177
***n*-docosanol** *see* docosanol *on page* 304

nebivolol (ne BIV oh lole)

Synonyms nebivolol hydrochloride

U.S. Brand Names Bystolic®

Therapeutic Category Beta-Blocker, Beta-1 Selective

Use Treatment of hypertension, alone or in combination with other agents

General Dosage Range Dosage adjustment recommended in patients with hepatic or renal impairment

Oral: *Adults:* Initial: 5 mg once daily; Maintenance: 5-40 mg once daily

Dosage Forms

Tablet, oral:

Bystolic®: 2.5 mg, 5 mg, 10 mg, 20 mg

nebivolol hydrochloride *see* nebivolol *on page* 631
Nebupent® *see* pentamidine *on page* 704
NebuSal™ *see* sodium chloride *on page* 840
Necon® 0.5/35 *see* ethinyl estradiol and norethindrone *on page* 359
Necon® 1/35 *see* ethinyl estradiol and norethindrone *on page* 359
Necon® 1/50 *see* norethindrone and mestranol *on page* 649
Necon® 7/7/7 *see* ethinyl estradiol and norethindrone *on page* 359
Necon® 10/11 *see* ethinyl estradiol and norethindrone *on page* 359

nedocromil (ne doe KROE mil)

Synonyms nedocromil sodium

U.S. Brand Names Alocril®

Canadian Brand Names Alocril®

Therapeutic Category Mast Cell Stabilizer

Use Treatment of itching associated with allergic conjunctivitis

General Dosage Range

Ophthalmic: *Children ≥3 years and Adults:* 1-2 drops in each eye twice daily

Dosage Forms

Solution, ophthalmic:

Alocril®: 2% (5 mL)

nedocromil sodium *see* nedocromil *on page* 631

Néevo® *see* vitamins (multiple/prenatal) *on page* 952

Néevo® DHA *see* vitamins (multiple/prenatal) *on page* 952

nefazodone (nef AY zoe done)

Medication Safety Issues

Sound-alike/look-alike issues:

Serzone® may be confused with selegiline, SEROquel®, sertraline

Synonyms nefazodone hydrochloride; Serzone

Therapeutic Category Antidepressant, Miscellaneous

Use Treatment of depression

General Dosage Range Oral:

Adults: Initial: 200 mg/day in 2 divided doses; Maintenance: 300-600 mg/day in 2 divided doses

Elderly: Initial: 50 mg twice daily; Maintenance: 200-400 mg/day in 2 divided doses

Dosage Forms

Tablet, oral: 50 mg, 100 mg, 150 mg, 200 mg, 250 mg

nefazodone hydrochloride *see* nefazodone *on page* 632

nelarabine (nel AY re been)

Medication Safety Issues

Sound-alike/look-alike issues:

Nelarabine may be confused with clofarabine

High alert medication:

This medication is in a class the Institute for Safe Medication Practices (ISMP) includes among its list of drug classes which have a heightened risk of causing significant patient harm when used in error.

Synonyms 2-amino-6-methoxypurine arabinoside; 506U78; GW506U78

U.S. Brand Names Arranon®

Canadian Brand Names Atriance™

Therapeutic Category Antineoplastic Agent, Antimetabolite

Use Treatment of relapsed or refractory T-cell acute lymphoblastic leukemia (ALL) and T-cell lymphoblastic lymphoma

General Dosage Range I.V.:

Children: 650 mg/m^2/dose on days 1 through 5; repeat every 21 days

Adults: 1500 mg/m^2/dose on days 1, 3, and 5; repeat every 21 days

Dosage Forms

Injection, solution:

Arranon®: 5 mg/mL (50 mL)

Dosage Forms - Canada

Injection, solution:

Atriance™: 5 mg/mL (50 mL)

nelfinavir (nel FIN a veer)

Medication Safety Issues

Sound-alike/look-alike issues:

Nelfinavir may be confused with nevirapine

Viracept® may be confused with Viramune®, Viramune® XR™

Synonyms NFV

U.S. Brand Names Viracept®

Canadian Brand Names Viracept®

Therapeutic Category Antiviral Agent

Use In combination with other antiretroviral therapy in the treatment of HIV infection

General Dosage Range Oral:

Children 2-13 years: 45-55 mg/kg twice daily **or** 25-35 mg/kg 3 times/day (maximum: 2500 mg/day)

Adults: 750 mg 3 times/day **or** 1250 mg twice daily

Dosage Forms

Tablet, oral:

Viracept®: 250 mg, 625 mg

Nembutal® *see* pentobarbital *on page 706*

Nembutal® Sodium (Can) *see* pentobarbital *on page 706*

Neo DM *see* brompheniramine, pseudoephedrine, and dextromethorphan *on page 144*

Neo DM [OTC] *see* chlorpheniramine, phenylephrine, and dextromethorphan *on page 201*

Neo-Fradin™ [DSC] *see* neomycin *on page 633*

Neofrin *see* phenylephrine (ophthalmic) *on page 716*

neomycin (nee oh MYE sin)

Synonyms neomycin sulfate

U.S. Brand Names Neo-Fradin™ [DSC]

Therapeutic Category Aminoglycoside (Antibiotic); Antibiotic, Topical

Use Orally to prepare GI tract for surgery; treatment of diarrhea caused by *E. coli*; adjunct in the treatment of hepatic encephalopathy

General Dosage Range Oral:

Children: Encephalopathy: 50-100 mg/kg/day divided every 6-8 hours **or** 2.5-7 g/m^2/day divided every 4-6 hours (maximum: 12 g/day); Preoperative GI preparation: 75-90 mg/kg/day

Adults: Encephalopathy/hepatic insufficiency: 500 mg to 12 g/day in divided doses every 4-8 hours; Preoperative GI preparation: 1 g for 3-9 doses

Dosage Forms

Tablet, oral: 500 mg

neomycin and polymyxin B (nee oh MYE sin & pol i MIKS in bee)

Synonyms polymyxin B and neomycin

U.S. Brand Names Neosporin® G.U. Irrigant

Canadian Brand Names Neosporin® Irrigating Solution

Therapeutic Category Antibiotic, Topical; Genitourinary Irrigant

Use Short-term as a continuous irrigant or rinse in the urinary bladder to prevent bacteriuria and gram-negative rod septicemia associated with the use of indwelling catheters

General Dosage Range Irrigation (bladder): *Children and Adults:* Add 1 mL irrigant to 1 L isotonic saline solution (maximum: Usually no more than 1 L irrigant/day)

Dosage Forms

Solution, irrigation: Neomycin 40 mg and polymyxin B sulfate 200,000 units per 1 mL (1 mL, 20 mL)

Neosporin® G.U. Irrigant: Neomycin 40 mg and polymyxin sulfate B 200,000 units per 1 mL (1 mL, 20 mL)

neomycin, bacitracin, and polymyxin B *see* bacitracin, neomycin, and polymyxin B *on page 111*

neomycin, bacitracin, polymyxin B, and hydrocortisone *see* bacitracin, neomycin, polymyxin B, and hydrocortisone *on page 112*

neomycin, bacitracin, polymyxin B, and pramoxine *see* bacitracin, neomycin, polymyxin B, and pramoxine *on page 112*

neomycin, colistin, hydrocortisone, and thonzonium

(nee oh MYE sin, koe LIS tin, hye droe KOR ti sone, & thon ZOE nee um)

Synonyms colistin, hydrocortisone, neomycin, and thonzonium; hydrocortisone, neomycin, colistin, and thonzonium; thonzonium, neomycin, colistin, and hydrocortisone

U.S. Brand Names Coly-Mycin® S; Cortisporin®-TC

Therapeutic Category Antibiotic/Corticosteroid, Otic

Use Treatment of superficial and susceptible bacterial infections of the external auditory canal; for treatment of susceptible bacterial infections of mastoidectomy and fenestration cavities

General Dosage Range Otic:

Children: 3-4 drops in affected ear 3-4 times/day

Adults: 4-5 drops in affected ear 3-4 times/day

Dosage Forms

Suspension, otic [drops]:

Coly-Mycin® S: Neomycin 0.33%, colistin 0.3%, hydrocortisone 1%, and thonzonium 0.05% (5 mL)

Cortisporin®-TC: Neomycin 0.33%, colistin 0.3%, hydrocortisone 1%, and thonzonium 0.05% (10 mL)

neomycin, polymyxin B, and dexamethasone

(nee oh MYE sin, pol i MIKS in bee, & deks a METH a sone)

Synonyms dexamethasone, neomycin, and polymyxin B; polymyxin B, neomycin, and dexamethasone

U.S. Brand Names Maxitrol®

Canadian Brand Names Dioptrol®; Maxitrol®

Therapeutic Category Antibiotic/Corticosteroid, Ophthalmic

Use Steroid-responsive inflammatory ocular conditions in which a corticosteroid is indicated and where bacterial infection or a risk of bacterial infection exists

General Dosage Range Ophthalmic:

Ointment: *Adults:* Place ~1/2" ribbon in the conjunctival sac of the affected eye(s) 3-4 times/day or at bedtime as an adjunct with suspension

Suspension: *Children ≥2 years and Adults:* Instill 1-2 drops in the conjunctival sac of the affected eye(s) 4-6 times/day

Dosage Forms

Ointment, ophthalmic: Neomycin 3.5 mg, polymyxin B 10,000 units, and dexamethasone 0.1% per g (3.5 g)

Maxitrol®: Neomycin 3.5 mg, polymyxin B 10,000 units, and dexamethasone 0.1% per g (3.5 g)

Suspension, ophthalmic: Neomycin 3.5 mg, polymyxin B 10,000 units, and dexamethasone 0.1% per 1 mL (5 mL)

Maxitrol®: Neomycin 3.5 mg, polymyxin B10,000 units, and dexamethasone 0.1% per 1 mL (5 mL)

neomycin, polymyxin B, and gramicidin

(nee oh MYE sin, pol i MIKS in bee, & gram i SYE din)

Synonyms gramicidin, neomycin, and polymyxin B; polymyxin B, neomycin, and gramicidin

U.S. Brand Names Neosporin® Ophthalmic Solution

Canadian Brand Names Neosporin®; Optimyxin Plus®

Therapeutic Category Antibiotic, Ophthalmic

Use Treatment of superficial ocular infection

General Dosage Range Ophthalmic: *Children and Adults:* Instill 1-2 drops 4-6 times/day

Dosage Forms

Solution, ophthalmic [drops]: Neomycin 1.75 mg, polymyxin B 10,000 units, and gramicidin 0.025 mg per 1 mL (10 mL)

Neosporin® Ophthalmic Solution: Neomycin 1.75 mg, polymyxin B 10,000 units, and gramicidin 0.025 mg per 1 mL (10 mL)

neomycin, polymyxin B, and hydrocortisone

(nee oh MYE sin, pol i MIKS in bee, & hye droe KOR ti sone)

Synonyms hydrocortisone, neomycin, and polymyxin B; polymyxin B, neomycin, and hydrocortisone

U.S. Brand Names Cortisporin®; Cortomycin

Canadian Brand Names Cortimyxin®; Cortisporin® Otic

Therapeutic Category Antibiotic/Corticosteroid, Ophthalmic; Antibiotic/Corticosteroid, Otic; Antibiotic/Corticosteroid, Topical

Use Steroid-responsive inflammatory condition for which a corticosteroid is indicated and where bacterial infection or a risk of bacterial infection exists

General Dosage Range

Ophthalmic: *Adults:* Instill 1-2 drops every 3-4 hours, or more frequently

Otic:

Children ≥2 years: Instill 3 drops into affected ear 3-4 times/day

Children ≥12 years and Adults: Instill 4 drops into affected ear 3-4 times/day

Topical: *Adults:* Apply a thin layer 1-4 times/day

Dosage Forms

Cream, topical:

Cortisporin®: Neomycin 3.5 mg, polymyxin B 10,000 units, and hydrocortisone 5 mg per g (7.5 g)

Solution, otic: Neomycin 3.5 mg, polymyxin B 10,000 units, and hydrocortisone 10 mg per mL (10 mL)

Cortisporin®, Cortomycin: Neomycin 3.5 mg, polymyxin B 10,000 units, and hydrocortisone 10 mg per mL (10 mL)

Suspension, ophthalmic [drops]: Neomycin 3.5 mg, polymyxin B 10,000 units, and hydrocortisone 10 mg per mL (7.5 mL)

Suspension, otic: Neomycin 3.5 mg, polymyxin B 10,000 units, and hydrocortisone 10 mg per mL (10 mL)

Cortomycin: Neomycin 3.5 mg, polymyxin B 10,000 units, and hydrocortisone 10 mg per mL (10 mL)

neomycin sulfate *see* neomycin *on page 633*

neonatal trace metals *see* trace elements *on page 908*

Neo-Polycin™ *see* bacitracin, neomycin, and polymyxin B *on page 111*

Neo-Polycin™ HC *see* bacitracin, neomycin, polymyxin B, and hydrocortisone *on page 112*

NeoProfen® *see* ibuprofen *on page 468*

Neoral® *see* cyclosporine (systemic) *on page 245*

Neosalus® *see* emollients *on page 328*

neosar *see* cyclophosphamide *on page 244*

Neosporin® (Can) *see* neomycin, polymyxin B, and gramicidin *on page 634*

Neosporin® AF [OTC] *see* miconazole (topical) *on page 599*

Neosporin® G.U. Irrigant *see* neomycin and polymyxin B *on page 633*

Neosporin® Irrigating Solution (Can) *see* neomycin and polymyxin B *on page 633*

Neosporin® Neo To Go® [OTC] *see* bacitracin, neomycin, and polymyxin B *on page 111*

Neosporin® Ophthalmic Solution *see* neomycin, polymyxin B, and gramicidin *on page 634*

Neosporin® + Pain Relief Ointment [OTC] *see* bacitracin, neomycin, polymyxin B, and pramoxine *on page 112*

Neosporin® Topical [OTC] *see* bacitracin, neomycin, and polymyxin B *on page 111*

neostigmine (nee oh STIG meen)

Medication Safety Issues

Sound-alike/look-alike issues:

Prostigmin® may be confused with physostigmine

Synonyms neostigmine bromide; neostigmine methylsulfate

U.S. Brand Names Prostigmin®

Canadian Brand Names Prostigmin®

Therapeutic Category Cholinergic Agent

Use Reversal of the effects of nondepolarizing neuromuscular-blocking agents; treatment of myasthenia gravis; prevention and treatment of postoperative bladder distention and urinary retention

General Dosage Range Dosage adjustment recommended in patients with renal impairment

I.M., SubQ:

Children: Myasthenia gravis: Diagnosis: 0.04 mg/kg as a single I.M. dose; Treatment: 0.01-0.04 mg/kg every 2-4 hours

Adults:

Bladder atony: Prevention: 0.25 mg every 4-6 hours; Treatment: 0.5-1 mg every 3 hours for 5 doses after bladder emptied

Myasthenia gravis: Diagnosis: 0.02 mg/kg as a single I.M. dose; Treatment: 0.5-2.5 mg every 1-3 hours (maximum: 10 mg/day)

I.V.:

Infants: 0.025-0.1 mg/kg/dose

Children: 0.01-0.04 mg/kg every 2-4 hours **or** 0.025-0.08 mg/kg/dose

Adults: 0.5-2.5 mg every 1-3 hours (maximum: 10 mg/day) **or** 0.5-2.5 mg as a single dose (maximum dose: 5 mg)

Oral:

Children: 2 mg/kg/day divided every 3-4 hours

Adults: 15 mg/dose every 3-4 hours (maximum: 375 mg/day)

Dosage Forms

Injection, solution: 0.5 mg/mL (1 mL, 10 mL); 1 mg/mL (10 mL)

Tablet, oral:

Prostigmin®: 15 mg

neostigmine bromide *see* neostigmine *on page* 635
neostigmine methylsulfate *see* neostigmine *on page* 635
NeoStrata® HQ (Can) *see* hydroquinone *on page* 461
NeoStrata® HQ Skin Lightening [OTC] *see* hydroquinone *on page* 461
Neo-Synephrine® (Can) *see* phenylephrine (nasal) *on page* 716
Neo-Synephrine® Extra Strength [OTC] *see* phenylephrine (nasal) *on page* 716
Neo-Synephrine® Mild Formula [OTC] *see* phenylephrine (nasal) *on page* 716
Neo-Synephrine® Nighttime12-Hour [OTC] *see* oxymetazoline (nasal) *on page* 681
Neo-Synephrine® Regular Strength [OTC] *see* phenylephrine (nasal) *on page* 716

nepafenac (ne pa FEN ak)

U.S. Brand Names Nevanac®

Canadian Brand Names Nevanac®

Therapeutic Category Nonsteroidal Antiinflammatory Drug (NSAID), Ophthalmic

Use Treatment of pain and inflammation associated with cataract surgery

General Dosage Range Ophthalmic: *Children ≥10 years and Adults:* Instill 1 drop into affected eye(s) 3 times/day

Dosage Forms

Suspension, ophthalmic:

Nevanac®: 0.1% (3 mL)

NephrAmine® *see* amino acid injection *on page* 61
Nephro-Calci® [OTC] *see* calcium carbonate *on page* 161
Neptazane™ *see* methazolamide *on page* 582
nerve agent antidote kit *see* atropine and pralidoxime *on page* 103
Nesacaine® *see* chloroprocaine *on page* 198
Nesacaine®-CE (Can) *see* chloroprocaine *on page* 198
Nesacaine®-MPF *see* chloroprocaine *on page* 198

nesiritide (ni SIR i tide)

Medication Safety Issues

High alert medication:

The Institute for Safe Medication Practices (ISMP) includes this medication among its list of drugs which have a heightened risk of causing significant patient harm when used in error.

International issues:

Natrecor [U.S., Canada, Argentina, Venezuela] may be confused with Nitrocor brand name for nitroglycerin [Italy, Russia, Venezuela]

Synonyms B-type natriuretic peptide (human); hBNP; natriuretic peptide

U.S. Brand Names Natrecor®

Canadian Brand Names Natrecor®

Therapeutic Category Natriuretic Peptide, B-type, Human; Vasodilator

Use Treatment of acutely decompensated heart failure (HF) with dyspnea at rest or with minimal activity

General Dosage Range I.V.: *Adults:* Bolus: 2 mcg/kg; Infusion: Initial: 0.01 mcg/kg/minute (maximum: 0.03 mcg/kg/minute)

Dosage Forms

Injection, powder for reconstitution:

Natrecor®: 1.5 mg

NESP *see* darbepoetin alfa *on page* 254
Neulasta® *see* pegfilgrastim *on page* 696
Neuleptil® (Can) *see* periciazine *(Canada only) on page* 708
Neumega® *see* oprelvekin *on page* 670
Neuotrogena T/Gel Therapeutic Shampoo [OTC] (Can) *see* coal tar *on page* 228

Neupogen® *see* filgrastim *on page* *384*
Neupro® *see* rotigotine *on page* *813*
Neurontin® *see* gabapentin *on page* *413*
Neut® *see* sodium bicarbonate *on page* *840*
NeutraCare® *see* fluoride *on page* *393*
NeutraGard® Advanced *see* fluoride *on page* *393*
Neutrahist PDX [OTC] *see* chlorpheniramine, pseudoephedrine, and dextromethorphan *on page* *202*
Neutrahist Pediatric [OTC] *see* chlorpheniramine and pseudoephedrine *on page* *200*
Neutra-Phos *see* potassium phosphate and sodium phosphate *on page* *747*
Neutra-Phos®-K [OTC] [DSC] *see* potassium phosphate *on page* *746*
NeutraSal® *see* saliva substitute *on page* *819*
Neutrogena® Acne Stress Control [OTC] *see* salicylic acid *on page* *816*
Neutrogena® Advanced Solutions™ [OTC] *see* salicylic acid *on page* *816*
Neutrogena® Blackhead Eliminating™ [OTC] *see* salicylic acid *on page* *816*
Neutrogena® Blackhead Eliminating™ 2-in-1 Foaming Pads [OTC] *see* salicylic acid *on page* *816*
Neutrogena® Blackhead Eliminating™ Daily Scrub [OTC] *see* salicylic acid *on page* *816*
Neutrogena® Body Clear® [OTC] *see* salicylic acid *on page* *816*
Neutrogena® Clear Pore™ Oil-Controlling Astringent [OTC] *see* salicylic acid *on page* *816*
Neutrogena® Maximum Strength T/Sal® [OTC] *see* salicylic acid *on page* *816*
Neutrogena® Oil-Free Acne [OTC] *see* salicylic acid *on page* *816*
Neutrogena® Oil-Free Acne Stress Control [OTC] *see* salicylic acid *on page* *816*
Neutrogena® Oil-Free Acne Wash [OTC] *see* salicylic acid *on page* *816*
Neutrogena® Oil-Free Acne Wash 60 Second Mask Scrub [OTC] *see* salicylic acid *on page* *816*
Neutrogena® Oil-Free Acne Wash Cream Cleanser [OTC] *see* salicylic acid *on page* *816*
Neutrogena® Oil-Free Acne Wash Foam Cleanser [OTC] *see* salicylic acid *on page* *816*
Neutrogena® Oil-Free Anti-Acne [OTC] *see* salicylic acid *on page* *816*
Neutrogena® On The Spot® Acne Treatment [OTC] *see* benzoyl peroxide *on page* *124*
Neutrogena® Rapid Clear® [OTC] *see* salicylic acid *on page* *816*
Neutrogena® Rapid Clear® Acne Defense [OTC] *see* salicylic acid *on page* *816*
Neutrogena® Rapid Clear® Acne Eliminating [OTC] *see* salicylic acid *on page* *816*
Neutrogena® T/Gel® [OTC] *see* coal tar *on page* *228*
Neutrogena® T/Gel® Extra Strength [OTC] *see* coal tar *on page* *228*
Neutrogena® T/Gel® Stubborn Itch Control [OTC] *see* coal tar *on page* *228*
Nevanac® *see* nepafenac *on page* *636*

nevirapine (ne VYE ra peen)

Medication Safety Issues

Sound-alike/look-alike issues:

Nevirapine may be confused with nelfinavir
Viramune®, Viramune® XR™ may be confused with Viracept®

Synonyms NVP

U.S. Brand Names Viramune®; Viramune® XR™

Canadian Brand Names Auro-Nevirapine; Viramune®; Viramune® XR

Therapeutic Category Antiviral Agent

Use In combination therapy with other antiretroviral agents for the treatment of HIV-1

General Dosage Range Dosage adjustment recommended in patients with renal impairment and who are receiving hemodialysis.

Oral, immediate release:

Infants and Children <8 years: Initial: 150-200 mg/m^2/dose once daily (maximum: 200 mg/day); Maintenance: 150-200 mg/m^2/dose twice daily (maximum: 400 mg/day).

Children ≥8 years: Initial: 120-150 mg/m^2/dose once daily (maximum: 200 mg/day); Maintenance: 120-150 mg/m^2/dose twice daily (maximum: 400 mg/day)

Adolescents and Adults: Initial: 200 mg once daily; Maintenance: 200 mg twice daily

Oral, extended release: *Adults:* Maintenance: 400 mg once daily

Dosage Forms

Suspension, oral: 50 mg/5 mL (240 mL)
Viramune®: 50 mg/5 mL (240 mL)

Tablet, oral: 200 mg
Viramune®: 200 mg

Tablet, extended release, oral:
Viramune® XR™: 400 mg

NexAVAR® *see* sorafenib *on page* 850
Nexavar® (Can) *see* sorafenib *on page* 850
Nexiclon™ XR *see* clonidine *on page* 224
NexIUM® *see* esomeprazole *on page* 346
Nexium® (Can) *see* esomeprazole *on page* 346
NexIUM® I.V. *see* esomeprazole *on page* 346
Nexplanon® *see* etonogestrel *on page* 366
Next Choice® *see* levonorgestrel *on page* 533
Next Choice™ One Dose *see* levonorgestrel *on page* 533
Nexterone® *see* amiodarone *on page* 63
NFV *see* nelfinavir *on page* 632
NGX-4010 *see* capsaicin *on page* 170

niacin (NYE a sin)

Medication Safety Issues

Sound-alike/look-alike issues:
Niacin may be confused with Minocin®, niacinamide, Niaspan®

Synonyms nicotinic acid; vitamin B_3

U.S. Brand Names Niacin-Time® [OTC]; Niacor®; Niaspan®; Slo-Niacin® [OTC]

Canadian Brand Names Niaspan®; Niaspan® FCT; Niodan

Therapeutic Category Vitamin, Water Soluble

Use Treatment of dyslipidemias (Fredrickson types IIa and IIb or primary hypercholesterolemia) as mono- or adjunctive therapy; to lower the risk of recurrent MI in patients with a history of MI and hyperlipidemia; to slow progression or promote regression of coronary artery disease; treatment of hypertriglyceridemia in patients at risk of pancreatitis; dietary supplement

General Dosage Range Oral:
Extended release: *Adults:* 500 mg to 2 g once daily
Regular release: *Adults:* 100-250 mg/day in 1-2 divided doses **or** 1.5-6 g/day in 2-3 divided doses (maximum dose: 6 g/day in 3 divided doses)
Sustained release: *Adults:* Usual: 1-2 g/day

Dosage Forms

Caplet, timed release, oral: 500 mg
Capsule, oral: 50 mg, 250 mg
Capsule, extended release, oral: 250 mg, 500 mg
Capsule, timed release, oral: 250 mg, 400 mg, 500 mg
Tablet, oral: 50 mg, 100 mg, 250 mg, 500 mg
Niacor®: 500 mg
Tablet, controlled release, oral:
Slo-Niacin® [OTC]: 250 mg, 500 mg, 750 mg
Tablet, extended release, oral:
Niaspan®: 500 mg, 750 mg, 1000 mg
Tablet, timed release, oral: 250 mg, 500 mg, 750 mg, 1000 mg
Niacin-Time® [OTC]: 500 mg

niacinamide (nye a SIN a mide)

Medication Safety Issues

Sound-alike/look-alike issues:
Niacinamide may be confused with niacin, niCARdipine

Synonyms Nicomide-T; nicotinamide; nicotinic acid amide; vitamin B_3

Therapeutic Category Vitamin, Water Soluble

Use Dietary supplement

General Dosage Range Oral:
Children: 10-50 mg every 6 hours
Adults: Initial: 100 mg every 6 hours; Maintenance: 50 mg every 8-12 hours

Dosage Forms
Tablet, oral: 100 mg, 250 mg, 500 mg

niacin and lovastatin (NYE a sin & LOE va sta tin)

Medication Safety Issues
Sound-alike/look-alike issues:
Advicor® may be confused with Adcirca®, Advair®

Synonyms lovastatin and niacin

U.S. Brand Names Advicor®

Canadian Brand Names Advicor®

Therapeutic Category HMG-CoA Reductase Inhibitor; Vitamin, Water Soluble

Use For use when treatment with both extended-release niacin and lovastatin is appropriate in combination with a standard cholesterol-lowering diet:
Extended-release niacin: Adjunctive treatment of dyslipidemias (types IIa and IIb or primary hypercholesterolemia) to lower the risk of recurrent MI and/or slow progression of coronary artery disease, including combination therapy with other antidyslipidemic agents when additional triglyceride-lowering or HDL-increasing effects are desired; treatment of hypertriglyceridemia in patients at risk of pancreatitis
Lovastatin: Treatment of primary hypercholesterolemia (Frederickson types IIa and IIb); primary and secondary prevention of cardiovascular disease

General Dosage Range Oral: *Adults:* Initial: Niacin 500 mg/lovastatin 20 mg at bedtime; Maintenance: Up to niacin 2000 mg/lovastatin 40 mg at bedtime

Dosage Forms
Tablet, variable release, oral:
Advicor®: 500/20: Niacin 500 mg [extended release] and lovastatin 20 mg [immediate release]; 750/20: Niacin 750 mg [extended release] and lovastatin 20 mg [immediate release]; 1000/20: Niacin 1000 mg [extended release] and lovastatin 20 mg [immediate release]; 1000/40: Niacin 1000 mg [extended release] and lovastatin 40 mg [immediate release]

niacin and simvastatin (NYE a sin & sim va STAT in)

Synonyms simvastatin and niacin

U.S. Brand Names Simcor®

Therapeutic Category Antilipemic Agent, HMG-CoA Reductase Inhibitor; Antilipemic Agent, Miscellaneous

Use Reduce total cholesterol, LDL, Apo B, non-HDL, TG, and/or increase HDL in patients with primary hypercholesterolemia, mixed dyslipidemia, or hypertriglyceridemia in combination with standard cholesterol-lowering diet when simvastatin or niacin monotherapy is inadequate

General Dosage Range Oral: *Adults:* Niacin 500-2000 mg/simvastatin 20-40 mg once daily

Dosage Forms
Tablet, variable release, oral:
Simcor®: 500/20: Niacin 500 mg [extended release] and simvastatin 20 mg [immediate release]; 500/40: Niacin 500 mg [extended release] and simvastatin 40 mg [immediate release]; 750/20: Niacin 750 mg [extended release] and simvastatin 20 mg [immediate release]; 1000/20: Niacin 1000 mg [extended release] and simvastatin 20 mg [immediate release]; 1000/40: Niacin 1000 mg [extended release] and simvastatin 40 mg [immediate release]

Niacin-Time® [OTC] *see* niacin *on page 638*

Niacor® *see* niacin *on page 638*

Niaspan® *see* niacin *on page 638*

Niaspan® FCT (Can) *see* niacin *on page 638*

Niastase® (Can) *see* factor VIIa (recombinant) *on page 371*

Niastase® RT (Can) *see* factor VIIa (recombinant) *on page 371*

nicardipine (nye KAR de peen)

Medication Safety Issues

Sound-alike/look-alike issues:

NiCARdipine may be confused with niacinamide, NIFEdipine, niMODipine

Cardene® may be confused with Cardizem®, Cardura®, codeine

Administration issues:

Significant differences exist between oral and I.V. dosing. Use caution when converting from one route of administration to another.

International issues:

Cardene [U.S., Great Britain, Netherlands] may be confused with Cardem brand name for celiprolol [Spain]; Cardin brand name for simvastatin [Poland]

Synonyms nicardipine hydrochloride

Tall-Man ni**CAR**dipine

U.S. Brand Names Cardene® I.V.; Cardene® SR

Therapeutic Category Calcium Channel Blocker

Use Chronic stable angina (immediate-release product only); management of hypertension (immediate and sustained release products); parenteral only for short-term use when oral treatment is not feasible

General Dosage Range Dosage adjustment recommended in patients with hepatic or renal impairment

I.V.: *Adults:* Initial: 5 mg/hour; Maintenance: 3-15 mg/hour

Oral:

Immediate release: *Adults:* Initial: 20 mg 3 times/day; Maintenance: 20-40 mg 3 times/day

Sustained release: *Adults:* Initial: 30 mg twice daily; Maintenance: Up to 60 mg twice daily

Dosage Forms

Capsule, oral: 20 mg, 30 mg

Capsule, sustained release, oral:

Cardene® SR: 30 mg, 45 mg, 60 mg

Infusion, premixed iso-osmotic dextrose solution:

Cardene® I.V.: 20 mg (200 mL); 40 mg (200 mL)

Infusion, premixed iso-osmotic sodium chloride solution:

Cardene® I.V.: 20 mg (200 mL); 40 mg (200 mL)

Injection, solution: 2.5 mg/mL (10 mL)

Cardene® I.V.: 2.5 mg/mL (10 mL)

nicardipine hydrochloride *see* nicardipine *on page* 640

Nicoderm® (Can) *see* nicotine *on page* 640

NicoDerm® CQ® [OTC] *see* nicotine *on page* 640

Nicomide-T *see* niacinamide *on page* 638

Nicorelief [OTC] *see* nicotine *on page* 640

Nicorette® [OTC] *see* nicotine *on page* 640

Nicorette® (Can) *see* nicotine *on page* 640

Nicorette® Plus (Can) *see* nicotine *on page* 640

nicotinamide *see* niacinamide *on page* 638

nicotine (nik oh TEEN)

Medication Safety Issues

Sound-alike/look-alike issues:

NicoDerm® may be confused with Nitroderm

Nicorette® may be confused with Nordette®

Other safety concerns:

Transdermal patch may contain conducting metal (eg, aluminum); remove patch prior to MRI.

Synonyms Habitrol; nicotine patch

U.S. Brand Names Commit® [OTC]; NicoDerm® CQ® [OTC]; Nicorelief [OTC]; Nicorette® [OTC]; Nicotrol® Inhaler; Nicotrol® NS; Thrive™ [OTC]

Canadian Brand Names Habitrol®; Nicoderm®; Nicorette®; Nicorette® Plus; Nicotrol®

Therapeutic Category Smoking Deterrent

Use Treatment to aid smoking cessation for the relief of nicotine withdrawal symptoms (including nicotine craving)

General Dosage Range Dosage adjustment recommended for transdermal route in patients on concomitant therapy

Inhalation:

Nasal: *Adults:* 1-2 sprays/hour (maximum: 10 sprays/hour; 80 sprays/day)

Oral: *Adults:* Usually 6 to 16 cartridges per day; best effect was achieved by frequent continuous puffing (20 minutes)

Oral: *Adults:* 2 mg or 4 mg every 1-2 hours (weeks 1-6); every 2-4 hours (weeks 7-9); and every 4-8 hours (weeks 10-12) (maximum: 24 pieces gum/day; 20 lozenges/day)

Transdermal:

Patients smoking >10 cigarettes/day: Begin with **step 1** (21 mg/day) for 6 weeks, followed by **step 2** (14 mg/day) for 2 weeks; finish with **step 3** (7 mg/day) for 2 weeks

Patients smoking ≤10 cigarettes/day: Begin with **step 2** (14 mg/day) for 6 weeks, followed by **step 3** (7 mg/day) for 2 weeks

Dosage Forms

Gum, chewing, oral: 2 mg (20s, 40s, 50s, 100s, 108s, 110s); 4 mg (20s, 40s, 48s, 50s, 100s, 108s, 110s)

Nicorelief [OTC]: 2 mg (50s, 110s); 4 mg (50s, 110s)

Nicorette® [OTC]: 2 mg (40s, 48s, 50s, 100s, 108s, 110s, 168s, 170s, 192s, 200s, 216s); 4 mg (40s, 48s, 50s, 100s, 108s, 110s, 168s, 170s, 192s, 200s, 216s)

Thrive™ [OTC]: 2 mg (40s); 4 mg (40s)

Lozenge, oral:

Commit® [OTC]: 2 mg (48s, 72s); 4 mg (48s, 72s)

Nicorette® [OTC]: 4 mg (50s)

Oral inhalation system, for oral inhalation:

Nicotrol® Inhaler: 10 mg (10 mL)

Patch, transdermal: 7 mg/24 hours (7s, 14s, 30s); 14 mg/24 hours (7s, 14s, 30s); 21 mg/24 hours (7s, 14s, 30s)

NicoDerm® CQ® [OTC]: 7 mg/24 hours (14s); 14 mg/24 hours (14s); 21 mg/24 hours (7s, 14s)

Solution, intranasal:

Nicotrol® NS: 10 mg/mL (10 mL)

nicotine patch *see* nicotine *on page 640*

nicotinic acid *see* niacin *on page 638*

nicotinic acid amide *see* niacinamide *on page 638*

Nicotrol® (Can) *see* nicotine *on page 640*

Nicotrol® Inhaler *see* nicotine *on page 640*

Nicotrol® NS *see* nicotine *on page 640*

Nidagel™ (Can) *see* metronidazole (topical) *on page 597*

Nifediac CC® *see* nifedipine *on page 641*

Nifedical XL® *see* nifedipine *on page 641*

nifedipine (nye FED i peen)

Medication Safety Issues

Sound-alike/look-alike issues:

NIFEdipine may be confused with niCARdipine, niMODipine, nisoldipine

Procardia XL® may be confused with Cartia XT®

BEERS Criteria medication:

This drug may be potentially inappropriate for use in geriatric patients (Quality of evidence - high; Strength of recommendation - strong).

International issues:

Depin [India] may be confused with Depen brand name for penicillamine [U.S.]; Depon brand name for acetaminophen [Greece]; Dipen brand name for diltiazem [Greece]

Nipin [Italy and Singapore] may be confused with Nipent brand name for pentostatin [U.S., Canada, and multiple international markets]

Tall-Man NIFEdipine

U.S. Brand Names Adalat® CC; Afeditab® CR; Nifediac CC®; Nifedical XL®; Procardia XL®; Procardia®

Canadian Brand Names Adalat® XL®; Apo-Nifed PA®; Mylan-Nifedipine Extended Release; Nu-Nifed; Nu-Nifedipine-PA; PMS-Nifedipine

Therapeutic Category Calcium Channel Blocker

Use Management of chronic stable or vasospastic angina; treatment of hypertension (sustained release products only)

General Dosage Range Oral:

Immediate release: *Adults:* Initial: 10 mg 3-4 times/day (maximum: 180 mg/day)

Extended release: *Adults:* Initial: 30 mg once daily; Maintenance: 30-60 mg once daily (maximum: 120-180 mg/day)

Dosage Forms

Capsule, softgel, oral: 10 mg, 20 mg

Procardia®: 10 mg

Tablet, extended release, oral: 30 mg, 60 mg, 90 mg

Adalat® CC: 30 mg, 60 mg, 90 mg

Afeditab® CR: 30 mg, 60 mg

Nifediac CC®: 30 mg, 60 mg, 90 mg

Nifedical XL®: 30 mg, 60 mg

Procardia XL®: 30 mg, 60 mg, 90 mg

Niferex® [OTC] [DSC] *see* polysaccharide-iron complex *on page 740*

Niftolid *see* flutamide *on page 399*

Night Time Multi-Symptom Cold/Flu Relief [OTC] *see* acetaminophen, dextromethorphan, and doxylamine *on page 27*

Nilandron® *see* nilutamide *on page 642*

nilotinib (nye LOE ti nib)

Medication Safety Issues

Sound-alike/look-alike issues:

Nilotinib may be confused with dasatinib, imatinib, nilutamide, SUNItinib, vandetanib

High alert medication:

This medication is in a class the Institute for Safe Medication Practices (ISMP) includes among its list of drug classes which have a heightened risk of causing significant patient harm when used in error.

Synonyms AMN107; nilotinib hydrochloride monohydrate

U.S. Brand Names Tasigna®

Canadian Brand Names Tasigna®

Therapeutic Category Antineoplastic Agent, Tyrosine Kinase Inhibitor

Use Treatment of newly-diagnosed Philadelphia chromosome-positive chronic myelogenous leukemia (Ph+ CML) in chronic phase; treatment of chronic and accelerated phase Ph+ CML refractory or intolerant to prior therapy (including imatinib)

General Dosage Range Dosage adjustment recommended in patients with hepatic impairment, on concomitant therapy, or who develop toxicities

Oral: *Adults:* 300-400 mg twice daily

Dosage Forms

Capsule, oral:

Tasigna®: 150 mg, 200 mg

nilotinib hydrochloride monohydrate *see* nilotinib *on page 642*

nilutamide (ni LOO ta mide)

Medication Safety Issues

Sound-alike/look-alike issues:

Nilutamide may be confused with nilotinib

Synonyms RU-23908

U.S. Brand Names Nilandron®

Canadian Brand Names Anandron®

Therapeutic Category Antineoplastic Agent

Use Treatment of metastatic prostate cancer (in combination with surgical castration)

General Dosage Range Oral: *Adults:* Initial: 300 mg once daily; Maintenance: 150 mg once daily

Dosage Forms

Tablet, oral:

Nilandron®: 150 mg

Nimbex® *see* cisatracurium *on page 212*

nimodipine (nye MOE di peen)

Medication Safety Issues

Sound-alike/look-alike issues:

NiMODipine may be confused with niCARdipine, NIFEdipine, nisoldipine

Administration issues:

For oral administration only. For patients unable to swallow a capsule, the drug should be dispensed in an oral syringe (preferably amber in color) labeled **"WARNING: For ORAL use only"** or **"Not for I.V. use."** Nimodipine has inadvertently been administered I.V. when withdrawn from capsules into a syringe for subsequent nasogastric tube administration. Severe cardiovascular adverse events, including fatalities, have resulted. Employ precautions against such an event.

Tall-Man niMODipine

Canadian Brand Names Nimotop®

Therapeutic Category Calcium Channel Blocker

Use Vasospasm following subarachnoid hemorrhage from ruptured intracranial aneurysms

General Dosage Range Dosage adjustment recommended in patients with hepatic impairment

Oral: *Adults:* 60 mg every 4 hours

Dosage Forms

Capsule, liquid filled, oral: 30 mg

Capsule, softgel, oral: 30 mg

Nimotop® (Can) *see* nimodipine *on page 643*

Niodan (Can) *see* niacin *on page 638*

Nipent® *see* pentostatin *on page 707*

Nipride® (Can) *see* nitroprusside *on page 646*

Niravam™ *see* alprazolam *on page 52*

nisoldipine (nye SOL di peen)

Medication Safety Issues

Sound-alike/look-alike issues:

Nisoldipine may be confused with NIFEdipine, niMODipine

U.S. Brand Names Sular®

Therapeutic Category Calcium Channel Blocker

Use Management of hypertension, alone or in combination with other antihypertensive agents

General Dosage Range Dosage adjustment recommended in patients with hepatic impairment

Oral:

Adults:

Sular® (Geomatrix® delivery system): Initial: 17 mg once daily; Maintenance: 17-34 mg once daily (maximum: 34 mg/day)

Nisoldipine extended-release (original formulation): Initial: 20 mg once daily; Maintenance: 10-40 mg once daily (maximum: 60 mg/day)

Elderly: Sular® (Geomatrix® delivery system): Initial: 8.5 mg once daily; Nisoldipine extended-release (original formulation): Initial: 10 mg once daily

Dosage Forms

Tablet, extended release, oral: 8.5 mg, 17 mg, 20 mg, 25.5 mg, 30 mg, 34 mg, 40 mg

Sular®: 8.5 mg, 17 mg, 34 mg

nitalapram *see* citalopram *on page 213*

nitazoxanide (nye ta ZOX a nide)

Synonyms NTZ

U.S. Brand Names Alinia®

Therapeutic Category Antiprotozoal

Use Treatment of diarrhea caused by *Cryptosporidium parvum* or *Giardia lamblia*

General Dosage Range Oral:

Children 1-3 years: 100 mg every 12 hours

Children 4-11 years: 200 mg every 12 hours

Children ≥12 years and Adults: 500 mg every 12 hours

Dosage Forms

Powder for suspension, oral:

Alinia®: 100 mg/5 mL (60 mL)

Tablet, oral:

Alinia®: 500 mg

Nithiodote™ *see* sodium nitrite and sodium thiosulfate *on page* 843

nitisinone (ni TIS i known)

Synonyms NTBC

U.S. Brand Names Orfadin®

Therapeutic Category 4-Hydroxyphenylpyruvate Dioxygenase Inhibitor

Use Treatment of hereditary tyrosinemia type 1 (HT-1) as an adjunct to dietary restriction of tyrosine and phenylalanine

General Dosage Range Oral: *Infants, Children, and Adults:* 1-2 mg/kg/day in 2 divided doses

Dosage Forms

Capsule, oral:

Orfadin®: 2 mg, 5 mg, 10 mg

Nitoman™ (Can) *see* tetrabenazine *on page* 883

Nitrazadon® (Can) *see* nitrazepam *(Canada only) on page* 644

nitrazepam *(Canada only)* (nye TRA ze pam)

Synonyms nitrozepamum

Canadian Brand Names Apo-Nitrazepam®; Mogadon; Nitrazadon®; Sandoz-Nitrazepam

Therapeutic Category Benzodiazepine

Controlled Substance CDSA IV

Use Short-term management of insomnia; treatment of myoclonic seizures

General Dosage Range Oral:

Children ≤30 kg: 0.3-1 mg/kg/day in 3 divided doses

Adults: 5-10 mg once daily

Elderly: 2.5-5 mg once daily

Product Availability Not available in U.S.

Dosage Forms - Canada

Tablet, oral:

Apo-Nitrazepam®, Mogadon, Nitrazadon, Nitrazepam (Pro-Doc), Sandoz-Nitrazepam: 5 mg, 10 mg

nitric oxide (NYE trik OKS ide)

U.S. Brand Names INOmax®

Canadian Brand Names INOmax®

Therapeutic Category Vasodilator, Pulmonary

Use Treatment of term and near-term (>34 weeks) neonates with hypoxic respiratory failure associated with pulmonary hypertension; used concurrently with ventilatory support and other agents

General Dosage Range Inhalation: *Neonates (up to 14 days old):* 20 ppm

Dosage Forms

Gas, for inhalation:

INOmax®: 100 ppm (353 L, 1963 L); 800 ppm (353 L, 1963 L)

Nitro-Bid® *see* nitroglycerin *on page* 645

Nitro-Dur® *see* nitroglycerin *on page* 645

nitrofurantoin (nye troe fyoor AN toyn)

Medication Safety Issues

Sound alike/look alike issues:

Macrobid® may be confused with microK®, Nitro-Bid®

Nitrofurantoin may be confused with Neurontin®, nitroglycerin

BEERS Criteria medication:

This drug may be potentially inappropriate for use in geriatric patients (Quality of evidence - moderate; Strength of recommendation - strong).

U.S. Brand Names Furadantin®; Macrobid®; Macrodantin®

Canadian Brand Names Apo-Nitrofurantoin®; Macrobid®; Macrodantin®; Novo-Furantoin; Teva-Nitrofurantoin

Therapeutic Category Antibiotic, Miscellaneous

Use Prevention and treatment of urinary tract infections caused by susceptible strains of *E. coli, S. aureus, Enterococcus, Klebsiella,* and *Enterobacter*

General Dosage Range Oral:

Children >1 month: Furadantin®, Macrodantin®: 5-7 mg/kg/day divided every 6 hours (maximum: 400 mg/day) **or** 1-2 mg/kg/day divided every 12-24 hours (maximum: 100 mg/day)

Children >12 years: Macrobid®: 100 mg twice daily

Adults: Furadantin®, Macrodantin®: 50-100 mg every 6 hours **or** once daily; Macrobid®: 100 mg twice daily

Dosage Forms

Capsule, oral: 50 mg, 100 mg

Macrobid®: 100 mg

Macrodantin®: 25 mg, 50 mg, 100 mg

Suspension, oral: 25 mg/5 mL (230 mL)

Furadantin®: 25 mg/5 mL (230 mL)

nitrogen mustard *see* mechlorethamine *on page 566*

nitroglycerin (nye troe GLI ser in)

Medication Safety Issues

Sound-alike/look-alike issues:

Nitroglycerin may be confused with nitrofurantoin, nitroprusside

Nitro-Bid® may be confused with Macrobid®

Nitroderm may be confused with NicoDerm®

Nitrol may be confused with Nizoral®

Nitrostat® may be confused with Nilstat, nystatin

Other safety concerns:

Transdermal patch may contain conducting metal (eg, aluminum); remove patch prior to MRI.

International issues:

Nitrocor [Italy, Russia, and Venezuela] may be confused with Natrecor brand name for nesiritide [U.S., Canada, and multiple international markets]; Nutracort brand name for hydrocortisone in the [U.S. and multiple international markets]; Nitro-Dur [U.S., Canada, and multiple international markets]

Synonyms glyceryl trinitrate; nitroglycerol; NTG; Tridil

U.S. Brand Names Minitran™; Nitro-Bid®; Nitro-Dur®; Nitro-Time®; Nitrolingual®; NitroMist®; Nitrostat®; Rectiv™

Canadian Brand Names Minitran™; Mylan-Nitro Sublingual Spray; Nitro-Dur®; Nitroglycerin Injection, USP; Nitrol®; Nitrostat®; Rho®-Nitro Pump Spray; Transderm-Nitro®; Trinipatch®

Therapeutic Category Vasodilator

Use Treatment or prevention of angina pectoris

Intravenous (I.V.) administration: Treatment or prevention of angina pectoris; acute decompensated heart failure (especially when associated with acute myocardial infarction); perioperative hypertension (especially during cardiovascular surgery); induction of intraoperative hypotension

Intra-anal administration (Rectiv™ ointment): Treatment of moderate-to-severe pain associated with chronic anal fissure

General Dosage Range

I.V.: *Adults:* Initial: 5 mcg/minute; Maintenance: 20-200 mcg/minute (maximum: 400 mcg/minute)

Intra-anal: *Adults:* 1 inch every 12 hours

Oral: *Adults:* 2.5-6.5 mg 3-4 times/day; Maintenance: Up to 26 mg 4 times/day

Sublingual: *Adults:* 0.3-0.6 mg every 5 minutes for maximum of 3 doses in 15 minutes **or** 5-10 minutes prior to activities which may provoke an attack

Topical: *Adults:*

Ointment: Apply 0.5" to 2" every 6 hours with a daily nitrate-free interval of ~10-12 hours

Patch: Initial: 0.2-0.4 mg/hour for 12-14 hours/day; Maintenance: 0.2-0.8 mg/hour for 12-14 hours

Translingual: *Adults:* 1-2 sprays under tongue every 3-5 minutes for maximum of 3 doses in 15 minutes **or** 5-10 minutes prior to activities which may provoke an attack

Dosage Forms

Aerosol, spray, translingual:
NitroMist®: 0.4 mg/spray (8.5 g)

Capsule, extended release, oral: 2.5 mg, 6.5 mg, 9 mg
Nitro-Time®: 2.5 mg, 6.5 mg, 9 mg

Infusion, premixed in D_5W: 25 mg (250 mL); 50 mg (250 mL, 500 mL); 100 mg (250 mL)

Injection, solution: 5 mg/mL (5 mL, 10 mL)

Ointment, rectal:
Rectiv™: 0.4% (30 g)

Ointment, topical:
Nitro-Bid®: 2% (1 g, 30 g, 60 g)

Patch, transdermal: 0.1 mg/hr (30s); 0.2 mg/hr (30s); 0.4 mg/hr (30s); 0.6 mg/hr (30s)
Minitran™: 0.1 mg/hr (30s); 0.2 mg/hr (30s); 0.4 mg/hr (30s); 0.6 mg/hr (30s)
Nitro-Dur®: 0.1 mg/hr (30s); 0.2 mg/hr (30s); 0.3 mg/hr (30s); 0.4 mg/hr (30s); 0.6 mg/hr (30s); 0.8 mg/hr (30s)

Solution, translingual: 0.4 mg/spray (4.9 g, 12 g)
Nitrolingual®: 0.4 mg/spray (4.9 g, 12 g)

Tablet, sublingual:
Nitrostat®: 0.3 mg, 0.4 mg, 0.6 mg

Nitroglycerin Injection, USP (Can) *see* nitroglycerin *on page* 645
nitroglycerol *see* nitroglycerin *on page* 645
Nitrol® (Can) *see* nitroglycerin *on page* 645
Nitrolingual® *see* nitroglycerin *on page* 645
NitroMist® *see* nitroglycerin *on page* 645
Nitropress® *see* nitroprusside *on page* 646

nitroprusside (nye troe PRUS ide)

Medication Safety Issues

Sound-alike/look-alike issues:
Nitroprusside may be confused with nitroglycerin

High alert medication:
The Institute for Safe Medication Practices (ISMP) includes this medication among its list of drugs which have a heightened risk of causing significant patient harm when used in error.

Synonyms nitroprusside sodium; sodium nitroferricyanide; sodium nitroprusside

U.S. Brand Names Nitropress®

Canadian Brand Names Nipride®

Therapeutic Category Vasodilator

Use Management of hypertensive crises; acute decompensated heart failure (HF); used for controlled hypotension to reduce bleeding during surgery

General Dosage Range I.V.: *Children and Adults:* Initial: 0.3 mcg/kg/minute; Usual dose: 3 mcg/kg/minute (maximum: 10 mcg/kg/minute)

Dosage Forms

Injection, solution:
Nitropress®: 25 mg/mL (2 mL)

nitroprusside sodium *see* nitroprusside *on page* 646
Nitrostat® *see* nitroglycerin *on page* 645
Nitro-Time® *see* nitroglycerin *on page* 645
4′-nitro-3′-trifluoromethylisobutyrantide *see* flutamide *on page* 399

nitrous oxide (NYE trus OKS ide)

Medication Safety Issues

High alert medication:
The Institute for Safe Medication Practices (ISMP) includes this medication among its list of drug classes which have a heightened risk of causing significant patient harm when used in error.

Therapeutic Category Anesthetic, Gas

Use Sedation, analgesia, and amnesia; principal adjunct to inhalation and intravenous general anesthesia

General Dosage Range Inhalation: *Children and Adults:* Dental: Concentrations of 25% to 50%; Surgical: Concentrations of 25% to 70%

Dosage Forms

Supplied in blue cylinders

nitrozepamum *see* nitrazepam *(Canada only) on page 644*

Nix® (Can) *see* permethrin *on page 709*

Nix® Complete Lice Treatment System [OTC] *see* permethrin *on page 709*

Nix® Creme Rinse [OTC] *see* permethrin *on page 709*

Nix® Creme Rinse Lice Treatment [OTC] *see* permethrin *on page 709*

Nix® Lice Control Spray [OTC] *see* permethrin *on page 709*

nizatidine (ni ZA ti deen)

Medication Safety Issues

Sound-alike/look-alike issues:

Axid® may be confused with Ansaid®

International issues:

Tazac [Australia] may be confused with Tazact brand name for piperacillin/tazobactam [India]; Tiazac brand name for diltiazem [U.S., Canada]

U.S. Brand Names Axid®

Canadian Brand Names Apo-Nizatidine®; Axid®; Gen-Nizatidine; Novo-Nizatidine; Nu-Nizatidine; PMS-Nizatidine

Therapeutic Category Histamine H_2 Antagonist

Use Treatment and maintenance of duodenal ulcer; treatment of benign gastric ulcer; treatment of gastroesophageal reflux disease (GERD)

General Dosage Range Dosage adjustment recommended in patients with renal impairment

Oral:

Children ≥12 years: 150 mg twice daily

Adults: 300 mg/day in 1-2 divided doses **or** 75 mg twice daily (OTC dosing)

Dosage Forms

Capsule, oral: 150 mg, 300 mg

Solution, oral: 15 mg/mL (473 mL)

Axid®: 15 mg/mL (480 mL)

Nizoral® *see* ketoconazole (topical) *on page 512*

Nizoral® A-D [OTC] *see* ketoconazole (topical) *on page 512*

N-methylhydrazine *see* procarbazine *on page 760*

N-methylnaltrexone bromide *see* methylnaltrexone *on page 590*

NN2211 *see* liraglutide *on page 543*

No Doz® Maximum Strength [OTC] *see* caffeine *on page 157*

NoHist [OTC] *see* chlorpheniramine and phenylephrine *on page 200*

NoHist DM [OTC] *see* chlorpheniramine, phenylephrine, and dextromethorphan *on page 201*

NoHist LQ [OTC] *see* chlorpheniramine and phenylephrine *on page 200*

Nolvadex *see* tamoxifen *on page 868*

Nolvadex®-D (Can) *see* tamoxifen *on page 868*

Non-Aspirin Pain Reliever [OTC] *see* acetaminophen *on page 20*

nonoxynol 9 (non OKS i nole nine)

Medication Safety Issues

Sound-alike/look-alike issues:

Delfen® may be confused with Delsym®

Synonyms N-9

U.S. Brand Names Conceptrol® [OTC]; Delfen® [OTC]; Encare® [OTC]; Gynol II® Extra Strength [OTC]; Gynol II® [OTC]; Today® [OTC]; VCF® [OTC]

Therapeutic Category Spermicide

Use Prevention of pregnancy

General Dosage Range Intravaginal: *Adolescents and Adults:* Insert 1 applicatorful, film, suppository, or sponge 10 minutes to 3 hours prior to intercourse [product specific]

Dosage Forms

Aerosol, foam, vaginal:
Delfen® [OTC]: 12.5% (18 g)
VCF® [OTC]: 12.5% (40 g)

Film, vaginal:
VCF® [OTC]: 28% (3s, 6s, 12s)

Gel, vaginal:
Conceptrol® [OTC]: 4% (2.7 g)
Encare® [OTC]: 4% (2.7 g)
Gynol II® [OTC]: 2% (108 g)
Gynol II® Extra Strength [OTC]: 3% (81 g)

Sponge, vaginal:
Today® [OTC]: 1 g (3s, 12s)

Suppository, vaginal:
Encare® [OTC]: 100 mg (12s, 18s)

Nora-BE® *see* norethindrone *on page 648*
noradrenaline *see* norepinephrine *on page 648*
noradrenaline acid tartrate *see* norepinephrine *on page 648*
Norco® *see* hydrocodone and acetaminophen *on page 454*
Norcuron *see* vecuronium *on page 940*
Norcuron® (Can) *see* vecuronium *on page 940*
nordeoxyguanosine *see* ganciclovir (ophthalmic) *on page 419*
nordeoxyguanosine *see* ganciclovir (systemic) *on page 418*
Nordette® 28 *see* ethinyl estradiol and levonorgestrel *on page 357*
Norditropin FlexPro® *see* somatropin *on page 849*
Norditropin® NordiFlex® *see* somatropin *on page 849*
norelgestromin and ethinyl estradiol *see* ethinyl estradiol and norelgestromin *on page 359*
norel® SR *see* acetaminophen, chlorpheniramine, phenylephrine, and phenyltoloxamine *on page 27*

norepinephrine (nor ep i NEF rin)

Medication Safety Issues

Sound-alike/look-alike issues:
Levophed® may be confused with levofloxacin

High alert medication:
The Institute for Safe Medication Practices (ISMP) includes this medication among its list of drugs which have a heightened risk of causing significant patient harm when used in error.

Synonyms levarterenol bitartrate; noradrenaline; noradrenaline acid tartrate; norepinephrine bitartrate

U.S. Brand Names Levophed®

Canadian Brand Names Levophed®

Therapeutic Category Adrenergic Agonist Agent

Use Treatment of shock which persists after adequate fluid volume replacement; severe hypotension

General Dosage Range I.V.:
Children: Initial: 0.05-0.1 mcg/kg/minute; Maintenance: Titrate to desired effect (maximum: 2 mcg/kg/minute)
Adults: Initial: 8-12 mcg/minute; Maintenance: Titrate to desired effect (usual maintenance range: 2-4 mcg/minute)

Dosage Forms

Injection, solution: 1 mg/mL (4 mL)
Levophed®: 1 mg/mL (4 mL)

norepinephrine bitartrate *see* norepinephrine *on page 648*

norethindrone (nor ETH in drone)

Medication Safety Issues

Sound-alike/look-alike issues:
Micronor® may be confused with miconazole, Micronase

Synonyms norethindrone acetate; norethisterone

U.S. Brand Names Aygestin®; Camila®; Errin®; Heather; Jolivette®; Nor-QD®; Nora-BE®; Ortho Micronor®

Canadian Brand Names Micronor®; Norlutate®

Therapeutic Category Contraceptive, Progestin Only; Progestin

Use Treatment of amenorrhea; abnormal uterine bleeding; endometriosis; prevention of pregnancy

General Dosage Range Oral:

Norethindrone: *Children (postmenarche) and Adults:* 0.35 mg every day

Norethindrone acetate: *Adolescents and Adults:* 2.5-15 mg once daily for 5-14 days of menstrual cycle

Dosage Forms

Tablet, oral: 0.35 mg, 5 mg

Aygestin®: 5 mg

Camila®: 0.35 mg

Errin®: 0.35 mg

Heather: 0.35 mg

Jolivette®: 0.35 mg

Nor-QD®: 0.35 mg

Nora-BE®: 0.35 mg

Ortho Micronor®: 0.35 mg

norethindrone acetate *see* norethindrone *on page 648*

norethindrone acetate and ethinyl estradiol *see* ethinyl estradiol and norethindrone *on page 359*

norethindrone and estradiol *see* estradiol and norethindrone *on page 349*

norethindrone and mestranol (nor eth IN drone & MES tra nole)

Medication Safety Issues

Sound-alike/look-alike issues:

Norinyl® may be confused with Nardil®

Synonyms mestranol and norethindrone; Ortho Novum 1/50

U.S. Brand Names Necon® 1/50; Norinyl® 1+50

Canadian Brand Names Ortho-Novum® 1/50

Therapeutic Category Contraceptive, Oral

Use Prevention of pregnancy

General Dosage Range Oral:

21-tablet package: *Children (menarche) and Adults:* 1 tablet daily for 21 days, followed by 7 days off

28-tablet package: *Children (menarche) and Adults:* 1 tablet daily

Dosage Forms

Tablet, monophasic formulations:

Necon® 1/50: Norethindrone 1 mg and mestranol 0.05 mg [21 light blue tablets and 7 white inactive tablets] (28s)

Norinyl® 1+50: Norethindrone 1 mg and mestranol 0.05 mg [21 white tablets and 7 orange inactive tablets] (28s)

norethisterone *see* norethindrone *on page 648*

Norflex™ *see* orphenadrine *on page 671*

norfloxacin (nor FLOKS a sin)

Medication Safety Issues

Sound-alike/look-alike issues:

Norfloxacin may be confused with Norflex™, Noroxin®

Noroxin® may be confused with Neurontin®, Norflex™

U.S. Brand Names Noroxin®

Canadian Brand Names Apo-Norflox®; CO Norfloxacin; Norfloxacine®; Novo-Norfloxacin; PMS-Norfloxacin; Riva-Norfloxacin

Therapeutic Category Quinolone

Use Uncomplicated and complicated urinary tract infections caused by susceptible gram-negative and gram-positive bacteria; sexually-transmitted disease (eg, uncomplicated urethral and cervical gonorrhea) caused by *N. gonorrhoeae*; prostatitis due to *E. coli*

Note: As of April 2007, the CDC no longer recommends the use of fluoroquinolones for the treatment of gonococcal disease.

General Dosage Range Dosage adjustment recommended in patients with renal impairment

Oral: *Adults:* 400 mg every 12 hours **or** 800 mg as a single dose

Dosage Forms

Tablet, oral:

Noroxin®: 400 mg

Norfloxacine® (Can) *see* norfloxacin *on page 649*

Norgesic *see* orphenadrine, aspirin, and caffeine *on page 672*

norgestimate and estradiol *see* estradiol and norgestimate *on page 350*

norgestimate and ethinyl estradiol *see* ethinyl estradiol and norgestimate *on page 361*

norgestrel and ethinyl estradiol *see* ethinyl estradiol and norgestrel *on page 362*

Norinyl® 1+35 *see* ethinyl estradiol and norethindrone *on page 359*

Norinyl® 1+50 *see* norethindrone and mestranol *on page 649*

Noritate® *see* metronidazole (topical) *on page 597*

Norlevo (Can) *see* levonorgestrel *on page 533*

Norlutate® (Can) *see* norethindrone *on page 648*

normal human serum albumin *see* albumin *on page 41*

normal saline *see* sodium chloride *on page 840*

normal serum albumin (human) *see* albumin *on page 41*

Normlshield® *see* emollients *on page 328*

Normocarb HF® 25 *see* electrolyte solution, renal replacement *on page 325*

Normocarb HF® 35 *see* electrolyte solution, renal replacement *on page 325*

Normodyne® (Can) *see* labetalol *on page 516*

Noroxin® *see* norfloxacin *on page 649*

Norpace® *see* disopyramide *on page 301*

Norpace® CR *see* disopyramide *on page 301*

Norpramin® *see* desipramine *on page 262*

Nor-QD® *see* norethindrone *on page 648*

Nortemp Children's [OTC] *see* acetaminophen *on page 20*

North American antisnake-bite serum, FAB (ovine) *see* crotalidae polyvalent immune FAB (ovine) *on page 241*

North American coral snake antivenin *see* antivenin *(Micrurus fulvius) on page 81*

North American coral snake antivenom *see* antivenin *(Micrurus fulvius) on page 81*

Nortrel® 0.5/35 *see* ethinyl estradiol and norethindrone *on page 359*

Nortrel® 1/35 *see* ethinyl estradiol and norethindrone *on page 359*

Nortrel® 7/7/7 *see* ethinyl estradiol and norethindrone *on page 359*

nortriptyline (nor TRIP ti leen)

Medication Safety Issues

Sound-alike/look-alike issues:

Aventyl® HCl may be confused with Bentyl®

Nortriptyline may be confused with amitriptyline, desipramine, Norpramin®

Pamelor™ may be confused with Demerol®, Tambocor™

BEERS Criteria medication:

This drug may be potentially inappropriate for use in geriatric patients (SIADH: Quality of evidence - moderate; Strength of recommendation - strong).

Synonyms nortriptyline hydrochloride

U.S. Brand Names Pamelor™

Canadian Brand Names Apo-Nortriptyline®; Ava-Nortriptyline; Aventyl®; Dom-Nortriptyline; Norventyl; Nu-Nortriptyline; PMS-Nortriptyline; Teva-Nortriptyline

Therapeutic Category Antidepressant, Tricyclic (Secondary Amine)

Use Treatment of symptoms of depression

General Dosage Range Oral:

Adults: 25 mg 3-4 times/day (maximum: 150 mg/day)

Elderly: Initial: 10-25 mg once daily; Maintenance: 75 mg/day in 1-2 divided doses

Dosage Forms

Capsule, oral: 10 mg, 25 mg, 50 mg, 75 mg

Pamelor™: 10 mg, 25 mg, 50 mg, 75 mg

Solution, oral: 10 mg/5 mL (473 mL)

Novo-Cloxin (Can) *see* cloxacillin *(Canada only) on page* 227
Novo-Cycloprine (Can) *see* cyclobenzaprine *on page* 243
Novo-Cyproterone (Can) *see* cyproterone *(Canada only) on page* 246
Novo-Cyproterone/Ethinyl Estradiol (Can) *see* cyproterone and ethinyl estradiol *(Canada only) on page* 247
Novo-Desipramine (Can) *see* desipramine *on page* 262
Novo-Desmopressin (Can) *see* desmopressin *on page* 264
Novo-Diflunisal (Can) *see* diflunisal *on page* 284
Novo-Dimenate [OTC] (Can) *see* dimenhydrinate *on page* 289
Novo-Dipam (Can) *see* diazepam *on page* 277
Novo-Divalproex (Can) *see* divalproex *on page* 302
Novo-Docusate Calcium (Can) *see* docusate *on page* 304
Novo-Docusate Sodium (Can) *see* docusate *on page* 304
Novo-Doxazosin (Can) *see* doxazosin *on page* 311
Novo-Doxepin (Can) *see* doxepin (systemic) *on page* 312
Novo-Doxylin (Can) *see* doxycycline *on page* 314
Novo-Enalapril (Can) *see* enalapril *on page* 330
Novo-Etidronatecal (Can) *see* etidronate and calcium carbonate *(Canada only) on page* 364
Novo-Famotidine (Can) *see* famotidine *on page* 372
Novo-Fenofibrate (Can) *see* fenofibrate *on page* 375
Novo-Fenofibrate Micronized (Can) *see* fenofibrate *on page* 375
Novo-Fenofibrate-S (Can) *see* fenofibrate *on page* 375
Novo-Fentanyl (Can) *see* fentanyl *on page* 377
Novo-Ferrogluc (Can) *see* ferrous gluconate *on page* 380
Novo-Finasteride (Can) *see* finasteride *on page* 384
Novo-Fluconazole (Can) *see* fluconazole *on page* 388
Novo-Flunarizine (Can) *see* flunarizine *(Canada only) on page* 391
Novo-Fluoxetine (Can) *see* fluoxetine *on page* 396
Novo-Flurprofen (Can) *see* flurbiprofen (systemic) *on page* 399
Novo-Flutamide (Can) *see* flutamide *on page* 399
Novo-Fluvoxamine (Can) *see* fluvoxamine *on page* 403
Novo-Furantoin (Can) *see* nitrofurantoin *on page* 644
Novo-Gemfibrozil (Can) *see* gemfibrozil *on page* 422
Novo-Gesic (Can) *see* acetaminophen *on page* 20
Novo-Gliclazide (Can) *see* gliclazide *(Canada only) on page* 425
Novo-Glimepiride (Can) *see* glimepiride *on page* 426
Novo-Glyburide (Can) *see* glyburide *on page* 428
Novo-Hydrazide (Can) *see* hydrochlorothiazide *on page* 452
Novo-Hydroxyzin (Can) *see* hydroxyzine *on page* 464
Novo-Hylazin (Can) *see* hydralazine *on page* 451
Novo-Indapamide (Can) *see* indapamide *on page* 479
Novo-Ipramide (Can) *see* ipratropium (oral inhalation) *on page* 499
Novo-Ketoconazole (Can) *see* ketoconazole (systemic) *on page* 511
Novo-Ketorolac (Can) *see* ketorolac (systemic) *on page* 512
Novo-Ketotifen (Can) *see* ketotifen (systemic) *(Canada only) on page* 514
Novo-Lamotrigine (Can) *see* lamotrigine *on page* 521
Novo-Leflunomide (Can) *see* leflunomide *on page* 525
Novo-Levobunolol (Can) *see* levobunolol *on page* 529
Novo-Levofloxacin (Can) *see* levofloxacin (systemic) *on page* 531
Novo-Lexin (Can) *see* cephalexin *on page* 189
NovoLIN® 70/30 *see* insulin NPH and insulin regular *on page* 489
Novolin® ge 30/70 (Can) *see* insulin NPH and insulin regular *on page* 489
Novolin® ge 40/60 (Can) *see* insulin NPH and insulin regular *on page* 489

Nu-Tetra (Can) *see* tetracycline *on page 884*
Nu-Tiaprofenic (Can) *see* tiaprofenic acid *(Canada only) on page 895*
Nu-Ticlopidine (Can) *see* ticlopidine *on page 895*
Nu-Timolol (Can) *see* timolol (systemic) *on page 896*
nutracort *see* hydrocortisone (topical) *on page 457*
Nutralox® [OTC] *see* calcium carbonate *on page 161*
Nutraplus® [OTC] *see* urea *on page 930*
Nu-Trazodone (Can) *see* trazodone *on page 912*
Nu-Trazodone D (Can) *see* trazodone *on page 912*
Nu-Triazide (Can) *see* hydrochlorothiazide and triamterene *on page 453*
Nutrimin-Plus [OTC] *see* vitamins (multiple/oral) *on page 951*
Nu-Trimipramine (Can) *see* trimipramine *on page 921*
Nutropin® *see* somatropin *on page 849*
Nutropin AQ® *see* somatropin *on page 849*
Nutropin® AQ (Can) *see* somatropin *on page 849*
Nutropin AQ® NuSpin™ *see* somatropin *on page 849*
Nutropin AQ Pen® *see* somatropin *on page 849*
NuvaRing® *see* ethinyl estradiol and etonogestrel *on page 357*
Nu-Verap (Can) *see* verapamil *on page 942*
Nu-Verap SR (Can) *see* verapamil *on page 942*
Nuvigil® *see* armodafinil *on page 91*
Nu-Zopiclone (Can) *see* zopiclone *(Canada only) on page 967*
NVP *see* nevirapine *on page 637*
Nyaderm (Can) *see* nystatin (topical) *on page 657*
Nyamyc® *see* nystatin (topical) *on page 657*
Nycoff [OTC] *see* dextromethorphan *on page 272*

nystatin (oral) (nye STAT in)

Medication Safety Issues

Sound-alike/look-alike issues:

Nystatin may be confused with HMG-CoA reductase inhibitors (also known as "statins"; eg, atorvaSTATin, fluvastatin, lovastatin, pitavastatin, pravastatin, rosuvastatin, simvastatin), Nitrostat®

Canadian Brand Names PMS-Nystatin

Therapeutic Category Antifungal Agent, Oral Nonabsorbed

Use Treatment of susceptible cutaneous, mucocutaneous, and oral cavity fungal infections normally caused by the *Candida* species

General Dosage Range Oral:

Premature infants: 100,000 units 4 times/day
Infants: 200,000 units 4 times/day
Children: 400,000-600,000 units 4 times/day
Adults: 400,000-1,000,000 units/day in 3-4 divided doses

Dosage Forms

Powder, for prescription compounding: 50 million units (10 g); 150 million units (30 g); 500 million units (100 g)
Suspension, oral: 100,000 units/mL (5 mL, 60 mL, 3 mL, 480 mL)
Tablet, oral: 500,000 units

nystatin (topical) (nye STAT in)

Medication Safety Issues

Sound-alike/look-alike issues:

Nystatin may be confused with HMG-CoA reductase inhibitors (also known as "statins"; eg, atorvaSTATin, fluvastatin, lovastatin, pitavastatin, pravastatin, rosuvastatin, simvastatin), Nitrostat®

U.S. Brand Names Nyamyc®; Nystop®; Pedi-Dri®; Pediaderm™ AF

Canadian Brand Names Candistatin®; Nyaderm

Therapeutic Category Antifungal Agent, Topical; Antifungal Agent, Vaginal

Use Treatment of susceptible cutaneous and mucocutaneous fungal infections normally caused by the *Candida* species

General Dosage Range

Intravaginal: *Adults:* Insert 1 vaginal tablet/day at bedtime

Topical: *Children and Adults:* Apply 2-3 times/day to affected areas

Dosage Forms

Cream, topical: 100,000 units/g (15 g, 30 g)

Pediaderm™ AF: 100,000 units/g (30 g)

Ointment, topical: 100,000 units/g (15 g, 30 g)

Powder, topical: 100,000 units/g (15 g, 30 g, 60 g)

Nyamyc®: 100,000 units/g (15 g, 30 g, 60 g)

Nystop®: 100,000 units/g (15 g, 30 g, 60 g)

Pedi-Dri®: 100,000 units/g (56.7 g)

Tablet, vaginal: 100,000 units

nystatin and metronidazole *see* metronidazole and nystatin *(Canada only) on page* 597

nystatin and triamcinolone (nye STAT in & trye am SIN oh lone)

Synonyms triamcinolone and nystatin

Therapeutic Category Antifungal/Corticosteroid

Use Treatment of cutaneous candidiasis

General Dosage Range

Topical:

Children: Apply sparingly 2-4 times/day

Adults: Apply sparingly 2-4 times/day

Dosage Forms

Cream: Nystatin 100,000 units and triamcinolone 0.1% (15 g, 30 g, 60 g)

Ointment: Nystatin 100,000 units and triamcinolone 0.1% (15 g, 30 g, 60 g)

Nystop® *see* nystatin (topical) *on page* 657

Nytol® (Can) *see* diphenhydramine (systemic) *on page* 292

Nytol® Extra Strength (Can) *see* diphenhydramine (systemic) *on page* 292

Nytol® Quick Caps [OTC] *see* diphenhydramine (systemic) *on page* 292

Nytol® Quick Gels [OTC] *see* diphenhydramine (systemic) *on page* 292

Oasis® *see* saliva substitute *on page* 819

OCBZ *see* oxcarbazepine *on page* 676

Occlusal™-HP (Can) *see* salicylic acid *on page* 816

Ocean® [OTC] *see* sodium chloride *on page* 840

Ocean® for Kids [OTC] *see* sodium chloride *on page* 840

Ocella™ *see* ethinyl estradiol and drospirenone *on page* 356

Octagam® *see* immune globulin *on page* 477

Octaplex® (Can) *see* prothrombin complex (human) [(factors II, VII, IX, X), protein C, and protein S] *(Canada only) on page* 770

Octostim® (Can) *see* desmopressin *on page* 264

OctreoScan® *see* indium in-111 pentetreotide *on page* 480

OctreoScan® (Prep Kit) *see* indium in-111 pentetreotide *on page* 480

octreotide (ok TREE oh tide)

Medication Safety Issues

Sound-alike/look-alike issues:

SandoSTATIN® may be confused with SandIMMUNE®, SandoSTATIN LAR®, sargramostim, simvastatin

Synonyms longastatin; octreotide acetate

U.S. Brand Names SandoSTATIN LAR®; SandoSTATIN®

Canadian Brand Names Octreotide Acetate Injection; Octreotide Acetate Omega; Sandostatin LAR®; Sandostatin®

Therapeutic Category Somatostatin Analog

Use Control of symptoms (diarrhea and flushing) in patients with metastatic carcinoid tumors; treatment of watery diarrhea associated with vasoactive intestinal peptide-secreting tumors (VIPomas); treatment of acromegaly

General Dosage Range Dosage adjustment recommended in patients with hepatic or renal impairment

I.M.: *Adults:* Depot: 20 mg every 4 weeks (maximum: 40 mg every 2 weeks)

I.V., SubQ: *Adults:* 50-1500 mcg/day in 2-4 divided doses

Dosage Forms

Injection, microspheres for suspension:
SandoSTATIN LAR®: 10 mg, 20 mg, 30 mg

Injection, solution: 100 mcg/mL (1 mL); 200 mcg/mL (5 mL); 1000 mcg/mL (5 mL)
SandoSTATIN®: 200 mcg/mL (5 mL); 1000 mcg/mL (5 mL)

Injection, solution [preservative free]: 50 mcg/mL (1 mL); 100 mcg/mL (1 mL); 200 mcg/mL (5 mL); 500 mcg/mL (1 mL)
SandoSTATIN®: 50 mcg/mL (1 mL); 100 mcg/mL (1 mL); 500 mcg/mL (1 mL)

octreotide acetate *see* octreotide *on page 658*

Octreotide Acetate Injection (Can) *see* octreotide *on page 658*

Octreotide Acetate Omega (Can) *see* octreotide *on page 658*

Ocudox™ *see* doxycycline *on page 314*

Ocufen® *see* flurbiprofen (ophthalmic) *on page 399*

Ocuflox® *see* ofloxacin (ophthalmic) *on page 660*

Ocuvite® [OTC] *see* vitamins (multiple/oral) *on page 951*

Ocuvite® Adult 50+ [OTC] *see* vitamins (multiple/oral) *on page 951*

Ocuvite® Extra® [OTC] *see* vitamins (multiple/oral) *on page 951*

Ocuvite® Lutein [OTC] *see* vitamins (multiple/oral) *on page 951*

Odans Liquor Carbonis Detergens [OTC] (Can) *see* coal tar *on page 228*

O-desmethylvenlafaxine *see* desvenlafaxine *on page 266*

ODV *see* desvenlafaxine *on page 266*

Oesclim® (Can) *see* estradiol (systemic) *on page 347*

ofatumumab (oh fa TOOM yoo mab)

Medication Safety Issues

Sound-alike/look-alike issues:
Ofatumumab may be confused with omalizumab

High alert medication:
This medication is in a class the Institute for Safe Medication Practices (ISMP) includes among its list of drug classes which have a heightened risk of causing significant patient harm when used in error.

Synonyms huMax-CD20

U.S. Brand Names Arzerra™

Therapeutic Category Antineoplastic Agent, Monoclonal Antibody; Monoclonal Antibody

Use Treatment of refractory chronic lymphocytic leukemia (CLL)

General Dosage Range Dosage adjustment recommended in patients who develop toxicities

I.V.: *Adults:* 300 mg week 1, followed 1 week later by 2000 mg once weekly for 7 doses (doses 2-8), followed 4 weeks later by 2000 mg once every 4 weeks for 4 doses (doses 9-12; for a total of 12 doses)

Dosage Forms

Injection, solution [preservative free]:
Arzerra™: 20 mg/mL (5 mL, 50 mL)

Ofirmev™ *see* acetaminophen *on page 20*

ofloxacin (systemic) (oh FLOKS a sin)

Canadian Brand Names Apo-Oflox®; Novo-Ofloxacin

Therapeutic Category Antibiotic, Quinolone

Use Quinolone antibiotic for the treatment of acute exacerbations of chronic bronchitis, community-acquired pneumonia, skin and skin structure infections (uncomplicated), urethral and cervical gonorrhea (acute, uncomplicated), urethritis and cervicitis (nongonococcal), mixed infections of the urethra and cervix, pelvic inflammatory disease (acute), cystitis (uncomplicated), urinary tract infections (complicated), prostatitis

Note: As of April 2007, the CDC no longer recommends the use of fluoroquinolones for the treatment of gonococcal disease.

General Dosage Range Dosage adjustment recommended in patients with hepatic or renal impairment

Oral: *Adults:* 200-400 mg every 12 hours

Dosage Forms

Tablet, oral: 200 mg, 300 mg, 400 mg

ofloxacin (ophthalmic) (oh FLOKS a sin)

Medication Safety Issues

Sound-alike/look-alike issues:

Ocuflox® may be confused with Occlusal™-HP, Ocufen®

U.S. Brand Names Ocuflox®

Canadian Brand Names Ocuflox®

Therapeutic Category Antibiotic, Ophthalmic; Antibiotic, Quinolone

Use Treatment of superficial ocular infections involving the conjunctiva or cornea due to strains of susceptible organisms

General Dosage Range Ophthalmic: *Children >1 year and Adults:* Initial: 1-2 drops every 30 minutes to 4 hours; Maintenance: 1-2 drops every 4-6 hours

Dosage Forms

Solution, ophthalmic: 0.3% (5 mL, 10 mL)

Ocuflox®: 0.3% (5 mL)

ofloxacin (otic) (oh FLOKS a sin)

Medication Safety Issues

Sound-alike/look-alike issues:

Floxin may be confused with Flexeril®

International issues:

Floxin: Brand name for ofloxacin [U.S., Canada], but also the brand name for flunarizine [Thailand], norfloxacin [South Africa], and perfloxacin [Philippines]

Floxin [U.S., Canada] may be confused with Flexin brand name for diclofenac [Argentina], cyclobenzaprine [Chile], and orphenadrine [Israel]; Flogen brand name for naproxen [Mexico]

Synonyms Floxin Otic Singles

Therapeutic Category Antibiotic, Quinolone

Use Otitis externa, chronic suppurative otitis media, acute otitis media

General Dosage Range

Otic:

Children <6 months: Dosage not established

Children ≥6 months to 12 years: 5 drops daily

Children >12 years: 10 drops once or twice daily

Adults: 10 drops once or twice daily

Dosage Forms

Solution, otic: 0.3% (5 mL, 10 mL)

Oforta™ [DSC] *see* fludarabine *on page 389*

Ogen® (Can) *see* estropipate *on page 353*

Ogestrel® *see* ethinyl estradiol and norgestrel *on page 362*

OGMT *see* metyrosine *on page 598*

OGT-918 *see* miglustat *on page 603*

17OHPC *see* hydroxyprogesterone caproate *on page 463*

9-OH-risperidone *see* paliperidone *on page 685*

olanzapine (oh LAN za peen)

Medication Safety Issues

Sound-alike/look-alike issues:

OLANZapine may be confused with olsalazine, QUEtiapine

ZyPREXA® may be confused with CeleXA®, Reprexain™, Zestril®, ZyrTEC®

ZyPREXA® Zydis® may be confused with Zelapar®, zolpidem

ZyPREXA® Relprevv™ may be confused with ZyPREXA® IntraMuscular

BEERS Criteria medication:

This drug may be potentially inappropriate for use in geriatric patients (Quality of evidence - moderate; Strength of recommendation - strong).

Synonyms LY170053; olanzapine pamoate

Tall-Man **OLANZ**apine

U.S. Brand Names ZyPREXA®; ZyPREXA® IntraMuscular; ZyPREXA® Relprevv™; ZyPREXA® Zydis®

Canadian Brand Names Apo-Olanzapine ODT®; Apo-Olanzapine®; Ava-Olanzapine; CO Olanzapine; CO Olanzapine ODT; Mylan-Olanzapine; Olanzapine ODT; PHL-Olanzapine; PHL-Olanzapine ODT; PMS-Olanzapine; PMS-Olanzapine ODT; Riva-Olanzapine; Riva-Olanzapine ODT; Sandoz-Olanzapine; Sandoz-Olanzapine ODT; Teva-Olanzapine; Teva-Olanzapine OD; Zyprexa®; Zyprexa® Intramuscular; Zyprexa® Zydis®

Therapeutic Category Antipsychotic Agent

Use

Oral: Treatment of the manifestations of schizophrenia; treatment of acute or mixed mania episodes associated with bipolar I disorder (as monotherapy or in combination with lithium or valproate); maintenance treatment of bipolar disorder; in combination with fluoxetine for treatment-resistant or bipolar I depression

I.M., extended-release (Zyprexa® Relprevv™): Treatment of schizophrenia

I.M., short-acting (Zyprexa® IntraMuscular): Treatment of acute agitation associated with schizophrenia and bipolar I mania

General Dosage Range

I.M.: *Adults:*

Extended release: 150-300 mg every 2 weeks **or** 300-405 mg every 4 weeks (maximum: 300 mg every 2 weeks; 405 mg every 4 weeks)

Short-acting: Initial: 10 mg/dose; 2-4 hours between doses (maximum: 30 mg/day)

Oral:

Adolescents ≥13 years: Initial: 2.5-5 mg once daily; dosing range: 2.5-20 mg/day

Adults: Initial: 5-15 mg once daily; Maintenance: 5-20 mg once daily

Elderly: Initial: 2.5-5 mg/day

Dosage Forms

Injection, powder for reconstitution: 10 mg

ZyPREXA® IntraMuscular: 10 mg

Injection, powder for suspension, extended release:

ZyPREXA® Relprevv™: 210 mg, 300 mg, 405 mg

Tablet, oral: 2.5 mg, 5 mg, 7.5 mg, 10 mg, 15 mg, 20 mg

ZyPREXA®: 2.5 mg, 5 mg, 7.5 mg, 10 mg, 15 mg, 20 mg

Tablet, orally disintegrating, oral: 5 mg, 10 mg, 15 mg, 20 mg

ZyPREXA® Zydis®: 5 mg, 10 mg, 15 mg, 20 mg

olanzapine and fluoxetine (oh LAN za peen & floo OKS e teen)

Medication Safety Issues

Sound-alike/look-alike issues:

Symbyax® may be confused with Cymbalta®

BEERS Criteria medication:

This drug may be potentially inappropriate for use in geriatric patients (Quality of evidence - moderate; Strength of recommendation - strong).

Synonyms fluoxetine and olanzapine; olanzapine and fluoxetine hydrochloride

U.S. Brand Names Symbyax®

Therapeutic Category Antidepressant, Selective Serotonin Reuptake Inhibitor; Antipsychotic Agent, Thienobenzodiaepine

Use Treatment of depressive episodes associated with bipolar I disorder; treatment-resistant depression (unresponsive to 2 trials of different antidepressants in the current episode)

General Dosage Range Dosage adjustment recommended in patients with hepatic impairment

Oral:

Adults: Initial: Olanzapine 6 mg and fluoxetine 25 mg once daily; Maintenance: Olanzapine 6-12 mg and fluoxetine 25-50 mg once daily

Elderly >65 years: Initial: Olanzapine 3-6 mg and fluoxetine 25 mg once daily

Dosage Forms

Capsule, oral: 6/25: Olanzapine 6 mg and fluoxetine 25 mg; 6/50: Olanzapine 6 mg and fluoxetine 50 mg; 12/25: Olanzapine 12 mg and fluoxetine 25 mg; 12/50: Olanzapine 12 mg and fluoxetine 50 mg

Symbyax®:

3/25: Olanzapine 3 mg and fluoxetine 25 mg
6/25: Olanzapine 6 mg and fluoxetine 25 mg
6/50: Olanzapine 6 mg and fluoxetine 50 mg
12/25: Olanzapine 12 mg and fluoxetine 25 mg
12/50: Olanzapine 12 mg and fluoxetine 50 mg

olanzapine and fluoxetine hydrochloride *see* olanzapine and fluoxetine *on page* 661
Olanzapine ODT (Can) *see* olanzapine *on page* 660
olanzapine pamoate *see* olanzapine *on page* 660
oleovitamin A *see* vitamin A *on page* 949
Oleptro™ *see* trazodone *on page* 912
Olestyr (Can) *see* cholestyramine resin *on page* 205
oleum ricini *see* castor oil *on page* 180

olmesartan (ole me SAR tan)

Medication Safety Issues

Sound-alike/look-alike issues:

Benicar® may be confused with Mevacor®

Synonyms olmesartan medoxomil

U.S. Brand Names Benicar®

Canadian Brand Names Olmetec®

Therapeutic Category Angiotensin II Receptor Antagonist

Use Treatment of hypertension with or without concurrent use of other antihypertensive agents

General Dosage Range Oral:

Children 6-16 years:

20 kg to <35 kg: Initial: 10 mg once daily (maximum: 20 mg once daily)

≥35 kg: Initial: 20 mg once daily (maximum: 40 mg once daily)

Adolescents >16 years and Adults: Initial: 20 mg once daily; Maintenance: 20-40 mg once daily

Elderly: Initial: 5-20 mg once daily

Dosage Forms

Tablet, oral:

Benicar®: 5 mg, 20 mg, 40 mg

olmesartan, amlodipine, and hydrochlorothiazide

(ole me SAR tan, am LOE di peen, & hye droe klor oh THYE a zide)

Synonyms amlodipine besylate, olmesartan medoxomil, and hydrochlorothiazide; amlodipine, hydrochlorothiazide, and olmesartan; hydrochlorothiazide, olmesartan, and amlodipine; olmesartan, hydrochlorothiazide, and amlodipine

U.S. Brand Names Tribenzor™

Therapeutic Category Angiotensin II Receptor Blocker; Calcium Channel Blocker; Calcium Channel Blocker, Dihydropyridine; Diuretic, Thiazide

Use Treatment of hypertension (not for initial therapy)

General Dosage Range Oral: *Adults:* Amlodipine 5-10 mg and olmesartan 20-40 mg and hydrochlorothiazide 12.5-25 mg once daily (maximum: 10 mg/day [amlodipine]; 25 mg/day [hydrochlorothiazide]; 40 mg/day [olmesartan])

Dosage Forms

Tablet, oral:

Tribenzor™: Olmesartan medoxomil 40 mg, amlodipine 5 mg, and hydrochlorothiazide 25 mg, olmesartan medoxomil 40 mg, amlodipine 10 mg, and hydrochlorothiazide 25 mg, olmesartan medoxomil 20 mg, amlodipine 5 mg, and hydrochlorothiazide 12.5 mg, olmesartan medoxomil 40 mg, amlodipine 5 mg, and hydrochlorothiazide 12.5 mg, olmesartan medoxomil 40 mg, amlodipine 10 mg, and hydrochlorothiazide 12.5 mg

olmesartan and amlodipine *see* amlodipine and olmesartan *on page* 67

olmesartan and hydrochlorothiazide (ole me SAR tan & hye droe klor oh THYE a zide)

Synonyms hydrochlorothiazide and olmesartan medoxomil; olmesartan medoxomil and hydrochlorothiazide

U.S. Brand Names Benicar HCT®

Canadian Brand Names Olmetec Plus®

Therapeutic Category Angiotensin II Receptor Antagonist; Diuretic, Thiazide

Use Treatment of hypertension (not recommended for initial treatment)

General Dosage Range Oral: *Adults:* Olmesartan 20-40 mg and hydrochlorothiazide 12.5-25 mg once daily (maximum: 25 mg/day [hydrochlorothiazide]; 40 mg/day [olmesartan])

Dosage Forms

Tablet:

Benicar HCT®: 20/12.5: Olmesartan 20 mg and hydrochlorothiazide 12.5 mg; 40/12.5: Olmesartan 40 mg and hydrochlorothiazide 12.5 mg; 40/25: Olmesartan 40 mg and hydrochlorothiazide 25 mg

olmesartan, hydrochlorothiazide, and amlodipine *see* olmesartan, amlodipine, and hydrochlorothiazide *on page* 662

olmesartan medoxomil *see* olmesartan *on page* 662

olmesartan medoxomil and hydrochlorothiazide *see* olmesartan and hydrochlorothiazide *on page* 663

Olmetec® (Can) *see* olmesartan *on page* 662

Olmetec Plus® (Can) *see* olmesartan and hydrochlorothiazide *on page* 663

olopatadine (nasal) (oh la PAT a deen)

Synonyms olopatadine hydrochloride

U.S. Brand Names Patanase®

Therapeutic Category Histamine H_1 Antagonist; Histamine H_1 Antagonist, Second Generation

Use Treatment of the symptoms of seasonal allergic rhinitis

General Dosage Range Intranasal:

Children 6-11 years: 1 spray into each nostril twice daily

Children ≥12 years, Adolescents, and Adults: 2 sprays into each nostril twice daily

Dosage Forms

Solution, intranasal:

Patanase®: 0.6% (30.5 g)

olopatadine (ophthalmic) (oh la PAT a deen)

Medication Safety Issues

Sound-alike/look-alike issues:

Patanol® may be confused with Platinol

International issues:

Patanol [U.S., Canada, and multiple international markets] may be confused with Bétanol brand name for metipranolol [Monaco]

Synonyms olopatadine hydrochloride

U.S. Brand Names Pataday™; Patanol®

Canadian Brand Names Pataday™; Patanol®

Therapeutic Category Histamine H_1 Antagonist; Histamine H_1 Antagonist, Second Generation

Use Treatment of the signs and symptoms of allergic conjunctivitis

General Dosage Range Ophthalmic:

Children ≥3 years, Adolescents, and Adults: Patanol®: Instill 1 drop into each affected eye twice daily

Children ≥2 years, Adolescents, and Adults: Pataday™: Instill 1 drop into each affected eye once daily

Dosage Forms

Solution, ophthalmic:

Pataday™: 0.2% (2.5 mL)

Patanol®: 0.1% (5 mL)

olopatadine hydrochloride *see* olopatadine (nasal) *on page* 663

olopatadine hydrochloride *see* olopatadine (ophthalmic) *on page* 663

olsalazine (ole SAL a zeen)

Medication Safety Issues

Sound-alike/look-alike issues:

Olsalazine may be confused with OLANZapine

Dipentum® may be confused with Dilantin®

Synonyms olsalazine sodium

U.S. Brand Names Dipentum®

Canadian Brand Names Dipentum®

Therapeutic Category 5-Aminosalicylic Acid Derivative

Use Maintenance of remission of ulcerative colitis in patients intolerant to sulfasalazine

General Dosage Range Oral: *Adults:* 1 g/day in 2 divided doses

Dosage Forms

Capsule, oral:

Dipentum®: 250 mg

olsalazine sodium *see* olsalazine *on page* 664

Olux® *see* clobetasol *on page* 221

Olux-E™ *see* clobetasol *on page* 221

omalizumab (oh mah lye ZOO mab)

Medication Safety Issues

Sound-alike/look-alike issues:

Omalizumab may be confused with ofatumumab

Synonyms rhuMAb-E25

U.S. Brand Names Xolair®

Canadian Brand Names Xolair®

Therapeutic Category Monoclonal Antibody

Use Treatment of moderate-to-severe, persistent allergic asthma not adequately controlled with inhaled corticosteroids

General Dosage Range SubQ:

IgE ≥30-100 units/mL:

Children ≥12 years and Adults 30-90 kg: 150 mg every 4 weeks

Children ≥12 years and Adults >90-150 kg: 300 mg every 4 weeks

IgE >100-200 units/mL:

Children ≥12 years and Adults 30-90 kg: 300 mg every 4 weeks

Children ≥12 years and Adults >90-150 kg: 225 mg every 2 weeks

IgE >200-300 units/mL:

Children ≥12 years and Adults 30-60 kg: 300 mg every 4 weeks

Children ≥12 years and Adults >60-90 kg: 225 mg every 2 weeks

Children ≥12 years and Adults >90-150 kg: 300 mg every 2 weeks

IgE >300-400 units/mL:

Children ≥12 years and Adults 30-70 kg: 225 mg every 2 weeks

Children ≥12 years and Adults >70-90 kg: 300 mg every 2 weeks

IgE >400-500 units/mL:

Children ≥12 years and Adults 30-70 kg: 300 mg every 2 weeks

Children ≥12 years and Adults >70-90 kg: 375 mg every 2 weeks

IgE >500-600 units/mL:

Children ≥12 years and Adults 30-60 kg: 300 mg every 2 weeks

Children ≥12 years and Adults >60-70 kg: 375 mg every 2 weeks

IgE >600-700 units/mL: *Children ≥12 years and Adults 30-60 kg:* 375 mg every 2 weeks

Dosage Forms

Injection, powder for reconstitution:

Xolair®: 150 mg

Omeclamox-Pak® *see* omeprazole, clarithromycin, and amoxicillin *on page* 666

omega 3 *see* omega-3-acid ethyl esters *on page* 665

omega-3-acid ethyl esters (oh MEG a three AS id ETH il ES ters)

Medication Safety Issues

Sound-alike/look-alike issues:

Lovaza® may be confused with LORazepam

International issues:

Omacor [multiple international markets] may be confused with Amicar brand name for aminocaproic acid [U.S.]

Other safety concerns:

The Institute for Safe Medication Practices (ISMP) reported a case of a foam plastic cup dissolving after contact with the liquid contents from a Lovaza® capsule. ISMP is requesting the manufacturer to add warnings to its labeling and that healthcare providers add Lovaza® to their list of medications to not crush.

Synonyms ethyl esters of omega-3 fatty acids; fish oil; omega 3; P-OM3

U.S. Brand Names Lovaza®

Therapeutic Category Antilipemic Agent, Miscellaneous

Use Lovaza®: Adjunct to diet therapy in the treatment of hypertriglyceridemia (≥500 mg/dL)

Note: A number of OTC formulations containing omega-3 fatty acids are marketed as nutritional supplements; these do not have FDA-approved indications and may not contain the same amounts of the active ingredient.

General Dosage Range Oral: *Adults:* 4 g/day in 1-2 divided doses

Dosage Forms

Capsule, liquid gel, oral:

Lovaza®: 1 g

omeprazole (oh MEP ra zole)

Medication Safety Issues

Sound-alike/look-alike issues:

Omeprazole may be confused with aripiprazole, fomepizole

PriLOSEC® may be confused with Plendil®, Prevacid®, predniSONE, prilocaine, Prinivil®, Proventil®, PROzac®

International issues:

Losec [multiple international markets] may be confused with Lasix brand name for furosemide [U.S., Canada, and multiple international markets]

Medral [Mexico] may be confused with Medrol brand name for methylprednisolone [U.S., Canada, and multiple international markets]

Norpramin: Brand name for omeprazole [Spain], but also the brand name for desipramine [U.S., Canada] and enalapril/hydrochlorothiazide [Portugal]

Synonyms omeprazole magnesium

U.S. Brand Names First®-Omeprazole; PriLOSEC OTC® [OTC]; PriLOSEC®

Canadian Brand Names Apo-Omeprazole®; Losec®; Mylan-Omeprazole; PMS-Omeprazole; PMS-Omeprazole DR; ratio-Omeprazole; Sandoz-Omeprazole

Therapeutic Category Gastric Acid Secretion Inhibitor; Proton Pump Inhibitor

Use Short-term (4-8 weeks) treatment of active duodenal ulcer disease or active benign gastric ulcer; treatment of heartburn and other symptoms associated with gastroesophageal reflux disease (GERD); short-term (4-8 weeks) treatment of endoscopically-diagnosed erosive esophagitis; maintenance healing of erosive esophagitis; long-term treatment of pathological hypersecretory conditions; as part of a multidrug regimen for *H. pylori* eradication to reduce the risk of duodenal ulcer recurrence

OTC labeling: Short-term treatment of frequent, uncomplicated heartburn occurring ≥2 days/week

General Dosage Range Oral:

Children 1-16 years and 5 kg to <10 kg: 5 mg once daily

Children 1-16 years and 10 kg to <20 kg: 10 mg once daily

Children 1-16 years and ≥20 kg: 20 mg once daily

Adults: 20-40 mg/day (may be given in 2 divided doses); doses up to 360 mg/day [pathological hypersecretory syndrome]

Dosage Forms

Capsule, delayed release, oral: 10 mg, 20 mg, 40 mg

PriLOSEC®: 10 mg, 20 mg, 40 mg

Granules for suspension, delayed release, oral:

PriLOSEC®: 2.5 mg/packet (30s); 10 mg/packet (30s)

Powder for suspension, oral:
First®-Omeprazole: 2 mg/mL (90 mL, 150 mL, 300 mL)
Tablet, delayed release, oral: 20 mg
PriLOSEC OTC® [OTC]: 20 mg

omeprazole, amoxicillin, and clarithromycin *see* omeprazole, clarithromycin, and amoxicillin *on page 666*

omeprazole and sodium bicarbonate (oh MEP ra zole & SOW dee um bye KAR bun ate)

Medication Safety Issues
Sound-alike/look-alike issues:
Zegerid® may be confused with Zestril®

Synonyms sodium bicarbonate and omeprazole

U.S. Brand Names Zegerid OTC™ [OTC]; Zegerid®

Therapeutic Category Proton Pump Inhibitor; Substituted Benzimidazole

Use Short-term (4-8 weeks) treatment of active duodenal ulcer or active benign gastric ulcer; treatment of heartburn and other symptoms associated with gastroesophageal reflux disease (GERD); short-term (4-8 weeks) treatment of endoscopically-diagnosed erosive esophagitis; maintenance healing of erosive esophagitis; reduction of risk of upper gastrointestinal bleeding in critically-ill patients

OTC labeling: Short-term (2 weeks) treatment of frequent (2 days/week), uncomplicated heartburn

General Dosage Range Oral: *Adults:* 20-40 mg/day in 1-2 divided doses

Dosage Forms
Capsule, oral: Omeprazole 20 mg [immediate release] and sodium bicarbonate 1100 mg; omeprazole 40 mg [immediate release] and sodium bicarbonate 1100 mg
Zegerid®: Omeprazole 20 mg [immediate release] and sodium bicarbonate 1100 mg
Zegerid®: Omeprazole 40 mg [immediate release] and sodium bicarbonate 1100 mg
Zegerid OTC™ [OTC]: Omeprazole 20 mg [immediate release] and sodium bicarbonate 1100 mg
Powder for suspension, oral:
Zegerid®: Omeprazole 20 mg and sodium bicarbonate 1680 mg per packet
Zegerid®: Omeprazole 40 mg and sodium bicarbonate 1680 mg per packet

omeprazole, clarithromycin, and amoxicillin

(oh MEP ra zole, kla RITH roe mye sin, & a moks i SIL in)

Synonyms amoxicillin, clarithromycin, and omeprazole; clarithromycin, amoxicillin, and omeprazole; omeprazole, amoxicillin, and clarithromycin

U.S. Brand Names Omeclamox-Pak®

Therapeutic Category Antibiotic, Macrolide Combination; Antibiotic, Penicillin; Gastrointestinal Agent, Miscellaneous; Proton Pump Inhibitor; Substituted Benzimidazole

Use Eradication of *H. pylori* infection in patients with duodenal ulcer disease (active or a history of up to 1 year)

General Dosage Range Oral: *Adults:* Omeprazole 20 mg, clarithromycin 500 mg, and amoxicillin 1000 mg twice daily

Dosage Forms
Combination package, oral [each administration card contains]:
Omeclamox-Pak™:
Capsule, delayed release: Omeprazole: 20 mg (2s)
Tablet: Clarithromycin: 500 mg (2s)
Capsule: Amoxicillin: 500 mg (4s) [contains sodium ≤0.0052 mEq (0.119 mg)/capsule]

omeprazole magnesium *see* omeprazole *on page 665*
Omnaris® *see* ciclesonide (nasal) *on page 207*
Omnicef® [DSC] *see* cefdinir *on page 182*
Omni Gel™ [OTC] *see* fluoride *on page 393*
Omnipaque™ (Can) *see* iohexol *on page 495*
Omnipaque™ 140 [DSC] *see* iohexol *on page 495*
Omnipaque™ 180 *see* iohexol *on page 495*
Omnipaque™ 240 *see* iohexol *on page 495*
Omnipaque™ 300 *see* iohexol *on page 495*
Omnipaque™ 350 *see* iohexol *on page 495*

Omnipred™ *see* prednisolone (ophthalmic) *on page 754*
Omniscan® *see* gadodiamide *on page 415*
Omnitarg *see* pertuzumab *on page 710*
Omnitrope® *see* somatropin *on page 849*
Omontys® *see* peginesatide *on page 696*

onabotulinumtoxinA (oh nuh BOT yoo lin num TOKS in aye)

Medication Safety Issues

Other safety concerns:

Botulinum products are not interchangeable; potency differences may exist between the products.

Synonyms botulinum toxin type A; BTX-A

U.S. Brand Names Botox®; Botox® Cosmetic

Canadian Brand Names Botox®; Botox® Cosmetic

Therapeutic Category Ophthalmic Agent, Toxin

Use Treatment of strabismus and blepharospasm associated with dystonia (including benign essential blepharospasm or VII nerve disorders) in patients ≥12 years of age; treatment of cervical dystonia (spasmodic torticollis) in patients ≥16 years of age; temporary improvement in the appearance of lines/ wrinkles of the face (moderate-to-severe glabellar lines associated with corrugator and/or procerus muscle activity) in adult patients ≤65 years of age; treatment of severe primary axillary hyperhidrosis in adults not adequately controlled with topical treatments; treatment of focal spasticity (specifically upper limb spasticity) in adults; prophylaxis of chronic migraine headache (≥15 days/month with ≥4 hours/day headache duration) in adults; treatment of urinary incontinence due to detrusor overactivity associated with neurologic conditions

Canadian labeling: Additional use (not in U.S. labeling): Dynamic equinus foot deformity in pediatric cerebral palsy patients; treatment of forehead, lateral canthus, and glabellar lines in adults >65 years of age

General Dosage Range

I.M.: *Children ≥12 years and Adults:* Dosage varies greatly depending on indication

Intradermal: *Adults:* 50 units/axilla evenly distributed into multiple sites (10-15), in 0.1-0.2 mL aliquots, ~1-2 cm apart

Intradetrusor: *Adults:* 200 units/30 mL, in 1 mL aliquots, ~1 cm apart

Dosage Forms

Injection, powder for reconstitution [preservative free]:

Botox®: *Clostridium botulinum* type A neurotoxin complex 100 units, *Clostridium botulinum* type A neurotoxin complex 200 units

Botox® Cosmetic: *Clostridium botulinum* type A neurotoxin complex 100 units, *Clostridium botulinum* type A neurotoxin complex 50 units

Dosage Forms - Canada

Injection, powder for reconstitution [preservative free]:

Botox®: Botulinum toxin A 50 units, 100 units, 200 units

Botox Cosmetic®: Botulinum toxin A 50 unit, 100 units, 200 units

Onbrez® Breezhaler® (Can) *see* indacaterol *on page 479*
Oncaspar® *see* pegaspargase *on page 696*
Oncotice™ (Can) *see* BCG *on page 116*
Oncovin *see* vincristine *on page 946*

ondansetron (on DAN se tron)

Medication Safety Issues

Sound-alike/look-alike issues:

Ondansetron may be confused with dolasetron, granisetron, palonosetron

Zofran® may be confused with Zantac®, Zosyn®

Synonyms GR38032R; ondansetron hydrochloride

U.S. Brand Names Zofran®; Zofran® ODT; Zuplenz®

Canadian Brand Names Apo-Ondansetron®; CO Ondansetron; Dom-Ondansetron; JAMP-Ondansetron; Mint-Ondansetron; Mylan-Ondansetron; Ondansetron Injection; Ondansetron Injection USP; Ondansetron-Odan; Ondansetron-Omega; PHL-Ondansetron; PMS-Ondansetron; RAN™-Ondansetron; ratio-Ondansetron; Sandoz-Ondansetron; Teva-Ondansetron; Zofran®; Zofran® ODT; ZYM-Ondansetron

Therapeutic Category Selective 5-HT_3 Receptor Antagonist

Use

I.V.: Prevention of nausea and vomiting associated with initial and repeat courses of emetogenic cancer chemotherapy (including high-dose cisplatin); prevention of postoperative nausea and/or vomiting (PONV); treatment of PONV if no prophylactic dose of ondansetron received

Oral: Prevention of nausea and vomiting associated with highly emetogenic cancer chemotherapy (including high-dose cisplatin); prevention of nausea and vomiting associated with initial and repeat courses of moderately emetogenic cancer chemotherapy; prevention of nausea and vomiting associated with radiotherapy (either total body irradiation, single high-dose fraction to the abdomen, or daily fractions to the abdomen); prevention of PONV

General Dosage Range Dosage adjustment recommended in patients with hepatic impairment

I.M.: *Adults:* 4 mg as a single dose

I.V.:

Infants 1-6 months: 0.1 mg/kg as a single dose

Children 6 months to 12 years and ≤40 kg: 0.1 mg/kg as a single dose **or** 0.15 mg/kg/dose (maximum: 16 mg/dose) for 3 doses

Children 6 months to 12 years and >40 kg and Children >12 years to 18 years: 4 mg as a single dose **or** 0.15 mg/kg/dose (maximum: 16 mg/dose) for 3 doses

Adults: 0.15 mg/kg/dose (maximum: 16 mg/dose) for 3 doses **or** 4 mg as a single dose

Oral:

Children 4-11 years: 4 mg every 4 hours for 3 doses (day 1), then 4 mg every 8 hours for 1-2 days

Children ≥12 years and Adults: 16 mg or 24 mg as a single dose **or** 8 mg every 8-12 hours

Dosage Forms

Film, soluble, oral:

Zuplenz®: 4 mg (10s); 8 mg (10s)

Infusion, premixed in D_5W [preservative free]: 32 mg (50 mL)

Infusion, premixed in NS [preservative free]: 32 mg (50 mL)

Injection, solution: 2 mg/mL (2 mL, 20 mL)

Zofran®: 2 mg/mL (20 mL)

Injection, solution [preservative free]: 2 mg/mL (2 mL)

Solution, oral: 4 mg/5 mL (5 mL, 50 mL)

Zofran®: 4 mg/5 mL (50 mL)

Tablet, oral: 4 mg, 8 mg

Zofran®: 4 mg, 8 mg

Tablet, orally disintegrating, oral: 4 mg, 8 mg

Zofran® ODT: 4 mg, 8 mg

ondansetron hydrochloride *see* ondansetron *on page 667*

Ondansetron Injection (Can) *see* ondansetron *on page 667*

Ondansetron Injection USP (Can) *see* ondansetron *on page 667*

Ondansetron-Odan (Can) *see* ondansetron *on page 667*

Ondansetron-Omega (Can) *see* ondansetron *on page 667*

One A Day® Cholesterol Plus [OTC] *see* vitamins (multiple/oral) *on page 951*

One A Day® Energy [OTC] *see* vitamins (multiple/oral) *on page 951*

One A Day® Essential [OTC] *see* vitamins (multiple/oral) *on page 951*

One A Day® Kids Jolly Rancher™ Gummies [OTC] *see* vitamins (multiple/pediatric) *on page 952*

One A Day® Kids Jolly Rancher™ Sour Gummies [OTC] *see* vitamins (multiple/pediatric) *on page 952*

One A Day® Kids Scooby-Doo!™ Complete [OTC] *see* vitamins (multiple/pediatric) *on page 952*

One A Day® Kids Scooby-Doo!™ Gummies [OTC] *see* vitamins (multiple/pediatric) *on page 952*

One A Day® Maximum [OTC] *see* vitamins (multiple/oral) *on page 951*

One A Day® Men's 50+ Advantage [OTC] *see* vitamins (multiple/oral) *on page 951*

One A Day® Men's Health Formula [OTC] *see* vitamins (multiple/oral) *on page 951*

One A Day® Teen Advantage for Her [OTC] *see* vitamins (multiple/oral) *on page 951*

One A Day® Teen Advantage for Him [OTC] *see* vitamins (multiple/oral) *on page 951*

One A Day® Weight Smart® Advanced [OTC] *see* vitamins (multiple/oral) *on page 951*

One A Day® Women's 50+ Advantage [OTC] *see* vitamins (multiple/oral) *on page 951*

One A Day® Women's [OTC] *see* vitamins (multiple/oral) *on page 951*

One A Day® Women's Active Mind & Body [OTC] *see* vitamins (multiple/oral) *on page 951*

One A Day® Women's Prenatal [OTC] *see* vitamins (multiple/prenatal) *on page 952*

One-Alpha® (Can) *see* alfacalcidol *(Canada only) on page 46*
One Gram C [OTC] *see* ascorbic acid *on page 94*
One Tab™ Allergy & Sinus [OTC] *see* acetaminophen, diphenhydramine, and phenylephrine *on page 29*
One Tab™ Cold & Flu [OTC] *see* acetaminophen, diphenhydramine, and phenylephrine *on page 29*
OneTab™ Congestion & Cold [OTC] *see* guaifenesin and phenylephrine *on page 435*
Onfi™ *see* clobazam *on page 220*
Onglyza™ *see* saxagliptin *on page 825*
Onsolis® *see* fentanyl *on page 377*
ONTAK® *see* denileukin diftitox *on page 260*
Opana® *see* oxymorphone *on page 682*
Opana® ER *see* oxymorphone *on page 682*
OPC-13013 *see* cilostazol *on page 209*
OPC-14597 *see* aripiprazole *on page 90*
OPC-41061 *see* tolvaptan *on page 905*
OP-CCK *see* sincalide *on page 835*
Opcon-A® [OTC] *see* naphazoline and pheniramine *on page 627*
o,p′-DDD *see* mitotane *on page 607*
Operand® Chlorhexidine Gluconate [OTC] *see* chlorhexidine gluconate *on page 196*
Operand® Povidone-Iodine [OTC] *see* povidone-iodine (topical) *on page 747*
Ophtho-Dipivefrin™ (Can) *see* dipivefrin *on page 300*
Ophtho-Tate® (Can) *see* prednisolone (ophthalmic) *on page 754*
opium and belladonna *see* belladonna and opium *on page 118*

opium tincture (OH pee um TING chur)

Medication Safety Issues

Sound-alike/look-alike issues:

Opium tincture may be confused with camphorated tincture of opium (paregoric)

High alert medication:

The Institute for Safe Medication Practices (ISMP) includes this medication among its list of drugs which have a heightened risk of causing significant patient harm when used in error.

Administration issues:

Use care when prescribing opium tincture; opium tincture is 25 times more concentrated than paregoric, each undiluted mL of opium tincture contains the equivalent of morphine 10 mg/mL.

If opium tincture is used in neonates, a 25-fold dilution should be prepared (final concentration: 0.4 mg/mL morphine). Of note, paregoric (which contains the equivalent of morphine 0.4 mg/mL) is **not** recommended for use in neonates due to the high alcohol content (~45%) and the presence of other additives; as an alternative to the use of diluted opium tincture or paregoric, ISMP recommends using a diluted preservative free injectable morphine solution orally.

Although historically opium tincture is dosed as mL/kg, the preferred dosing units are **mg**/kg (Levine, 2001). ISMP suggests hospitals evaluate the need for this product at their institution.

Other safety concerns:

DTO is an error-prone abbreviation and should never be used as an abbreviation for opium tincture (also known as *Deodorized* Tincture of Opium) due to potential for being mistaken as *Diluted* Tincture of Opium

Synonyms deodorized tincture of opium (error-prone synonym); DTO (error-prone abbreviation); opium tincture, deodorized; tincture of opium

Therapeutic Category Analgesic, Narcotic

Controlled Substance C-II

Use Treatment of diarrhea in adults

General Dosage Range

Oral: Opium tincture 10% contains morphine 10 mg/mL. Use caution in ordering, dispensing, and/or administering. The following doses are expressed in **mg** (milligram) dosing units of morphine.

Adults: Usual: 6 **mg** of undiluted opium tincture (10 mg/mL) 4 times daily

Dosage Forms

Tincture, oral: Anhydrous morphine 10 mg/mL (118 mL, 120 mL, 473 mL, 480 mL)

opium tincture, deodorized *see* opium tincture *on page 669*

oprelvekin (oh PREL ve kin)

Medication Safety Issues

Sound-alike/look-alike issues:

Oprelvekin may be confused with aldesleukin, Proleukin®

Neumega® may be confused with Neulasta®, Neupogen®

Synonyms IL-11; interleukin-11; recombinant human interleukin-11; recombinant interleukin-11; rhIL-11

U.S. Brand Names Neumega®

Therapeutic Category Platelet Growth Factor

Use Prevention of severe thrombocytopenia; reduce the need for platelet transfusions following myelosuppressive chemotherapy for nonmyeloid malignancy

General Dosage Range Dosage adjustment recommended in patients with renal impairment

SubQ: *Adults:* 50 mcg/kg once daily

Dosage Forms

Injection, powder for reconstitution [preservative free]:

Neumega®: 5 mg

OPT-80 *see* fidaxomicin *on page* 383
Optase™ *see* trypsin, balsam Peru, and castor oil *on page* 925
Optho-Bunolol® (Can) *see* levobunolol *on page* 529
Opti-Clear [OTC] *see* tetrahydrozoline (ophthalmic) *on page* 885
Opticrom® (Can) *see* cromolyn (ophthalmic) *on page* 241
OptiMARK® *see* gadoversetamide *on page* 417
Optimyxin® (Can) *see* bacitracin and polymyxin B *on page* 111
Optimyxin Plus® (Can) *see* neomycin, polymyxin B, and gramicidin *on page* 634
OptiNate® *see* vitamins (multiple/prenatal) *on page* 952
OptiPranolol® *see* metipranolol *on page* 593
Optiray® 240 *see* ioversol *on page* 497
Optiray® 300 *see* ioversol *on page* 497
Optiray® 320 *see* ioversol *on page* 497
Optiray® 350 *see* ioversol *on page* 497
Optivar® *see* azelastine (ophthalmic) *on page* 107
Optive™ [OTC] *see* carboxymethylcellulose *on page* 176
Optivite® P.M.T. [OTC] *see* vitamins (multiple/oral) *on page* 951
Orabase® with Benzocaine [OTC] *see* benzocaine *on page* 121
Orabloc™™ *see* articaine and epinephrine *on page* 92
Oracea® *see* doxycycline *on page* 314
Oracort (Can) *see* triamcinolone (topical) *on page* 916
Orajel® [OTC] *see* benzocaine *on page* 121
Orajel® Baby Daytime and Nighttime [OTC] *see* benzocaine *on page* 121
Orajel® Baby Teething [OTC] *see* benzocaine *on page* 121
Orajel® Baby Teething Nighttime [OTC] *see* benzocaine *on page* 121
Orajel® Cold Sore [OTC] *see* benzocaine *on page* 121
Orajel® Denture Plus [OTC] *see* benzocaine *on page* 121
Orajel® Dry Mouth [OTC] *see* glycerin *on page* 429
Orajel® Maximum Strength [OTC] *see* benzocaine *on page* 121
Orajel® Medicated Mouth Sore [OTC] *see* benzocaine *on page* 121
Orajel® Medicated Toothache [OTC] *see* benzocaine *on page* 121
Orajel® Mouth Sore [OTC] *see* benzocaine *on page* 121
Orajel® Multi-Action Cold Sore [OTC] *see* benzocaine *on page* 121
Orajel® PM Maximum Strength [OTC] *see* benzocaine *on page* 121
Orajel® Ultra Mouth Sore [OTC] *see* benzocaine *on page* 121
oral cholera vaccine *see* traveler's diarrhea and cholera vaccine *(Canada only) on page* 911
Oralone® *see* triamcinolone (topical) *on page* 916
Oral Purgative (Can) *see* sodium picosulfate, magnesium oxide, and citric acid *on page* 846
Oramorph® SR *see* morphine (systemic) *on page* 612

Oranyl [OTC] *see* pseudoephedrine *on page* 771
Orap® *see* pimozide *on page* 723
Orapred® *see* prednisolone (systemic) *on page* 754
Orapred ODT® *see* prednisolone (systemic) *on page* 754
Oraqix® *see* lidocaine and prilocaine *on page* 538
OraVerse™ *see* phentolamine *on page* 715
Oravig® [DSC] *see* miconazole (oral) *on page* 599
Oraxyl™ *see* doxycycline *on page* 314
Orazinc® 110 [OTC] *see* zinc sulfate *on page* 963
Orazinc® 220 [OTC] *see* zinc sulfate *on page* 963
Orbivan™ *see* butalbital, acetaminophen, and caffeine *on page* 153
orciprenaline sulfate *see* metaproterenol *on page* 579
Orencia® *see* abatacept *on page* 16
Orfadin® *see* nitisinone *on page* 644
ORG 946 *see* rocuronium *on page* 808
Orgalutran® (Can) *see* ganirelix *on page* 419
Organ-I NR [OTC] *see* guaifenesin *on page* 433
Orgaran® (Can) *see* danaparoid *(Canada only) on page* 252
ORG NC 45 *see* vecuronium *on page* 940
Orinase *see* tolbutamide *on page* 903

orlistat (OR li stat)

Medication Safety Issues

Sound-alike/look-alike issues:

Xenical® may be confused with Xeloda®

U.S. Brand Names Alli® [OTC]; Xenical®

Canadian Brand Names Xenical®

Therapeutic Category Lipase Inhibitor

Use Management of obesity, including weight loss and weight management, when used in conjunction with a reduced-calorie and low-fat diet; reduce the risk of weight regain after prior weight loss; indicated for obese patients with an initial body mass index (BMI) ≥30 kg/m^2 or ≥27 kg/m^2 in the presence of other risk factors (eg, diabetes, dyslipidemia, hypertension)

General Dosage Range Oral:

Children ≥12 years and Adults: Xenical®: 120 mg 3 times/day
Adults: Alli™ (OTC labeling): 60 mg 3 times/day

Dosage Forms

Capsule, oral:
Alli® [OTC]: 60 mg
Xenical®: 120 mg

Ornex® [OTC] *see* acetaminophen and pseudoephedrine *on page* 25
Ornex® Maximum Strength [OTC] *see* acetaminophen and pseudoephedrine *on page* 25
ORO-Clense (Can) *see* chlorhexidine gluconate *on page* 196
Orphenace® (Can) *see* orphenadrine *on page* 671

orphenadrine (or FEN a dreen)

Medication Safety Issues

Sound-alike/look-alike issues:

Norflex™ may be confused with norfloxacin, Noroxin®

BEERS Criteria medication:

This drug may be potentially inappropriate for use in geriatric patients (Quality of evidence - moderate; Strength of recommendation - strong).

International issues:

Flexin: Brand name for orphenadrine [Israel] but is also the brand name for cyclobenzaprine [Chile] and diclofenac [Argentina]

Flexin [Israel] may be confused with Floxin which is a brand name for flunarizine [Thailand], norfloxacin [South Africa], ofloxacin [U.S., Canada], and perfloxacin [Philippines]

Synonyms orphenadrine citrate
U.S. Brand Names Norflex™
Canadian Brand Names Norflex™; Orphenace®; Rhoxal-orphendrine
Therapeutic Category Skeletal Muscle Relaxant
Use Treatment of muscle spasm associated with acute painful musculoskeletal conditions
General Dosage Range
I.M., I.V.: *Adults:* 60 mg every 12 hours
Oral: *Adults:* 100 mg twice daily
Dosage Forms
Injection, solution: 30 mg/mL (2 mL)
Norflex™: 30 mg/mL (2 mL)
Injection, solution [preservative free]: 30 mg/mL (2 mL)
Tablet, extended release, oral: 100 mg

orphenadrine, aspirin, and caffeine (or FEN a dreen, AS pir in, & KAF een)

Medication Safety Issues
BEERS Criteria medication:
This drug may be potentially inappropriate for use in geriatric patients (Quality of evidence - moderate; Strength of recommendation - strong).
Synonyms aspirin, caffeine, and orphenadrine; aspirin, orphenadrine, and caffeine; caffeine, orphenadrine, and aspirin; Norgesic
Therapeutic Category Analgesic, Nonnarcotic; Skeletal Muscle Relaxant
Use Relief of discomfort associated with skeletal muscular conditions
General Dosage Range Oral: *Adults:* 1-2 tablets 3-4 times/day
Dosage Forms
Tablet: Orphenadrine 25 mg, aspirin 385 mg, and caffeine 30 mg; orphenadrine 50 mg, aspirin 770 mg, and caffeine 60 mg

orphenadrine citrate *see* orphenadrine *on page 671*
Orsythia™ *see* ethinyl estradiol and levonorgestrel *on page 357*
Ortho® 0.5/35 (Can) *see* ethinyl estradiol and norethindrone *on page 359*
Ortho® 1/35 (Can) *see* ethinyl estradiol and norethindrone *on page 359*
Ortho® 7/7/7 (Can) *see* ethinyl estradiol and norethindrone *on page 359*
Ortho-Cept® *see* ethinyl estradiol and desogestrel *on page 356*
Ortho-Cyclen® *see* ethinyl estradiol and norgestimate *on page 361*
Ortho Est *see* estropipate *on page 353*
Ortho Evra® *see* ethinyl estradiol and norelgestromin *on page 359*
Ortho Micronor® *see* norethindrone *on page 648*
Ortho Novum *see* ethinyl estradiol and norethindrone *on page 359*
Ortho-Novum® 1/35 *see* ethinyl estradiol and norethindrone *on page 359*
Ortho Novum 1/50 *see* norethindrone and mestranol *on page 649*
Ortho-Novum® 1/50 (Can) *see* norethindrone and mestranol *on page 649*
Ortho-Novum® 7/7/7 *see* ethinyl estradiol and norethindrone *on page 359*
ortho,para-DDD *see* mitotane *on page 607*
Ortho Prefest *see* estradiol and norgestimate *on page 350*
Ortho Tri-Cyclen® *see* ethinyl estradiol and norgestimate *on page 361*
Ortho Tri-Cyclen® Lo *see* ethinyl estradiol and norgestimate *on page 361*
Orthovisc® *see* hyaluronate and derivatives *on page 450*
OrthoVisc® (Can) *see* hyaluronate and derivatives *on page 450*
OrthoWash™ *see* fluoride *on page 393*
Orviban® CF *see* butalbital and acetaminophen *on page 154*
oscal *see* calcium carbonate *on page 161*
Os-Cal® (Can) *see* calcium carbonate *on page 161*
Os-Cal® 500+D [OTC] *see* calcium and vitamin D *on page 161*
Oscimin *see* hyoscyamine *on page 465*

oseltamivir (oh sel TAM i vir)

Medication Safety Issues

Sound-alike/look-alike issues:

Tamiflu® may be confused with Tambocor™, Thera-Flu®

Other safety concerns:

Oseltamivir (Tamiflu®) oral suspension is packaged with an oral syringe. When dispensing commercially prepared oseltamivir oral suspension, verify the intended concentration to be dispensed and the correct dose, dosing instructions, and oral dosing device provided for the patient. Oseltamivir oral suspension is available in a 6 mg/mL concentration. The previous concentration (12 mg/mL) has been discontinued, but may be still be on the market until product expires. The 6 mg/mL concentration is packaged with an oral syringe calibrated in **milliliters** up to a total of 10 mL. The previous, discontinued concentration (12 mg/mL) was packaged with an oral syringe calibrated in mg (30 mg, 45 mg, and 60 mg graduations). **When the oral syringe is dispensed, instructions to the patient should be provided based on these units of measure (ie, mL or mg). Do NOT dispense an oral syringe with units of measure in milligrams when providing oseltamivir suspension for children <1 year of age** instead supply an oral syringe capable of measuring mL doses. Patients should always be provided with a measuring device calibrated the same way as their labeled instructions.

When commercially-prepared oseltamivir oral suspension is not available, an extemporaneously prepared suspension may be compounded to provide a 6 mg/mL concentration (to match the preferred, currently manufactured commercially available oral suspension concentration).

U.S. Brand Names Tamiflu®

Canadian Brand Names Tamiflu®

Therapeutic Category Antiviral Agent, Oral

Use Treatment of uncomplicated acute illness due to influenza (A or B) infection in children ≥1 year of age and adults who have been symptomatic for no more than 2 days; prophylaxis against influenza (A or B) infection in children ≥1 year of age and adults

The Advisory Committee on Immunization Practices (ACIP) recommends that **treatment** be considered for the following:

- Persons with severe, complicated or progressive illness
- Hospitalized persons
- Persons at higher risk for influenza complications:
  - Children <2 years of age (highest risk in children <6 months of age)
  - Adults ≥65 years of age
  - Persons with chronic disorders of the pulmonary (including asthma) or cardiovascular systems (except hypertension)
  - Persons with chronic metabolic diseases (including diabetes mellitus), hepatic disease, renal dysfunction, hematologic disorders (including sickle cell disease), or immunosuppression (including immunosuppression caused by medications or HIV)
  - Persons with neurologic/neuromuscular conditions (including conditions such as spinal cord injuries, seizure disorders, cerebral palsy, stroke, mental retardation, moderate to severe developmental delay, or muscular dystrophy) which may compromise respiratory function, the handling of respiratory secretions, or that can increase the risk of aspiration
  - Pregnant or postpartum women (≤2 weeks after delivery)
  - Persons <19 years of age on long-term aspirin therapy
  - American Indians and Alaskan Natives
  - Persons who are morbidly obese (BMI ≥40)
  - Residents of nursing homes or other chronic care facilities
- Use may also be considered for previously healthy, nonhigh-risk outpatients with confirmed or suspected influenza based on clinical judgment when treatment can be started within 48 hours of illness onset.

The ACIP recommends that **prophylaxis** be considered for the following:

- Postexposure prophylaxis may be considered for family or close contacts of suspected or confirmed cases, who are at higher risk of influenza complications, and who have not been vaccinated against the circulating strain at the time of the exposure.
- Postexposure prophylaxis may be considered for unvaccinated healthcare workers who had occupational exposure without protective equipment.
- Preexposure prophylaxis should only be used for persons at very high risk of influenza complications who cannot be otherwise protected at times of high risk for exposure.
- Prophylaxis should also be administered to all eligible residents of institutions that house patients at high risk when needed to control outbreaks.

The ACIP recommends that treatment and prophylaxis be given to children <1 year of age when indicated.

General Dosage Range Dosage adjustment recommended in patients with renal impairment

Oral:

Children <1 year: 3 mg/kg/dose once daily

Children 1-12 years and ≤15 kg: 30 mg once or twice daily

Children 1-12 years and >15 to ≤23 kg: 45 mg once or twice daily

Children 1-12 years and >23 to ≤40 kg: 60 mg once or twice daily

Children 1-12 years and >40 kg, Children ≥13 years, and Adults: 75 mg once or twice daily

Dosage Forms

Capsule, oral:

Tamiflu®: 30 mg, 45 mg, 75 mg

Powder for suspension, oral:

Tamiflu®: 6 mg/mL (60 mL)

OSI-774 *see* erlotinib *on page* 341
Osmitrol *see* mannitol *on page* 561
Osmitrol® (Can) *see* mannitol *on page* 561
OsmoPrep® *see* sodium phosphates *on page* 845
Osmovist® (Can) *see* iotrolan *(Canada only) on page* 497
Osteocit® (Can) *see* calcium citrate *on page* 164
Ostoforte® (Can) *see* ergocalciferol *on page* 339
OTFC (oral transmucosal fentanyl citrate) *see* fentanyl *on page* 377
Otix® [OTC] *see* carbamide peroxide *on page* 173
Outgro® [OTC] *see* benzocaine *on page* 121
Ovace® *see* sulfacetamide (topical) *on page* 858
Ovace® Plus *see* sulfacetamide (topical) *on page* 858
Ovcon® 35 *see* ethinyl estradiol and norethindrone *on page* 359
Ovcon® 50 [DSC] *see* ethinyl estradiol and norethindrone *on page* 359
Ovide® *see* malathion *on page* 561
Ovidrel® *see* chorionic gonadotropin (recombinant) *on page* 206
ovine corticotrophin-releasing hormone (oCRH) *see* corticorelin *on page* 237
Ovol® (Can) *see* simethicone *on page* 834
Ovral® (Can) *see* ethinyl estradiol and norgestrel *on page* 362

oxacillin (oks a SIL in)

Synonyms methylphenyl isoxazolyl penicillin; oxacillin sodium

Therapeutic Category Penicillin

Use Treatment of infections such as osteomyelitis, septicemia, endocarditis, and CNS infections caused by susceptible strains of *Staphylococcus*

General Dosage Range I.M., I.V.:

Children: 100-200 mg/kg/day in divided doses every 6 hours (maximum: 12 g/day)

Adults: 250-2000 mg every 4-6 hours

Dosage Forms

Infusion, premixed iso-osmotic solution: 1 g (50 mL); 2 g (50 mL)

Injection, powder for reconstitution: 1 g, 2 g, 10 g

oxacillin sodium *see* oxacillin *on page* 674
oxalatoplatin *see* oxaliplatin *on page* 674
oxalatoplatinum *see* oxaliplatin *on page* 674

oxaliplatin (ox AL i pla tin)

Medication Safety Issues

Sound-alike/look-alike issues:

Oxaliplatin may be confused with Aloxi®, carboplatin, cisplatin

High alert medication:

This medication is in a class the Institute for Safe Medication Practices (ISMP) includes among its list of drug classes which have a heightened risk of causing significant patient harm when used in error.

Synonyms diaminocyclohexane oxalatoplatinum; L-OHP; oxalatoplatin; oxalatoplatinum

U.S. Brand Names Eloxatin®

Canadian Brand Names Eloxatin®

Therapeutic Category Antineoplastic Agent, Alkylating Agent

Use Treatment of stage III colon cancer (adjuvant) after complete resection of primary tumor; treatment of advanced colorectal cancer

General Dosage Range Dosage adjustment recommended in patients with renal impairment or who develop toxicities

I.V.: *Adults:* 85 mg/m^2 every 2 weeks

Dosage Forms

Injection, solution [preservative free]:

Eloxatin®: 5 mg/mL (10 mL, 20 mL, 40 mL)

Dosage Forms - Canada

Injection, powder for reconstitution:

Eloxatin®: 50 mg, 100 mg

Oxandrin® *see* oxandrolone *on page* 675

oxandrolone (oks AN droe lone)

U.S. Brand Names Oxandrin®

Therapeutic Category Androgen

Controlled Substance C-III

Use Adjunctive therapy to promote weight gain after weight loss following extensive surgery, chronic infections, or severe trauma, and in some patients who, without definite pathophysiologic reasons, fail to gain or to maintain normal weight; to offset protein catabolism with prolonged corticosteroid administration; relief of bone pain associated with osteoporosis

General Dosage Range Oral:

Children: ≤0.1 mg/kg/day or ≤0.045 mg/lb/day

Adults: 2.5-20 mg/day in 2-4 divided doses

Elderly: 5 mg twice daily

Dosage Forms

Tablet, oral: 2.5 mg, 10 mg

Oxandrin®: 2.5 mg, 10 mg

oxaprozin (oks a PROE zin)

Medication Safety Issues

Sound-alike/look-alike issues:

Oxaprozin may be confused with oxazepam

BEERS Criteria medication:

This drug may be potentially inappropriate for use in geriatric patients (Quality of evidence - moderate; Strength of recommendation - strong).

U.S. Brand Names Daypro®

Canadian Brand Names Apo-Oxaprozin®; Daypro®

Therapeutic Category Analgesic, Nonnarcotic; Nonsteroidal Antiinflammatory Drug (NSAID)

Use Management of signs and symptoms of osteoarthritis, rheumatoid arthritis, and juvenile idiopathic arthritis (JIA)

General Dosage Range Dosage adjustment recommended in patients with renal impairment

Oral:

Children 6-16 years and 22-31 kg: 600 mg once daily

Children 6-16 years and 32-54 kg: 900 mg once daily

Children 6-16 years and ≥55 kg: 1200 mg once daily

Adults: 600-1800 mg once daily (maximum: 1200 mg daily [<50 kg]; 1800 mg daily or 26 mg/kg/day (whichever lower) [>50 kg])

Dosage Forms

Caplet, oral:

Daypro®: 600 mg

Tablet, oral: 600 mg

oxazepam (oks A ze pam)

Medication Safety Issues

Sound-alike/look-alike issues:

Oxazepam may be confused with oxaprozin, quazepam

Serax may be confused with Eurax®, Urex, ZyrTEC®

BEERS Criteria medication:

This drug may be potentially inappropriate for use in geriatric patients (Quality of evidence - high; Strength of recommendation - strong).

International issues:

Murelax [Australia] may be confused with MiraLax brand name for polyethylene glycol 3350 [U.S.]

Synonyms Serax

Canadian Brand Names Apo-Oxazepam®; Bio-Oxazepam; Novoxapram®; Oxpam®; Oxpram®; PMS-Oxazepam; Riva-Oxazepam

Therapeutic Category Anticonvulsant; Benzodiazepine

Controlled Substance C-IV

Use Treatment of anxiety; management of ethanol withdrawal

General Dosage Range Oral:

Adults: 10-30 mg 3-4 times/day

Elderly: Initial: 10 mg 2-3 times/day; Maintenance: 30-45 mg/day

Dosage Forms

Capsule, oral: 10 mg, 15 mg, 30 mg

oxcarbazepine (ox car BAZ e peen)

Medication Safety Issues

Sound-alike/look-alike issues:

OXcarbazepine may be confused with carBAMazepine

Trileptal® may be confused with TriLipix®

Synonyms GP 47680; OCBZ

Tall-Man **OX**carbazepine

U.S. Brand Names Trileptal®

Canadian Brand Names Apo-Oxcarbazepine®; Trileptal®

Therapeutic Category Anticonvulsant

Use Monotherapy or adjunctive therapy in the treatment of partial seizures in adults and children ≥4 years of age with epilepsy; adjunctive therapy in the treatment of partial seizures in children ≥2 years of age with epilepsy

General Dosage Range Dosage adjustment recommended in patients with renal impairment

Oral:

Children 2-3 years and <20 kg: Initial: 8-20 mg/kg/day (maximum: 600 mg/day) in 2 divided doses; Maintenance: maximum of 60 mg/kg/day in 2 divided doses

Children 2-3 years and ≥20 kg: Initial: 8-10 mg/kg/day (maximum: 600 mg/day) in 2 divided doses; Maintenance: maximum of 60 mg/kg/day in 2 divided doses

Children 4-16 years and <25 kg: Initial: 8-10 mg/kg/day (maximum: 600 mg/day) in 2 divided doses; Maintenance: up to 900 mg/day

Children 4-16 years and 25-30 kg: Initial: 8-10 mg/kg/day (maximum: 600 mg/day) in 2 divided doses; Maintenance: up to 1200 mg/day

Children 4-16 years and 31-45 kg: Initial: 8-10 mg/kg/day (maximum: 600 mg/day) in 2 divided doses; Maintenance: up to 1500 mg/day

Children 4-16 years and 46-55 kg: Initial: 8-10 mg/kg/day (maximum: 600 mg/day) in 2 divided doses; Maintenance: up to 1800 mg/day

Children 4-16 years and >56 kg: Initial: 8-10 mg/kg/day (maximum: 600 mg/day) in 2 divided doses; Maintenance: up to 2100 mg/day

Children >16 years and Adults: Initial: 300 mg twice daily; Maintenance: 1200-2400 mg/day in 2 divided doses (maximum: 2400 mg/day)

Dosage Forms

Suspension, oral: 300 mg/5 mL (250 mL)

Trileptal®: 300 mg/5 mL (250 mL)

Tablet, oral: 150 mg, 300 mg, 600 mg

Trileptal®: 150 mg, 300 mg, 600 mg

Oxecta™ *see* oxycodone *on page 678*

Oxeze® Turbuhaler® (Can) *see* formoterol *on page 406*

oxiconazole (oks i KON a zole)

Synonyms oxiconazole nitrate

U.S. Brand Names Oxistat®

Canadian Brand Names Oxistat®

Therapeutic Category Antifungal Agent

Use Treatment of tinea pedis (athlete's foot), tinea cruris (jock itch), tinea corporis (ringworm), and tinea (pityriasis) versicolor

General Dosage Range Topical: *Children and Adults:* Apply to affected areas 1-2 times daily

Dosage Forms

Cream, topical:

Oxistat®: 1% (30 g, 60 g)

Lotion, topical:

Oxistat®: 1% (30 mL, 60 mL)

oxiconazole nitrate *see* oxiconazole *on page 677*

oxidized regenerated cellulose *see* cellulose, oxidized regenerated *on page 188*

Oxilan® 300 *see* ioxilan *on page 498*

Oxilan® 350 *see* ioxilan *on page 498*

oxilapine succinate *see* loxapine *on page 554*

Oxipor® VHC [OTC] *see* coal tar *on page 228*

Oxistat® *see* oxiconazole *on page 677*

Oxpam® (Can) *see* oxazepam *on page 676*

oxpentifylline *see* pentoxifylline *on page 707*

Oxpram® (Can) *see* oxazepam *on page 676*

Oxsoralen® *see* methoxsalen (topical) *on page 586*

Oxsoralen® Capsule (Can) *see* methoxsalen (systemic) *on page 586*

Oxsoralen® Lotion (Can) *see* methoxsalen (topical) *on page 586*

Oxsoralen-Ultra® *see* methoxsalen (systemic) *on page 586*

OXY® [OTC] *see* salicylic acid *on page 816*

oxybate *see* sodium oxybate *on page 844*

OXY® Body Wash [OTC] *see* salicylic acid *on page 816*

Oxybutyn (Can) *see* oxybutynin *on page 677*

oxybutynin (oks i BYOO ti nin)

Medication Safety Issues

Sound-alike/look-alike issues:

Oxybutynin may be confused with OxyCONTIN®

Ditropan may be confused with Detrol®, diazepam, Diprivan®, dithranol

BEERS Criteria medication:

This drug may be potentially inappropriate for use in geriatric patients (Quality of evidence - varies based on comorbidity; Strength of recommendation - varies based on comorbidity)

Other safety concerns:

Transdermal patch may contain conducting metal (eg, aluminum); remove patch prior to MRI.

Synonyms Ditropan; oxybutynin chloride

U.S. Brand Names Ditropan XL®; Gelnique 3%™; Gelnique®; Oxytrol®

Canadian Brand Names Apo-Oxybutynin®; Ditropan XL®; Dom-Oxybutynin; Gelnique®; Mylan-Oxybutynin; Novo-Oxybutynin; Nu-Oxybutyn; Oxybutyn; Oxybutynine; Oxytrol®; PHL-Oxybutynin; PMS-Oxybutynin; Riva-Oxybutynin; Uromax®

Therapeutic Category Antispasmodic Agent, Urinary

Use Antispasmodic for neurogenic bladder (urgency, frequency, leakage, urge incontinence, dysuria); extended release formulation also indicated for treatment of symptoms associated with detrusor overactivity due to a neurological condition (eg, spina bifida)

General Dosage Range

Oral:

Extended release:

Children ≥6 years: 5 mg once daily (maximum: 20 mg/day)

Adults: Initial: 5-10 mg once daily; Maintenance: 5-30 mg once daily (maximum: 30 mg/day)

Immediate release:

Children ≥5 years: 5 mg 2-3 times/day (maximum: 15 mg/day)

Adults: 5 mg 2-4 times/day (maximum: 20 mg/day)

Elderly: 2.5 mg 2-3 times/day

Topical gel: *Adults:* Gelnique 3%™: Apply 3 pumps (84 mg) once daily; Gelnique® 10%: Apply contents of 1 sachet (100 mg/g) once daily

Transdermal: *Adults:* Apply one 3.9 mg/day patch twice weekly

Dosage Forms

Gel, topical:

Gelnique 3%™: 3% (92 g)

Gelnique®: 10% (1 g)

Patch, transdermal:

Oxytrol®: 3.9 mg/24 hours (8s)

Syrup, oral: 5 mg/5 mL (5 mL, 473 mL, 480 mL)

Tablet, oral: 5 mg

Tablet, extended release, oral: 5 mg, 10 mg, 15 mg

Ditropan XL®: 5 mg, 10 mg, 15 mg

oxybutynin chloride *see* oxybutynin *on page* 677

Oxybutynine (Can) *see* oxybutynin *on page* 677

OXY® Chill Factor® [OTC] *see* salicylic acid *on page* 816

oxychlorosene (oks i KLOR oh seen)

Synonyms oxychlorosene sodium

U.S. Brand Names Clorpactin® WCS-90 [OTC]

Therapeutic Category Antibiotic, Topical

Use Treatment of localized infections

General Dosage Range **Topical:** *Adults:* Apply by irrigation, instillation, spray, soaks, or wet compresses

Dosage Forms

Powder for solution, topical:

Clorpactin® WCS-90 [OTC]: 2 g/bottle

oxychlorosene sodium *see* oxychlorosene *on page* 678

OXY® Clinical Clearing Treatment [OTC] *see* benzoyl peroxide *on page* 124

Oxycocet® (Can) *see* oxycodone and acetaminophen *on page* 679

Oxycodan® (Can) *see* oxycodone and aspirin *on page* 680

oxycodone (oks i KOE done)

Medication Safety Issues

Sound-alike/look-alike issues:

OxyCODONE may be confused with HYDROcodone, OxyCONTIN®, oxymorphone

OxyCONTIN® may be confused with MS Contin®, oxybutynin

OxyFast® may be confused with Roxanol

Roxicodone® may be confused with Roxanol

High alert medication:

The Institute for Safe Medication Practices (ISMP) includes this medication among its list of drug classes which have a heightened risk of causing significant patient harm when used in error.

Synonyms dihydrohydroxycodeinone; oxycodone hydrochloride

Tall-Man oxy**CODONE**

U.S. Brand Names Oxecta™; OxyCONTIN®; Roxicodone®

Canadian Brand Names Oxy.IR®; OxyContin®; OxyNEO™; PMS-Oxycodone; Supeudol®

Therapeutic Category Analgesic, Narcotic

Controlled Substance C-II

Use Management of moderate-to-severe pain, normally used in combination with nonopioid analgesics

OxyContin® is indicated for around-the-clock management of moderate-to-severe pain when an analgesic is needed for an extended period of time.

General Dosage Range Dosage adjustment recommended in patients with hepatic impairment or on concomitant therapy

Oral:

Controlled release: *Adults:* 10-160 mg every 12 hours

Immediate release: *Adults:* 5-20 mg every 4-6 hours as needed

Dosage Forms

Capsule, oral: 5 mg

Solution, oral: 5 mg/5 mL (5 mL, 500 mL); 20 mg/mL (30 mL)

Tablet, oral: 5 mg, 10 mg, 15 mg, 20 mg, 30 mg

Oxecta™: 5 mg, 7.5 mg

Roxicodone®: 5 mg, 15 mg, 30 mg

Tablet, controlled release, oral:

OxyCONTIN®: 10 mg, 15 mg, 20 mg, 30 mg, 40 mg, 60 mg, 80 mg

oxycodone and acetaminophen (oks i KOE done & a seet a MIN oh fen)

Medication Safety Issues

Sound-alike/look-alike issues:

Endocet® may be confused with Indocid®

Percocet® may be confused with Fioricet®, Percodan®

Roxicet™ may be confused with Roxanol

Tylox® may be confused with Trimox, Tylenol®, Xanax®

High alert medication:

The Institute for Safe Medication Practices (ISMP) includes this medication among its list of drug classes which have a heightened risk of causing significant patient harm when used in error.

Other safety concerns:

Duplicate therapy issues: This product contains acetaminophen, which may be a component of other combination products. Do not exceed the maximum recommended daily dose of acetaminophen.

Synonyms acetaminophen and oxycodone

U.S. Brand Names Endocet®; Percocet®; Primlev™; Roxicet™; Roxicet™ 5/500; Tylox®

Canadian Brand Names Endocet®; Novo-Oxycodone Acet; Oxycocet®; Percocet®; Percocet®-Demi; PMS-Oxycodone-Acetaminophen

Therapeutic Category Analgesic, Narcotic

Controlled Substance C-II

Use Management of moderate-to-severe pain

General Dosage Range Dosage adjustment recommended in patients with hepatic impairment

Oral:

Acetaminophen:

Children <45 kg: 10-15 mg/kg every 4-6 hours as needed (maximum: 90 mg/kg/day)

Children ≥45 kg: 10-15 mg/kg every 4-6 hours (maximum: 4 g/day)

Adults: 325-650 mg every 4-6 hours (maximum: 4 g/day)

Oxycodone:

Children: 0.05-0.3 mg/kg every 4-6 hours as needed

Adults: 2.5-30 mg/dose every 4-6 hours as needed

Elderly: Initial: 2.5-5 mg every 6 hours as needed

Dosage Forms

Caplet: Oxycodone 5 mg and acetaminophen 500 mg

Roxicet™ 5/500: Oxycodone 5 mg and acetaminophen 500 mg

Capsule: Oxycodone 5 mg and acetaminophen 500 mg

Tylox®: Oxycodone 5 mg and acetaminophen 500 mg

Solution, oral: Oxycodone 5 mg and acetaminophen 325 mg per 5 mL

Roxicet™: Oxycodone 5 mg and acetaminophen 325 mg per 5 mL

Tablet:
Generics:
Oxycodone 2.5 mg and acetaminophen 325 mg
Oxycodone 5 mg and acetaminophen 325 mg
Oxycodone 7.5 mg and acetaminophen 325 mg
Oxycodone 7.5 mg and acetaminophen 500 mg
Oxycodone 10 mg and acetaminophen 325 mg
Oxycodone 10 mg and acetaminophen 650 mg
Brands:
Endocet®:
5/325 [scored]: Oxycodone 5 mg and acetaminophen 325 mg
7.5/325: Oxycodone 7.5 mg and acetaminophen 325 mg
7.5/500: Oxycodone 7.5 mg and acetaminophen 500 mg
10/325: Oxycodone 10 mg and acetaminophen 325 mg
10/650: Oxycodone 10 mg and acetaminophen 650 mg
Percocet®:
2.5/325: Oxycodone 2.5 mg and acetaminophen 325 mg
5/325 [scored]: Oxycodone 5 mg and acetaminophen 325 mg
7.5/325: Oxycodone 7.5 mg and acetaminophen 325 mg
7.5/500: Oxycodone 7.5 mg and acetaminophen 500 mg
10/325: Oxycodone 10 mg and acetaminophen 325 mg
10/650: Oxycodone 10 mg and acetaminophen 650 mg
Primlev™:
5/300: Oxycodone 5 mg and acetaminophen 300 mg
7.5/300: Oxycodone 7.5 mg and acetaminophen 300 mg
10/300: Oxycodone 10 mg and acetaminophen 300 mg
Roxicet™ [scored]: Oxycodone 5 mg and acetaminophen 325 mg

oxycodone and aspirin (oks i KOE done & AS pir in)

Medication Safety Issues
Sound-alike/look-alike issues:
Percodan® may be confused with Decadron, Percocet®, Percogesic®, Periactin
High alert medication:
The Institute for Safe Medication Practices (ISMP) includes this medication among its list of drug classes which have a heightened risk of causing significant patient harm when used in error.

Synonyms aspirin and oxycodone

U.S. Brand Names Endodan®; Percodan®

Canadian Brand Names Endodan®; Oxycodan®; Percodan®

Therapeutic Category Analgesic, Narcotic

Controlled Substance C-II

Use Management of moderate- to moderately-severe pain

General Dosage Range Oral:
Children: 0.1-0.2 mg/kg/dose (based on oxycodone content) every 4-6 hours as needed (maximum: 5 mg/dose [oxycodone]; 4 g/day [aspirin])
Adults: 1 tablet every 6 hours as needed (maximum: 4 g/day [aspirin])

Dosage Forms
Tablet: Oxycodone hydrochloride 4.8355 mg and aspirin 325 mg
Endodan®, Percodan®: Oxycodone hydrochloride 4.8355 mg and aspirin 325 mg

oxycodone and ibuprofen (oks i KOE done & eye byoo PROE fen)

Medication Safety Issues
High alert medication:
The Institute for Safe Medication Practices (ISMP) includes this medication among its list of drug classes which have a heightened risk of causing significant patient harm when used in error.

Synonyms ibuprofen and oxycodone

Therapeutic Category Analgesic, Opioid; Nonsteroidal Antiinflammatory Drug (NSAID), Oral

Controlled Substance C-II

Use Short-term (≤7 days) management of acute, moderate-to-severe pain

General Dosage Range Oral: *Adults:* 1 tablet as needed (maximum: 4 tablets/day; 7 days)

Dosage Forms

Tablet: Oxycodone 5 mg and ibuprofen 400 mg

oxycodone hydrochloride *see* oxycodone *on page 678*
OxyCONTIN® *see* oxycodone *on page 678*
OxyContin® (Can) *see* oxycodone *on page 678*
OXY® Daily [OTC] *see* salicylic acid *on page 816*
OXY® Daily Cleansing [OTC] *see* salicylic acid *on page 816*
Oxyderm™ (Can) *see* benzoyl peroxide *on page 124*
OXY® Face Wash [OTC] *see* salicylic acid *on page 816*
Oxy.IR® (Can) *see* oxycodone *on page 678*
OXY® Maximum [OTC] *see* salicylic acid *on page 816*
OXY® Maximum Daily Cleansing [OTC] *see* salicylic acid *on page 816*
OXY® Maximum Face Wash [OTC] *see* benzoyl peroxide *on page 124*
OXY® Maximum Spot Treatment [OTC] *see* benzoyl peroxide *on page 124*

oxymetazoline (nasal) (oks i met AZ oh leen)

Medication Safety Issues

Sound-alike/look-alike issues:

Oxymetazoline may be confused with oxymetholone
Afrin® may be confused with aspirin
Afrin® (oxymetazoline) may be confused with Afrin® (saline)
Neo-Synephrine® (oxymetazoline) may be confused with Neo-Synephrine® (phenylephrine, nasal)

Synonyms oxymetazoline hydrochloride

U.S. Brand Names 12 Hour Nasal Relief [OTC]; 4-Way® 12 Hour [OTC]; Afrin® Extra Moisturizing [OTC]; Afrin® Original [OTC]; Afrin® Severe Congestion [OTC]; Afrin® Sinus [OTC]; Dristan® [OTC]; Duramist Plus [OTC]; Neo-Synephrine® Nighttime12-Hour [OTC]; Nostrilla® [OTC]; NRS® [OTC]; Vicks® Sinex® VapoSpray 12-Hour; Vicks® Sinex® VapoSpray 12-Hour UltraFine Mist [OTC]; Vicks® Sinex® VapoSpray Moisturizing 12-Hour UltraFine Mist [OTC]

Canadian Brand Names Claritin® Allergic Decongestant; Dristan® Long Lasting Nasal; Drixoral® Nasal

Therapeutic Category Adrenergic Agonist Agent; Imidazoline Derivative

Use Adjunctive therapy for nasal congestion, associated with acute or chronic rhinitis, the common cold, sinusitis, hay fever, or other allergies

General Dosage Range Intranasal: *Children ≥6 years and Adults:* Instill 2-3 sprays into each nostril twice daily

Dosage Forms

Solution, intranasal: 0.05% (15 mL, 30 mL)
12 Hour Nasal Relief [OTC]: 0.05% (15 mL, 30 mL)
4-Way® 12 Hour [OTC]: 0.05% (15 mL)
Afrin® Extra Moisturizing [OTC]: 0.05% (15 mL)
Afrin® Original [OTC]: 0.05% (15 mL, 30 mL)
Afrin® Severe Congestion [OTC]: 0.05% (15 mL)
Afrin® Sinus [OTC]: 0.05% (15 mL)
Dristan® [OTC]: 0.05% (15 mL)
Duramist Plus [OTC]: 0.05% (15 mL)
Neo-Synephrine® Nighttime12-Hour [OTC]: 0.05% (15 mL)
Nostrilla® [OTC]: 0.05% (15 mL)
NRS® [OTC]: 0.05% (15 mL, 30 mL)
Vicks® Sinex® VapoSpray 12-Hour: 0.05% (15 mL)
Vicks® Sinex® VapoSpray 12-Hour UltraFine Mist [OTC]: 0.05% (15 mL)
Vicks® Sinex® VapoSpray Moisturizing 12-Hour UltraFine Mist [OTC]: 0.05% (15 mL)

oxymetazoline (ophthalmic) (oks i met AZ oh leen)

Medication Safety Issues

Sound-alike/look-alike issues:

Oxymetazoline may be confused with oxymetholone
Visine® may be confused with Visken®

Synonyms oxymetazoline hydrochloride

U.S. Brand Names Visine® L.R.® [OTC]

Therapeutic Category Vasoconstrictor

Use Relief of redness of eye due to minor eye irritations

General Dosage Range **Ophthalmic:** *Children ≥6 years and Adults:* Instill 1-2 drops in affected eye(s) every 6 hours as needed

Dosage Forms

Solution, ophthalmic:

Visine® L.R.® [OTC]: 0.025% (15 mL, 30 mL)

oxymetazoline hydrochloride *see* oxymetazoline (nasal) *on page* 681

oxymetazoline hydrochloride *see* oxymetazoline (ophthalmic) *on page* 681

oxymetholone (oks i METH oh lone)

Medication Safety Issues

Sound-alike/look-alike issues:

Oxymetholone may be confused with oxymetazoline, oxymorphone

U.S. Brand Names Anadrol®-50

Therapeutic Category Anabolic Steroid

Controlled Substance C-III

Use Treatment of anemias caused by deficient red cell production

General Dosage Range **Oral:** *Children and Adults:* 1-5 mg/kg once daily

Dosage Forms

Tablet, oral:

Anadrol®-50: 50 mg

oxymorphone (oks i MOR fone)

Medication Safety Issues

Sound-alike/look-alike issues:

Oxymorphone may be confused with oxycodone, oxymetholone

High alert medication:

The Institute for Safe Medication Practices (ISMP) includes this medication among its list of drug classes which have a heightened risk of causing significant patient harm when used in error.

Synonyms oxymorphone hydrochloride

U.S. Brand Names Opana®; Opana® ER

Therapeutic Category Analgesic, Narcotic

Controlled Substance C-II

Use

Parenteral: Management of moderate-to-severe acute pain; relief of anxiety in patients with dyspnea associated with pulmonary edema secondary to acute left ventricular failure

Oral, regular release: Management of moderate-to-severe acute pain

Oral, extended release: Management of moderate-to-severe pain in patients requiring around-the-clock opioid treatment for an extended period of time

General Dosage Range Dosage adjustment recommended in patients with hepatic or renal impairment

I.M., SubQ: *Adults:* Initial: 0.5 mg; Maintenance: 1-1.5 mg every 4-6 hours as needed

I.V.: *Adults:* Initial: 0.5 mg

Oral:

Extended release: *Adults (opioid-naive):* Initial: 5 mg every 12 hours; Maintenance: Titrate upward with 5-10 mg every 12 hours at 3-7 day intervals until desired response

Immediate release: *Adults (opioid-naive):* Initial: 5-20 mg every 4-6 hours; Maintenance: Titrate upward to desired response

Dosage Forms

Injection, solution:

Opana®: 1 mg/mL (1 mL)

Tablet, oral: 5 mg, 10 mg

Opana®: 5 mg, 10 mg

Tablet, extended release, oral: 7.5 mg, 15 mg

Opana® ER: 5 mg, 10 mg, 20 mg, 30 mg, 40 mg

oxymorphone hydrochloride *see* oxymorphone *on page* 682

OxyNEO™ (Can) *see* oxycodone *on page* 678

OXY® Post-Shave [OTC] *see* salicylic acid *on page 816*
OXY® Spot Treatment [OTC] *see* salicylic acid *on page 816*

oxytocin (oks i TOE sin)

Medication Safety Issues

High alert medication:

The Institute for Safe Medication Practices (ISMP) includes this medication among its list of drugs which have a heightened risk of causing significant patient harm when used in error.

Synonyms pit

U.S. Brand Names Pitocin®

Canadian Brand Names Oxytocin for injection

Therapeutic Category Oxytocic Agent

Use Induction of labor in patients with a medical indication; stimulation or reinforcement of labor; adjunctive therapy in management of abortion; to produce uterine contractions during the third stage of labor; control of postpartum bleeding

General Dosage Range

I.M.: *Adults:* Total dose of 10 units after delivery of the placenta
I.V.: *Adults:* Dosage varies greatly depending on indication

Dosage Forms

Injection, solution: 10 units/mL (1 mL, 10 mL, 30 mL)
Pitocin®: 10 units/mL (1 mL, 10 mL)

Oxytocin for injection (Can) *see* oxytocin *on page 683*
Oxytrol® *see* oxybutynin *on page 677*
Oysco D [OTC] *see* calcium and vitamin D *on page 161*
Oysco 500 [OTC] *see* calcium carbonate *on page 161*
Oysco 500+D [OTC] *see* calcium and vitamin D *on page 161*
Oyst-Cal-D 500 [OTC] *see* calcium and vitamin D *on page 161*
Oystercal™ 500 [OTC] *see* calcium carbonate *on page 161*
Ozurdex® *see* dexamethasone (ophthalmic) *on page 267*
P01BE03 *see* artesunate *on page 92*
P32 *see* chromic phosphate P 32 *on page 207*
P-071 *see* cetirizine *on page 190*
P-1202 *see* methyl aminolevulinate *on page 587*
Pacerone® *see* amiodarone *on page 63*

paclitaxel (pac li TAKS el)

Medication Safety Issues

Sound-alike/look-alike issues:

PACLitaxel may be confused with DOCEtaxel, PARoxetine, Paxil®
PACLitaxel (conventional) may be confused with PACLitaxel (protein-bound)
Taxol® may be confused with Abraxane®, Paxil®, Taxotere®

High alert medication:

This medication is in a class the Institute for Safe Medication Practices (ISMP) includes among its list of drug classes which have a heightened risk of causing significant patient harm when used in error.

Synonyms conventional paclitaxel; paclitaxel (conventional); Taxol

Tall-Man PACLitaxel

Canadian Brand Names Apo-Paclitaxel®; Paclitaxel For Injection; Taxol®

Therapeutic Category Antineoplastic Agent

Use Treatment of breast, nonsmall cell lung, and ovarian cancers; treatment of AIDS-related Kaposi sarcoma (KS)

General Dosage Range Dosage adjustment recommended in patients with hepatic impairment or who develop toxicities

I.V.: *Adults:* Dosage varies greatly depending on indication

Dosage Forms

Injection, solution: 6 mg/mL (5 mL, 16.7 mL, 25 mL, 50 mL)

paclitaxel (protein bound) (pac li TAKS el PROE teen bownd)

Medication Safety Issues

Sound-alike/look-alike issues:

PACLitaxel may be confused with DOCEtaxel

PACLitaxel (protein bound) may be confused with PACLitaxel (conventional)

Abraxane® may be confused with Paxil®, Taxol®, Taxotere®

High alert medication:

This medication is in a class the Institute for Safe Medication Practices (ISMP) includes among its list of drug classes which have a heightened risk of causing significant patient harm when used in error.

Synonyms ABI-007; albumin-bound paclitaxel; albumin-stabilized nanoparticle paclitaxel; nab-paclitaxel; nanoparticle albumin-bound paclitaxel; paclitaxel, albumin-bound; protein-bound paclitaxel

Tall-Man PACLitaxel

U.S. Brand Names Abraxane®

Canadian Brand Names Abraxane® for Injectable Suspension

Therapeutic Category Antineoplastic Agent, Antimicrotubular; Antineoplastic Agent, Natural Source (Plant) Derivative

Use Treatment of refractory (metastatic) or relapsed (within 6 months of adjuvant therapy) breast cancer

General Dosage Range Dosage adjustment recommended in patients with hepatic impairment or who develop toxicities

I.V.: *Adults:* 260 mg/m^2 every 3 weeks

Dosage Forms

Injection, powder for reconstitution:

Abraxane®: 100 mg

paclitaxel, albumin-bound *see* paclitaxel (protein bound) *on page 684*

paclitaxel (conventional) *see* paclitaxel *on page 683*

Paclitaxel For Injection (Can) *see* paclitaxel *on page 683*

Pacnex® *see* benzoyl peroxide *on page 124*

Pacnex® MX *see* benzoyl peroxide *on page 124*

Pacnex® HP *see* benzoyl peroxide *on page 124*

Pacnex® LP *see* benzoyl peroxide *on page 124*

Pain-A-Lay® [OTC] *see* phenol *on page 713*

Pain Eze [OTC] *see* acetaminophen *on page 20*

Pain & Fever Children's [OTC] *see* acetaminophen *on page 20*

Pain-Off [OTC] *see* acetaminophen, aspirin, and caffeine *on page 26*

Paire OB™ Plus DHA *see* vitamins (multiple/prenatal) *on page 952*

Palafer® (Can) *see* ferrous fumarate *on page 379*

Palgic® *see* carbinoxamine *on page 175*

palifermin (pal ee FER min)

Synonyms AMJ 9701; keratinocyte growth factor, recombinant human; rhKGF; rhu keratinocyte growth factor; rHu-KGF

U.S. Brand Names Kepivance®

Canadian Brand Names Kepivance®

Therapeutic Category Keratinocyte Growth Factor

Use Decrease the incidence and duration of severe oral mucositis associated with hematologic malignancies in patients receiving myelotoxic therapy requiring hematopoietic stem cell support (when the preparative regimen is expected to result in mucositis ≥grade 3 in most patients)

Note: Use (safety and efficacy) is not established for nonhematologic malignancies; use is not recommended with conditioning regimens containing melphalan 200 mg/m^2

General Dosage Range I.V.: *Adults:* 60 mcg/kg/day for 3 consecutive days before and after myelotoxic therapy

Dosage Forms

Injection, powder for reconstitution [preservative free]:

Kepivance®: 6.25 mg

paliperidone (pal ee PER i done)

Medication Safety Issues

BEERS Criteria medication:

This drug may be potentially inappropriate for use in geriatric patients (Quality of evidence - moderate; Strength of recommendation - strong).

Synonyms 9-hydroxy-risperidone; 9-OH-risperidone; paliperidone palmitate

U.S. Brand Names Invega®; Invega® Sustenna®

Canadian Brand Names Invega®; Invega® Sustenna®

Therapeutic Category Antipsychotic Agent, Atypical

Use

Oral: Acute and maintenance treatment of schizophrenia; acute treatment of schizoaffective disorder (monotherapy or adjunctive therapy to mood stabilizers and/or antidepressants)

Injection: Acute and maintenance treatment of schizophrenia

General Dosage Range Dosage adjustment recommended in patients with renal impairment

I.M.: *Adults:* Initial: 234 mg, then 156 mg 1 week later; Maintenance: 39-234 mg/month

Oral: *Adolescents 12-17 years and Adults:* 3-12 mg once daily (maximum: 12 mg/day)

Dosage Forms

Injection, suspension, extended release:

Invega® Sustenna®: 39 mg/0.25 mL (0.25 mL); 78 mg/0.5 mL (0.5 mL); 117 mg/0.75 mL (0.75 mL); 156 mg/mL (1 mL); 234 mg/1.5 mL (1.5 mL)

Tablet, extended release, oral:

Invega®: 1.5 mg, 3 mg, 6 mg, 9 mg

Dosage Forms - Canada

Injection, suspension, extended release:

Invega® Sustenna™: 25 mg/0.25 mL, 50 mg/0.5 mL, 75 mg/0.75 mL, 100mg/1 mL, and 150 mg/1.5 mL

paliperidone palmitate *see* paliperidone *on page 685*

palivizumab (pah li VIZ u mab)

Medication Safety Issues

Sound-alike/look-alike issues:

Synagis® may be confused with Synalgos®-DC, Synflorix™, Synvisc®

U.S. Brand Names Synagis®

Canadian Brand Names Synagis®

Therapeutic Category Monoclonal Antibody

Use Prevention of serious lower respiratory tract disease caused by respiratory syncytial virus (RSV) in infants and children at high risk of RSV disease

The American Academy of Pediatrics recommends RSV prophylaxis with palivizumab during RSV season for:

- Infants <3 months of age who were born between 32 and 34 6/7 weeks gestational age and have one of the following:
  - Day care attendance
  - One or more siblings <5 years of age living in the same household
- Infants <6 months of age who were born between 29 and 31 6/7 weeks gestational age
- Infants <12 months of age who were born <28 weeks gestational age
- Infants <12 months of age with congenital airway abnormality or neuromuscular disorder that decreases the ability to manage airway secretions
- Infants and children <24 months of age with chronic lung disease (CLD) necessitating medical therapy within 6 month prior to the beginning of RSV season
- Infants and children ≤24 months of age with congenital heart disease and one of the following:
  - Receiving medication to treat congestive heart failure
  - Moderate-to-severe pulmonary hypertension
  - Cyanotic heart disease

General Dosage Range I.M.: *Children <2 years:* 15 mg/kg monthly

Dosage Forms

Injection, solution [preservative free]:

Synagis®: 100 mg/mL (0.5 mL, 1 mL)

Palmer's® Skin Success Acne Cleanser [OTC] *see* salicylic acid *on page 816*

Palmer's® Skin Success® Eventone® Fade Cream [OTC] *see* hydroquinone *on page 461*

Palmer's® Skin Success® Eventone® Fade Milk [OTC] *see* hydroquinone *on page 461*

Palmer's® Skin Success® Eventone® Ultra Fade Serum [OTC] *see* hydroquinone *on page 461*

palonosetron (pal oh NOE se tron)

Medication Safety Issues

Sound-alike/look-alike issues:

Aloxi® may be confused with Eloxatin®, oxaliplatin

Palonosetron may be confused with dolasetron, granisetron, ondansetron

Synonyms palonosetron hydrochloride; RS-25259; RS-25259-197

U.S. Brand Names Aloxi®

Therapeutic Category Antiemetic; Selective 5-HT_3 Receptor Antagonist

Use Prevention of chemotherapy-associated nausea and vomiting; indicated for prevention of acute (highly-emetogenic therapy) as well as acute and delayed (moderately-emetogenic therapy) nausea and vomiting; prevention of postoperative nausea and vomiting (PONV)

General Dosage Range I.V.: *Adults:* 0.25 mg **or** 0.075 mg as a single dose

Dosage Forms

Injection, solution:

Aloxi®: 0.05 mg/mL (5 mL)

palonosetron hydrochloride *see* palonosetron *on page 686*

2-PAM *see* pralidoxime *on page 749*

pamabrom (PAM a brom)

U.S. Brand Names Aqua-Ban® Maximum Strength [OTC]; diurex® Aquagels® [OTC]; diurex® Maximum Relief [OTC]; diurex® [OTC]

Therapeutic Category Diuretic

Use Temporary relief of symptoms associated with premenstrual and menstrual periods (eg, bloating, water-weight gain, swelling, full feeling)

General Dosage Range Oral: *Adults:* 50 mg every 6 hours as needed (maximum: 200 mg/day)

Dosage Forms

Caplet, oral:

diurex® Maximum Relief [OTC]: 50 mg

Capsule, oral:

diurex® [OTC]: 50 mg

Capsule, softgel, oral:

diurex® Aquagels® [OTC]: 50 mg

Tablet, oral:

Aqua-Ban® Maximum Strength [OTC]: 50 mg

pamabrom and acetaminophen *see* acetaminophen and pamabrom *on page 24*

Pamelor™ *see* nortriptyline *on page 650*

pamidronate (pa mi DROE nate)

Medication Safety Issues

Sound-alike/look-alike issues:

Aredia® may be confused with Adriamycin®

Pamidronate may be confused with papaverine

Synonyms pamidronate disodium

U.S. Brand Names Aredia®

Canadian Brand Names Aredia®; Pamidronate Disodium Omega; Pamidronate Disodium®; PMS-Pamidronate

Therapeutic Category Bisphosphonate Derivative

Use Treatment of moderate or severe hypercalcemia associated with malignancy (in conjunction with adequate hydration) with or without bone metastases; treatment of osteolytic bone lesions associated with multiple myeloma or metastatic breast cancer; moderate-to-severe Paget disease of bone

General Dosage Range Dosage adjustment recommended in patients with renal impairment

I.V.: *Adults:* 60-90 mg as a single dose, may repeat every 3-4 weeks **or** 30 mg daily for 3 consecutive days

Dosage Forms

Injection, powder for reconstitution: 30 mg, 90 mg

Aredia®: 30 mg

Injection, solution: 3 mg/mL (10 mL); 6 mg/mL (10 mL); 9 mg/mL (10 mL)

Injection, solution [preservative free]: 3 mg/mL (10 mL); 9 mg/mL (10 mL)

pamidronate disodium *see* pamidronate *on page 686*

Pamidronate Disodium® (Can) *see* pamidronate *on page 686*

Pamidronate Disodium Omega (Can) *see* pamidronate *on page 686*

Pamine® *see* methscopolamine *on page 587*

Pamine® Forte *see* methscopolamine *on page 587*

p-amino-benzenesulfonamide *see* sulfanilamide *on page 861*

p-aminoclonidine *see* apraclonidine *on page 88*

Pamprin® Maximum Strength All Day Relief [OTC] *see* naproxen *on page 628*

Pancrease® MT (Can) *see* pancrelipase *on page 687*

pancreatic enzymes *see* pancrelipase *on page 687*

Pancreaze™ *see* pancrelipase *on page 687*

pancrelipase (pan kre LYE pase)

Medication Safety Issues

Sound-alike/look-alike issues:

Pancrelipase may be confused with pancreatin

Synonyms amylase, lipase, and protease; lipancreatin; lipase, protease, and amylase; pancreatic enzymes; protease, lipase, and amylase; Ultresa™

U.S. Brand Names Creon®; Pancreaze™; Pancrelipase™; Pertzye™; Ultresa™; Viokace™; Zenpep®

Canadian Brand Names Cotazym®; Creon®; Pancrease® MT; Ultrase®; Ultrase® MT; Viokase®

Therapeutic Category Enzyme

Use Treatment of exocrine pancreatic insufficiency (EPI) due to conditions such as cystic fibrosis (Creon®, Pancreaze™, Pertzye™, Ultresa™, Zenpep®); chronic pancreatitis (Creon®, Viokace™); or pancreatectomy (Creon®, Viokace™)

Note: Viokace™ must be administered with a proton pump inhibitor (PPI) since it is not enteric coated.

General Dosage Range Oral:

Infants ≤1 year: Lipase 2000-4000 units per 120 mL of formula or per breast-feeding

Children >1 and <4 years: Lipase 1000-2500 units/kg/meal; Maximum: Lipase ≤2500 units/kg/**meal or** lipase ≤10,000 units/kg/**day or** lipase <4000 units/g of fat daily

Children ≥4 years, Adolescents, and Adults: Lipase 500-2500 units/kg/meal **or** lipase 72,000 units/meal (while consuming ≥100 g of fat per day); Maximum: Lipase ≤2500 units/kg/**meal or** lipase ≤10,000 units/kg/**day or** lipase <4000 units/g of fat daily

Dosage Forms

Capsule, delayed release, bicarbonate buffered enteric coated microspheres [porcine derived]:

Pertzye™: Lipase 8,000 units, protease 28,750 units, and amylase 30,250 units

Pertzye™: Lipase 16,000 units, protease 57,500 units, and amylase 60,500 units

Capsule, delayed release, enteric coated beads, oral [porcine derived]:

Pancrelipase™: Lipase 5000 units, protease 17,000 units, and amylase 27,000 units

Zenpep®: Lipase 3000 units, protease 10,000 units, and amylase 16,000 units

Zenpep®: Lipase 5000 units, protease 17,000 units, and amylase 27,000 units

Zenpep®: Lipase 10,000 units, protease 34,000 units, and amylase 55,000 units

Zenpep®: Lipase 15,000 units, protease 51,000 units, and amylase 82,000 units

Zenpep®: Lipase 20,000 units, protease 68,000 units, and amylase 109,000 units

Zenpep®: Lipase 25,000 units, protease 85,000 units, and amylase 136,000 units

Capsule, delayed release, enteric coated microspheres, oral [new formulation; porcine derived]:

Creon®: Lipase 3000 units, protease 9500 units, and amylase 15,000 units

Creon®: Lipase 6000 units, protease 19,000 units, and amylase 30,000 units

Creon®: Lipase 12000 units, protease 38,000 units, and amylase 60,000 units

Creon®: Lipase 24,000 units, protease 76,000 units, and amylase 120,000 units

Capsule, delayed release, enteric coated microtablets, oral [porcine derived]:
Pancreaze™: Lipase 4200 units, protease 10,000 units, and amylase 17,500 units
Pancreaze™: Lipase 10,500 units, protease 25,000 units, and amylase 43,750 units
Pancreaze™: Lipase 16,800 units, protease 40,000 units, and amylase 70,000 units
Pancreaze™: Lipase 21,000 units, protease 37,000 units, and amylase 61,000 units
Tablet, oral [porcine derived]:
Viokace™: Lipase 10,440 units, protease 39,150 units, and amylase 39,150 units
Viokace™: Lipase 20,880 units, protease 78,300 units, and amylase 78,300 units

Pancrelipase™ *see* pancrelipase *on page 687*

pancuronium (pan kyoo ROE nee um)

Medication Safety Issues
High alert medication:
The Institute for Safe Medication Practices (ISMP) includes this medication among its list of drugs which have a heightened risk of causing significant patient harm when used in error.
Other safety concerns:
United States Pharmacopeia (USP) 2006: The Interdisciplinary Safe Medication Use Expert Committee of the USP has recommended the following:
- Hospitals, clinics, and other practice sites should institute special safeguards in the storage, labeling, and use of these agents and should include these safeguards in staff orientation and competency training.
- Healthcare professionals should be on high alert (especially vigilant) whenever a neuromuscular-blocking agent (NMBA) is stocked, ordered, prepared, or administered.

Synonyms pancuronium bromide; Pavulon [DSC]

Canadian Brand Names Pancuronium Bromide®

Therapeutic Category Skeletal Muscle Relaxant

Use Facilitation of endotracheal intubation and relaxation of skeletal muscles during surgery; facilitation of mechanical ventilation in ICU patients; does not relieve pain or produce sedation

General Dosage Range Dosage adjustment recommended in patients with renal impairment
I.V.: *Children >1 month and Adults:*
ICU paralysis: 0.06-0.1 mg/kg bolus followed by 1-2 mcg/kg/minute infusion **or** 0.1-0.2 mg/kg every 1-3 hours
Surgery: Intubation: Initial: 0.06-1 mg/kg **or** 0.05 mg/kg after succinylcholine; Maintenance: 0.01 mg/kg administered 60-100 minutes after initial dose and then every 25-60 minutes

Dosage Forms
Injection, solution: 1 mg/mL (10 mL)

pancuronium bromide *see* pancuronium *on page 688*
Pancuronium Bromide® (Can) *see* pancuronium *on page 688*
Pandel® *see* hydrocortisone (topical) *on page 457*
panglobulin *see* immune globulin *on page 477*
Panhematin® *see* hemin *on page 442*

panitumumab (pan i TOOM yoo mab)

Medication Safety Issues
Sound-alike/look-alike issues:
Panitumumab may be confused with pertuzumab

Synonyms ABX-EGF; MOAB ABX-EGF; monoclonal antibody ABX-EGF; rHuMAb-EGFr

U.S. Brand Names Vectibix®

Canadian Brand Names Vectibix®

Therapeutic Category Antineoplastic Agent, Monoclonal Antibody; Epidermal Growth Factor Receptor (EGFR) Inhibitor

Use Monotherapy in treatment of EGFR-expressing refractory metastatic colorectal cancer with disease progression on or following fluoropyrimidine-, oxaliplatin-, and irinotecan-based regimens
Panitumumab is not indicated for the treatment of patients with *KRAS* mutation-positive metastatic colorectal cancer or patients in which *KRAS* mutation status is unknown. Subset analyses (retrospective) in metastatic colorectal cancer trials have not shown a benefit with EGFR inhibitor treatment in patients whose tumors have codon 12 or 13 *KRAS* mutations.

General Dosage Range Dosage adjustment recommended in patients who develop toxicities

I.V.: *Adults:* 6 mg/kg every 14 days

Dosage Forms

Injection, solution [preservative free]:

Vectibix®: 20 mg/mL (5 mL, 20 mL)

PanOxyl® [OTC] *see* benzoyl peroxide *on page 124*

PanOxyl® (Can) *see* benzoyl peroxide *on page 124*

PanOxyl®-4 [OTC] *see* benzoyl peroxide *on page 124*

PanOxyl®-8 [OTC] *see* benzoyl peroxide *on page 124*

PanOxyl® Bar [OTC] *see* benzoyl peroxide *on page 124*

Panretin® *see* alitretinoin *on page 49*

Panto-250 [OTC] *see* pantothenic acid *on page 690*

Panto™ I.V. (Can) *see* pantoprazole *on page 689*

Pantoloc® (Can) *see* pantoprazole *on page 689*

pantoprazole (pan TOE pra zole)

Medication Safety Issues

Sound-alike/look-alike issues:

Pantoprazole may be confused with ARIPiprazole

Protonix® may be confused with Lotronex®, Lovenox®, protamine

Administration issues:

Vials containing Protonix® I.V. for injection are not recommended for use with spiked I.V. system adaptors. Nurses and pharmacists have reported breakage of the glass vials during attempts to connect spiked I.V. system adaptors, which may potentially result in injury to healthcare professionals.

International issues:

Protonix [U.S., Canada] may be confused with Pretanix brand name for indapamide [Hungary]

Synonyms pantoprazole magnesium; pantoprazole sodium

U.S. Brand Names Protonix®; Protonix® I.V.

Canadian Brand Names Apo-Pantoprazole®; Ava-Pantoprazole; CO Pantoprazole; Mylan-Pantoprazole; Pantoloc®; Pantoprazole for Injection; Panto™ I.V.; PMS-Pantoprazole; Q-Pantoprazole; RAN™-Pantoprazole; ratio-Pantoprazole; Riva-Pantoprazole; Sandoz-Pantoprazole; Tecta®; Teva-Pantoprazole

Therapeutic Category Proton Pump Inhibitor

Use

Oral: Treatment and maintenance of healing of erosive esophagitis associated with GERD; reduction in relapse rates of daytime and nighttime heartburn symptoms in GERD; hypersecretory disorders associated with Zollinger-Ellison syndrome or other GI hypersecretory disorders

I.V.: Short-term treatment (7-10 days) of patients with gastroesophageal reflux disease (GERD) and a history of erosive esophagitis; hypersecretory disorders associated with Zollinger-Ellison syndrome or other neoplastic disorders

Canadian labeling: Additional use (not in U.S. labeling): Oral: Peptic ulcer disease (eg, duodenal or gastric ulcer); adjunct treatment with antibiotics for *Helicobacter pylori* eradication; prevention of GI lesions in patients receiving prolonged NSAID therapy

General Dosage Range

I.V.: *Adults:* Erosive gastritis: 40 mg once daily; Hypersecretory disorders: 160-240 mg/day in divided doses

Oral:

Children ≥5 years: ≥15 to <40 kg: 20 mg once daily; ≥40 kg: 40 mg once daily

Adults: 20-40 mg once or twice daily (maximum: 240 mg/day normally reserved for treatment of hypersecretory conditions)

Dosage Forms

Granules for suspension, delayed release, enteric coated, oral:

Protonix®: 40 mg/packet (30s)

Injection, powder for reconstitution:

Protonix® I.V.: 40 mg

Tablet, delayed release, oral: 20 mg, 40 mg

Protonix®: 20 mg, 40 mg

Dosage Forms - Canada

Tablet, enteric coated:

Tecta®: 40 mg

Pantoprazole for Injection (Can) *see* pantoprazole *on page 689*

pantoprazole magnesium *see* pantoprazole *on page 689*

pantoprazole sodium *see* pantoprazole *on page 689*

pantothenic acid (pan toe THEN ik AS id)

Synonyms calcium pantothenate; vitamin B_5

U.S. Brand Names Panto-250 [OTC]

Therapeutic Category Vitamin, Water Soluble

Use Dietary supplement

General Dosage Range Oral:

Children 1-6 months: 1.7 mg/day
Children 7-12 months: 1.8 mg/day
Children 1-3 years: 2 mg/day
Children 4-8 years: 3 mg/day
Children 9-13 years: 4 mg/day
Children ≥14 years and Adults: 5 mg/day
Pregnancy: 6 mg/day
Lactation: 7 mg/day

Dosage Forms

Capsule, oral:
Panto-250 [OTC]: 250 mg

Liquid, oral: 200 mg/5 mL (240 mL)

Tablet, oral: 100 mg, 200 mg, 250 mg, 500 mg

Tablet, sustained release, oral: 500 mg

pantothenyl alcohol *see* dexpanthenol *on page 269*

papaverine (pa PAV er een)

Medication Safety Issues

Sound-alike/look-alike issues:

Papaverine may be confused with pamidronate

Synonyms papaverine hydrochloride; Pavabid

Therapeutic Category Vasodilator

Use Oral: Relief of peripheral and cerebral ischemia associated with arterial spasm and myocardial ischemia complicated by arrhythmias

General Dosage Range

I.M., I.V.:

Children: 6 mg/kg/day in 4 divided doses
Adults: 30-65 mg, may repeat every 3 hours

Oral: *Adults:* 150-300 mg every 12 hours **or** 150 mg every 8 hours

Dosage Forms

Injection, solution: 30 mg/mL (2 mL, 10 mL)

papaverine hydrochloride *see* papaverine *on page 690*

papillomavirus (types 6, 11, 16, 18) vaccine (human, recombinant)

(pap ih LO ma VYE rus typs six e LEV en SIX teen AYE teen vak SEEN YU man ree KOM be nant)

Medication Safety Issues

Sound-alike/look-alike issues:

Papillomavirus vaccine types 6, 11, 16, 18 (Gardasil®) may be confused with Papillomavirus vaccine types 16, 18 (Cervarix®)

Synonyms HPV vaccine; HPV4; human papillomavirus vaccine; papillomavirus vaccine, recombinant; quadrivalent human papillomavirus vaccine

U.S. Brand Names Gardasil®

Canadian Brand Names Gardasil®

Therapeutic Category Vaccine

Use

U.S. labeling:

Females ≥9 years and ≤26 years of age: Prevention of cervical, vulvar, vaginal, and anal cancer caused by HPV types 16 and 18; genital warts caused by HPV types 6 and 11; cervical adenocarcinoma *in situ*, and vulvar, vaginal, cervical, or anal intraepithelial neoplasia caused by HPV types 6, 11, 16, and 18

Males ≥9 years and ≤26 years of age: Prevention of genital warts caused by human papillomavirus (HPV) types 6 and 11; anal cancer caused by HPV types 16 and 18, and anal intraepithelial neoplasia caused by HPV types 6, 11, 16, and 18

Canadian labeling:

Females ≥9 years and ≤26 years of age: Prevention of anal cancer caused by HPV types 16 and 18; anal intraepithelial neoplasia caused by HPV types 6, 11, 16, and 18

Females ≥9 years and ≤45 years of age: Prevention of cervical, vulvar, and vaginal cancer caused by HPV types 16 and 18; genital warts caused by HPV types 6 and 11; cervical adenocarcinoma *in situ*, vulvar, vaginal, or cervical intraepithelial neoplasia caused by HPV types 6, 11, 16, and 18

Males ≥9 years and ≤26 years of age: Prevention of anal cancer caused by HPV types 16 and 18; anal intraepithelial neoplasia caused by HPV types 6, 11, 16, and 18; genital warts caused by HPV types 6 and 11

The Advisory Committee on Immunization Practices (ACIP) recommends routine vaccination for females and males 11-12 years of age; catch-up vaccination is recommended for females 13-26 years of age and males 13-21 years of age. Males 22-26 years may also be vaccinated. The ACIP also recommends routine vaccination for men who have sex with men (MSM) through 26 years of age (CDC, 59[20], 2010; CDC, 60[50], 2011). Vaccination is also recommended for immunocompromised persons or MSM through 26 years of age who were not previously vaccinated when they were younger. Although not specifically recommended for their profession, health care providers within the recommended age groups should also receive the HPV vaccine (CDC, 61[4], 2012).

General Dosage Range I.M.: *Children ≥9 years and Adults ≤26 years:* 0.5 mL initial dose, followed by 0.5 mL 2 and 6 months later

Dosage Forms

Injection, suspension [preservative free]:

Gardasil®: HPV 6 L1 protein 20 mcg, HPV 11 L1 protein 40 mcg, HPV 16 L1 protein 40 mcg, and HPV 18 L1 protein 20 mcg per 0.5 mL (0.5 mL)

papillomavirus (types 16, 18) vaccine (human, recombinant)

(pap ih LO ma VYE rus typs SIX teen AYE teen vak SEEN YU man ree KOM be nant)

Medication Safety Issues

Sound-alike/look-alike issues:

Papillomavirus vaccine types 16, 18 (Cervarix®) may be confused with Papillomavirus vaccine types 6, 11, 16, 18 (Gardasil®)

Cervarix® may be confused with Cerebyx®, CeleBREX®

Synonyms bivalent human papillomavirus vaccine; GSK-580299; HPV 16/18 L1 VLP/AS04 VAC; HPV vaccine; HPV2; human papillomavirus vaccine; papillomavirus vaccine, recombinant

U.S. Brand Names Cervarix®

Canadian Brand Names Cervarix®

Therapeutic Category Vaccine, Inactivated (Viral)

Use Females 9 through 25 years of age: Prevention of cervical cancer, cervical adenocarcinoma *in situ*, and cervical intraepithelial neoplasia caused by human papillomavirus (HPV) types 16, 18

The Advisory Committee on Immunization Practices (ACIP) recommends routine vaccination for females 11-12 years of age; catch-up vaccination is recommended for females 13-25 years of age (CDC, 59[20], 2010). Vaccination is also recommended for immunocompromised females through 26 years of age who were not previously vaccinated when they were younger. Although not specifically recommended for their profession, female health care providers within the recommended age groups should also receive the HPV vaccine (CDC, 61[4], 2012).

General Dosage Range I.M.: *Children ≥9 years and Adults ≤25 years (females):* 0.5 mL initial dose, followed by 0.5 mL 1 and 6 months later

Dosage Forms

Injection, suspension [preservative free]:

Cervarix®: HPV 16 L1 protein 20 mcg and HPV 18 L1 protein 20 mcg per 0.5 mL (0.5 mL)

papillomavirus vaccine, recombinant *see* papillomavirus (types 6, 11, 16, 18) vaccine (human, recombinant) *on page 690*

papillomavirus vaccine, recombinant *see* papillomavirus (types 16, 18) vaccine (human, recombinant) *on page 691*
PAR-101 *see* fidaxomicin *on page 383*
para-aminosalicylate sodium *see* aminosalicylic acid *on page 63*
paracetamol *see* acetaminophen *on page 20*
Parafon Forte® (Can) *see* chlorzoxazone *on page 204*
Parafon Forte® DSC *see* chlorzoxazone *on page 204*
Paraldahyde Injection BP (Can) *see* paraldehyde *(Canada only) on page 692*

paraldehyde *(Canada only)* (par AL de hyde)

Canadian Brand Names Paraldahyde Injection BP

Therapeutic Category Anticonvulsant, Miscellaneous; Anxiolytics, Sedatives, and Hypnotics, Miscellaneous

Use Alternative agent (only when conventional treatment is ineffective, inappropriate, or unavailable) in the treatment of convulsive seizure episodes associated with status epilepticus, tetanus, and convulsant drug toxicity. Historically, has also been used as a sedative/hypnotic, as an anxiolytic during withdrawal from narcotics or barbiturates, and in the management of acute agitation or delirium due to alcohol withdrawal; however, these uses are not recommended due to the availability of safer and more efficacious agents.

General Dosage Range I.M.:
Children: 0.15-0.3 mL/kg/daily **or** 0.1-0.15 mL/kg/dose every 4-8 hours
Adults: 5-10 mL **or** 5 mL every 4-6 hours (maximum: 30 mL on day 1; 20 mL/day thereafter)

Product Availability Not available in the U.S.

paraplatin *see* carboplatin *on page 176*
parathyroid hormone (1-34) *see* teriparatide *on page 880*
Parcaine™ [DSC] *see* proparacaine *on page 766*
Parcopa® *see* carbidopa and levodopa *on page 174*

paregoric (par e GOR ik)

Medication Safety Issues

Sound-alike/look-alike issues:
Camphorated tincture of opium is an error-prone synonym (mistaken as opium tincture)
Paregoric may be confused with Percogesic®

High alert medication:
The Institute for Safe Medication Practices (ISMP) includes this medication among its list of drug classes which have a heightened risk of causing significant patient harm when used in error.

Administration issues:
Use care when prescribing opium tincture; each mL contains the equivalent of morphine 10 mg; paregoric contains the equivalent of morphine 0.4 mg/mL

Synonyms camphorated tincture of opium (error-prone synonym)

Therapeutic Category Analgesic, Narcotic

Controlled Substance C-III

Use Treatment of diarrhea or relief of pain

General Dosage Range Oral:
Children: 0.25-0.5 mL/kg 1-4 times/day
Adults: 5-10 mL 1-4 times/day

Dosage Forms
Liquid, oral: Morphine equivalent 2 mg/5 mL (473 mL)

Paremyd® *see* hydroxyamphetamine and tropicamide *on page 462*
parenteral nutrition *see* total parenteral nutrition *on page 908*

paricalcitol (pah ri KAL si tole)

Medication Safety Issues

Sound alike/look alike issues:
Paricalcitol may be confused with calcitriol
Zemplar® may be confused with zaleplon, Zelapar®, zolpidem, ZyPREXA® Zydis®

U.S. Brand Names Zemplar®

Canadian Brand Names Zemplar®

Therapeutic Category Vitamin D Analog

Use

I.V.: Prevention and treatment of secondary hyperparathyroidism associated with stage 5 chronic kidney disease (CKD)

Oral: Prevention and treatment of secondary hyperparathyroidism associated with stage 3 and 4 CKD and stage 5 CKD patients on hemodialysis or peritoneal dialysis

General Dosage Range Dosage adjustment recommended in patients with renal impairment

I.V.: *Children ≥5 years and Adults:* 0.04-0.24 mcg/kg (2.8-16.8 mcg) every other day during dialysis

Oral: *Adults:* 1-2 mcg/day **or** 2-4 mcg 3 times/week

Dosage Forms

Capsule, soft gelatin, oral:

Zemplar®: 1 mcg, 2 mcg, 4 mcg

Injection, solution:

Zemplar®: 2 mcg/mL (1 mL); 5 mcg/mL (1 mL, 2 mL)

Pariet® (Can) *see* rabeprazole *on page* 784

pariprazole *see* rabeprazole *on page* 784

Parlodel® *see* bromocriptine *on page* 143

Parlodel® SnapTabs® *see* bromocriptine *on page* 143

Parnate® *see* tranylcypromine *on page* 911

paromomycin (par oh moe MYE sin)

Synonyms paromomycin sulfate

Canadian Brand Names Humatin®

Therapeutic Category Amebicide

Use Treatment of acute and chronic intestinal amebiasis; hepatic coma

General Dosage Range Oral: *Children and Adults:* Dosage varies greatly depending on indication

Dosage Forms

Capsule, oral: 250 mg

paromomycin sulfate *see* paromomycin *on page* 693

paroxetine (pa ROKS e teen)

Medication Safety Issues

Sound-alike/look-alike issues:

PARoxetine may be confused with FLUoxetine, PACLitaxel, piroxicam, pyridoxine

Paxil® may be confused with Doxil®, PACLitaxel, Plavix®, PROzac®, Taxol®

BEERS Criteria medication:

This drug may be potentially inappropriate for use in geriatric patients (SIADH: Quality of evidence - moderate; Strength of recommendation - strong).

Synonyms paroxetine hydrochloride; paroxetine mesylate

Tall-Man PARoxetine

U.S. Brand Names Paxil CR®; Paxil®; Pexeva®

Canadian Brand Names Apo-Paroxetine®; CO Paroxetine; Dom-Paroxetine; Mylan-Paroxetine; Novo-Paroxetine; Paxil CR®; Paxil®; PHL-Paroxetine; PMS-Paroxetine; ratio-Paroxetine; Riva-Paroxetine; Sandoz-Paroxetine; Teva-Paroxetine

Therapeutic Category Antidepressant, Selective Serotonin Reuptake Inhibitor

Use Treatment of major depressive disorder (MDD); treatment of panic disorder with or without agoraphobia; obsessive-compulsive disorder (OCD); social anxiety disorder (social phobia); generalized anxiety disorder (GAD); posttraumatic stress disorder (PTSD); premenstrual dysphoric disorder (PMDD)

General Dosage Range Dosage adjustment recommended in patients with hepatic or renal impairment

Oral:

Controlled release:

Adults: Initial: 12.5-25 mg once daily; Maintenance: 12.5-75 mg once daily (maximum: 75 mg/day)

Elderly: Initial: 12.5 mg once daily; Maintenance: 12.5-50 mg/day (maximum: 50 mg/day)

Immediate release:

Adults: Initial: 10-20 mg once daily: Maintenance: 10-60 mg once daily (maximum: 60 mg/day)

Elderly: Initial: 10 mg once daily; Maintenance: 10-40 mg once daily (maximum: 40 mg/day)

Dosage Forms

Suspension, oral:
Paxil®: 10 mg/5 mL (250 mL)
Tablet, oral: 10 mg, 20 mg, 30 mg, 40 mg
Paxil®: 10 mg, 20 mg, 30 mg, 40 mg
Pexeva®: 10 mg, 20 mg, 30 mg, 40 mg
Tablet, controlled release, enteric coated, oral: 12.5 mg, 25 mg, 37.5 mg
Paxil CR®: 12.5 mg, 25 mg, 37.5 mg
Tablet, extended release, enteric coated, oral: 12.5 mg, 25 mg

paroxetine hydrochloride *see* paroxetine *on page 693*
paroxetine mesylate *see* paroxetine *on page 693*
Parvolex® (Can) *see* acetylcysteine *on page 32*
PAS *see* aminosalicylic acid *on page 63*
Paser® *see* aminosalicylic acid *on page 63*
Pataday™ *see* olopatadine (ophthalmic) *on page 663*
Patanase® *see* olopatadine (nasal) *on page 663*
Patanol® *see* olopatadine (ophthalmic) *on page 663*
PAT-Galantamine ER (Can) *see* galantamine *on page 417*
Pat-Rabeprazole (Can) *see* rabeprazole *on page 784*
Pavabid *see* papaverine *on page 690*
Pavulon [DSC] *see* pancuronium *on page 688*
Paxil® *see* paroxetine *on page 693*
Paxil CR® *see* paroxetine *on page 693*

pazopanib (paz OH pa nib)

Medication Safety Issues

Sound-alike/look-alike issues:
Pazopanib may be confused with axitinib, SUNItinib, vandetanib
Votrient™ may be confused with vorinostat
High alert medication:
This medication is in a class the Institute for Safe Medication Practices (ISMP) includes among its list of drug classes which have a heightened risk of causing significant patient harm when used in error.

Synonyms GW786034; pazopanib hydrochloride

U.S. Brand Names Votrient™

Canadian Brand Names Votrient™

Therapeutic Category Antineoplastic Agent, Tyrosine Kinase Inhibitor; Vascular Endothelial Growth Factor (VEGF) Inhibitor

Use Treatment of advanced renal cell cancer (RCC); treatment of advanced soft tissue sarcoma (STS) (in patients previously treated with chemotherapy)

General Dosage Range Dosage adjustment recommended in patients with hepatic impairment, on concomitant therapy, or who develop toxicities
Oral: *Adults:* 800 mg once daily

Dosage Forms

Tablet, oral:
Votrient™: 200 mg

pazopanib hydrochloride *see* pazopanib *on page 694*
PCA (error-prone abbreviation) *see* procainamide *on page 759*
PCC *see* factor IX complex (human) *on page 371*
PCE® *see* erythromycin (systemic) *on page 342*
PCEC *see* rabies vaccine *on page 784*
PCV-13 *see* pneumococcal conjugate vaccine (13-valent) *on page 734*
PDX *see* pralatrexate *on page 748*
pectin, gelatin, and methylcellulose *see* gelatin, pectin, and methylcellulose *on page 421*
PediaCare® Children's Allergy [OTC] *see* diphenhydramine (systemic) *on page 292*
PediaCare® Children's Decongestant [OTC] *see* phenylephrine (systemic) *on page 715*
PediaCare® Children's Long-Acting Cough [OTC] *see* dextromethorphan *on page 272*

PediaCare® Children's NightTime Cough [OTC] *see* diphenhydramine (systemic) *on page* 292
PediaCare® Children's Multi-Symptom Cold [OTC] *see* dextromethorphan and phenylephrine *on page* 273
Pediacel® (Can) *see* diphtheria and tetanus toxoids, acellular pertussis, poliovirus and *Haemophilus* b conjugate vaccine *on page* 298
Pediaderm™ AF *see* nystatin (topical) *on page* 657
Pediaderm™ HC *see* hydrocortisone (topical) *on page* 457
Pediaderm™ TA *see* triamcinolone (topical) *on page* 916
PediaHist DM *see* brompheniramine, pseudoephedrine, and dextromethorphan *on page* 144
Pediapred® *see* prednisolone (systemic) *on page* 754
Pedia Relief Cough and Cold [OTC] *see* pseudoephedrine and dextromethorphan *on page* 772
Pedia Relief™ Cough-Cold [OTC] *see* chlorpheniramine, pseudoephedrine, and dextromethorphan *on page* 202
Pediarix® *see* diphtheria, tetanus toxoids, acellular pertussis, hepatitis B (recombinant), and poliovirus (inactivated) vaccine *on page* 300
Pediatex® TD *see* triprolidine and pseudoephedrine *on page* 922
Pediatric Cough & Cold [OTC] *see* chlorpheniramine, pseudoephedrine, and dextromethorphan *on page* 202
Pediatric Digoxin CSD (Can) *see* digoxin *on page* 285
Pediatrix (Can) *see* acetaminophen *on page* 20
Pediazole® (Can) *see* erythromycin and sulfisoxazole *on page* 344
Pedi-Boro® [OTC] *see* aluminum sulfate and calcium acetate *on page* 57
Pedi-Dri® *see* nystatin (topical) *on page* 657
Pedipirox™ -4 Kit *see* ciclopirox *on page* 207
PedvaxHIB® *see* *Haemophilus* B conjugate vaccine *on page* 439
PEG *see* polyethylene glycol 3350 *on page* 737
PEG-L-asparaginase *see* pegaspargase *on page* 696

pegademase (bovine) (peg A de mase BOE vine)

U.S. Brand Names Adagen®
Canadian Brand Names Adagen®
Therapeutic Category Enzyme
Use Enzyme replacement therapy for adenosine deaminase (ADA) deficiency in patients with severe combined immunodeficiency disease (SCID) who are not candidates for or who have failed bone marrow transplant
General Dosage Range I.M.: *Children:* First dose: 10 units/kg; Second dose: 15 units/kg 7 days after first dose; Third dose: 20 units/kg 7 days after second dose; Maintenance: 20 units/kg/week (maximum: 30 units/kg/week)
Dosage Forms
Injection, solution [preservative free]:
Adagen®: 250 units/mL (1.5 mL)

Peganone® *see* ethotoin *on page* 364

pegaptanib (peg AP ta nib)

Medication Safety Issues
Sound-alike/look-alike issues:
Pegaptanib may be confused with peginesatide, pegaspargase, pegfilgrastim, peginterferon, pegvisomant
Synonyms EYE001; pegaptanib sodium
U.S. Brand Names Macugen®
Canadian Brand Names Macugen®
Therapeutic Category Ophthalmic Agent; Vaccine, Recombinant
Use Treatment of neovascular (wet) age-related macular degeneration (AMD)
General Dosage Range Intravitreous: *Adults:* 0.3 mg into affected eye every 6 weeks

Dosage Forms

Injection, solution [preservative free]:

Macugen®: 0.3 mg/0.09 mL (0.09 mL)

pegaptanib sodium *see* pegaptanib *on page 695*

PEG-ASP *see* pegaspargase *on page 696*

PEG-asparaginase *see* pegaspargase *on page 696*

pegaspargase (peg AS par jase)

Medication Safety Issues

Sound-alike/look-alike issues:

Oncaspar® may be confused with Elspar®

Pegaspargase may be confused with asparaginase, peginesatide

High alert medication:

The Institute for Safe Medication Practices (ISMP) includes this medication among its list of drugs which have a heightened risk of causing significant harm when used in error.

Synonyms L-asparaginase with polyethylene glycol; PEG-ASP; PEG-asparaginase; PEG-L-asparaginase; PEGLA; polyethylene glycol-L-asparaginase

U.S. Brand Names Oncaspar®

Therapeutic Category Antineoplastic Agent

Use Treatment of acute lymphocytic leukemia (ALL); treatment of ALL with previous hypersensitivity to native L-asparaginase

General Dosage Range I.M., I.V.: *Children and Adults:* 2500 units/m^2 every 14 days

Dosage Forms

Injection, solution [preservative free]:

Oncaspar®: 750 units/mL (5 mL)

Pegasys® *see* peginterferon alfa-2a *on page 697*

Pegasys® RBV (Can) *see* peginterferon alfa-2a and ribavirin *(Canada only) on page 697*

Pegetron® (Can) *see* peginterferon alfa-2b and ribavirin *(Canada only) on page 699*

Pegetron® RediPen® (Can) *see* peginterferon alfa-2b and ribavirin *(Canada only) on page 699*

pegfilgrastim (peg fil GRA stim)

Medication Safety Issues

Sound-alike/look-alike issues:

Neulasta® may be confused with Neumega®, Neupogen®, and Lunesta®

Synonyms G-CSF (PEG conjugate); granulocyte colony stimulating factor (PEG conjugate); pegylated G-CSF; SD/01

U.S. Brand Names Neulasta®

Canadian Brand Names Neulasta®

Therapeutic Category Colony-Stimulating Factor

Use To decrease the incidence of infection, by stimulation of granulocyte production, in patients with nonmyeloid malignancies receiving myelosuppressive therapy associated with a significant risk of febrile neutropenia

General Dosage Range SubQ:

Children: 100 mcg/kg (maximum dose: 6 mg) once per chemotherapy cycle

Adolescents >45 kg and Adults: 6 mg once per chemotherapy cycle

Dosage Forms

Injection, solution [preservative free]:

Neulasta®: 6 mg/0.6 mL (0.6 mL)

PEG-IFN Alfa-2a *see* peginterferon alfa-2a *on page 697*

PEG-IFN Alfa-2b *see* peginterferon alfa-2b *on page 698*

peginesatide (peg in ESS a tide)

Medication Safety Issues

Sound-alike/look-alike issues:

Peginesatide may be confused with pegaptanib, pegaspargase, pegfilgrastim, peginterferon, pegvisomant

Synonyms erythropoiesis-stimulating agent (ESA); hematide

U.S. Brand Names Omontys®

Therapeutic Category Colony Stimulating Factor; Erythropoiesis-Stimulating Agent (ESA); Growth Factor

Use Treatment of anemia due to chronic kidney disease (CKD) in patients receiving dialysis

Note: Peginesatide is **not** indicated for use under the following conditions:

- CKD patients not receiving dialysis
- Cancer patients with anemia that is not due to CKD
- As a substitute for RBC transfusion in patients requiring immediate correction of anemia

Note: Peginesatide has not demonstrated improved symptoms, physical functioning, or health-related quality of life.

General Dosage Range **I.V., SubQ:** *Adults:* Initial: 0.04 mg/kg once monthly; maintenance: 2-20 mg/month

Dosage Forms

Injection, solution:

Omontys®: 10 mg/mL (1 mL, 2 mL)

peginterferon alfa-2a (peg in ter FEER on AL fa too aye)

Synonyms interferon alfa-2a (PEG conjugate); PEG-IFN Alfa-2a; pegylated interferon alfa-2a

U.S. Brand Names Pegasys®

Canadian Brand Names Pegasys®

Therapeutic Category Interferon

Use Treatment of chronic hepatitis C (CHC), in combination with ribavirin (unless contraindicated or significant intolerance to ribavirin), in patients ≥5 years of age with compensated liver disease and not previously treated with alfa interferons, in patients with histological evidence of cirrhosis (Child-Pugh class A) and compensated liver disease; treatment of adults coinfected with CHC and clinically-stable HIV disease (CD4 count >100 cells/mm^3); treatment (monotherapy) of adults with HBeAg-positive and HBeAg-negative chronic hepatitis B with compensated liver disease and evidence of viral replication and liver inflammation

General Dosage Range Dosage adjustment recommended in patients with hepatic or renal impairment or who develop toxicities

SubQ:

Children ≥ 5 years: 180 mcg/1.73 m^2 x BSA once weekly (maximum dose: 180 mcg)

Adults: 180 mcg once weekly

Dosage Forms

Injection, solution:

Pegasys®: 180 mcg/mL (1 mL); 135 mcg/0.5 mL (0.5 mL); 180 mcg/0.5 mL (0.5 mL)

peginterferon alfa-2a and ribavirin *(Canada only)*

(peg in ter FEER on AL fa too aye & rye ba VYE rin)

Synonyms ribavirin and peginterferon alfa-2a

Canadian Brand Names Pegasys® RBV

Therapeutic Category Antiviral Agent; Interferon

Use Combination therapy for the treatment of chronic hepatitis C (HCV) in patients without cirrhosis and patients with compensated cirrhosis; includes patients coinfected with stable HIV disease

General Dosage Range Dosage adjustment recommended in patients with hepatic or renal impairment or who develop toxicities

SubQ: Peginterferon Alfa-2a: *Adults:* 180 mcg/week

Oral: Ribavirin:

Adults <75kg: 800-1000 mg/day in 2 divided doses

Adults ≥75 kg: 800-1200 mg/day in 2 divided doses

Product Availability Not available in U.S.

Dosage Forms - Canada

Combination package:

Pegasys RBV® [1-week package]:

Tablet, oral: Ribavirin 200 mg (28s)

Injection, solution: Peginterferon alfa-2a: 180 mcg/0.5 mL (0.5 mL) (1s)

Tablet, oral: Ribavirin 200 mg (35s)
Injection, solution: Peginterferon alfa-2a: 180 mcg/0.5 mL (0.5 mL) (1s)

Tablet, oral: Ribavirin 200 mg (42s)
Injection, solution: Peginterferon alfa-2a: 180 mcg/0.5 mL (0.5 mL) (1s

Pegasys RBV® [1-week package]:
Tablet, oral: Ribavirin 200 mg (28s)
Injection, solution: Peginterferon alfa-2a: 180 mcg/mL (1 mL) (1s)

Tablet, oral: Ribavirin 200 mg (35s)
Injection, solution: Peginterferon alfa-2a: 180 mcg/mL (1 mL) (1s)

Tablet, oral: Ribavirin 200 mg (42s)
Injection, solution: Peginterferon alfa-2a: 180 mcg/mL (1 mL) (1s)

Pegasys RBV® [4-week package]:
Tablet, oral: Ribavirin 200 mg (112s)
Injection, solution: Peginterferon alfa-2a: 180 mcg/0.5 mL (0.5 mL) (4s)

Tablet, oral: Ribavirin 200 mg (140s)
Injection, solution: Peginterferon alfa-2a: 180 mcg/0.5 mL (0.5 mL) (4s)

Tablet, oral: Ribavirin 200 mg (168s)
Injection, solution: Peginterferon alfa-2a: 180 mcg/0.5 mL (0.5 mL) (4s)

Tablet, oral: Ribavirin 200 mg (168s + 28s)
Injection, solution: Peginterferon alfa-2a: 180 mcg/0.5 mL (0.5 mL) (4s)

Pegasys RBV® [4-week package]:
Tablet, oral: Ribavirin 200 mg (112s)
Injection, solution: Peginterferon alfa-2a: 180 mcg/mL (1 mL) (4s

Tablet, oral: Ribavirin 200 mg (140s)
Injection, solution: Peginterferon alfa-2a: 180 mcg/mL (1 mL) (4s)

Tablet, oral: Ribavirin 200 mg (168s)
Injection, solution: Peginterferon alfa-2a: 180 mcg/mL (1 mL) (4s)

peginterferon alfa-2b (peg in ter FEER on AL fa too bee)

Medication Safety Issues

Sound-alike/look-alike issues:

Peginterferon alfa-2b may be confused with interferon alfa-2a, interferon alfa-2b, interferon alfa-n3, peginterferon alfa-2a

PegIntron® may be confused with Intron® A

International issues:

Peginterferon alfa-2b may be confused with interferon alpha multi-subtype which is available in international markets

Synonyms interferon alfa-2b (PEG conjugate); PEG-IFN Alfa-2b; pegylated interferon alfa-2b; polyethylene glycol interferon alfa-2b

U.S. Brand Names PegIntron®; PegIntron™ Redipen®; Sylatron™

Canadian Brand Names PegIntron®

Therapeutic Category Interferon

Use

PegIntron®: Treatment of chronic hepatitis C (CHC; in combination with ribavirin) in patients who have compensated liver disease; treatment of chronic hepatitis C (as monotherapy) in adult patients with compensated liver disease who have never received alfa interferons

Sylatron™: Adjuvant treatment of melanoma (with microscopic or gross nodal involvement within 84 days of definitive surgical resection, including lymphadenectomy)

General Dosage Range Dosage adjustment recommended in patients with renal impairment or who develop toxicities

SubQ: Melanoma:

Adults: Initial: 6 mcg/kg/week; Maintenance: 3 mcg/kg/week

SubQ: Chronic hepatitis C:

Children ≥3 years: 60 mcg/m²/week (in combination with ribavirin)

Adults: Peginterferon monotherapy (based on average weekly dose of 1 mcg/kg):
Adults ≤45 kg: 40 mcg once weekly
Adults 46-56 kg: 50 mcg once weekly
Adults 57-72 kg: 64 mcg once weekly
Adults 73-88 kg: 80 mcg once weekly
Adults 89-106 kg: 96 mcg once weekly
Adults 107-136 kg: 120 mcg once weekly
Adults 137-160 kg: 150 mcg once weekly
Adults: Combination therapy with ribavirin (based on average weekly dose of 1.5 mcg/kg):
Adults <40 kg: 50 mcg once weekly (with ribavirin 800 mg/day)
Adults 40-50 kg: 64 mcg once weekly (with ribavirin 800 mg/day)
Adults 51-60 kg: 80 mcg once weekly (with ribavirin 800 mg/day)
Adults 61-65 kg: 96 mcg once weekly (with ribavirin 800 mg/day)
Adults 66-75 kg: 96 mcg once weekly (with ribavirin 1000 mg/day)
Adults 76-80 kg: 120 mcg once weekly (with ribavirin 1000 mg/day)
Adults 81-85 kg: 120 mcg once weekly (with ribavirin 1200 mg/day)
Adults 86-105 kg: 150 mcg once weekly (with ribavirin 1200 mg/day)
Adults >105 kg: 1.5 mcg/kg once weekly (with ribavirin 1400 mg/day)

Dosage Forms
Injection, powder for reconstitution:
Sylatron™: 296 mcg, 444 mcg, 888 mcg
Injection, powder for reconstitution [preservative free]:
PegIntron®: 50 mcg, 80 mcg, 120 mcg, 150 mcg
PegIntron™ Redipen®: 50 mcg, 80 mcg, 120 mcg, 150 mcg

peginterferon alfa-2b and ribavirin *(Canada only)*

(peg in ter FEER on AL fa too bee & rye ba VYE rin)

Synonyms ribavirin and peginterferon alfa-2b
Canadian Brand Names Pegetron®; Pegetron® RediPen®
Therapeutic Category Antiviral Agent; Interferon
Use Combination therapy for the treatment of chronic hepatitis C in patients with compensated liver disease, including treatment-naive patients and those who have failed prior treatment with pegylated or nonpegylated interferon alpha and ribavirin combination therapy
General Dosage Range Dosage varies based on HCV genotype, weight, response to treatment, and therapy related toxicity.
Product Availability Not available in U.S.

Dosage Forms - Canada
Combination package:
Pegetron®:
Capsule: Ribavirin 200 mg (56s)
Injection, powder for reconstitution: Peginterferon alfa-2b: 50 mcg
Pegetron®:
Capsule: Ribavirin 200 mg (56s)
Injection, powder for reconstitution: Peginterferon alfa-2b: 80 mcg
Pegetron®:
Capsule: Ribavirin 200 mg (56s)
Injection, powder for reconstitution: Peginterferon alfa-2b: 100 mcg
Pegetron®:
Capsule: Ribavirin 200 mg (70s)
Injection, powder for reconstitution: Peginterferon alfa-2b: 120 mcg
Pegetron®:
Capsule: Ribavirin 200 mg (84s, 98s)
Injection, powder for reconstitution: Peginterferon alfa-2b: 150 mcg

PegIntron® *see* peginterferon alfa-2b *on page 698*
PegIntron™ Redipen® *see* peginterferon alfa-2b *on page 698*
PEGLA *see* pegaspargase *on page 696*

pegloticase (peg LOE ti kase)

Synonyms PEG-uricase; pegylated urate oxidase; polyethylene glycol-conjugated uricase; recombinant urate oxidase, pegylated; urate oxidase, pegylated

U.S. Brand Names Krystexxa™
Therapeutic Category Enzyme; Enzyme, Urate-Oxidase (Recombinant)
Use Treatment of chronic gout refractory to conventional therapy
General Dosage Range I.V.: *Adults:* 8 mg every 2 weeks
Dosage Forms
Injection, solution:
Krystexxa™: Uricase protein 8 mg/mL (2 mL)

PegLyte® (Can) *see* polyethylene glycol-electrolyte solution *on page 738*
PEG-uricase *see* pegloticase *on page 699*

pegvisomant (peg VI soe mant)

Medication Safety Issues
Sound-alike/look-alike issues:
Pegvisomant may be confused with peginesatide
Synonyms B2036-PEG
U.S. Brand Names Somavert®
Canadian Brand Names Somavert®
Therapeutic Category Growth Hormone Receptor Antagonist
Use Treatment of acromegaly in patients resistant to or unable to tolerate other therapies
General Dosage Range SubQ: *Adults:* Initial loading dose: 40 mg; Maintenance: 10-30 mg/day (maximum: 30 mg/day)
Dosage Forms
Injection, powder for reconstitution:
Somavert®: 10 mg, 15 mg, 20 mg

pegylated DOXOrubicin liposomal *see* doxorubicin (liposomal) *on page 314*
pegylated G-CSF *see* pegfilgrastim *on page 696*
pegylated interferon alfa-2a *see* peginterferon alfa-2a *on page 697*
pegylated interferon alfa-2b *see* peginterferon alfa-2b *on page 698*
pegylated liposomal DOXOrubicin *see* doxorubicin (liposomal) *on page 314*
pegylated urate oxidase *see* pegloticase *on page 699*
PE-Hist-DM [OTC] *see* chlorpheniramine, phenylephrine, and dextromethorphan *on page 201*

pemetrexed (pem e TREKS ed)

Medication Safety Issues
Sound-alike/look-alike issues:
PEMEtrexed may be confused with methotrexate, PRALAtrexate
High alert medication:
This medication is in a class the Institute for Safe Medication Practices (ISMP) includes among its list of drug classes which have a heightened risk of causing significant patient harm when used in error.
Synonyms LY231514; pemetrexed disodium
Tall-Man PEMEtrexed
U.S. Brand Names Alimta®
Canadian Brand Names Alimta®
Therapeutic Category Antineoplastic Agent, Antimetabolite; Antineoplastic Agent, Antimetabolite (Antifolate)
Use Treatment of unresectable malignant pleural mesothelioma (in combination with cisplatin); treatment of locally advanced or metastatic **non**squamous nonsmall cell lung cancer (NSCLC; as initial treatment in combination with cisplatin, as single-agent maintenance treatment after 4 cycles of initial platinum-based double therapy, and single-agent treatment after prior chemotherapy)

Note: Not indicated for the treatment of **squamous** cell NSCLC
General Dosage Range Dosage adjustment recommended in patients with hepatic impairment, on concomitant therapy, or who develop toxicities
I.V.: *Adults:* 500 mg/m^2 on day 1 of each 21-day cycle
Dosage Forms
Injection, powder for reconstitution:
Alimta®: 100 mg, 500 mg

pemetrexed disodium *see* pemetrexed *on page* 700

pemirolast (pe MIR oh last)

U.S. Brand Names Alamast®

Canadian Brand Names Alamast®

Therapeutic Category Mast Cell Stabilizer; Ophthalmic Agent, Miscellaneous

Use Prevention of itching of the eye due to allergic conjunctivitis

General Dosage Range Ophthalmic: *Children ≥3 years and Adults:* Instill 1-2 drops in affected eye(s) 4 times/day

Dosage Forms

Solution, ophthalmic:

Alamast®: 0.1% (10 mL)

penbutolol (pen BYOO toe lole)

Medication Safety Issues

Sound-alike/look-alike issues:

Levatol® may be confused with Lipitor®

International issues:

Levatol [U.S.] may be confused with Lovacol brand name for lovastatin [Chile and Finland]

Synonyms penbutolol sulfate

U.S. Brand Names Levatol®

Canadian Brand Names Levatol®

Therapeutic Category Beta-Adrenergic Blocker

Use Treatment of mild-to-moderate arterial hypertension

General Dosage Range Oral: *Adults:* Initial: 20 mg once daily; Maintenance: 10-40 mg once daily (maximum: 80 mg/day)

Dosage Forms

Tablet, oral:

Levatol®: 20 mg

penbutolol sulfate *see* penbutolol *on page* 701

penciclovir (pen SYE kloe veer)

Medication Safety Issues

Sound-alike/look-alike issues:

Denavir® may be confused with indinavir

U.S. Brand Names Denavir®

Therapeutic Category Antiviral Agent

Use Topical treatment of recurrent herpes simplex labialis (cold sores)

General Dosage Range Topical: *Children ≥12 years and Adults:* Apply every 2 hours during waking hours

Dosage Forms

Cream, topical:

Denavir®: 1% (1.5 g, 5 g)

penicillamine (pen i SIL a meen)

Medication Safety Issues

Sound-alike/look-alike issues:

Penicillamine may be confused with penicillin

International issues:

Depen [U.S.] may be confused with Depin brand name for nifedipine [India]; Depon brand name for acetaminophen [Greece]; Dipen brand name for diltiazem [Greece]

Pemine [Italy] may be confused with Pamine brand name for methscopolamine [U.S., Canada]

Synonyms D-3-mercaptovaline; D-penicillamine; β,β-dimethylcysteine

Tall-Man Penicill**AMINE**

U.S. Brand Names Cuprimine®; Depen®

Canadian Brand Names Cuprimine®

Therapeutic Category Chelating Agent

Use Treatment of Wilson disease, cystinuria; adjunctive treatment of severe, active rheumatoid arthritis

Canadian labeling: Additional use (not in U.S. labeling): Treatment of chronic lead poisoning

General Dosage Range Dosage adjustment recommended in patients with renal impairment

Oral:

Children: 30 mg/kg/day in 4 divided doses

Adults: Dosage varies greatly depending on indication

Dosage Forms

Capsule, oral:

Cuprimine®: 250 mg

Tablet, oral:

Depen®: 250 mg

penicillin G benzathine (pen i SIL in jee BENZ a theen)

Medication Safety Issues

Sound-alike/look-alike issues:

Penicillin may be confused with penicillamine

Bicillin® may be confused with Wycillin®

Administration issues:

Penicillin G benzathine may only be administered by deep intramuscular injection; intravenous administration of penicillin G benzathine has been associated with cardiopulmonary arrest and death.

Other safety concerns:

Bicillin® C-R (penicillin G benzathine and penicillin G procaine) may be confused with Bicillin® L-A (penicillin G benzathine). Penicillin G benzathine is the only product currently approved for the treatment of syphilis. Administration of penicillin G benzathine and penicillin G procaine combination instead of Bicillin® L-A may result in inadequate treatment response.

Synonyms benzathine benzylpenicillin; benzathine penicillin G; benzylpenicillin benzathine

U.S. Brand Names Bicillin® L-A

Canadian Brand Names Bicillin® L-A

Therapeutic Category Penicillin

Use Active against some gram-positive organisms, few gram-negative organisms such as *Neisseria gonorrhoeae*, and some anaerobes and spirochetes; used in the treatment of syphilis; used only for the treatment of mild to moderately-severe upper respiratory tract infections caused by organisms susceptible to low concentrations of penicillin G or for prophylaxis of infections caused by these organisms; primary and secondary prevention of rheumatic fever

General Dosage Range I.M.:

Children ≤27 kg: 600,000 units/dose

Children >27 kg: 1.2 million units/dose

Adults: 1.2-2.4 million units as a single dose

Dosage Forms

Injection, suspension:

Bicillin® L-A: 600,000 units/mL (1 mL, 2 mL, 4 mL)

penicillin G benzathine and penicillin G procaine

(pen i SIL in jee BENZ a theen & pen i SIL in jee PROE kane)

Medication Safety Issues

Sound-alike/look-alike issues:

Penicillin may be confused with penicillamine

Bicillin® may be confused with Wycillin®

Administration issues:

Penicillin G benzathine may only be administered by deep intramuscular injection; intravenous administration of penicillin G benzathine has been associated with cardiopulmonary arrest and death.

Other safety concerns:

Bicillin® C-R (penicillin G benzathine and penicillin G procaine) may be confused with Bicillin® L-A (penicillin G benzathine). Penicillin G benzathine is the only product currently approved for the treatment of syphilis. Administration of penicillin G benzathine and penicillin G procaine combination instead of Bicillin® L-A may result in inadequate treatment response.

Synonyms penicillin G procaine and benzathine combined

U.S. Brand Names Bicillin® C-R; Bicillin® C-R 900/300

Therapeutic Category Penicillin

Use May be used in specific situations in the treatment of streptococcal infections; primary prevention of rheumatic fever

General Dosage Range I.M.:

Children <14 kg: 600,000 units/dose

Children 14-27 kg: 900,000 units to 1.2 million units as a single dose

Children >27 kg and Adults: 2.4 million units/dose

Dosage Forms

Injection, suspension [prefilled syringe]:

Bicillin® C-R: 1,200,000 units: Penicillin G benzathine 600,000 units and penicillin G procaine 600,000 units per 2 mL (2 mL)

Bicillin® C-R 900/300: 1,200,000 units: Penicillin G benzathine 900,000 units and penicillin G procaine 300,000 units per 2 mL (2 mL)

penicillin G (parenteral/aqueous) (pen i SIL in jee, pa REN ter al, AYE kwee us)

Medication Safety Issues

Sound-alike/look-alike issues:

Penicillin may be confused with penicillamine

Synonyms benzylpenicillin potassium; benzylpenicillin sodium; crystalline penicillin; penicillin G potassium; penicillin G sodium

U.S. Brand Names Pfizerpen®

Canadian Brand Names Crystapen®

Therapeutic Category Penicillin

Use Treatment of infections (including sepsis, pneumonia, pericarditis, endocarditis, meningitis, anthrax) caused by susceptible organisms; active against some gram-positive organisms, generally not *Staphylococcus aureus*; some gram-negative organisms such as *Neisseria gonorrhoeae*, and some anaerobes and spirochetes

General Dosage Range Dosage adjustment recommended in patients with renal impairment

I.M., I.V.:

Infants ≥1 month and Children: 100,000-400,000 units/kg/day in divided doses every 4-6 hours (maximum: 24 million units/day)

Adults: 2-30 million units/day in divided doses every 4-6 hours

Dosage Forms

Infusion, premixed iso-osmotic dextrose solution: 1 million units (50 mL); 2 million units (50 mL); 3 million units (50 mL)

Injection, powder for reconstitution: 5 million units, 20 million units

Pfizerpen®: 5 million units, 20 million units

penicillin G potassium *see* penicillin G (parenteral/aqueous) *on page 703*

penicillin G procaine (pen i SIL in jee PROE kane)

Medication Safety Issues

Sound-alike/look-alike issues:

Penicillin G procaine may be confused with penicillin V potassium

Wycillin® may be confused with Bicillin®

Synonyms APPG; aqueous procaine penicillin G; procaine benzylpenicillin; procaine penicillin G; Wycillin [DSC]

Canadian Brand Names Pfizerpen-AS®; Wycillin®

Therapeutic Category Penicillin

Use Treatment of moderately-severe infections due to *Treponema pallidum* and other penicillin G-sensitive microorganisms that are susceptible to low, but prolonged serum penicillin concentrations; anthrax due to *Bacillus anthracis* (postexposure) to reduce the incidence or progression of disease following exposure to aerolized *Bacillus anthracis*

General Dosage Range Dosage adjustment recommended in patients with renal impairment

I.M.:

Children: 25,000-50,000 units/kg/day in divided doses 1-2 times/day (maximum: 4.8 million units/day)

Adults: 0.6-4.8 million units/day in divided doses every 12-24 hours

Dosage Forms

Injection, suspension: 600,000 units/mL (1 mL, 2 mL)

penicillin G procaine and benzathine combined *see* penicillin G benzathine and penicillin G procaine *on page 702*

penicillin G sodium *see* penicillin G (parenteral/aqueous) *on page 703*

penicillin V potassium (pen i SIL in vee poe TASS ee um)

Medication Safety Issues

Sound-alike/look-alike issues:

Penicillin V procaine may be confused with penicillin G potassium

Synonyms pen VK; phenoxymethyl penicillin

Canadian Brand Names Apo-Pen VK®; Novo-Pen-VK; Nu-Pen-VK

Therapeutic Category Penicillin

Use Treatment of infections caused by susceptible organisms involving the respiratory tract, otitis media, sinusitis, skin, and urinary tract; prophylaxis in rheumatic fever

General Dosage Range Dosage adjustment recommended in patients with renal impairment

Oral:

Children <12 years: 25-50 mg/kg/day divided every 6-8 hours (maximum: 3 g/day)

Children ≥12 years and Adults: 125-500 mg every 6-8 hours

Dosage Forms

Powder for solution, oral: 125 mg/5 mL (100 mL, 200 mL); 250 mg/5 mL (100 mL, 200 mL)

Tablet, oral: 250 mg, 500 mg

penicilloyl-polylysine *see* benzylpenicilloyl polylysine *on page 127*

Penlac® *see* ciclopirox *on page 207*

Pennsaid® *see* diclofenac (topical) *on page 280*

Pentacel® *see* diphtheria and tetanus toxoids, acellular pertussis, poliovirus and *Haemophilus* b conjugate vaccine *on page 298*

pentahydrate *see* sodium thiosulfate *on page 848*

Pentam® 300 *see* pentamidine *on page 704*

pentamidine (pen TAM i deen)

Synonyms pentamidine isethionate

U.S. Brand Names Nebupent®; Pentam® 300

Therapeutic Category Antiprotozoal

Use

I.M., I.V.: Treatment of pneumonia caused by *Pneumocystis jirovecii* pneumonia (PCP)

Inhalation: Prevention of PCP in high-risk, HIV-infected patients either with a history of PCP or with a CD4+ count ≤200/mm^3

General Dosage Range Dosage adjustment recommended in patients with renal impairment

I.M.: *Children >4 months and Adults:* 4 mg/kg once daily for 14-21 days

I.V.:

*Children >4 months and Adults:*4 mg/kg once daily for 14-21 days

Inhalation: *Children >16 years and Adults:* 300 mg/dose every 4 weeks

Dosage Forms

Injection, powder for reconstitution:

Pentam® 300: 300 mg

Powder for solution, for nebulization:

Nebupent®: 300 mg

pentamidine isethionate *see* pentamidine *on page 704*

Pentamycetin® (Can) *see* chloramphenicol *on page 195*

Pentasa® *see* mesalamine *on page 577*

pentasodium colistin methanesulfonate *see* colistimethate *on page 233*

Pentaspan® (Can) *see* pentastarch *(Canada only) on page 704*

pentastarch *(Canada only)* (PEN ta starch)

Synonyms HES; HES 200/0.5; hydroxyethyl starch

Canadian Brand Names Pentaspan®

Therapeutic Category Blood Modifiers

Use Adjunctive treatment in the management of shock

General Dosage Range I.V.: *Adults:* 500-2000 mL/day (maximum daily dose: 28 mL/kg or 2000 mL)

Product Availability Not available in U.S.

Dosage Forms - Canada

Infusion, premixed in NS:

Pentaspan®: 10% (250 mL, 500 mL)

pentavalent human-bovine reassortant rotavirus vaccine (PRV) *see* rotavirus vaccine *on page 813*

pentazocine (pen TAZ oh seen)

Medication Safety Issues

High alert medication:

The Institute for Safe Medication Practices (ISMP) includes this medication among its list of drug classes which have a heightened risk of causing significant patient harm when used in error.

BEERS Criteria medication:

This drug may be potentially inappropriate for use in geriatric patients (Quality of evidence - low; Strength of recommendation - strong).

Synonyms pentazocine lactate

U.S. Brand Names Talwin®

Canadian Brand Names Talwin®

Therapeutic Category Analgesic, Narcotic

Controlled Substance C-IV

Use Relief of moderate-to-severe pain; has also been used as a sedative prior to surgery and as a supplement to surgical anesthesia

General Dosage Range Dosage adjustment recommended in patients with renal impairment

I.M.:

Children 1-16 years: 0.5 mg/kg preoperatively

Adults: 30-60 mg every 3-4 hours (maximum: 360 mg/day; 60 mg/dose) **or** 30 mg once

I.V.: *Adults:* 30 mg every 3-4 hours (maximum: 360 mg/day; 30 mg/dose) **or** 20 mg every 2-3 hours as needed (maximum total dose: 60 mg)

SubQ: *Adults:* 30 mg every 3-4 hours (maximum: 360 mg/day; 60 mg/dose)

Dosage Forms

Injection, solution:

Talwin®: 30 mg/mL (1 mL, 10 mL)

pentazocine and acetaminophen (pen TAZ oh seen & a seet a MIN oh fen)

Medication Safety Issues

Sound-alike/look-alike issues:

Talacen may be confused with Timoptic®, Tinactin®

High alert medication:

The Institute for Safe Medication Practices (ISMP) includes this medication among its list of drug classes which have a heightened risk of causing significant patient harm when used in error.

Other safety concerns:

Duplicate therapy issues: This product contains acetaminophen, which may be a component of other combination products. Do not exceed the maximum recommended daily dose of acetaminophen.

Synonyms acetaminophen and pentazocine; pentazocine hydrochloride and acetaminophen; Talacen

Therapeutic Category Analgesic Combination (Opioid)

Controlled Substance C-IV

Use Relief of mild-to-moderate pain

General Dosage Range Oral: *Children ≥12 years and Adults:* One caplet (pentazocine 25 mg/acetaminophen 650 mg) every 4 hours as needed (maximum: 6 caplets/day)

Dosage Forms

Tablet: Pentazocine 25 mg and acetaminophen 650 mg

pentazocine and naloxone (pen TAZ oh seen & nal OKS one)

Medication Safety Issues

High alert medication:

The Institute for Safe Medication Practices (ISMP) includes this medication among its list of drug classes which have a heightened risk of causing significant patient harm when used in error.

Synonyms naloxone hydrochloride and pentazocine; pentazocine hydrochloride and naloxone hydrochloride; Talwin NX

Therapeutic Category Analgesic, Opioid

Controlled Substance C-IV

Use Relief of moderate-to-severe pain; indicated for oral use only

General Dosage Range Dosage adjustment recommended in patients with renal impairment

Oral: *Children ≥12 years and Adults:* Based upon pentazocine: 50-100 mg every 3-4 hours (maximum: 600 mg/day)

Dosage Forms

Tablet: Pentazocine 50 mg and naloxone 0.5 mg

pentazocine hydrochloride and acetaminophen *see* pentazocine and acetaminophen *on page 705*

pentazocine hydrochloride and naloxone hydrochloride *see* pentazocine and naloxone *on page 705*

pentazocine lactate *see* pentazocine *on page 705*

pentetate calcium trisodium *see* diethylene triamine penta-acetic acid *on page 283*

pentetate indium disodium in 111

(PEN te tate IN dee um dye SOW dee um eye en won e LEV en)

Medication Safety Issues

Other safety concerns:

Radiopharmaceutical: Use appropriate precaution for handling, disposal, and minimizing exposure to patients and healthcare personnel. Use under supervision of experienced personnel. Should be stored in original lead container or adequate radiation shield.

Synonyms ^{111}in-DTPA; ^{111}in-pentetate; DTPA; indium IN-111 pentetate disodium

U.S. Brand Names Indium DTPA In 111

Therapeutic Category Radiopharmaceutical

Use Radionuclide cisternography

pentetate zinc trisodium *see* diethylene triamine penta-acetic acid *on page 283*

pentobarbital (pen toe BAR bi tal)

Medication Safety Issues

Sound-alike/look-alike issues:

PENTobarbital may be confused with PHENobarbital

Nembutal® may be confused with Myambutol®

BEERS Criteria medication:

This drug may be potentially inappropriate for use in geriatric patients (Quality of evidence - high; Strength of recommendation - strong).

Synonyms pentobarbital sodium

Tall-Man PENTobarbital

U.S. Brand Names Nembutal®

Canadian Brand Names Nembutal® Sodium

Therapeutic Category Barbiturate

Controlled Substance C-II

Use Sedative/hypnotic; refractory status epilepticus

General Dosage Range

I.M.:

Children: 2-6 mg/kg (maximum: 100 mg/dose)

Adults: 150-200 mg

I.V.:

Children:

Hypnotic/sedative: 1-6 mg/kg

Refractory status epilepticus: Loading dose: 5-15 mg/kg; Maintenance infusion: 0.5-5 mg/kg/hour

Adults:

Hypnotic/sedative: 100 mg; may repeat (maximum total dose: 500 mg)

Refractory status epilepticus: Loading dose: 10-15 mg/kg; Maintenance infusion: 0.5-10 mg/kg/hour

Dosage Forms

Injection, solution:

Nembutal®: 50 mg/mL (20 mL, 50 mL)

pentobarbital sodium *see* pentobarbital *on page 706*

pentosan polysulfate sodium (PEN toe san pol i SUL fate SOW dee um)

Medication Safety Issues

Sound-alike/look-alike issues:

Pentosan may be confused with pentostatin

Elmiron® may be confused with Imuran®

Synonyms PPS

U.S. Brand Names Elmiron®

Canadian Brand Names Elmiron®

Therapeutic Category Analgesic, Urinary

Use Relief of bladder pain or discomfort due to interstitial cystitis

General Dosage Range Oral: *Children ≥16 years and Adults:* 100 mg 3 times/day

Dosage Forms

Capsule, oral:

Elmiron®: 100 mg

pentostatin (pen toe STAT in)

Medication Safety Issues

Sound-alike/look-alike issues:

Pentostatin may be confused with pentamidine, pentosan

High alert medication:

The Institute for Safe Medication Practices (ISMP) includes this medication among its list of drug classes which have a heightened risk of causing significant patient harm when used in error.

International issues:

Nipent [U.S., Canada, and multiple international markets] may be confused with Nipin brand name for nifedipine [Italy, Singapore]

Synonyms 2′-deoxycoformycin; co-vidarabine; dCF; deoxycoformycin; NSC-218321

U.S. Brand Names Nipent®

Canadian Brand Names Nipent®

Therapeutic Category Antineoplastic Agent

Use Treatment of hairy cell leukemia

General Dosage Range Dosage adjustment recommended in patients with renal impairment

I.V.: *Adults:* 4 mg/m^2 every 2 weeks

Dosage Forms

Injection, powder for reconstitution:

Nipent®: 10 mg

Injection, powder for reconstitution [preservative free]: 10 mg

Pentothal® [DSC] *see* thiopental *on page 891*

pentoxifylline (pen toks IF i lin)

Medication Safety Issues

Sound-alike/look-alike issues:

Pentoxifylline may be confused with tamoxifen

TRENtal® may be confused with Bentyl®, TEGretol®, Trandate®

Synonyms oxpentifylline

U.S. Brand Names TRENtal®

Canadian Brand Names Albert® Pentoxifylline; Apo-Pentoxifylline SR®; Nu-Pentoxifylline SR; ratio-Pentoxifylline; Trental®

Therapeutic Category Blood Viscosity Reducer Agent

Use Treatment of intermittent claudication on the basis of chronic occlusive arterial disease of the limbs; may improve function and symptoms, but not intended to replace more definitive therapy

Note: The American College of Chest Physicians (ACCP) discourages the use of pentoxifylline for the treatment of intermittent claudication refractory to exercise therapy (and smoking cessation) (Guyatt, 2012).

General Dosage Range Dosage adjustment recommended in patients with renal impairment

Oral: *Adults:* 400 mg 2-3 times/day

Dosage Forms

Tablet, controlled release, oral:

TRENtal®: 400 mg

Tablet, extended release, oral: 400 mg

Pentrax® [OTC] *see* coal tar *on page 228*

Pentrax Gold Shampoo [OTC] (Can) *see* coal tar *on page 228*

Pentrax Tar Shampoo [OTC] (Can) *see* coal tar *on page 228*

pen VK *see* penicillin V potassium *on page 704*

PEP005 *see* ingenol mebutate *on page 484*

Pepcid® *see* famotidine *on page 372*

Pepcid® AC [OTC] *see* famotidine *on page 372*

Pepcid® AC (Can) *see* famotidine *on page 372*

Pepcid® AC Maximum Strength [OTC] *see* famotidine *on page 372*

Pepcid® Complete® [OTC] *see* famotidine, calcium carbonate, and magnesium hydroxide *on page 373*

Pepcid® I.V. (Can) *see* famotidine *on page 372*

Peptic Relief [OTC] *see* bismuth *on page 135*

Pepto-Bismol® [OTC] *see* bismuth *on page 135*

Pepto-Bismol® Maximum Strength [OTC] *see* bismuth *on page 135*

Pepto Relief [OTC] *see* bismuth *on page 135*

Peranex™ HC *see* lidocaine and hydrocortisone *on page 538*

Peranex™ HC Medi-Pad *see* lidocaine and hydrocortisone *on page 538*

Percocet® *see* oxycodone and acetaminophen *on page 679*

Percocet®-Demi (Can) *see* oxycodone and acetaminophen *on page 679*

Percodan® *see* oxycodone and aspirin *on page 680*

Percogesic® Extra Strength [OTC] *see* acetaminophen and diphenhydramine *on page 23*

Perdiem® Overnight Relief [OTC] *see* senna *on page 829*

perflutren lipid microspheres (per FLOO tren LIPid MI kro SFIRS)

U.S. Brand Names Definity®

Canadian Brand Names Definity®

Therapeutic Category Diagnostic Agent

Use Opacification of left ventricular chamber and improvement of delineation of the left ventricular endocardial border in patients with suboptimal echocardiograms

General Dosage Range I.V.: *Adults:* Bolus: 10 microliters (µL)/kg of activated product, followed by 10 mL saline flush; may repeat in 30 minutes if needed; Infusion: Initial: 4 mL/minute (or 240 mL/hour) of prepared infusion; titrate to achieve optimal image; Maximum rate: 10 mL/minute (or 600 mL/hour)

Dosage Forms

Injection, solution [preservative free]:

Definity®: OFP 6.52 mg/mL and lipid blend 0.75 mg/mL (2 mL)

Perforomist® *see* formoterol *on page 406*

Periactin *see* cyproheptadine *on page 246*

periciazine *(Canada only)* (per ee CYE ah zeen)

Synonyms pericyazine

Canadian Brand Names Neuleptil®

Therapeutic Category Phenothiazine Derivative

Use Adjunctive therapy in selected psychotic patients to control prevailing hostility, impulsivity, or aggression

General Dosage Range Oral:
Children ≥5 years: Initial: 2.5-10 mg in the morning, followed by 5-30 mg in the evening
Adults: Initial: 5-20 mg in the morning, followed by 10-40 mg in the evening
Elderly: Initial: 5 mg/day; may increase dose gradually based on effect and tolerance. Doses >30 mg/day are rarely needed.

Product Availability Not available in U.S.

Dosage Forms - Canada

Capsule, oral:
Neuleptil®: 5 mg, 10 mg, 20 mg

Solution, oral [drops]:
Neuleptil®: 10 mg/mL

Peri-Colace® [OTC] *see* docusate and senna *on page* 305
pericyazine *see* periciazine *(Canada only) on page* 708
Peridex® *see* chlorhexidine gluconate *on page* 196
Peridex® Oral Rinse (Can) *see* chlorhexidine gluconate *on page* 196
perindopril and indapamide *see* perindopril erbumine and indapamide *(Canada only) on page* 709

perindopril erbumine (per IN doe pril er BYOO meen)

U.S. Brand Names Aceon®

Canadian Brand Names Apo-Perindopril®; Coversyl®

Therapeutic Category Miscellaneous Product

Use Treatment of hypertension; reduction of cardiovascular mortality or nonfatal myocardial infarction in patients with stable coronary artery disease

Canadian labeling: Additional use (unlabeled use in U.S.): Treatment of mild-moderate (NYHA I-III) heart failure

General Dosage Range Dosage adjustment recommended in patients with renal impairment
Oral: *Adults:* Initial: 2-4 mg once daily; Maintenance: 4-8 mg/day in 1-2 divided doses (maximum: 16 mg/day)

Dosage Forms

Tablet, oral: 2 mg, 4 mg, 8 mg
Aceon®: 2 mg, 4 mg, 8 mg

perindopril erbumine and indapamide *(Canada only)*
(per IN doe pril er BYOO meen & in DAP a mide)

Synonyms indapamide and perindopril erbumine; perindopril and indapamide

Canadian Brand Names Coversyl® Plus; Coversyl® Plus HD; Coversyl® Plus LD

Therapeutic Category Angiotensin-Converting Enzyme (ACE) Inhibitor; Antihypertensive Agent, Combination; Diuretic, Thiazide-Related

Use Treatment of hypertension
Note: Coversyl® Plus LD may be used as initial treatment; Coversyl® Plus and Coversyl® Plus HD are not indicated for initial treatment of hypertension.

General Dosage Range Oral: *Adults:* Perindopril 2-8 mg/indapamide 0.625-2.5 mg once daily

Product Availability Not available in U.S.

Dosage Forms - Canada

Tablet, oral:
Coversyl® Plus: Perindopril erbumine 4 mg and indapamide 1.25 mg
Coversyl® Plus HD: Perindopril erbumine 8 mg and indapamide 2.5 mg
Coversyl® Plus LD: Perindopril erbumine 2 mg and indapamide 0.625 mg

periochip® *see* chlorhexidine gluconate *on page* 196
PerioGard® [OTC] *see* chlorhexidine gluconate *on page* 196
PerioMed™ *see* fluoride *on page* 393
Periostat® *see* doxycycline *on page* 314
Perjeta™ *see* pertuzumab *on page* 710
Perlane® *see* hyaluronate and derivatives *on page* 450

permethrin (per METH rin)

Synonyms Elimite

U.S. Brand Names A200® Lice [OTC]; Nix® Complete Lice Treatment System [OTC]; Nix® Creme Rinse Lice Treatment [OTC]; Nix® Creme Rinse [OTC]; Nix® Lice Control Spray [OTC]; Rid® [OTC]

Canadian Brand Names Kwellada-P™; Nix®

Therapeutic Category Scabicides/Pediculicides

Use Single-application treatment of infestation with *Pediculus humanus capitis* (head louse) and its nits or *Sarcoptes scabiei* (scabies); indicated for prophylactic use during epidemics of lice

General Dosage Range Topical:

Cream: *Children and Adults:* Apply from head to toe, leave on 8-14 hours before washing off with water; May reapply in 1 week if live mites appear

Liquid (lotion or cream rinse): *Children >2 months and Adults:* Apply a sufficient volume to saturate the hair and scalp, leave on for 10 minutes before rinsing off with water; May reapply in 1 week if lice or nits still present

Dosage Forms

Cream, topical: 5% (60 g)

Liquid, topical:

Nix® Complete Lice Treatment System [OTC]: 1% (1s)
Nix® Creme Rinse [OTC]: 1% (60 mL)
Nix® Creme Rinse Lice Treatment [OTC]: 1% (60 mL)
Nix® Lice Control Spray [OTC]: 0.25% (150 mL)

Lotion, topical: 1% (60 mL)

Solution, topical:

A200® Lice [OTC]: 0.5% (170.1 g)
Rid® [OTC]: 0.5% (150 mL)

Pernox® Lemon [OTC] *see* sulfur and salicylic acid *on page 861*

Pernox® Regular [OTC] *see* sulfur and salicylic acid *on page 861*

perphenazine (per FEN a zeen)

Medication Safety Issues

Sound-alike/look-alike issues:

Trilafon may be confused with Tri-Levlen®

BEERS Criteria medication:

This drug may be potentially inappropriate for use in geriatric patients (Quality of evidence - moderate; Strength of recommendation - strong).

Synonyms Trilafon

Canadian Brand Names Apo-Perphenazine®

Therapeutic Category Phenothiazine Derivative

Use Treatment of schizophrenia; severe nausea and vomiting

General Dosage Range Oral: *Adults:* 4-16 mg 2-4 times/day (maximum: 64 mg/day)

Dosage Forms

Tablet, oral: 2 mg, 4 mg, 8 mg, 16 mg

perphenazine and amitriptyline hydrochloride *see* amitriptyline and perphenazine *on page 65*

Persantine® *see* dipyridamole *on page 300*

pertussis, acellular (adsorbed) *see* diphtheria and tetanus toxoids, acellular pertussis, poliovirus and *Haemophilus* b conjugate vaccine *on page 298*

pertuzumab (per TU zoo mab)

Medication Safety Issues

Sound-alike/look-alike issues:

Pertuzumab may be confused with panitumumab, trastuzumab

High alert medication:

This medication is in a class the Institute for Safe Medication Practices (ISMP) includes among its list of drug classes which have a heightened risk of causing significant patient harm when used in error.

Synonyms 2C4 antibody; MOAB 2C4; monoclonal antibody 2C4; Omnitarg; rhuMAb-2C4

U.S. Brand Names Perjeta™

Therapeutic Category Antineoplastic Agent, Anti-HER2; Antineoplastic Agent, Monoclonal Antibody

Use Treatment of HER2-positive metastatic breast cancer (in combination with trastuzumab and docetaxel) in patients who have not received prior anti-HER2 therapy or chemotherapy to treat metastatic disease

General Dosage Range I.V.: *Adults:* Initial: 840 mg; Maintenance: 420 mg every 3 weeks

Dosage Forms

Injection, solution [preservative free]:

Perjeta™: 30 mg/mL (14 mL)

Pertzye™ *see* pancrelipase *on page 687*

pethidine hydrochloride *see* meperidine *on page 574*

Pexeva® *see* paroxetine *on page 693*

PF-02341066 *see* crizotinib *on page 240*

PFA *see* foscarnet *on page 408*

Pfizerpen® *see* penicillin G (parenteral/aqueous) *on page 703*

Pfizerpen-AS® (Can) *see* penicillin G procaine *on page 703*

PGE_1 *see* alprostadil *on page 53*

PGE_2 *see* dinoprostone *on page 291*

PGI_2 *see* epoprostenol *on page 338*

PGX *see* epoprostenol *on page 338*

Pharmorubicin® (Can) *see* epirubicin *on page 336*

Phazyme™ (Can) *see* simethicone *on page 834*

Phazyme® Ultra Strength [OTC] *see* simethicone *on page 834*

Phenadoz® *see* promethazine *on page 763*

Phenaseptic [OTC] *see* phenol *on page 713*

Phenazo [OTC] *see* phenazopyridine *on page 711*

phenazopyridine (fen az oh PEER i deen)

Medication Safety Issues

Sound-alike/look-alike issues:

Phenazopyridine may be confused with phenoxybenzamine

Pyridium® may be confused with Dyrenium®, Perdiem®, pyridoxine, pyrithione

Synonyms phenazopyridine hydrochloride; phenylazo diamino pyridine hydrochloride

U.S. Brand Names AZO Standard® Maximum Strength [OTC] [DSC]; AZO Standard® [OTC] [DSC]; AZO Urinary Pain Relief™ Maximum Strength [OTC]; AZO Urinary Pain Relief™ [OTC]; Azo-Gesic™ [OTC]; Baridium [OTC]; Phenazo [OTC]; Pyridium®; Urinary Pain Relief [OTC]

Therapeutic Category Analgesic, Urinary

Use Symptomatic relief of urinary burning, itching, frequency, and urgency in association with urinary tract infection or following urologic procedures

General Dosage Range Dosage adjustment recommended in patients with renal impairment

Oral:

Children: 12 mg/kg/day in 3 divided doses

Adults: 100-200 mg 3 times/day

Dosage Forms

Tablet, oral: 100 mg, 200 mg

AZO Urinary Pain Relief™ [OTC]: 95 mg

AZO Urinary Pain Relief™ Maximum Strength [OTC]: 97.5 mg

Azo-Gesic™ [OTC]: 95 mg

Baridium [OTC]: 97.2 mg

Phenazo [OTC]: 95 mg

Pyridium®: 100 mg, 200 mg

Urinary Pain Relief [OTC]: 95 mg

phenazopyridine hydrochloride *see* phenazopyridine *on page 711*

phendimetrazine (fen dye ME tra zeen)

Medication Safety Issues

Sound-alike/look-alike issues:

Bontril PDM® may be confused with Bentyl®

Synonyms phendimetrazine tartrate

U.S. Brand Names Bontril® PDM; Bontril® Slow-Release

Canadian Brand Names Bontril®; Plegine®; Statobex®

Therapeutic Category Anorexiant

Controlled Substance C-III

Use Short-term (few weeks) adjunct in exogenous obesity

Pharmacotherapy for weight loss is recommended only for obese patients with a body mass index ≥30 kg/m^2, or ≥27 kg/m^2 in the presence of other risk factors such as hypertension, diabetes, and/or dyslipidemia or a high waist circumference; therapy should be used in conjunction with a comprehensive weight management program.

General Dosage Range Oral:

Capsule: *Adolescents 17 years and Adults:* 105 mg once daily before breakfast

Tablet: *Adults:* 17.5-35 mg 2-3 times/day, 1 hour before meals (maximum: 70 mg 3 times/day)

Dosage Forms

Capsule, slow release, oral: 105 mg

Bontril® Slow-Release: 105 mg

Tablet, oral: 35 mg

Bontril® PDM: 35 mg

phendimetrazine tartrate *see* phendimetrazine *on page* 711

phenelzine (FEN el zeen)

Medication Safety Issues

Sound-alike/look-alike issues:

Phenelzine may be confused with phenytoin

Nardil® may be confused with Norinyl®

Synonyms phenelzine sulfate

U.S. Brand Names Nardil®

Canadian Brand Names Nardil®

Therapeutic Category Antidepressant, Monoamine Oxidase Inhibitor

Use Symptomatic treatment of atypical, nonendogenous, or neurotic depression

General Dosage Range Oral: *Adults:* Initial: 45 mg/day in 3 divided doses; Maintenance: 15-90 mg/day in 1-3 divided doses

Dosage Forms

Tablet, oral: 15 mg

Nardil®: 15 mg

phenelzine sulfate *see* phenelzine *on page* 712

Phenergan *see* promethazine *on page* 763

pheniramine and naphazoline *see* naphazoline and pheniramine *on page* 627

phenobarbital (fee noe BAR bi tal)

Medication Safety Issues

Sound-alike/look-alike issues:

PHENobarbital may be confused with PENTobarbital, Phenergan®, phenytoin

BEERS Criteria medication:

This drug may be potentially inappropriate for use in geriatric patients (Quality of evidence - high; Strength of recommendation - strong).

Synonyms luminal sodium; phenobarbital sodium; phenobarbitone; phenylethylmalonylurea

Tall-Man PHENobarbital

Canadian Brand Names PMS-Phenobarbital

Therapeutic Category Anticonvulsant; Barbiturate

Controlled Substance C-IV

Use Management of generalized tonic-clonic (grand mal), status epilepticus, and partial seizures; sedative/hypnotic

Note: Use to treat insomnia is not recommended (Schutte-Rodin, 2008)

General Dosage Range Dosage adjustment recommended in patients with renal impairment

I.M.:

Children: 3-5 mg/kg at bedtime or 1-3 mg/kg 1-1.5 hours before procedure

Adults: Dosage varies greatly depending on indication

I.V.:

Infants: Loading dose: 10-20 mg/kg in a single or divided dose; Maintenance: 5-8 mg/kg/day in 1-2 divided doses

Children: Loading dose: 15-20 mg/kg in a single or divided dose; Maintenance: Dosage varies greatly depending on indication

Adults: Loading dose: 10-20 mg/kg; may repeat dose in 20-minute intervals as needed (maximum total dose: 30 mg/kg); Maintenance: Dosage varies greatly depending on indication

Oral:

Infants: 5-8 mg/kg/day in 1-2 divided doses

Children and Adults: Dosage varies greatly depending on indication

Dosage Forms

Elixir, oral: 20 mg/5 mL (5 mL, 7.5 mL, 15 mL, 473 mL, 480 mL)

Injection, solution: 65 mg/mL (1 mL); 130 mg/mL (1 mL)

Tablet, oral: 15 mg, 16.2 mg, 30 mg, 32.4 mg, 60 mg, 100 mg

phenobarbital, hyoscyamine, atropine, and scopolamine *see* hyoscyamine, atropine, scopolamine, and phenobarbital *on page 467*

phenobarbital sodium *see* phenobarbital *on page 712*

phenobarbitone *see* phenobarbital *on page 712*

phenol (FEE nol)

Medication Safety Issues

Sound-alike/look-alike issues:

Cēpastat® may be confused with Capastat®

Synonyms carbolic acid

U.S. Brand Names Castellani Paint Modified [OTC]; Cepastat® Extra Strength [OTC]; Cepastat® [OTC]; Cheracol® Spray [OTC]; Chloraseptic® Kids Sore Throat Spray [OTC]; Chloraseptic® Mouth Pain [OTC]; Chloraseptic® Sore Throat Gargle [OTC]; Chloraseptic® Sore Throat Spray [OTC]; Pain-A-Lay® [OTC]; Phenaseptic [OTC]; Phenol EZ® [OTC]; Ulcerease® [OTC]; Vicks® Formula 44® Sore Throat [OTC]

Canadian Brand Names P & S™ Liquid Phenol

Therapeutic Category Pharmaceutical Aid

Use Relief of sore throat pain, mouth, gum, and throat irritations; antiseptic; topical anesthetic

General Dosage Range

Oral:

Children 2-12 years:

Chloraseptic®: 3 sprays onto throat or affected area; may repeat every 2 hours

Chloraseptic® for Kids: 5 sprays onto throat or affected area; may repeat every 2 hours

Children >3 years: Ulcerease®: Gargle or swish for 15 seconds, then expectorate; may repeat every 2 hours

Children 6-12 years:

Cēpastat® Extra Strength: Up to 1 lozenge every 2 hours as needed (maximum: 10 lozenges/24 hours)

Cēpastat®: Up to 1 lozenge every 2 hours as needed (maximum: 18 lozenges/24 hours)

Pain-A-Lay® Gargle: Using gauze pad, apply 10 mL to affected area, or gargle or swish for 15 seconds, then expectorate

Children ≥12 years and Adults:

Cēpastat® Extra Strength, Cēpastat®: Up to 2 lozenges every 2 hours as needed

Cheracol®, Pain-A-Lay® Spray: Spray directly in throat; rinse for 15 seconds then expectorate; may repeat every 2 hours

Chloraseptic®: 5 sprays onto throat or affected area; may repeat every 2 hours

Chloraseptic® Gargle, Cēpastat® Mouth Pain, Pain-A-Lay® Gargle, Ulcerease®: Gargle or swish for 15 seconds, then expectorate; may repeat every 2 hours

Topical: *Adults:* Apply small amount to affected area 1-3 times/day

Dosage Forms

Lozenge, oral:

Cepastat® [OTC]: 14.5 mg (18s)

Cepastat® Extra Strength [OTC]: 29 mg (18s)

Solution, oral: 1.4% (177 mL)
Cheracol® Spray [OTC]: 1.4% (177 mL)
Chloraseptic® Kids Sore Throat Spray [OTC]: 0.5% (177 mL)
Chloraseptic® Mouth Pain [OTC]: 1.4% (29 mL)
Chloraseptic® Sore Throat Gargle [OTC]: 1.4% (296 mL)
Chloraseptic® Sore Throat Spray [OTC]: 1.4% (20 mL, 177 mL)
Pain-A-Lay® [OTC]: 1.4% (177 mL, 236 mL, 532 mL)
Phenaseptic [OTC]: 1.4% (177 mL)
Ulcerease® [OTC]: 0.6% (30 mL, 180 mL)
Vicks® Formula 44® Sore Throat [OTC]: 1.4% (177 mL)

Solution, topical:
Castellani Paint Modified [OTC]: 1.5% (30 mL)

Swab, topical:
Phenol EZ® [OTC]: 89% (30s)

phenol and camphor *see* camphor and phenol *on page* 167
Phenol EZ® [OTC] *see* phenol *on page* 713
phenoptin *see* sapropterin *on page* 823

phenoxybenzamine (fen oks ee BEN za meen)

Medication Safety Issues
Sound-alike/look-alike issues:
Phenoxybenzamine may be confused with phenazopyridine
Synonyms phenoxybenzamine hydrochloride
U.S. Brand Names Dibenzyline®
Therapeutic Category Alpha-Adrenergic Blocking Agent
Use Symptomatic management of pheochromocytoma
General Dosage Range Oral: *Adults:* Initial: 10 mg twice daily; Maintenance: 10-40 mg 1-3 times/day (maximum: 240 mg/day)
Dosage Forms
Capsule, oral:
Dibenzyline®: 10 mg

phenoxybenzamine hydrochloride *see* phenoxybenzamine *on page* 714
phenoxymethyl penicillin *see* penicillin V potassium *on page* 704

phentermine (FEN ter meen)

Medication Safety Issues
Sound-alike/look-alike issues:
Phentermine may be confused with phentolamine, phenytoin
Synonyms phentermine hydrochloride
U.S. Brand Names Adipex-P®; Suprenza™
Therapeutic Category Anorexiant
Controlled Substance C-IV
Use Short-term (few weeks) adjunct therapy in obese patients with an initial body mass index (BMI) ≥30 kg/m^2 or ≥27 kg/m^2 in the presence of other risk factors (eg, diabetes, hyperlipidemia, controlled hypertension); therapy should be used in conjunction with a comprehensive weight management program.
General Dosage Range Oral: *Children >16 years and Adults:* 15-37.5 mg/day
Dosage Forms
Capsule, oral: 15 mg, 30 mg, 37.5 mg
Adipex-P®: 37.5 mg
Tablet, oral: 37.5 mg
Adipex-P®: 37.5 mg
Tablet, orally disintegrating, oral:
Suprenza™: 15 mg, 30 mg

phentermine and topiramate (FEN ter meen & toe PYRE a mate)

Synonyms Qnexa; Qsymia™; topiramate and phentermine
U.S. Brand Names Qsymia™

Therapeutic Category Anorexiant; Anticonvulsant, Miscellaneous; Sympathomimetic

Controlled Substance C-IV

Use Chronic weight management, as an adjunct to a reduced-calorie diet and increased physical activity, in patients with either an initial body mass index (BMI) of ≥30 kg/m^2 **or** an initial BMI of ≥27 kg/m^2 and at least one weight-related comorbid condition (eg, hypertension, dyslipidemia, type 2 diabetes)

General Dosage Range Dosage adjustment recommended in patients with renal impairment or hepatic impairment.

Oral: *Adults:* Phentermine 3.75-15 mg/topiramate 23-92 mg once daily.

phentermine hydrochloride *see* phentermine *on page 714*

phentolamine (fen TOLE a meen)

Medication Safety Issues

Sound-alike/look-alike issues:

Phentolamine may be confused with phentermine, Ventolin®

Synonyms phentolamine mesylate; Regitine [DSC]

U.S. Brand Names OraVerse™

Canadian Brand Names Regitine®; Rogitine®

Therapeutic Category Alpha-Adrenergic Blocking Agent; Diagnostic Agent

Use Diagnosis of pheochromocytoma and treatment of hypertension associated with pheochromocytoma or other forms of hypertension caused by excess sympathomimetic amines; treatment of dermal necrosis after extravasation of drugs with alpha-adrenergic effects (ie, dopamine, epinephrine, norepinephrine, phenylephrine)

OraVerse™: Reversal of soft tissue anesthesia and the associated functional deficits resulting from a local dental anesthetic containing a vasoconstrictor

General Dosage Range

I.M., I.V.:

Children: 0.05-0.1 mg/kg/dose as a single dose 1-2 hours before procedure, repeat as needed every 2-4 hours (maximum: 5 mg/dose)

Adults: 5 mg as a single dose 1-2 hours before procedure, may repeat as needed every 2-4 hours **or** 5-20 mg (hypertensive crisis)

Submucosal injection:

Children 15-30 kg and <12 years: 0.2 mg (maximum)

Children >30 kg and <12 years: 0.4 mg (maximum)

Children >30 kg and ≥12 years and Adults: 0.2 mg to 0.8 mg (depending on number of cartridges of anesthesia)

SubQ: *Children and Adults:* Infiltrate area with a small amount (eg, 1 mL) of solution (made by diluting 5-10 mg in 10 mL of NS) within 12 hours of extravasation; in general, do not exceed 0.1-0.2 mg/kg (5 mg total); typically doses of ≤5 mg are effective

Dosage Forms

Injection, powder for reconstitution: 5 mg

Injection, solution [preservative free]:

OraVerse™: 0.4 mg/1.7 mL (1.7 mL)

phentolamine mesylate *see* phentolamine *on page 715*

phenylalanine mustard *see* melphalan *on page 570*

phenylazo diamino pyridine hydrochloride *see* phenazopyridine *on page 711*

phenylephrine (systemic) (fen il EF rin)

Medication Safety Issues

Sound-alike/look-alike issues:

Sudafed PE® may be confused with Sudafed®

High alert medication:

The Institute for Safe Medication Practices (ISMP) includes this medication among its list of drugs which have a heightened risk of causing significant patient harm when used in error.

Synonyms phenylephrine hydrochloride

U.S. Brand Names Medi-First® Sinus Decongestant [OTC]; Medi-Phenyl [OTC]; PediaCare® Children's Decongestant [OTC]; Sudafed PE® Children's [OTC]; Sudafed PE® Congestion [OTC]; Sudafed PE™ Nasal Decongestant [OTC]; Sudogest™ PE [OTC]; Triaminic Thin Strips® Children's Cold with Stuffy Nose [OTC]

Therapeutic Category Alpha/Beta Agonist

Use Treatment of hypotension, vascular failure in shock; as a vasoconstrictor in regional analgesia; supraventricular tachycardia (**Note:** Not for routine use in treatment of supraventricular tachycardias); as a decongestant [OTC]

General Dosage Range

I.V.:

Children: Bolus: 5-20 mcg/kg/dose every 10-15 minutes as needed; Infusion: 0.1-0.5 mcg/kg/minute

Adults: Bolus: 100-500 mcg/dose every 10-15 minutes as needed (maximum: 500 mcg); Infusion: Initial: 100-180 mcg/minute

Oral:

Children 4 to <6 years: 2.5 mg every 4 hours as needed (maximum: 15 mg/24 hours)

Children 6 to <12 years: 5 mg every 4 hours as needed (maximum: 30 mg/24 hours)

Children ≥12 years and Adults: 10 mg every 4 hours as needed (maximum: 60 mg/24 hours)

Dosage Forms

Injection, solution: 1% [10 mg/mL] (1 mL, 2 mL, 5 mL, 10 mL)

Liquid, oral:

PediaCare® Children's Decongestant [OTC]: 2.5 mg/5 mL (118 mL)

Sudafed PE® Children's [OTC]: 2.5 mg/5 mL (118 mL)

Strip, orally disintegrating, oral:

Triaminic Thin Strips® Children's Cold with Stuffy Nose [OTC]: 2.5 mg (14s)

Tablet, oral: 10 mg

Medi-First® Sinus Decongestant [OTC]: 10 mg

Medi-Phenyl [OTC]: 5 mg

Sudafed PE® Congestion [OTC]: 10 mg

Sudafed PE™ Nasal Decongestant [OTC]: 10 mg

Sudogest™ PE [OTC]: 10 mg

phenylephrine (nasal) (fen il EF rin)

Medication Safety Issues

Sound-alike/look-alike issues:

Neo-Synephrine® (phenylephrine, nasal) may be confused with Neo-Synephrine® (oxymetazoline)

Synonyms phenylephrine hydrochloride

U.S. Brand Names 4 Way® Fast Acting [OTC]; 4 Way® Menthol [OTC]; Little Noses® Decongestant [OTC]; Neo-Synephrine® Extra Strength [OTC]; Neo-Synephrine® Mild Formula [OTC]; Neo-Synephrine® Regular Strength [OTC]; Rhinall® [OTC]

Canadian Brand Names Neo-Synephrine®

Therapeutic Category Alpha/Beta Agonist

Use For OTC use as symptomatic relief of nasal and nasopharyngeal mucosal congestion

General Dosage Range Intranasal:

Children 2-6 years: 0.125% solution: Instill 1 drop in each nostril every 2-4 hours as needed for ≤3 days

Children 6-12 years: 0.25% solution: Instill 2-3 sprays in each nostril every 4 hours as needed for ≤3 days

Children >12 years: 0.25% to 0.5% solution: Instill 2-3 sprays or 2-3 drops in each nostril every 4 hours as needed for ≤3 days

Adults: 0.25% to 1% solution: Instill 2-3 sprays or 2-3 drops in each nostril every 4 hours as needed for ≤3 days

Dosage Forms

Solution, intranasal:

4 Way® Fast Acting [OTC]: 1% (15 mL, 30 mL, 37 mL)

4 Way® Menthol [OTC]: 1% (15 mL, 30 mL)

Little Noses® Decongestant [OTC]: 0.125% (15 mL)

Neo-Synephrine® Extra Strength [OTC]: 1% (15 mL)

Neo-Synephrine® Mild Formula [OTC]: 0.25% (15 mL)

Neo-Synephrine® Regular Strength [OTC]: 0.5% (15 mL)

Rhinall® [OTC]: 0.25% (30 mL, 40 mL)

phenylephrine (ophthalmic) (fen il EF rin)

Medication Safety Issues

Sound-alike/look-alike issues:

Mydfrin® may be confused with Midrin®

Synonyms phenylephrine hydrochloride

U.S. Brand Names AK-Dilate™; Altafrin; Mydfrin®; Neofrin

Canadian Brand Names Dionephrine®; Mydfrin®

Therapeutic Category Alpha/Beta Agonist; Ophthalmic Agent, Antiglaucoma; Ophthalmic Agent, Mydriatic

Use Used as a mydriatic in ophthalmic procedures and treatment of wide-angle glaucoma; OTC use as symptomatic relief of redness of the eye due to irritation

General Dosage Range Ophthalmic:

Infants <1 year: Instill 1 drop of 2.5% solution 15-30 minutes before procedures

Children ≥1 year and Adults: Instill 1 drop of 2.5% or 10% solution; may repeat in 10-60 minutes as needed **or** 1-2 drops of 0.12% solution up to 4 times/day [OTC dosing] (maximum: 72 hours)

Dosage Forms

Solution, ophthalmic: 2.5% (2 mL, 3 mL, 5 mL, 15 mL)

AK-Dilate™: 2.5% (2 mL, 15 mL); 10% (5 mL)

Altafrin: 2.5% (15 mL); 10% (5 mL)

Mydfrin®: 2.5% (3 mL, 5 mL)

Neofrin: 2.5% (15 mL); 10% (5 mL)

phenylephrine (topical) (fen il EF rin)

Synonyms phenylephrine hydrochloride

U.S. Brand Names Anu-Med [OTC]; Formulation R™ [OTC]; Medicone® Suppositories [OTC]; Preparation H® [OTC]; Rectacaine [OTC]; Tronolane® Suppository [OTC]

Therapeutic Category Alpha/Beta Agonist

Use For OTC use as treatment of hemorrhoids

General Dosage Range Rectal: *Children >12 years and Adults:* Ointment: Apply up to 4 times/day; Suppository: Insert 1 up to 4 times/day

Dosage Forms

Ointment, rectal: 0.25% (60 g)

Formulation R™ [OTC]: 0.25% (30 g, 60 g)

Preparation H® [OTC]: 0.25% (30 g, 60 g)

Suppository, rectal: 0.25% (1s); 0.25% (12s)

Anu-Med [OTC]: 0.25% (12s)

Medicone® Suppositories [OTC]: 0.25% (12s, 24s)

Preparation H® [OTC]: 0.25% (12s, 24s, 48s)

Rectacaine [OTC]: 0.25% (12s)

Tronolane® Suppository [OTC]: 0.25% (12s, 24s)

phenylephrine, acetaminophen, and dextromethorphan *see* acetaminophen, dextromethorphan, and phenylephrine *on page* 28

phenylephrine and brompheniramine *see* brompheniramine and phenylephrine *on page* 144

phenylephrine and chlorpheniramine *see* chlorpheniramine and phenylephrine *on page* 200

phenylephrine and cyclopentolate *see* cyclopentolate and phenylephrine *on page* 244

phenylephrine and dextromethorphan *see* dextromethorphan and phenylephrine *on page* 273

phenylephrine and diphenhydramine *see* diphenhydramine and phenylephrine *on page* 294

phenylephrine and promethazine *see* promethazine and phenylephrine *on page* 764

phenylephrine and pyrilamine (fen il EF rin & peer IL a meen)

Synonyms pyrilamine and phenylephrine; pyrilamine maleate and phenylephrine hydrochloride

U.S. Brand Names Ru-Hist-D

Therapeutic Category Antihistamine; Antihistamine/Decongestant Combination; Sympathomimetic

Use Symptomatic relief of nasal congestion and discharge associated with the common cold, sinusitis, allergic rhinitis, and other respiratory tract conditions

General Dosage Range Oral: *Children ≥6 years and Adults:* Dosage varies greatly depending on product

Dosage Forms

Liquid, oral:

Ru-Hist-D: Phenylephrine 10 mg and pyrilamine 30 mg per 5 mL (480 mL)

Tablet, oral:

Ru-Hist-D: Phenylephrine 10 mg and pyrilamine 30 mg

phenylephrine and zinc sulfate *(Canada only)* (fen il EF rin & zingk SUL fate)

Synonyms zinc sulfate and phenylephrine

Canadian Brand Names Zincfrin®

Therapeutic Category Adrenergic Agonist Agent

Use Soothe, moisturize, and remove redness due to minor eye irritation

General Dosage Range Ophthalmic: *Adults:* Instill 1-2 drops in eye(s) 2-4 times/day as needed

Product Availability Not available in U.S.

Dosage Forms - Canada

Solution, ophthalmic:

Zincfrin® [OTC]: Phenylephrine 0.12% and zinc sulfate 0.25% (15 mL)

phenylephrine, chlorpheniramine, acetaminophen, and phenyltoloxamine *see* acetaminophen, chlorpheniramine, phenylephrine, and phenyltoloxamine *on page 27*

phenylephrine, chlorpheniramine, and dextromethorphan *see* chlorpheniramine, phenylephrine, and dextromethorphan *on page 201*

phenylephrine, chlorpheniramine, and dihydrocodeine *see* dihydrocodeine, chlorpheniramine, and phenylephrine *on page 287*

phenylephrine, chlorpheniramine, and pyrilamine *see* chlorpheniramine, pyrilamine, and phenylephrine *on page 203*

phenylephrine, dextromethorphan, and acetaminophen *see* acetaminophen, dextromethorphan, and phenylephrine *on page 28*

phenylephrine hydrochloride *see* phenylephrine (nasal) *on page 716*

phenylephrine hydrochloride *see* phenylephrine (ophthalmic) *on page 716*

phenylephrine hydrochloride *see* phenylephrine (systemic) *on page 715*

phenylephrine hydrochloride *see* phenylephrine (topical) *on page 717*

phenylephrine hydrochloride, acetaminophen, and diphenhydramine *see* acetaminophen, diphenhydramine, and phenylephrine *on page 29*

phenylephrine hydrochloride and acetaminophen *see* acetaminophen and phenylephrine *on page 24*

phenylephrine hydrochloride and diphenhydramine hydrochloride *see* diphenhydramine and phenylephrine *on page 294*

phenylephrine hydrochloride and guaifenesin *see* guaifenesin and phenylephrine *on page 435*

phenylephrine hydrochloride, guaifenesin, and dextromethorphan hydrobromide *see* guaifenesin, dextromethorphan, and phenylephrine *on page 437*

phenylephrine, promethazine, and codeine *see* promethazine, phenylephrine, and codeine *on page 765*

phenylephrine, pyrilamine, and dextromethorphan

(fen il EF rin, peer IL a meen, & deks troe meth OR fan)

Synonyms dextrmethorphan, pyrilamine, and phenylephrine; pyrilamine maleate, dextromethorphan hydrobromide, and phenylephrine hydrochloride

U.S. Brand Names Codituss DM [OTC]; Pyril DM [OTC]; Ru-Hist Plus [OTC]

Therapeutic Category Antihistamine; Antihistamine/Decongestant/Antitussive; Antitussive; Sympathomimetic

Use Symptomatic relief of cough, nasal congestion, and discharge associated with the common cold, sinusitis, allergic rhinitis, and other respiratory tract conditions

General Dosage Range Oral: *Children ≥6 years and Adults:* Dosage varies greatly depending on product

Dosage Forms

Liquid, oral:

Ru-Hist Plus [OTC]: Phenylephrine 10 mg, pyrilamine 30 mg, and dextromethorphan 20 mg per 5 mL (480 mL)

Suspension, oral:

Pyril DM [OTC]: Phenylephrine 5 mg, pyrilamine 16 mg, and dextromethorphan 15 mg per 5 mL (473 mL)

Syrup, oral:
Coditus DM [OTC]: Phenylephrine 5 mg, pyrilamine 8.33 mg, and dextromethorphan 10 mg per 5 mL (118 mL)

Tablet, oral:
Ru-Hist Plus [OTC]: Phenylephrine 10 mg, pyrilamine 30 mg, and dextromethorphan 20 mg

phenylephrine tannate and diphenhydramine tannate *see* diphenhydramine and phenylephrine *on page 294*

phenylethylmalonylurea *see* phenobarbital *on page 712*

Phenylhistine DH [OTC] *see* chlorpheniramine, pseudoephedrine, and codeine *on page 202*

phenyl salicylate, methenamine, methylene blue, benzoic acid, and hyoscyamine *see* methenamine, phenyl salicylate, methylene blue, benzoic acid, and hyoscyamine *on page 583*

phenyltoloxamine, chlorpheniramine, phenylephrine, and acetaminophen *see* acetaminophen, chlorpheniramine, phenylephrine, and phenyltoloxamine *on page 27*

phenyltoloxamine citrate and acetaminophen *see* acetaminophen and phenyltoloxamine *on page 25*

Phenytek® *see* phenytoin *on page 719*

phenytoin (FEN i toyn)

Medication Safety Issues

Sound-alike/look-alike issues:
Phenytoin may be confused with phenelzine, phentermine, PHENobarbital
Dilantin® may be confused with Dilaudid®, diltiazem, Dipentum®

High alert medication:
The Institute for Safe Medication Practices (ISMP) includes this medication (I.V. formulation) among its list of drug classes which have a heightened risk of causing significant patient harm when used in error.

International issues:
Dilantin [U.S., Canada, and multiple international markets] may be confused with Dolantine brand name for pethidine [Belgium]

Synonyms diphenylhydantoin; DPH; phenytoin sodium; phenytoin sodium, extended; phenytoin sodium, prompt

U.S. Brand Names Dilantin-125®; Dilantin®; Phenytek®

Canadian Brand Names Dilantin®; Novo-Phenytoin; Taro-Phenytoin; Tremytoine Inj

Therapeutic Category Antiarrhythmic Agent, Class I-B; Hydantoin

Use Management of generalized tonic-clonic (grand mal), complex partial seizures; prevention of seizures following neurosurgery

General Dosage Range

I.V.:
Children 6 months to 3 years: Loading dose: 15-20 mg/kg; Maintenance: 5-10 mg/kg/day in 2 divided doses
Children 4-6 years: Loading dose: 15-20 mg/kg; Maintenance: 5-9 mg/kg/day in 2 divided doses
Children 7-9 years: Loading dose: 15-20 mg/kg; Maintenance: 5-8 mg/kg/day in 2 divided doses
Children 10-16 years: Loading dose: 15-20 mg/kg; Maintenance: 5-7 mg/kg/day in 2 divided doses
Adolescents >16 years and Adults: Loading dose: 10-20 mg/kg; Maintenance: 300-400 mg/day in 3 or 4 divided doses

Oral:
Children: Loading dose: 15-20 mg/kg in divided doses; Maintenance: 4-8 mg/kg/day in divided doses
Adults: Loading dose: 15-20 mg/kg in 3 divided doses every 2-4 hours; Maintenance: 300 mg/day in 1-3 divided doses **or** 5-6 mg/kg/day in 1-3 divided doses **or** 100 mg every 6-8 hours (range: 300-600 mg/day)

Dosage Forms

Capsule, extended release, oral: 100 mg, 200 mg, 300 mg
Dilantin®: 30 mg, 100 mg
Phenytek®: 200 mg, 300 mg

Injection, solution: 50 mg/mL (2 mL, 5 mL)

Suspension, oral: 100 mg/4 mL (4 mL); 125 mg/5 mL (237 mL, 240 mL)
Dilantin-125®: 125 mg/5 mL (240 mL)

Tablet, chewable, oral:
Dilantin®: 50 mg

phenytoin sodium *see* phenytoin *on page 719*

phenytoin sodium, extended *see* phenytoin *on page* 719
phenytoin sodium, prompt *see* phenytoin *on page* 719
PHiD-CV *see* pneumococcal conjugate vaccine (10-valent) *(Canada only) on page* 733
Phillips'® M-O [OTC] *see* magnesium hydroxide and mineral oil *on page* 559
Phillips'® Laxative Dietary Supplement Cramp-Free [OTC] *see* magnesium oxide *on page* 559
Phillips'® Liquid-Gels® [OTC] *see* docusate *on page* 304
Phillips'® Milk of Magnesia [OTC] *see* magnesium hydroxide *on page* 558
Phillips'® Stool Softener Laxative [OTC] *see* docusate *on page* 304
pHisoHex® *see* hexachlorophene *on page* 447
PHL-Alendronate (Can) *see* alendronate *on page* 45
PHL-Amantadine (Can) *see* amantadine *on page* 58
PHL-Amiodarone (Can) *see* amiodarone *on page* 63
PHL-Amlodipine (Can) *see* amlodipine *on page* 65
PHL-Amoxicillin (Can) *see* amoxicillin *on page* 69
PHL-Azithromycin (Can) *see* azithromycin (systemic) *on page* 108
PHL-Baclofen (Can) *see* baclofen *on page* 112
PHL-Bethanechol (Can) *see* bethanechol *on page* 131
PHL-Bicalutamide (Can) *see* bicalutamide *on page* 133
PHL-Bisoprolol (Can) *see* bisoprolol *on page* 136
PHL-Cilazapril (Can) *see* cilazapril *(Canada only) on page* 208
PHL-Ciprofloxacin (Can) *see* ciprofloxacin (systemic) *on page* 210
PHL-Citalopram (Can) *see* citalopram *on page* 213
PHL-Clonazepam (Can) *see* clonazepam *on page* 223
PHL-Cyclobenzaprine (Can) *see* cyclobenzaprine *on page* 243
PHL-Dexamethasone (Can) *see* dexamethasone (systemic) *on page* 266
PHL-Divalproex (Can) *see* divalproex *on page* 302
PHL-Domperidone (Can) *see* domperidone *(Canada only) on page* 308
PHL-Doxycycline (Can) *see* doxycycline *on page* 314
PHL-Fenofibrate Micro (Can) *see* fenofibrate *on page* 375
PHL-Fenofibrate Supra (Can) *see* fenofibrate *on page* 375
PHL-Fluconazole (Can) *see* fluconazole *on page* 388
PHL-Fluoxetine (Can) *see* fluoxetine *on page* 396
PHL-Gabapentin (Can) *see* gabapentin *on page* 413
PHL-Indapamide (Can) *see* indapamide *on page* 479
PHL-Leflunomide (Can) *see* leflunomide *on page* 525
PHL-Levetiracetam (Can) *see* levetiracetam *on page* 528
PHL-Lithium Carbonate (Can) *see* lithium *on page* 544
PHL-Lorazepam (Can) *see* lorazepam *on page* 550
PHL-Lovastatin (Can) *see* lovastatin *on page* 553
PHL-Loxapine (Can) *see* loxapine *on page* 554
PHL-Meloxicam (Can) *see* meloxicam *on page* 569
PHL-Metformin (Can) *see* metformin *on page* 579
PHL-Methimazole (Can) *see* methimazole *on page* 583
PHL-Methylphenidate (Can) *see* methylphenidate *on page* 590
PHL-Minocycline (Can) *see* minocycline *on page* 604
PHL-Olanzapine (Can) *see* olanzapine *on page* 660
PHL-Olanzapine ODT (Can) *see* olanzapine *on page* 660
PHL-Ondansetron (Can) *see* ondansetron *on page* 667
PHL-Oxybutynin (Can) *see* oxybutynin *on page* 677
PHL-Paroxetine (Can) *see* paroxetine *on page* 693
PHL-Pioglitazone (Can) *see* pioglitazone *on page* 725
PHL-Pravastatin (Can) *see* pravastatin *on page* 752
PHL-Procyclidine (Can) *see* procyclidine *(Canada only) on page* 761

physostigmine (fye zoe STIG meen)

Medication Safety Issues

Sound-alike/look-alike issues:

Physostigmine may be confused with Prostigmin®, pyridostigmine

Synonyms eserine salicylate; physostigmine salicylate; physostigmine sulfate

Therapeutic Category Cholinesterase Inhibitor

Use Reverse toxic, life-threatening delirium caused by atropine, diphenhydramine, dimenhydrinate, *Atropa belladonna* (deadly nightshade), or jimsonweed (*Datura* spp)

General Dosage Range

I.M.: *Adults:* Initial: 0.5-2 mg, repeat every 20 minutes until response or adverse effects occur; repeat 1-4 mg every 30-60 minutes as life-threatening symptoms recur

I.V.:

Children: 0.01-0.03 mg/kg/dose, may repeat after 5-10 minutes (maximum total dose: 2 mg)

Adults: Initial: 0.5-2 mg, repeat every 20 minutes until response or adverse effects occur; repeat 1-4 mg every 30-60 minutes as life-threatening symptoms recur

Dosage Forms

Injection, solution: 1 mg/mL (2 mL)

physostigmine salicylate *see* physostigmine *on page* 721

physostigmine sulfate *see* physostigmine *on page* 721

phytomenadione *see* phytonadione *on page* 722

phytonadione (fye toe na DYE one)

Medication Safety Issues

Sound-alike/look-alike issues:

Mephyton® may be confused with melphalan, methadone

Synonyms methylphytyl napthoquinone; phylloquinone; phytomenadione; vitamin K_1

U.S. Brand Names Mephyton®

Canadian Brand Names AquaMEPHYTON®; Konakion; Mephyton®

Therapeutic Category Vitamin, Fat Soluble

Use Prevention and treatment of hypoprothrombinemia caused by coumarin derivative-induced or other drug-induced vitamin K deficiency, hypoprothrombinemia caused by malabsorption or inability to synthesize vitamin K; hemorrhagic disease of the newborn

General Dosage Range

I.M.:

Newborns: Prophylaxis: 0.5-1 mg within 1 hour of birth; Treatment: 1 mg/dose/day

Adults: Initial: 2.5-25 mg/dose (usual: 5-10 mg; maximum: 50 mg)

I.V.: *Adults:* Initial: 2.5-25 mg/dose (usual: 5-10 mg; maximum: 50 mg)

Oral:

Children 1-3 years: RDA: 30 mcg/day

Children 4-8 years: RDA: 55 mcg/day

Children 9-13 years: RDA: 60 mcg/day

Children 14-18 years: RDA: 75 mcg/day

Adults: Initial: 2.5-25 mg/dose (usual: 5-10 mg; maximum: 50 mg)

SubQ:

Newborns: 1 mg/dose/day

Adults: Initial: 2.5-25 mg/dose (usual: 5-10 mg; maximum: 50 mg)

Dosage Forms

Injection, aqueous colloidal: 1 mg/0.5 mL (0.5 mL); 10 mg/mL (1 mL)

Injection, aqueous colloidal [preservative free]: 1 mg/0.5 mL (0.5 mL)

Tablet, oral: 100 mcg

Mephyton®: 5 mg

α_1-PI *see* alpha$_1$-proteinase inhibitor *on page* 51

Picato® *see* ingenol mebutate *on page* 484

Picodan (Can) *see* sodium picosulfate, magnesium oxide, and citric acid *on page* 846

Picoflo (Can) *see* sodium picosulfate, magnesium oxide, and citric acid *on page* 846

Pico-Salax® (Can) *see* sodium picosulfate, magnesium oxide, and citric acid *on page* 846

pidorubicin *see* epirubicin *on page* 336

pidorubicin hydrochloride *see* epirubicin *on page* 336

pilocarpine (systemic) (pye loe KAR peen)

Medication Safety Issues

Sound-alike/look-alike issues:

Salagen® may be confused with selegiline

Synonyms pilocarpine hydrochloride

U.S. Brand Names Salagen®

Canadian Brand Names Salagen®

Therapeutic Category Cholinergic Agonist

Use Symptomatic treatment of xerostomia caused by salivary gland hypofunction resulting from radiotherapy for cancer of the head and neck or Sjögren syndrome

General Dosage Range Dosage adjustment recommended in patients with hepatic impairment

Oral: *Adults:* 5 mg 3-4 times/day (maximum: 30 mg/day)

Dosage Forms

Tablet, oral: 5 mg, 7.5 mg

Salagen®: 5 mg, 7.5 mg

pilocarpine (ophthalmic) (pye loe KAR peen)

Medication Safety Issues

Sound-alike/look-alike issues:

Isopto® Carpine may be confused with Isopto® Carbachol

Synonyms pilocarpine hydrochloride

U.S. Brand Names Isopto® Carpine; Pilopine HS®

Canadian Brand Names Diocarpine; Isopto® Carpine; Pilopine HS®

Therapeutic Category Ophthalmic Agent, Antiglaucoma; Ophthalmic Agent, Miotic

Use Management of chronic simple glaucoma, chronic and acute angle-closure glaucoma

General Dosage Range Ophthalmic: *Adults:* Gel: Instill 0.5" ribbon once daily at bedtime; Solution: Instill 1-2 drops up to 6 times/day

Dosage Forms

Gel, ophthalmic:

Pilopine HS®: 4% (4 g)

Solution, ophthalmic: 1% (2 mL, 15 mL); 2% (2 mL, 15 mL); 4% (2 mL, 15 mL)

Isopto® Carpine: 1% (15 mL); 2% (15 mL); 4% (15 mL)

pilocarpine hydrochloride *see* pilocarpine (ophthalmic) *on page 723*

pilocarpine hydrochloride *see* pilocarpine (systemic) *on page 722*

Pilopine HS® *see* pilocarpine (ophthalmic) *on page 723*

pimaricin *see* natamycin *on page 630*

pimecrolimus (pim e KROE li mus)

Medication Safety Issues

Sound-alike/look-alike issues:

Pimecrolimus may be confused with tacrolimus

U.S. Brand Names Elidel®

Canadian Brand Names Elidel®

Therapeutic Category Immunosuppressant Agent; Topical Skin Product

Use Short-term and intermittent long-term treatment of mild-to-moderate atopic dermatitis in patients not responsive to conventional therapy or when conventional therapy is not appropriate

General Dosage Range Topical: *Children >2 years and Adults:* Apply thin layer to affected area twice daily

Dosage Forms

Cream, topical:

Elidel®: 1% (30 g, 60 g, 100 g)

pimozide (PI moe zide)

Medication Safety Issues

BEERS Criteria medication:

This drug may be potentially inappropriate for use in geriatric patients (Quality of evidence - moderate; Strength of recommendation - strong).

U.S. Brand Names Orap®

Canadian Brand Names Apo-Pimozide®; Orap®; PMS-Pimozide

Therapeutic Category Neuroleptic Agent

Use Suppression of severe motor and phonic tics in patients with Tourette disorder who have failed to respond satisfactorily to standard treatment

General Dosage Range Dosage adjustment recommended in patients who develop toxicities or those with a CYP2D6 poor metabolizer status.

Oral:

Children 2-12 years: Initial: 0.05 mg/kg once daily (preferably bedtime); Maintenance: 2-4 mg once daily (maximum: 10 mg/day [0.2 mg/kg/day])

Children >12 years and Adults: Initial: 1-2 mg in divided doses (maximum: 10 mg/day [0.2 mg/kg/day])

Dosage Forms
Tablet, oral:
Orap®: 1 mg, 2 mg

Pin-X® [OTC] *see* pyrantel pamoate *on page 775*

pinaverium bromide *see* pinaverium *(Canada only) on page 724*

pinaverium *(Canada only)* (pin ah VEER ee um)

Synonyms pinaverium bromide

Canadian Brand Names Dicetel®

Therapeutic Category Calcium Antagonist; Gastrointestinal Agent, Miscellaneous

Use Treatment and relief of symptoms associated with irritable bowel syndrome (IBS); treatment of symptoms related to functional disorders of the biliary tract

General Dosage Range Oral: *Adults:* 50 mg 3 times/day (maximum: 300 mg/day)

Product Availability Not available in U.S.

Dosage Forms - Canada
Tablet, oral:
Dicetel®: 50 mg, 100 mg

pindolol (PIN doe lole)

Medication Safety Issues
Sound-alike/look-alike issues:
Pindolol may be confused with Parlodel®, Plendil®
Visken® may be confused with Visine®, Viskazide®

Canadian Brand Names Apo-Pindol®; Dom-Pindolol; Mylan-Pindolol; Novo-Pindol; Nu-Pindol; PMS-Pindolol; Sandoz-Pindolol; Teva-Pindolol; Visken®

Therapeutic Category Beta-Adrenergic Blocker

Use Treatment of hypertension, alone or in combination with other agents

General Dosage Range Dosage adjustment recommended in patients with hepatic impairment
Oral:
Adults: Initial: 5 mg twice daily; Maintenance: 10-40 mg twice daily (maximum: 60 mg/day)
Elderly: Initial: 5 mg once daily

Dosage Forms
Tablet, oral: 5 mg, 10 mg

pindolol and hydrochlorothiazide *(Canada only)*
(PIN doe lole & hye droe klor oh THYE a zide)

Medication Safety Issues
Sound-alike/look-alike issues:
Viskazide® may be confused with hydrochlorothiazide, Visken®

Synonyms hydrochlorothiazide and pindolol

Canadian Brand Names Viskazide®

Therapeutic Category Beta-Blocker With Intrinsic Sympathomimetic Activity; Diuretic, Thiazide

Use Treatment of hypertension; not for initial therapy

General Dosage Range Oral: *Adults:* Usual dose: Pindolol 10-20 mg and hydrochlorothiazide 25-100 mg once daily (maximum daily dose: Pindolol 20 mg/hydrochlorothiazide 100 mg)

Product Availability Not available in U.S.

Dosage Forms - Canada
Tablet, oral:
Viskazide® 10/25: Pindolol 10 mg and hydrochlorothiazide 25 mg
Viskazide® 10/50: Pindolol 10 mg and hydrochlorothiazide 50 mg

pink bismuth *see* bismuth *on page 135*

pioglitazone (pye oh GLI ta zone)

Medication Safety Issues

Sound-alike/look-alike issues:

Actos® may be confused with Actidose®, Actonel®

High alert medication:

The Institute for Safe Medication Practices (ISMP) includes this medication among its list of drug classes which have a heightened risk of causing significant patient harm when used in error.

International issues:

Tiazac: Brand name for pioglitazone [Chile], but also the brand name for diltiazem [U.S, Canada]

U.S. Brand Names Actos®

Canadian Brand Names Accel-Pioglitazone; Actos®; Apo-Pioglitazone®; Ava-Pioglitazone; CO Pioglitazone; Dom-Pioglitazone; JAMP-Pioglitazone; Mint-Pioglitazone; Mylan-Pioglitazone; Novo-Pioglitazone; PHL-Pioglitazone; PMS-Pioglitazone; PRO-Pioglitazone; ratio-Pioglitazone; Sandoz-Pioglitazone; Teva-Pioglitazone; ZYM-Pioglitazone

Therapeutic Category Antidiabetic Agent, Oral; Thiazolidinedione Derivative

Use

Type 2 diabetes mellitus (noninsulin-dependent, NIDDM), monotherapy: Adjunct to diet and exercise, to improve glycemic control

Type 2 diabetes mellitus (noninsulin-dependent, NIDDM), combination therapy with sulfonylurea, metformin, or insulin: When diet, exercise, and a single agent alone does not result in adequate glycemic control

General Dosage Range Dosage adjustment recommended in patients on concomitant therapy.

Oral: *Adults:* Initial: 15-30 mg once daily; Maintenance: 15-45 mg once daily (maximum: 45 mg/day)

Dosage Forms

Tablet, oral: 15 mg, 30 mg, 45 mg

Actos®: 15 mg, 30 mg, 45 mg

pioglitazone and glimepiride (pye oh GLI ta zone & GLYE me pye ride)

Medication Safety Issues

High alert medication:

The Institute for Safe Medication Practices (ISMP) includes this medication among its list of drugs which have a heightened risk of causing significant patient harm when used in error.

Synonyms glimepiride and pioglitazone; glimepiride and pioglitazone hydrochloride

U.S. Brand Names Duetact™

Therapeutic Category Antidiabetic Agent, Sulfonylurea; Antidiabetic Agent, Thiazolidinedione; Hypoglycemic Agent, Oral

Use Management of type 2 diabetes mellitus (noninsulin-dependent, NIDDM) as an adjunct to diet and exercise

General Dosage Range Dosage adjustment recommended in patients with renal impairment

Oral:

Adults:

Patients inadequately controlled on **glimepiride** alone: Initial dose: Pioglitazone 30 mg and glimepiride 2-4 mg once daily (maximum: 45 mg/day [pioglitazone]; 8 mg/day [glimepiride])

Patients inadequately controlled on **pioglitazone** alone: Initial dose: Pioglitazone 30 mg and glimepiride 2 mg once daily (maximum: 45 mg/day [pioglitazone]; 8 mg/day [glimepiride])

Elderly: Initial: Glimepiride 1 mg/day prior to initiating Duetact™

Dosage Forms

Tablet:

Duetact™: 30 mg/2 mg: Pioglitazone 30 mg and glimepiride 2 mg; 30 mg/4 mg: Pioglitazone 30 mg and glimepiride 4 mg

pioglitazone and metformin (pye oh GLI ta zone & met FOR min)

Medication Safety Issues

High alert medication:

The Institute for Safe Medication Practices (ISMP) includes this medication among its list of drug classes which have a heightened risk of causing significant patient harm when used in error.

Synonyms metformin hydrochloride and pioglitazone hydrochloride

U.S. Brand Names Actoplus Met®; Actoplus Met® XR

Therapeutic Category Antidiabetic Agent, Biguanide; Antidiabetic Agent, Thiazolidinedione

Use Management of type 2 diabetes mellitus (noninsulin-dependent, NIDDM)

General Dosage Range Oral: *Adults:*

Immediate release tablet: Pioglitazone 15-45 mg/day and metformin 500-2550 mg/day (maximum: 45 mg/day [pioglitazone]; 2550 mg/day [metformin])

Variable release tablet: Pioglitazone 15-45 mg/day and metformin 1000-2000 mg/day (maximum: 45 mg/day [pioglitazone]; 2000 mg/day [metformin])

Dosage Forms

Tablet, oral: 15/500: Pioglitazone 15 mg and metformin hydrochloride 500 mg; 15/850: Pioglitazone 15 mg and metformin hydrochloride 850 mg

Actoplus Met®: 15/500: Pioglitazone 15 mg and metformin 500 mg; 15/850: Pioglitazone 15 mg and metformin 850 mg

Tablet, variable release, oral:

Actoplus Met® XR: 15/1000: Pioglitazone 15 mg and metformin 1000 mg; 30/1000: Pioglitazone 30 mg and metformin 1000 mg

piperacillin (pi PER a sil in)

Synonyms piperacillin sodium

Canadian Brand Names Piperacillin for Injection, USP

Therapeutic Category Penicillin

Use Treatment of susceptible infections such as septicemia, acute and chronic respiratory tract infections, skin and soft tissue infections, and urinary tract infections due to susceptible strains of *Pseudomonas*, *Proteus*, and *Escherichia coli* and *Enterobacter*; active against some streptococci and some anaerobic bacteria; febrile neutropenia (as part of combination regimen)

General Dosage Range Dosage adjustment recommended in patients with renal impairment

I.M., I.V.:

Children: 200-300 mg/kg/day in divided doses every 4-6 hours

Adults: 2-4 g/dose every 4-6 hours (maximum: 24 g/day)

piperacillin and tazobactam (pi PER a sil in & ta zoe BAK tam)

Medication Safety Issues

Sound-alike/look-alike issues:

Zosyn® may be confused with Zofran®, Zyvox®

International issues:

Tazact [India] may be confused with Tazac brand name for nizatidine [Australia]; Tiazac brand name for diltiazem [U.S., Canada]

Synonyms piperacillin and tazobactam sodium; piperacillin sodium and tazobactam sodium; tazobactam and piperacillin

U.S. Brand Names Zosyn®

Canadian Brand Names Piperacillin and Tazobactam for Injection; Tazocin®

Therapeutic Category Penicillin

Use Treatment of moderate-to-severe infections caused by susceptible organisms, including infections of the lower respiratory tract (community-acquired pneumonia, nosocomial pneumonia); uncomplicated and complicated skin and skin structures (including diabetic foot infections); gynecologic (endometritis, pelvic inflammatory disease); and intraabdominal infections (appendicitis with rupture/abscess, peritonitis). Tazobactam expands activity of piperacillin to include beta-lactamase producing strains of *S. aureus*, *H. influenzae*, *E. coli*, *Bacteroides* spp, and other gram-positive and gram-negative aerobic and anaerobic bacteria.

General Dosage Range Dosage adjustment recommended in patients with renal impairment

I.V.:

Children 2-8 months: 80 mg/kg every 8 hours

Children ≥9 months and ≤40 kg: 100 mg/kg every 8 hours

Children >40 kg: 4.5 g every 8 hours **or** 3.375 g every 6 hours

Adults: 3.375 g every 6 hours **or** 4.5 g every 6-8 hours (maximum: 18 g/day)

Dosage Forms 8:1 ratio of piperacillin sodium/tazobactam sodium

Infusion [premixed iso-osmotic solution, frozen]:

Zosyn®:

2.25 g: Piperacillin 2 g and tazobactam 0.25 g (50 mL)

3.375 g: Piperacillin 3 g and tazobactam 0.375 g (50 mL)

4.5 g: Piperacillin 4 g and tazobactam 0.5 g (100 mL)

Injection, powder for reconstitution: 2.25 g: Piperacillin 2 g and tazobactam 0.25 g; 3.375 g: Piperacillin 3 g and tazobactam 0.375 g; 4.5 g: Piperacillin 4 g and tazobactam 0.5 g; 40.5 g: Piperacillin 36 g and tazobactam 4.5 g

Zosyn®:

2.25 g: Piperacillin 2 g and tazobactam 0.25 g

3.375 g: Piperacillin 3 g and tazobactam 0.375 g

4.5 g: Piperacillin 4 g and tazobactam 0.5 g

40.5 g: Piperacillin 36 g and tazobactam 4.5 g

Piperacillin and Tazobactam for Injection (Can) *see* piperacillin and tazobactam *on page* 726

piperacillin and tazobactam sodium *see* piperacillin and tazobactam *on page* 726

Piperacillin for Injection, USP (Can) *see* piperacillin *on page* 726

piperacillin sodium *see* piperacillin *on page* 726

piperacillin sodium and tazobactam sodium *see* piperacillin and tazobactam *on page* 726

piperazine estrone sulfate *see* estropipate *on page* 353

piperonyl butoxide and pyrethrins *see* pyrethrins and piperonyl butoxide *on page* 776

pirbuterol (peer BYOO ter ole)

Synonyms pirbuterol acetate

U.S. Brand Names Maxair® Autohaler®

Therapeutic Category Adrenergic Agonist Agent

Use Prevention and treatment of reversible bronchospasm including asthma

General Dosage Range **Inhalation:** *Children ≥12 years and Adults:* Prevention: 2 inhalations every 4-6 hours; Treatment: 2 inhalations at an interval of at least 1-3 minutes, followed by a third inhalation (maximum: 12 inhalations/day)

Dosage Forms

Aerosol, for oral inhalation:

Maxair® Autohaler®: 200 mcg/actuation (14 g)

pirbuterol acetate *see* pirbuterol *on page* 727

piroxicam (peer OKS i kam)

Medication Safety Issues

Sound-alike/look-alike issues:

Feldene® may be confused with FLUoxetine

Piroxicam may be confused with PARoxetine

BEERS Criteria medication:

This drug may be potentially inappropriate for use in geriatric patients (Quality of evidence - moderate; Strength of recommendation - strong).

International issues:

Flogene [Brazil] may be confused with Flogen brand name for naproxen [Mexico]; Florone brand name for diflorasone [Germany, Greece]; Flovent brand name for fluticasone [U.S., Canada]

U.S. Brand Names Feldene®

Canadian Brand Names Apo-Piroxicam®; Dom-Piroxicam; Novo-Pirocam; Nu-Pirox; PMS-Piroxicam

Therapeutic Category Analgesic, Nonnarcotic; Nonsteroidal Antiinflammatory Drug (NSAID)

Use Symptomatic treatment of acute and chronic rheumatoid arthritis and osteoarthritis

Canadian labeling: Additional use (not in U.S. labeling): Symptomatic treatment of ankylosing spondylitis

General Dosage Range Dosage adjustment recommended in patients with hepatic impairment

Oral: *Adults:* 10-20 mg/day in 1-2 divided doses (maximum: 20 mg/day)

Dosage Forms

Capsule, oral: 10 mg, 20 mg

Feldene®: 10 mg, 20 mg

***p*-isobutylhydratropic acid** *see* ibuprofen *on page* 468

pit *see* oxytocin *on page* 683

pitavastatin (pi TA va sta tin)

Medication Safety Issues

Sound-alike/look-alike issues:

Pitavastatin may be confused with atorvaSTATin, fluvastatin, lovastatin, nystatin, pravastatin, rosuvastatin, simvastatin

Synonyms pitavastatin calcium

U.S. Brand Names Livalo®

Therapeutic Category Antilipemic Agent, HMG-CoA Reductase Inhibitor

Use Adjunct to dietary therapy to reduce elevations in total cholesterol (TC), LDL-C, apolipoprotein B (Apo B), and triglycerides (TG), and to increase low HDL-C in patients with primary hyperlipidemia and mixed dyslipidemia

General Dosage Range Dosage adjustment recommended in patients with renal impairment or on concomitant therapy

Oral: *Adults:* Initial: 2 mg once daily; Maintenance: 2-4 mg once daily (maximum: 4 mg/day)

Dosage Forms

Tablet, oral:

Livalo®: 1 mg, 2 mg, 4 mg

pitavastatin calcium *see* pitavastatin *on page 728*
Pitocin® *see* oxytocin *on page 683*
Pitressin® *see* vasopressin *on page 940*
Pitrex (Can) *see* tolnaftate *on page 904*
pix carbonis *see* coal tar *on page 228*

pizotifen *(Canada only)* (pi ZOE ti fen)

Synonyms pizotifen malate

Canadian Brand Names Sandomigran DS®; Sandomigran®

Therapeutic Category Antimigraine Agent

Use Migraine prophylaxis

General Dosage Range Oral: *Children ≥12 years and Adults:* Initial: 0.5 mg at bedtime; Maintenance: 1-6 mg/day in 1-3 divided doses

Product Availability Not available in U.S.

Dosage Forms - Canada

Tablet:

Sandomigran®: 0.5 mg

Tablet, double strength:

Sandomigran® DS: 1 mg

pizotifen malate *see* pizotifen *(Canada only) on page 728*
Plan B *see* levonorgestrel *on page 533*
Plan B® (Can) *see* levonorgestrel *on page 533*
Plan B® One Step *see* levonorgestrel *on page 533*
plantago seed *see* psyllium *on page 774*
plantain seed *see* psyllium *on page 774*
Plaquenil® *see* hydroxychloroquine *on page 462*
Plasbumin®-5 *see* albumin *on page 41*
Plasbumin®-25 *see* albumin *on page 41*
Plasmanate® *see* plasma protein fraction *on page 728*

plasma protein fraction (PLAS mah PROE teen FRAK shun)

U.S. Brand Names Plasmanate®

Therapeutic Category Blood Product Derivative

Use Plasma volume expansion and maintenance of cardiac output in the treatment of certain types of shock or impending shock

General Dosage Range I.V.: *Adults:* Usual minimum dose: 250-500 mL; adjust dose based on response

Dosage Forms

Injection, solution [preservative free]:

Plasmanate®: 5% (50 mL, 250 mL)

plerixafor (pler IX a fore)

Synonyms AMD3100; LM3100

U.S. Brand Names Mozobil™

Therapeutic Category Hematopoietic Stem Cell Mobilizer

Use Mobilization of hematopoietic stem cells (HSC) for collection and subsequent autologous transplantation (in combination with filgrastim) in patients with non-Hodgkin lymphoma (NHL) and multiple myeloma (MM)

General Dosage Range Dosage adjustment recommended in patients with renal impairment

SubQ: *Adults:* 0.24 mg/kg/day (maximum dose: 40 mg/day)

Dosage Forms

Injection, solution [preservative free]:

Mozobil™: 20 mg/mL (1.2 mL)

pneumococcal conjugate vaccine (10-valent) *(Canada only)*

(noo moe KOK al KON ju gate vak SEEN, ten vay lent)

Medication Safety Issues

Sound-alike/look-alike issues:

Synflorix™ may be confused with Synagis®

Synonyms 10-valent pneumococcal nontypeable *Haemophilus influenzae* protein D conjugate vaccine; PHiD-CV; pneumococcal conjugate vaccine (nontypeable *Haemophilus influenzae* [NTHi] protein D, diphtheria or tetanus toxoid conjugates) adsorbed

Canadian Brand Names Synflorix™

Therapeutic Category Vaccine, Inactivated (Bacterial)

Use Immunization of infants and children against *Streptococcus pneumoniae* infection and invasive diseases caused by serotypes included in the vaccine

General Dosage Range I.M.:

Infants 6 weeks to 6 months: 0.5 mL dose at 2, 4, and 6 months (minimum interval of 1 month between each of the first 3 doses), followed by booster dose of 0.5 mL administered at 12-15 months (minimum interval of 6 months between doses 3 and 4) **or** 0.5 mL dose at 2 and 4 months (minimum interval of 2 months between doses 1 and 2), followed by an additional 0.5 mL dose at 11-12 months (minimum interval of 6 months between doses 2 and 3)

Infants 7-11 months (previously unvaccinated): 0.5 mL for 2 doses administered at least 1 month apart, followed by a third dose administered after 1 year of age (minimum interval of 2 months between doses 2 and 3)

Children 12 months to <6 years (previously unvaccinated): 0.5 mL for a total of 2 doses administered at least 2 months apart

Product Availability Not available in the U.S.

Dosage Forms - Canada

Injection, suspension:

Synflorix™: 1 mcg of each capsular saccharide for serotypes 1, 5, 6B, 7F, 9V, 14, and 23F, and 3 mcg each of serotypes 4, 18C, and 19F (bound to protein D [from nontypeable *H. Influenzae*], tetanus toxoid, or diphtheria toxoid) per 0.5 mL (0.5 mL)

pneumococcal 13-valent conjugate vaccine *see* pneumococcal conjugate vaccine (13-valent) *on page 734*

pneumococcal conjugate vaccine (13-valent)

(noo moe KOK al KON ju gate vak SEEN, thur TEEN vay lent)

Medication Safety Issues

Sound-alike/look-alike issues:

Pneumococcal 13-Valent Conjugate Vaccine (Prevnar 13®) may be confused with Pneumococcal 7-Valent Conjugate Vaccine (Prevnar®) or with Pneumococcal 23-Valent Polysaccharide Vaccine (Pneumovax® 23)

Synonyms PCV-13; PCV13; pneumococcal 13-valent conjugate vaccine

U.S. Brand Names Prevnar 13®

Canadian Brand Names Prevnar 13®

Therapeutic Category Vaccine, Inactivated (Bacterial)

Use

Immunization of infants and children against *Streptococcus pneumoniae* infection caused by serotypes included in the vaccine

Immunization of infants and children against otitis media caused by *Streptococcus pneumoniae* serotypes 4, 6B, 9V, 14, 18C, 19F, and 23F

Immunization of adults ≥50 years against pneumococcal pneumonia and invasive disease caused by *Streptococcus pneumoniae* serotypes included in the vaccine

The Advisory Committee on Immunization Practices (ACIP) recommends routine vaccination for the following:

All children age 2-59 months

Children 60-71 months with underlying medical conditions including: Cochlear implants, functional or anatomic asplenia (includes sickle cell disease and other hemoglobinopathies, congenital or acquired asplenia, or splenic dysfunction); immunocompromising conditions (includes HIV infection, congenital immunodeficiencies [excluding chronic granulomatous disease], chronic renal failure, nephrotic syndrome, diseases associated with immunosuppressive or radiation therapy, solid organ transplant); chronic illnesses (cardiac disease, cerebrospinal fluid leaks, diabetes mellitus, pulmonary disease [excluding asthma unless on high dose oral corticosteroids])

Children who received ≥1 dose of PCV7

Children 6-18 years of age at increased risk for invasive pneumococcal disease due to anatomic or functional asplenia (including sickle cell disease), HIV infection or other immunocompromising conditions, cochlear implant, or cerebrospinal fluid leaks (regardless of prior receipt of PCV7 or PPSV23). Routine use is not recommended for healthy children ≥5 years of age.

General Dosage Range I.M.:

Infants 2-6 months: 0.5 mL at approximately 2-month intervals for 3 consecutive doses, followed by a fourth dose of 0.5 mL at 12-15 months of age

Infants 7-11 months (previously unvaccinated): 0.5 mL for a total of 3 doses, 2 doses at least 4 weeks apart, followed by a third dose at 12-15 months (at least 2 months after second dose)

Children 12-23 months (previously unvaccinated) and Children 24-71 months (previously unvaccinated) with underlying conditions: 0.5 mL for a total of 2 doses, separated by at least 2 months

Healthy Children 24-59 months (previously unvaccinated) and Children 6-18 years at high risk for invasive pneumococcal disease: 0.5 mL as a single dose

Children 14 months-71 months (previously completing vaccination with PCV7): 0.5 mL supplemental dose

Adults ≥50 years: 0.5 mL as a single dose

Dosage Forms

Injection, suspension:

Prevnar 13®: 2 mcg of each capsular saccharide for serotypes 1, 3, 4, 5, 6A, 7F, 9V, 14, 18C, 19A, 19F, and 23F, and 4 mcg of serotype 6B [bound to diphtheria CRM_{197} protein ~34 mcg] per 0.5 mL (0.5 mL)

pneumococcal conjugate vaccine (nontypeable *Haemophilus influenzae* [NTHi] protein D, diphtheria or tetanus toxoid conjugates) adsorbed *see* pneumococcal conjugate vaccine (10-valent) *(Canada only) on page 733*

pneumococcal polysaccharide vaccine (polyvalent)

(noo moe KOK al pol i SAK a ride vak SEEN, pol i VAY lent)

Medication Safety Issues

Sound-alike/look-alike issues:

Pneumococcal 23-Valent Polysaccharide Vaccine (Pneumovax® 23) may be confused with Pneumococcal 7-Valent Conjugate Vaccine (Prevnar®) or with Pneumococcal 13-Valent Conjugate Vaccine (Prevnar 13®)

Synonyms 23-valent pneumococcal polysaccharide vaccine; 23PS; PPSV; PPSV23; PPV23

U.S. Brand Names Pneumovax® 23

Canadian Brand Names Pneumo 23™; Pneumovax® 23

Therapeutic Category Vaccine, Inactivated Bacteria

Use Immunization against pneumococcal disease caused by serotypes included in the vaccine. Routine vaccination is recommended for persons ≥50 years of age and persons ≥2 years in certain situations.

The Advisory Committee on Immunization Practices (ACIP) recommends routine vaccination for the following (CDC, 59[34], 2010; CDC, 59[11], 2010):

Patients ≥65 years of age without a history of vaccination (CDC, 61[4], 2012)

Patients 2-18 years of age with certain high-risk condition(s):

- Chronic heart disease (particularly cyanotic congenital heart disease and cardiac failure)
- Chronic lung disease (including asthma if treated with high-dose oral corticosteroids)

Patients 2-64 years of age with certain high-risk condition(s):

- Diabetes mellitus
- Cochlear implants
- Cerebrospinal fluid leaks
- Functional or anatomic asplenia (including sickle cell disease and other hemoglobinopathies, splenic dysfunction, or splenectomy)
- Immunocompromising conditions including congenital immunodeficiency (includes B- or T-lymphocyte deficiency, complement deficiencies, and phagocytic disorders [excluding chronic granulomatous disease]); HIV infection; leukemia, lymphoma, Hodgkin disease, multiple myeloma, generalized malignancy; chronic renal failure, nephrotic syndrome; patients requiring treatment with immunosuppressive therapy, including chemotherapy, long-term systemic corticosteroids, or radiation therapy; patients who have received a solid organ transplant

Patients 19-64 years of age with certain high-risk condition(s):

- Chronic heart disease (including heart failure and cardiomyopathy, and excluding hypertension)
- Chronic lung disease (including COPD, emphysema, and asthma)
- Persons who smoke cigarettes
- Alcoholism
- Chronic liver disease (including cirrhosis)
- Residents of nursing homes or long term care facilities (CDC, 61[4], 2012)

Routine vaccination is not recommended for Alaska Natives or American Indian persons unless they have underlying conditions which are indications for vaccination; in special situations, vaccination may be recommended when living in an area at increased risk of invasive pneumococcal disease.

General Dosage Range I.M., SubQ: *Children ≥2 years and Adults:* 0.5 mL

Dosage Forms

Injection, solution:

Pneumovax® 23: 25 mcg each of 23 capsular polysaccharide isolates/0.5 mL (0.5 mL, 2.5 mL)

Pneumovax® 23 *see* pneumococcal polysaccharide vaccine (polyvalent) *on page 735*

PNU-140690E *see* tipranavir *on page 899*

Podactin Cream [OTC] *see* miconazole (topical) *on page 599*

Podactin Powder [OTC] *see* tolnaftate *on page 904*

Podocon-25® *see* podophyllum resin *on page 736*

Podofilm® (Can) *see* podophyllum resin *on page 736*

podofilox (poe DOF il oks)

U.S. Brand Names Condylox®

Canadian Brand Names Condyline™; Wartec®

Therapeutic Category Keratolytic Agent

Use Treatment of external genital warts

General Dosage Range Topical: *Adults:* Apply twice daily for 3 consecutive days, then withhold use for 4 consecutive days; May repeat cycle up to 4 times

Dosage Forms

Gel, topical:

Condylox®: 0.5% (3.5 g)

Solution, topical: 0.5% (3.5 mL)

Condylox®: 0.5% (3.5 mL)

podophyllin *see* podophyllum resin *on page* 736

podophyllum resin (po DOF fil um REZ in)

Synonyms mandrake; may apple; podophyllin

U.S. Brand Names Podocon-25®

Canadian Brand Names Podofilm®

Therapeutic Category Keratolytic Agent

Use Topical treatment of soft external genital (venereal) warts (condylomata acuminata); compound benzoin tincture generally is used as the medium for topical application

General Dosage Range Topical: *Children and Adults:* Applied by physician only

Dosage Forms

Liquid, topical:

Podocon-25®: 25% (15 mL)

Polibar® ACB *see* barium *on page* 114

polidocanol (pol i DOE kuh nol)

U.S. Brand Names Asclera™

Therapeutic Category Sclerosing Agent

Use Treatment of small, uncomplicated varicose veins of the lower extremities

General Dosage Range I.V.: *Adults:* 0.1-0.3 mL injection (0.5% or 1% solution) per session (maximum: 10 mL/session)

Dosage Forms

Injection, solution [preservative free]:

Asclera™: 0.5% (2 mL); 1% (2 mL)

polio vaccine *see* poliovirus vaccine (inactivated) *on page* 736

poliovirus, inactivated (IPV) *see* diphtheria and tetanus toxoids, acellular pertussis, and poliovirus vaccine *on page* 296

poliovirus, inactivated (IPV) *see* diphtheria and tetanus toxoids, acellular pertussis, poliovirus and *Haemophilus* b conjugate vaccine *on page* 298

poliovirus vaccine (inactivated) (POE lee oh VYE rus vak SEEN, in ak ti VAY ted)

Medication Safety Issues

Administration issues:

Poliovirus vaccine (inactivated) may be confused with tuberculin products. Medication errors have occurred when poliovirus vaccine (IPV) has been inadvertently administered instead of ttuberculin skin tests (PPD). These products are refrigerated and often stored in close proximity to each other.

Synonyms enhanced-potency inactivated poliovirus vaccine; IPV; polio vaccine; salk vaccine

U.S. Brand Names IPOL®

Canadian Brand Names Imovax® Polio

Therapeutic Category Vaccine, Live Virus and Inactivated Virus

Use Active immunization against poliomyelitis caused by poliovirus types 1, 2 and 3. **Note:** Combination products containing polio vaccine are also available and may be preferred in certain age groups if recipients are likely to be susceptible to the agents contained within each vaccine.

The Advisory Committee on Immunization Practices (ACIP) recommends routine vaccination for the following:

- All children (first dose given at 2 months of age)

Routine immunization of adults in the United States is generally not recommended. Adults with previous wild poliovirus disease, who have never been immunized, or those who are incompletely immunized may receive inactivated poliovirus vaccine if they fall into one of the following categories:

- Travelers to regions or countries where poliomyelitis is endemic or epidemic
- Healthcare workers in close contact with patients who may be excreting poliovirus
- Laboratory workers handling specimens that may contain poliovirus
- Members of communities or specific population groups with diseases caused by wild poliovirus
- Incompletely vaccinated or unvaccinated adults in a household or with other close contact with children receiving oral poliovirus (may be at increased risk of vaccine associated paralytic poliomyelitis)

General Dosage Range I.M., SubQ:

Children: Primary immunization: Administer three 0.5 mL doses at 2, 4, and 6-18 months of age; do not administer more frequently than 4 weeks apart (preferably given more than 8 weeks apart). Booster dose: 0.5 mL at 4-6 years of age; Minimum interval between booster and previous dose is 6 months.

Adults (previously unvaccinated): Two 0.5 mL doses administered at 1- to 2-month intervals followed by a third dose 6-12 months later.

Dosage Forms

Injection, suspension:

IPOL®: Type 1 poliovirus 40 D-antigen units, type 2 poliovirus 8 D-antigen units, and type 3 poliovirus 32 D-antigen units per 0.5 mL (0.5 mL, 5 mL)

Polocaine® *see* mepivacaine *on page* 575

Polocaine® 2% and Levonordefrin 1:20,000 (Can) *see* mepivacaine and levonordefrin *on page* 576

Polocaine® Dental with Levonordefrin *see* mepivacaine and levonordefrin *on page* 576

Polocaine® MPF *see* mepivacaine *on page* 575

polycarbophil (pol i KAR boe fil)

U.S. Brand Names Equalactin® [OTC]; Fiber-Lax [OTC]; Fiber-Tabs™ [OTC]; FiberCon® [OTC]; Fibertab [OTC]; Konsyl® Fiber [OTC]

Therapeutic Category Gastrointestinal Agent, Miscellaneous; Laxative

Use Treatment of constipation or diarrhea

General Dosage Range Oral:

Children 6-12 years: 625 mg calcium polycarbophil 1-4 times/day

Children ≥12 years and Adults: 1250 mg calcium polycarbophil 1-4 times/day

Dosage Forms

Caplet, oral: Calcium polycarbophil 625 mg

FiberCon® [OTC]: Calcium polycarbophil 625 mg

Konsyl® Fiber [OTC]: Calcium polycarbophil 625 mg

Captab, oral:

Fiber-Lax [OTC]: Calcium polycarbophil 625 mg

Tablet, oral:

Fiber-Tabs™ [OTC]: Calcium polycarbophil 625 mg

Fibertab [OTC]: Calcium polycarbophil 625 mg

Tablet, chewable, oral:

Equalactin® [OTC]: Calcium polycarbophil 625 mg

Polycin™ *see* bacitracin and polymyxin B *on page* 111

Polycitra *see* citric acid, sodium citrate, and potassium citrate *on page* 214

Polycitra K *see* potassium citrate and citric acid *on page* 745

Polycose® [OTC] *see* glucose polymers *on page* 428

polyethylene glycol-L-asparaginase *see* pegaspargase *on page* 696

polyethylene glycol 3350 (pol i ETH i leen GLY kol 3350)

Medication Safety Issues

Sound-alike/look-alike issues:

MiraLax® may be confused with Mirapex®

Polyethylene glycol 3350 may be confused with polyethylene glycol electrolyte solution

International issues:

MiraLax may be confused with Murelax brand name for oxazepam [Australia]

Synonyms PEG

U.S. Brand Names Dulcolax Balance® [OTC]; MiraLAX® [OTC]

Therapeutic Category Laxative, Osmotic

Use Treatment of occasional constipation in adults

General Dosage Range Oral: *Adults:* 17 g of powder (~1 heaping tablespoon) dissolved in 4-8 ounces of beverage once daily (maximum use: 1 week)

Dosage Forms

Powder for solution, oral: 17 g/dose (119 g, 238 g, 255 g, 510 g, 527 g); 17 g/packet (14s, 30s)

Dulcolax Balance® [OTC]: 17 g/dose (119 g, 238 g, 510 g)

MiraLAX® [OTC]: 17 g/dose (119 g, 238 g, 510 g); 17 g/packet (10s)

polyethylene glycol-conjugated uricase *see* pegloticase *on page* 699

polyethylene glycol-electrolyte solution

(pol i ETH i leen GLY kol ee LEK troe lite soe LOO shun)

Medication Safety Issues

Sound-alike/look-alike issues:

GoLYTELY® may be confused with NuLYTELY®

TriLyte® may be confused with TriLipix®

Synonyms electrolyte lavage solution

U.S. Brand Names Colyte®; GaviLyte™-C; GaviLyte™-G; GaviLyte™-N; GoLYTELY®; MoviPrep®; NuLYTELY®; TriLyte®

Canadian Brand Names Colyte™; Klean-Prep®; PegLyte®

Therapeutic Category Laxative

Use Bowel cleansing prior to GI examination

General Dosage Range

Nasogastric tube:

Children ≥6 months: 25 mL/kg/hour until rectal effluent is clear

Adults: 20-30 mL/minute (1.2-1.8 L/hour) until rectal effluent is clear

Oral:

Children ≥6 months: (GaviLyte™-N, NuLYTELY®, TriLyte®): 25 mL/kg/hour (some studies have used up to 40 mL/kg/hour) for 4-10 hours until rectal effluent is clear (maximum total dose: 4 L)

Adults: CoLyte®, GaviLyte™-C, GaviLyte™-G, GaviLyte™-N, GoLYTELY®, NuLYTELY®, TriLyte®: 240 mL (8 oz) every 10 minutes, until 4 L are consumed or the rectal effluent is clear; MoviPrep®: 240 mL (8 oz) every 15 minutes until 1 L consumed; repeat 1 time

Dosage Forms

Powder, for solution, oral: PEG 3350 240 g, sodium sulfate 22.72 g, sodium bicarbonate 6.72 g, sodium chloride 5.84 g, and potassium 2.98 g (4000 mL); PEG 3350 236 g, sodium sulfate 22.74 g, sodium bicarbonate 6.74 g, sodium chloride 5.86 g, and potassium chloride 2.97 g (4000 mL); PEG 3350 240 g, sodium bicarbonate 5.72 g, sodium chloride 11.2 g, and potassium chloride 1.48 g (4000 mL)

Colyte®: PEG 3350 227.1 g, sodium sulfate 21.5 g, sodium bicarbonate 6.36 g, sodium chloride 5.53 g, and potassium chloride 2.82 g (3785 mL)

Colyte®: PEG 3350 240 g, sodium sulfate 22.72 g, sodium bicarbonate 6.72 g, sodium chloride 5.84 g, and potassium 2.98 g (4000 mL)

GaviLyte™-C: PEG 3350 240 g, sodium sulfate 22.72 g, sodium bicarbonate 6.72 g, sodium chloride 5.84 g, and potassium chloride 2.98 g (4000 mL)

GaviLyte™-G: PEG 3350 236 g, sodium sulfate 22.74 g, sodium bicarbonate 6.74 g, sodium chloride 5.86 g, and potassium chloride 2.97 g (4000 mL)

GaviLyte™-N: PEG 3350 420 g, sodium bicarbonate 5.72 g, sodium chloride 11.2 g, and potassium chloride 1.48 g (4000 mL)

GoLYTELY®: PEG 3350 227.1 g, sodium sulfate 21.5 g, sodium bicarbonate 6.36 g, sodium chloride 5.53 g, and potassium 2.82 g per packet (1s)

GoLYTELY®: PEG 3350 236 g, sodium sulfate 22.74 g, sodium bicarbonate 6.74 g, sodium chloride 5.86 g, and potassium 2.97 g (4000 mL)

MoviPrep®: Pouch A: PEG 3350 100g, sodium sulfate 7.5 g, sodium chloride 2.69 g, potassium chloride 1.015 g; Pouch B: Ascorbic acid 4.7 g, sodium ascorbate 5.9 g

NuLYTELY®: PEG 3350 420 g, sodium bicarbonate 5.72 g, sodium chloride 11.2 g, and potassium 1.48 g

TriLyte®: PEG 3350 420 g, sodium bicarbonate 5.72 g, sodium chloride 11.2 g, and potassium 1.48 g

polyethylene glycol-electrolyte solution and bisacodyl

(pol i ETH i leen GLY kol ee LEK troe lite soe LOO shun & bis a KOE dil)

Synonyms bisacodyl and polyethylene glycol-electrolyte solution; electrolyte lavage solution

U.S. Brand Names HalfLytely® and Bisacodyl

Therapeutic Category Laxative, Bowel Evacuant; Laxative, Stimulant

Use Bowel cleansing prior to colonoscopy

General Dosage Range Oral: *Adults:* 5 mg of bisacodyl as a single dose, after bowel movement or 6 hours (whichever occurs first) initiate 8 ounces of polyethylene glycol-electrolyte solution every 10 minutes until 2 L are consumed

Dosage Forms

Kit [each kit contains]:

HalfLytely® and Bisacodyl:

Powder for solution, oral (HalfLytely®): PEG 3350 210 g, sodium bicarbonate 2.86 g, sodium chloride 5.6 g, potassium chloride 0.74 g (2000 mL) [contains 4 flavor packs (each 1 g) cherry, lemon-lime, orange, pineapple flavors]

Tablet, delayed release (Bisacodyl): 5 mg (1s)

polyethylene glycol interferon alfa-2b *see* peginterferon alfa-2b *on page 698*

Poly-Iron 150 [OTC] *see* polysaccharide-iron complex *on page 740*

Poly-Iron 150 Forte *see* polysaccharide-iron complex, vitamin B12, and folic acid *on page 741*

polymyxin B (pol i MIKS in bee)

Medication Safety Issues

High alert medication:

The Institute for Safe Medication Practices (ISMP) includes this medication (intrathecal administration) among its list of drug classes which have a heightened risk of causing significant patient harm when used in error.

Synonyms polymyxin B sulfate

U.S. Brand Names Poly-Rx [DSC]

Therapeutic Category Antibiotic, Irrigation; Antibiotic, Miscellaneous

Use Treatment of acute infections caused by susceptible strains of *Pseudomonas aeruginosa*; used occasionally for gut decontamination; parenteral use of polymyxin B has mainly been replaced by less toxic antibiotics, reserved for life-threatening infections caused by organisms resistant to the preferred drugs (eg, pseudomonal meningitis - intrathecal administration)

General Dosage Range Dosage adjustment recommended in patients with renal impairment

I.M.:

Children <2 years: Up to 40,000 units/kg/day divided every 6 hours

Children ≥2 years and Adults: 25,000-30,000 units/kg/day divided every 4-6 hours (maximum: 2,000,000 units/day)

I.V.:

Children <2 years: Up to 40,000 units/kg/day divided every 12 hours

Children ≥2 years and Adults: 15,000-25,000 units/kg/day divided every 12 hours (maximum: 2,000,000 units/day)

Intrathecal:

Children <2 years: 20,000 units/day for 3-4 days, then 25,000 units every other day

Children ≥2 years and Adults: 50,000 units/day for 3-4 days, then every other day

Irrigation: *Adults:*

Bladder: 20 mg (equal to 200,000 units) added to 1 L of normal saline as continuous irrigant or rinse

Topical: 500,000 units/L of normal saline (maximum: 2 million units/day)

Ophthalmic: *Children ≥2 years and Adults:* Initial: 1-3 drops/hour; Reduce to 1-2 drops 4-6 times/day based on response

Otic: *Children and Adults:* 1-2 drops 3-4 times/day

Dosage Forms

Injection, powder for reconstitution: 500,000 units

polymyxin B and bacitracin *see* bacitracin and polymyxin B *on page 111*

polymyxin B and neomycin *see* neomycin and polymyxin B *on page 633*

polymyxin B and trimethoprim *see* trimethoprim and polymyxin B *on page 921*

polymyxin B, bacitracin, and neomycin *see* bacitracin, neomycin, and polymyxin B *on page 111*

polymyxin B, bacitracin, neomycin, and hydrocortisone *see* bacitracin, neomycin, polymyxin B, and hydrocortisone *on page 112*

polymyxin B, neomycin, and dexamethasone *see* neomycin, polymyxin B, and dexamethasone *on page 634*

polymyxin B, neomycin, and gramicidin *see* neomycin, polymyxin B, and gramicidin *on page 634*

polymyxin B, neomycin, and hydrocortisone *see* neomycin, polymyxin B, and hydrocortisone *on page 634*

polymyxin B, neomycin, bacitracin, and pramoxine *see* bacitracin, neomycin, polymyxin B, and pramoxine *on page 112*

polymyxin B sulfate *see* polymyxin B *on page 739*

polymyxin E *see* colistimethate *on page 233*

polyphenols *see* sinecatechins *on page 836*

polyphenon E *see* sinecatechins *on page 836*

Poly-Rx [DSC] *see* polymyxin B *on page 739*

Polysaccharide Iron 150 Forte *see* polysaccharide-iron complex, vitamin B12, and folic acid *on page 741*

polysaccharide-iron complex (pol i SAK a ride-EYE ern KOM pleks)

Medication Safety Issues

Sound-alike/look-alike issues:

Niferex® may be confused with Nephrox®

Synonyms iron-polysaccharide complex

U.S. Brand Names Ferrex™ 150 Plus [OTC]; Ferrex™ 150 [OTC]; Niferex® [OTC] [DSC]; Nu-Iron® 150 [OTC]; Poly-Iron 150 [OTC]; ProFe [OTC]

Therapeutic Category Electrolyte Supplement, Oral

Use Prevention and treatment of iron-deficiency anemias

General Dosage Range Oral:

Children ≥6 years: 50-100 mg once daily or in divided doses

Adults: 100-300 mg/day in 1-2 divided doses

Dosage Forms

Capsule, oral:

Ferrex™ 150 [OTC]: Elemental iron 150 mg

Ferrex™ 150 Plus [OTC]: Elemental iron 150 mg (50 mg as ferrous asparto glycinate)

Nu-Iron® 150 [OTC]: Elemental iron 150 mg

Poly-Iron 150 [OTC]: Elemental iron 150 mg

ProFe [OTC]: Elemental iron 180 mg

polysaccharide-iron complex and folic acid

(pol i SAK a ride-EYE ern KOM pleks & FOE lik AS id)

Synonyms folic acid and polysaccharide-iron complex; iron-polysaccharide complex and folic acid

U.S. Brand Names NovaFerrum®

Therapeutic Category Iron Salt

Use Prevention and treatment of iron-deficiency anemias

General Dosage Range Oral: *Children >12 years and Adults:* Iron deficiency: 5 mL daily

Dosage Forms

Powder for solution, oral:

NovaFerrum®: Elemental iron 100 mg and folic acid 1 mg per 5 mL (120 mL)

polysaccharide-iron complex, vitamin B12, and folic acid

(pol i SAK a ride-EYE ern KOM pleks, VYE ta min bee twelve & FOE lik AS id)

Synonyms iron-polysaccharide complex, vitamin B12, and folic acid

U.S. Brand Names Ferrex™ 150 Forte; Ferrex™ 150 Forte Plus; Maxaron® Forte; Poly-Iron 150 Forte; Polysaccharide Iron 150 Forte

Therapeutic Category Iron Salt

Use Prevention and treatment of iron-deficiency anemias and/or nutritional megaloblastic anemias

General Dosage Range Oral: *Adults:* 1-2 capsules daily

Dosage Forms

Capsule, oral:

Ferrex™ 150 Forte: Elemental iron 150 mg, cyanocobalamin 25 mcg, and folic acid 1 mg

Ferrex™ 150 Forte Plus: Elemental iron 150 mg (50 mg as ferrous asparto glycinate), cyanocobalamin 25 mcg, and folic acid 1 mg

Maxaron® Forte: Elemental iron 150 mg (80 mg as ferrous bisglycinate), cyanocobalamin 25 mcg, and folic acid 1 mg

Poly-Iron 150 Forte: Elemental iron 150 mg, cyanocobalamin 25 mcg, and folic acid 1 mg

Polysaccharide Iron 150 Forte: Elemental iron 150 mg, cyanocobalamin 25 mcg, and folic acid 1 mg

Polysporin® [OTC] *see* bacitracin and polymyxin B *on page 111*
Polytrim® *see* trimethoprim and polymyxin B *on page 921*
Polytrim™ (Can) *see* trimethoprim and polymyxin B *on page 921*
polyvinyl alcohol *see* artificial tears *on page 93*
polyvinylpyrrolidone with iodine *see* povidone-iodine (ophthalmic) *on page 747*
polyvinylpyrrolidone with iodine *see* povidone-iodine (topical) *on page 747*
Poly-Vi-Sol® [OTC] *see* vitamins (multiple/pediatric) *on page 952*
Poly-Vi-Sol® With Iron [OTC] *see* vitamins (multiple/pediatric) *on page 952*
P-OM3 *see* omega-3-acid ethyl esters *on page 665*
Ponstan® (Can) *see* mefenamic acid *on page 568*
Ponstel® *see* mefenamic acid *on page 568*
Pontocaine® [DSC] *see* tetracaine (topical) *on page 884*
Pontocaine® (Can) *see* tetracaine (ophthalmic) *on page 883*
Pontocaine® (Can) *see* tetracaine (systemic) *on page 883*
Pontocaine® (Can) *see* tetracaine (topical) *on page 884*

poractant alfa (por AKT ant AL fa)

Synonyms porcine lung surfactant

U.S. Brand Names Curosurf®

Canadian Brand Names Curosurf®

Therapeutic Category Lung Surfactant

Use Treatment of respiratory distress syndrome (RDS) in premature infants

General Dosage Range Intratracheal: *Premature infants:* Initial: 2.5 mL/kg of birth weight, up to 2 subsequent doses of 1.25 mL/kg birth weight can be administered at 12-hour intervals if needed; Maximum total dose: 5 mL/kg

Dosage Forms

Suspension, intratracheal [preservative free]:

Curosurf®: 80 mg/mL (1.5 mL, 3 mL)

porcine lung surfactant *see* poractant alfa *on page 741*

porfimer (POR fi mer)

Medication Safety Issues

High alert medication:

This medication is in a class the Institute for Safe Medication Practices (ISMP) includes among its list of drug classes which have a heightened risk of causing significant patient harm when used in error.

Synonyms CL-184116; dihematoporphyrin ether; porfimer sodium

U.S. Brand Names Photofrin®

Canadian Brand Names Photofrin®

Therapeutic Category Antineoplastic Agent

Use Palliation in patients with obstructing (partial or complete) esophageal cancer; treatment of microinvasive endobronchial nonsmall cell lung cancer (NSCLC); reduction of obstruction and palliation in patients with obstructing (partial or complete) NSCLC; ablation of high-grade dysplasia in Barrett esophagus

Canadian labeling (additional use; not in U.S. labeling): Second-line treatment of recurrent, superficial papillary bladder cancer

General Dosage Range I.V.: *Adults:* 2 mg/kg, followed by endoscopic exposure to the appropriate laser light

Dosage Forms

Injection, powder for reconstitution:

Photofrin®: 75 mg

Dosage Forms - Canada

Injection, powder for reconstitution, as sodium:

Photofrin®: 15 mg

porfimer sodium *see* porfimer *on page* *741*

Portia® *see* ethinyl estradiol and levonorgestrel *on page* *357*

posaconazole (poe sa KON a zole)

Medication Safety Issues

Sound-alike/look-alike issues:

Noxafil® may be confused with minoxidil

International issues:

Noxafil [U.S. and multiple international markets] may be confused with Noxidil brand name for minoxidil [Thailand]

Synonyms SCH 56592

U.S. Brand Names Noxafil®

Canadian Brand Names Posanol™

Therapeutic Category Antifungal Agent, Oral

Use

U.S. labeling: Prophylaxis of invasive *Aspergillus* and *Candida* infections in severely-immunocompromised patients (eg, hematopoietic stem cell transplant [HSCT] recipients with graft-versus-host disease [GVHD] or those with prolonged neutropenia secondary to chemotherapy for hematologic malignancies); treatment of oropharyngeal candidiasis (including patients refractory to itraconazole and/or fluconazole)

Canadian labeling: Prophylaxis of invasive *Aspergillus* and *Candida* infections in severely-immunocompromised patients (eg, hematopoietic stem cell transplant [HSCT] recipients with graft-versus-host disease [GVHD] or those with prolonged neutropenia); treatment of invasive aspergillosis in patients refractory to or intolerant of itraconazole or amphotericin B; treatment of oropharyngeal candidiasis

General Dosage Range Oral: *Children ≥13 years, Adolescents, and Adults:* 100-800 mg/day; doses >100 mg/day are given in 2-3 divided doses

Dosage Forms

Suspension, oral:

Noxafil®: 40 mg/mL (123 mL)

Posanol™ (Can) *see* posaconazole *on page* *742*

Posicaine N (Can) *see* articaine and epinephrine *on page* *92*

Posicaine SP (Can) *see* articaine and epinephrine *on page* *92*

Posture® [OTC] *see* calcium phosphate (tribasic) *on page* *166*

potassium acetate (poe TASS ee um AS e tate)

Medication Safety Issues

Other safety concerns:

Consider special storage requirements for intravenous potassium salts; I.V. potassium salts have been administered IVP in error, leading to fatal outcomes.

Therapeutic Category Electrolyte Supplement, Oral

Use Potassium deficiency; to avoid chloride when high concentration of potassium is needed, source of bicarbonate

General Dosage Range I.V.:

Children: 2-5 mEq/kg/day; Intermittent infusion: 0.5-1 mEq/kg/dose (maximum: 30 mEq/dose) to infuse at 0.3-0.5 mEq/kg/hour (maximum: 1 mEq/kg/hour)

Adults: 40-100 mEq/day; Intermittent infusion: 5-10 mEq/dose (maximum: 40 mEq/dose) to infuse over 2-3 hours (maximum: 40 mEq over 1 hour)

Dosage Forms

Injection, solution: 2 mEq/mL (20 mL, 50 mL, 100 mL)

Injection, solution [preservative free]: 2 mEq/mL (20 mL, 50 mL, 100 mL); 4 mEq/mL (50 mL)

potassium acid phosphate (poe TASS ee um AS id FOS fate)

U.S. Brand Names K-Phos® Original

Therapeutic Category Urinary Acidifying Agent

Use Acidifies urine and lowers urinary calcium concentration; reduces odor and rash caused by ammoniacal urine; increases the antibacterial activity of methenamine

General Dosage Range Oral: *Adults:* 1000 mg dissolved in 6-8 oz of water 4 times/day

Dosage Forms

Tablet, oral:

K-Phos® Original: 500 mg

potassium bicarbonate (poe TASS ee um bye KAR bun ate)

U.S. Brand Names K-Effervescent

Therapeutic Category Electrolyte Supplement, Oral

Use Potassium deficiency, hypokalemia

General Dosage Range Oral:

Children: 1-4 mEq/kg/day

Adults: 25 mEq 2-4 times/day

Dosage Forms

Tablet for solution, oral: Potassium 25 mEq

K-Effervescent: Potassium 25 mEq

potassium bicarbonate and potassium chloride
(poe TASS ee um bye KAR bun ate & poe TASS ee um KLOR ide)

Synonyms K-Lyte/Cl; potassium bicarbonate and potassium chloride (effervescent)

Therapeutic Category Electrolyte Supplement, Oral

Use Treatment or prevention of hypokalemia

General Dosage Range

Oral:

Children: 1-4 mEq/kg/day in divided doses

Adults: Prevention: 16-24 mEq/day in 2-4 divided doses; Treatment: 40-100 mEq/day in 2-4 divided doses

Dosage Forms

Tablet for solution, oral [effervescent]: Potassium chloride 25 mEq

potassium bicarbonate and potassium chloride (effervescent) *see* potassium bicarbonate and potassium chloride *on page 743*

potassium bicarbonate and potassium citrate
(poe TASS ee um bye KAR bun ate & poe TASS ee um SIT rate)

Medication Safety Issues

Sound-alike/look-alike issues:

Klor-Con® may be confused with Klaron®

Synonyms potassium bicarbonate and potassium citrate (effervescent)

U.S. Brand Names Effer-K®; Klor-Con®/EF

Therapeutic Category Electrolyte Supplement, Oral

Use Treatment or prevention of hypokalemia

General Dosage Range

Oral:

Children: 1-4 mEq/kg/day in divided doses

Adults: Prevention: 16-24 mEq/day in 2-4 divided doses; Treatment: 40-100 mEq/day in 2-4 divided doses

Dosage Forms

Tablet for solution, oral [effervescent]:

Effer-K®: Potassium 10 mEq; potassium 20 mEq; potassium 25 mEq

Klor-Con®/EF: Potassium 25 mEq

potassium bicarbonate and potassium citrate (effervescent) *see* potassium bicarbonate and potassium citrate *on page* 743

potassium chloride (poe TASS ee um KLOR ide)

Medication Safety Issues

Sound-alike/look-alike issues:

Kaon-Cl-10® may be confused with kaolin

KCl may be confused with HCl

Klor-Con® may be confused with Klaron®

microK® may be confused with Macrobid®, Micronase

High alert medication:

The Institute for Safe Medication Practices (ISMP) includes this medication (I.V. formulation) among its list of drugs which have a heightened risk of causing significant patient harm when used in error.

Other safety concerns:

Per JCAHO recommendations, concentrated electrolyte solutions should not be available in patient care areas.

Consider special storage requirements for intravenous potassium salts; I.V. potassium salts have been administered IVP in error, leading to fatal outcomes.

Synonyms KCl; kdur

U.S. Brand Names Epiklor™; Epiklor™/25; K-Tab®; Kaon-CL® 10; Klor-Con®; Klor-Con® 10; Klor-Con® 8; Klor-Con® M10; Klor-Con® M15; Klor-Con® M20; Klor-Con®/25; microK®; microK® 10

Canadian Brand Names Apo-K®; K-10®; K-Dur®; Micro-K Extencaps®; Roychlor®; Slo-Pot; Slow-K®

Therapeutic Category Electrolyte Supplement, Oral

Use Treatment or prevention of hypokalemia

General Dosage Range

I.V.:

Children: Initial: 0.5-1 mEq/kg/dose (maximum dose: 40 mEq); repeat as needed based on lab values

Adults: Intermittent infusion: ≤10 mEq/hour; repeat as needed based on lab values (maximum: 200 mEq/day)

Oral:

Children: 1-2 mEq/kg/day in 1-2 divided doses or as needed based on lab values

Adults: Initial: 6-10 mEq/dose (maximum: 40 mEq/dose); Maintenance: 40-100 mEq/day in divided doses or as needed based on lab values

Dosage Forms

Capsule, extended release, microencapsulated, oral: 8 mEq, 10 mEq

microK®: 8 mEq

microK® 10: 10 mEq

Infusion, premixed in 1/2 NS: 20 mEq (1000 mL)

Infusion, premixed in D_5 1/2 NS: 10 mEq (500 mL, 1000 mL); 20 mEq (1000 mL); 30 mEq (1000 mL); 40 mEq (1000 mL)

Infusion, premixed in D_5 1/3 NS: 20 mEq (1000 mL)

Infusion, premixed in D_5 1/4 NS: 5 mEq (250 mL); 10 mEq (500 mL, 1000 mL); 20 mEq (1000 mL)

Infusion, premixed in D_5LR: 20 mEq (1000 mL)

Infusion, premixed in D_5NS: 20 mEq (1000 mL); 40 mEq (1000 mL)

Infusion, premixed in D_5W: 20 mEq (500 mL, 1000 mL); 40 mEq (1000 mL)

Infusion, premixed in NS: 20 mEq (1000 mL); 40 mEq (1000 mL)

Infusion, premixed in water for injection: 10 mEq (50 mL, 100 mL); 20 mEq (50 mL, 100 mL); 30 mEq (100 mL); 40 mEq (100 mL)

Injection, solution: 2 mEq/mL (5 mL, 10 mL, 15 mL, 20 mL, 30 mL, 250 mL, 500 mL)

Injection, solution [preservative free]: 2 mEq/mL (5 mL, 10 mL, 15 mL, 20 mL)

Powder for solution, oral:
Epiklor™: 20 mEq/packet (30s, 100s)
Epiklor™/25: 25 mEq/packet (30s, 100s)
Klor-Con®: 20 mEq/packet (30s, 100s)
Klor-Con®/25: 25 mEq/packet (30s, 100s)
Solution, oral: 20 mEq/15 mL (15 mL, 30 mL, 473 mL, 480 mL); 40 mEq/15 mL (15 mL, 473 mL, 480 mL)
Tablet, extended release, oral: 10 mEq
Tablet, extended release, microencapsulated, oral: 8 mEq, 10 mEq, 20 mEq
Klor-Con® M10: 10 mEq
Klor-Con® M15: 15 mEq
Klor-Con® M20: 20 mEq
Tablet, extended release, wax matrix, oral: 8 mEq, 10 mEq
K-Tab®: 10 mEq
Kaon-CL® 10: 10 mEq
Klor-Con® 8: 8 mEq
Klor-Con® 10: 10 mEq

potassium citrate (poe TASS ee um SIT rate)

Medication Safety Issues
Sound-alike/look-alike issues:
Urocit®-K may be confused with Urised

U.S. Brand Names Urocit®-K

Canadian Brand Names Urocit®-K

Therapeutic Category Alkalinizing Agent

Use Prevention of uric acid nephrolithiasis; prevention of calcium renal stones in patients with hypocitraturia; urinary alkalinizer when sodium citrate is contraindicated

General Dosage Range Oral: *Adults:*
Immediate release: 10-20 mEq 3 times/day or 15 mEq 4 times/day (maximum: 100 mEq/day)
Extended release: 15-30 mEq 2 times/day or 10-20 mEq 3 times/day (maximum: 100 mEq/day)

Dosage Forms
Tablet, extended release, oral: 540 mg, 1080 mg
Urocit®-K: 540 mg, 1080 mg, 1620 mg

potassium citrate and citric acid (poe TASS ee um SIT rate & SI trik AS id)

Synonyms citric acid and potassium citrate; Polycitra K

U.S. Brand Names Cytra-K

Therapeutic Category Alkalinizing Agent

Use Treatment of metabolic acidosis; alkalinizing agent in conditions where long-term maintenance of an alkaline urine is desirable

General Dosage Range Oral:
Children: 5-15 mL after meals and at bedtime
Adults: 15-30 mL **or** 1 packet dissolved in water after meals and at bedtime

Dosage Forms
Powder for solution, oral:
Cytra-K: Potassium citrate monohydrate 3300 mg and citric acid monohydrate 1002 mg per packet (100s) [sugar free; fruit-punch flavor; each packet contains potassium 30 mEq equivalent to bicarbonate 30 mEq]
Solution, oral:
Cytra-K: Potassium citrate monohydrate 1100 mg and citric acid monohydrate 334 mg per 5 mL (480 mL) [ethanol free, sugar free; contains propylene glycol; cherry flavor; contains potassium 2 mEq/mL equivalent to bicarbonate 2 mEq /mL]

potassium citrate, citric acid, and sodium citrate *see* citric acid, sodium citrate, and potassium citrate *on page* 214

potassium gluconate (poe TASS ee um GLOO coe nate)

Therapeutic Category Electrolyte Supplement, Oral

Use Dietary supplement

General Dosage Range Oral: *Adults:* One tablet daily

Dosage Forms

Caplet, oral: 595 mg
Capsule, oral: 99 mg
Tablet, oral: 99 mg, 550 mg, 595 mg
Tablet, timed release, oral: 95 mg

potassium iodide (poe TASS ee um EYE oh dide)

Medication Safety Issues

Sound-alike/look-alike issues:

Potassium iodide products, including saturated solution of potassium iodide (SSKI®) may be confused with potassium iodide and iodine (Strong Iodide Solution or Lugol's solution)

Synonyms KI

U.S. Brand Names iOSAT™ [OTC]; SSKI®; ThyroSafe® [OTC]; Thyroshield® [OTC]

Therapeutic Category Antithyroid Agent; Expectorant

Use Expectorant for the symptomatic treatment of chronic pulmonary diseases complicated by mucous; block thyroidal uptake of radioactive isotopes of iodine in a radiation emergency

General Dosage Range Oral:

Infants 1-12 months and Children 1-3 years: Iosat™, ThyroSafe®, ThyroShield®: 32.5 mg once daily
Children 3-18 years: Iosat™, ThyroSafe®, ThyroShield®: 65-130 mg once daily
Adults: Iosat™, ThyroSafe®, ThyroShield®: 130 mg once daily; SSKI®: 300-600 mg (6-12 drops) 3-4 times/day

Dosage Forms

Solution, oral:
SSKI®: 1 g/mL (30 mL, 237 mL)
Thyroshield® [OTC]: 65 mg/mL (30 mL)

Tablet, oral:
iOSAT™ [OTC]: 130 mg
ThyroSafe® [OTC]: 65 mg

potassium phosphate (poe TASS ee um FOS fate)

Medication Safety Issues

High alert medication:

The Institute for Safe Medication Practices (ISMP) includes this medication (I.V. formulation) among its list of drugs which have a heightened risk of causing significant patient harm when used in error.

Other safety concerns:

Per JCAHO recommendations, concentrated electrolyte solutions should not be available in patient care areas.

Consider special storage requirements for intravenous potassium salts; I.V. potassium salts have been administered IVP in error, leading to fatal outcomes.

Safe Prescribing: Because inorganic phosphate exists as monobasic and dibasic anions, with the mixture of valences dependent on pH, ordering by mEq amounts is unreliable and may lead to large dosing errors. In addition, I.V. phosphate is available in the sodium and potassium salt; therefore, the content of these cations must be considered when ordering phosphate. The most reliable method of ordering I.V. phosphate is by millimoles, then specifying the potassium or sodium salt. For example, an order for 15 mmol of phosphate as potassium phosphate in one liter of normal saline.

Synonyms phosphate, potassium

U.S. Brand Names Neutra-Phos®-K [OTC] [DSC]

Therapeutic Category Electrolyte Supplement, Oral

Use Treatment and prevention of hypophosphatemia; **Note:** The concomitant amount of potassium must be calculated into the total electrolyte content. For each 1 mmol of phosphate, ~1.5 mEq of potassium will be administered. Therefore, if ordering 30 mmol of potassium phosphate, the patient will receive ~45 mEq of potassium.

General Dosage Range

I.V.:

Children: 0.08-1 mmol phosphate/kg **or** Parenteral nutrition Infusion: 0.5-2 mmol/kg/24 hours
Adults: 0.08-1 mmol phosphate/kg **or** Parenteral nutrition: Infusion: 20-40 mmol/24 hours

Dosage Forms

Injection, solution: Potassium 4.4 mEq and phosphorus 3 mmol per mL (5 mL, 15 mL, 50 mL)

potassium phosphate and sodium phosphate

(poe TASS ee um FOS fate & SOW dee um FOS fate)

Medication Safety Issues

Sound-alike/look-alike issues:

K-Phos® Neutral may be confused with Neutra-Phos-K®

Synonyms Neutra-Phos; sodium phosphate and potassium phosphate

U.S. Brand Names K-Phos® MF; K-Phos® Neutral; K-Phos® No. 2; Phos-NaK; Phospha 250™ Neutral

Therapeutic Category Electrolyte Supplement, Oral

Use Treatment of conditions associated with excessive renal phosphate loss or inadequate GI absorption of phosphate; to acidify the urine to lower calcium concentrations; to increase the antibacterial activity of methenamine; reduce odor and rash caused by ammonia in urine

General Dosage Range Oral: *Children ≥4 years and Adults:* Elemental phosphorus 250 mg 4 times/day after meals and at bedtime

Dosage Forms

Powder for solution, oral:

Phos-NaK: Dibasic potassium phosphate, monobasic potassium phosphate, dibasic sodium phosphate, and monobasic sodium phosphate per packet (100s)

Tablet, oral:

K-Phos® MF: Potassium phosphate 155 mg and sodium phosphate 350 mg

K-Phos® Neutral: Monobasic potassium phosphate 155 mg, dibasic sodium phosphate 852 mg, and monobasic sodium phosphate 130 mg

K-Phos® No. 2: Potassium phosphate 305 mg and sodium phosphate 700 mg

Phospha 250™ Neutral: Monobasic potassium phosphate 155 mg, dibasic sodium phosphate 852 mg, and monobasic sodium phosphate 130 mg

potassium sulfate, magnesium sulfate, and sodium sulfate *see* sodium sulfate, potassium sulfate, and magnesium sulfate *on page 847*

potassium sulfate, sodium sulfate, and magnesium sulfate *see* sodium sulfate, potassium sulfate, and magnesium sulfate *on page 847*

Potiga™ *see* ezogabine *on page 370*

Povidine™ [OTC] *see* povidone-iodine (topical) *on page 747*

povidone-iodine (ophthalmic) (POE vi done EYE oh dyne)

Medication Safety Issues

Sound-alike/look-alike issues:

Betadine® may be confused with Betagan®, betaine

Synonyms polyvinylpyrrolidone with iodine; PVP-I

U.S. Brand Names Betadine®

Therapeutic Category Antiseptic, Ophthalmic

Use Prepping the periocular region (lids, brows, and cheeks) and irrigation of the ocular surface

General Dosage Range Topical: *Adults:* Ophthalmic solution: Eyelids: Apply to area (repeat once); Periocular area: Apply to area (repeat 3 times); Ocular area: Irrigate once

Dosage Forms

Solution, ophthalmic:

Betadine®: 5% (30 mL)

povidone-iodine (topical) (POE vi done EYE oh dyne)

Medication Safety Issues

Sound-alike/look-alike issues:

Betadine® may be confused with Betagan®, betaine

Synonyms polyvinylpyrrolidone with iodine; PVP-I

U.S. Brand Names Betadine® Swab Aids [OTC]; Betadine® [OTC]; Operand® Povidone-Iodine [OTC]; Povidine™ [OTC]; Summer's Eve® Medicated Douche [OTC]; Vagi-Gard® [OTC]

Canadian Brand Names Betadine®; Proviodine

Therapeutic Category Antiseptic, Topical; Antiseptic, Vaginal; Topical Skin Product

Use External antiseptic with broad microbicidal spectrum for the prevention or treatment of topical infections associated with surgery, burns, minor cuts/scrapes; relief of minor vaginal irritation

General Dosage Range

Intravaginal: *Adults:* Insert 0.3% solution vaginally once daily

Topical: *Adults:* Apply to affected area as needed **or** apply to wet skin or hands, scrub for ~5 minutes, then rinse

Dosage Forms

Gel, topical: 10% (120 mL)

Operand® Povidone-Iodine [OTC]: 10% (118 mL)

Liquid, topical: 10% (0.65 mL)

Ointment, topical: 10% (1 g, 30 g)

Povidine™ [OTC]: 10% (30 g)

Pad, topical: 10% (200s)

Betadine® Swab Aids [OTC]: 10% (100s)

Solution, perineal:

Operand® Povidone-Iodine [OTC]: 10% (240 mL)

Solution, topical: 7.5% (60 mL, 120 mL); 10% (22 mL, 30 mL, 59 mL, 60 mL, 90 mL, 120 mL, 237 mL, 240 mL, 473 mL, 480 mL, 3840 mL, 50s)

Betadine® [OTC]: 5% (88.7 mL); 10% (15 mL, 120 mL, 237 mL, 473 mL, 960 mL, 3840 mL); 7.5% (118 mL, 473 mL, 960 mL, 3840 mL)

Operand® Povidone-Iodine [OTC]: 7.5% (59 mL, 118 mL, 237 mL, 473 mL, 946 mL, 3785 mL); 10% (59 mL, 118 mL, 237 mL, 473 mL, 946 mL, 3785 mL)

Povidine™ [OTC]: 10% (240 mL)

Solution, vaginal:

Operand® Povidone-Iodine [OTC]: 10% (240 mL)

Summer's Eve® Medicated Douche [OTC]: 0.3% (135 mL)

Vagi-Gard® [OTC]: 10% (180 mL, 240 mL)

Swabsticks, topical: 7.5% (50s, 75s, 1000s); 10% (50s, 75s, 1000s)

Betadine® [OTC]: 10% (150s, 200s)

PPD *see* tuberculin tests *on page* 925

PPI-0903 *see* ceftaroline fosamil *on page* 185

PPI-0903M *see* ceftaroline fosamil *on page* 185

PPL *see* benzylpenicilloyl polylysine *on page* 127

PPS *see* pentosan polysulfate sodium *on page* 707

PPSV *see* pneumococcal polysaccharide vaccine (polyvalent) *on page* 735

PPSV23 *see* pneumococcal polysaccharide vaccine (polyvalent) *on page* 735

PPV23 *see* pneumococcal polysaccharide vaccine (polyvalent) *on page* 735

PR-171 *see* carfilzomib *on page* 177

Pradax™ (Can) *see* dabigatran etexilate *on page* 250

Pradaxa® *see* dabigatran etexilate *on page* 250

pralatrexate (pral a TREX ate)

Medication Safety Issues

Sound-alike/look-alike issues:

PRALAtrexate may be confused with methotrexate, PEMEtrexed, raltitrexed

Folotyn® may be confused with Focalin®

High alert medication:

This medication is in a class the Institute for Safe Medication Practices (ISMP) includes among its list of drug classes which have a heightened risk of causing significant patient harm when used in error.

Synonyms PDX

Tall-Man **PRALA**trexate

U.S. Brand Names Folotyn®

Therapeutic Category Antineoplastic Agent, Antimetabolite (Antifolate)

Use Treatment of relapsed or refractory peripheral T-cell lymphoma (PTCL)

General Dosage Range Dosage adjustment recommended in patients with renal impairment, hepatic impairment, or who develop toxicities.

I.V.: *Adults:* 30 mg/m^2 once weekly for 6 weeks of a 7-week treatment cycle

Dosage Forms

Injection, solution [preservative free]:

Folotyn®: 20 mg/mL (1 mL, 2 mL)

pralidoxime (pra li DOKS eem)

Medication Safety Issues

Sound-alike/look-alike issues:

Pralidoxime may be confused with pramoxine, pyridoxine

Protopam® may be confused with protamine

Synonyms 2-PAM; 2-pyridine aldoxime methochloride; pralidoxime chloride

U.S. Brand Names Protopam®

Therapeutic Category Antidote

Use Treatment of muscle weakness and/or respiratory depression secondary to poisoning due to organophosphate anticholinesterase pesticides and chemicals (eg, nerve agents); control of overdose of anticholinesterase medications used to treat myasthenia gravis (ambenonium, neostigmine, pyridostigmine)

General Dosage Range Dosage adjustment recommended in patients with renal impairment

I.M.:

Children <40 kg: 15 mg/kg; repeat twice to deliver a total dose of 45 mg/kg

Children ≥40 kg and Adults: 600 mg; repeat twice to deliver a total dose of 1800 mg

I.V.:

Children ≤16 years: Loading dose: 20-50 mg/kg (maximum: 2000 mg/dose); Maintenance infusion: 10-20 mg/kg/hour or repeat bolus of 20-50 mg/kg (maximum: 2000 mg/dose)

Children >16 years and Adults: Loading dose: 1000-2000 mg; Maintenance: Repeat bolus of 1000-2000 mg after 1 hour and every 10-12 hours thereafter, as needed **or** 1000-2000 mg, followed by increments of 250 mg every 5 minutes as needed

Dosage Forms

Injection, powder for reconstitution:

Protopam®: 1 g

Injection, solution: 300 mg/mL (2 mL)

pralidoxime and atropine *see* atropine and pralidoxime *on page 103*

pralidoxime chloride *see* pralidoxime *on page 749*

pramipexole (pra mi PEKS ole)

Medication Safety Issues

Sound-alike/look-alike issues:

Mirapex® may be confused with Hiprex®, Mifeprex®, MiraLax®

Synonyms pramipexole dihydrochloride monohydrate

U.S. Brand Names Mirapex®; Mirapex® ER®

Canadian Brand Names Apo-Pramipexole®; Ava-Pramipexole; CO Pramipexole; Mirapex®; PMS-Pramipexole; Sandoz-Pramipexole; Teva-Pramipexole

Therapeutic Category Anti-Parkinson Agent (Dopamine Agonist)

Use

Immediate release: Treatment of the signs and symptoms of idiopathic Parkinson disease; treatment of moderate-to-severe primary Restless Legs Syndrome (RLS)

Extended release: Treatment of the signs and symptoms of idiopathic Parkinson disease

General Dosage Range Dosage adjustment recommended in patients with renal impairment

Oral: Immediate release: *Adults:* Initial: 0.125 mg 3 times daily **or** 0.125 mg once daily before bedtime; Maintenance: 0.5-1.5 mg 3 times daily **or** 0.125-0.5 mg once daily before bedtime

Oral: Extended release: *Adults:* 0.375-4.5 mg once daily

Dosage Forms

Tablet, oral: 0.125 mg, 0.25 mg, 0.5 mg, 0.75 mg, 1 mg, 1.5 mg

Mirapex®: 0.125 mg, 0.25 mg, 0.5 mg, 0.75 mg, 1 mg, 1.5 mg

Tablet, extended release, oral:

Mirapex® ER®: 0.375 mg, 0.75 mg, 1.5 mg, 2.25 mg, 3 mg, 3.75 mg, 4.5 mg

pramipexole dihydrochloride monohydrate *see* pramipexole *on page 749*

pramlintide (PRAM lin tide)

Medication Safety Issues

High alert medication:

The Institute for Safe Medication Practices (ISMP) includes this medication among its list of drug classes which have a heightened risk of causing significant patient harm when used in error.

Administration issues:

Use caution when drawing up doses from the vial (concentration 600 micrograms (mcg)/mL). Manufacturer recommended dosing ranges from 15 mcg to 120 mcg, which corresponds to injectable volumes of 0.025 mL to 0.2 mL. Patients and healthcare providers should exercise caution when administering this product to avoid inadvertent calculation of the dose based on "units," which could result in a sixfold overdose.

Synonyms pramlintide acetate

U.S. Brand Names SymlinPen®; Symlin® [DSC]

Therapeutic Category Antidiabetic Agent, Oral

Use

Adjunctive treatment with mealtime insulin in type 1 diabetes mellitus (insulin-dependent, IDDM) patients who have failed to achieve desired glucose control despite optimal insulin therapy

Adjunctive treatment with mealtime insulin in type 2 diabetes mellitus (noninsulin-dependent, NIDDM) patients who have failed to achieve desired glucose control despite optimal insulin therapy, with or without concurrent sulfonylurea and/or metformin

General Dosage Range SubQ: *Adults:*

Type 1 diabetes mellitus (insulin-dependent, IDDM): Initial: 15 mcg immediately prior to meals; Target dose: 30-60 mcg prior to meals

Type 2 diabetes mellitus (noninsulin-dependent, NIDDM): Initial: 60 mcg immediately prior to meals; after 3-7 days increase to 120 mcg prior to meals

Dosage Forms

Injection, solution:

SymlinPen®: 1000 mcg/mL (1.5 mL, 2.7 mL)

pramlintide acetate *see* pramlintide *on page 750*

Pramosone® *see* pramoxine and hydrocortisone *on page 751*

Pramosone E™ *see* pramoxine and hydrocortisone *on page 751*

Pramox® HC (Can) *see* pramoxine and hydrocortisone *on page 751*

pramoxine (pra MOKS een)

Medication Safety Issues

Sound-alike/look-alike issues:

Pramoxine may be confused with pralidoxime

Anusol® may be confused with Anusol-HC®, Aplisol®, Aquasol®

Synonyms pramoxine hydrochloride

U.S. Brand Names Caladryl® Clear™ [OTC]; Callergy Clear [OTC]; Curasore® [OTC]; Dermarest® Eczema Medicated Moisturizer [OTC]; Itch-X® [OTC]; Prax® [OTC]; Proctofoam® NS [OTC]; Sarna® Sensitive [OTC]; Soothing Care™ Itch Relief [OTC]; Summer's Eve® Anti-Itch Maximum Strength [OTC]; Tronolane® Cream [OTC]; Tucks® Hemorrhoidal [OTC]

Therapeutic Category Local Anesthetic

Use Temporary relief of pain and itching associated with hemorrhoids, burns, minor cuts, scrapes, or minor skin irritations

General Dosage Range Topical:

Children ≥2 years and Adults: Lotion, cream: Apply up to 3-4 times daily

Children ≥12 years and Adults: Hemorrhoidal foam, ointment, wipes: Apply up to 5 times daily

Dosage Forms

Aerosol, foam, topical:

Proctofoam® NS [OTC]: 1% (15 g)

Cream, topical:

Dermarest® Eczema Medicated Moisturizer [OTC]: 1% (56.6 g)

Tronolane® Cream [OTC]: 1% (30 g, 57 g)

Gel, topical:

Itch-X® [OTC]: 1% (35.4 g)

Summer's Eve® Anti-Itch Maximum Strength [OTC]: 1% (30 mL)

Liquid, topical:
Curasore® [OTC]: 1% (15 mL)
Lotion, topical:
Caladryl® Clear™ [OTC]: 1% (177 mL)
Callergy Clear [OTC]: 1% (177 mL)
Prax® [OTC]: 1% (15 mL, 120 mL, 240 mL)
Sarna® Sensitive [OTC]: 1% (222 mL)
Ointment, rectal:
Tucks® Hemorrhoidal [OTC]: 1% (28.3 g)
Solution, topical:
Itch-X® [OTC]: 1% (60 mL)
Soothing Care™ Itch Relief [OTC]: 1% (74 mL)
Wipe, topical:
Prax® [OTC]: 1% (12s)

pramoxine and hydrocortisone (pra MOKS een & hye droe KOR ti sone)

Medication Safety Issues
Sound-alike/look-alike issues:
Pramosone® may be confused with predniSONE

Synonyms hydrocortisone and pramoxine; pramoxine hydrochloride and hydrocortisone acetate

U.S. Brand Names Analpram E™; Analpram HC®; Epifoam®; Pramosone E™; Pramosone®; ProCort®; ProctoFoam® HC; Zypram™

Canadian Brand Names Pramox® HC; Proctofoam™-HC

Therapeutic Category Anesthetic/Corticosteroid

Use Relief of inflammatory and pruritic manifestations of corticosteroid-responsive dermatoses

General Dosage Range Rectal, topical: *Adults:* Apply to affected areas 3-4 times/day

Dosage Forms
Aerosol, foam, rectal:
ProctoFoam® HC: Pramoxine 1% and hydrocortisone 1% (10 g)
Aerosol, foam, topical:
Epifoam®: Pramoxine 1% and hydrocortisone 1% (10 g)
Cream, topical: Pramoxine 1% and hydrocortisone 1% (30 g); pramoxine 1% and hydrocortisone 2.5% (4 g, 30 g)
Analpram Advanced™ Kit: Pramoxine 1% and hydrocortisone 2.5% (1s) [kit includes Analpram HC® cream (4 g x 30), diosmiplex (Vasculera™) tablets, AloeClean™ wipes, and applicators]
Analpram Advanced™ Kit: Pramoxine 1% and hydrocortisone 2.5% (1s) [kit includes Analpram HC® cream (30 g), diosmiplex (Vasculera™) tablets, AloeClean™ wipes, and applicator]
Analpram E™: Pramoxine 1% and hydrocortisone 2.5% (4 g, 30 g)
Analpram HC®: Pramoxine 1% and hydrocortisone 1% (4 g, 30 g); pramoxine 1% and hydrocortisone 2.5% (4 g, 30 g)
Pramosone®: Pramoxine 1% and hydrocortisone 1% (30 g, 60 g); pramoxine 1% and hydrocortisone 2.5% (30 g, 60 g)
Pramosone E™: Pramoxine 1% and hydrocortisone 2.5% (30 g, 60 g)
ProCort®: Pramoxine 1.15% and hydrocortisone 1.85% (60 g)
Zypram™: Pramoxine 1% and hydrocortisone 2.35% (30 g)
Lotion, topical:
Analpram HC®: Pramoxine 1% and hydrocortisone 2.5% (60 mL)
Pramosone®: Pramoxine 1% and hydrocortisone 1% (60 mL, 120 mL, 240 mL); pramoxine 1% and hydrocortisone 2.5% (60 mL, 120 mL)
Ointment, topical:
Pramosone®: Pramoxine 1% and hydrocortisone 1% (30 g); pramoxine 1% and hydrocortisone 2.5% (30 g)

pramoxine hydrochloride *see* pramoxine *on page* *750*

pramoxine hydrochloride and hydrocortisone acetate *see* pramoxine and hydrocortisone *on page* *751*

pramoxine, neomycin, bacitracin, and polymyxin B *see* bacitracin, neomycin, polymyxin B, and pramoxine *on page* *112*

PrandiMet® *see* repaglinide and metformin *on page* *794*

Prandin® *see* repaglinide *on page* *794*

Prascion® *see* sulfur and sulfacetamide *on page* *862*

Prascion® FC *see* sulfur and sulfacetamide *on page 862*
Prascion® RA *see* sulfur and sulfacetamide *on page 862*

prasugrel (PRA soo grel)

Medication Safety Issues

Sound-alike/look-alike issues:

Prasugrel may be confused with pravastatin, propranolol

BEERS Criteria medication:

This drug may be potentially inappropriate for use in geriatric patients (Quality of evidence - moderate; Strength of recommendation - weak).

Synonyms CS-747; LY-640315; prasugrel hydrochloride

U.S. Brand Names Effient®

Canadian Brand Names Effient®

Therapeutic Category Antiplatelet Agent

Use Reduces rate of thrombotic cardiovascular events (eg, stent thrombosis) in patients who are to be managed with percutaneous coronary intervention (PCI) for unstable angina (UA), non-ST-segment elevation MI (NSTEMI), or ST-elevation MI (STEMI)

General Dosage Range Oral: *Adults:* Loading dose: 60 mg; Maintenance dose: 10 mg once daily (in combination with aspirin 81-325 mg/day)

Dosage Forms

Tablet, oral:

Effient®: 5 mg, 10 mg

prasugrel hydrochloride *see* prasugrel *on page 752*
Pravachol® *see* pravastatin *on page 752*

pravastatin (prav a STAT in)

Medication Safety Issues

Sound-alike/look-alike issues:

Pravachol® may be confused with atorvaSTATin, Prevacid®, Prinivil®, propranolol
Pravastatin may be confused with nystatin, pitavastatin, prasugrel

Synonyms pravastatin sodium

U.S. Brand Names Pravachol®

Canadian Brand Names Apo-Pravastatin®; CO Pravastatin; Dom-Pravastatin; JAMP-Pravastatin; Mint-Pravastatin; Mylan-Pravastatin; Novo-Pravastatin; Nu-Pravastatin; PHL-Pravastatin; PMS-Pravastatin; Pravachol®; RAN™-Pravastatin; ratio-Pravastatin; Riva-Pravastatin; Sandoz-Pravastatin; Teva-Pravastatin; ZYM-Pravastatin

Therapeutic Category HMG-CoA Reductase Inhibitor

Use Use with dietary therapy for the following:

Primary prevention of coronary events: In hypercholesterolemic patients without established coronary heart disease to reduce cardiovascular morbidity (myocardial infarction, coronary revascularization procedures) and mortality.

Secondary prevention of cardiovascular events in patients with established coronary heart disease: To slow the progression of coronary atherosclerosis; to reduce cardiovascular morbidity (myocardial infarction, coronary vascular procedures) and to reduce mortality; to reduce the risk of stroke and transient ischemic attacks

Hyperlipidemias: Reduce elevations in total cholesterol, LDL-C, apolipoprotein B, and triglycerides (elevations of 1 or more components are present in Fredrickson type IIa, IIb, III, and IV hyperlipidemias)

Heterozygous familial hypercholesterolemia (HeFH): In pediatric patients, 8-18 years of age, with HeFH having LDL-C ≥190 mg/dL **or** LDL ≥160 mg/dL with positive family history of premature cardiovascular disease (CVD) or 2 or more CVD risk factors in the pediatric patient

General Dosage Range Dosage adjustment recommended in patients with hepatic or renal impairment or on concomitant therapy

Oral:

Children 8-13 years: 20 mg once daily
Children 14-18 years: 40 mg once daily
Adults: Initial: 10-40 mg once daily; Maintenance: 10-80 mg once daily (maximum: 80 mg/day)

Dosage Forms

Tablet, oral: 10 mg, 20 mg, 40 mg, 80 mg

Pravachol®: 10 mg, 20 mg, 40 mg, 80 mg

pravastatin sodium *see* pravastatin *on page* 752
Prax® [OTC] *see* pramoxine *on page* 750
Praxis ASA EC 81 Mg Daily Dose (Can) *see* aspirin *on page* 96

praziquantel (pray zi KWON tel)

U.S. Brand Names Biltricide®
Canadian Brand Names Biltricide®
Therapeutic Category Anthelmintic
Use Treatment of all stages of schistosomiasis caused by all *Schistosoma* species; treatment of infection (clonorchiasis and opisthorchiasis) due to liver flukes
General Dosage Range Oral: *Children ≥4 years and Adults:* 20 mg/kg/dose 2-3 times/day for 1 day at 4- to 6-hour intervals **or** 25 mg/kg 3 times/day for 1 day
Dosage Forms
Tablet, oral:
Biltricide®: 600 mg

prazosin (PRAZ oh sin)

Medication Safety Issues
Sound-alike/look-alike issues:
Prazosin may be confused with predniSONE
BEERS Criteria medication:
This drug may be potentially inappropriate for use in geriatric patients (Quality of evidence - moderate; Strength of recommendation - strong).
Synonyms furazosin; prazosin hydrochloride
U.S. Brand Names Minipress®
Canadian Brand Names Apo-Prazo®; Minipress®; Novo-Prazin; Nu-Prazo; Teva-Prazosin
Therapeutic Category Alpha-Adrenergic Blocking Agent
Use Treatment of hypertension
General Dosage Range Oral: *Adults:* Initial: 1 mg/dose 2-3 times/day; Maintenance: 2-20 mg/day in divided doses 2-3 times/day (maximum: 20 mg/day) (JNC 7)
Dosage Forms
Capsule, oral: 1 mg, 2 mg, 5 mg
Minipress®: 1 mg, 2 mg, 5 mg

prazosin hydrochloride *see* prazosin *on page* 753
PR™ Cream *see* emollients *on page* 328
PreCare® *see* vitamins (multiple/prenatal) *on page* 952
Precedex® *see* dexmedetomidine *on page* 268
Precise® [OTC] *see* methyl salicylate and menthol *on page* 592
Precose® *see* acarbose *on page* 19
Pred Forte® *see* prednisolone (ophthalmic) *on page* 754
Pred-G® *see* prednisolone and gentamicin *on page* 755
Pred Mild® *see* prednisolone (ophthalmic) *on page* 754

prednicarbate (pred ni KAR bate)

Medication Safety Issues
Sound-alike/look-alike issues:
Dermatop® may be confused with Dimetapp®
U.S. Brand Names Dermatop®
Canadian Brand Names Dermatop®
Therapeutic Category Corticosteroid, Topical
Use Relief of the inflammatory and pruritic manifestations of corticosteroid-responsive dermatoses (medium-potency topical corticosteroid)
General Dosage Range Topical:
Children ≥1 year and Adults: Cream: Apply a thin film to affected area twice daily
Children ≥10 year and Adults: Ointment: Apply a thin film to affected area twice daily

Dosage Forms
Cream, topical: 0.1% (15 g, 60 g)
Dermatop®: 0.1% (60 g)
Ointment, topical: 0.1% (15 g, 60 g)
Dermatop®: 0.1% (60 g)

prednisolone (systemic) (pred NISS oh lone)

Medication Safety Issues
Sound-alike/look-alike issues:
PrednisoLONE may be confused with predniSONE
Pediapred® may be confused with Pediazole®
Prelone® may be confused with PROzac®

Synonyms prednisolone sodium phosphate

Tall-Man predniso**LONE**

U.S. Brand Names Flo-Pred™; Millipred™; Millipred™ DP; Orapred ODT®; Orapred®; Pediapred®; Veripred™ 20

Canadian Brand Names Hydeltra T.B.A.®; Novo-Prednisolone; Pediapred®

Therapeutic Category Corticosteroid, Systemic

Use Treatment of endocrine disorders, rheumatic disorders, collagen diseases, allergic states, respiratory diseases, hematologic disorders, neoplastic diseases, edematous states, and gastrointestinal diseases; resolution of acute exacerbations of multiple sclerosis; management of fulminating or disseminated tuberculosis and trichinosis; acute or chronic solid organ rejection

General Dosage Range Oral:
Children: Dosage varies greatly depending on indication
Adults: 5-60 mg/day **or** 200 mg/day for 1 week followed by 80 mg every other day for 1 month

Dosage Forms
Solution, oral: 5 mg/5 mL (5 mL, 10 mL, 20 mL, 118 mL, 120 mL); 15 mg/5 mL (237 mL, 240 mL, 473 mL, 480 mL)
Millipred™: 10 mg/5 mL (237 mL)
Orapred®: 15 mg/5 mL (20 mL, 237 mL)
Pediapred®: 5 mg/5 mL (120 mL)
Veripred™ 20: 20 mg/5 mL (237 mL)
Suspension, oral:
Flo-Pred™: 15 mg/5 mL (52 mL)
Tablet, oral:
Millipred™: 5 mg
Millipred™ DP: 5 mg
Tablet, orally disintegrating, oral:
Orapred ODT®: 10 mg, 15 mg, 30 mg

prednisolone (ophthalmic) (pred NISS oh lone)

Medication Safety Issues
Sound-alike/look-alike issues:
PrednisoLONE may be confused with predniSONE

Synonyms Econopred; prednisolone acetate, ophthalmic; prednisolone sodium phosphate, ophthalmic

Tall-Man predniso**LONE**

U.S. Brand Names Omnipred™; Pred Forte®; Pred Mild®

Canadian Brand Names Diopred®; Ophtho-Tate®; Pred Forte®; Pred Mild®

Therapeutic Category Corticosteroid, Ophthalmic

Use Treatment of palpebral and bulbar conjunctivitis; corneal injury from chemical, radiation, thermal burns, or foreign body penetration; steroid-responsive inflammatory ophthalmic diseases

General Dosage Range Ophthalmic: *Children and Adults:* Initial: Instill 1-2 drops into conjunctival sac every hour during day, every 2 hours at night; Maintenance: 1 drop every 4 hours

Dosage Forms
Solution, ophthalmic: 1% (5 mL, 10 mL, 15 mL)
Suspension, ophthalmic: 1% (5 mL, 10 mL, 15 mL)
Omnipred™: 1% (5 mL, 10 mL)
Pred Forte®: 1% (1 mL, 5 mL, 10 mL, 15 mL)
Pred Mild®: 0.12% (5 mL, 10 mL)

prednisolone acetate, ophthalmic *see* prednisolone (ophthalmic) *on page 754*

prednisolone and gentamicin (pred NIS oh lone & jen ta MYE sin)

Synonyms gentamicin and prednisolone

U.S. Brand Names Pred-G®

Therapeutic Category Antibiotic/Corticosteroid, Ophthalmic

Use Treatment of steroid responsive inflammatory conditions where either a superficial bacterial ocular infection or the risk of bacterial ocular infection exists

General Dosage Range Ophthalmic: *Adults:*

Ointment: Apply 1/2" ribbon into the conjunctival sac of the affected eye(s) 1-3 times/day

Suspension: Initial: Instill 1 drop into the conjunctival sac of the affected eye(s) every hour for 1-2 days; Maintenance: 1 drop 2-4 times/day

Dosage Forms

Ointment, ophthalmic:

Pred-G®: Prednisolone 0.6% and gentamicin 0.3% (3.5 g)

Suspension, ophthalmic:

Pred-G®: Prednisolone 1% and gentamicin 0.3% (5 mL)

prednisolone and sulfacetamide *see* sulfacetamide and prednisolone *on page 859*

prednisolone sodium phosphate *see* prednisolone (systemic) *on page 754*

prednisolone sodium phosphate, ophthalmic *see* prednisolone (ophthalmic) *on page 754*

prednisone (PRED ni sone)

Medication Safety Issues

Sound-alike/look-alike issues:

PredniSONE may be confused with methylPREDNISolone, Pramosone®, prazosin, prednisoLONE, PriLOSEC®, primidone, promethazine

Synonyms deltacortisone; deltadehydrocortisone; Rayos®

Tall-Man predni**SONE**

U.S. Brand Names PredniSONE Intensol™

Canadian Brand Names Apo-Prednisone®; Novo-Prednisone; Winpred™

Therapeutic Category Adrenal Corticosteroid

Use Treatment of a variety of diseases, including:

Allergic states (including adjunctive treatment of anaphylaxis)
Autoimmune disorders (including systemic lupus erythematosus [SLE])
Collagen diseases
Dermatologic conditions/diseases
Edematous states (including nephrotic syndrome)
Endocrine disorders
Gastrointestinal diseases
Hematologic disorders (including idiopathic thrombocytopenia purpura [ITP])
Multiple sclerosis exacerbations
Neoplastic diseases
Ophthalmic diseases
Respiratory diseases (including acute asthma exacerbation)
Rheumatic disorders (including rheumatoid arthritis)
Trichinosis with neurologic or myocardial involvement
Tuberculous meningitis

General Dosage Range Oral: *Children:* Initial: 5-60 mg/day

Product Availability Rayos® (prednisone delayed-release tablets): FDA approved July 2012; availability anticipated September 2012. Please consult prescribing information for additional information.

Dosage Forms

Solution, oral: 1 mg/mL (5 mL, 120 mL, 500 mL)

PredniSONE Intensol™: 5 mg/mL (30 mL)

Tablet, oral: 1 mg, 2.5 mg, 5 mg, 10 mg, 20 mg, 50 mg

PredniSONE Intensol™ *see* prednisone *on page 755*

PreferaOB® *see* vitamins (multiple/prenatal) *on page 952*

PreferaOB® + DHA *see* vitamins (multiple/prenatal) *on page 952*

PreferaOB® One™ *see* vitamins (multiple/prenatal) *on page 952*

Prefest™ *see* estradiol and norgestimate *on page* 350

pregabalin (pre GAB a lin)

Medication Safety Issues

Sound-alike/look-alike issues:

Lyrica® may be confused with Lopressor®

Other safety concerns:

Pregabalin (Lyrica®) oral solution (20 mg/mL): Prescriptions should be written in terms of mg. The pharmacist will calculate the appropriate dose in mL for dispensing.

Synonyms CI-1008; S-(+)-3-isobutylgaba

U.S. Brand Names Lyrica®

Canadian Brand Names Lyrica®

Therapeutic Category Analgesic, Miscellaneous; Anticonvulsant, Miscellaneous

Controlled Substance C-V

Use Management of neuropathic pain associated with diabetic peripheral neuropathy or with spinal cord injury; management of postherpetic neuralgia; adjunctive therapy for partial-onset seizure disorder; management of fibromyalgia

General Dosage Range Dosage adjustment recommended in patients with renal impairment

Oral: *Adults:* Initial: 150 mg daily in 2-3 divided doses; Maintenance: 150-600 mg daily in 2-3 divided doses (maximum: 600 mg daily)

Dosage Forms

Capsule, oral:

Lyrica®: 25 mg, 50 mg, 75 mg, 100 mg, 150 mg, 200 mg, 225 mg, 300 mg

Solution, oral:

Lyrica®: 20 mg/mL (473 mL)

pregnenedione *see* progesterone *on page* 762

Pregnyl® *see* chorionic gonadotropin (human) *on page* 206

Premarin® *see* estrogens (conjugated/equine, systemic) *on page* 351

Premarin® *see* estrogens (conjugated/equine, topical) *on page* 352

PremaSol™ *see* amino acid injection *on page* 61

Premium Activated Charcoal [OTC] (Can) *see* charcoal, activated *on page* 193

Premjact® *see* lidocaine (topical) *on page* 535

Premphase® *see* estrogens (conjugated/equine) and medroxyprogesterone *on page* 352

Premplus® (Can) *see* estrogens (conjugated/equine) and medroxyprogesterone *on page* 352

Prempro® *see* estrogens (conjugated/equine) and medroxyprogesterone *on page* 352

Prenatabs FA *see* vitamins (multiple/prenatal) *on page* 952

Prenatal One Daily [OTC] *see* vitamins (multiple/prenatal) *on page* 952

Prenatal Rx 1 *see* vitamins (multiple/prenatal) *on page* 952

prenatal vitamins *see* vitamins (multiple/prenatal) *on page* 952

Prenatal With Beta Carotene [OTC] *see* vitamins (multiple/prenatal) *on page* 952

Prenate DHA™ *see* vitamins (multiple/prenatal) *on page* 952

Prenate Elite® *see* vitamins (multiple/prenatal) *on page* 952

Prenate Essential™ *see* vitamins (multiple/prenatal) *on page* 952

PreNexa® Premier *see* vitamins (multiple/prenatal) *on page* 952

Preparation H® [OTC] *see* phenylephrine (topical) *on page* 717

Preparation H® Cleansing Pads (Can) *see* witch hazel *on page* 956

Preparation H® Hydrocortisone [OTC] *see* hydrocortisone (topical) *on page* 457

Preparation H® Medicated Wipes [OTC] *see* witch hazel *on page* 956

Pre-Pen® *see* benzylpenicilloyl polylysine *on page* 127

Prepidil® *see* dinoprostone *on page* 291

Prepopik™ *see* sodium picosulfate, magnesium oxide, and citric acid *on page* 846

PreserVision® AREDS [OTC] *see* vitamins (multiple/oral) *on page* 951

PreserVision® Lutein [OTC] *see* vitamins (multiple/oral) *on page* 951

Pressyn® (Can) *see* vasopressin *on page* 940

Pressyn® AR (Can) *see* vasopressin *on page* 940

Pretz® [OTC] *see* sodium chloride *on page 840*
Prevacare® [OTC] *see* alcohol (ethyl) *on page 43*
Prevacid® *see* lansoprazole *on page 522*
Prevacid® 24 HR [OTC] *see* lansoprazole *on page 522*
Prevacid® FasTab (Can) *see* lansoprazole *on page 522*
Prevacid® SoluTab™ *see* lansoprazole *on page 522*
Prevalite® *see* cholestyramine resin *on page 205*
Prevex® B (Can) *see* betamethasone *on page 129*
Prevex® HC (Can) *see* hydrocortisone (topical) *on page 457*
PreviDent® *see* fluoride *on page 393*
PreviDent® 5000 Booster *see* fluoride *on page 393*
PreviDent® 5000 Dry Mouth *see* fluoride *on page 393*
PreviDent® 5000 Plus® *see* fluoride *on page 393*
PreviDent® 5000 Sensitive *see* fluoride *on page 393*
Previfem® *see* ethinyl estradiol and norgestimate *on page 361*
Prevnar 13® *see* pneumococcal conjugate vaccine (13-valent) *on page 734*
Prevpac® *see* lansoprazole, amoxicillin, and clarithromycin *on page 523*
Prezista® *see* darunavir *on page 255*
Prialt® *see* ziconotide *on page 961*
Priftin® *see* rifapentine *on page 800*

prilocaine (PRIL oh kane)

Medication Safety Issues

Sound-alike/look-alike issues:

Prilocaine may be confused with Polocaine®, PriLOSEC®

U.S. Brand Names Citanest® Plain Dental

Canadian Brand Names Citanest® Plain

Therapeutic Category Local Anesthetic

Use Amide-type anesthetic used for local infiltration anesthesia; injection near nerve trunks to produce nerve block

General Dosage Range Dental (infiltration or conduction block):

Children <10 years: Doses >40 mg (1 mL) as a 4% solution per procedure rarely needed

Children ≥10 years and Adults: Initial: 40-80 mg (1-2 mL) as a 4% solution, up to a maximum of 400 mg (10 mL) as a 4% solution within a 2-hour period (maximum: 600 mg/dose [per manufacturer])

Dosage Forms

Injection, solution:

Citanest® Plain Dental: 4% [40 mg/mL] (1.8 mL)

prilocaine and lidocaine *see* lidocaine and prilocaine *on page 538*
PriLOSEC® *see* omeprazole *on page 665*
PriLOSEC OTC® [OTC] *see* omeprazole *on page 665*
PrimaCare® One *see* vitamins (multiple/prenatal) *on page 952*
primaclone *see* primidone *on page 758*
Primacor® (Can) *see* milrinone *on page 603*

primaquine (PRIM a kween)

Medication Safety Issues

Sound-alike/look-alike issues:

Primaquine may be confused with primidone

Synonyms primaquine phosphate; prymaccone

Therapeutic Category Aminoquinoline (Antimalarial)

Use Prevention of relapse of *P. vivax* malaria

General Dosage Range Oral:

Children: 0.5 mg/kg once daily for 14 days (maximum dose: 30 mg/day)

Adults: 30 mg once daily for 14 days; Alternative regimen (recommended for mild G6PD deficiency): 45 mg once weekly for 8 weeks

Dosage Forms
Tablet, oral: 26.3 mg

primaquine phosphate *see* primaquine *on page* 757
Primatene® Mist [OTC] [DSC] *see* epinephrine (systemic, oral inhalation) *on page* 334
Primaxin® I.M. [DSC] *see* imipenem and cilastatin *on page* 475
Primaxin® I.V. *see* imipenem and cilastatin *on page* 475
Primaxin® I.V. Infusion (Can) *see* imipenem and cilastatin *on page* 475
Primene® (Can) *see* amino acid injection *on page* 61

primidone (PRI mi done)

Medication Safety Issues
Sound-alike/look-alike issues:
Primidone may be confused with predniSONE, primaquine, pyridoxine
Synonyms desoxyphenobarbital; primaclone
U.S. Brand Names Mysoline®
Canadian Brand Names Apo-Primidone®
Therapeutic Category Anticonvulsant; Barbiturate
Use Management of grand mal, psychomotor, and focal seizures
General Dosage Range Dosage adjustment recommended in patients with renal impairment
Oral:
Children <8 years: Initial: 50 mg once daily at bedtime; Maintenance: 375-750 mg/day (10-25 mg/kg/day) in 3-4 divided doses
Children ≥8 years and Adults: Initial: 100-125 mg/day at bedtime; Maintenance: 750-1500 mg/day in 3-4 divided doses (maximum: 2 g/day)
Dosage Forms
Tablet, oral: 50 mg, 250 mg
Mysoline®: 50 mg, 250 mg
Dosage Forms - Canada
Tablet:
Apo-Primidone®: 125 mg, 250 mg

Primlev™ *see* oxycodone and acetaminophen *on page* 679
Primovist (Can) *see* gadoxetate *on page* 417
Primsol® *see* trimethoprim *on page* 920
Prinivil® *see* lisinopril *on page* 544
Prinzide® *see* lisinopril and hydrochlorothiazide *on page* 544
Priorix™ (Can) *see* measles, mumps, and rubella virus vaccine *on page* 564
Priorix-Tetra™ (Can) *see* measles, mumps, rubella, and varicella virus vaccine *on page* 564
PrismaSol *see* electrolyte solution, renal replacement *on page* 325
Pristiq® *see* desvenlafaxine *on page* 266
Privigen® *see* immune globulin *on page* 477
Privine® [OTC] *see* naphazoline (nasal) *on page* 626
ProAir® HFA *see* albuterol *on page* 41
ProAmatine *see* midodrine *on page* 601
PRO-Amiodarone (Can) *see* amiodarone *on page* 63
Pro-Amox-250 (Can) *see* amoxicillin *on page* 69
Pro-Amox-500 (Can) *see* amoxicillin *on page* 69
PRO-Azithromycin (Can) *see* azithromycin (systemic) *on page* 108

probenecid (proe BEN e sid)

Medication Safety Issues
Sound-alike/look-alike issues:
Probenecid may be confused with Procanbid
Synonyms Benemid [DSC]
Canadian Brand Names Benuryl™
Therapeutic Category Uricosuric Agent

Use Treatment of hyperuricemia associated with gout or gouty arthritis; prolongation and elevation of beta-lactam plasma levels (eg, uncomplicated gonococcal infection)

General Dosage Range Avoid use if Cl_{cr} <30 mL/minute.

Oral:

Children 2-14 years: Prolong penicillin serum levels: Initial: 25 mg/kg then 40 mg/kg/day given 4 times/day (maximum: 500 mg/dose)

Children >50 kg and Adults:

Gonorrhea, PID: 1 g as a single dose

Gout: Initial: 250 mg twice daily (maximum: 2 g/day)

Neurosyphilis: 500 mg 4 times/day for 10-14 days

Prolong PCN levels: 500 mg 4 times/day

Dosage Forms

Tablet, oral: 500 mg

probenecid and colchicine *see* colchicine and probenecid *on page 232*

PRO-Bicalutamide (Can) *see* bicalutamide *on page 133*

PRO-Bisoprolol (Can) *see* bisoprolol *on page 136*

procainamide (pro KANE a mide)

Medication Safety Issues

Sound-alike/look-alike issues:

Procanbid may be confused with probenecid, Procan SR®

Pronestyl may be confused with Ponstel®

High alert medication:

The Institute for Safe Medication Practices (ISMP) includes this medication among its list of drugs which have a heightened risk of causing significant patient harm when used in error.

BEERS Criteria medication:

This drug may be potentially inappropriate for use in geriatric patients (Quality of evidence - high; Strength of recommendation - strong).

Administration issues:

Procainamide hydrochloride is available in 10 mL vials of 100 mg/mL and in 2 mL vials with 500 mg/mL. Note that **BOTH** vials contain 1 gram of drug; confusing the strengths can lead to massive overdoses or underdoses.

Other safety concerns:

PCA is an error-prone abbreviation (mistaken as patient controlled analgesia)

Synonyms PCA (error-prone abbreviation); procainamide hydrochloride; procaine amide hydrochloride; Procanbid; Pronestyl

Canadian Brand Names Apo-Procainamide®; Procainamide Hydrochloride Injection, USP; Procan SR®

Therapeutic Category Antiarrhythmic Agent, Class I-A

Use

Intravenous: Treatment of life-threatening ventricular arrhythmias

Oral (Canadian labeling; not available in U.S.): Treatment of supraventricular arrhythmias. **Note:** In the treatment of atrial fibrillation, use only when preferred treatment is ineffective or cannot be used. Use in paroxysmal atrial tachycardia when reflex stimulation or other measures are ineffective.

General Dosage Range Dosage adjustment recommended in patients with hepatic or renal impairment

I.M.:

Children: 20-30 mg/kg/day divided every 4-6 hours (maximum: 4 g/day)

Adults: 50 mg/kg/day divided every 3-6 hours **or** 0.5-1 g every 4-8 hours

I.V.:

Children: Loading dose: 3-6 mg/kg/dose over 5 minutes (maximum: 100 mg/dose), may repeat every 5-10 minutes to maximum of 15 mg/kg/load; Infusion: 20-80 mcg/kg/minute (maximum: 2 g/day)

Adults: Loading dose: 15-18 mg/kg administered as slow infusion over 25-30 minutes **or** 100 mg/dose at a rate not to exceed 50 mg/minute repeated every 5 minutes as needed (maximum total dose: 1 g); Infusion: 1-4 mg/minute

Dosage Forms

Injection, solution: 100 mg/mL (10 mL); 500 mg/mL (2 mL)

Dosage Forms - Canada

Tablet, sustained release, oral:

Procan SR®: 250 mg, 500 mg, 750 mg

procainamide hydrochloride *see* procainamide *on page 759*

procarbazine (proe KAR ba zeen)

Medication Safety Issues

Sound-alike/look-alike issues:

Procarbazine may be confused with dacarbazine

High alert medication:

The Institute for Safe Medication Practices (ISMP) includes this medication among its list of drugs which have a heightened risk of causing significant patient harm when used in error.

Synonyms benzmethyzin; N-methylhydrazine; procarbazine hydrochloride

U.S. Brand Names Matulane®

Canadian Brand Names Matulane®; Natulan®

Therapeutic Category Antineoplastic Agent

Use Treatment of Hodgkin disease

General Dosage Range Dosage adjustment recommended in patients with hepatic impairment

Oral:

Children: 100 mg/m^2/day for 14 days and repeated every 4 weeks

Adults: Initial: 2-4 mg/kg/day in single or divided doses for 7 days, then increase dose to 4-6 mg/kg/day; Maintenance: 1-2 mg/kg/day

Dosage Forms

Capsule, oral:

Matulane®: 50 mg

prochlorperazine (proe klor PER a zeen)

Medication Safety Issues

Sound-alike/look-alike issues:

Prochlorperazine may be confused with chlorproMAZINE

Compazine may be confused with Copaxone®, Coumadin®

BEERS Criteria medication:

This drug may be potentially inappropriate for use in geriatric patients (Quality of evidence - varies based on comorbidity; Strength of recommendation - varies based on comorbidity)

Other safety concerns:

CPZ (occasional abbreviation for Compazine) is an error-prone abbreviation (mistaken as chlorpromazine)

Synonyms chlormeprazine; Compazine; prochlorperazine edisylate; prochlorperazine maleate; prochlorperazine mesylate

U.S. Brand Names Compro®

Canadian Brand Names Apo-Prochlorperazine®; Nu-Prochlor; PMS-Prochlorperazine; Sandoz-Prochlorperazine

Therapeutic Category Phenothiazine Derivative

Use Management of nausea and vomiting; psychotic disorders, including schizophrenia and anxiety; nonpsychotic anxiety

General Dosage Range

I.M. (as edisylate):

Children ≥2 years and ≥9 kg: 0.13 mg/kg/dose; change to oral as soon as possible

Adults:

Antiemetic: 5-10 mg every 3-4 hours **or** 5-10 mg as a single dose with surgery, may repeat (maximum: 40 mg/day)

Antipsychotic: Initial: 10-20 mg every 2-4 hours to gain control (more than 3-4 doses are rarely needed); Maintenance: 10-20 mg every 4-6 hours

I.V. (as edisylate): *Adults:* 2.5-10 mg every 3-4 hours as needed (maximum: 40 mg/day) **or** 5-10 mg as a single dose with surgery, may repeat

Oral, rectal:

Children ≥2 years and ≥9 kg: Antiemetic:

9-13 kg: 2.5 mg 1-2 times/day as needed (maximum: 7.5 mg/day)

>13-18 kg: 2.5 mg 2-3 times/day as needed (maximum: 10 mg/day)

>18-39 kg: 2.5 mg 3 times/day or 5 mg 2 times/day as needed (maximum: 15 mg/day)

Children 2-12 years: Antipsychotic: Initial: 2.5 mg 2-3 times/day; Maintenance: Increase as needed to maximum of 20 mg/day for 2-5 years and 25 mg/day for 6-12 years

Adults:

Antiemetic: 5-10 mg 3-4 times/day (maximum: 40 mg/day)

Antipsychotic: Initial: 5-10 mg 3-4 times/day; Maintenance: Up to 150 mg/day

Nonpsychotic anxiety: 15-20 mg/day in divided doses; do not give doses >20 mg/day or for longer than 12 weeks

Dosage Forms

Injection, solution: 5 mg/mL (2 mL, 10 mL)

Suppository, rectal: 25 mg (12s)

Compro®: 25 mg (12s)

Tablet, oral: 5 mg, 10 mg

Dosage Forms - Canada

Injection, solution 5 mg/mL (2 mL)

Suppository, rectal: 10 mg (10s)

prochlorperazine edisylate *see* prochlorperazine *on page* *760*
prochlorperazine maleate *see* prochlorperazine *on page* *760*
prochlorperazine mesylate *see* prochlorperazine *on page* *760*
PRO-Ciprofloxacin (Can) *see* ciprofloxacin (systemic) *on page* *210*
PRO-Clonazepam (Can) *see* clonazepam *on page* *223*
ProCort® *see* pramoxine and hydrocortisone *on page* *751*
Procrit® *see* epoetin alfa *on page* *337*
Proctocort® *see* hydrocortisone (topical) *on page* *457*
ProctoCream®-HC *see* hydrocortisone (topical) *on page* *457*
proctofene *see* fenofibrate *on page* *375*
ProctoFoam® HC *see* pramoxine and hydrocortisone *on page* *751*
Proctofoam™-HC (Can) *see* pramoxine and hydrocortisone *on page* *751*
Proctofoam® NS [OTC] *see* pramoxine *on page* *750*
Procto-Pak™ *see* hydrocortisone (topical) *on page* *457*
Proctosol-HC® *see* hydrocortisone (topical) *on page* *457*
Proctozone-HC 2.5%™ *see* hydrocortisone (topical) *on page* *457*

procyclidine *(Canada only)* (proe SYE kli deen)

Synonyms procyclidine hydrochloride

Canadian Brand Names PHL-Procyclidine; PMS-Procyclidine

Therapeutic Category Anti-Parkinson Agent; Anticholinergic Agent

Use Relieves symptoms of parkinsonian syndrome and drug-induced extrapyramidal symptoms

General Dosage Range Oral:

Adults: Initial: 2.5 mg 3 times/day; Maintenance: Up to 30 mg/day in 3-4 divided doses

Elderly: Initial: 2.5 mg 1-2 times/day

Product Availability Not available in U.S.

Dosage Forms - Canada

Tablet, oral: 2.5 mg, 5 mg

Elixir, oral: 2.5 mg/5 mL

procyclidine hydrochloride *see* procyclidine *(Canada only) on page* 761
Procytox® (Can) *see* cyclophosphamide *on page* 244
PRO-Dexamethasone (Can) *see* dexamethasone (systemic) *on page* 266
PRO-Diclo-Rapide (Can) *see* diclofenac (systemic) *on page* 279
PRO-Doc Limitee Bromazepam (Can) *see* bromazepam *(Canada only) on page* 142
PRO-Enalapril (Can) *see* enalapril *on page* 330
ProFe [OTC] *see* polysaccharide-iron complex *on page* 740
PRO-Feno-Super (Can) *see* fenofibrate *on page* 375
Profilnine® SD *see* factor IX complex (human) *on page* 371
Proflavanol C™ (Can) *see* ascorbic acid *on page* 94
PRO-Fluconazole (Can) *see* fluconazole *on page* 388
PRO-Fluoxetine (Can) *see* fluoxetine *on page* 396
PRO-Gabapentin (Can) *see* gabapentin *on page* 413

progesterone (proe JES ter one)

Synonyms pregnenedione; progestin

U.S. Brand Names Crinone®; Endometrin®; First™-Progesterone VGS 100; First™-Progesterone VGS 200; First™-Progesterone VGS 25; First™-Progesterone VGS 400; First™-Progesterone VGS 50; Prometrium®

Canadian Brand Names Crinone®; Prometrium®

Therapeutic Category Progestin

Use

Oral: Prevention of endometrial hyperplasia in nonhysterectomized, postmenopausal women who are receiving conjugated estrogen tablets; secondary amenorrhea

I.M.: Amenorrhea; abnormal uterine bleeding due to hormonal imbalance

Intravaginal gel: Part of assisted reproductive technology (ART) for infertile women with progesterone deficiency; secondary amenorrhea

Vaginal tablet: Part of ART for infertile women with progesterone deficiency

General Dosage Range

I.M.: *Adults (females):* 5-10 mg/day for 6 doses

Intravaginal: *Adults (females):*

ART: 90 mg (8% gel) once or twice daily or 100 mg (vaginal tablet) 2-3 times/day

Secondary amenorrhea: 45 mg (4% gel) every other day, may increase to 90 mg (8% gel) every other day if needed (maximum: 6 doses)

Oral: *Adults (females):*

Amenorrhea: 400 mg once daily in the evening for 10 days

Endometrial hyperplasia prevention: 200 mg once daily in the evening for 12 days sequentially per 28-day cycle

Dosage Forms

Capsule, oral: 100 mg, 200 mg

Prometrium®: 100 mg, 200 mg

Gel, vaginal:

Crinone®: 4% (1.45 g); 8% (1.45 g)

Injection, oil: 50 mg/mL (10 mL)

Suppository, vaginal:

First™-Progesterone VGS 25: 25 mg (30s)
First™-Progesterone VGS 50: 50 mg (30s)
First™-Progesterone VGS 100: 100 mg (30s)
First™-Progesterone VGS 200: 200 mg (30s)
First™-Progesterone VGS 400: 400 mg (30s)

Tablet, vaginal:

Endometrin®: 100 mg

progestin *see* progesterone *on page* 762
PRO-Glyburide (Can) *see* glyburide *on page* 428
Proglycem® *see* diazoxide *on page* 278

promethazine (proe METH a zeen)

Medication Safety Issues

Sound-alike/look-alike issues:

Promethazine may be confused with chlorproMAZINE, predniSONE

Phenergan® may be confused with PHENobarbital, Phrenilin®, Theragran

High alert medication:

The Institute for Safe Medication Practices (ISMP) includes this medication (I.V. formulation) among its list of drugs which have a heightened risk of causing significant patient harm when used in error.

BEERS Criteria medication:

This drug may be potentially inappropriate for use in geriatric patients (Quality of evidence - high; Strength of recommendation - strong).

Administration issues:

To prevent or minimize tissue damage during I.V. administration, the Institute for Safe Medication Practices (ISMP) has the following recommendations:

- Limit concentration available to the 25 mg/mL product
- Consider limiting initial doses to 6.25-12.5 mg
- Further dilute the 25 mg/mL strength into 10-20 mL NS
- Administer through a large bore vein (not hand or wrist)
- Administer via running I.V. line at port farthest from patient's vein
- Consider administering over 10-15 minutes
- Instruct patients to report immediately signs of pain or burning

International issues:

Sominex: Brand name for promethazine in Great Britain, but also is a brand name for diphenhydrAMINE in the U.S.

Synonyms promethazine hydrochloride

U.S. Brand Names Phenadoz®; Phenergan; Promethegan™

Canadian Brand Names Bioniche Promethazine; Histantil; Phenergan; PMS-Promethazine

Therapeutic Category Antiemetic; Phenothiazine Derivative

Use Symptomatic treatment of various allergic conditions; antiemetic; motion sickness; sedative; adjunct to postoperative analgesia and anesthesia

General Dosage Range

I.M., I.V.:

Children ≥2 years: 0.25-1 mg/kg 4-6 times/day as needed (maximum: 25 mg/dose; sedation: 50 mg/dose)

Adults: 12.5-75 mg/dose as a single dose **or** 12.5-50 mg every 4-6 hours as needed

Oral, rectal:

Children ≥2 years:

Allergic reactions: 0.1 mg/kg every 6 hours (maximum: 12.5 mg) during the day and 0.5 mg/kg (maximum: 25 mg/dose) at bedtime as needed

Antiemetic: 0.25-1 mg/kg 4-6 times/day as needed (maximum: 25 mg/dose)

Motion sickness: 0.5 mg/kg 30 minutes to 1 hour before departure, then every 12 hours as needed (maximum: 25 mg twice daily)

Sedation: 0.5-1 mg/kg every 6 hours as needed (maximum: 50 mg/dose)

Adults: 6.25-25 mg every 4-8 hours as needed **or** 12.5-50 mg as a single dose **or** 25 mg 30-60 minutes before departure, then every 12 hours as needed

Dosage Forms

Injection, solution: 25 mg/mL (1 mL, 10 mL); 50 mg/mL (1 mL)

Phenergan: 25 mg/mL (1 mL); 50 mg/mL (1 mL)

Suppository, rectal: 12.5 mg (12s); 25 mg (12s)

Phenadoz®: 12.5 mg (12s); 25 mg (12s)

Promethegan™: 12.5 mg (12s); 25 mg (12s); 50 mg (12s)

Syrup, oral: 6.25 mg/5 mL (118 mL, 473 mL)

Tablet, oral: 12.5 mg, 25 mg, 50 mg

promethazine and codeine (proe METH a zeen & KOE deen)

Medication Safety Issues

High alert medication:

The Institute for Safe Medication Practices (ISMP) includes this medication among its list of drug classes which have a heightened risk of causing significant patient harm when used in error.

Synonyms codeine and promethazine

Therapeutic Category Antihistamine/Antitussive

Controlled Substance C-V

Use Temporary relief of coughs and upper respiratory symptoms associated with allergy or the common cold

General Dosage Range Oral:

Children 6-11 years: 2.5-5 mL every 4-6 hours (maximum: 30 mL/day)

Children ≥12 years and Adults: 5 mL every 4-6 hours (maximum: 30 mL/day)

Dosage Forms

Syrup: Promethazine 6.25 mg and codeine 10 mg per 5 mL

promethazine and dextromethorphan (proe METH a zeen & deks troe meth OR fan)

Synonyms dextromethorphan and promethazine

Therapeutic Category Antihistamine/Antitussive

Use Temporary relief of coughs and upper respiratory symptoms associated with allergy or the common cold

General Dosage Range Oral:

Children 2-6 years: 1.25-2.5 mL every 4-6 hours (maximum: 10 mL/day)

Children 6-12 years: 2.5-5 mL every 4-6 hours (maximum: 20 mL/day)

Adults: 5 mL every 4-6 hours (maximum: 30 mL/day)

Dosage Forms

Syrup: Promethazine 6.25 mg and dextromethorphan 15 mg per 5 mL

promethazine and phenylephrine (proe METH a zeen & fen il EF rin)

Synonyms phenylephrine and promethazine

U.S. Brand Names Promethazine VC

Therapeutic Category Antihistamine/Decongestant Combination

Use Temporary relief of upper respiratory symptoms associated with allergy or the common cold

General Dosage Range Oral:
Children 2-6 years: 1.25-2.5 mL every 4-6 hours (maximum: 7.5 mL/day)
Children 6-12 years: 2.5-5 mL every 4-6 hours (maximum: 30 mL/day)
Children >12 years and Adults: 5 mL every 4-6 hours (maximum: 30 mL/day)

Dosage Forms

Syrup, oral:
Promethazine VC: Promethazine 6.25 mg and phenylephrine 5 mg per 5 mL (118 mL, 473 mL)

promethazine hydrochloride *see* promethazine *on page 763*

promethazine, phenylephrine, and codeine

(proe METH a zeen, fen il EF rin, & KOE deen)

Synonyms codeine, phenylephrine, and promethazine; phenylephrine, promethazine, and codeine

Therapeutic Category Antihistamine/Decongestant/Antitussive

Controlled Substance C-V

Use Temporary relief of coughs and upper respiratory symptoms including nasal congestion associated with allergy or the common cold

General Dosage Range Oral:
Children 6-11 years: 2.5-5 mL every 4-6 hours (maximum: 30 mL/day)
Children ≥12 years and Adults: 5 mL every 4-6 hours (maximum: 30 mL/day)

Dosage Forms

Syrup: Promethazine 6.25 mg, phenylephrine 5 mg, and codeine 10 mg per 5 mL

Promethazine VC *see* promethazine and phenylephrine *on page 764*

Promethegan™ *see* promethazine *on page 763*

Prometrium® *see* progesterone *on page 762*

PRO-Mirtazapine (Can) *see* mirtazapine *on page 606*

Promiseb™ *see* emollients *on page 328*

PRO-Naproxen EC (Can) *see* naproxen *on page 628*

Pronestyl *see* procainamide *on page 759*

Pronto® Complete Lice Removal System [OTC] *see* pyrethrins and piperonyl butoxide *on page 776*

Pronto® Lice Control (Can) *see* pyrethrins and piperonyl butoxide *on page 776*

Pronto® Plus Lice Killing Mousse Plus Vitamin E [OTC] *see* pyrethrins and piperonyl butoxide *on page 776*

Pronto® Plus Lice Killing Mousse Shampoo Plus Natural Extracts and Oils [OTC] *see* pyrethrins and piperonyl butoxide *on page 776*

Pronto® Plus Warm Oil Treatment and Conditioner [OTC] *see* pyrethrins and piperonyl butoxide *on page 776*

propafenone (pro PAF en one)

Medication Safety Issues

BEERS Criteria medication:
This drug may be potentially inappropriate for use in geriatric patients (Quality of evidence - high; Strength of recommendation - strong).

Synonyms propafenone hydrochloride

U.S. Brand Names Rythmol®; Rythmol® SR

Canadian Brand Names Apo-Propafenone®; Mylan-Propafenone; PMS-Propafenone; Rythmol® Gen-Propafenone

Therapeutic Category Antiarrhythmic Agent, Class I-C

Use Treatment of life-threatening ventricular arrhythmias; treatment of paroxysmal atrial fibrillation/flutter (PAF) or paroxysmal supraventricular tachycardia (PSVT) in patients with disabling symptoms and without structural heart disease

Extended release capsule: Prolong the time to recurrence of symptomatic atrial fibrillation in patients without structural heart disease

General Dosage Range Dosage adjustment recommended in patients with hepatic impairment

Oral:
Extended release: *Adults:* Initial: 225 mg every 12 hours; Maintenance: 225-425 mg every 12 hours
Immediate release: *Adults:* Initial: 150 mg every 8 hours; Maintenance: 150-300 mg every 8 hours

Dosage Forms

Capsule, extended release, oral: 225 mg, 325 mg, 425 mg

Rythmol® SR: 225 mg, 325 mg, 425 mg

Tablet, oral: 150 mg, 225 mg, 300 mg

Rythmol®: 150 mg, 225 mg

propafenone hydrochloride *see* propafenone *on page* *765*

propantheline (proe PAN the leen)

Medication Safety Issues

BEERS Criteria medication:

This drug may be potentially inappropriate for use in geriatric patients (Quality of evidence - moderate; Strength of recommendation - strong).

Synonyms propantheline bromide

Therapeutic Category Anticholinergic Agent

Use Adjunctive treatment of peptic ulcer

General Dosage Range Oral:

Children: 1-3 mg/kg/day in 3-6 divided doses

Adults: 15 mg 3 times/day and 30 mg at bedtime

Dosage Forms

Tablet, oral: 15 mg

propantheline bromide *see* propantheline *on page* *766*

proparacaine (proe PAR a kane)

Synonyms proparacaine hydrochloride; proxymetacaine

U.S. Brand Names Alcaine®; Parcaine™ [DSC]

Canadian Brand Names Alcaine®; Diocaine®

Therapeutic Category Local Anesthetic

Use Anesthesia for tonometry, gonioscopy; suture removal from cornea; removal of corneal foreign body; cataract extraction, glaucoma surgery; short operative procedure involving the cornea and conjunctiva

General Dosage Range Ophthalmic: *Children and Adults:* Instill 1-2 drops of 0.5% solution in eye once **or** instill 1 drop of 0.5% solution in eye every 5-10 minutes for 5-7 doses

Dosage Forms

Solution, ophthalmic: 0.5% (15 mL)

Alcaine®: 0.5% (15 mL)

proparacaine and fluorescein (proe PAR a kane & FLURE e seen)

Synonyms fluorescein and proparacaine

U.S. Brand Names Flucaine

Therapeutic Category Diagnostic Agent; Local Anesthetic

Use Anesthesia for tonometry, gonioscopy; suture removal from cornea; removal of corneal foreign body; cataract extraction, glaucoma surgery

General Dosage Range Ophthalmic: *Children and Adults:* Instill 1 drop in each eye every 5-10 minutes for 5-7 doses **or** instill 1-2 drops in each eye once

Dosage Forms

Solution, ophthalmic: Proparacaine 0.5% and fluorescein 0.25% (5 mL)

Flucaine: Proparacaine 0.5% and fluorescein 0.25% (5 mL)

proparacaine hydrochloride *see* proparacaine *on page* *766*

Propecia® *see* finasteride *on page* *384*

Propine® (Can) *see* dipivefrin *on page* *300*

PRO-Pioglitazone (Can) *see* pioglitazone *on page* *725*

propofol (PROE po fole)

Medication Safety Issues

Sound-alike/look-alike issues:

Diprivan® may be confused with Diflucan®, Ditropan

Propofol may be confused with fospropofol

High alert medication:

The Institute for Safe Medication Practices (ISMP) includes this medication among its list of drugs which have a heightened risk of causing significant patient harm when used in error.

Administration issues:

Propofol may be confused with bupivacaine liposome injectable suspension (Exparel™) in operating rooms and other surgical areas due to their similar white, milky appearance especially when prepared in syringes. Bupivacaine liposome injectable suspension (Exparel™) is intended only for administration via infiltration into the surgical site (and **not** for systemic use). Confusion with propofol may lead to accidental intravenous administration of Exparel™ instead of the intended propofol. Therefore, to avoid potential confusion ISMP recommends that all vials be separated when stocked in common areas and all prepared syringes be labeled.

U.S. Brand Names Diprivan®

Canadian Brand Names Diprivan®

Therapeutic Category General Anesthetic

Use Induction of anesthesia in patients ≥3 years of age; maintenance of anesthesia in patients >2 months of age; in adults, for monitored anesthesia care sedation during procedures; sedation in intubated, mechanically-ventilated ICU patients

General Dosage Range I.V.: *Children and Adults:* Dosage varies greatly depending on indication

Dosage Forms

Injection, emulsion: 10 mg/mL (20 mL, 50 mL, 100 mL)

Diprivan®: 10 mg/mL (20 mL, 50 mL, 100 mL)

propranolol (proe PRAN oh lole)

Medication Safety Issues

Sound-alike/look-alike issues:

Propranolol may be confused with prasugrel, Pravachol®, Propulsid®

Inderal® may be confused with Adderall®, Enduron, Imdur®, Imuran®, Inderide, Isordil®, Toradol®

High alert medication:

The Institute for Safe Medication Practices (ISMP) includes this medication among its list of drugs which have a heightened risk of causing significant patient harm when used in error.

Administration issues:

Significant differences exist between oral and I.V. dosing. Use caution when converting from one route of administration to another.

International issues:

Inderal [Canada and multiple international markets] and Inderal LA [U.S.] may be confused with Indiaral brand name for loperamide [France]

Synonyms propranolol hydrochloride

U.S. Brand Names Inderal® LA; InnoPran XL®

Canadian Brand Names Apo-Propranolol®; Dom-Propranolol; Inderal®; Inderal® LA; Novo-Pranol; Nu-Propranolol; PMS-Propranolol; Propranolol Hydrochloride Injection, USP; Teva-Propranolol

Therapeutic Category Antiarrhythmic Agent, Class II; Beta-Adrenergic Blocker

Use Management of hypertension; angina pectoris; pheochromocytoma; essential tremor; supraventricular arrhythmias (such as atrial fibrillation and flutter, AV nodal reentrant tachycardias), ventricular tachycardias (catecholamine-induced arrhythmias, digoxin toxicity); prevention of myocardial infarction; migraine headache prophylaxis; symptomatic treatment of hypertrophic subaortic stenosis (hypertrophic obstructive cardiomyopathy)

General Dosage Range

I.V.: *Adults:* 1-3 mg, repeat every 2-5 minutes up to a total of 5 mg **or** 0.1 mg/kg divided into 3 equal doses given at 2- to 3-minute intervals; may repeat total dose in 2 minutes if needed

Oral:

Extended release: *Adults:* Initial: 80 mg once daily; Maintenance: 60-320 mg once daily (maximum: 640 mg/day)

Regular release: *Adults:* 30-320 mg/day in 2-4 divided doses (maximum: 640 mg/day)

Dosage Forms

Capsule, extended release, oral: 60 mg, 80 mg, 120 mg, 160 mg

InnoPran XL®: 80 mg, 120 mg

Capsule, sustained release, oral:

Inderal® LA: 60 mg, 80 mg, 120 mg, 160 mg

Injection, solution: 1 mg/mL (1 mL)

Injection, solution [preservative free]: 1 mg/mL (1 mL)
Solution, oral: 4 mg/mL (500 mL); 8 mg/mL (500 mL)
Tablet, oral: 10 mg, 20 mg, 40 mg, 60 mg, 80 mg

propranolol and hydrochlorothiazide (proe PRAN oh lole & hye droe klor oh THYE a zide)

Medication Safety Issues
Sound-alike/look-alike issues:
Inderide may be confused with Inderal®
Synonyms hydrochlorothiazide and propranolol; Inderide
Therapeutic Category Antihypertensive Agent, Combination
Use Management of hypertension
General Dosage Range Oral: *Adults:* Propranolol 80-160 mg/day and hydrochlorothiazide 12.5-50 mg/day in 2 divided doses
Dosage Forms
Tablet: Propranolol 40 mg and hydrochlorothiazide 25 mg; propranolol 80 mg and hydrochlorothiazide 25 mg

propranolol hydrochloride *see* propranolol *on page* 767
Propranolol Hydrochloride Injection, USP (Can) *see* propranolol *on page* 767
Proprinal® [OTC] *see* ibuprofen *on page* 468
Proprinal® Cold and Sinus [OTC] *see* pseudoephedrine and ibuprofen *on page* 773
Propulsid® *see* cisapride *on page* 212
propylene glycol diacetate, acetic acid, and hydrocortisone *see* acetic acid, propylene glycol diacetate, and hydrocortisone *on page* 31

propylhexedrine (proe pil HEKS e dreen)

U.S. Brand Names Benzedrex® [OTC]
Therapeutic Category Adrenergic Agonist Agent
Use Topical nasal decongestant
General Dosage Range Oral: *Children ≥6 years and Adults:* 2 inhalations in each nostril, not more frequently than every 2 hours
Dosage Forms
Inhaler, nasal:
Benzedrex® [OTC]: 0.4-0.5 mg/inhalation (1s)

2-propylpentanoic acid *see* valproic acid *on page* 934

propylthiouracil (proe pil thye oh YOOR a sil)

Medication Safety Issues
Sound-alike/look-alike issues:
Propylthiouracil may be confused with Purinethol®
PTU is an error-prone abbreviation (mistaken as mercaptopurine [Purinethol®; 6-MP])
Synonyms PTU (error-prone abbreviation)
Canadian Brand Names Propyl-Thyracil®
Therapeutic Category Antithyroid Agent
Use Adjunctive therapy in patients intolerant of methimazole to ameliorate hyperthyroidism symptoms in preparation for surgical treatment or radioactive iodine therapy; treatment of hyperthyroidism in patients intolerant of methimazole and not candidates for surgical/radiotherapy
General Dosage Range Oral:
Children 6-10 years: 50-150 mg/day
Children >10 years: 150-300 mg/day
Adults: Initial: 300-900 mg/day in 3 divided doses; Maintenance: 100-150 mg/day
Dosage Forms
Tablet, oral: 50 mg

Propyl-Thyracil® (Can) *see* propylthiouracil *on page* 768
2-propylvaleric acid *see* valproic acid *on page* 934
ProQuad® *see* measles, mumps, rubella, and varicella virus vaccine *on page* 564
PRO-Quetiapine (Can) *see* quetiapine *on page* 781

PRO-Rabeprazole (Can) *see* rabeprazole *on page 784*
PRO-Risperidone (Can) *see* risperidone *on page 803*
Proscar® *see* finasteride *on page 384*
Prosed®/DS *see* methenamine, phenyl salicylate, methylene blue, benzoic acid, and hyoscyamine *on page 583*
Prosol *see* amino acid injection *on page 61*
ProSom *see* estazolam *on page 347*
PRO-Sotalol (Can) *see* sotalol *on page 851*
prostacyclin *see* epoprostenol *on page 338*
prostacyclin PGI_2 *see* iloprost *on page 474*
prostaglandin E_1 *see* alprostadil *on page 53*
prostaglandin E_2 *see* dinoprostone *on page 291*
prostaglandin F_2 *see* carboprost tromethamine *on page 176*
prostate cancer vaccine, cell-based *see* sipuleucel-T *on page 836*
Prostigmin® *see* neostigmine *on page 635*
Prostin E2® *see* dinoprostone *on page 291*
Prostin E_2® (Can) *see* dinoprostone *on page 291*
Prostin® VR (Can) *see* alprostadil *on page 53*
Prostin VR Pediatric® *see* alprostadil *on page 53*

protamine (PROE ta meen)

Medication Safety Issues

Sound-alike/look-alike issues:

Protamine may be confused with ProAmatine, Protonix®, Protopam®

Synonyms protamine sulfate

Therapeutic Category Antidote

Use Treatment of heparin overdosage; neutralize heparin during surgery or dialysis procedures

General Dosage Range I.V.: *Children and Adults:* 1 mg of protamine neutralizes ~100 units of heparin (maximum dose: 50 mg)

Dosage Forms

Injection, solution [preservative free]: 10 mg/mL (5 mL, 25 mL)

protamine sulfate *see* protamine *on page 769*
protease, lipase, and amylase *see* pancrelipase *on page 687*
Protection Plus® [OTC] *see* alcohol (ethyl) *on page 43*
protein C *see* protein C concentrate (human) *on page 769*
protein C (activated), human, recombinant *see* drotrecogin alfa (activated) *on page 318*
protein-bound paclitaxel *see* paclitaxel (protein bound) *on page 684*

protein C concentrate (human) (PROE teen cee KON suhn trate HYU man)

Medication Safety Issues

Sound-alike/look-alike issues:

Ceprotin may be confused with aprotinin, Cipro®

Protein C concentrate (human) may be confused with activated protein C (human, recombinant) which refers to drotrecogin alfa

Synonyms protein C

U.S. Brand Names Ceprotin

Therapeutic Category Anticoagulant

Use Replacement therapy for severe congenital protein C deficiency for the prevention and/or treatment of venous thromboembolism and purpura fulminans

General Dosage Range I.V.: *Children and Adults:* Initial: 100-120 units, followed by 60-80 units every 6 hours for 3 doses; maintenance: 45-60 units every 6 hours (short-term) or every 12 hours (short-to-long term)

Dosage Forms

Injection, powder for reconstitution [preservative free]:

Ceprotin: ~500 units, ~1000 units

prothrombin complex concentrate *see* factor IX complex (human) *on page 371*

prothrombin complex concentrate *see* prothrombin complex (human) [(factors II, VII, IX, X), protein C, and protein S] *(Canada only) on page 770*

prothrombin complex (human) [(factors II, VII, IX, X), protein C, and protein S] *(Canada only)*

(PRO throm bin KOM pleks HYU man FAK ters too SEV en nyne ten PROE teen cee & PROE teen ess)

Synonyms prothrombin complex concentrate

Canadian Brand Names Octaplex®

Therapeutic Category Hemostatic Agent

Use Prophylaxis (perioperative) and treatment of bleeding due to acquired deficiency (eg, overdose of vitamin K antagonist) of one or more of the prothrombin complex coagulation factors II, VII, IX, and X, when rapid correction of factor deficiency is necessary

General Dosage Range I.V.: *Adults:* Maximum dose not to exceed 120 mL. Approximate doses required for normalization of INR (≤1.2 within 1 hour): Initial INR: 2-2.5: Administer 0.9-1.3 mL/kg; 2.5-3: Administer 1.3-1.6 mL/kg; 3-3.5: Administer 1.6-1.9 mL/kg; >3.5: Administer >1.9 mL/kg

Product Availability Not available in U.S.

Dosage Forms - Canada

Injection, powder for reconstitution:

Octaplex®: Human coagulation factor II: 11-38 units/mL; factor VII: 9-24 units/mL; factor IX: 20-31 units/mL; factor X: 18-30 units/mL: protein C: 7-31 units/mL; protein S: 7-32 units/mL (20 mL)

Protonix® *see* pantoprazole *on page 689*

Protonix® I.V. *see* pantoprazole *on page 689*

Protopam® *see* pralidoxime *on page 749*

Protopic® *see* tacrolimus (topical) *on page 866*

PRO-Topiramate (Can) *see* topiramate *on page 906*

Pro-Triazide (Can) *see* hydrochlorothiazide and triamterene *on page 453*

protriptyline (proe TRIP ti leen)

Medication Safety Issues

Sound-alike/look-alike issues:

Vivactil® may be confused with Vyvanse®

BEERS Criteria medication:

This drug may be potentially inappropriate for use in geriatric patients (SIADH: Quality of evidence - moderate; Strength of recommendation - strong).

Synonyms protriptyline hydrochloride

U.S. Brand Names Vivactil®

Therapeutic Category Antidepressant, Tricyclic (Secondary Amine)

Use Treatment of depression

General Dosage Range Oral:

Adolescents: 15-20 mg/day

Adults: 15-60 mg/day in 3-4 divided doses

Elderly: Initial: 5-10 mg/day; Maintenance: 15-20 mg/day

Dosage Forms

Tablet, oral: 5 mg, 10 mg

Vivactil®: 5 mg, 10 mg

protriptyline hydrochloride *see* protriptyline *on page 770*

Protylol (Can) *see* dicyclomine *on page 282*

PRO-Valacyclovir (Can) *see* valacyclovir *on page 933*

Provenge® *see* sipuleucel-T *on page 836*

Proventil® HFA *see* albuterol *on page 41*

Provera® *see* medroxyprogesterone *on page 567*

Provera-Pak (Can) *see* medroxyprogesterone *on page 567*

PRO-Verapamil SR (Can) *see* verapamil *on page 942*

Provigil® *see* modafinil *on page 609*

Proviodine (Can) *see* povidone-iodine (topical) *on page 747*

Provisc® *see* hyaluronate and derivatives *on page 450*
Provocholine® *see* methacholine *on page 580*
proxymetacaine *see* proparacaine *on page 766*
PROzac® *see* fluoxetine *on page 396*
Prozac® (Can) *see* fluoxetine *on page 396*
PROzac® Weekly™ *see* fluoxetine *on page 396*
PRO-Zopiclone (Can) *see* zopiclone *(Canada only) on page 967*
PRP-OMP *see Haemophilus* B conjugate vaccine *on page 439*
PRP-T *see Haemophilus* B conjugate vaccine *on page 439*

prucalopride *(Canada only)* (proo KAL oh pride)

Medication Safety Issues

Sound-alike/look-alike issues:

Resotran™ may be confused with Restoril™

Synonyms prucalopride succinate; R093877; R108512

Canadian Brand Names Resotran™

Therapeutic Category Serotonin 5-HT_4 Receptor Agonist

Use Treatment of chronic idiopathic constipation in adult females with inadequate response to laxatives

General Dosage Range Dosage adjustment recommended in patients with renal impairment.

Oral:

Adults (females ≥18 years): 2 mg once daily
Elderly (females >65 years): Initial: 1 mg once daily; maintenance: 1-2 mg once daily

Product Availability Not available in U.S.

Dosage Forms - Canada

Tablet, oral:

Resotran™: 1 mg, 2 mg [contains lactose]

prucalopride succinate *see* prucalopride *(Canada only) on page 771*
PruClair™ *see* emollients *on page 328*
Prudoxin™ *see* doxepin (topical) *on page 312*
PruMyx™ *see* emollients *on page 328*
prussian blue *see* ferric hexacyanoferrate *on page 379*
PruTect™ *see* emollients *on page 328*
PR™ Wash *see* benzoyl peroxide *on page 124*
prymaccone *see* primaquine *on page 757*
P&S® [OTC] *see* salicylic acid *on page 816*
23PS *see* pneumococcal polysaccharide vaccine (polyvalent) *on page 735*
PS-341 *see* bortezomib *on page 139*

pseudoephedrine (soo doe e FED rin)

Medication Safety Issues

Sound-alike/look-alike issues:

Sudafed® may be confused with sotalol, Sudafed PE®, Sufenta®

Synonyms *d*-isoephedrine hydrochloride; pseudoephedrine hydrochloride; pseudoephedrine sulfate; Sudafed

U.S. Brand Names Children's Nasal Decongestant [OTC]; Contac® Cold + Flu Maximum Strength Non-Drowsy [OTC]; Oranyl [OTC]; Silfedrine Children's [OTC]; Sudafed® 12 Hour [OTC]; Sudafed® 24 Hour [OTC]; Sudafed® Children's [OTC]; Sudafed® Maximum Strength Nasal Decongestant [OTC]; Sudo-Tab® [OTC]; SudoGest 12 Hour [OTC]; SudoGest Children's [OTC] [DSC]; SudoGest [OTC]

Canadian Brand Names Balminil Decongestant; Benylin® D for Infants; Contac® Cold 12 Hour Relief Non Drowsy; Drixoral® ND; Eltor®; PMS-Pseudoephedrine; Pseudofrin; Robidrine®; Sudafed® Decongestant

Therapeutic Category Adrenergic Agonist Agent

Use Temporary symptomatic relief of nasal congestion due to common cold, upper respiratory allergies, and sinusitis; also promotes nasal or sinus drainage

General Dosage Range Oral:
Immediate release:
Children 4-5 years: 15 mg every 4-6 hours (maximum: 60 mg/day)
Children 6-12 years: 30 mg every 4-6 hours (maximum: 120 mg/day)
Adults: 60 mg every 4-6 hours (maximum: 240 mg/day)
Extended release: *Adults:* 120 mg every 12 hours or 240 mg every 24 hours (maximum: 240 mg/day)

Dosage Forms

Caplet, oral:
Contac® Cold + Flu Maximum Strength Non-Drowsy [OTC]: Acetaminophen 500 mg and phenylephrine hydrochloride 5 mg

Caplet, extended release, oral:
Sudafed® 12 Hour [OTC]: 120 mg

Liquid, oral: 30 mg/5 mL (473 mL)
Children's Nasal Decongestant [OTC]: 30 mg/5 mL (118 mL)
Silfedrine Children's [OTC]: 15 mg/5 mL (118 mL, 237 mL)
Sudafed® Children's [OTC]: 15 mg/5 mL (118 mL)

Syrup, oral: 30 mg/5 mL (118 mL)

Tablet, oral: 30 mg
Oranyl [OTC]: 30 mg
Sudafed® Maximum Strength Nasal Decongestant [OTC]: 30 mg
Sudo-Tab® [OTC]: 30 mg
SudoGest [OTC]: 30 mg, 60 mg

Tablet, extended release, oral:
Sudafed® 24 Hour [OTC]: 240 mg
SudoGest 12 Hour [OTC]: 120 mg

pseudoephedrine and acetaminophen *see* acetaminophen and pseudoephedrine *on page 25*

pseudoephedrine and brompheniramine *see* brompheniramine and pseudoephedrine *on page 144*

pseudoephedrine and chlorpheniramine *see* chlorpheniramine and pseudoephedrine *on page 200*

pseudoephedrine and codeine (soo doe e FED rin & KOE deen)

Medication Safety Issues

High alert medication:
The Institute for Safe Medication Practices (ISMP) includes this medication among its list of drug classes which have a heightened risk of causing significant patient harm when used in error.

Synonyms codeine and pseudoephedrine; codeine phosphate and pseudoephedrine hydrochloride; pseudoephedrine hydrochloride and codeine phosphate

U.S. Brand Names Codar® D; EndaCof-DC; Notuss®-DC

Therapeutic Category Antitussive/Decongestant

Controlled Substance Liquid: C-V

Use Temporary symptomatic relief of congestion and cough due to upper respiratory infections including common cold, bronchitis, sinusitis, and influenza

General Dosage Range Oral:
Children 6-11 years: 2.5-5 mL every 4-6 hours as needed (maximum: 20 mL/24 hours)
Children ≥12 years and Adults: 5-10 mL every 4-6 hours as needed (maximum: 40 mL/24 hours)

Dosage Forms

Liquid, oral:
Codar® D: Pseudoephedrine 30 mg and codeine 8 mg per 5 mL
EndaCof-DC, Notuss®-DC: Pseudoephedrine 30 mg and codeine 10 mg per 5 mL

pseudoephedrine and desloratadine *see* desloratadine and pseudoephedrine *on page 263*

pseudoephedrine and dextromethorphan (soo doe e FED rin & deks troe meth OR fan)

Synonyms dextromethorphan and pseudoephedrine

U.S. Brand Names Pedia Relief Cough and Cold [OTC]; Sudafed® Children's Cold & Cough [OTC]

Canadian Brand Names Balminil DM D; Benylin® DM-D; Koffex DM-D; Novahistex® DM Decongestant; Novahistine® DM Decongestant; Robitussin® Childrens Cough & Cold

Therapeutic Category Antitussive/Decongestant

Use Temporary symptomatic relief of nasal congestion and cough due to common cold, hay fever, upper respiratory allergies

General Dosage Range Oral:

Children 2-6 years: 15 mg (based on pseudoephedrine) every 4-6 hours (maximum: 60 mg/day)

Children 6-12 years: 30 mg (based on pseudoephedrine) every 4-6 hours (maximum: 120 mg/day)

Children ≥12 years and Adults: 60 mg (based on pseudoephedrine) every 4-6 hours (maximum: 240 mg/day)

Dosage Forms

Liquid:

Sudafed® Children's Cold & Cough [OTC]: Pseudoephedrine 15 mg and dextromethorphan 5 mg per 5 mL

Syrup:

Pedia Relief Cough and Cold [OTC]: Pseudoephedrine 15 mg and dextromethorphan 7.5 mg per 5 mL

pseudoephedrine and fexofenadine *see* fexofenadine and pseudoephedrine *on page* 382

pseudoephedrine and guaifenesin *see* guaifenesin and pseudoephedrine *on page* 436

pseudoephedrine and hydrocodone *see* hydrocodone and pseudoephedrine *on page* 456

pseudoephedrine and ibuprofen (soo doe e FED rin & eye byoo PROE fen)

Synonyms ibuprofen and pseudoephedrine

U.S. Brand Names Advil® Cold & Sinus [OTC]; Proprinal® Cold and Sinus [OTC]

Canadian Brand Names Advil® Cold & Sinus; Advil® Cold & Sinus Daytime; Children's Advil® Cold; Sudafed® Sinus Advance

Therapeutic Category Decongestant/Analgesic

Use For temporary relief of cold, sinus, and flu symptoms (including nasal congestion, sinus pressure, headache, minor body aches and pains, and fever)

General Dosage Range Oral: *Children ≥12 years and Adults:* 1-2 doses (ibuprofen 200 mg and pseudoephedrine 30 mg per dose) every 4-6 hours as needed (maximum: 6 doses/day)

Dosage Forms

Caplet:

Advil® Cold & Sinus [OTC], Proprinal® Cold and Sinus [OTC]: Pseudoephedrine 30 mg and ibuprofen 200 mg

Capsule, liquid filled:

Advil® Cold & Sinus [OTC]: Pseudoephedrine 30 mg and ibuprofen 200 mg

pseudoephedrine and loratadine *see* loratadine and pseudoephedrine *on page* 550

pseudoephedrine and naproxen *see* naproxen and pseudoephedrine *on page* 629

pseudoephedrine and triprolidine *see* triprolidine and pseudoephedrine *on page* 922

pseudoephedrine, chlorpheniramine, and codeine *see* chlorpheniramine, pseudoephedrine, and codeine *on page* 202

pseudoephedrine, chlorpheniramine, and dextromethorphan *see* chlorpheniramine, pseudoephedrine, and dextromethorphan *on page* 202

pseudoephedrine, chlorpheniramine, and dihydrocodeine *see* pseudoephedrine, dihydrocodeine, and chlorpheniramine *on page* 773

pseudoephedrine, chlorpheniramine, and ibuprofen *see* ibuprofen, pseudoephedrine, and chlorpheniramine *on page* 470

pseudoephedrine, codeine, and triprolidine *see* triprolidine, pseudoephedrine, and codeine *(Canada only) on page* 922

pseudoephedrine, dextromethorphan, and guaifenesin *see* guaifenesin, pseudoephedrine, and dextromethorphan *on page* 437

pseudoephedrine, dihydrocodeine, and chlorpheniramine

(soo doe e FED rin, dye hye droe KOE deen, & klor fen IR a meen)

Medication Safety Issues

High alert medication:

The Institute for Safe Medication Practices (ISMP) includes this medication among its list of drug classes which have a heightened risk of causing significant patient harm when used in error.

Synonyms chlorpheniramine, dihydrocodeine, and pseudoephedrine; dihydrocodeine bitartrate, pseudoephedrine hydrochloride, and chlorpheniramine maleate; pseudoephedrine, chlorpheniramine, and dihydrocodeine

U.S. Brand Names DiHydro-CP

Therapeutic Category Antihistamine/Decongestant/Antitussive

Controlled Substance C-III

Use Temporary relief of cough, congestion, and sneezing due to colds, respiratory infections, or hay fever

General Dosage Range Oral:

Children 2-6 years: 1.25-2.5 mL every 4-6 hours (maximum: 4 doses/day)

Children 6-12 years: 2.5-5 mL every 4-6 hours (maximum: 4 doses/day)

Children >12 years and Adults: 5-10 mL every 4-6 hours (maximum: 4 doses/day)

Dosage Forms

Syrup:

DiHydro-CP: Pseudoephedrine 15 mg, dihydrocodeine 7.5 mg, and chlorpheniramine 2 mg per 5 mL

pseudoephedrine, guaifenesin, and codeine *see* guaifenesin, pseudoephedrine, and codeine *on page* 437

pseudoephedrine hydrochloride *see* pseudoephedrine *on page* 771

pseudoephedrine hydrochloride and acetaminophen *see* acetaminophen and pseudoephedrine *on page* 25

pseudoephedrine hydrochloride and acrivastine *see* acrivastine and pseudoephedrine *on page* 33

pseudoephedrine hydrochloride and cetirizine hydrochloride *see* cetirizine and pseudoephedrine *on page* 191

pseudoephedrine hydrochloride and codeine phosphate *see* pseudoephedrine and codeine *on page* 772

pseudoephedrine hydrochloride and hydrocodone bitartrate *see* hydrocodone and pseudoephedrine *on page* 456

pseudoephedrine hydrochloride, hydrocodone bitartrate, and chlorpheniramine maleate *see* hydrocodone, chlorpheniramine, and pseudoephedrine *on page* 457

pseudoephedrine, hydrocodone, and chlorpheniramine *see* hydrocodone, chlorpheniramine, and pseudoephedrine *on page* 457

pseudoephedrine sulfate *see* pseudoephedrine *on page* 771

pseudoephedrine tannate, dextromethorphan tannate, and brompheniramine tannate *see* brompheniramine, pseudoephedrine, and dextromethorphan *on page* 144

pseudoephedrine, triprolidine, and codeine *see* triprolidine, pseudoephedrine, and codeine *(Canada only) on page* 922

Pseudofrin (Can) *see* pseudoephedrine *on page* 771

pseudomonic acid A *see* mupirocin *on page* 618

P & S™ Liquid Phenol (Can) *see* phenol *on page* 713

Psoriasin [OTC] (Can) *see* coal tar *on page* 228

psyllium (SIL i yum)

Medication Safety Issues

Sound-alike/look-alike issues:

Fiberall® may be confused with Feverall®

Synonyms plantago seed; plantain seed; psyllium husk; psyllium hydrophilic mucilloid

U.S. Brand Names Bulk-K [OTC]; Fiberall® [OTC]; Fibro-Lax [OTC]; Fibro-XL [OTC]; Hydrocil® Instant [OTC]; Konsyl-D™ [OTC]; Konsyl® Easy Mix™ [OTC]; Konsyl® Orange [OTC]; Konsyl® Original [OTC]; Konsyl® [OTC]; Metamucil® Plus Calcium [OTC]; Metamucil® Smooth Texture [OTC]; Metamucil® [OTC]; Natural Fiber Therapy Smooth Texture [OTC]; Natural Fiber Therapy [OTC]; Reguloid [OTC]

Canadian Brand Names Metamucil®

Therapeutic Category Laxative

Use OTC labeling: Dietary fiber supplement; treatment of occasional constipation; reduce risk of coronary heart disease (CHD)

General Dosage Range Oral:

Children 6-11 years: Psyllium 1.25-15 g/day in divided doses

Children ≥12 years and Adults: Psyllium 2.5-30 g/day in divided doses

Dosage Forms

Capsule, oral: 500 mg
- Fibro-XL [OTC]: 0.675 g
- Konsyl® [OTC]: 0.52 g
- Metamucil® [OTC]: 0.52 g
- Metamucil® Plus Calcium [OTC]: 0.52 g
- Reguloid [OTC]: 0.52 g

Powder, oral: (454 g)
- Bulk-K [OTC]: (392 g)
- Fiberall® [OTC]: (454 g)
- Fibro-Lax [OTC]: (140 g, 392 g)
- Hydrocil® Instant [OTC]: (300 g); 3.5 g/packet (30s, 500s)
- Konsyl-D™ [OTC]: (325 g, 397 g, 500 g); 3.4 g/packet (100s, 500s)
- Konsyl® Easy Mix™ [OTC]: (250 g); 6 g/packet (500s)
- Konsyl® Orange [OTC]: (425 g, 538 g); 3.4 g/packet (30s)
- Konsyl® Original [OTC]: (300 g, 450 g); 6 g/packet (30s, 100s, 500s)
- Metamucil® [OTC]: (390 g, 570 g, 870 g, 1254 g)
- Metamucil® Smooth Texture [OTC]: (173 g, 283 g, 288 g, 300 g, 425 g, 432 g, 450 g, 609 g, 660 g, 684 g, 690 g, 912 g, 1020 g, 1368 g); 3.4 g/packet (30s)
- Natural Fiber Therapy [OTC]: (390 g, 539 g)
- Natural Fiber Therapy Smooth Texture [OTC]: (300 g)
- Reguloid [OTC]: (284 g, 369 g, 426 g, 540 g)

Wafer, oral:
- Metamucil® [OTC]: 3.4 g/2 wafers (24s)

psyllium husk *see* psyllium *on page 774*

psyllium hydrophilic mucilloid *see* psyllium *on page 774*

pteroylglutamic acid *see* folic acid *on page 403*

PTG *see* teniposide *on page 877*

PTU (error-prone abbreviation) *see* propylthiouracil *on page 768*

Pulmicort Flexhaler® *see* budesonide (systemic, oral inhalation) *on page 145*

Pulmicort Respules® *see* budesonide (systemic, oral inhalation) *on page 145*

Pulmicort® Turbuhaler® (Can) *see* budesonide (systemic, oral inhalation) *on page 145*

Pulmophylline (Can) *see* theophylline *on page 888*

Pulmozyme® *see* dornase alfa *on page 310*

Puregon® (Can) *see* follitropin beta *on page 405*

Purell® [OTC] *see* alcohol (ethyl) *on page 43*

Purell® 2 in 1 [OTC] *see* alcohol (ethyl) *on page 43*

Purell® Lasting Care [OTC] *see* alcohol (ethyl) *on page 43*

Purell® Moisture Therapy [OTC] *see* alcohol (ethyl) *on page 43*

Purell® with Aloe [OTC] *see* alcohol (ethyl) *on page 43*

Purg-Odan™ (Can) *see* sodium picosulfate, magnesium oxide, and citric acid *on page 846*

purified chick embryo cell *see* rabies vaccine *on page 784*

Purinethol® *see* mercaptopurine *on page 576*

PVP-I *see* povidone-iodine (ophthalmic) *on page 747*

PVP-I *see* povidone-iodine (topical) *on page 747*

Pylera™ *see* bismuth, metronidazole, and tetracycline *on page 136*

pyrantel pamoate (pi RAN tel PAM oh ate)

U.S. Brand Names Pin-X® [OTC]; Reese's Pinworm Medicine [OTC]

Canadian Brand Names Combantrin™

Therapeutic Category Anthelmintic

Use Treatment of pinworms caused by *Enterobius vermicularis* (alternative agent; not preferred therapy)

General Dosage Range Oral: *Children ≥2 years and Adults:* 11 mg/kg as a single dose (maximum: 1 g/dose)

Dosage Forms

Suspension, oral:

Pin-X® [OTC]: 144 mg/mL (30 mL, 60 mL)

Reese's Pinworm Medicine [OTC]: 144 mg/mL (30 mL, 60 mL, 240 mL)

Tablet, chewable, oral:

Pin-X® [OTC]: 720.5 mg

pyrazinamide (peer a ZIN a mide)

Synonyms pyrazinoic acid amide

Canadian Brand Names Tebrazid™

Therapeutic Category Antitubercular Agent

Use Adjunctive treatment of tuberculosis in combination with other antituberculosis agents

General Dosage Range Dosage adjustment recommended in patients with renal impairment

Oral:

Children: 15-30 mg/kg once daily (maximum: 2 g/day) **or** 50 mg/kg/dose twice weekly (maximum: 2 g/dose)

Adults 40-55 kg: 1000 mg once daily **or** 2000 mg twice weekly **or** 1500 mg 3 times/week

Adults 56-75 kg: 1500 mg once daily **or** 3000 mg twice weekly **or** 2500 mg 3 times/week

Adults 76-90 kg: 2000 mg once daily (maximum dose regardless of weight) **or** 4000 mg twice weekly (maximum dose regardless of weight) **or** 3000 mg 3 times/week (maximum dose regardless of weight)

Dosage Forms

Tablet, oral: 500 mg

pyrazinamide, rifampin, and isoniazid *see* rifampin, isoniazid, and pyrazinamide *on page 800*

pyrazinoic acid amide *see* pyrazinamide *on page 776*

pyrethrins and piperonyl butoxide (pye RE thrins & pi PER oh nil byo TOKS ide)

Synonyms piperonyl butoxide and pyrethrins

U.S. Brand Names A-200® Lice Treatment Kit [OTC]; A-200® Maximum Strength [OTC]; Licide® [OTC]; Pronto® Complete Lice Removal System [OTC]; Pronto® Plus Lice Killing Mousse Plus Vitamin E [OTC]; Pronto® Plus Lice Killing Mousse Shampoo Plus Natural Extracts and Oils [OTC]; Pronto® Plus Warm Oil Treatment and Conditioner [OTC]; RID® Maximum Strength [OTC]

Canadian Brand Names Pronto® Lice Control; R & C™ II; R & C™ Shampoo/Conditioner; RID® Mousse

Therapeutic Category Scabicides/Pediculicides

Use Treatment of *Pediculus humanus* infestations (head lice, body lice, pubic lice, and their eggs)

General Dosage Range Topical: *Children and Adults:* Apply to infested area, keep on for 10 minutes, wash, and rinse; may repeat once in a 24-hour period and then again in 7-10 days

Dosage Forms

Kit:

A-200® Lice Treatment Kit [OTC]:

Shampoo: Pyrethrins 0.33% and piperonyl butoxide 4% (120 mL)

Solution: Permethrin 0.5% (180 mL)

Pronto® Complete Lice Removal System [OTC]:

Shampoo: Pyrethrins 0.33% and piperonyl butoxide 4% (60 mL)

Solution, topical: Benzalkonium chloride 0.1% (60 mL)

Oil, topical:

Pronto® Plus Warm Oil Treatment and Conditioner [OTC]: Pyrethrins 0.33% and piperonyl butoxide 4% (36 mL)

Shampoo:

A-200® Maximum Strength [OTC]: Pyrethrins 0.33% and piperonyl butoxide 4% (60 mL, 120 mL)

Licide® [OTC], Pronto® Plus Lice Killing Mousse Shampoo Plus Vitamin E [OTC]: Pyrethrins 0.33% and piperonyl butoxide 4% (120 mL)

Pronto® Plus Lice Killing Mousse Shampoo Plus Natural Extracts and Oils [OTC]: Pyrethrins 0.33% and piperonyl butoxide 4% (60 mL)

Pronto® Plus Lice Killing Mousse Shampoo Plus Vitamin E [OTC]: Pyrethrins 0.33% and piperonyl butoxide 4% (120 mL)

RID® Maximum Strength [OTC]: Pyrethrins 0.33% and piperonyl butoxide 4% (60 mL, 120 mL, 180 mL, 240 mL)

Pyri-500 [OTC] *see* pyridoxine *on page 777*

2-pyridine aldoxime methochloride *see* pralidoxime *on page* 749

Pyridium® *see* phenazopyridine *on page* 711

pyridostigmine (peer id oh STIG meen)

Medication Safety Issues

Sound-alike/look-alike issues:

Pyridostigmine may be confused with physostigmine

Regonol® may be confused with Reglan®, Renagel®

Synonyms pyridostigmine bromide

U.S. Brand Names Mestinon®; Mestinon® Timespan®; Regonol®

Canadian Brand Names Mestinon®; Mestinon®-SR

Therapeutic Category Cholinergic Agent

Use Symptomatic treatment of myasthenia gravis; antagonism of nondepolarizing neuromuscular blockers

Military use: Pretreatment for Soman nerve gas exposure

General Dosage Range

I.M.:

Children: 0.05-0.15 mg/kg/dose

Adults: ~1/30th of oral dose

I.V.:

Children: 0.05-0.25 mg/kg/dose

Adults: IVP: ~1/30th of oral dose **or** 0.1-0.25 mg/kg/dose (usual: 10-20 mg); Infusion: 2 mg/hour with gradual titration in increments of 0.5-1 mg/hour (maximum: 4 mg/hour)

Oral:

Immediate release:

Children: 7 mg/kg/day divided into 5-6 doses

Adults: 60-1500 mg/day in 5-6 divided doses (usual: 600 mg/day)

Sustained release: *Adults:* 180-540 mg once or twice daily (doses separated by at least 6 hours)

Dosage Forms

Injection, solution:

Regonol®: 5 mg/mL (2 mL)

Syrup, oral:

Mestinon®: 60 mg/5 mL (480 mL)

Tablet, oral: 60 mg

Mestinon®: 60 mg

Tablet, sustained release, oral:

Mestinon® Timespan®: 180 mg

pyridostigmine bromide *see* pyridostigmine *on page* 777

pyridoxine (peer i DOKS een)

Medication Safety Issues

Sound-alike/look-alike issues:

Pyridoxine may be confused with paroxetine, pralidoxime, Pyridium®

International issues:

Doxal [Brazil] may be confused with Doxil brand name for DOXOrubicin [U.S.]

Doxal: Brand name for pyridoxine/thiamine combination [Brazil], but also the brand name for doxepin [Finland]

Synonyms B6; B_6; pyridoxine hydrochloride; vitamin B_6

U.S. Brand Names Aminoxin® [OTC]; Pyri-500 [OTC]

Therapeutic Category Vitamin, Water Soluble

Use Prevention and treatment of vitamin B_6 deficiency

General Dosage Range

I.M., I.V.: *Adults:* 10-20 mg/day

Oral:

Infants 1-6 months: Adequate intake: 0.1 mg/day
Infants 7-12 months: Adequate intake: 0.3 mg/day
Children 1-3 years: RDA: 0.5 mg
Children 4-8 years: RDA: 0.6 mg
Children 9-13 years: RDA: 1 mg
Children 14-18 years: RDA: 1.2 mg (females); 1.3 mg (males)
Adults 19-50 years: RDA: 1.3 mg
Adults ≥51 years: RDA: 1.5 mg (females); 1.7 mg (males)
Pregnancy: RDA: 1.9 mg
Lactation: RDA: 2 mg

Dosage Forms

Capsule, oral: 50 mg, 250 mg
Aminoxin® [OTC]: 20 mg
Injection, solution: 100 mg/mL (1 mL)
Liquid, oral: 200 mg/5 mL (120 mL)
Tablet, oral: 25 mg, 50 mg, 100 mg, 250 mg, 500 mg
Tablet, sustained release, oral:
Pyri-500 [OTC]: 500 mg

pyridoxine and doxylamine *see* doxylamine and pyridoxine *(Canada only) on page 316*

pyridoxine, folic acid, and cyanocobalamin *see* folic acid, cyanocobalamin, and pyridoxine *on page 404*

pyridoxine hydrochloride *see* pyridoxine *on page 777*

pyrilamine and phenylephrine *see* phenylephrine and pyrilamine *on page 717*

pyrilamine, chlorpheniramine, and phenylephrine *see* chlorpheniramine, pyrilamine, and phenylephrine *on page 203*

pyrilamine maleate and phenylephrine hydrochloride *see* phenylephrine and pyrilamine *on page 717*

pyrilamine maleate, dextromethorphan hydrobromide, and phenylephrine hydrochloride *see* phenylephrine, pyrilamine, and dextromethorphan *on page 718*

Pyril DM [OTC] *see* phenylephrine, pyrilamine, and dextromethorphan *on page 718*

pyrimethamine (peer i METH a meen)

Medication Safety Issues

Sound-alike/look-alike issues:
Daraprim® may be confused with Dantrium®, Daranide®

U.S. Brand Names Daraprim®

Canadian Brand Names Daraprim®

Therapeutic Category Folic Acid Antagonist (Antimalarial)

Use Prophylaxis of malaria due to susceptible strains of plasmodia; used in conjunction with a sulfonamide for the treatment of uncomplicated malaria due to susceptible strains of plasmodia (alternative agent; not preferred therapy); synergistic combination with sulfonamide in treatment of toxoplasmosis

General Dosage Range Oral:

Children <4 years: Malaria prophylaxis: 6.25 mg once weekly (maximum: 25 mg/dose)
Children 4-10 years: Malaria prophylaxis: 12.5 mg once weekly (maximum: 25 mg/dose); Malaria treatment: 25 mg daily
Children >10 years: Malaria prophylaxis: 25 mg once weekly; Malaria treatment: 25 mg daily
Children: Toxoplasmosis treatment: Loading dose: 1 mg/kg/day divided into 2 equal doses for 2-4 days; Maintenance: 0.5 mg/kg/day divided into 2 doses (maximum: 25 mg/day)
Adults: Malaria prophylaxis: 25 mg once weekly; Malaria treatment: 25-50 mg daily; Toxoplasmosis treatment: Initial: 50-75 mg/day; Maintenance: 12.5-37.5 mg/day

Dosage Forms

Tablet, oral:
Daraprim®: 25 mg

pyrimethamine and sulfadoxine *see* sulfadoxine and pyrimethamine *on page 860*

pyrithione zinc (peer i THYE one zingk)

Medication Safety Issues

Sound-alike/look-alike issues:

Pyrithione may be confused with Pyridium®

U.S. Brand Names BetaMed™ [OTC]; DermaZinc™ [OTC]; DHS™ Zinc [OTC]; Head & Shoulders® Citrus Breeze 2-in-1 [OTC]; Head & Shoulders® Citrus Breeze [OTC]; Head & Shoulders® Classic Clean 2-in-1 [OTC]; Head & Shoulders® Classic Clean [OTC]; Head & Shoulders® Dry Scalp 2-in-1 [OTC]; Head & Shoulders® Dry Scalp Care 2-in-1 [OTC]; Head & Shoulders® Dry Scalp Care [OTC]; Head & Shoulders® Dry Scalp [OTC]; Head & Shoulders® Extra Volume [OTC]; Head & Shoulders® intensive solutions 2 in 1 [OTC]; Head & Shoulders® intensive solutions for dry/damaged hair [OTC]; Head & Shoulders® intensive solutions for fine/oily hair [OTC]; Head & Shoulders® intensive solutions for normal hair [OTC]; Head & Shoulders® Ocean Lift 2-in-1 [OTC]; Head & Shoulders® Ocean Lift [OTC]; Head & Shoulders® Refresh 2-in-1 [OTC]; Head & Shoulders® Refresh [OTC]; Head & Shoulders® Restoring Shine 2 in 1 [OTC]; Head & Shoulders® Restoring Shine [OTC]; Head & Shoulders® Sensitive Care 2 in 1 [OTC]; Head & Shoulders® Sensitive Care [OTC]; Head & Shoulders® Smooth & Silky 2-in-1 [OTC]; Head & Shoulders® Smooth & Silky [OTC]; Selsun blue® Itchy Dry Scalp [OTC]; Selsun® Salon™ Classic [OTC] [DSC]; Selsun® Salon™ Dandruff 2-in-1 [OTC] [DSC]; Selsun® Salon™ Dandruff Volumizing [OTC] [DSC]; Skin Care™ [OTC]; T/Gel® Daily Control 2 in 1 Dandruff Shampoo Plus Conditioner [OTC]; T/Gel® Daily Control Dandruff Shampoo [OTC]; Zincon® [OTC]; ZNP® [OTC]

Therapeutic Category Antiseborrheic Agent, Topical

Use Relieves the itching, irritation, and scalp flaking associated with dandruff and/or seborrheal dermatitis

General Dosage Range **Topical:** *Adults:* Apply at least twice weekly

Dosage Forms

Bar, topical:

DermaZinc™ [OTC]: 2% (112.5 g)
ZNP® [OTC]: 2% (119 g)

Conditioner, topical:

Head & Shoulders® Classic Clean [OTC]: 0.5% (400 mL)
Head & Shoulders® Dry Scalp Care [OTC]: 0.5% (400 mL)

Cream, topical:

DermaZinc™ [OTC]: 0.25% (120 g)

Lotion, topical:

Skin Care™ [OTC]: 0.25% (120 mL)

Shampoo, topical:

BetaMed™ [OTC]: 2% (480 mL)
DermaZinc™ [OTC]: 2% (240 mL)
DHS™ Zinc [OTC]: 2% (240 mL, 360 mL)
Head & Shoulders® Citrus Breeze [OTC]: 1% (420 mL, 700 mL)
Head & Shoulders® Citrus Breeze 2-in-1 [OTC]: 1% (420 mL)
Head & Shoulders® Classic Clean [OTC]: 1% (50 mL, 420 mL, 700 mL, 1000 mL, 1200 mL)
Head & Shoulders® Classic Clean 2-in-1 [OTC]: 1% (420 mL, 700 mL)
Head & Shoulders® Dry Scalp [OTC]: 1% (420 mL)
Head & Shoulders® Dry Scalp 2-in-1 [OTC]: 1% (420 mL)
Head & Shoulders® Dry Scalp Care [OTC]: 1% (340 mL, 700 mL, 1200 mL)
Head & Shoulders® Dry Scalp Care 2-in-1 [OTC]: 1% (700 mL)
Head & Shoulders® Extra Volume [OTC]: 1% (420 mL, 700 mL)
Head & Shoulders® intensive solutions 2 in 1 [OTC]: 2% (241 mL)
Head & Shoulders® intensive solutions for dry/damaged hair [OTC]: 2% (251 mL)
Head & Shoulders® intensive solutions for fine/oily hair [OTC]: 2% (251 mL)
Head & Shoulders® intensive solutions for normal hair [OTC]: 2% (251 mL)
Head & Shoulders® Ocean Lift [OTC]: 1% (420 mL, 700 mL)
Head & Shoulders® Ocean Lift 2-in-1 [OTC]: 1% (420 mL, 700 mL)
Head & Shoulders® Refresh [OTC]: 1% (420 mL, 700 mL, 1000 mL, 1200 mL)
Head & Shoulders® Refresh 2-in-1 [OTC]: 1% (420 mL)
Head & Shoulders® Restoring Shine [OTC]: 1% (420 mL, 700 mL)
Head & Shoulders® Restoring Shine 2 in 1 [OTC]: 1% (420 mL)
Head & Shoulders® Sensitive Care [OTC]: 1% (420 mL, 700 mL)
Head & Shoulders® Sensitive Care 2 in 1 [OTC]: 1% (420 mL, 700 mL)
Head & Shoulders® Smooth & Silky [OTC]: 1% (420 mL, 700 mL)
Head & Shoulders® Smooth & Silky 2-in-1 [OTC]: 1% (420 mL)
Selsun blue® Itchy Dry Scalp [OTC]: 1% (207 mL, 325 mL)

T/Gel® Daily Control 2 in 1 Dandruff Shampoo Plus Conditioner [OTC]: 1% (250 mL)
T/Gel® Daily Control Dandruff Shampoo [OTC]: 1% (250 mL)
Zincon® [OTC]: 1% (120 mL, 240 mL)

Solution, topical:
DermaZinc™ [OTC]: 0.25% (120 mL)

QAB149 *see* indacaterol *on page 479*
Q-Alendronate (Can) *see* alendronate *on page 45*
Q-Amlodipine (Can) *see* amlodipine *on page 65*
Q-Citalopram (Can) *see* citalopram *on page 213*
Q-Cyclobenzaprine (Can) *see* cyclobenzaprine *on page 243*
Q-dryl [OTC] *see* diphenhydramine (systemic) *on page 292*
Q-Fluoxetine (Can) *see* fluoxetine *on page 396*
qinghao derivative *see* artesunate *on page 92*
qinghaosu derivative *see* artesunate *on page 92*
Q-Metformin (Can) *see* metformin *on page 579*
Qnasl™ *see* beclomethasone (nasal) *on page 117*
Qnexa *see* phentermine and topiramate *on page 714*
Q-Pantoprazole (Can) *see* pantoprazole *on page 689*
Q-Pap [OTC] *see* acetaminophen *on page 20*
Q-Pap Children's [OTC] *see* acetaminophen *on page 20*
Q-Pap Extra Strength [OTC] *see* acetaminophen *on page 20*
Q-Pap Infant's [OTC] *see* acetaminophen *on page 20*
Q-Simvastatin (Can) *see* simvastatin *on page 835*
Qsymia™ *see* phentermine and topiramate *on page 714*
Q-Tapp Cold & Allergy [OTC] *see* brompheniramine and pseudoephedrine *on page 144*
Q-Tapp Cold & Cough [OTC] *see* brompheniramine, pseudoephedrine, and dextromethorphan *on page 144*
Q-Terbinafine (Can) *see* terbinafine (systemic) *on page 878*
Q-Tussin [OTC] *see* guaifenesin *on page 433*
Q-Tussin DM [OTC] *see* guaifenesin and dextromethorphan *on page 434*
Quadramet® *see* samarium Sm 153 lexidronam *on page 821*
quadrivalent human papillomavirus vaccine *see* papillomavirus (types 6, 11, 16, 18) vaccine (human, recombinant) *on page 690*
Qualaquin® *see* quinine *on page 783*
Quasense® *see* ethinyl estradiol and levonorgestrel *on page 357*
quaternium-18 bentonite *see* bentoquatam *on page 120*

quazepam (KWAZ e pam)

Medication Safety Issues

Sound-alike/look-alike issues:
Quazepam may be confused with oxazepam

BEERS Criteria medication:
This drug may be potentially inappropriate for use in geriatric patients (Quality of evidence - high; Strength of recommendation - strong).

U.S. Brand Names Doral®

Canadian Brand Names Doral®

Therapeutic Category Benzodiazepine

Controlled Substance C-IV

Use Treatment of insomnia

General Dosage Range Oral:
Adults: 7.5-15 mg at bedtime
Elderly: Initial: 7.5 mg at bedtime

Dosage Forms

Tablet, oral:
Doral®: 15 mg

Quelicin® *see* succinylcholine *on page 855*
Quenalin [OTC] *see* diphenhydramine (systemic) *on page 292*
Questran® *see* cholestyramine resin *on page 205*
Questran® Light *see* cholestyramine resin *on page 205*
Questran® Light Sugar Free (Can) *see* cholestyramine resin *on page 205*

quetiapine (kwe TYE a peen)

Medication Safety Issues

Sound-alike/look-alike issues:

QUEtiapine may be confused with OLANZapine
SEROquel® may be confused with Serzone, SINEquan®

BEERS Criteria medication:

This drug may be potentially inappropriate for use in geriatric patients (Quality of evidence - moderate; Strength of recommendation - strong).

Synonyms quetiapine fumarate

Tall-Man QUEtiapine

U.S. Brand Names SEROquel XR®; SEROquel®

Canadian Brand Names Apo-Quetiapine®; CO Quetiapine; Dom-Quetiapine; JAMP-Quetiapine; Mylan-Quetiapine; PHL-Quetiapine; PMS-Quetiapine; PRO-Quetiapine; ratio-Quetiapine; Riva-Quetiapine; Sandoz-Quetiapine; Seroquel XR®; Seroquel®; Teva-Quetiapine

Therapeutic Category Antipsychotic Agent

Use Treatment of schizophrenia; treatment of acute manic or mixed episodes associated with bipolar I disorder (as monotherapy or in combination with lithium or divalproex); maintenance treatment of bipolar I disorder (in combination with lithium or divalproex); treatment of acute depressive episodes associated with bipolar disorder; adjunctive treatment of major depressive disorder

General Dosage Range Dosage adjustment recommended in patients with hepatic impairment

Oral:

Immediate release:

Children ≥10 years: Initial: 25 mg twice daily; Maintenance: Titrate to 50-800 mg/day
Adults: Initial: 25-50 mg twice daily; Maintenance: 150-800 mg/day in 2-3 divided doses
Elderly: Initial: 25 mg/day

Extended release:

Adults: Initial: 50-300 mg once daily; Maintenance: Titrate to 150-800 mg/day
Elderly: Initial: 50 mg/day

Dosage Forms

Tablet, oral: 25 mg, 50 mg, 100 mg, 150 mg, 200 mg, 300 mg, 400 mg
SEROquel®: 25 mg, 50 mg, 100 mg, 200 mg, 300 mg, 400 mg

Tablet, extended release, oral:
SEROquel XR®: 50 mg, 150 mg, 200 mg, 300 mg, 400 mg

quetiapine fumarate *see* quetiapine *on page 781*
quinalbarbitone sodium *see* secobarbital *on page 827*

quinapril (KWIN a pril)

Medication Safety Issues

Sound-alike/look-alike issues:

Accupril® may be confused with Accolate®, Accutane®, AcipHex®, Monopril®

International issues:

Accupril [U.S., Canada] may be confused with Acepril which is a brand name for captopril [Great Britain]; enalapril [Hungary, Switzerland]; lisinopril [Malaysia]

Synonyms quinapril hydrochloride

U.S. Brand Names Accupril®

Canadian Brand Names Accupril®

Therapeutic Category Angiotensin-Converting Enzyme (ACE) Inhibitor

Use Treatment of hypertension; treatment of heart failure

General Dosage Range Dosage adjustment recommended in patients with renal impairment

Oral:

Adults: Initial: 5-20 mg/day in 1-2 divided doses; Maintenance: 10-40 mg/day in 1-2 divided doses
Elderly: Initial: 2.5-5 mg/day

Dosage Forms

Tablet, oral: 5 mg, 10 mg, 20 mg, 40 mg

Accupril®: 5 mg, 10 mg, 20 mg, 40 mg

quinapril and hydrochlorothiazide (KWIN a pril & hye droe klor oh THYE a zide)

Synonyms hydrochlorothiazide and quinapril; Quinaretic

U.S. Brand Names Accuretic®

Canadian Brand Names Accuretic®

Therapeutic Category Antihypertensive Agent, Combination

Use Treatment of hypertension (not for initial therapy)

General Dosage Range Oral: *Adults:* Initial: 10-20 mg quinapril and 12.5 mg hydrochlorothiazide once daily; Maintenance: 5-40 mg quinapril and 6.25-25 mg hydrochlorothiazide once daily

Dosage Forms

Tablet, oral: 10/12.5: Quinapril 10 mg and hydrochlorothiazide 12.5 mg; 20/12.5: Quinapril 20 mg and hydrochlorothiazide 12.5 mg; 20/25: Quinapril 20 mg and hydrochlorothiazide 25 mg

Accuretic®: 10/12.5: Quinapril 10 mg and hydrochlorothiazide 12.5 mg; 20/12.5: Quinapril 20 mg and hydrochlorothiazide 12.5 mg; 20/25: Quinapril 20 mg and hydrochlorothiazide 25 mg

quinapril hydrochloride *see* quinapril *on page* 781

Quinaretic *see* quinapril and hydrochlorothiazide *on page* 782

Quinate® (Can) *see* quinidine *on page* 782

quinidine (KWIN i deen)

Medication Safety Issues

Sound-alike/look-alike issues:

QuiNIDine may be confused with cloNIDine, quiNINE

High alert medication:

The Institute for Safe Medication Practices (ISMP) includes this medication (I.V. formulation) among its list of drug classes which have a heightened risk of causing significant patient harm when used in error.

BEERS Criteria medication:

This drug may be potentially inappropriate for use in geriatric patients (Quality of evidence - high; Strength of recommendation - strong).

Synonyms quinidine gluconate; quinidine polygalacturonate; quinidine sulfate

Tall-Man qui**NID**ine

Canadian Brand Names Apo-Quinidine®; BioQuin® Durules™; Novo-Quinidin; Quinate®

Therapeutic Category Antiarrhythmic Agent, Class I-A

Use

Quinidine gluconate and sulfate salts: Conversion and prevention of relapse into atrial fibrillation and/or flutter; suppression of ventricular arrhythmias. **Note:** Due to proarrhythmic effects, use should be reserved for life-threatening arrhythmias. Moreover, the use of quinidine has largely been replaced by more effective/safer antiarrhythmic agents and/or nonpharmacologic therapies (eg, radiofrequency ablation).

Quinidine gluconate (I.V. formulation): Conversion of atrial fibrillation/flutter and ventricular tachycardia. **Note:** The use of I.V. quinidine gluconate for these indications has been replaced by more effective/safer antiarrhythmic agents (eg, amiodarone and procainamide).

Quinidine gluconate (I.V. formulation) and quinidine sulfate: Treatment of malaria (*Plasmodium falciparum*)

General Dosage Range Dosages expressed in terms of the salt. Dosage adjustment recommended in patients with renal impairment.

I.V.: Quinidine gluconate: *Children and Adults:* 10 mg/kg bolus followed by 0.02 mg/kg/minute **or** 24 mg/kg bolus followed by 12 mg/kg every 8 hours

Oral:

Immediate release: Quinidine sulfate: *Adults:* Initial: 200-400 mg/dose every 6 hours

Extended release:

Quinidine gluconate: *Adults:* Initial: 324 mg every 8-12 hours

Quinidine sulfate: *Adults:* Initial: 300 mg every 8-12 hours

Dosage Forms

Injection, solution: 80 mg/mL (10 mL)

Tablet, oral: 200 mg, 300 mg

Tablet, extended release, oral: 300 mg, 324 mg

quinidine and dextromethorphan *see* dextromethorphan and quinidine *on page 274*
quinidine gluconate *see* quinidine *on page 782*
quinidine polygalacturonate *see* quinidine *on page 782*
quinidine sulfate *see* quinidine *on page 782*

quinine (KWYE nine)

Medication Safety Issues
Sound-alike/look-alike issues:
QuiNINE may be confused with quiNIDine
Synonyms quinine sulfate
Tall-Man quiNINE
U.S. Brand Names Qualaquin®
Canadian Brand Names Apo-Quinine®; Novo-Quinine; Quinine-Odan
Therapeutic Category Antimalarial Agent
Use In conjunction with other antimalarial agents, treatment of uncomplicated chloroquine-resistant *P. falciparum* malaria
General Dosage Range Dosage adjustment recommended in patients with renal impairment
Oral:
Children: 30 mg/kg/day divided every 8 hours
Adults: 648 mg every 8 hours
Dosage Forms
Capsule, oral: 324 mg
Qualaquin®: 324 mg

Quinine-Odan (Can) *see* quinine *on page 783*
quinine sulfate *see* quinine *on page 783*
Quinnostik *see* urea *on page 930*
quinol *see* hydroquinone *on page 461*
Quintabs [OTC] *see* vitamins (multiple/oral) *on page 951*
Quintabs-M [OTC] *see* vitamins (multiple/oral) *on page 951*
Quintabs-M Iron-Free [OTC] *see* vitamins (multiple/oral) *on page 951*

quinupristin and dalfopristin (kwi NYOO pris tin & dal FOE pris tin)

Synonyms dalfopristin and quinupristin; RP-59500
U.S. Brand Names Synercid®
Canadian Brand Names Synercid®
Therapeutic Category Antibiotic, Streptogramin
Use Treatment of complicated skin and skin structure infections caused by methicillin-susceptible *Staphylococcus aureus* or *Streptococcus pyogenes*
General Dosage Range I.V.: *Children ≥12 years and Adults:* 7.5 mg/kg every 12 hours
Dosage Forms
Injection, powder for reconstitution:
Synercid®: 500 mg: Quinupristin 150 mg and dalfopristin 350 mg

Quixin® *see* levofloxacin (ophthalmic) *on page 532*
Qutenza™ *see* capsaicin *on page 170*
QVAR® *see* beclomethasone (oral inhalation) *on page 117*
R & C™ II (Can) *see* pyrethrins and piperonyl butoxide *on page 776*
R & C™ Shampoo/Conditioner (Can) *see* pyrethrins and piperonyl butoxide *on page 776*
R-1569 *see* tocilizumab *on page 902*
R093877 *see* prucalopride *(Canada only) on page 771*
R108512 *see* prucalopride *(Canada only) on page 771*
RabAvert® *see* rabies vaccine *on page 784*

rabeprazole (ra BEP ra zole)

Medication Safety Issues

Sound-alike/look-alike issues:

AcipHex® may be confused with Acephen™, Accupril®, Aricept®, pHisoHex®

RABEprazole may be confused with ARIPiprazole, donepezil, lansoprazole, omeprazole, raloxifene

Synonyms pariprazole

Tall-Man **RABE**prazole

U.S. Brand Names AcipHex®

Canadian Brand Names Apo-Rabeprazole®; Pariet®; Pat-Rabeprazole; PMS-Rabeprazole EC; PRO-Rabeprazole; Rabeprazole EC; RAN™-Rabeprazole; Riva-Rabeprazole EC; Sandoz-Rabeprazole; Teva-Rabeprazole EC

Therapeutic Category Gastric Acid Secretion Inhibitor

Use Short-term (4-8 weeks) treatment and maintenance of erosive or ulcerative gastroesophageal reflux disease (GERD); symptomatic GERD; short-term (up to 4 weeks) treatment of duodenal ulcers; long-term treatment of pathological hypersecretory conditions, including Zollinger-Ellison syndrome; *H. pylori* eradication (in combination therapy)

Canadian labeling: Additional uses (not in U.S. labeling): Treatment of nonerosive reflux disease (NERD); treatment of gastric ulcers

General Dosage Range Oral:

Children ≥12 years: 20 mg/day

Adults: 10-20 mg once to twice daily **or** 60 mg once daily

Dosage Forms

Tablet, delayed release, enteric coated, oral:

AcipHex®: 20 mg

Dosage Forms - Canada

Tablet, delayed release, enteric coated:

Pariet®: 10 mg, 20 mg

Rabeprazole EC (Can) *see* rabeprazole *on page 784*

rabies immune globulin (human) (RAY beez i MYUN GLOB yoo lin, HYU man)

Synonyms HRIG; RIG

U.S. Brand Names HyperRAB® S/D; Imogam® Rabies-HT

Canadian Brand Names HyperRAB® S/D; Imogam® Rabies Pasteurized

Therapeutic Category Immune Globulin

Use Part of postexposure prophylaxis of persons with rabies exposure. Provides passive immunity until active immunity with rabies vaccine is established. Not for use in persons with a history of preexposure vaccination, history of postexposure prophylaxis, or previous vaccination with rabies vaccine and documentation of antibody response.

General Dosage Range Local wound infiltration/I.M.: *Children and Adults:* 20 units/kg in a single dose

Dosage Forms

Injection, solution [preservative free]:

HyperRAB® S/D: 150 units/mL (2 mL, 10 mL)

Imogam® Rabies-HT: 150 units/mL (2 mL, 10 mL)

rabies vaccine (RAY beez vak SEEN)

Synonyms HDCV; human diploid cell cultures rabies vaccine; PCEC; purified chick embryo cell

U.S. Brand Names Imovax® Rabies; RabAvert®

Canadian Brand Names Imovax® Rabies; RabAvert®

Therapeutic Category Vaccine, Inactivated Virus

Use Preexposure and postexposure vaccination against rabies

The Advisory Committee on Immunization Practices (ACIP) recommends a primary course of prophylactic immunization (preexposure vaccination) for the following:

- Persons with continuous risk of infection, including rabies research laboratory and biologics production workers
- Persons with frequent risk of infection in areas where rabies is enzootic, including rabies diagnostic laboratory workers, cavers, veterinarians and their staff, and animal control and wildlife workers; persons who frequently handle bats

- Persons with infrequent risk of infection, including veterinarians and animal control staff with terrestrial animals in areas where rabies infection is rare, veterinary students, and travelers visiting areas where rabies is enzootic and immediate access to medical care and biologicals is limited

The ACIP recommends the use of postexposure vaccination for a particular person be assessed by the severity and likelihood versus the actual risk of acquiring rabies. Consideration should include the type of exposure, epidemiology of rabies in the area, species of the animal, circumstances of the incident, and the availability of the exposing animal for observation or rabies testing. Postexposure vaccination is used in both previously vaccinated and previously unvaccinated individuals.

General Dosage Range I.M.: *Children and Adults:* 1 mL

Dosage Forms

Injection, powder for reconstitution [preservative free]:

Imovax® Rabies: ≥2.5 units

RabAvert®: ≥2.5 units

racemic epinephrine *see* epinephrine (systemic, oral inhalation) *on page 334*

racepinephrine *see* epinephrine (systemic, oral inhalation) *on page 334*

RAD001 *see* everolimus *on page 367*

Radiogardase® *see* ferric hexacyanoferrate *on page 379*

rAHF *see* antihemophilic factor (recombinant) *on page 78*

RAL *see* raltegravir *on page 785*

R-albuterol *see* levalbuterol *on page 528*

Ralivia™ (Can) *see* tramadol *on page 909*

raloxifene (ral OKS i feen)

Medication Safety Issues

Sound-alike/look-alike issues:

Evista® may be confused with AVINza®, Eovist®

Synonyms keoxifene hydrochloride; raloxifene hydrochloride

U.S. Brand Names Evista®

Canadian Brand Names Apo-Raloxifene®; Evista®; Novo-Raloxifene; Teva-Raloxifene

Therapeutic Category Selective Estrogen Receptor Modulator (SERM)

Use Prevention and treatment of osteoporosis in postmenopausal women; risk reduction for invasive breast cancer in postmenopausal women with osteoporosis and in postmenopausal women with high risk for invasive breast cancer

General Dosage Range Oral: *Adults (females):* 60 mg/day

Dosage Forms

Tablet, oral:

Evista®: 60 mg

raloxifene hydrochloride *see* raloxifene *on page 785*

raltegravir (ral TEG ra vir)

Synonyms MK-0518; RAL

U.S. Brand Names Isentress®

Canadian Brand Names Isentress®

Therapeutic Category Antiretroviral Agent, Integrase Inhibitor

Use Treatment of HIV-1 infection in combination with other antiretroviral agents

General Dosage Range Dosage adjustment recommended in patients on concomitant therapy

Oral:

Children 2 to <6 years: Chewable tablet: Weight-based dosing: 75-300 mg twice daily

Children 6 to <12 years: Chewable tablet: Weight-based dosing: 75-300 mg twice daily; if ≥25 kg, refer to weight-based dosing or adult dosing

Adolescents ≥12 years and Adults: Film-coated tablet: 400 mg twice daily

Product Availability Isentress® chewable tablets (25 mg, 100 mg): FDA approved December 2011; availability anticipated mid-2012

Dosage Forms

Tablet, oral:

Isentress®: 400 mg

raltitrexed *(Canada only)* (ral ti TREX ed)

Medication Safety Issues

Sound-alike/look-alike issues:

Raltitrexed may be confused with methotrexate, PEMEtrexed, PRALAtrexate

High alert medication:

This medication is in a class the Institute for Safe Medication Practices (ISMP) includes among its list of drug classes which have a heightened risk of causing significant patient harm when used in error.

Synonyms D1694; ICI-D1694; raltitrexed disodium; TDX; ZD1694

Canadian Brand Names Tomudex®

Therapeutic Category Antineoplastic Agent

Use Treatment of advanced colorectal cancer

General Dosage Range Dosage adjustment recommended in patients with renal impairment or who develop toxicities

I.V.: *Adults:* 3 mg/m^2 every 3 weeks

Product Availability Not available in U.S.

Dosage Forms - Canada

Injection, powder for reconstitution, as disodium:

Tomudex®: 2 mg

raltitrexed disodium *see* raltitrexed *(Canada only) on page 786*

ramelteon (ra MEL tee on)

Medication Safety Issues

Sound-alike/look-alike issues:

Ramelteon may be confused with Remeron®

Rozerem® may be confused with Razadyne®, Remeron®

Synonyms TAK-375

U.S. Brand Names Rozerem®

Therapeutic Category Hypnotic, Miscellaneous

Use Treatment of insomnia characterized by difficulty with sleep onset

General Dosage Range Oral: *Adults:* 8 mg at bedtime

Dosage Forms

Tablet, oral:

Rozerem®: 8 mg

ramipril (RA mi pril)

Medication Safety Issues

Sound-alike/look-alike issues:

Ramipril may be confused with enalapril, Monopril®

Altace® may be confused with Altace® HCT, alteplase, Amaryl®, Amerge®, Artane

U.S. Brand Names Altace®

Canadian Brand Names Altace®; Apo-Ramipril®; Ava-Ramipril; CO Ramipril; Dom-Ramipril; JAMP-Ramipril; Mylan-Ramipril; PHL-Ramipril; PMS-Ramipril; RAN™-Ramipril; ratio-Ramipril; Sandoz-Ramipril; Teva-Ramipril

Therapeutic Category Angiotensin-Converting Enzyme (ACE) Inhibitor

Use Treatment of hypertension, alone or in combination with thiazide diuretics; treatment of left ventricular dysfunction after MI; to reduce risk of MI, stroke, and death in patients at increased risk for these events

General Dosage Range Dosage adjustment recommended in patients with renal impairment

Oral: *Adults:* 2.5-20 mg/day (maximum: 20 mg/day)

Dosage Forms

Capsule, oral: 1.25 mg, 2.5 mg, 5 mg, 10 mg

Altace®: 1.25 mg, 2.5 mg, 5 mg, 10 mg

ramipril and felodipine *(Canada only)* (RA mi pril & fe LOE di peen)

Synonyms felodipine and ramipril; ramipril and felodipine ER

Canadian Brand Names Altace® Plus Felodipine

Therapeutic Category Antihypertensive Agent, Combination

Use Treatment of hypertension when combination therapy is appropriate (not for initial therapy)

General Dosage Range Dosage adjustment recommended in patients with hepatic or renal impairment

Oral:

Adults: Ramipril 2.5-10 mg and felodipine ER 2.5-10 mg once daily

Elderly: Initial: Felodipine ER: 2.5 mg daily (maximum: 10 mg/day)

Product Availability Not available in U.S.

Dosage Forms - Canada

Tablet, variable release, oral:

Altace® Plus Felodipine 2.5/2.5: Ramipril 2.5 mg [immediate release] and felodipine 2.5 mg [extended release]

Altace® Plus Felodipine 5/5: Ramipril 5 mg [immediate release] and felodipine 5 mg [extended release]

ramipril and felodipine ER *see* ramipril and felodipine *(Canada only) on page 786*

ramipril and hydrochlorothiazide *(Canada only)*

(RA mi pril & hye droe klor oh THYE a zide)

Medication Safety Issues

Sound-alike/look-alike issues:

Altace® HCT may be confused with alteplase, Artane, Altace®

Synonyms hydrochlorothiazide and ramipril

Canadian Brand Names Altace® HCT; PMS-Ramipril HCTZ

Therapeutic Category Angiotensin-Converting Enzyme (ACE) Inhibitor; Antihypertensive Agent, Combination; Diuretic, Thiazide

Use Treatment of essential hypertension (not for initial therapy)

General Dosage Range Dosage adjustment recommended in patients with renal impairment

Oral: *Adults:* Ramipril 2.5 mg/hydrochlorothiazide 12.5 mg once daily (maximum: Ramipril 10 mg/hydrochlorothiazide 50 mg once daily)

Product Availability Not available in U.S.

Dosage Forms - Canada

Tablet, oral:

Altace® HCT: 2.5/12.5: Ramipril 2.5 mg and hydrochlorothiazide 12.5 mg; 5/12.5: Ramipril 5 mg and hydrochlorothiazide 12.5 mg; 5/25: Ramipril 5 mg and hydrochlorothiazide 25 mg; 10/12.5: Ramipril 10 mg and hydrochlorothiazide 12.5 mg;10/25: Ramipril 10 mg and hydrochlorothiazide 25 mg

RAN™-Amlodipine (Can) *see* amlodipine *on page 65*

RAN™-Atenolol (Can) *see* atenolol *on page 99*

RAN™-Atorvastatin (Can) *see* atorvastatin *on page 100*

RAN™-Carvedilol (Can) *see* carvedilol *on page 179*

RAN™-Cefprozil (Can) *see* cefprozil *on page 185*

RAN™-Ciprofloxacin (Can) *see* ciprofloxacin (systemic) *on page 210*

RAN™-Citalo (Can) *see* citalopram *on page 213*

RAN™-Clarithromycin (Can) *see* clarithromycin *on page 215*

RAN™-Domperidone (Can) *see* domperidone *(Canada only) on page 308*

RAN™-Enalapril (Can) *see* enalapril *on page 330*

Ranexa® *see* ranolazine *on page 789*

RAN™-Fentanyl Matrix Patch (Can) *see* fentanyl *on page 377*

RAN™-Fentanyl Transdermal System (Can) *see* fentanyl *on page 377*

RAN™-Fosinopril (Can) *see* fosinopril *on page 409*

RAN™-Gabapentin (Can) *see* gabapentin *on page 413*

ranibizumab (ra ni BIZ oo mab)

Synonyms rhuFabV2

U.S. Brand Names Lucentis®

Canadian Brand Names Lucentis®

Therapeutic Category Monoclonal Antibody; Ophthalmic Agent; Vascular Endothelial Growth Factor (VEGF) Inhibitor

Use Treatment of neovascular (wet) age-related macular degeneration (AMD); treatment of macular edema following retinal vein occlusion (RVO); diabetic macular edema (DME)

General Dosage Range **Intravitreal:** *Adults:* 0.3 mg or 0.5 mg once every 1-3 months

Dosage Forms

Injection, solution [preservative free]:

Lucentis®: 0.3 mg/0.05 mL (0.05 mL); 0.5 mg/0.05 mL (0.05 mL)

Dosage Forms - Canada

Injection, solution [preservative free]:

Lucentis®: 10 mg/mL (0.3 mL)

RAN™-Imipenem-Cilastatin (Can) *see* imipenem and cilastatin *on page 475*
Ran™-Irbesartan HCTZ (Can) *see* irbesartan and hydrochlorothiazide *on page 501*

ranitidine (ra NI ti deen)

Medication Safety Issues

Sound-alike/look-alike issues:

Ranitidine may be confused with amantadine, rimantadine

Zantac® may be confused with Xanax®, Zarontin®, Zofran®, ZyrTEC®

Synonyms ranitidine hydrochloride

U.S. Brand Names Zantac 150® [OTC]; Zantac 75® [OTC]; Zantac®; Zantac® EFFERdose®

Canadian Brand Names Acid Reducer; Apo-Ranitidine®; CO Ranitidine; Dom-Ranitidine; Myl-Ranitidine; Mylan-Ranitidine; Nu-Ranit; PHL-Ranitidine; PMS-Ranitidine; Ranitidine Injection, USP; RAN™-Ranitidine; ratio-Ranitidine; Riva-Ranitidine; Sandoz-Ranitidine; ScheinPharm Ranitidine; Teva-Ranitidine; Zantac 75®; Zantac Maximum Strength Non-Prescription; Zantac®

Therapeutic Category Histamine H_2 Antagonist

Use

Zantac®: Short-term and maintenance therapy of duodenal ulcer, gastric ulcer, gastroesophageal reflux disease (GERD), active benign ulcer, erosive esophagitis, and pathological hypersecretory conditions; as part of a multidrug regimen for *H. pylori* eradication to reduce the risk of duodenal ulcer recurrence

Zantac 75® [OTC]: Relief of heartburn, acid indigestion, and sour stomach

General Dosage Range Dosage adjustment recommended in patients with renal impairment

I.M.: *Children >16 years and Adults:* 50 mg every 6-8 hours

I.V.:

Children 1 month to 16 years: 2-4 mg/kg/day divided every 6-8 hours (maximum: 200 mg/day) **or** 1 mg/kg/dose for one dose followed by infusion of 0.08-0.17 mg/kg/hour

Children >16 years and Adults: 50 mg every 6-8 hours **or** Infusion: 6.25 mg/hour **or** 1-2.5 mg/kg/hour

Oral:

Children 1 month to 11 years: 2-4 mg/kg/dose once or twice daily **or** 5-10 mg/kg/day in 2 divided doses (maximum: 300 mg/day)

Children ≥12 to 16 years: 2-4 mg/kg once or twice daily **or** 5-10 mg/kg/day in 2 divided doses (maximum: 300 mg/day); OTC dosing: 75 mg 30-60 minutes before eating or drinking (maximum: 150 mg/day)

Children >16 years and Adults: 150 mg 1-4 times/day **or** 300 mg once daily; OTC dosing: 75 mg 30-60 minutes before eating or drinking (maximum: 150 mg/day)

Dosage Forms

Capsule, oral: 150 mg, 300 mg

Infusion, premixed in 1/2 NS [preservative free]:

Zantac®: 50 mg (50 mL)

Injection, solution: 25 mg/mL (2 mL, 6 mL, 40 mL)

Zantac®: 25 mg/mL (2 mL, 6 mL, 40 mL)

Syrup, oral: 15 mg/mL (1 mL, 5 mL, 10 mL, 120 mL, 473 mL, 474 mL, 480 mL)

Zantac®: 15 mg/mL (480 mL)

Tablet, oral: 75 mg, 150 mg, 300 mg

Zantac 150® [OTC]: 150 mg

Zantac 75® [OTC]: 75 mg

Zantac®: 150 mg, 300 mg

Tablet for solution, oral:

Zantac® EFFERdose®: 25 mg

ranitidine hydrochloride *see* ranitidine *on page 788*
Ranitidine Injection, USP (Can) *see* ranitidine *on page 788*
RAN™-Lisinopril (Can) *see* lisinopril *on page 544*
RAN™-Lovastatin (Can) *see* lovastatin *on page 553*
RAN™-Metformin (Can) *see* metformin *on page 579*

ranolazine (ra NOE la zeen)

Medication Safety Issues

Sound-alike/look-alike issues:

Ranexa® may be confused with CeleXA®

U.S. Brand Names Ranexa®

Therapeutic Category Cardiovascular Agent, Miscellaneous

Use Treatment of chronic angina

General Dosage Range Dosage adjustment recommended in patients on concomitant therapy

Oral: *Adults:* Initial: 500 mg twice daily; Maintenance: 500-1000 mg twice daily (maximum: 2000 mg/day)

Dosage Forms

Tablet, extended release, oral:

Ranexa®: 500 mg, 1000 mg

RAN™-Ondansetron (Can) *see* ondansetron *on page 667*
RAN™-Pantoprazole (Can) *see* pantoprazole *on page 689*
RAN™-Pravastatin (Can) *see* pravastatin *on page 752*
RAN™-Rabeprazole (Can) *see* rabeprazole *on page 784*
RAN™-Ramipril (Can) *see* ramipril *on page 786*
RAN™-Ranitidine (Can) *see* ranitidine *on page 788*
RAN™-Risperidone (Can) *see* risperidone *on page 803*
RAN™-Ropinirole (Can) *see* ropinirole *on page 810*
RAN™-Rosuvastatin (Can) *see* rosuvastatin *on page 812*
RAN™-Simvastatin (Can) *see* simvastatin *on page 835*
RAN™-Tamsulosin (Can) *see* tamsulosin *on page 868*
Ran-Valsartan (Can) *see* valsartan *on page 935*
Ran-Venlafaxine XR (Can) *see* venlafaxine *on page 942*
RAN™-Zopiclone (Can) *see* zopiclone *(Canada only) on page 967*
Rapaflo® *see* silodosin *on page 833*
Rapamune® *see* sirolimus *on page 836*
rapamycin *see* sirolimus *on page 836*
RapiMed® Children's [OTC] *see* acetaminophen *on page 20*
RapiMed® Junior [OTC] *see* acetaminophen *on page 20*

rasagiline (ra SA ji leen)

Medication Safety Issues

Sound-alike/look-alike issues:

Azilect® may be confused with Aricept®

Synonyms AGN 1135; rasagiline mesylate; TVP-1012

U.S. Brand Names Azilect®

Canadian Brand Names Azilect®

Therapeutic Category Anti-Parkinson Agent, MAO Type B Inhibitor

Use Treatment of idiopathic Parkinson disease (initial monotherapy or as adjunct to levodopa)

General Dosage Range Dosage adjustment recommended in patients with hepatic impairment or on concomitant therapy

Oral: *Adults:* 0.5-1 mg once daily

Dosage Forms

Tablet, oral:

Azilect®: 0.5 mg, 1 mg

rasagiline mesylate *see* rasagiline *on page 789*

rasburicase (ras BYOOR i kayse)

Synonyms recombinant urate oxidase; urate oxidase

U.S. Brand Names Elitek®

Canadian Brand Names Fasturtec®

Therapeutic Category Enzyme

Use Initial management of uric acid levels in patients with leukemia, lymphoma, and solid tumor malignancies receiving chemotherapy expected to result in tumor lysis and elevation of plasma uric acid

General Dosage Range I.V.: *Children and Adults:* 0.2 mg/kg once daily

Dosage Forms

Injection, powder for reconstitution:

Elitek®: 1.5 mg, 7.5 mg

Rasilez® (Can) *see* aliskiren *on page* 47
Rasilez HCT® (Can) *see* aliskiren and hydrochlorothiazide *on page* 48
rATG *see* antithymocyte globulin (rabbit) *on page* 80
ratio-Aclavulanate (Can) *see* amoxicillin and clavulanate *on page* 70
ratio-Acyclovir (Can) *see* acyclovir (systemic) *on page* 34
ratio-Alendronate (Can) *see* alendronate *on page* 45
ratio-Amcinonide (Can) *see* amcinonide *on page* 59
ratio-Amiodarone (Can) *see* amiodarone *on page* 63
ratio-Amlodipine (Can) *see* amlodipine *on page* 65
ratio-Atenolol (Can) *see* atenolol *on page* 99
ratio-Atorvastatin (Can) *see* atorvastatin *on page* 100
ratio-Azithromycin (Can) *see* azithromycin (systemic) *on page* 108
ratio-Baclofen (Can) *see* baclofen *on page* 112
ratio-Bicalutamide (Can) *see* bicalutamide *on page* 133
ratio-Bisacodyl [OTC] (Can) *see* bisacodyl *on page* 134
ratio-Brimonidine (Can) *see* brimonidine *on page* 141
ratio-Bupropion SR (Can) *see* bupropion *on page* 150
ratio-Carvedilol (Can) *see* carvedilol *on page* 179
ratio-Cefuroxime (Can) *see* cefuroxime *on page* 187
ratio-Ciprofloxacin (Can) *see* ciprofloxacin (systemic) *on page* 210
ratio-Citalopram (Can) *see* citalopram *on page* 213
ratio-Clarithromycin (Can) *see* clarithromycin *on page* 215
ratio-Clobetasol (Can) *see* clobetasol *on page* 221
ratio-Clonazepam (Can) *see* clonazepam *on page* 223
ratio-Codeine (Can) *see* codeine *on page* 230
ratio-Cotridin (Can) *see* triprolidine, pseudoephedrine, and codeine *(Canada only) on page* 922
ratio-Cyclobenzaprine (Can) *see* cyclobenzaprine *on page* 243
ratio-Dexamethasone (Can) *see* dexamethasone (systemic) *on page* 266
ratio-Diltiazem CD (Can) *see* diltiazem *on page* 288
ratio-Domperidone (Can) *see* domperidone *(Canada only) on page* 308
ratio-Ectosone (Can) *see* betamethasone *on page* 129
ratio-Emtec (Can) *see* acetaminophen and codeine *on page* 22
ratio-Enalapril (Can) *see* enalapril *on page* 330
ratio-Fenofibrate MC (Can) *see* fenofibrate *on page* 375
ratio-Fentanyl (Can) *see* fentanyl *on page* 377
ratio-Finasteride (Can) *see* finasteride *on page* 384
ratio-Fluoxetine (Can) *see* fluoxetine *on page* 396
ratio-Fluticasone (Can) *see* fluticasone (nasal) *on page* 400
ratio-Gabapentin (Can) *see* gabapentin *on page* 413
ratio-Gentamicin (Can) *see* gentamicin (topical) *on page* 424
ratio-Glimepiride (Can) *see* glimepiride *on page* 426
ratio-Glyburide (Can) *see* glyburide *on page* 428
ratio-Indomethacin (Can) *see* indomethacin *on page* 480
ratio-Ipra-Sal (Can) *see* albuterol *on page* 41
ratio-Ipra Sal UDV (Can) *see* ipratropium and albuterol *on page* 499
ratio-Irbesartan (Can) *see* irbesartan *on page* 500
ratio-Irbesartan HCTZ (Can) *see* irbesartan and hydrochlorothiazide *on page* 501

regadenoson (re ga DEN of son)

Synonyms CVT-3146
U.S. Brand Names Lexiscan®

Therapeutic Category Diagnostic Agent

Use Radionuclide myocardial perfusion imaging (MPI) in patients unable to undergo adequate exercise stress testing

General Dosage Range I.V.: *Adults:* 0.4 mg (5 mL) as a single dose

Dosage Forms

Injection, solution [preservative free]:

Lexiscan®: 0.08 mg/mL (5 mL)

Regenecare® *see* lidocaine (topical) *on page* 535
Regenecare® HA [OTC] *see* lidocaine (topical) *on page* 535
Regitine [DSC] *see* phentolamine *on page* 715
Regitine® (Can) *see* phentolamine *on page* 715
Reglan® *see* metoclopramide *on page* 594
Regonol® *see* pyridostigmine *on page* 777
Regranex® *see* becaplermin *on page* 117
regular insulin *see* insulin regular *on page* 489
Regulex® (Can) *see* docusate *on page* 304
Reguloid [OTC] *see* psyllium *on page* 774
Rejuva-A® (Can) *see* tretinoin (topical) *on page* 914
Relafen *see* nabumetone *on page* 623
Relafen® (Can) *see* nabumetone *on page* 623
Relenza® *see* zanamivir *on page* 959
Relistor® *see* methylnaltrexone *on page* 590
Relpax® *see* eletriptan *on page* 326
Remeron® *see* mirtazapine *on page* 606
Remeron® RD (Can) *see* mirtazapine *on page* 606
Remeron SolTab® *see* mirtazapine *on page* 606
Remeven™ *see* urea *on page* 930
Remicade® *see* infliximab *on page* 481

remifentanil (rem i FEN ta nil)

Medication Safety Issues

Sound-alike/look-alike issues:

Remifentanil may be confused with alfentanil

High alert medication:

The Institute for Safe Medication Practices (ISMP) includes this medication among its list of drug classes which have a heightened risk of causing significant patient harm when used in error.

Synonyms GI87084B

U.S. Brand Names Ultiva®

Canadian Brand Names Ultiva®

Therapeutic Category Analgesic, Narcotic

Controlled Substance C-II

Use Analgesic for use during the induction and maintenance of general anesthesia; for continued analgesia into the immediate postoperative period; analgesic component of monitored anesthesia

General Dosage Range I.V.:

Infants Birth to 2 months: Infusion: 0.4-1 mcg/kg/minute; Supplemental bolus dose: ≤1 mcg/kg
Children 1-12 years: Infusion: 0.05-1.3 mcg/kg/minute; Bolus: 1 mcg/kg every 2-5 minutes
Adults: Infusion: 0.025-4 mcg/kg/minute; Bolus: 0.5-1 mcg/kg every 2-5 minutes
Elderly: Doses should be decreased by 50% and titrated

Dosage Forms

Injection, powder for reconstitution:

Ultiva®: 1 mg, 2 mg, 5 mg

Reminyl® (Can) *see* galantamine *on page* 417
Reminyl® ER (Can) *see* galantamine *on page* 417
Remodulin® *see* treprostinil *on page* 913
Renacidin® *see* citric acid, magnesium carbonate, and glucono-delta-lactone *on page* 214

Renagel® *see* sevelamer *on page 831*
renal replacement solution *see* electrolyte solution, renal replacement *on page 325*
Renax® *see* vitamins (multiple/oral) *on page 951*
Renax® 5.5 *see* vitamins (multiple/oral) *on page 951*
Renedil® (Can) *see* felodipine *on page 374*
Renova® *see* tretinoin (topical) *on page 914*
Renvela® *see* sevelamer *on page 831*
Reopro® *see* abciximab *on page 17*
ReoPro® (Can) *see* abciximab *on page 17*

repaglinide (re PAG li nide)

Medication Safety Issues

Sound-alike/look-alike issues:

Prandin® may be confused with Avandia®

High alert medication:

The Institute for Safe Medication Practices (ISMP) includes this medication among its list of drug classes which have a heightened risk of causing significant patient harm when used in error.

U.S. Brand Names Prandin®

Canadian Brand Names CO-Repaglinide; GlucoNorm®; PMS-Repaglinide; Sandoz-Repaglinide

Therapeutic Category Hypoglycemic Agent, Oral

Use Management of type 2 diabetes mellitus (noninsulin-dependent, NIDDM) as an adjunct to diet and exercise; may be used in combination with metformin or thiazolidinediones

General Dosage Range Dosage adjustment recommended in patients with renal impairment

Oral: *Adults:* Initial: 0.5-2 mg before each meal; Maintenance: 0.5-4 mg before each meal (maximum: 16 mg/day)

Dosage Forms

Tablet, oral:

Prandin®: 0.5 mg, 1 mg, 2 mg

repaglinide and metformin (re PAG li nide & met FOR min)

Medication Safety Issues

Sound-alike/look-alike issues:

PrandiMet® may be confused with Avandamet®, Prandin®

High alert medication:

The Institute for Safe Medication Practices (ISMP) includes this medication among its list of drug classes which have a heightened risk of causing significant patient harm when used in error.

Synonyms metformin and repaglinide; repaglinide and metformin hydrochloride

U.S. Brand Names PrandiMet®

Therapeutic Category Antidiabetic Agent, Biguanide; Antidiabetic Agent, Meglitinide Derivative; Hypoglycemic Agent, Oral

Use Management of type 2 diabetes mellitus (noninsulin-dependent, NIDDM), as an adjunct to diet and exercise, in patients currently receiving or not adequately controlled on metformin and/or a meglitinide

General Dosage Range Oral: *Adults:* Repaglinide 1-2 mg and metformin 500 mg 2-3 times daily with meals (maximum single dose: 4 mg/dose [repaglinide], 1000 mg/dose [metformin]; maximum daily dose: 10 mg/day [repaglinide], 2500 mg/day [metformin])

Dosage Forms

Tablet:

PrandiMet®: 1/500: Repaglinide 1 mg and metformin hydrochloride 500 mg; 2/500: Repaglinide 2 mg and metformin hydrochloride 500 mg

repaglinide and metformin hydrochloride *see* repaglinide and metformin *on page 794*
Repan® *see* butalbital, acetaminophen, and caffeine *on page 153*
Replace [OTC] *see* vitamins (multiple/oral) *on page 951*
Replace Without Iron [OTC] *see* vitamins (multiple/oral) *on page 951*
Replagal® (Can) *see* agalsidase alfa *(Canada only) on page 39*
Repliva 21/7® *see* vitamins (multiple/oral) *on page 951*
Reprexain™ *see* hydrocodone and ibuprofen *on page 456*
Repronex® *see* menotropins *on page 573*

Requa® Activated Charcoal [OTC] *see* charcoal, activated *on page* 193
Requip® *see* ropinirole *on page* 810
Requip® XL™ *see* ropinirole *on page* 810
Rescon DM [OTC] *see* chlorpheniramine, pseudoephedrine, and dextromethorphan *on page* 202
Rescon GG [OTC] *see* guaifenesin and phenylephrine *on page* 435
Rescriptor® *see* delavirdine *on page* 259

reserpine (re SER peen)

Medication Safety Issues

Sound-alike/look-alike issues:

Reserpine may be confused with RisperDAL®, risperiDONE

BEERS Criteria medication:

This drug may be potentially inappropriate for use in geriatric patients (Quality of evidence - low; Strength of recommendation - strong).

Therapeutic Category Rauwolfia Alkaloid

Use Management of mild-to-moderate hypertension; treatment of agitated psychotic states (schizophrenia)

General Dosage Range Oral:

Adults: Initial: 0.5 mg once daily; Maintenance: 0.05-0.5 mg once daily
Elderly: Initial: 0.05 mg once daily

Dosage Forms

Tablet, oral: 0.1 mg, 0.25 mg

resistant dextrin *see* wheat dextrin *on page* 955
resistant maltodextrin *see* wheat dextrin *on page* 955
Resonium Calcium® (Can) *see* calcium polystyrene sulfonate *(Canada only) on page* 166
Resotran™ (Can) *see* prucalopride *(Canada only) on page* 771
Resperal-DM *see* brompheniramine, pseudoephedrine, and dextromethorphan *on page* 144
Restasis® *see* cyclosporine (ophthalmic) *on page* 246
Restoril™ *see* temazepam *on page* 875
Restylane® *see* hyaluronate and derivatives *on page* 450

retapamulin (re te PAM ue lin)

U.S. Brand Names Altabax™

Therapeutic Category Antibiotic, Pleuromutilin; Antibiotic, Topical

Use Treatment of impetigo caused by susceptible strains of *S. pyogenes* or methicillin-susceptible *S. aureus*

General Dosage Range Topical: *Children ≥9 months and Adults:* Apply to affected area twice daily. Total treatment area should not exceed 2% of total body surface area.

Dosage Forms

Ointment, topical:

Altabax™: 1% (15 g)

Retavase® (Can) *see* reteplase *on page* 795
Retavase® Half-Kit *see* reteplase *on page* 795
Retavase® Kit *see* reteplase *on page* 795

reteplase (RE ta plase)

Medication Safety Issues

High alert medication:

The Institute for Safe Medication Practices (ISMP) includes this medication (I.V.) among its list of drugs which have a heightened risk of causing significant patient harm when used in error.

Synonyms r-PA; recombinant plasminogen activator

U.S. Brand Names Retavase® Half-Kit; Retavase® Kit

Canadian Brand Names Retavase®

Therapeutic Category Thrombolytic Agent

Use Management of ST-elevation myocardial infarction (STEMI); improvement of ventricular function; reduction of the incidence of CHF and the reduction of mortality following AMI

Recommended criteria for treatment (Antman, 2004): STEMI: Chest pain ≥20 minutes duration, onset of chest pain within 12 hours of treatment (or within prior 12-24 hours in patients with continuing ischemic symptoms), and ST-segment elevation >0.1 mV in at least two contiguous precordial leads or two adjacent limb leads on ECG or new or presumably new left bundle branch block (LBBB)

General Dosage Range I.V.: *Adults:* 10 units; repeat after 30 minutes

Dosage Forms

Injection, powder for reconstitution [preservative free]:
Retavase® Half-Kit: 10.4 units
Retavase® Kit: 10.4 units

Rhinocort® Turbuhaler® (Can) *see* budesonide (nasal) *on page 146*
RhinoFlex™ [DSC] *see* acetaminophen and phenyltoloxamine *on page 25*
RhinoFlex™-650 [DSC] *see* acetaminophen and phenyltoloxamine *on page 25*
r-hirudin *see* desirudin *on page 263*
rhKGF *see* palifermin *on page 684*
r-hLH *see* lutropin alfa *on page 556*
Rho(D) immune globulin (human) *see* Rh_o(D) immune globulin *on page 797*

Rh_o(D) immune globulin (ar aych oh (dee) i MYUN GLOB yoo lin)

Synonyms anti-D immunoglobulin; RhIG; Rho(D) immune globulin (human); RhoIGIV; RhoIVIM

U.S. Brand Names HyperRHO™ S/D Full Dose; HyperRHO™ S/D Mini-Dose; MICRhoGAM® UF Plus; RhoGAM® UF Plus; Rhophylac®; WinRho® SDF

Canadian Brand Names WinRho® SDF

Therapeutic Category Immune Globulin

Use

Suppression of Rh isoimmunization: Use in the following situations when an Rh_o(D)-negative individual is exposed to Rh_o(D)-positive blood: During delivery of an Rh_o(D)-positive infant; abortion; amniocentesis; chorionic villus sampling; ruptured tubal pregnancy; abdominal trauma; hydatidiform mole; transplacental hemorrhage. Used when the mother is Rh_o(D)-negative, the father of the child is either Rh_o(D)-positive or Rh_o(D)-unknown, or the baby is either Rh_o(D)-positive or Rh_o(D)-unknown.

Transfusion: Suppression of Rh isoimmunization in Rh_o(D)-negative individuals transfused with Rh_o(D) antigen-positive RBCs or blood components containing Rh_o(D) antigen-positive RBCs

Treatment of idiopathic thrombocytopenic purpura (ITP): Used intravenously in the following non-splenectomized Rh_o(D)-positive individuals: Children with acute or chronic ITP, adults with chronic ITP, and children and adults with ITP secondary to HIV infection

General Dosage Range I.M., I.V.: *Children and Adults:* Dosage varies greatly depending on indication

Dosage Forms

Injection, solution [preservative free]:

HyperRHO™ S/D Full Dose: ≥300 mcg/mL (1 mL)
HyperRHO™ S/D Mini-Dose: ≥50 mcg/0.17 mL (0.17 mL)
MICRhoGAM® UF Plus: ~50 mcg/0.75 mL (0.75 mL)
RhoGAM® UF Plus: ~300 mcg/0.75 mL (0.75 mL)
Rhophylac®: ≥ 300 mcg/2 mL (2 mL)
WinRho® SDF: 300 mcg/~1.3 mL (1.3 mL); 3000 mcg/~13 mL (13 mL); 500 mcg/~2.2 mL (2.2 mL); 1000 mcg/~4.4 mL (4.4 mL)

RhoGAM® UF Plus *see* Rh_o(D) immune globulin *on page 797*
RhoIGIV *see* Rh_o(D) immune globulin *on page 797*
RhoIVIM *see* Rh_o(D) immune globulin *on page 797*
Rho®-Loperamine (Can) *see* loperamide *on page 547*
Rho®-Nitro Pump Spray (Can) *see* nitroglycerin *on page 645*
Rhophylac® *see* Rh_o(D) immune globulin *on page 797*
Rhotral (Can) *see* acebutolol *on page 19*
Rhotrimine® (Can) *see* trimipramine *on page 921*
Rhovane® (Can) *see* zopiclone *(Canada only) on page 967*
Rhoxal-cyclosporine (Can) *see* cyclosporine (systemic) *on page 245*
Rhoxal-fluvoxamine (Can) *see* fluvoxamine *on page 403*
Rhoxal-glimepiride (Can) *see* glimepiride *on page 426*
Rhoxal-loperamide (Can) *see* loperamide *on page 547*
Rhoxal-nabumetone (Can) *see* nabumetone *on page 623*
Rhoxal-orphendrine (Can) *see* orphenadrine *on page 671*
Rhoxal-sotalol (Can) *see* sotalol *on page 851*
Rhoxal-valproic (Can) *see* valproic acid *on page 934*
rhPTH(1-34) *see* teriparatide *on page 880*
Rh-TSH *see* thyrotropin alpha *on page 894*
***r*HuEPO** *see* epoetin alfa *on page 337*
rhuFabV2 *see* ranibizumab *on page 787*

ribavirin (rye ba VYE rin)

Medication Safety Issues

Sound-alike/look-alike issues:

Ribavirin may be confused with riboflavin, rifampin, Robaxin®

Synonyms RTCA; tribavirin

U.S. Brand Names Copegus®; Rebetol®; Ribasphere®; Ribasphere® RibaPak®; Virazole®

Canadian Brand Names Virazole®

Therapeutic Category Antiviral Agent

Use

Inhalation: Treatment of hospitalized infants and young children with respiratory syncytial virus (RSV) infections; specially indicated for treatment of severe lower respiratory tract RSV infections in patients with an underlying compromising condition (prematurity, cardiopulmonary disease, or immunosuppression)

Oral capsule:

In combination with interferon alfa-2b (Intron® A) injection for the treatment of chronic hepatitis C in patients with compensated liver disease who have relapsed after alpha interferon therapy or were previously untreated with alpha interferons

In combination with peginterferon alfa-2b (PEG-Intron®) injection for the treatment of chronic hepatitis C in patients with compensated liver disease who were previously untreated with alpha interferons

Oral solution: In combination with interferon alfa-2b (Intron® A) injection for the treatment of chronic hepatitis C in patients with compensated liver disease who were previously untreated with alpha interferons or patients who have relapsed after alpha interferon therapy

Oral tablet: In combination with peginterferon alfa-2a (Pegasys®) injection for the treatment of chronic hepatitis C in patients with compensated liver disease who were previously untreated with alpha interferons (includes patients with histological evidence of cirrhosis [Child-Pugh class A] and patients with clinically-stable HIV disease)

General Dosage Range Dosage adjustment recommended in patients with renal impairment and in patients who develop toxicities.

Inhalation: *Children:* 20 mg/mL (6 g in 300 mL) solution; continuous: 12-18 hours/day

Oral:

Children ≥3 years and ≤25 kg: 15 mg/kg/day in 2 divided doses
Children ≥3 years and 26-36 kg: 400 mg/day in 2 divided doses
Children ≥3 years and 37-49 kg: 600 mg/day in 2 divided doses
Children ≥3 years and 50-61 kg: 800 mg/day in 2 divided doses
Children ≥3 years and >61 kg to <75 kg: 1000 mg/day in 2 divided doses
Adults ≤75 kg: 800-1000 mg/day in 2 divided doses
Adults >75 kg: 800-1200 mg/day in 2 divided doses

Dosage Forms

Capsule, oral: 200 mg
Rebetol®: 200 mg
Ribasphere®: 200 mg

Powder for solution, for nebulization:
Virazole®: 6 g

Solution, oral:
Rebetol®: 40 mg/mL (100 mL)

Tablet, oral: 200 mg
Copegus®: 200 mg
Ribasphere®: 200 mg, 400 mg, 600 mg

Tablet, oral [dose-pack]:
Ribasphere® RibaPak® 600: 200 mg AM dose, 400 mg PM dose (14s, 56s)
Ribasphere® RibaPak® 800: 400 mg AM dose, 400 mg PM dose (14s, 56s)
Ribasphere® RibaPak® 1000: 600 mg AM dose, 400 mg PM dose (14s, 56s)
Ribasphere® RibaPak® 1200: 600 mg AM dose, 600 mg PM dose (14s, 56s)

ribavirin and peginterferon alfa-2a *see* peginterferon alfa-2a and ribavirin *(Canada only)* *on page 697*

ribavirin and peginterferon alfa-2b *see* peginterferon alfa-2b and ribavirin *(Canada only)* *on page 699*

Ribo-100 [OTC] *see* riboflavin *on page 799*

riboflavin (RYE boe flay vin)

Medication Safety Issues

Sound-alike/look-alike issues:
Riboflavin may be confused with ribavirin

Synonyms lactoflavin; vitamin B_2; vitamin G

U.S. Brand Names Ribo-100 [OTC]

Therapeutic Category Vitamin, Water Soluble

Use Dietary supplement

General Dosage Range Oral: *Adults:* 100 mg once or twice daily

Dosage Forms

Tablet, oral: 25 mg, 50 mg, 100 mg
Ribo-100 [OTC]: 100 mg

Rid® [OTC] *see* permethrin *on page 709*

Rid-A-Pain Dental [OTC] *see* benzocaine *on page 121*

Ridaura® *see* auranofin *on page 103*

RID® Maximum Strength [OTC] *see* pyrethrins and piperonyl butoxide *on page 776*

RID® Mousse (Can) *see* pyrethrins and piperonyl butoxide *on page 776*

rifabutin (rif a BYOO tin)

Medication Safety Issues

Sound-alike/look-alike issues:
Rifabutin may be confused with rifampin

Synonyms ansamycin

U.S. Brand Names Mycobutin®

Canadian Brand Names Mycobutin®

Therapeutic Category Antibiotic, Miscellaneous

Use Prevention of disseminated *Mycobacterium avium* complex (MAC) in patients with advanced HIV infection

General Dosage Range Dosage adjustment recommended in patients with renal impairment or on concomitant therapy

Oral:
Children <6 years: 5 mg/kg once daily
Children ≥6 years and Adults: 300 mg once daily

Dosage Forms

Capsule, oral:
Mycobutin®: 150 mg

Rifadin® *see* rifampin *on page 799*

Rifamate® *see* rifampin and isoniazid *on page 800*

rifampicin *see* rifampin *on page 799*

rifampin (rif AM pin)

Medication Safety Issues

Sound-alike/look-alike issues:
Rifadin® may be confused with Rifater®, Ritalin®
Rifampin may be confused with ribavirin, rifabutin, Rifamate®, rifapentine, rifaximin

Synonyms rifampicin

U.S. Brand Names Rifadin®
Canadian Brand Names Rifadin®; Rofact™
Therapeutic Category Antibiotic, Miscellaneous
Use Management of active tuberculosis in combination with other agents; elimination of meningococci from the nasopharynx in asymptomatic carriers
General Dosage Range I.V., oral:
Children <12 years: 10-20 mg/kg/day in 1-2 divided doses **or** 10-20 mg/kg twice weekly (maximum: 600 mg/day)
Children ≥12 years and Adults: 10 mg/kg/day **or** 10 mg/kg 2-3 times/week **or** 600 mg every 12-24 hours
Dosage Forms
Capsule, oral: 150 mg, 300 mg
Rifadin®: 150 mg, 300 mg
Injection, powder for reconstitution: 600 mg
Rifadin®: 600 mg

rifampin and isoniazid (rif AM pin & eye soe NYE a zid)

Medication Safety Issues
Sound-alike/look-alike issues:
Rifamate® may be confused with rifampin
Synonyms isoniazid and rifampin
U.S. Brand Names IsonaRif™; Rifamate®
Canadian Brand Names Rifamate®
Therapeutic Category Antibiotic, Miscellaneous
Use Management of active tuberculosis; see individual agents for additional information
General Dosage Range Oral: *Adults:* 2 capsules (rifampin 300 mg/isoniazid 150 mg/capsule) once daily
Dosage Forms
Capsule, oral:
IsonaRif™, Rifamate®: Rifampin 300 mg and isoniazid 150 mg

rifampin, isoniazid, and pyrazinamide
(rif AM pin, eye soe NYE a zid, & peer a ZIN a mide)

Medication Safety Issues
Sound-alike/look-alike issues:
Rifater® may be confused with Rifadin®
Synonyms isoniazid, pyrazinamide, and rifampin; pyrazinamide, rifampin, and isoniazid
U.S. Brand Names Rifater®
Canadian Brand Names Rifater®
Therapeutic Category Antibiotic, Miscellaneous
Use Initial phase, short-course treatment of pulmonary tuberculosis; see individual agents for additional information
General Dosage Range Oral:
Children ≥15 years and Adults ≤44 kg: 4 tablets (rifampin 120 mg/isoniazid 50 mg/pyrazinamide 300 mg per tablet) once daily
Children ≥15 years and Adults 45-54 kg: 5 tablets (rifampin 120 mg/isoniazid 50 mg/pyrazinamide 300 mg per tablet) once daily
Children ≥15 years and Adults ≥55 kg: 6 tablets (rifampin 120 mg/isoniazid 50 mg/pyrazinamide 300 mg per tablet) once daily
Dosage Forms
Tablet, oral:
Rifater®: Rifampin 120 mg, isoniazid 50 mg, and pyrazinamide 300 mg

rifapentine (rif a PEN teen)

Medication Safety Issues
Sound-alike/look-alike issues:
Rifapentine may be confused with rifampin
U.S. Brand Names Priftin®
Canadian Brand Names Priftin®
Therapeutic Category Antitubercular Agent

Use Treatment of pulmonary tuberculosis; rifapentine must always be used in conjunction with at least one other antituberculosis drug to which the isolate is susceptible; it may also be necessary to add a third agent (either streptomycin or ethambutol) until susceptibility is known.

General Dosage Range Oral: *Adults:* 600 mg once or twice weekly

Dosage Forms

Tablet, oral:

Priftin®: 150 mg

Rifater® *see* rifampin, isoniazid, and pyrazinamide *on page 800*

rifaximin (rif AX i min)

Medication Safety Issues

Sound-alike/look-alike issues:

Rifaximin may be confused with rifampin

U.S. Brand Names Xifaxan®

Therapeutic Category Antibiotic, Miscellaneous

Use Treatment of traveler's diarrhea caused by noninvasive strains of *E. coli*; reduction in the risk of overt hepatic encephalopathy (HE) recurrence

General Dosage Range Oral:

Children ≥12 years: 200 mg 3 times/day

Adults: 200 mg 3 times/day **or** 550 mg 2 times/day

Dosage Forms

Tablet, oral:

Xifaxan®: 200 mg, 550 mg

rIFN beta-1a *see* interferon beta-1a *on page 492*

rIFN beta-1b *see* interferon beta-1b *on page 492*

RIG *see* rabies immune globulin (human) *on page 784*

rilonacept (ri LON a sept)

U.S. Brand Names Arcalyst®

Therapeutic Category Interleukin-1 Inhibitor

Use Treatment of cryopyrin-associated periodic syndromes (CAPS) including familial cold auto-inflammatory syndrome (FCAS) and Muckle-Wells syndrome (MWS)

General Dosage Range SubQ:

Children ≥12 years: Loading dose 4.4 mg/kg (maximum dose: 320 mg); Maintenance dose: 2.2 mg/kg once weekly (maximum dose: 160 mg)

Adults: Loading dose: 320 mg; Maintenance dose: 160 mg once weekly

Dosage Forms

Injection, powder for reconstitution:

Arcalyst®: 220 mg

rilpivirine (ril pi VIR een)

Synonyms TMC278

U.S. Brand Names Edurant™

Canadian Brand Names Edurant™

Therapeutic Category Antiretroviral Agent, Non-nucleoside Reverse Transcriptase Inhibitor (NNRTI)

Use Treatment of HIV-1 infections in combination with at least two other antiretroviral agents

General Dosage Range Oral: *Adults:* 25 mg once daily

Dosage Forms

Tablet, oral:

Edurant™: 25 mg

rilpivirine, emtricitabine, and tenofovir *see* emtricitabine, rilpivirine, and tenofovir *on page 329*

Rilutek® *see* riluzole *on page 801*

riluzole (RIL yoo zole)

Synonyms 2-amino-6-trifluoromethoxy-benzothiazole; RP-54274

U.S. Brand Names Rilutek®

Canadian Brand Names Rilutek®

Therapeutic Category Miscellaneous Product

Use Treatment of amyotrophic lateral sclerosis (ALS); riluzole can extend survival or time to tracheostomy

General Dosage Range Oral: *Adults:* 50 mg every 12 hours

Dosage Forms

Tablet, oral:

Rilutek®: 50 mg

rimabotulinumtoxinB (rime uh BOT yoo lin num TOKS in bee)

Medication Safety Issues

Other safety concerns:

Botulinum products are not interchangeable; potency differences may exist between the products.

Synonyms botulinum toxin type B

U.S. Brand Names Myobloc®

Therapeutic Category Neuromuscular Blocker Agent, Toxin

Use Treatment of cervical dystonia (spasmodic torticollis)

General Dosage Range I.M.: *Adults:* Initial: 2500-5000 units divided among the affected muscles

Dosage Forms

Injection, solution [preservative free]:

Myobloc®: 5000 units/mL (0.5 mL, 1 mL, 2 mL)

rimantadine (ri MAN ta deen)

Medication Safety Issues

Sound-alike/look-alike issues:

Rimantadine may be confused with amantadine, ranitidine, Rimactane

Flumadine® may be confused with fludarabine, flunisolide, flutamide

Synonyms rimantadine hydrochloride

U.S. Brand Names Flumadine®

Canadian Brand Names Flumadine®

Therapeutic Category Antiviral Agent

Use Prophylaxis (adults and children >1 year of age) and treatment (adults) of influenza A viral infection (per manufacturer labeling; also refer to current ACIP guidelines for recommendations during current flu season)

Note: In certain circumstances, the ACIP recommends use of rimantadine in combination with oseltamivir for the treatment or prophylaxis of influenza A infection when resistance to oseltamivir is suspected.

General Dosage Range Dosage adjustment recommended in patients with hepatic or renal impairment

Oral:

Children 1-9 years: 5 mg/kg/day in 1-2 divided doses (maximum: 150 mg/day)

Children ≥10 years and <40 kg: 5 mg/kg/day in 2 divided doses

Children ≥10 years and Adults: 100 mg twice daily

Elderly: 100 mg daily

Dosage Forms

Tablet, oral: 100 mg

Flumadine®: 100 mg

rimantadine hydrochloride *see* rimantadine *on page* 802

rimexolone (ri MEKS oh lone)

Medication Safety Issues

Sound-alike/look-alike issues:

Vexol® may be confused with VoSoL®

U.S. Brand Names Vexol®

Canadian Brand Names Vexol®

Therapeutic Category Adrenal Corticosteroid

Use Treatment of inflammation after ocular surgery and the treatment of anterior uveitis

General Dosage Range Ophthalmic: *Adults:* Instill 1-2 drops 4 times/day **or** instill 1-2 drops every 1-2 hours during waking hours

Dosage Forms

Suspension, ophthalmic:

Vexol®: 1% (5 mL, 10 mL)

Rimso-50® *see* dimethyl sulfoxide *on page* 290
Riomet® *see* metformin *on page* 579
Riopan Plus *see* magaldrate and simethicone *on page* 557
Risamine™ [OTC] *see* menthol and zinc oxide (topical) *on page* 574
RisaQuad™ [OTC] *see* Lactobacillus *on page* 518
RisaQuad®-2 [OTC] *see* Lactobacillus *on page* 518

risedronate (ris ED roe nate)

Medication Safety Issues

Sound-alike/look-alike issues:

Actonel® may be confused with Actos®
Risedronate may be confused with alendronate

Synonyms risedronate sodium

U.S. Brand Names Actonel®; Atelvia™

Canadian Brand Names Actonel®; Actonel® DR; Apo-Risedronate®; Dom-Risedronate; Novo-Risedronate; PMS-Risedronate; ratio-Risedronate; Riva-Risedronate; Sandoz-Risedronate; Teva-Risedronate

Therapeutic Category Bisphosphonate Derivative

Use

Actonel®: Treatment of Paget disease of the bone; treatment and prevention of glucocorticoid-induced osteoporosis; treatment and prevention of osteoporosis in postmenopausal women; treatment of osteoporosis in men

Atelvia™: Treatment of osteoporosis in postmenopausal women

General Dosage Range Oral: *Adults:* 5 mg or 30 mg once daily **or** 35 mg once weekly **or** 150 mg once a month

Dosage Forms

Tablet, oral:

Actonel®: 5 mg, 30 mg, 35 mg, 150 mg

Tablet, delayed release, oral:

Atelvia™: 35 mg

risedronate sodium *see* risedronate *on page* 803
RisperDAL® *see* risperidone *on page* 803
Risperdal® (Can) *see* risperidone *on page* 803
Risperdal M-Tab *see* risperidone *on page* 803
RisperDAL® M-Tab® *see* risperidone *on page* 803
Risperdal® M-Tab® (Can) *see* risperidone *on page* 803
RisperDAL® Consta® *see* risperidone *on page* 803
Risperdal® Consta® (Can) *see* risperidone *on page* 803

risperidone (ris PER i done)

Medication Safety Issues

Sound-alike/look-alike issues:

RisperiDONE may be confused with reserpine, rOPINIRole
RisperDAL® may be confused with lisinopril, reserpine, Restoril™

BEERS Criteria medication:

This drug may be potentially inappropriate for use in geriatric patients (Quality of evidence - moderate; Strength of recommendation - strong).

Synonyms Risperdal M-Tab

Tall-Man risperi**DONE**

U.S. Brand Names RisperDAL®; RisperDAL® Consta®; RisperDAL® M-Tab®

Canadian Brand Names Apo-Risperidone®; Ava-Risperidone; CO Risperidone; Dom-Risperidone; JAMP-Risperidone; Mint-Risperidon; Mylan-Risperidone; Novo-Risperidone; PHL-Risperidone; PMS-Risperidone; PMS-Risperidone ODT; PRO-Risperidone; RAN™-Risperidone; ratio-Risperidone; Risperdal®; Risperdal® Consta®; Risperdal® M-Tab®; Riva-Risperidone; Sandoz-Risperidone

Therapeutic Category Antipsychotic Agent, Benzisoxazole

Use

Oral: Treatment of schizophrenia; treatment of acute mania or mixed episodes associated with bipolar I disorder (as monotherapy in children or adults, or in combination with lithium or valproate in adults); treatment of irritability/aggression associated with autistic disorder

Injection: Treatment of schizophrenia; maintenance treatment of bipolar I disorder in adults as monotherapy or in combination with lithium or valproate

General Dosage Range Dosage adjustment recommended in patients with hepatic or renal impairment

I.M.:

Adults: 25 mg every 2 weeks (range: 12.5-50 mg every 2 weeks; maximum: 50 mg every 2 weeks)

Elderly: 12.5-25 mg every 2 weeks

Oral:

Children ≥5 years: Autism: Initial: 0.25 mg/day (<20 kg) or 0.5 mg/day (≥20 kg); Maximum dose: 1 mg/day (<20 kg) or 2.5 mg/day (≥20 kg) (3 mg/day in children >45 kg)

Children 10-17 years: Bipolar disorder: Initial: 0.5 mg once daily; Recommended target dose: 2.5 mg/day; dosing range 0.5-6 mg/day

Children: 13-17 years: Schizophrenia: Initial: 0.5 mg once daily; Recommended target dose: 3 mg/day; dosing range 1-6 mg/day

Adults: Initial: 2-3 mg/day in 1-2 divided doses; Maintenance: 1-8 mg/day in 1-2 divided doses

Elderly: Initial: 0.5 mg twice daily

Dosage Forms

Injection, microspheres for reconstitution, extended release:

RisperDAL® Consta®: 12.5 mg, 25 mg, 37.5 mg, 50 mg

Solution, oral: 1 mg/mL (30 mL)

RisperDAL®: 1 mg/mL (30 mL)

Tablet, oral: 0.25 mg, 0.5 mg, 1 mg, 2 mg, 3 mg, 4 mg

RisperDAL®: 0.25 mg, 0.5 mg, 1 mg, 2 mg, 3 mg, 4 mg

Tablet, orally disintegrating, oral: 0.25 mg, 0.5 mg, 1 mg, 2 mg, 3 mg, 4 mg

RisperDAL® M-Tab®: 0.5 mg, 1 mg, 2 mg, 3 mg, 4 mg

Ritalin® *see* methylphenidate *on page 590*

Ritalin LA® *see* methylphenidate *on page 590*

Ritalin-SR® *see* methylphenidate *on page 590*

Ritalin® SR (Can) *see* methylphenidate *on page 590*

ritonavir (ri TOE na veer)

Medication Safety Issues

Sound-alike/look-alike issues:

Ritonavir may be confused with Retrovir®

Norvir® may be confused with Norvasc®

U.S. Brand Names Norvir®

Canadian Brand Names Norvir®; Norvir® SEC

Therapeutic Category Antiviral Agent

Use Treatment of HIV infection; should always be used as part of a multidrug regimen (at least three antiretroviral agents); may be used as a pharmacokinetic "booster" for other protease inhibitors

General Dosage Range Dosage adjustment recommended in patients on concurrent therapy

Oral:

Children >1 month: Initial: 250 mg/m^2 twice daily; Maintenance: 350-400 mg/m^2 twice daily (maximum dose: 1200 mg/day)

Adults: 300-600 mg twice daily (maximum: 1200 mg/day)

Dosage Forms

Capsule, soft gelatin, oral:

Norvir®: 100 mg

Solution, oral:

Norvir®: 80 mg/mL (240 mL)

Tablet, oral:

Norvir®: 100 mg

ritonavir and lopinavir *see* lopinavir and ritonavir *on page 548*

Rituxan® *see* rituximab *on page 805*

rituximab (ri TUK si mab)

Medication Safety Issues

Sound-alike/look-alike issues:

Rituxan® may be confused with Remicade®

RiTUXimab may be confused with brentuximab, bevacizumab, inFLIXimab, ruxolitinib

High alert medication:

The medication is in a class the Institute for Safe Medication Practices (ISMP) includes among its list of drug classes which have a heightened risk of causing significant patient harm when used in error.

Administration issues:

The rituximab dose for rheumatoid arthritis is a flat dose (1000 mg) and is not based on body surface area (BSA).

Synonyms anti-CD20 monoclonal antibody; C2B8 monoclonal antibody; IDEC-C2B8

Tall-Man riTUXimab

U.S. Brand Names Rituxan®

Canadian Brand Names Rituxan®

Therapeutic Category Antineoplastic Agent

Use

Treatment of CD20-positive non-Hodgkin lymphomas (NHL):

Relapsed or refractory, low-grade or follicular B-cell NHL (as a single agent)

Follicular B-cell NHL, previously untreated (in combination with first-line chemotherapy, and as single-agent maintenance therapy if response to first-line rituximab with chemotherapy)

Nonprogressing, low-grade B-cell NHL (as a single agent after first-line CVP treatment)

Diffuse large B-cell NHL, previously untreated (in combination with CHOP chemotherapy [or other anthracycline-based regimen])

Treatment of CD20-positive chronic lymphocytic leukemia (CLL) (in combination with fludarabine and cyclophosphamide)

Treatment of moderately- to severely-active rheumatoid arthritis (in combination with methotrexate) in adult patients with inadequate response to one or more TNF antagonists

Treatment of Wegener granulomatosis (WG) (in combination with glucocorticoids)

Treatment of microscopic polyangiitis (MPA) (in combination with glucocorticoids)

General Dosage Range I.V.: *Adults:* Dosage varies greatly depending on indication

Dosage Forms

Injection, solution [preservative free]:

Rituxan®: 10 mg/mL (10 mL, 50 mL)

Riva-Alendronate (Can) *see* alendronate *on page* 45
Riva-Amiodarone (Can) *see* amiodarone *on page* 63
Riva-Amlodipine (Can) *see* amlodipine *on page* 65
Riva-Atenolol (Can) *see* atenolol *on page* 99
Riva-Azithromycin (Can) *see* azithromycin (systemic) *on page* 108
Riva-Baclofen (Can) *see* baclofen *on page* 112
Riva-Buspirone (Can) *see* buspirone *on page* 152
Riva-Ciprofloxacin (Can) *see* ciprofloxacin (systemic) *on page* 210
Riva-Citalopram (Can) *see* citalopram *on page* 213
Riva-Clarithromycin (Can) *see* clarithromycin *on page* 215
Riva-Clindamycin (Can) *see* clindamycin (systemic) *on page* 218
Riva-Clonazepam (Can) *see* clonazepam *on page* 223
Riva-Cycloprine (Can) *see* cyclobenzaprine *on page* 243
Riva-Dicyclomine (Can) *see* dicyclomine *on page* 282
Riva-Enalapril (Can) *see* enalapril *on page* 330
Riva-Fenofibrate Micro (Can) *see* fenofibrate *on page* 375
Riva-Fluconazole (Can) *see* fluconazole *on page* 388
Riva-Fluoxetine (Can) *see* fluoxetine *on page* 396
Riva-Fluvox (Can) *see* fluvoxamine *on page* 403
Riva-Fosinopril (Can) *see* fosinopril *on page* 409
Riva-Gabapentin (Can) *see* gabapentin *on page* 413
Riva-Glyburide (Can) *see* glyburide *on page* 428

Riva-Hydroxyzine (Can) *see* hydroxyzine *on page 464*
Riva-Indapamide (Can) *see* indapamide *on page 479*
Riva-Lisinopril (Can) *see* lisinopril *on page 544*
Riva-Loperamide (Can) *see* loperamide *on page 547*
Riva-Lovastatin (Can) *see* lovastatin *on page 553*
Riva-Memantine (Can) *see* memantine *on page 570*
Riva-Metformin (Can) *see* metformin *on page 579*
Riva-Metoprolol-L (Can) *see* metoprolol *on page 595*
Riva-Minocycline (Can) *see* minocycline *on page 604*
Riva-Mirtazapine (Can) *see* mirtazapine *on page 606*
Riva-Naproxen (Can) *see* naproxen *on page 628*
Riva-Naproxen Sodium (Can) *see* naproxen *on page 628*
Riva-Naproxen Sodium DS (Can) *see* naproxen *on page 628*
Rivanase AQ (Can) *see* beclomethasone (nasal) *on page 117*
Riva-Norfloxacin (Can) *see* norfloxacin *on page 649*
Riva-Olanzapine (Can) *see* olanzapine *on page 660*
Riva-Olanzapine ODT (Can) *see* olanzapine *on page 660*
Riva-Oxazepam (Can) *see* oxazepam *on page 676*
Riva-Oxybutynin (Can) *see* oxybutynin *on page 677*
Riva-Pantoprazole (Can) *see* pantoprazole *on page 689*
Riva-Paroxetine (Can) *see* paroxetine *on page 693*
Riva-Pravastatin (Can) *see* pravastatin *on page 752*
Riva-Quetiapine (Can) *see* quetiapine *on page 781*
Riva-Rabeprazole EC (Can) *see* rabeprazole *on page 784*
Riva-Ranitidine (Can) *see* ranitidine *on page 788*
Riva-Risedronate (Can) *see* risedronate *on page 803*
Riva-Risperidone (Can) *see* risperidone *on page 803*

rivaroxaban (riv a ROX a ban)

Medication Safety Issues

High alert medication:

The Institute for Safe Medication Practices (ISMP) includes this medication among its list of drug classes which have a heightened risk of causing significant patient harm when used in error.

Synonyms BAY 59-7939

U.S. Brand Names Xarelto®

Canadian Brand Names Xarelto®

Therapeutic Category Factor Xa Inhibitor

Use Postoperative thromboprophylaxis in patients who have undergone hip or knee replacement surgery; prevention of stroke and systemic embolism in patients with nonvalvular atrial fibrillation

Canadian labeling: Additional use (not in U.S. labeling): Treatment of deep vein thrombosis (DVT) without symptomatic pulmonary embolism

General Dosage Range Oral: *Adults:* 10-20 mg/day

Dosage Forms

Tablet, oral:

Xarelto®: 10 mg, 15 mg, 20 mg

Riva-Sertraline (Can) *see* sertraline *on page 831*
Riva-Simvastatin (Can) *see* simvastatin *on page 835*
Rivasol (Can) *see* zinc sulfate *on page 963*
Rivasone (Can) *see* betamethasone *on page 129*
Riva-Sotalol (Can) *see* sotalol *on page 851*

rivastigmine (ri va STIG meen)

Synonyms ENA 713; rivastigmine tartrate; SDZ ENA 713

U.S. Brand Names Exelon®

Canadian Brand Names Apo-Rivastigmine®; Exelon®; Mylan-Rivastigmine; Novo-Rivastigmine; PMS-Rivastigmine; ratio-Rivastigmine; Sandoz-Rivastigmine

Therapeutic Category Acetylcholinesterase Inhibitor; Cholinergic Agent

Use Treatment of mild-to-moderate dementia associated with Alzheimer disease or Parkinson disease

General Dosage Range

Oral: *Adults:* Initial: 1.5 mg twice daily; Maintenance: 1.5-6 mg twice daily (maximum: 12 mg/day)

Transdermal patch: *Adults:* Initial: 4.6 mg/24 hours; Maintenance: 9.5 mg/24 hours (maximum dose: 9.5 mg/24 hours)

Dosage Forms

Capsule, oral: 1.5 mg, 3 mg, 4.5 mg, 6 mg

Exelon®: 1.5 mg, 3 mg, 4.5 mg, 6 mg

Patch, transdermal:

Exelon®: 4.6 mg/24 hours (30s); 9.5 mg/24 hours (30s)

Solution, oral:

Exelon®: 2 mg/mL (120 mL)

rivastigmine tartrate *see* rivastigmine *on page 806*

Riva-Sumatriptan (Can) *see* sumatriptan *on page 863*

Riva-Terbinafine (Can) *see* terbinafine (systemic) *on page 878*

Riva-Valacyclovir (Can) *see* valacyclovir *on page 933*

Riva-Venlafaxine XR (Can) *see* venlafaxine *on page 942*

Riva-Verapamil SR (Can) *see* verapamil *on page 942*

Riva-Zide (Can) *see* hydrochlorothiazide and triamterene *on page 453*

Riva-Zopiclone (Can) *see* zopiclone *(Canada only) on page 967*

Rivotril® (Can) *see* clonazepam *on page 223*

rizatriptan (rye za TRIP tan)

Synonyms MK462

U.S. Brand Names Maxalt-MLT®; Maxalt®

Canadian Brand Names CO Rizatriptan ODT; JAMP-Rizatriptan; Maxalt RPD™; Maxalt™; Sandoz-Rizatriptan ODT

Therapeutic Category Antimigraine Agent; Serotonin Agonist

Use Acute treatment of migraine with or without aura

General Dosage Range Oral:

Children 6-17 years: <40 kg: 5 mg as a single dose; ≥40 kg: 10 mg as a single dose

Adults: 5-10 mg once, repeat if needed (maximum: 30 mg/day)

Dosage Forms

Tablet, oral:

Maxalt®: 5 mg, 10 mg

Tablet, orally disintegrating, oral:

Maxalt-MLT®: 5 mg, 10 mg

rLFN-α2 *see* interferon alfa-2b *on page 490*

R-modafinil *see* armodafinil *on page 91*

Ro 5488 *see* tretinoin (systemic) *on page 913*

RO5185426 *see* vemurafenib *on page 941*

RoActemra® *see* tocilizumab *on page 902*

Robafen [OTC] *see* guaifenesin *on page 433*

Robafen AC *see* guaifenesin and codeine *on page 434*

Robafen CF Cough & Cold [OTC] *see* guaifenesin, dextromethorphan, and phenylephrine *on page 437*

Robafen Cough [OTC] *see* dextromethorphan *on page 272*

Robafen DM [OTC] *see* guaifenesin and dextromethorphan *on page 434*

Robafen DM Clear [OTC] *see* guaifenesin and dextromethorphan *on page 434*

Robaxin® *see* methocarbamol *on page 583*

Robaxin®-750 *see* methocarbamol *on page 583*

Robidrine® (Can) *see* pseudoephedrine *on page 771*

Robinul® *see* glycopyrrolate *on page 429*

Robinul® Forte *see* glycopyrrolate *on page 429*
Robitussin® (Can) *see* guaifenesin *on page 433*
Robitussin AC *see* guaifenesin and codeine *on page 434*
Robitussin® Childrens Cough & Cold (Can) *see* pseudoephedrine and dextromethorphan *on page 772*
Robitussin® Children's Cough & Cold CF [OTC] *see* guaifenesin, dextromethorphan, and phenylephrine *on page 437*
Robitussin® Children's Cough Long-Acting [OTC] *see* dextromethorphan *on page 272*
Robitussin® Children's Cough & Cold Long-Acting [OTC] *see* dextromethorphan and chlorpheniramine *on page 273*
Robitussin® Cough & Cold CF [OTC] [DSC] *see* guaifenesin, dextromethorphan, and phenylephrine *on page 437*
Robitussin® Cough & Cold CF Max [OTC] [DSC] *see* guaifenesin, dextromethorphan, and phenylephrine *on page 437*
Robitussin® Cough & Cold Long-Acting [OTC] [DSC] *see* dextromethorphan and chlorpheniramine *on page 273*
Robitussin® CoughGels™ Long-Acting [OTC] [DSC] *see* dextromethorphan *on page 272*
Robitussin® Cough Long Acting [OTC] [DSC] *see* dextromethorphan *on page 272*
Robitussin® Lingering Cold Long-Acting Cough [OTC] *see* dextromethorphan *on page 272*
Robitussin® Lingering Cold Long-Acting CoughGels® [OTC] *see* dextromethorphan *on page 272*
Robitussin® Night Time Cough & Cold [OTC] [DSC] *see* diphenhydramine and phenylephrine *on page 294*
Robitussin® Peak Cold Cough + Chest Congestion DM [OTC] *see* guaifenesin and dextromethorphan *on page 434*
Robitussin® Peak Cold Maximum Strength Cough + Chest Congestion DM [OTC] *see* guaifenesin and dextromethorphan *on page 434*
Robitussin® Peak Cold Maximum Strength Multi-Symptom Cold [OTC] *see* guaifenesin, dextromethorphan, and phenylephrine *on page 437*
Robitussin® Peak Cold Multi-Symptom Cold [OTC] *see* guaifenesin, dextromethorphan, and phenylephrine *on page 437*
Robitussin® Peak Cold Nasal Relief [OTC] *see* acetaminophen and phenylephrine *on page 24*
Robitussin® Peak Cold Nighttime Multi-Symptom Cold [OTC] *see* acetaminophen, diphenhydramine, and phenylephrine *on page 29*
Robitussin® Peak Cold Sugar-Free Cough + Chest Congestion DM [OTC] *see* guaifenesin and dextromethorphan *on page 434*
Rocaltrol® *see* calcitriol *on page 160*
Rocephin® *see* ceftriaxone *on page 186*

rocuronium (roe kyoor OH nee um)

Medication Safety Issues

Sound-alike/look-alike issues:

Zemuron® may be confused with Remeron®

High alert medication:

The Institute for Safe Medication Practices (ISMP) includes this medication among its list of drugs which have a heightened risk of causing significant patient harm when used in error.

Other safety concerns:

United States Pharmacopeia (USP) 2006: The Interdisciplinary Safe Medication Use Expert Committee of the USP has recommended the following:

- Hospitals, clinics, and other practice sites should institute special safeguards in the storage, labeling, and use of these agents and should include these safeguards in staff orientation and competency training.
- Healthcare professionals should be on high alert (especially vigilant) whenever a neuromuscular-blocking agent (NMBA) is stocked, ordered, prepared, or administered.

Synonyms ORG 946; rocuronium bromide

U.S. Brand Names Zemuron®

Canadian Brand Names Rocuronium Bromide Injection; Zemuron®

Therapeutic Category Skeletal Muscle Relaxant

Use Facilitate both rapid sequence and routine endotracheal intubation and to relax skeletal muscles during surgery; to facilitate mechanical ventilation in ICU patients

General Dosage Range I.V.:

Infants ≥28 days and Children: Initial: 0.45-0.6 mg/kg; Maintenance: 0.075-0.15 mg/kg **or** 7-10 **mcg**/kg/minute

Adults: 0.03-1.2 mg/kg; Infusion: 8-12 **mcg**/kg/minute

Dosage Forms

Injection, solution: 10 mg/mL (5 mL, 10 mL)

Zemuron®: 10 mg/mL (5 mL, 10 mL)

Injection, solution [preservative free]: 10 mg/mL (5 mL, 10 mL)

rocuronium bromide *see* rocuronium *on page 808*

Rocuronium Bromide Injection (Can) *see* rocuronium *on page 808*

Rofact™ (Can) *see* rifampin *on page 799*

roflumilast (roe FLUE mi last)

U.S. Brand Names Daliresp®

Canadian Brand Names Daxas™

Therapeutic Category Phosphodiesterase-4 Enzyme Inhibitor

Use Adjunct to bronchodilator therapy in the maintenance treatment of severe chronic obstructive pulmonary disease (COPD) associated with chronic bronchitis

General Dosage Range Oral: *Adults:* 500 mcg once daily

Dosage Forms

Tablet, oral:

Daliresp®: 500 mcg

Dosage Forms - Canada

Tablet, oral:

Daxas™: 500 mcg

Rogaine® (Can) *see* minoxidil (topical) *on page 605*

Rogaine® Extra Strength for Men [OTC] *see* minoxidil (topical) *on page 605*

Rogaine® for Men [OTC] *see* minoxidil (topical) *on page 605*

Rogaine® for Women [OTC] *see* minoxidil (topical) *on page 605*

Rogitine® (Can) *see* phentolamine *on page 715*

Rolaids® [OTC] *see* calcium carbonate and magnesium hydroxide *on page 163*

Rolaids® Extra Strength [OTC] *see* calcium carbonate *on page 161*

Rolaids® Extra Strength [OTC] *see* calcium carbonate and magnesium hydroxide *on page 163*

Rolene (Can) *see* betamethasone *on page 129*

Romazicon® *see* flumazenil *on page 390*

romidepsin (roe mi DEP sin)

Medication Safety Issues

Sound-alike/look-alike issues:

RomiDEPsin may be confused with romiPLOStim

High alert medication:

This medication is in a class the Institute for Safe Medication Practices (ISMP) includes among its list of drug classes which have a heightened risk of causing significant patient harm when used in error.

Synonyms depsipeptide; FK228; FR901228

Tall-Man romi**DEP**sin

U.S. Brand Names Istodax®

Therapeutic Category Antineoplastic Agent, Histone Deacetylase Inhibitor

Use Treatment of refractory cutaneous T-cell lymphoma (CTCL) and refractory peripheral T-cell lymphoma (PTCL)

General Dosage Range Dosage adjustment recommended in patients who develop toxicities

I.V.: *Adults:* 14 mg/m^2 days 1, 8, and 15 of a 28-day treatment cycle

Dosage Forms

Injection, powder for reconstitution:

Istodax®: 10 mg

romiplostim (roe mi PLOE stim)

Medication Safety Issues

Sound-alike/look-alike issues:

RomiPLOStim may be confused with romiDEPsin

Synonyms AMG 531

Tall-Man romi**PLOS**tim

U.S. Brand Names Nplate®

Canadian Brand Names Nplate®

Therapeutic Category Colony-Stimulating Factor; Thrombopoietic Agent

Use Treatment of thrombocytopenia in patients with chronic immune (idiopathic) thrombocytopenia purpura (ITP) who have had insufficient response to corticosteroids, immune globulin, or splenectomy

Note: Should be used only when the degree of thrombocytopenia and clinical condition increase the risk for bleeding; should not be used in attempt to normalize platelet counts; **not** indicated for the treatment of thrombocytopenia due to myelodysplastic syndrome.

General Dosage Range SubQ: *Adults:* Initial: 1 mcg/kg once weekly; adjust dose by 1 mcg/kg/week to achieve platelet count ≥50,000/mm^3 and reduce the risk of bleeding; Maximum: 10 mcg/kg/week

Dosage Forms

Injection, powder for reconstitution:

Nplate®: 250 mcg, 500 mcg

ropinirole (roe PIN i role)

Medication Safety Issues

Sound-alike/look-alike issues:

Requip® may be confused with Reglan®

ROPINIRole may be confused with RisperDAL®, risperiDONE, ropivacaine

Synonyms ropinirole hydrochloride

Tall-Man r**OPINIR**ole

U.S. Brand Names Requip®; Requip® XL™

Canadian Brand Names CO Ropinirole; JAMP-Ropinirole; PMS-Ropinirole; RAN™-Ropinirole; Requip®

Therapeutic Category Anti-Parkinson Agent (Dopamine Agonist)

Use Treatment of idiopathic Parkinson disease; in patients with early Parkinson disease who were not receiving concomitant levodopa therapy as well as in patients with advanced disease on concomitant levodopa; treatment of moderate-to-severe primary restless legs syndrome (RLS)

General Dosage Range Oral: *Adults:*

Parkinson:

Immediate release: Initial: 0.25 mg 3 times/day; Maintenance: 0.75-24 mg/day in 3 divided doses

Extended release: Initial: 2 mg once daily; Maintenance: 2-24 mg once daily (maximum: 24 mg/day)

Restless legs: Immediate release: Initial: 0.25 mg prior to bedtime; Maintenance: 0.25-4 mg prior to bedtime

Dosage Forms

Tablet, oral: 0.25 mg, 0.5 mg, 1 mg, 2 mg, 3 mg, 4 mg, 5 mg

Requip®: 0.25 mg, 0.5 mg, 1 mg, 2 mg, 3 mg, 4 mg, 5 mg

Tablet, extended release, oral: 2 mg, 4 mg, 6 mg, 8 mg, 12 mg

Requip® XL™: 2 mg, 4 mg, 6 mg, 8 mg, 12 mg

ropinirole hydrochloride *see* ropinirole *on page* 810

ropivacaine (roe PIV a kane)

Medication Safety Issues

Sound-alike/look-alike issues:

Ropivacaine may be confused with bupivacaine, rOPINIRole

High alert medication:

The Institute for Safe Medication Practices (ISMP) includes this medication (epidural administration) among its list of drug classes which have a heightened risk of causing significant patient harm when used in error.

Synonyms ropivacaine hydrochloride

U.S. Brand Names Naropin®

Canadian Brand Names Naropin®

Therapeutic Category Local Anesthetic

Use Local anesthetic for use in surgery, postoperative pain management, and obstetrical procedures when local or regional anesthesia is needed

General Dosage Range

Epidural:

Lumbar: *Adults:* 10-30 mL of 0.2% to 1% solution **or** 15-20 mL of 0.75% solution; Infusion: 6-14 mL/hour of 0.2% solution, with incremental injections of 10-15 mL/hour of 0.2% solution

Thoracic: *Adults:* 5-15 mL of 0.5% or 0.75% solution; Infusion: 6-14 mL/hour of 0.2% solution

Field Block: *Adults:* 1-40 mL (5-200 mg) of 0.5% solution

Infiltration: *Adults:* 1-100 mL of 0.2% solution **or** 1-40 mL of 0.5% solution

Nerve Block: *Adults:* Major: 35-50 mL (175-250 mg) of 0.5 % solution **or** 10-40 mL (75-300 mg) of 0.75% solution; Minor: 1-100 mL of 0.2% solution **or** 1-40 mL of 0.5% solution

Dosage Forms

Injection, solution [preservative free]:

Naropin®: 2 mg/mL (10 mL, 20 mL, 100 mL, 200 mL); 5 mg/mL (20 mL, 30 mL, 100 mL, 200 mL); 7.5 mg/mL (20 mL); 10 mg/mL (10 mL, 20 mL)

ropivacaine hydrochloride *see* ropivacaine *on page 810*

Rosadan™ *see* metronidazole (topical) *on page 597*

Rosanil® *see* sulfur and sulfacetamide *on page 862*

Rosasol® (Can) *see* metronidazole (topical) *on page 597*

rosiglitazone (roh si GLI ta zone)

Medication Safety Issues

Sound-alike/look-alike issues:

Avandia® may be confused with Avalide®, Coumadin®, Prandin®

High alert medication:

The Institute for Safe Medication Practices (ISMP) includes this medication among its list of drug classes which have a heightened risk of causing significant patient harm when used in error.

International issues:

Avandia [U.S., Canada, and multiple international markets] may be confused with Avanza brand name for mirtazapine [Australia]

U.S. Brand Names Avandia®

Canadian Brand Names Avandia®

Therapeutic Category Hypoglycemic Agent, Oral; Thiazolidinedione Derivative

Use Type 2 diabetes mellitus (noninsulin-dependent, NIDDM):

Monotherapy: Improve glycemic control as an adjunct to diet and exercise

Note: Canadian labeling approves use as monotherapy only when metformin is contraindicated or not tolerated.

Combination therapy: **Note:** Use when diet, exercise, and a single agent do not result in adequate glycemic control.

U.S. labeling: In combination with a sulfonylurea, metformin, or sulfonylurea plus metformin

Canadian labeling: In combination with metformin; in combination with a sulfonylurea only when metformin use is contraindicated or not tolerated

General Dosage Range Oral: *Adults:* Initial: 4 mg/day in 1-2 divided doses; Maintenance: 4-8 mg/day in 1-2 divided doses

Dosage Forms

Tablet, oral:

Avandia®: 2 mg, 4 mg, 8 mg

rosiglitazone and glimepiride (roh si GLI ta zone & GLYE me pye ride)

Medication Safety Issues

High alert medication:

The Institute for Safe Medication Practices (ISMP) includes this medication among its list of drugs which have a heightened risk of causing significant patient harm when used in error.

Synonyms glimepiride and rosiglitazone maleate

U.S. Brand Names Avandaryl®

Canadian Brand Names Avandaryl®

Therapeutic Category Antidiabetic Agent, Sulfonylurea; Antidiabetic Agent, Thiazolidinedione

Use Management of type 2 diabetes mellitus (noninsulin-dependent, NIDDM) as an adjunct to diet and exercise

General Dosage Range Dosage adjustment recommended in patients with hepatic or renal impairment

Oral:

Adults: Initial: Rosiglitazone 4 mg and glimepiride 1-2 mg once daily; Maintenance: Rosiglitazone 4-8 mg and glimepiride 1-4 mg once daily

Elderly: Initial: Rosiglitazone 4 mg and glimepiride 1 mg once daily

Dosage Forms

Tablet:

Avandaryl®: 4 mg/1 mg: Rosiglitazone 4 mg and glimepiride 1 mg; 4 mg/2 mg: Rosiglitazone 4 mg and glimepiride 2 mg; 4 mg/4 mg: Rosiglitazone 4 mg and glimepiride 4 mg; 8 mg/2 mg: Rosiglitazone 8 mg and glimepiride 2 mg; 8 mg/4 mg: Rosiglitazone 8 mg and glimepiride 4 mg

rosiglitazone and metformin (roh si GLI ta zone & met FOR min)

Medication Safety Issues

Sound-alike/look-alike issues:

Avandamet® may be confused with Anzemet®

High alert medication:

The Institute for Safe Medication Practices (ISMP) includes this medication among its list of drug classes which have a heightened risk of causing significant patient harm when used in error.

Synonyms metformin and rosiglitazone; metformin hydrochloride and rosiglitazone maleate; rosiglitazone maleate and metformin hydrochloride

U.S. Brand Names Avandamet®

Canadian Brand Names Avandamet®

Therapeutic Category Antidiabetic Agent (Biguanide); Antidiabetic Agent (Thiazolidinedione)

Use Management of type 2 diabetes mellitus (noninsulin-dependent, NIDDM) as an adjunct to diet and exercise in patients where dual rosiglitazone and metformin therapy is appropriate

General Dosage Range **Oral:** *Adults:* Initial: Rosiglitazone 2 mg and metformin 500 mg once or twice daily; may increase by 2 mg/500 mg per day after 4 weeks (maximum: rosiglitazone 8 mg/day; metformin 2000 mg/day)

Dosage Forms

Tablet:

Avandamet®: 2/500: Rosiglitazone 2 mg and metformin 500 mg; 4/500: Rosiglitazone 4 mg and metformin 500 mg; 2/1000: Rosiglitazone 2 mg and metformin 1000 mg; 4/1000: Rosiglitazone 4 mg and metformin 1000 mg

rosiglitazone maleate and metformin hydrochloride *see* rosiglitazone and metformin *on page 812*

Rosone (Can) *see* betamethasone *on page 129*

rosuvastatin (roe soo va STAT in)

Medication Safety Issues

Sound-alike/look-alike issues:

Rosuvastatin may be confused with atorvaSTATin, nystatin, pitavastatin

Synonyms rosuvastatin calcium

U.S. Brand Names Crestor®

Canadian Brand Names Apo-Rosuvastatin; CO Rosuvastatin; Crestor®; Mylan-Rosuvastatin; PMS-Rosuvastatin; RAN™-Rosuvastatin; Sandoz-Rosuvastatin; Teva-Rosuvastatin

Therapeutic Category Antilipemic Agent, HMG-CoA Reductase Inhibitor

Use

Treatment of dyslipidemias:

Used with dietary therapy for hyperlipidemias to reduce elevations in total cholesterol (TC), LDL-C, apolipoprotein B, nonHDL-C, and triglycerides (TG) in patients with primary hypercholesterolemia (elevations of 1 or more components are present in Fredrickson type IIa, IIb, and IV hyperlipidemias); increase HDL-C; treatment of primary dysbetalipoproteinemia (Fredrickson type III hyperlipidemia); treatment of homozygous familial hypercholesterolemia (FH); to slow progression of atherosclerosis as an adjunct to diet to lower TC and LDL-C

Heterozygous familial hypercholesterolemia (HeFH): In adolescent patients (10-17 years of age, females >1 year postmenarche) with HeFH having LDL-C >190 mg/dL or LDL >160 mg/dL with positive family history of premature cardiovascular disease (CVD), or ≥2 other CVD risk factors.

Primary prevention of cardiovascular disease: To reduce the risk of stroke, myocardial infarction, or arterial revascularization procedures in patients without clinically evident coronary heart disease or lipid abnormalities but with all of the following: 1) an increased risk of cardiovascular disease based on age ≥50 years old in men and ≥60 years old in women, 2) hsCRP ≥2 mg/L, and 3) the presence of at least one additional cardiovascular disease risk factor such as hypertension, low HDL-C, smoking, or a family history of premature coronary heart disease.

Secondary prevention of cardiovascular disease: To slow progression of atherosclerosis

General Dosage Range Dosage adjustment recommended in patients with renal impairment, on concomitant therapy, or who develop toxicities

Oral:

Children 10-17 years (females >1 year postmenarche): Initial: 5-20 mg once daily (maximum: 20 mg/day)

Adults: Initial: 5-20 mg once daily; Maintenance: 5-40 mg once daily (maximum: 40 mg/day)

Dosage Forms

Tablet, oral:

Crestor®: 5 mg, 10 mg, 20 mg, 40 mg

rosuvastatin calcium *see* rosuvastatin *on page 812*

Rotarix® *see* rotavirus vaccine *on page 813*

RotaTeq® *see* rotavirus vaccine *on page 813*

rotavirus vaccine (ROE ta vye rus vak SEEN)

Synonyms human rotavirus vaccine, attenuated (HRV); pentavalent human-bovine reassortant rotavirus vaccine (PRV); rotavirus vaccine, pentavalent; RV1 (RotaTeq®); RV5 (Rotarix®)

U.S. Brand Names Rotarix®; RotaTeq®

Canadian Brand Names Rotarix®; RotaTeq®

Therapeutic Category Vaccine

Use Prevention of rotavirus gastroenteritis in infants and children

The Advisory Committee on Immunization Practices (ACIP) recommends routine vaccination of all infants.

General Dosage Range Oral:

Infants 6-24 weeks: Rotarix®: A total of two 1 mL doses administered at 2 and 4 months of age

Infants 6-32 weeks: RotaTeq®: A total of three 2 mL doses given at 2, 4, and 6 months of age

Dosage Forms

Powder, for suspension, oral [preservative free; human derived]:

Rotarix®: G1P[8] ≥10^6 $CCID_{50}$ per 1 mL

Suspension, oral [preservative free]:

RotaTeq®: G1 ≥2.2 x 10^6 infectious units, G2 ≥2.8 x 10^6 infectious units, G3 ≥2.2 x 10^6 infectious units, G4 ≥2 x 10^6 infectious units, and P1A [8] ≥2.3 x 10^6 infectious units per 2 mL (2 mL)

rotavirus vaccine, pentavalent *see* rotavirus vaccine *on page 813*

rotigotine (roe TIG oh teen)

Medication Safety Issues

Sound-alike/look-alike issues:

Neupro® may be confused with Neupogen®

Transdermal patch contains metal (eg, aluminum); remove patch prior to MRI or cardioversion

Synonyms N-0923

U.S. Brand Names Neupro®

Therapeutic Category Anti-Parkinson Agent (Dopamine Agonist)

Use Treatment of the signs and symptoms of idiopathic Parkinson disease (early-stage to advanced-stage disease); treatment of moderate-to-severe primary restless legs syndrome (RLS)

General Dosage Range

Transdermal: *Adults:* 1-4 mg/24 hours; Maintenance (usual): 1-8 mg/24 hours (maximum: varies by indication)

Dosage Forms

Patch, transdermal:

Neupro®: 1 mg/24 hours (30s); 2 mg/24 hours (30s); 3 mg/24 hours (30s); 4 mg/24 hours (30s); 6 mg/24 hours (30s); 8 mg/24 hours (30s)

rufinamide (roo FIN a mide)

Synonyms CGP 33101; E 2080; RUF 331; xilep

U.S. Brand Names Banzel®

Canadian Brand Names Banzel™

Therapeutic Category Anticonvulsant, Triazole Derivative

Use Adjunctive therapy in the treatment of generalized seizures of Lennox-Gastaut syndrome

General Dosage Range Oral:

Children ≥4 years: Initial: 10 mg/kg/day in 2 equally divided doses (maximum: 45 mg/kg/day or 3200 mg/day)

Adults: Initial: 400-800 mg/day in 2 equally divided doses (maximum: 3200 mg/day)

Dosage Forms

Suspension, oral:

Banzel®: 40 mg/mL (460 mL)

Tablet, oral:

Banzel®: 200 mg, 400 mg

Dosage Forms - Canada

Tablet, oral:

Banzel™: 100 mg

ruxolitinib (rux oh LI ti nib)

Medication Safety Issues

Sound-alike/look-alike issues:

Ruxolitinib may be confused with riTUXimab

Synonyms INCB 18424; INCB018424; INCB424; ruxolitinib phosphate

U.S. Brand Names Jakafi™

Canadian Brand Names Jakavi™

Therapeutic Category Antineoplastic Agent, Janus Associated Kinase Inhibitor; Antineoplastic Agent, Tyrosine Kinase Inhibitor; Janus Associated Kinase Inhibitor

Use Treatment of intermediate or high-risk myelofibrosis, including primary myelofibrosis, post-polycythemia vera (post-PV) myelofibrosis and post-essential thrombocythemia (post-ET) myelofibrosis

General Dosage Range Dosage adjustment recommended in patients with hepatic impairment, renal impairment, on concomitant strong CYP3A4 inhibitor therapy, or who develop toxicities.

Oral: *Adults:* 15-20 mg twice daily; maximum dose: 25 mg twice daily

Dosage Forms

Tablet, oral:

Jakafi™: 5 mg, 10 mg, 15 mg, 20 mg, 25 mg

ruxolitinib phosphate *see* ruxolitinib *on page 815*
RV1 (RotaTeq®) *see* rotavirus vaccine *on page 813*
RV5 (Rotarix®) *see* rotavirus vaccine *on page 813*
Rybix™ ODT *see* tramadol *on page 909*
Rylosol (Can) *see* sotalol *on page 851*
Rynex PE *see* brompheniramine and phenylephrine *on page 144*
Rythmodan® (Can) *see* disopyramide *on page 301*
Rythmodan®-LA (Can) *see* disopyramide *on page 301*
Rythmol® *see* propafenone *on page 765*
Rythmol® Gen-Propafenone (Can) *see* propafenone *on page 765*
Rythmol® SR *see* propafenone *on page 765*
Ryzolt™ *see* tramadol *on page 909*
S2® [OTC] *see* epinephrine (systemic, oral inhalation) *on page 334*
S-(+)-3-isobutylgaba *see* pregabalin *on page 756*
6(S)-5-methyltetrahydrofolate *see* methylfolate *on page 589*
6(S)-5-MTHF *see* methylfolate *on page 589*
S-4661 *see* doripenem *on page 309*
Sabril® *see* vigabatrin *on page 945*

Saccharomyces boulardii (sak roe MYE sees boo LAR dee)

Medication Safety Issues

International issues:

Codex: Brand name for *saccharomyces boulardii* [Italy], but also the brand name for acetaminophen/codeine [Brazil]

Codex [Italy] may be confused with Cedax brand name for ceftibuten [U.S. and multiple international markets]; Clobex brand name for clobetasol [U.S., Canada, and multiple international markets]

Precosa [Finland, Norway, Sweden] may be confused with Precose brand name for acarbose [U.S.]

Synonyms *S. boulardii*; *Saccharomyces boulardii lyo*

U.S. Brand Names Florastor® Kids [OTC]; Florastor® [OTC]

Therapeutic Category Dietary Supplement; Probiotic

Use Promote maintenance of normal microflora in the gastrointestinal tract; used in management of bloating, gas, and diarrhea, particularly to decrease the incidence of diarrhea associated with antibiotic use

General Dosage Range Oral: *Children and Adults:* 250 mg twice daily

Dosage Forms

Capsule, oral:

Florastor® [OTC]: *S. boulardii* lyo 250 mg

Powder, oral:

Florastor® Kids [OTC]: *S. boulardii* lyo 250 mg/packet (10s)

Saccharomyces boulardii lyo *see* Saccharomyces boulardii *on page 815*

sacrosidase (sak ROE si dase)

U.S. Brand Names Sucraid®

Canadian Brand Names Sucraid®

Therapeutic Category Enzyme

Use Orphan drug: Oral replacement therapy in sucrase deficiency, as seen in congenital sucrase-isomaltase deficiency (CSID)

General Dosage Range Oral:

Infants and Children ≥5 and <15 kg: 8500 units (1 mL) per meal or snack

Children >15 kg and Adults: 17,000 units (2 mL) per meal or snack

Dosage Forms

Solution, oral:

Sucraid®: 8500 units/mL (118 mL)

Safetussin® CD [OTC] *see* dextromethorphan and phenylephrine *on page 273*
Safe Tussin® DM [OTC] *see* guaifenesin and dextromethorphan *on page 434*
Safe Wash™ [OTC] *see* sodium chloride *on page 840*
Safyral™ *see* ethinyl estradiol, drospirenone, and levomefolate *on page 363*
SAHA *see* vorinostat *on page 954*
Saizen® *see* somatropin *on page 849*
Salactic® [OTC] *see* salicylic acid *on page 816*
Salagen® *see* pilocarpine (systemic) *on page 722*
Salazopyrin® (Can) *see* sulfasalazine *on page 861*
Salazopyrin En-Tabs® (Can) *see* sulfasalazine *on page 861*
salbutamol *see* albuterol *on page 41*
salbutamol and ipratropium *see* ipratropium and albuterol *on page 499*
salbutamol sulphate *see* albuterol *on page 41*
Salex® *see* salicylic acid *on page 816*
Salflex® (Can) *see* salsalate *on page 820*
salicylazosulfapyridine *see* sulfasalazine *on page 861*

salicylic acid (sal i SIL ik AS id)

Medication Safety Issues

Sound-alike/look-alike issues:

Occlusal™-HP may be confused with Ocuflox®

Other safety concerns:

Transdermal patch may contain conducting metal (eg, aluminum); remove patch prior to MRI.

U.S. Brand Names Aliclen™; Beta Sal® [OTC]; Clean & Clear® Advantage® Acne Cleanser [OTC]; Clean & Clear® Advantage® Acne Spot Treatment [OTC]; Clean & Clear® Advantage® Invisible Acne Patch [OTC]; Clean & Clear® Advantage® Oil-Free Acne [OTC]; Clean & Clear® Blackhead Clearing Daily Cleansing [OTC]; Clean & Clear® Blackhead Clearing Scrub [OTC]; Clean & Clear® Deep Cleaning [OTC]; Clean & Clear® Dual Action Moisturizer [OTC]; Clean & Clear® Invisible Blemish Treatment [OTC]; Compound W® One Step Invisible Strip [OTC]; Compound W® One Step Wart Remover for Feet [OTC]; Compound W® One-Step Wart Remover for Kids [OTC]; Compound W® One-Step Wart Remover [OTC]; Compound W® [OTC]; Curad® Mediplast® [OTC]; Denorex® Extra Strength Protection 2-in-1 [OTC]; Denorex® Extra Strength Protection [OTC]; Dermarest® Psoriasis Medicated Moisturizer [OTC]; Dermarest® Psoriasis Medicated Scalp Treatment [OTC]; Dermarest® Psoriasis Medicated Shampoo/Conditioner [OTC]; Dermarest® Psoriasis Medicated Skin Treatment [OTC]; Dermarest® Psoriasis Overnight Treatment [OTC]; DHS™ Sal [OTC]; Dr. Scholl's® Callus Removers [OTC]; Dr. Scholl's® Clear Away® One Step Wart Remover [OTC]; Dr. Scholl's® Clear Away® Plantar Wart Remover For Feet [OTC]; Dr. Scholl's® Clear Away® Wart Remover Fast-Acting [OTC]; Dr. Scholl's® Clear Away® Wart Remover Invisible Strips [OTC]; Dr. Scholl's® Clear Away® Wart Remover [OTC]; Dr. Scholl's® Corn Removers [OTC]; Dr. Scholl's® Corn/Callus Remover [OTC]; Dr. Scholl's® Extra Thick Corn Removers [OTC]; Dr. Scholl's® Extra-Thick Callus Removers [OTC]; Dr. Scholl's® For Her Corn Removers [OTC]; Dr. Scholl's® OneStep Callus Removers [OTC]; Dr. Scholl's® OneStep Corn Removers [OTC]; Dr. Scholl's® Small Corn Removers [OTC]; Dr. Scholl's® Ultra-Thin Corn Removers [OTC]; DuoFilm® [OTC]; Freezone® [OTC]; Fung-O® [OTC]; Gets-It® [OTC]; Gordofilm [OTC]; Hydrisalic® [OTC]; Ionil Plus® [OTC]; Ionil® [OTC]; Keralyt®; Keralyt® [OTC]; LupiCare® Dandruff [OTC]; LupiCare® Psoriasis [OTC];

MG217® Sal-Acid [OTC]; Mosco® Callus & Corn Remover [OTC]; Mosco® One Step Corn Remover [OTC]; Neutrogena® Acne Stress Control [OTC]; Neutrogena® Advanced Solutions™ [OTC]; Neutrogena® Blackhead Eliminating™ 2-in-1 Foaming Pads [OTC]; Neutrogena® Blackhead Eliminating™ Daily Scrub [OTC]; Neutrogena® Blackhead Eliminating™ [OTC]; Neutrogena® Body Clear® [OTC]; Neutrogena® Clear Pore™ Oil-Controlling Astringent [OTC]; Neutrogena® Maximum Strength T/Sal® [OTC]; Neutrogena® Oil-Free Acne Stress Control [OTC]; Neutrogena® Oil-Free Acne Wash 60 Second Mask Scrub [OTC]; Neutrogena® Oil-Free Acne Wash Cream Cleanser [OTC]; Neutrogena® Oil-Free Acne Wash Foam Cleanser [OTC]; Neutrogena® Oil-Free Acne Wash [OTC]; Neutrogena® Oil-Free Acne [OTC]; Neutrogena® Oil-Free Anti-Acne [OTC]; Neutrogena® Rapid Clear® Acne Defense [OTC]; Neutrogena® Rapid Clear® Acne Eliminating [OTC]; Neutrogena® Rapid Clear® [OTC]; OXY® Body Wash [OTC]; OXY® Chill Factor® [OTC]; OXY® Daily Cleansing [OTC]; OXY® Daily [OTC]; OXY® Face Wash [OTC]; OXY® Maximum Daily Cleansing [OTC]; OXY® Maximum [OTC]; OXY® Post-Shave [OTC]; OXY® Spot Treatment [OTC]; OXY® [OTC]; P&S® [OTC]; Palmer's® Skin Success Acne Cleanser [OTC]; Sal-Plant® [OTC]; Salactic® [OTC]; Salex®; Salvax; Scalpicin® Anti-Itch [OTC]; Selsun blue® Deep Cleaning Micro-Bead Scrub [OTC]; Selsun blue® Naturals Island Breeze [OTC]; Selsun blue® Naturals Itchy Dry Scalp [OTC]; Stridex® Essential Care® [OTC]; Stridex® Facewipes To Go® [OTC]; Stridex® Maximum Strength [OTC]; Stridex® Sensitive Skin [OTC]; Thera-Sal [OTC] [DSC]; Tinamed® Corn and Callus Remover [OTC]; Tinamed® Wart Remover [OTC]; Trans-Ver-Sal® [OTC]; Virasal®; Wart-Off® Maximum Strength [OTC]; Zapzyt® Acne Wash [OTC]; Zapzyt® Pore Treatment [OTC]

Canadian Brand Names Duofilm®; Duoforte® 27; Occlusal™-HP; Sebcur®; Soluver®; Soluver® Plus; Trans-Plantar®; Trans-Ver-Sal®

Therapeutic Category Keratolytic Agent

Use Topically for its keratolytic effect in controlling seborrheic dermatitis or psoriasis of body and scalp, dandruff, and other scaling dermatoses; also used to remove warts, corns, and calluses; acne

General Dosage Range Topical: *Children and Adults:* Dosage varies greatly depending on product

Dosage Forms

Aerosol, foam, topical: 6% (70 g)
- Salvax: 6% (70 g, 200 g)

Bar, topical: 2% (113 g)
- OXY® [OTC]: 0.5% (119 g)

Cloth, topical:
- Neutrogena® Oil-Free Acne Wash [OTC]: 2% (30s)

Cream, topical: 6% (400 g, 480 g)
- Clean & Clear® Advantage® Acne Cleanser [OTC]: 2% (148 mL)
- Clean & Clear® Advantage® Acne Spot Treatment [OTC]: 2% (22 g)
- Clean & Clear® Blackhead Clearing Scrub [OTC]: 2% (141 g, 226 g)
- Clean & Clear® Dual Action Moisturizer [OTC]: 0.5% (120 mL)
- LupiCare® Psoriasis [OTC]: 2% (227 g)
- Neutrogena® Acne Stress Control [OTC]: 2% (125 g)
- Neutrogena® Oil-Free Acne [OTC]: 2% (125 mL)
- Neutrogena® Oil-Free Acne Stress Control [OTC]: 2% (172 g)
- Neutrogena® Oil-Free Acne Wash Cream Cleanser [OTC]: 2% (200 mL)
- Neutrogena® Oil-Free Anti-Acne [OTC]: 0.5% (50 g)
- Salex®: 6% (454 g)

Gel, topical: 6% (40 g)
- Clean & Clear® Advantage® Invisible Acne Patch [OTC]: 2% (1.9 mL)
- Clean & Clear® Invisible Blemish Treatment [OTC]: 2% (22 mL)
- Compound W® [OTC]: 17.6% (7 g)
- Dermarest® Psoriasis Medicated Scalp Treatment [OTC]: 3% (118 mL)
- Dermarest® Psoriasis Medicated Skin Treatment [OTC]: 3% (118 mL)
- Dermarest® Psoriasis Overnight Treatment [OTC]: 3% (56.7 g)
- Hydrisalic® [OTC]: 6% (28 g)
- Keralyt® [OTC]: 3% (30 g); 6% (40 g, 100 g)
- Neutrogena® Advanced Solutions™ [OTC]: 2% (40 g)
- Neutrogena® Oil-Free Acne Wash [OTC]: 2% (177 mL, 296 mL)
- Neutrogena® Rapid Clear® Acne Eliminating [OTC]: 2% (15 mL)
- OXY® [OTC]: 2% (355 mL)
- OXY® Body Wash [OTC]: 2% (355 mL)
- OXY® Chill Factor® [OTC]: 2% (142 g)
- OXY® Face Wash [OTC]: 2% (177 mL)
- OXY® Maximum [OTC]: 2% (142 g)

OXY® Spot Treatment [OTC]: 1% (14.7 g)
Sal-Plant® [OTC]: 17% (14 g)
Zapzyt® Acne Wash [OTC]: 2% (188.5 g)
Zapzyt® Pore Treatment [OTC]: 2% (22 mL)

Liquid, topical:
Clean & Clear® Advantage® Oil-Free Acne [OTC]: 0.5% (120 mL)
Clean & Clear® Deep Cleaning [OTC]: 2% (240 mL)
Compound W® [OTC]: 17.6% (9 mL)
Dr. Scholl's® Clear Away® Wart Remover Fast-Acting [OTC]: 17% (9.8 mL)
Dr. Scholl's® Corn/Callus Remover [OTC]: 12.6% (9.8 mL)
DuoFilm® [OTC]: 17% (9.8 mL)
Freezone® [OTC]: 17.6% (9.3 mL)
Fung-O® [OTC]: 17% (15 mL)
Gets-It® [OTC]: 13.9% (15 mL)
Gordofilm [OTC]: 16.7% (15 mL)
Mosco® Callus & Corn Remover [OTC]: 17.6% (9 mL)
Neutrogena® Blackhead Eliminating™ Daily Scrub [OTC]: 2% (125 mL)
Neutrogena® Body Clear® [OTC]: 2% (250 mL)
Neutrogena® Clear Pore™ Oil-Controlling Astringent [OTC]: 2% (236 mL)
Neutrogena® Oil-Free Acne Stress Control [OTC]: 0.5% (177 mL); 2% (50 mL)
Neutrogena® Oil-Free Acne Wash 60 Second Mask Scrub [OTC]: 1% (170 g)
Neutrogena® Oil-Free Acne Wash Foam Cleanser [OTC]: 2% (150 mL)
Palmer's® Skin Success Acne Cleanser [OTC]: 0.5% (240 mL)
Salactic® [OTC]: 17% (15 mL)
Scalpicin® Anti-Itch [OTC]: 3% (44 mL, 74 mL)
Tinamed® Corn and Callus Remover [OTC]: 17% (15 mL)
Tinamed® Wart Remover [OTC]: 17% (15 mL)
Virasal®: 27.5% (10 mL)
Wart-Off® Maximum Strength [OTC]: 17.5% (14.8 mL)

Lotion, topical: 6% (414 mL, 420 mL); 6% (400 g)
Dermarest® Psoriasis Medicated Moisturizer [OTC]: 2% (118 mL)
Neutrogena® Rapid Clear® Acne Defense [OTC]: 2% (50 mL)
OXY® Post-Shave [OTC]: 0.5% (50 g)
Salex®: 6% (237 mL)

Ointment, topical:
MG217® Sal-Acid [OTC]: 3% (57 g)

Pad, topical:
Clean & Clear® Blackhead Clearing Daily Cleansing [OTC]: 1% (70s)
Curad® Mediplast® [OTC]: 40% (25s)
Neutrogena® Blackhead Eliminating™ [OTC]: 0.5% (28s)
Neutrogena® Blackhead Eliminating™ 2-in-1 Foaming Pads [OTC]: 0.5% (28s)
Neutrogena® Rapid Clear® [OTC]: 2% (60s)
OXY® Chill Factor® [OTC]: 2% (90s)
OXY® Daily [OTC]: 0.2% (90s)
OXY® Daily Cleansing [OTC]: 0.5% (90s)
OXY® Maximum Daily Cleansing [OTC]: 2% (55s, 90s)
Stridex® Essential Care® [OTC]: 1% (55s)
Stridex® Facewipes To Go® [OTC]: 0.5% (32s)
Stridex® Maximum Strength [OTC]: 2% (55s, 90s)
Stridex® Sensitive Skin [OTC]: 0.5% (55s, 90s)

Patch, topical:
Compound W® One Step Invisible Strip [OTC]: 14% (14s)
Compound W® One Step Wart Remover for Feet [OTC]: 40% (20s)
Compound W® One-Step Wart Remover [OTC]: 40% (14s)
Compound W® One-Step Wart Remover for Kids [OTC]: 40% (12s)
Dr. Scholl's® Callus Removers [OTC]: 40% (4s)
Dr. Scholl's® Clear Away® One Step Wart Remover [OTC]: 40% (14s)
Dr. Scholl's® Clear Away® Plantar Wart Remover For Feet [OTC]: 40% (24s)
Dr. Scholl's® Clear Away® Wart Remover [OTC]: 40% (18s)
Dr. Scholl's® Clear Away® Wart Remover Invisible Strips [OTC]: 40% (18s)
Dr. Scholl's® Corn Removers [OTC]: 40% (9s)
Dr. Scholl's® Extra Thick Corn Removers [OTC]: 40% (9s)

Dr. Scholl's® Extra-Thick Callus Removers [OTC]: 40% (4s)
Dr. Scholl's® For Her Corn Removers [OTC]: 40% (6s)
Dr. Scholl's® OneStep Callus Removers [OTC]: 40% (4s)
Dr. Scholl's® OneStep Corn Removers [OTC]: 40% (6s)
Dr. Scholl's® Small Corn Removers [OTC]: 40% (9s)
Dr. Scholl's® Ultra-Thin Corn Removers [OTC]: 40% (9s)
Mosco® One Step Corn Remover [OTC]: 40% (8s)
Trans-Ver-Sal® [OTC]: 15% (10s, 12s, 15s, 25s, 40s)

Shampoo, topical: 6% (177 mL)
Aliclen™: 6% (177 mL)
Beta Sal® [OTC]: 3% (480 mL)
Denorex® Extra Strength Protection [OTC]: 3% (118 mL, 355 mL)
DHS™ Sal [OTC]: 3% (120 mL)
Ionil Plus® [OTC]: 2% (240 mL)
Ionil® [OTC]: 2% (120 mL)
LupiCare® Dandruff [OTC]: 2% (237 mL)
LupiCare® Psoriasis [OTC]: 2% (237 mL)
Neutrogena® Maximum Strength T/Sal® [OTC]: 3% (135 mL)
P&S® [OTC]: 2% (118 mL, 236 mL)
Salex®: 6% (177 mL)
Selsun blue® Deep Cleaning Micro-Bead Scrub [OTC]: 3% (325 mL)
Selsun blue® Naturals Island Breeze [OTC]: 3% (325 mL)
Selsun blue® Naturals Itchy Dry Scalp [OTC]: 3% (207 mL, 325 mL)

Shampoo/Conditioner, topical:
Denorex® Extra Strength Protection 2-in-1 [OTC]: 3% (118 mL, 355 mL)
Dermarest® Psoriasis Medicated Shampoo/Conditioner [OTC]: 3% (236 mL)

salicylic acid and coal tar *see* coal tar and salicylic acid *on page 229*
salicylic acid and sulfur *see* sulfur and salicylic acid *on page 861*
salicylsalicylic acid *see* salsalate *on page 820*
saline *see* sodium chloride *on page 840*
Saline Mist [OTC] *see* sodium chloride *on page 840*

saliva substitute (sa LYE va SUB stee tute)

Synonyms artificial saliva

U.S. Brand Names Aquoral™; Biotene® Moisturizing Mouth Spray [OTC]; Biotene® Oral Balance® [OTC]; Caphosol®; Entertainer's Secret® [OTC]; Moi-Stir® [OTC]; Mouth Kote® [OTC]; NeutraSal®; Numoisyn™; Oasis®; SalivaSure™ [OTC]

Therapeutic Category Gastrointestinal Agent, Miscellaneous

Use Relief of dry mouth and throat in xerostomia or hyposalivation; adjunct to standard oral care in relief of symptoms associated with chemotherapy or radiation therapy-induced mucositis

General Dosage Range Oral: *Adults:* Dosage varies greatly depending on product

Dosage Forms

Liquid, oral:
Biotene® Oral Balance® [OTC]: Water, starch, sunflower oil, propylene glycol, xylitol, glycerine, purified milk extract
Numoisyn™: Water, sorbitol, linseed extract, *Chondrus crispus*, methylparaben, sodium benzoate, potassium sorbate, dipotassium phosphate, propylparaben

Lozenge, oral:
Numoisyn™: Sorbitol 0.3 g/lozenge, polyethylene glycol, malic acid, sodium citrate, calcium phosphate dibasic, hydrogenated cottonseed oil, citric acid, magnesium stearate, silicon dioxide
SalivaSure™ [OTC]: Xylitol, citric acid, apple acid, sodium citrate dihydrate, sodium carboxymethylcellulose, dibasic calcium phosphate, silica colloidal, magnesium stearate, stearic acid

Powder, for reconstitution, oral:
NeutraSal®: Sodium, phosphates, calcium, chloride, bicarbonate, silicon dioxide

Solution, oral:
Caphosol®: Dibasic sodium phosphate 0.032%, monobasic sodium phosphate 0.009%, calcium chloride 0.052%, sodium chloride 0.569%, purified water
Entertainer's Secret® [OTC]: Sodium carboxymethylcellulose, aloe vera gel, glycerin (60 mL)

Solution, oral [mouthwash/gargle]:
Oasis®: Water, glycerin, sorbitol, poloxamer 338, PEG-60, hydrogenated castor oil, copovidone, sodium benzoate, carboxymethylcellulose
Solution, oral [spray]:
Aquoral™: Oxidized glycerol triesters and silicon dioxide
Biotene® Moisturizing Mouth Spray [OTC]: Water, polyglycitol, propylene glycol, sunflower oil, xylitol, milk protein extract, potassium sorbate, acesulfame K, potassium thiocyanate, lysozyme, lactoferrin, lactoperoxidase
Moi-Stir® [OTC]: Water, sorbitol, sodium carboxymethylcellulose, methylparaben, propylparaben, potassium chloride, dibasic sodium phosphate, calcium chloride, magnesium chloride, sodium chloride
Mouth Kote® [OTC]: Water, xylitol, sorbitol, yerba santa, citric acid, ascorbic acid, sodium saccharin, sodium benzoate
Oasis®: Glycerin, cetylpyridinium, copovidone

SalivaSure™ [OTC] *see* saliva substitute *on page 819*
Saljet® [OTC] *see* sodium chloride *on page 840*
salk vaccine *see* poliovirus vaccine (inactivated) *on page 736*

salmeterol (sal ME te role)

Medication Safety Issues
Sound-alike/look-alike issues:
Salmeterol may be confused with Salbutamol, Solu-Medrol®
Serevent® may be confused with Atrovent®, Combivent®, sertraline, Sinemet®, Spiriva®, Zoloft®

Synonyms salmeterol xinafoate
U.S. Brand Names Serevent® Diskus®
Canadian Brand Names Serevent® Diskhaler® Disk; Serevent® Diskus®
Therapeutic Category Adrenergic Agonist Agent
Use Maintenance treatment of asthma and prevention of bronchospasm (as concomitant therapy) in patients with reversible obstructive airway disease, including patients with symptoms of nocturnal asthma; prevention of exercise-induced bronchospasm (monotherapy may be indicated in patients without persistent asthma); maintenance treatment of bronchospasm associated with COPD
General Dosage Range Inhalation: *Children ≥4 years and Adults:* 1 inhalation (50 mcg) twice daily
Dosage Forms
Powder, for oral inhalation:
Serevent® Diskus®: 50 mcg (28s, 60s)
Dosage Forms - Canada
Powder for oral inhalation:
Serevent® Diskhaler® Disk: 50 mcg (60s)

salmeterol and fluticasone *see* fluticasone and salmeterol *on page 401*
salmeterol xinafoate *see* salmeterol *on page 820*
Salofalk® (Can) *see* mesalamine *on page 577*
Salofalk® 5-ASA (Can) *see* mesalamine *on page 577*
Salonpas® [OTC] *see* methyl salicylate and menthol *on page 592*
Salonpas® Arthritis Pain® [OTC] *see* methyl salicylate and menthol *on page 592*
Salonpas® Gel-Patch Hot [OTC] *see* capsaicin *on page 170*
Salonpas® Hot [OTC] *see* capsaicin *on page 170*
Salonpas® Jet Spray [OTC] *see* methyl salicylate and menthol *on page 592*
Salonpas® Massage Foam [OTC] *see* methyl salicylate and menthol *on page 592*
Salonpas® Pain Relief Patch® [OTC] *see* methyl salicylate and menthol *on page 592*
Sal-Plant® [OTC] *see* salicylic acid *on page 816*

salsalate (SAL sa late)

Medication Safety Issues
Sound-alike/look-alike issues:
Salsalate may be confused with sucralfate, sulfaSALAzine

Synonyms disalicylic acid; salicylsalicylic acid
Canadian Brand Names Amigesic®; Salflex®
Therapeutic Category Analgesic, Nonnarcotic; Antipyretic; Nonsteroidal Antiinflammatory Drug (NSAID)

Use Treatment of rheumatoid arthritis, osteoarthritis, and related rheumatic disorders

General Dosage Range Dosage adjustment recommended in patients with renal impairment

Oral: *Adults:* 3 g/day in 2-3 divided doses

Dosage Forms

Tablet, oral: 500 mg, 750 mg

salt *see* sodium chloride *on page 840*

salt-poor albumin *see* albumin *on page 41*

Salvax *see* salicylic acid *on page 816*

samarium Sm 153 lexidronam (sa MAR ee um es em won fif tee three lex ID roe nam)

Medication Safety Issues

Other safety concerns:

Radiopharmaceutical: Use appropriate precaution for handling, disposal, and minimizing exposure to patients and healthcare personnel. Use under supervision of experienced personnel. Should be stored in original lead container or adequate radiation shield.

Synonyms ^{153}Sm-lexidronam

U.S. Brand Names Quadramet®

Therapeutic Category Radiopharmaceutical

Use Relief of pain associated with osteoblastic metastatic bone lesions that demonstrate increased localization on radionuclide bone scans

Samsca™ *see* tolvaptan *on page 905*

Sanctura® *see* trospium *on page 924*

Sanctura® XR *see* trospium *on page 924*

Sancuso® *see* granisetron *on page 432*

SandIMMUNE® *see* cyclosporine (systemic) *on page 245*

Sandimmune® I.V. (Can) *see* cyclosporine (systemic) *on page 245*

Sandomigran® (Can) *see* pizotifen *(Canada only) on page 728*

Sandomigran DS® (Can) *see* pizotifen *(Canada only) on page 728*

SandoSTATIN® *see* octreotide *on page 658*

Sandostatin® (Can) *see* octreotide *on page 658*

SandoSTATIN LAR® *see* octreotide *on page 658*

Sandostatin LAR® (Can) *see* octreotide *on page 658*

Sandoz-Acebutolol (Can) *see* acebutolol *on page 19*

Sandoz-Alendronate (Can) *see* alendronate *on page 45*

Sandoz-Alfuzosin (Can) *see* alfuzosin *on page 47*

Sandoz-Amiodarone (Can) *see* amiodarone *on page 63*

Sandoz Amlodipine (Can) *see* amlodipine *on page 65*

Sandoz-Anagrelide (Can) *see* anagrelide *on page 74*

Sandoz-Atenolol (Can) *see* atenolol *on page 99*

Sandoz-Atomoxetine (Can) *see* atomoxetine *on page 99*

Sandoz-Atorvastatin (Can) *see* atorvastatin *on page 100*

Sandoz-Azithromycin (Can) *see* azithromycin (systemic) *on page 108*

Sandoz-Betaxolol (Can) *see* betaxolol (ophthalmic) *on page 131*

Sandoz-Bicalutamide (Can) *see* bicalutamide *on page 133*

Sandoz-Bisoprolol (Can) *see* bisoprolol *on page 136*

Sandoz-Bosentan (Can) *see* bosentan *on page 139*

Sandoz-Brimonidine (Can) *see* brimonidine *on page 141*

Sandoz-Bupropion SR (Can) *see* bupropion *on page 150*

Sandoz-Calcitonin (Can) *see* calcitonin *on page 159*

Sandoz-Candesartan (Can) *see* candesartan *on page 168*

Sandoz-Carbamazepine (Can) *see* carbamazepine *on page 172*

Sandoz-Cefprozil (Can) *see* cefprozil *on page 185*

Sandoz-Ciprofloxacin (Can) *see* ciprofloxacin (systemic) *on page 210*

Sandoz-Citalopram (Can) *see* citalopram *on page 213*

sapropterin (sap roe TER in)

Medication Safety Issues

Sound-alike/look-alike issues:

Sapropterin may be confused with cyproterone

Synonyms 6R-BH4; phenoptin; sapropterin dihydrochloride

U.S. Brand Names Kuvan™

Therapeutic Category Enzyme Cofactor

Use Adjunct to dietary management in the treatment of tetrahydrobiopterin (BH4) responsive phenylketonuria (PKU)

General Dosage Range Oral: *Children ≥4 years and Adults:* 10 mg/kg once daily; Maintenance range: 5-20 mg/kg/day

Dosage Forms

Tablet, oral:

Kuvan™: 100 mg

sapropterin dihydrochloride *see* sapropterin *on page 823*

saquinavir (sa KWIN a veer)

Medication Safety Issues

Sound-alike/look-alike issues:

Saquinavir may be confused with SINEquan®

Synonyms saquinavir mesylate; SQV

U.S. Brand Names Invirase®

Canadian Brand Names Invirase®

Therapeutic Category Antiviral Agent

Use Treatment of HIV infection; used in combination with at least two other antiretroviral agents

General Dosage Range Dosage adjustment recommended in patients on concomitant therapy

Oral: *Children >16 years and Adults:* 1000 mg twice daily

Dosage Forms

Capsule, oral:

Invirase®: 200 mg

Tablet, oral:

Invirase®: 500 mg

saquinavir mesylate *see* saquinavir *on page 824*

Sarafem® *see* fluoxetine *on page 396*

sargramostim (sar GRAM oh stim)

Medication Safety Issues

Sound-alike/look-alike issues:

Leukine® may be confused with Leukeran®, leucovorin

Synonyms GM-CSF; granulocyte-macrophage colony-stimulating factor; NSC-613795; rGM-CSF

U.S. Brand Names Leukine®

Canadian Brand Names Leukine®

Therapeutic Category Colony-Stimulating Factor

Use

Acute myelogenous leukemia (AML) following induction chemotherapy in older adults (≥55 years of age) to shorten time to neutrophil recovery and to reduce the incidence of severe and life-threatening infections and infections resulting in death

Bone marrow transplant (allogeneic or autologous) failure or engraftment delay

Myeloid reconstitution after allogeneic bone marrow transplantation

Myeloid reconstitution after autologous bone marrow transplantation: Non-Hodgkin lymphoma (NHL), acute lymphoblastic leukemia (ALL), Hodgkin lymphoma

Peripheral stem cell transplantation: Mobilization and myeloid reconstitution following autologous peripheral stem cell transplantation

General Dosage Range

I.V.: *Children and Adults:* Infusion: 250 mcg/m^2/day (maximum: 500 mcg/m^2/day)

SubQ: *Children and Adults:* 250 mcg/m^2 once daily

Dosage Forms

Injection, powder for reconstitution:

Leukine®: 250 mcg

Injection, solution:

Leukine®: 500 mcg/mL (1 mL)

Sarna® HC (Can) *see* hydrocortisone (topical) *on page 457*

Sarna® Sensitive [OTC] *see* pramoxine *on page 750*

Sativex® (Can) *see* tetrahydrocannabinol and cannabidiol *(Canada only) on page 884*

Savella® *see* milnacipran *on page 603*

saxagliptin (sax a GLIP tin)

Medication Safety Issues

Sound-alike/look-alike issues:

Saxagliptin may be confused with sitaGLIPtin, SUMAtriptan

High alert medication:

The Institute for Safe Medication Practices (ISMP) includes this medication among its list of drug classes which have a heightened risk of causing significant patient harm when used in error.

Synonyms BMS-477118

U.S. Brand Names Onglyza™

Canadian Brand Names Onglyza™

Therapeutic Category Antidiabetic Agent, Dipeptidyl Peptidase IV (DPP-IV) Inhibitor

Use Treatment of type 2 diabetes mellitus (noninsulin-dependent, NIDDM) as an adjunct to diet and exercise as monotherapy or in combination therapy with other antidiabetic agents to improve glycemic control

General Dosage Range Dosage adjustment recommended in patients with renal impairment or on concomitant therapy

Oral: *Adults:* 2.5-5 mg once daily

Dosage Forms

Tablet, oral:

Onglyza™: 2.5 mg, 5 mg

saxagliptin and metformin (sax a GLIP tin & met FOR min)

Medication Safety Issues

Sound-alike/look-alike issues:

Saxagliptin and Metformin may be confused with sitaGLIPtin and Metformin

High alert medication:

The Institute for Safe Medication Practices (ISMP) includes this medication among its list of drug classes which have a heightened risk of causing significant patient harm when used in error.

Synonyms metformin and saxagliptin; metformin hydrochloride and saxagliptin; saxagliptin and metformin hydrochloride

U.S. Brand Names Kombiglyze™ XR

Therapeutic Category Antidiabetic Agent, Biguanide; Antidiabetic Agent, Dipeptidyl Peptidase IV (DPP-IV) Inhibitor

Use Management of type 2 diabetes mellitus (noninsulin dependent, NIDDM) as an adjunct to diet and exercise when treatment with both saxagliptin and metformin is appropriate

General Dosage Range Dosage adjustment recommended in patients on concomitant therapy

Oral: *Adults:* Saxagliptin 2.5-5 mg and metformin 500-2000 mg once daily (maximum: 5 mg/day [saxagliptin], 2000 mg/day [metformin])

Dosage Forms

Tablet, variable release, oral:

Kombiglyze™ XR 2.5/1000: Saxagliptin 2.5 mg [immediate release] and metformin hydrochloride 1000 mg [extended release]; 5/500: Saxagliptin 5 mg [immediate release] and metformin hydrochloride 500 mg [extended release]; 5/1000: Saxagliptin 5 mg [immediate release] and metformin hydrochloride 1000 mg [extended release]

saxagliptin and metformin hydrochloride *see* saxagliptin and metformin *on page 825*

SB-265805 *see* gemifloxacin *on page 422*

SB-497115 *see* eltrombopag *on page 327*

SB-497115-GR *see* eltrombopag *on page 327*

SB659746-A *see* vilazodone *on page 945*

S. boulardii *see Saccharomyces boulardii on page 815*

SC 33428 *see* idarubicin *on page 472*

Scalpana [OTC] *see* hydrocortisone (topical) *on page 457*

Scalpicin® Anti-Itch [OTC] *see* salicylic acid *on page 816*

Scandonest® 2% L *see* mepivacaine and levonordefrin *on page 576*

SCH 13521 *see* flutamide *on page 399*

SCH 52365 *see* temozolomide *on page 876*

SCH 56592 *see* posaconazole *on page 742*

SCH503034 *see* boceprevir *on page* 138
ScheinPharm Ranitidine (Can) *see* ranitidine *on page* 788
SCIG *see* immune globulin *on page* 477
S-citalopram *see* escitalopram *on page* 345
Sclerosol® *see* talc (sterile) *on page* 867

scopolamine (systemic) (skoe POL a meen)

Medication Safety Issues

BEERS Criteria medication:

This drug may be potentially inappropriate for use in geriatric patients (Quality of evidence - moderate; Strength of recommendation - strong).

Other safety concerns:

Transdermal patch may contain conducting metal (eg, aluminum); remove patch prior to MRI.

Synonyms hyoscine butylbromide; scopolamine base; scopolamine butylbromide; scopolamine hydrobromide

U.S. Brand Names Transderm Scōp®

Canadian Brand Names Buscopan®; Scopolamine Hydrobromide Injection; Transderm-V®

Therapeutic Category Anticholinergic Agent

Use

Scopolamine base: Transdermal: Prevention of nausea/vomiting associated with motion sickness and recovery from anesthesia and surgery

Scopolamine hydrobromide: Injection: Preoperative medication to produce amnesia, sedation, tranquilization, antiemetic effects, and decrease salivary and respiratory secretions

Scopolamine butylbromide [not available in the U.S.]: Oral/injection: Treatment of smooth muscle spasm of the genitourinary or gastrointestinal tract; injection may also be used prior to radiological/ diagnostic procedures to prevent spasm

General Dosage Range

I.M., I.V., SubQ:

Children 6 months to 3 years: 0.1-0.15 mg
Children 3-6 years: 0.2-0.3 mg
Adults: 0.3-0.65 mg (single dose) **or** 0.6 mg 3-4 times/day

Transdermal: *Adults:* Apply 1 patch every 3 days as needed

Dosage Forms

Injection, solution: 0.4 mg/mL (1 mL)

Patch, transdermal:

Transderm Scōp®: 1.5 mg (4s, 10s, 24s)

Dosage Forms - Canada

Tablet, oral:

Buscopan®: 10 mg

scopolamine (ophthalmic) (skoe POL a meen)

Synonyms hyoscine hydrobromide; scopolamine hydrobromide

U.S. Brand Names Isopto® Hyoscine

Therapeutic Category Anticholinergic Agent; Anticholinergic Agent, Ophthalmic; Ophthalmic Agent, Mydriatic

Use Produce cycloplegia and mydriasis; treatment of iridocyclitis

General Dosage Range Ophthalmic: *Adults:* Instill 1-2 drops to eye(s) up to 4 times/day

Dosage Forms

Solution, ophthalmic:

Isopto® Hyoscine: 0.25% (5 mL)

scopolamine base *see* scopolamine (systemic) *on page* 826
scopolamine butylbromide *see* scopolamine (systemic) *on page* 826
scopolamine hydrobromide *see* scopolamine (ophthalmic) *on page* 826
scopolamine hydrobromide *see* scopolamine (systemic) *on page* 826
Scopolamine Hydrobromide Injection (Can) *see* scopolamine (systemic) *on page* 826
scopolamine, hyoscyamine, atropine, and phenobarbital *see* hyoscyamine, atropine, scopolamine, and phenobarbital *on page* 467
scorpion antivenin *see* *Centruroides* immune $F(ab')_2$ (equine) *on page* 189

scorpion antivenom *see Centruroides* immune $F(ab')_2$ (equine) *on page 189*
Scot-Tussin® Diabetes [OTC] *see* dextromethorphan *on page 272*
Scot-Tussin® DM Maximum Strength [OTC] *see* dextromethorphan and chlorpheniramine *on page 273*
Scot-Tussin® Expectorant [OTC] *see* guaifenesin *on page 433*
Scot-Tussin® Senior [OTC] *see* guaifenesin and dextromethorphan *on page 434*
Scytera™ [OTC] *see* coal tar *on page 228*
SD/01 *see* pegfilgrastim *on page 696*
SDX-105 *see* bendamustine *on page 120*
SDZ ENA 713 *see* rivastigmine *on page 806*
Sea Soft Nasal Mist [OTC] *see* sodium chloride *on page 840*
Seasonale® [DSC] *see* ethinyl estradiol and levonorgestrel *on page 357*
Seasonale® (Can) *see* ethinyl estradiol and levonorgestrel *on page 357*
Seasonique® *see* ethinyl estradiol and levonorgestrel *on page 357*
Sebcur® (Can) *see* salicylic acid *on page 816*
Sebcur/T® (Can) *see* coal tar and salicylic acid *on page 229*
Sebex [OTC] *see* sulfur and salicylic acid *on page 861*
Sebivo® (Can) *see* telbivudine *on page 874*
SE BPO *see* benzoyl peroxide *on page 124*
Seb-Prev™ [DSC] *see* sulfacetamide (topical) *on page 858*
Sebulex® [OTC] *see* sulfur and salicylic acid *on page 861*

secobarbital (see koe BAR bi tal)

Medication Safety Issues

Sound-alike/look-alike issues:

Seconal® may be confused with Sectral®

BEERS Criteria medication:

This drug may be potentially inappropriate for use in geriatric patients (Quality of evidence - high; Strength of recommendation - strong).

Synonyms quinalbarbitone sodium; secobarbital sodium

U.S. Brand Names Seconal®

Therapeutic Category Barbiturate

Controlled Substance C-II

Use Preanesthetic agent; short-term treatment of insomnia

General Dosage Range Oral: *Adults:* 100 mg at bedtime **or** 200-300 mg 1-2 hours before procedure

Dosage Forms

Capsule, oral:

Seconal®: 100 mg

secobarbital sodium *see* secobarbital *on page 827*
Seconal® *see* secobarbital *on page 827*

secretin (SEE kr tin)

Synonyms secretin, human; secretin, porcine

U.S. Brand Names ChiRhoStim®

Therapeutic Category Diagnostic Agent

Use Secretin-stimulation testing to aid in diagnosis of pancreatic exocrine dysfunction; diagnosis of gastrinoma (Zollinger-Ellison syndrome); facilitation of endoscopic retrograde cholangiopancreatography (ERCP) visualization

General Dosage Range I.V.: *Adults:* Test dose: 0.1 mL (0.2-0.4 mcg); Diagnostic dose: 0.2-0.4 mcg/kg

Dosage Forms

Injection, powder for reconstitution:

ChiRhoStim®: 16 mcg

secretin, human *see* secretin *on page 827*
secretin, porcine *see* secretin *on page 827*
Sectral® *see* acebutolol *on page 19*

Secura® Antifungal Extra Thick [OTC] *see* miconazole (topical) *on page* 599
Secura® Antifungal Greaseless [OTC] *see* miconazole (topical) *on page* 599
Sedapap® *see* butalbital and acetaminophen *on page* 154
Selax® (Can) *see* docusate *on page* 304
Select™ 1/35 (Can) *see* ethinyl estradiol and norethindrone *on page* 359
Select-OB™ *see* vitamins (multiple/prenatal) *on page* 952

selegiline (se LE ji leen)

Medication Safety Issues

Sound-alike/look-alike issues:

Selegiline may be confused with Salagen®, sertraline, Serzone, Stelazine

Eldepryl® may be confused with Elavil®, enalapril

Zelapar® may be confused with zaleplon, Zemplar®, zolpidem, ZyPREXA® Zydis®

Synonyms deprenyl; L-deprenyl; selegiline hydrochloride

U.S. Brand Names Eldepryl®; Emsam®; Zelapar®

Canadian Brand Names Apo-Selegiline®; Gen-Selegiline; Mylan-Selegiline; Novo-Selegiline; Nu-Selegiline

Therapeutic Category Anti-Parkinson Agent; Dopaminergic Agent (Anti-Parkinson)

Use Adjunct in the management of parkinsonian patients in which levodopa/carbidopa therapy is deteriorating (oral products); treatment of major depressive disorder (transdermal product)

General Dosage Range

Oral:

Capsule/Tablet: *Adults:* 5 mg twice daily

Disintegrating tablet: *Adults:* Initial: 1.25 mg daily; Maintenance: 1.25-2.5 mg daily (maximum: 2.5 mg daily)

Transdermal:

Adults: Initial: 6 mg once daily; Maintenance: 6-12 mg once daily (maximum: 12 mg/day)

Elderly: 6 mg once daily

Dosage Forms

Capsule, oral: 5 mg

Eldepryl®: 5 mg

Patch, transdermal:

Emsam®: 6 mg/24 hours (30s); 9 mg/24 hours (30s); 12 mg/24 hours (30s)

Tablet, oral: 5 mg

Tablet, orally disintegrating, oral:

Zelapar®: 1.25 mg

selegiline hydrochloride *see* selegiline *on page* 828
selenium *see* trace elements *on page* 908

selenium sulfide (se LEE nee um SUL fide)

U.S. Brand Names Dandrex; Head & Shoulders® Clinical Strength [OTC]; Selsun blue® 2-in-1 [OTC]; Selsun blue® Medicated [OTC]; Selsun blue® Moisturizing [OTC]; Selsun blue® Normal to Oily [OTC]; Tersi

Canadian Brand Names Versel®

Therapeutic Category Antiseborrheic Agent, Topical

Use Treatment of itching and flaking of the scalp associated with dandruff, to control scalp seborrheic dermatitis; treatment of tinea versicolor

General Dosage Range Topical: *Adults:* Foam: Rub into affected skin twice daily; Lotion: Apply to affected area daily; Shampoo: Massage 5-10 mL into wet scalp

Dosage Forms

Aerosol, foam, topical:

Tersi: 2.25% (70 g)

Lotion, topical: 2.5% (118 mL, 120 mL)

Shampoo, topical: 1% (210 mL)
Dandrex: 1% (236 mL)
Head & Shoulders® Clinical Strength [OTC]: 1% (420 mL)
Selsun blue® 2-in-1 [OTC]: 1% (207 mL, 325 mL)
Selsun blue® Medicated [OTC]: 1% (120 mL, 207 mL, 325 mL)
Selsun blue® Moisturizing [OTC]: 1% (207 mL, 325 mL)
Selsun blue® Normal to Oily [OTC]: 1% (207 mL, 325 mL)

Selsun blue® 2-in-1 [OTC] *see* selenium sulfide *on page* 828
Selsun blue® Deep Cleaning Micro-Bead Scrub [OTC] *see* salicylic acid *on page* 816
Selsun blue® Itchy Dry Scalp [OTC] *see* pyrithione zinc *on page* 779
Selsun blue® Medicated [OTC] *see* selenium sulfide *on page* 828
Selsun blue® Moisturizing [OTC] *see* selenium sulfide *on page* 828
Selsun blue® Naturals Island Breeze [OTC] *see* salicylic acid *on page* 816
Selsun blue® Naturals Itchy Dry Scalp [OTC] *see* salicylic acid *on page* 816
Selsun blue® Normal to Oily [OTC] *see* selenium sulfide *on page* 828
Selsun® Salon™ Classic [OTC] [DSC] *see* pyrithione zinc *on page* 779
Selsun® Salon™ Dandruff 2-in-1 [OTC] [DSC] *see* pyrithione zinc *on page* 779
Selsun® Salon™ Dandruff Volumizing [OTC] [DSC] *see* pyrithione zinc *on page* 779
Selzentry® *see* maraviroc *on page* 562
Semprex®-D *see* acrivastine and pseudoephedrine *on page* 33
Senexon [OTC] *see* senna *on page* 829
Senexon-S [OTC] *see* docusate and senna *on page* 305

senna (SEN na)

Medication Safety Issues

Sound-alike/look-alike issues:
Perdiem® may be confused with Pyridium®
Senexon® may be confused with Cenestin®
Senokot® may be confused with Depakote®

Synonyms sennosides

U.S. Brand Names Black Draught® [OTC]; Evac-U-Gen® [OTC]; ex-lax® Maximum Strength [OTC]; ex-lax® [OTC]; Fleet® Pedia-Lax™ Quick Dissolve [OTC]; Fletcher's® [OTC]; Geri-kot [OTC]; Little Tummys® Laxative [OTC]; Perdiem® Overnight Relief [OTC]; Senexon [OTC]; Senna-Lax [OTC]; SennaGen [OTC]; Senokot® [OTC]

Therapeutic Category Laxative

Use Short-term treatment of constipation; evacuate the colon for bowel or rectal examinations

General Dosage Range Oral:
Children 2-6 years: Initial: 3.75 mg once daily; Maintenance: 3.75-15 mg/day in 1-2 divided doses (maximum: 15 mg/day) **or** 5-10 mL (33.3 mg/mL) up to twice daily
Children 6-12 years: Initial: 8.6 mg once daily; Maintenance: 8.6-50 mg/day in 1-2 divided doses (maximum: 50 mg/day) **or** 10-30 mL (33.3 mg/mL) up to twice daily
Children ≥12 years and Adults: Initial: 15 mg once daily; Maintenance: 15-100 mg/day in 1-2 divided doses (maximum: 100 mg/day) **or** 130 mg as a single dose

Dosage Forms

Liquid, oral:
Fletcher's® [OTC]: Senna concentrate 33.3 mg/mL (75 mL)
Little Tummys® Laxative [OTC]: Sennosides 8.8 mg/mL (30 mL)
Senexon [OTC]: Sennosides 8.8 mg/5 mL (237 mL)

Strip, orally disintegrating, oral:
Fleet® Pedia-Lax™ Quick Dissolve [OTC]: Sennosides 8.6 mg (12s)

Syrup, oral: Sennosides 8.8 mg/5 mL (237 mL, 240 mL)

Tablet, oral: Sennosides 8.6 mg, Sennosides 15 mg, Sennosides 25 mg
ex-lax® [OTC]: Sennosides USP 15 mg
ex-lax® Maximum Strength [OTC]: Sennosides USP 25 mg
Geri-kot [OTC]: Sennosides 8.6 mg
Perdiem® Overnight Relief [OTC]: Sennosides USP 15 mg
Senexon [OTC]: Sennosides 8.6 mg
Senna-Lax [OTC]: Sennosides 8.6 mg

SennaGen [OTC]: Sennosides 8.6 mg
Senokot® [OTC]: Sennosides 8.6 mg

Tablet, chewable, oral:
Black Draught® [OTC]: Sennosides 10 mg
Evac-U-Gen® [OTC]: Sennosides 10 mg
ex-lax® [OTC]: Sennosides USP 15 mg

senna and docusate *see* docusate and senna *on page* 305
SennaGen [OTC] *see* senna *on page* 829
Senna-Lax [OTC] *see* senna *on page* 829
SennaLax-S [OTC] *see* docusate and senna *on page* 305
Senna Plus [OTC] *see* docusate and senna *on page* 305
senna-S *see* docusate and senna *on page* 305
sennosides *see* senna *on page* 829
Senokot® [OTC] *see* senna *on page* 829
Senokot-S® [OTC] *see* docusate and senna *on page* 305
SenoSol™-SS [OTC] *see* docusate and senna *on page* 305
Sensatrast™ *see* barium *on page* 114
Sensipar® *see* cinacalcet *on page* 209
Sensorcaine® *see* bupivacaine *on page* 147
Sensorcaine®-MPF *see* bupivacaine *on page* 147
Sensorcaine®-MPF Spinal *see* bupivacaine *on page* 147
Sensorcaine®-MPF with Epinephrine *see* bupivacaine and epinephrine *on page* 148
Sensorcaine® with Epinephrine *see* bupivacaine and epinephrine *on page* 148
Sepasoothe® [OTC] *see* benzocaine *on page* 121
Septa-Amlodipine (Can) *see* amlodipine *on page* 65
Septa-Atenolol (Can) *see* atenolol *on page* 99
Septa-Citalopram (Can) *see* citalopram *on page* 213
Septanest® N (Can) *see* articaine and epinephrine *on page* 92
Septanest® SP (Can) *see* articaine and epinephrine *on page* 92
Septocaine® with epinephrine 1:100,000 *see* articaine and epinephrine *on page* 92
Septocaine® with epinephrine 1:200,000 *see* articaine and epinephrine *on page* 92
Septra *see* sulfamethoxazole and trimethoprim *on page* 860
Septra® DS *see* sulfamethoxazole and trimethoprim *on page* 860
Septra® Injection (Can) *see* sulfamethoxazole and trimethoprim *on page* 860
Serax *see* oxazepam *on page* 676
Serc® (Can) *see* betahistine *(Canada only) on page* 129
Serevent® Diskhaler® Disk (Can) *see* salmeterol *on page* 820
Serevent® Diskus® *see* salmeterol *on page* 820
Seromycin® *see* cycloserine *on page* 244
Serophene® *see* clomiphene *on page* 222
SEROquel® *see* quetiapine *on page* 781
Seroquel® (Can) *see* quetiapine *on page* 781
SEROquel XR® *see* quetiapine *on page* 781
Seroquel XR® (Can) *see* quetiapine *on page* 781
Serostim® *see* somatropin *on page* 849

sertaconazole (ser ta KOE na zole)

Synonyms sertaconazole nitrate

U.S. Brand Names Ertaczo®

Therapeutic Category Antifungal Agent, Topical

Use Topical treatment of tinea pedis (athlete's foot)

General Dosage Range Topical: *Children ≥12 years and Adults:* Apply twice daily

Dosage Forms

Cream, topical:

Ertaczo®: 2% (30 g, 60 g)

sertaconazole nitrate *see* sertaconazole *on page 830*

sertraline (SER tra leen)

Medication Safety Issues

Sound-alike/look-alike issues:

Sertraline may be confused with selegiline, Serevent®, Soriatane®

Zoloft® may be confused with Zocor®

BEERS Criteria medication:

This drug may be potentially inappropriate for use in geriatric patients (Quality of evidence - moderate; Strength of recommendation - strong).

Synonyms sertraline hydrochloride

U.S. Brand Names Zoloft®

Canadian Brand Names Apo-Sertraline®; CO Sertraline; Dom-Sertraline; GD-Sertraline; Mylan-Sertraline; Nu-Sertraline; PHL-Sertraline; PMS-Sertraline; ratio-Sertraline; Riva-Sertraline; Sandoz-Sertraline; Teva-Sertraline; Zoloft®

Therapeutic Category Antidepressant, Selective Serotonin Reuptake Inhibitor

Use Treatment of major depression; obsessive-compulsive disorder (OCD); panic disorder; posttraumatic stress disorder (PTSD); premenstrual dysphoric disorder (PMDD); social anxiety disorder

General Dosage Range Dosage adjustment recommended in patients with hepatic impairment

Oral:

Children 6-12 years: Initial: 25 mg once daily; Maintenance: 25-200 mg once daily (maximum: 200 mg/day)

Children 13-17 years: Initial: 50 mg once daily; Maintenance: 25-200 mg once daily (maximum: 200 mg/day)

Adults: Initial: 25-50 mg once daily; Maintenance: 50-200 mg once daily (maximum: 200 mg/day)

Elderly: Initial: 25 mg once daily in the morning; Maintenance: 50-100 mg once daily (maximum: 200 mg/day)

Dosage Forms

Solution, oral: 20 mg/mL (60 mL)

Zoloft®: 20 mg/mL (60 mL)

Tablet, oral: 25 mg, 50 mg, 100 mg

Zoloft®: 25 mg, 50 mg, 100 mg

sertraline hydrochloride *see* sertraline *on page 831*

Serzone *see* nefazodone *on page 632*

sevelamer (se VEL a mer)

Medication Safety Issues

Sound-alike/look-alike issues:

Renagel® may be confused with Reglan®, Regonol®, Renvela®

Renvela® may be confused with Reglan®, Regonol®, Renagel®

Sevelamer may be confused with Savella®

International issues:

Renagel [U.S., Canada, and multiple international markets] may be confused with Remegel brand name for aluminium hydroxide and magnesium carbonate [Netherlands] and for calcium carbonate [Hungary, Great Britain and Ireland] and with Remegel Wind Relief brand name for calcium carbonate and simethicone [Great Britain]

Synonyms sevelamer carbonate; sevelamer hydrochloride

U.S. Brand Names Renagel®; Renvela®

Canadian Brand Names Renagel®

Therapeutic Category Phosphate Binder

Use Reduction or control of serum phosphorous in patients with chronic kidney disease on hemodialysis

General Dosage Range Oral: *Adults:* Initial: 800-1600 mg 3 times/day; Maintenance: Up to 2400-14,000 mg/day in 3 divided doses

Dosage Forms

Powder for suspension, oral:

Renvela®: 0.8 g/packet (90s); 2.4 g/packet (90s)

Tablet, oral:

Renagel®: 400 mg, 800 mg

Renvela®: 800 mg

sevelamer carbonate *see* sevelamer *on page* 831

sevelamer hydrochloride *see* sevelamer *on page* 831

sevoflurane (see voe FLOO rane)

Medication Safety Issues

Sound-alike/look-alike issues:

Ultane® may be confused with Ultram®

High alert medication:

The Institute for Safe Medication Practices (ISMP) includes this medication among its list of drug classes which have a heightened risk of causing significant patient harm when used in error.

U.S. Brand Names Sojourn™; Ultane®

Canadian Brand Names Sevorane® AF; Sojourn Sevoflurane

Therapeutic Category General Anesthetic

Use Induction and maintenance of general anesthesia

General Dosage Range Inhalation:

Neonates 0-1 month (full-term): 3.3% in O_2

Infants 1 to <6 months: 3% in O_2

Children 6 months to <3 years: 2.8% in O_2; 2% in 60% N_20/40% O_2

Children 3-12 years: 2.5% in O_2

Adults 25 years: 2.6% in O_2; 1.4% in 65% N_20/35% O_2

Adults 40 years: 2.1% in O_2; 1.1% in 65% N_20/35% O_2

Adults 60 years: 1.7% in O_2; 0.9% in 65% N_20/35% O_2

Adults 80 years: 1.4% in O_2; 0.7% in 65% N_20/35% O_2

Dosage Forms

Liquid, for inhalation: 100% (250 mL)

Sojourn™: 100% (250 mL)

Ultane®: 100% (250 mL)

Sevorane® AF (Can) *see* sevoflurane *on page* 832

sfRowasa™ *see* mesalamine *on page* 577

SGN-35 *see* brentuximab vedotin *on page* 140

SH 714 *see* cyproterone *(Canada only) on page* 246

shingles vaccine *see* zoster vaccine *on page* 968

Sig-Enalapril (Can) *see* enalapril *on page* 330

Silace [OTC] *see* docusate *on page* 304

Siladryl Allergy [OTC] *see* diphenhydramine (systemic) *on page* 292

Silafed [OTC] *see* triprolidine and pseudoephedrine *on page* 922

Silapap Children's [OTC] *see* acetaminophen *on page* 20

Silapap Infant's [OTC] *see* acetaminophen *on page* 20

sildenafil (sil DEN a fil)

Medication Safety Issues

Sound-alike/look-alike issues:

Revatio® may be confused with ReVia®, Revonto®

Sildenafil may be confused with silodosin, tadalafil, vardenafil

Viagra® may be confused with Allegra®, Vaniqa®

Synonyms sildenafil citrate; UK92480

U.S. Brand Names Revatio®; Viagra®

Canadian Brand Names ratio-Sildenafil R; Revatio®; Viagra®

Therapeutic Category Phosphodiesterase (Type 5) Enzyme Inhibitor

Use

Revatio®: Treatment of pulmonary arterial hypertension (PAH) (WHO Group I) to improve exercise ability and delay clinical worsening. Efficacy established based upon short-term studies (12-16 weeks).

Viagra®: Treatment of erectile dysfunction (ED)

General Dosage Range Dosage adjustment recommended in patients with hepatic or renal impairment or on concomitant therapy

I.V.: *Adults:* Revatio®: 10 mg 3 times/day

Oral:

Adults: Revatio®: 20 mg 3 times/day; Viagra®: 25-100 mg once daily

Elderly: Viagra®: Initial: 25 mg

Dosage Forms

Injection, solution:

Revatio®: 0.8 mg/mL (12.5 mL)

Tablet, oral:

Revatio®: 20 mg

Viagra®: 25 mg, 50 mg, 100 mg

sildenafil citrate *see* sildenafil *on page* 832
Silenor® *see* doxepin (systemic) *on page* 312
Silexin [OTC] *see* guaifenesin and dextromethorphan *on page* 434
Silfedrine Children's [OTC] *see* pseudoephedrine *on page* 771

silodosin (SI lo doe sin)

Medication Safety Issues

Sound-alike/look-alike issues:

Rapaflo® may be confused with Rapamune®

Silodosin may be confused with sildenafil

Synonyms KMD 3213

U.S. Brand Names Rapaflo®

Canadian Brand Names Rapaflo®

Therapeutic Category $Alpha_1$ Blocker

Use Treatment of signs and symptoms of benign prostatic hyperplasia (BPH)

General Dosage Range Dosage adjustment recommended in patients with renal impairment

Oral: *Adults:* Males: 8 mg once daily

Dosage Forms

Capsule, oral:

Rapaflo®: 4 mg, 8 mg

Silphen [OTC] *see* diphenhydramine (systemic) *on page* 292
Silphen-DM [OTC] *see* dextromethorphan *on page* 272
Siltussin DM [OTC] *see* guaifenesin and dextromethorphan *on page* 434
Siltussin DM DAS [OTC] *see* guaifenesin and dextromethorphan *on page* 434
Siltussin SA [OTC] *see* guaifenesin *on page* 433
Silvadene® *see* silver sulfadiazine *on page* 833
Silver Bullet Suppository [OTC] (Can) *see* bisacodyl *on page* 134

silver nitrate (SIL ver NYE trate)

Synonyms $AgNO_3$

Therapeutic Category Topical Skin Product

Use Astringent, cauterization of wounds, germicidal, removal of granulation tissue, corns and warts

General Dosage Range Topical: *Children and Adults:* Solution: Apply to affected area 2-3 times/day; Sticks: Apply to area to be treated

Dosage Forms

Applicator sticks, topical: Silver nitrate 75% and potassium 25% (6", 12", 18")

Solution, topical: 0.5% (960 mL); 10% (30 mL); 25% (30 mL); 50% (30 mL)

silver sulfadiazine (SIL ver sul fa DYE a zeen)

U.S. Brand Names Silvadene®; SSD™; Thermazene®

Canadian Brand Names Flamazine®

Therapeutic Category Antibacterial, Topical

Use Prevention and treatment of infection in second and third degree burns

General Dosage Range Topical: *Children and Adults:* Apply to a thickness of 1/16" once or twice daily

Dosage Forms

Cream, topical: 1% (25 g, 50 g, 85 g, 400 g)
Silvadene®: 1% (20 g, 50 g, 85 g, 400 g, 1000 g)
SSD™: 1% (25 g, 50 g, 85 g, 400 g)
Thermazene®: 1% (20 g, 25 g, 50 g, 85 g, 400 g, 1000 g)

Simcor® *see* niacin and simvastatin *on page 639*

simethicone (sye METH i kone)

Medication Safety Issues

Sound-alike/look-alike issues:
Simethicone may be confused with cimetidine
Mylanta® may be confused with Mynatal®
Mylicon® may be confused with Modicon®, Myleran®

Synonyms activated dimethicone; activated methylpolysiloxane

U.S. Brand Names Equalizer Gas Relief [OTC]; Gas Free Extra Strength [OTC]; Gas Relief Ultra Strength [OTC]; Gas-X® Children's Tongue Twisters™ [OTC]; Gas-X® Extra Strength [OTC]; Gas-X® Maximum Strength [OTC]; Gas-X® Thin Strips™ [OTC]; Gas-X® [OTC]; Gax-X® Infant [OTC]; Infantaire Gas [OTC]; Infants Gas Relief Drops [OTC] [DSC]; Little Tummys® Gas Relief [OTC]; Mi-Acid Gas Relief [OTC]; Mylanta® Gas Maximum Strength [OTC]; Mylicon® Infants' [OTC]; Mytab Gas Maximum [OTC]; Mytab Gas [OTC]; Phazyme® Ultra Strength [OTC]

Canadian Brand Names Ovol®; Phazyme™

Therapeutic Category Antiflatulent

Use Postoperative gas pain or for use in endoscopic examination; relief of bloating, pressure, and discomfort of gas

General Dosage Range Oral:
Infants and Children <2 years or <11 kg: 20 mg 4 times/day, as needed
Children >2 years or >11 kg: 40 mg 4 times/day, as needed
Children >12 years and Adults: 40-360 mg after meals and at bedtime, as needed

Dosage Forms

Capsule, softgel, oral: 125 mg, 180 mg
Gas Free Extra Strength [OTC]: 125 mg
Gas Relief Ultra Strength [OTC]: 180 mg
Gas-X® Extra Strength [OTC]: 125 mg
Gas-X® Maximum Strength [OTC]: 166 mg
Mylanta® Gas Maximum Strength [OTC]: 125 mg
Phazyme® Ultra Strength [OTC]: 180 mg

Strip, orally disintegrating, oral:
Gas-X® Children's Tongue Twisters™ [OTC]: 40 mg (16s)
Gas-X® Thin Strips™ [OTC]: 62.5 mg (18s, 32s)

Suspension, oral: 40 mg/0.6 mL (30 mL)
Equalizer Gas Relief [OTC]: 40 mg/0.6 mL (30 mL)
Gax-X® Infant [OTC]: 40 mg/0.6 mL (30 mL)
Infantaire Gas [OTC]: 40 mg/0.6 mL (30 mL)
Little Tummys® Gas Relief [OTC]: 40 mg/0.6 mL (30 mL, 45 mL)
Mylicon® Infants' [OTC]: 40 mg/0.6 mL (15 mL, 30 mL)

Tablet, chewable, oral: 80 mg, 125 mg
Gas-X® [OTC]: 80 mg
Gas-X® Extra Strength [OTC]: 125 mg
Mi-Acid Gas Relief [OTC]: 80 mg
Mylanta® Gas Maximum Strength [OTC]: 125 mg
Mytab Gas [OTC]: 80 mg
Mytab Gas Maximum [OTC]: 125 mg

simethicone, aluminum hydroxide, and magnesium hydroxide *see* aluminum hydroxide, magnesium hydroxide, and simethicone *on page 56*

simethicone and calcium carbonate *see* calcium carbonate and simethicone *on page 163*

simethicone and loperamide hydrochloride *see* loperamide and simethicone *on page 548*

simethicone and magaldrate *see* magaldrate and simethicone *on page* *557*
Similac® Glucose [OTC] *see* dextrose *on page* *275*
Simply Saline® [OTC] *see* sodium chloride *on page* *840*
Simply Saline® Baby [OTC] *see* sodium chloride *on page* *840*
Simply Sleep® [OTC] *see* diphenhydramine (systemic) *on page* *292*
Simply Sleep® (Can) *see* diphenhydramine (systemic) *on page* *292*
Simponi® *see* golimumab *on page* *431*
Simulect® *see* basiliximab *on page* *115*

simvastatin (sim va STAT in)

Medication Safety Issues

Sound-alike/look-alike issues:

Simvastatin may be confused with atorvasSTATin, nystatin, pitavastatin

Zocor® may be confused with Cozaar®, Lipitor®, Zoloft®, ZyrTEC®

International issues:

Cardin [Poland] may be confused with Cardem brand name for celiprolol [Spain]; Cardene brand name for nicardipine [U.S., Great Britain, Netherlands]

U.S. Brand Names Zocor®

Canadian Brand Names Apo-Simvastatin®; Ava-Simvastatin; CO Simvastatin; Dom-Simvastatin; JAMP-Simvastatin; Mint-Simvastatin; Mylan-Simvastatin; Nu-Simvastatin; PHL-Simvastatin; PMS-Simvastatin; Q-Simvastatin; RAN™-Simvastatin; ratio-Simvastatin; Riva-Simvastatin; Sandoz-Simvastatin; Simvastatin-Odan; Taro-Simvastatin; Teva-Simvastatin; Zocor®; ZYM-Simvastatin

Therapeutic Category HMG-CoA Reductase Inhibitor

Use Used with dietary therapy for the following:

Secondary prevention of cardiovascular events in hypercholesterolemic patients with established coronary heart disease (CHD) or at high risk for CHD: To reduce cardiovascular morbidity (myocardial infarction, coronary/noncoronary revascularization procedures) and mortality; to reduce the risk of stroke

Hyperlipidemias: To reduce elevations in total cholesterol (total-C), LDL-C, apolipoprotein B, triglycerides, and VLDL-C, and to increase HDL-C in patients with primary hypercholesterolemia (elevations of 1 or more components are present in Fredrickson type IIa, IIb, III, and IV hyperlipidemias); treatment of homozygous familial hypercholesterolemia

Heterozygous familial hypercholesterolemia (HeFH): In adolescent patients (10-17 years of age, females >1 year postmenarche) with HeFH having LDL-C ≥190 mg/dL **or** LDL-C ≥160 mg/dL with positive family history of premature cardiovascular disease (CVD), or 2 or more CVD risk factors in the adolescent patient

General Dosage Range Dosage adjustment recommended in patients with renal impairment or on concomitant therapy

Oral:

Children 10-17 years (females >1 year postmenarche): Initial: 10 mg once daily; Maintenance: 10-40 mg once daily (maximum: 40 mg/day)

Adults: Initial: 10-20 mg once daily; Maintenance: 5-40 mg once daily (maximum: 40 mg/day)

Dosage Forms

Tablet, oral: 5 mg, 10 mg, 20 mg, 40 mg, 80 mg

Zocor®: 5 mg, 10 mg, 20 mg, 40 mg, 80 mg

simvastatin and ezetimibe *see* ezetimibe and simvastatin *on page* *370*
simvastatin and niacin *see* niacin and simvastatin *on page* *639*
simvastatin and sitagliptin *see* sitagliptin and simvastatin *on page* *838*
Simvastatin-Odan (Can) *see* simvastatin *on page* *835*

sincalide (SIN ka lide)

Synonyms C8-CCK; OP-CCK

U.S. Brand Names Kinevac®

Therapeutic Category Diagnostic Agent

Use Postevacuation cholecystography; gallbladder bile sampling; stimulate pancreatic secretion for analysis; accelerate the transit of barium through the small bowel

General Dosage Range

I.M.: *Adults:* 0.1 mcg/kg

I.V.: *Adults:* 0.02-0.04 mcg/kg as a single dose; may repeat 0.04 mcg/kg once **or** 0.12 mcg/kg as a single dose

Dosage Forms

Injection, powder for reconstitution:

Kinevac®: 5 mcg

sinecatechins (sin e KAT e kins)

Synonyms catechins; green tea extract; kunecatechins; polyphenols; polyphenon E

U.S. Brand Names Veregen®

Therapeutic Category Immunomodulator, Topical; Topical Skin Product

Use Treatment of external genital and perianal warts secondary to condylomata acuminata

General Dosage Range Topical: *Adults:* Apply a thin layer (~0.5 cm strand) 3 times/day

Dosage Forms

Ointment, topical:

Veregen®: 15% (15 g)

Sinemet® *see* carbidopa and levodopa *on page* *174*

Sinemet® CR *see* carbidopa and levodopa *on page* *174*

Sinequan® (Can) *see* doxepin (systemic) *on page* *312*

Singulair® *see* montelukast *on page* *612*

Sinografin® *see* diatrizoate meglumine and iodipamide meglumine *on page* *277*

Sinus Pain & Pressure [OTC] *see* acetaminophen and phenylephrine *on page* *24*

Sinutab® Non Drowsy (Can) *see* acetaminophen and pseudoephedrine *on page* *25*

SINUtuss® DM [DSC] *see* guaifenesin, dextromethorphan, and phenylephrine *on page* *437*

sipuleucel-T (si pu LOO sel tee)

Medication Safety Issues

Other safety concerns:

For autologous use only; patient identity must be matched to the patient identifiers on the infusion bag and on the "Cell Product Disposition Form" prior to infusion. Healthcare providers should apply universal precautions when handling both the initial leukapheresis product and the activated product.

Synonyms APC8015; prostate cancer vaccine, cell-based

U.S. Brand Names Provenge®

Therapeutic Category Cellular Immunotherapy, Autologous

Use Treatment of metastatic hormone-refractory prostate cancer in patients who are asymptomatic or minimally symptomatic

General Dosage Range I.V.: *Adults (males):* ≥50 million autologous CD54+ cells activated with PAP-GM-CSF; dose administered at ~2 week intervals for a total of 3 doses

Dosage Forms

Infusion, premixed in LR [preservative free]:

Provenge®: ≥50 million autologous $CD54^+$ cells activated with PAP-GM-CSF (250 mL)

Sirdalud® *see* tizanidine *on page* *900*

sirolimus (sir OH li mus)

Medication Safety Issues

Sound-alike/look-alike issues:

Rapamune® may be confused with Rapaflo®

Sirolimus may be confused with everolimus, pimecrolimus, tacrolimus, temsirolimus

Synonyms rapamycin

U.S. Brand Names Rapamune®

Canadian Brand Names Rapamune®

Therapeutic Category Immunosuppressant Agent

Use Prophylaxis of organ rejection in patients receiving renal transplants

General Dosage Range Dosage adjustment recommended in patients with hepatic impairment

Oral:

Children ≥13 years and Adults <40 kg: Low-to-moderate immunologic risk: Loading dose: 3 mg/m^2 on day 1; Maintenance: 1 mg/m^2/day

Children ≥13 years and Adults ≥40 kg: Low-to-moderate immunologic risk: Loading dose: 6 mg on day 1; Maintenance: 2 mg/day (maximum: 40 mg/day)

Adults: High risk: Loading dose: Up to 15 mg on day 1; Maintenance: 5 mg/day (maximum: 40 mg/day)

Dosage Forms

Solution, oral:

Rapamune®: 1 mg/mL (60 mL)

Tablet, oral:

Rapamune®: 0.5 mg, 1 mg, 2 mg

sitagliptin (sit a GLIP tin)

Medication Safety Issues

Sound-alike/look-alike issues:

Januvia® may be confused with Enjuvia™, Janumet®, Jantoven®

SitaGLIPtin may be confused with saxagliptin, SUMAtriptan

High alert medication:

The Institute for Safe Medication Practices (ISMP) includes this medication among its list of drug classes which have a heightened risk of causing significant patient harm when used in error.

Synonyms MK-0431; sitagliptin phosphate

Tall-Man sita**GLIP**tin

U.S. Brand Names Januvia®

Canadian Brand Names Januvia®

Therapeutic Category Antidiabetic Agent, Dipeptidyl Peptidase IV (DPP-IV) Inhibitor

Use Management of type 2 diabetes mellitus (noninsulin-dependent, NIDDM) as an adjunct to diet and exercise as monotherapy or in combination therapy with other antidiabetic agents

General Dosage Range Dosage adjustment recommended in patients with renal impairment

Oral: *Adults:* 100 mg once daily

Dosage Forms

Tablet, oral:

Januvia®: 25 mg, 50 mg, 100 mg

sitagliptin and metformin (sit a GLIP tin & met FOR min)

Medication Safety Issues

Sound-alike/look-alike issues:

Janumet® may be confused with Jantoven®, Januvia®

Sitagliptin and Metformin may be confused with Linagliptin and Metformin

Sitagliptin and Metformin may be confused with Saxagliptin and Metformin

High alert medication:

The Institute for Safe Medication Practices (ISMP) includes this medication among its list of drug classes which have a heightened risk of causing significant patient harm when used in error.

Synonyms metformin and sitagliptin; sitagliptin phosphate and metformin hydrochloride

U.S. Brand Names Janumet®; Janumet® XR

Canadian Brand Names Janumet®

Therapeutic Category Antidiabetic Agent, Biguanide; Antidiabetic Agent, Dipeptidyl Peptidase IV (DPP-IV) Inhibitor; Hypoglycemic Agent, Oral

Use Management of type 2 diabetes mellitus (noninsulin-dependent, NIDDM) as an adjunct to diet and exercise in patients not adequately controlled on metformin or sitagliptin monotherapy

General Dosage Range Oral: *Adults:*

Immediate release: Sitagliptin 50 mg and metformin 500-1000 mg twice daily (maximum: 100 mg/day [sitagliptin], 2000 mg/day [metformin])

Extended release: Sitagliptin 100 mg and metformin 1000-2000 mg once daily (maximum: 100 mg/day [sitagliptin], 2000 mg/day [metformin])

Dosage Forms

Tablet, oral:

Janumet®: 50/500: Sitagliptin 50 mg and metformin 500 mg; 50/1000: Sitagliptin 50 mg and metformin 1000 mg

Tablet, extended release, oral:
Janumet® XR: 50/500: Sitagliptin 50 mg and metformin 500 mg
Janumet® XR: 50/1000: Sitagliptin 50 mg and metformin 1000 mg
Janumet® XR: 100/1000: Sitagliptin 100 mg and metformin 1000 mg

Dosage Forms - Canada
Tablet, oral:
Janumet® 50/850: Sitagliptin 50 mg and metformin 850 mg

sitagliptin and simvastatin (sit a GLIP tin & sim va STAT in)

Medication Safety Issues
High alert medication:
The Institute for Safe Medication Practices (ISMP) includes this medication among its list of drug classes which have a heightened risk of causing significant patient harm when used in error.

Synonyms simvastatin and sitagliptin; sitagliptin phosphate and simvastatin

U.S. Brand Names Juvisync™

Therapeutic Category Antidiabetic Agent, Dipeptidyl Peptidase IV (DPP-IV) Inhibitor; Antilipemic Agent, HMG-CoA Reductase Inhibitor

Use For use when treatment with both sitagliptin and simvastatin is appropriate:
Sitagliptin: Management of type 2 diabetes mellitus (noninsulin dependent, NIDDM) as an adjunct to diet and exercise as monotherapy or in combination therapy with other antidiabetic agents
Simvastatin: Used with dietary therapy for the following:
Secondary prevention of cardiovascular events in hypercholesterolemic patients with established coronary heart disease (CHD) or at high risk for CHD: To reduce cardiovascular morbidity (myocardial infarction, coronary/noncoronary revascularization procedures) and mortality; to reduce the risk of stroke
Hyperlipidemias: To reduce elevations in total cholesterol (total-C), LDL-C, apolipoprotein B, triglycerides, and VLDL-C, and to increase HDL-C in patients with primary hypercholesterolemia (elevations of 1 or more components are present in Fredrickson type IIa, IIb, III, and IV hyperlipidemias); treatment of homozygous familial hypercholesterolemia

General Dosage Range Dosage adjustment recommended in patients on concomitant therapy.
Oral: *Adults:* Initial: Sitagliptin 100 mg and simvastatin 40 mg once daily

Dosage Forms Tablet, oral:
Juvisync™ 100/10: Sitagliptin 100 mg and simvastatin 10 mg
Juvisync™ 100/20: Sitagliptin 100 mg and simvastatin 20 mg
Juvisync™ 100/40: Sitagliptin 100 mg and simvastatin 40 mg

sitagliptin phosphate *see* sitagliptin *on page* 837
sitagliptin phosphate and metformin hydrochloride *see* sitagliptin and metformin *on page* 837
sitagliptin phosphate and simvastatin *see* sitagliptin and simvastatin *on page* 838
Skeeter Stik® [OTC] *see* benzocaine *on page* 121
Skelaxin® *see* metaxalone *on page* 579
Skelid® *see* tiludronate *on page* 896
SKF 104864 *see* topotecan *on page* 906
SKF 104864-A *see* topotecan *on page* 906
Skin Care™ [OTC] *see* pyrithione zinc *on page* 779
Sklice™ *see* ivermectin (topical) *on page* 507
Sleep-ettes D [OTC] *see* diphenhydramine (systemic) *on page* 292
Sleepinal® [OTC] *see* diphenhydramine (systemic) *on page* 292
Sleep-Tabs [OTC] *see* diphenhydramine (systemic) *on page* 292
S-leucovorin *see* LEVOleucovorin *on page* 532
6S-leucovorin *see* LEVOleucovorin *on page* 532
Slo-Niacin® [OTC] *see* niacin *on page* 638
Slo-Pot (Can) *see* potassium chloride *on page* 744
Slow FE® [OTC] *see* ferrous sulfate *on page* 380
Slow-K® (Can) *see* potassium chloride *on page* 744
Slow-Mag® [OTC] *see* magnesium chloride *on page* 557
Slow Release [OTC] *see* ferrous sulfate *on page* 380
SM-13496 *see* lurasidone *on page* 555

smallpox vaccine (SMAL poks vak SEEN)

Synonyms live smallpox vaccine; vaccinia vaccine

U.S. Brand Names ACAM2000®

Therapeutic Category Vaccine

Use Active immunization against smallpox disease in persons determined to be at high risk for smallpox infection.

The Advisory Committee on Immunization Practices (ACIP) recommends routine vaccination for the following:

- Laboratory workers at risk of exposure from cultures or contaminated animals which may be a source of vaccinia or related Orthopoxviruses capable of causing infections in humans (eg, monkeypox, cowpox, variola, vaccinia).
- Consideration may also be given for vaccination of healthcare workers having contact with clinical specimens, contaminated material, or patients receiving vaccinia or recombinant vaccinia viruses.

In a Pre-Event Vaccination Program, the ACIP recommends vaccination for the following:

- Persons designated by authorities to investigate smallpox cases with the likelihood of direct patient contact
- Persons responsible for administering smallpox vaccine

In the event of an intentional release of smallpox virus, the ACIP recommends vaccination for the following:

- Persons exposed to the initial release of the virus
- Persons who had close contact with a confirmed or suspected smallpox patient at any time from the onset of the patient's fever until all scabs have separated
- Healthcare providers involved in evaluation, care, or transport of confirmed or suspected smallpox patients
- Laboratory personnel involved in processing specimens of confirmed or suspected smallpox patients
- Persons likely to have increased contact with infectious materials from smallpox patients

General Dosage Range **Percutaneous:** *Children ≥12 months and Adults:* A single drop of vaccine suspension and 15 needle punctures into superficial skin for both primary vaccination and revaccination

Dosage Forms

Injection, powder for reconstitution [purified monkey cell source]:

ACAM2000®: 1-5 x 10^8 plaque-forming units per mL

smelling salts *see* ammonia spirit (aromatic) *on page 68*

^{153}Sm-lexidronam *see* samarium Sm 153 lexidronam *on page 821*

SMX-TMP *see* sulfamethoxazole and trimethoprim *on page 860*

SMZ-TMP *see* sulfamethoxazole and trimethoprim *on page 860*

snake antivenin, FAB (ovine) *see* crotalidae polyvalent immune FAB (ovine) *on page 241*

snake antivenom, FAB (ovine) *see* crotalidae polyvalent immune FAB (ovine) *on page 241*

(+)-(*S*)-*N*-methyl-γ-(1-naphthyloxy)-2-thiophenepropylamine hydrochloride *see* duloxetine *on page 319*

Sochlor™ [OTC] *see* sodium chloride *on page 840*

sodium 2-mercaptoethane sulfonate *see* mesna *on page 578*

sodium 4-hydroxybutyrate *see* sodium oxybate *on page 844*

sodium *L*-triiodothyronine *see* liothyronine *on page 541*

sodium acetate (SOW dee um AS e tate)

Therapeutic Category Alkalinizing Agent; Electrolyte Supplement, Oral

Use Sodium source in large volume I.V. fluids to prevent or correct hyponatremia in patients with restricted intake; used to counter acidosis through conversion to bicarbonate

General Dosage Range **I.V.:**

Children: TPN: 3-4 mEq/kg/24 hours

Adults: TPN: 3-4 mEq/kg/24 hours **or** 25-40 mEq/1000 kcal/24 hours (maximum: 100-150 mEq/24 hours)

Dosage Forms

Injection, solution [preservative free]: 2 mEq/mL (20 mL, 50 mL, 100 mL); 4 mEq/mL (50 mL, 100 mL)

sodium acid carbonate *see* sodium bicarbonate *on page 840*

sodium artesunate *see* artesunate *on page 92*

sodium aurothiomalate *see* gold sodium thiomalate *on page 430*

sodium benzoate and caffeine *see* caffeine *on page 157*

sodium benzoate and sodium phenylacetate *see* sodium phenylacetate and sodium benzoate *on page 844*

sodium bicarbonate (SOW dee um bye KAR bun ate)

Synonyms baking soda; $NaHCO_3$; sodium acid carbonate; sodium hydrogen carbonate

U.S. Brand Names Brioschi® [OTC]; Neut®

Therapeutic Category Alkalinizing Agent; Antacid; Electrolyte Supplement, Oral

Use Management of metabolic acidosis; gastric hyperacidity; as an alkalinization agent for the urine; treatment of hyperkalemia; management of overdose of certain drugs, including tricyclic antidepressants and aspirin

General Dosage Range

I.V.: *Children and Adults:* Dosage varies greatly depending on indication

Oral:

Children: 1-10 mEq/kg/day as a single dose **or** divided every 4-6 hours

Adults <60 years: 0.5-200 mEq/kg/day in 4-5 divided doses **or** 325 mg to 2 g 1-4 times/day (maximum: 16 g [200 mEq] day)

Adults ≥60 years: 0.5-100 mEq/kg/day in 4-6 divided doses **or** 325 mg to 2 g 1-4 times/day (maximum: 8 g [100 mEq] day)

Dosage Forms

Granules for solution, oral:

Brioschi® [OTC]: 2.69 g/capful (120 g, 240 g); 2.69 g/packet (12s)

Injection, solution: 4.2% [5 mEq/10 mL] (10 mL); 8.4% [10 mEq/10 mL] (50 mL)

Neut®: 4% [2.4 mEq/5 mL] (5 mL)

Injection, solution [preservative free]: 4.2% [5 mEq/10 mL] (5 mL); 7.5% [8.92 mEq/10 mL] (50 mL); 8.4% [10 mEq/10 mL] (10 mL, 50 mL)

Powder, oral: USP: 100% (120 g, 454 g, 480 g)

Tablet, oral: 325 mg, 650 mg

sodium bicarbonate and omeprazole *see* omeprazole and sodium bicarbonate *on page 666*

sodium chloride (SOW dee um KLOR ide)

Medication Safety Issues

High alert medication:

The Institute for Safe Medication Practices (ISMP) includes this medication (I.V. formulation >0.9% concentration) among its list of drugs which have a heightened risk of causing significant patient harm when used in error.

Other safety concerns:

Per The Joint Commission (TJC) recommendations, concentrated electrolyte solutions (eg, NaCl >0.9%) should not be available in patient care areas.

Inappropriate use of low sodium or sodium-free intravenous fluids (eg, D_5W, hypotonic saline) in pediatric patients can lead to significant morbidity and mortality due to hyponatremia (ISMP, 2009).

Synonyms hypertonic saline; NaCl; normal saline; saline; salt

U.S. Brand Names 4-Way® Saline Moisturizing Mist [OTC]; Altachlore [OTC]; Altamist [OTC]; Ayr® Allergy & Sinus [OTC]; Ayr® Baby Saline [OTC]; Ayr® Saline Nasal Gel [OTC]; Ayr® Saline No-Drip [OTC]; Ayr® Saline [OTC]; Deep Sea [OTC]; Entsol® [OTC]; HuMist® [OTC]; HyperSal®; Little Noses® Saline [OTC]; Little Noses® Sterile Saline Nasal Mist [OTC]; Little Noses® Stuffy Nose Kit [OTC]; Muro 128® [OTC]; Na-Zone® [OTC]; NebuSal™; Ocean® for Kids [OTC]; Ocean® [OTC]; Pretz® [OTC]; Rhinaris® [OTC]; Safe Wash™ [OTC]; Saline Mist [OTC]; Saljet® [OTC]; Sea Soft Nasal Mist [OTC]; Simply Saline® Baby [OTC]; Simply Saline® [OTC]; Sochlor™ [OTC]; Syrex; Wound Wash Saline™ [OTC]

Therapeutic Category Electrolyte Supplement, Oral; Lubricant, Ocular

Use

Parenteral: Restores sodium ion in patients with restricted oral intake (especially hyponatremia states or low salt syndrome).

Concentrated sodium chloride: Additive for parenteral fluid therapy

Hypertonic sodium chloride: For severe hyponatremia and hypochloremia

Hypotonic sodium chloride: Hydrating solution

Normal saline: Restores water/sodium losses

Ophthalmic: Reduces corneal edema
Inhalation: Restores moisture to pulmonary system; loosens and thins congestion caused by colds or allergies; diluent for bronchodilator solutions that require dilution before inhalation
Intranasal: Restores moisture to nasal membranes
Irrigation: Wound cleansing, irrigation, and flushing

General Dosage Range

I.V.: *Children and Adults:* Dosage varies greatly depending on indication
Inhalation: *Children ≥2 years and Adults:* 1-3 sprays (1-3 mL)
Intranasal: *Children ≥2 years and Adults:* 2-3 sprays in each nostril as needed
Irrigation: *Children ≥2 years and Adults:* 1-3 L/day **or** spray affected area
Ophthalmic: *Adults:* Ointment: Apply once or more daily; Solution: Instill 1-2 drops into affected eye(s) every 3-4 hours

Dosage Forms

Aerosol, spray, intranasal [preservative free]:
Entsol® [OTC]: 3% (100 mL)
Little Noses® Sterile Saline Nasal Mist [OTC]: 0.9% (50 mL)
Aerosol, spray, topical [preservative free]:
Safe Wash™ [OTC]: 0.9% (210 mL)
Gel, intranasal:
Ayr® Saline [OTC]: < 0.5% (14 g)
Ayr® Saline No-Drip [OTC]: < 0.5% (22 mL)
Rhinaris® [OTC]: 0.2% (28.4 g)
Injection, solution: 0.45% (25 mL, 50 mL, 100 mL, 250 mL, 500 mL, 1000 mL); 0.9% (10 mL, 20 mL, 25 mL, 30 mL, 50 mL, 100 mL, 150 mL, 250 mL, 500 mL, 1000 mL, 1s); 3% (500 mL); 5% (500 mL); 14.6% (20 mL, 40 mL, 250 mL); 23.4% (50 mL, 100 mL, 250 mL)
Injection, solution [preservative free]: 0.9% (1 mL, 2 mL, 2.5 mL, 3 mL, 5 mL, 6 mL, 10 mL, 20 mL, 50 mL, 100 mL, 125 mL); 14.6% (20 mL, 40 mL); 23.4% (30 mL, 100 mL, 200 mL)
Syrex: 0.9% (2.5 mL, 3 mL, 5 mL, 10 mL)
Ointment, ophthalmic: 5% (3.5 g)
Altachlore [OTC]: 5% (3.5 g)
Sochlor™ [OTC]: 5% (3.5 g)
Ointment, ophthalmic [preservative free]:
Muro 128® [OTC]: 5% (3.5 g)
Powder for solution, intranasal [preservative free]:
Pretz® [OTC]: 1 teaspoon/dose (360 g)
Solution, for blood processing: 0.9% (3000 mL)
Solution, for inhalation [preservative free]: 0.9% (3 mL, 5 mL, 15 mL); 3% (15 mL); 10% (15 mL)
Solution, for irrigation: 0.9% (250 mL, 500 mL, 1000 mL, 1500 mL, 2000 mL, 3000 mL, 4000 mL, 5000 mL)
Solution, for irrigation [preservative free]: 0.9% (250 mL, 500 mL, 1000 mL, 1500 mL, 2000 mL, 3000 mL)
Solution, for nebulization [preservative free]: 3% (4 mL); 7% (4 mL)
HyperSal®: 3.5% (4 mL); 7% (4 mL)
NebuSal™: 6% (4 mL)
Solution, intranasal: 0.65% (44 mL, 45 mL, 88 mL)
4-Way® Saline Moisturizing Mist [OTC]: 0.74% (29.6 mL)
Altamist [OTC]: 0.65% (60 mL)
Ayr® Allergy & Sinus [OTC]: 2.65% (50 mL)
Ayr® Baby Saline [OTC]: 0.65% (30 mL)
Ayr® Saline [OTC]: 0.65% (50 mL)
Deep Sea [OTC]: 0.65% (44 mL)
HuMist® [OTC]: 0.65% (45 mL)
Little Noses® Saline [OTC]: 0.65% (30 mL)
Little Noses® Stuffy Nose Kit [OTC]: 0.65% (15 mL)
Na-Zone® [OTC]: 0.65% (60 mL)
Ocean® [OTC]: 0.65% (45 mL, 104 mL, 473 mL)
Ocean® for Kids [OTC]: 0.65% (37.5 mL)
Pretz® [OTC]: 0.75% (50 mL, 960 mL)
Rhinaris® [OTC]: 0.2% (30 mL)
Saline Mist [OTC]: 0.65% (45 mL)
Sea Soft Nasal Mist [OTC]: 0.65% (45 mL)

Solution, intranasal [preservative free]:
Pretz® [OTC]: 0.75% (20 mL)
Simply Saline® [OTC]: 0.9% (44 mL, 90 mL); 3% (44 mL)
Simply Saline® Baby [OTC]: 0.9% (45 mL)
Solution, ophthalmic: 5% (15 mL)
Altachlore [OTC]: 5% (15 mL)
Muro 128® [OTC]: 2% (15 mL); 5% (15 mL, 30 mL)
Sochlor™ [OTC]: 5% (15 mL)
Solution, topical [preservative free]:
Saljet® [OTC]: 0.9% (30 mL)
Wound Wash Saline™ [OTC]: 0.9% (90 mL, 210 mL)
Swab, intranasal:
Ayr® Saline Nasal Gel [OTC]: 0.65% (20s)
Tablet, oral: 1 g
Tablet for solution, topical: 1000 mg

sodium chondroitin sulfate and sodium hyaluronate

(SOW de um kon DROY tin SUL fate & SOW de um hye al yoor ON ate)

Synonyms chondroitin sulfate and sodium hyaluronate; sodium hyaluronate and chondroitin sulfate

U.S. Brand Names DisCoVisc®; Viscoat®

Therapeutic Category Ophthalmic Agent, Viscoelastic

Use Ophthalmic surgical aid in the anterior segment during cataract extraction and intraocular lens implantation

General Dosage Range **Ophthalmic:** *Adults:* Carefully introduce into anterior chamber during surgery

Dosage Forms

Injection, solution, intraocular:
DisCoVisc®: Sodium chondroitin sulfate ≤4% and sodium hyaluronate ≤1.7% (0.5 mL, 1 mL)
Viscoat®: Sodium chondroitin sulfate ≤4% and sodium hyaluronate ≤3% (0.5 mL, 0.75 mL)

sodium citrate, citric acid, and potassium citrate *see* citric acid, sodium citrate, and potassium citrate *on page* *214*
Sodium Diuril® *see* chlorothiazide *on page* *198*
Sodium Edecrin® *see* ethacrynic acid *on page* *355*
sodium etidronate *see* etidronate *on page* *364*
sodium ferric gluconate *see* ferric gluconate *on page* *379*
sodium fluorescein *see* fluorescein *on page* *393*
sodium fluoride *see* fluoride *on page* *393*
sodium fusidate *see* fusidic acid *(Canada only) on page* *413*
sodium hyaluronate *see* hyaluronate and derivatives *on page* *450*
sodium hyaluronate and chondroitin sulfate *see* sodium chondroitin sulfate and sodium hyaluronate *on page* *842*
sodium hydrogen carbonate *see* sodium bicarbonate *on page* *840*

sodium hypochlorite solution

(SOW dee um hye poe KLOR ite soe LOO shun)

Medication Safety Issues

Administration issues:

A potential for confusion associated with labeling of strengths for Dakin's solution manufactured by Century Pharmaceuticals exists. The labels list strengths as full strength at 0.5%, half strength at 0.25%, and quarter strength at 0.125%. This terminology is confusing to healthcare providers who consider half strength and quarter strength to correspond to 0.5% and 0.25%, respectively. Of note, most hospitals use a modified Dakin's solution of 0.025% for wound care; studies have suggested that concentrations of Dakin's solution >0.025% may potentially be harmful for wound healing.

Synonyms modified Dakin's solution

U.S. Brand Names Atrapro™ Dermal; Dakin's Solution; Di-Dak-Sol

Therapeutic Category Disinfectant

Use

Atrapro™ Dermal (0.004%): Management (via debridement) of wounds such as stage I-IV pressure ulcers; partial and full thickness wounds; diabetic foot ulcers; post surgical and donor sites; first- and second-degree burns

Dakin's Solution (0.125%, 0.25%, 0.5%); Di-Dak-Sol (0.0125%): Prevention/treatment of skin and tissue infections, cuts, abrasions, skin ulcers; pre- and postsurgery

General Dosage Range

Topical: *Children and Adults:*

Atrapro™ Dermal spray: Apply to affected area 3 times daily.

Dakin's solution, Di-Dak-Sol: Via irrigation: Lightly-to-moderately exudative wounds: Apply once daily; Highly exudative or contaminated wounds: Apply twice daily

Dosage Forms

Solution, topical:

Atrapro™ Dermal: 0.004% (236 mL)

Dakin's Solution: 0.125% (473 mL); 0.25% (473 mL); 0.5% (473 mL)

Di-Dak-Sol: 0.0125% (473 mL)

sodium hyposulfate *see* sodium thiosulfate *on page 848*

^{123}I-sodium iodide *see* sodium iodide I^{123} *on page 843*

sodium iodide I^{123} (SOW dee um EYE oh dide eye one TWEN tee three)

Medication Safety Issues

Other safety concerns:

Radiopharmaceutical: Use appropriate precaution for handling, disposal, and minimizing exposure to patients and healthcare personnel. Use under supervision of experienced personnel. Should be stored in original lead container or adequate radiation shield.

Synonyms ^{123}I-sodium iodide; NaI I-123

Therapeutic Category Radiopharmaceutical

Use Evaluation of thyroid function and/or morphology

sodium lactate (SOW dee um LAK tate)

Therapeutic Category Alkalinizing Agent

Use Source of bicarbonate for prevention and treatment of mild-to-moderate metabolic acidosis

General Dosage Range I.V.: *Adults:* Dosage depends on degree of acidosis

Dosage Forms

Injection, solution [preservative free]: 560 mg/mL (10 mL)

sodium nafcillin *see* nafcillin *on page 624*

sodium nitrite (SOW dee um NYE trite)

Therapeutic Category Antidote

Use Acute, life-threatening cyanide poisoning in combination with sodium thiosulfate

General Dosage Range I.V.:

Children: 6 mg/kg (maximum: 300 mg); may repeat at one-half the original dose if needed

Adults: 300 mg; may repeat at one-half the original dose if needed

Dosage Forms

Injection, solution: 30 mg/mL (10 mL)

sodium nitrite and sodium thiosulfate

(SOW dee um NYE trite & SOW dee um thye oh SUL fate)

Synonyms sodium thiosulfate and sodium nitrite

U.S. Brand Names Nithiodote™

Therapeutic Category Antidote

Use Acute, life-threatening cyanide poisoning

General Dosage Range

I.V.:

Children:

Sodium nitrite: 6 mg/kg (maximum: 300 mg); may repeat at one-half the original dose if needed

Sodium thiosulfate: 7 g/m^2 (maximum: 12.5 g); may repeat at one-half the original dose if needed

Adults:

Sodium nitrite: 300 mg; may repeat at one-half the original dose if needed

Sodium thiosulfate: 12.5 g; may repeat at one-half the original dose if needed

Dosage Forms

Injection, solution [combination package]:

Nithiodote™: Sodium nitrite 300 mg/10 mL (10 mL) and sodium thiosulfate 12.5 g/50 mL (50 mL)

sodium nitrite, sodium thiosulfate, and amyl nitrite

(SOW dee um NYE trite, SOW dee um thye oh SUL fate, & AM il NYE trite)

Synonyms amyl nitrite, sodium nitrite, and sodium thiosulfate; cyanide antidote kit; sodium thiosulfate, sodium nitrite, and amyl nitrite

U.S. Brand Names Cyanide Antidote Package

Therapeutic Category Antidote

Use Treatment of cyanide poisoning

General Dosage Range

I.V.:

Sodium nitrite: Given after amyl nitrite and prior to sodium thiosulfate:

Children: 6 mg/kg (maximum: 300 mg); may repeat at one-half the original dose if needed

Adults: 300 mg; may repeat at one-half the original dose if needed

Sodium thiosulfate: Given after sodium nitrite:

Children: 7 g/m^2 (maximum: 12.5 g); may repeat at one-half the original dose if needed

Adults: 12.5 g; may repeat at one-half the original dose if needed

Inhalation: Amyl nitrite: Given prior to sodium nitrite: *Children and Adults:* 0.3 mL ampul crushed into a gauze pad and placed in front of the patient's mouth (or endotracheal tube if patient is intubated) to inhale over 15-30 seconds; repeat every minute until sodium nitrite can be administered.

Dosage Forms Kit [each kit contains]:

Cyanide Antidote Package:

Injection, solution:

Sodium nitrite 300 mg/10 mL (2)

Sodium thiosulfate 12.5 g/50 mL (2)

Inhalant: Amyl nitrite 0.3 mL (12)

sodium nitroferricyanide *see* nitroprusside *on page 646*

sodium nitroprusside *see* nitroprusside *on page 646*

sodium oxybate (SOW dee um ox i BATE)

Synonyms 4-hydroxybutyrate; gamma hydroxybutyric acid; GHB; oxybate; sodium 4-hydroxybutyrate

U.S. Brand Names Xyrem®

Canadian Brand Names Xyrem®

Therapeutic Category Central Nervous System Depressant

Controlled Substance C-I (illicit use); C-III (medical use)

Use Treatment of cataplexy and daytime sleepiness in patients with narcolepsy

General Dosage Range Dosage adjustment recommended in patients with hepatic impairment

Oral: *Children ≥16 years and Adults:* Initial: 4.5 g/day in 2 equal doses given at bedtime and 2.5-4 hours later; Maintenance: 4.5-9 g/day (maximum: 9 g/day)

Dosage Forms

Solution, oral:

Xyrem®: 500 mg/mL (180 mL)

sodium PAS *see* aminosalicylic acid *on page 63*

sodium-PCA and lactic acid *see* lactic acid *on page 517*

sodium phenylacetate and sodium benzoate

(SOW dee um fen il AS e tate & SOW dee um BENZ oh ate)

Synonyms NAPA and NABZ; sodium benzoate and sodium phenylacetate

U.S. Brand Names Ammonul®

Therapeutic Category Ammonium Detoxicant

Use Adjunct to treatment of acute hyperammonemia and encephalopathy in patients with urea cycle disorders involving partial or complete deficiencies of carbamyl-phosphate synthetase (CPS), ornithine transcarbamoylase (OTC), argininosuccinate lysase (ASL), or argininosuccinate synthetase (ASS); for use with hemodialysis in acute neonatal hyperammonemic coma, moderate-to-severe hyperammonemic encephalopathy and hyperammonemia which fails to respond to initial therapy

General Dosage Range I.V.:

Children ≤20 kg: Loading dose: Ammonul® 2.5 mL/kg (sodium phenylacetate 250 mg/kg and sodium benzoate 250 mg/kg); Maintenance: Repeat same loading dose over 24 hours

Children >20 kg and Adults: Loading dose: Ammonul® 55 mL/m^2 (sodium phenylacetate 5.5 g/$m^2$and sodium benzoate 5.5 g/m^2); Maintenance: Repeat same loading dose over 24 hours

Dosage Forms

Injection, solution [concentrate]:

Ammonul®: Sodium phenylacetate 100 mg and sodium benzoate 100 mg per 1 mL (50 mL)

sodium phenylbutyrate (SOW dee um fen il BYOO ti rate)

Synonyms ammonapse

U.S. Brand Names Buphenyl®

Therapeutic Category Miscellaneous Product

Use Adjunctive therapy in the chronic management of patients with urea cycle disorder involving deficiencies of carbamoylphosphate synthetase, ornithine transcarbamylase, or argininosuccinic acid synthetase

General Dosage Range Oral:

Children <20 kg: Powder: 450-600 mg/kg/day administered in equally divided amounts with each meal or feeding, 3-6 times daily (maximum: 20 g/day)

Children ≥20 kg and Adults: 9.9-13 g/m^2/day, administered in equally divided amounts with each meal, 3-6 times daily (maximum: 20 g/day)

Dosage Forms

Powder for solution, oral:

Buphenyl®: (250 g)

Tablet, oral:

Buphenyl®: 500 mg

sodium phosphate and potassium phosphate *see* potassium phosphate and sodium phosphate *on page 747*

sodium phosphates (SOW dee um FOS fates)

Medication Safety Issues

Sound-alike/look-alike issues:

Visicol® may be confused with Asacol®, VESIcare®

Administration issues:

Enemas and oral solution are available in pediatric and adult sizes; prescribe by "volume" not by "bottle."

Because inorganic phosphate exists as monobasic and dibasic anions, with the mixture of valences dependent on pH, ordering by mEq amounts is unreliable and may lead to large dosing errors. In addition, I.V. phosphate is available in the sodium and potassium salt; therefore, the content of these cations must be considered when ordering phosphate. The most reliable method of ordering I.V. phosphate is by millimoles, then specifying the potassium or sodium salt.

Synonyms phosphates, sodium

U.S. Brand Names Fleet® Enema Extra® [OTC]; Fleet® Enema [OTC]; Fleet® Pedia-Lax™ Enema [OTC]; LaCrosse Complete [OTC]; OsmoPrep®; Visicol®

Canadian Brand Names Fleet Enema®

Therapeutic Category Electrolyte Supplement, Oral; Laxative

Use

Oral solution, rectal: Short-term treatment of constipation

Oral tablets (OsmoPrep®, Visicol®): Bowel cleansing prior to colonoscopy

I.V.: Source of phosphate in large volume I.V. fluids and parenteral nutrition; treatment and prevention of hypophosphatemia

General Dosage Range

I.V.:

Children: 0.08-1 mmol phosphate/kg **or** Parenteral nutrition: Infusion: 0.5-2 mmol/kg/24 hours

Adults: 0.08-1 mmol phosphate/kg **or** Parenteral nutrition: Infusion: 20-40 mmol/24 hours

Oral:

Solution:

Children 5-9 years: 7.5 mL as a single dose (maximum single daily dose: 7.5 mL)

Children 10-11 years: 15 mL as a single dose (maximum single daily dose: 15 mL)

Children ≥12 years and Adults: 15 mL as a single dose (maximum single daily dose: 45 mL)

Tablet: *Adults*:

Visicol®: 40 tablets in divided doses as directed beginning evening before colonoscopy

OsmoPrep®: 32 tablets in divided doses as directed beginning evening before colonoscopy

Rectal:

Children 2-4 years: One-half contents of one 2.25 oz pediatric enema

Children 5-11 years: Contents of one 2.25 oz pediatric enema

Children ≥12 years and Adults: Contents of one 4.5-ounce enema as a single dose

Dosage Forms

Injection, solution [concentrate; preservative free]: Phosphorus 3 mmol and sodium 4 mEq per 1 mL (5 mL, 15 mL, 50 mL)

Solution, oral: Monobasic sodium phosphate 2.4 g and dibasic sodium phosphate 0.9 g per 5 mL (45 mL)

Solution, rectal [enema]: Monobasic sodium phosphate 19 g and dibasic sodium phosphate 7 g per 118 mL delivered dose (133 mL)

Fleet® Enema [OTC], LaCrosse Complete [OTC]: Monobasic sodium phosphate 19 g and dibasic sodium phosphate 7 g per 118 mL delivered dose (133 mL)

Fleet® Enema Extra® [OTC]: Monobasic sodium phosphate 19 g and dibasic sodium phosphate 7 g per 197 mL delivered dose (230 mL)

Fleet® Pedia-Lax™ Enema [OTC]: Monobasic sodium phosphate 9.5 g and dibasic sodium phosphate 3.5 g per 59 mL delivered dose (66 mL)

Tablet, oral [scored]:

OsmoPrep®, Visicol®: Monobasic sodium phosphate 1.102 g and dibasic sodium phosphate 0.398 g

sodium picosulfate, magnesium oxide, and citric acid

(SOW dee um pye ko SUL fate mag NEE zhum OKS ide & SI trik AS id)

Synonyms citric acid, sodium picosulfate, and magnesium oxide; magnesium oxide, sodium picosulfate, and citric acid; Prepopik™; sodium picosulphate, magnesium oxide, and citric acid

Canadian Brand Names Oral Purgative; Pico-Salax®; Picodan; Picoflo; Purg-Odan™

Therapeutic Category Laxative, Osmotic; Laxative, Stimulant

Use Bowel cleansing prior to colonoscopy

Canadian labeling: Additional uses (not in U.S. labeling): Bowel cleansing prior to x-ray examination, endoscopy, or surgery

General Dosage Range Oral: *Adults:* Two 150 mL (5 oz) doses

Product Availability Prepopik™: FDA approved July 2012; availability anticipated October 2012. Consult prescribing information for additional information.

Dosage Forms

Powder for solution, oral [kit]:

Prepopik™: Sodium picosulfate 10 mg, magnesium oxide 3.5 g, and citric acid 12 g per packet (2s)

Dosage Forms - Canada

Powder for solution, oral [kit]:

Pico-Salex®: Sodium picosulphate 10 mg, magnesium oxide 3.5 g, and citric acid 12 g per sachet (1s, 2s) [orange or cranberry flavor]

Purg-Odan™: Sodium picosulphate 10 mg, magnesium oxide 3.5 g, and citric acid 12 g per sachet (1s, 2s) [orange flavor]

sodium picosulphate, magnesium oxide, and citric acid *see* sodium picosulfate, magnesium oxide, and citric acid *on page 846*

sodium polystyrene sulfonate (SOW dee um pol ee STYE reen SUL fon ate)

Medication Safety Issues

Sound-alike/look-alike issues:

Kayexalate® may be confused with Kaopectate®

Sodium polystyrene sulfonate may be confused with calcium polystyrene sulfonate

Administration issues:

Always prescribe either one-time doses or as a specific number of doses (eg, 15 g q6h x 2 doses). Scheduled doses with no dosage limit could be given for days leading to dangerous hypokalemia.

International issues:

Kionex [U.S.] may be confused with Kinex brand name for biperiden [Mexico]

U.S. Brand Names Kalexate; Kayexalate®; Kionex®; SPS®

Canadian Brand Names Kayexalate®; PMS-Sodium Polystyrene Sulfonate

Therapeutic Category Antidote

Use Treatment of hyperkalemia

General Dosage Range

Oral:

Children: 1 g/kg/dose every 6 hours
Adults: 15 g 1-4 times/day

Rectal:

Children: 1 g/kg/dose every 2-6 hours
Adults: 30-50 g every 6 hours

Dosage Forms

Powder for suspension, oral/rectal: (454 g)

Kalexate: (454 g)
Kayexalate®: (454 g)
Kionex®: (454 g)

Suspension, oral/rectal:

Kionex®: 15 g/60 mL (60 mL, 480 mL)
SPS®: 15 g/60 mL (60 mL, 120 mL, 473 mL)

Sodium Sulamyd (Can) *see* sulfacetamide (ophthalmic) *on page 858*

sodium sulfacetamide *see* sulfacetamide (ophthalmic) *on page 858*

sodium sulfacetamide *see* sulfacetamide (topical) *on page 858*

sodium sulfacetamide and sulfur *see* sulfur and sulfacetamide *on page 862*

sodium sulfate, magnesium sulfate, and potassium sulfate *see* sodium sulfate, potassium sulfate, and magnesium sulfate *on page 847*

sodium sulfate, potassium sulfate, and magnesium sulfate

(SOW dee um SUL fate, poe TASS ee um SUL fate, & mag NEE zhum SUL fate)

Synonyms magnesium sulfate, potassium sulfate, and sodium sulfate; magnesium sulfate, sodium sulfate, and potassium sulfate; potassium sulfate, magnesium sulfate, and sodium sulfate; potassium sulfate, sodium sulfate, and magnesium sulfate; sodium sulfate, magnesium sulfate, and potassium sulfate

U.S. Brand Names Suprep® Bowel Prep Kit

Therapeutic Category Laxative, Osmotic

Use Bowel cleansing prior to GI examination

General Dosage Range Oral: *Adults:* Contents of 2 bottles diluted as directed prior to colonoscopy; total volume of liquid to be consumed over the course of treatment: 2880 mL

Dosage Forms

Solution, oral:

Suprep® Bowel Prep Kit: Sodium sulfate 17.5 g, potassium sulfate 3.13 g, and magnesium sulfate 1.6 g per 180 mL (180 mL) [contains sodium benzoate]

sodium tetradecyl (SOW dee um tetra DEK il)

Synonyms sodium tetradecyl sulfate

U.S. Brand Names Sotradecol®

Canadian Brand Names Trombovar®

Therapeutic Category Sclerosing Agent

Use Treatment of small, uncomplicated varicose veins of the lower extremities

General Dosage Range I.V.: *Adults:* 0.5-2 mL in each vein (maximum: 10 mL per treatment session)

Dosage Forms

Injection, solution:

Sotradecol®: 1% (2 mL); 3% (2 mL)

sodium tetradecyl sulfate *see* sodium tetradecyl *on page 847*

sodium thiosulfate (SOW dee um thye oh SUL fate)

Synonyms disodium thiosulfate pentahydrate; pentahydrate; sodium hyposulfate; sodium thiosulphate; thiosulfuric acid disodium salt

Therapeutic Category Antidote; Antifungal Agent

Use Treatment of cyanide poisoning

General Dosage Range I.V.:

Children: 7 g/m^2 (maximum: 12.5 g); may repeat at one-half the original dose if needed

Adults: 12.5 g; may repeat at one-half the original dose if needed

Dosage Forms

Injection, solution: 250 mg/mL (50 mL)

Injection, solution [preservative free]: 100 mg/mL (10 mL); 250 mg/mL (50 mL)

sodium thiosulfate and sodium nitrite *see* sodium nitrite and sodium thiosulfate *on page 843*

sodium thiosulfate, sodium nitrite, and amyl nitrite *see* sodium nitrite, sodium thiosulfate, and amyl nitrite *on page 844*

sodium thiosulphate *see* sodium thiosulfate *on page 848*

Soflax [OTC] (Can) *see* bisacodyl *on page 134*

Soflax™ (Can) *see* docusate *on page 304*

Sojourn™ *see* sevoflurane *on page 832*

Sojourn Sevoflurane (Can) *see* sevoflurane *on page 832*

Solaquin® (Can) *see* hydroquinone *on page 461*

Solaquin Forte® (Can) *see* hydroquinone *on page 461*

Solaraze® *see* diclofenac (topical) *on page 280*

Solarcaine® cool aloe Burn Relief [OTC] *see* lidocaine (topical) *on page 535*

solifenacin (sol i FEN a sin)

Medication Safety Issues

Sound-alike/look-alike issues:

VESIcare® may be confused with Visicol®

BEERS Criteria medication:

This drug may be potentially inappropriate for use in geriatric patients (Quality of evidence - varies based on comorbidity; Strength of recommendation - varies based on comorbidity)

Synonyms solifenacin succinate; YM905

U.S. Brand Names VESIcare®

Therapeutic Category Anticholinergic Agent

Use Treatment of overactive bladder with symptoms of urinary frequency, urgency, or urge incontinence

General Dosage Range Dosage adjustment recommended in patients with hepatic or renal impairment and on concomitant therapy

Oral: *Adults:* 5-10 mg/day

Dosage Forms

Tablet, oral:

VESIcare®: 5 mg, 10 mg

solifenacin succinate *see* solifenacin *on page 848*

Soliris® *see* eculizumab *on page 322*

Solodyn® *see* minocycline *on page 604*

Soluble Fiber Therapy [OTC] *see* methylcellulose *on page 588*

soluble fluorescein *see* fluorescein *on page 393*

Solu-CORTEF® *see* hydrocortisone (systemic) *on page 457*

Solu-Cortef® (Can) *see* hydrocortisone (systemic) *on page 457*

Solugel® (Can) *see* benzoyl peroxide *on page 124*

Solumedrol *see* methylprednisolone *on page 591*

Solu-MEDROL® *see* methylprednisolone *on page 591*

Solu-Medrol® (Can) *see* methylprednisolone *on page 591*

Soluver® (Can) *see* salicylic acid *on page 816*

Soluver® Plus (Can) *see* salicylic acid *on page 816*

Solzira *see* gabapentin enacarbil *on page* 414

Soma® *see* carisoprodol *on page* 177

Soma Compound *see* carisoprodol and aspirin *on page* 178

soma compound w/codeine *see* carisoprodol, aspirin, and codeine *on page* 178

somatropin (soe ma TROE pin)

Medication Safety Issues

Sound-alike/look-alike issues:

Humatrope® may be confused with homatropine

Somatrem may be confused with somatropin

Somatropin may be confused with homatropine, sumatriptan

BEERS Criteria medication:

This drug may be potentially inappropriate for use in geriatric patients (Quality of evidence - high; Strength of recommendation - strong).

Synonyms growth hormone, human; hGH; human growth hormone

U.S. Brand Names Genotropin Miniquick®; Genotropin®; Humatrope®; Norditropin FlexPro®; Norditropin® NordiFlex®; Nutropin AQ Pen®; Nutropin AQ®; Nutropin AQ® NuSpin™; Nutropin®; Omnitrope®; Saizen®; Serostim®; Tev-Tropin®; Zorbtive®

Canadian Brand Names Humatrope®; Nutropin®; Nutropin® AQ; Omnitrope®; Saizen®; Serostim®

Therapeutic Category Growth Hormone

Use

Children:

Treatment of growth failure due to inadequate endogenous growth hormone secretion (Genotropin®, Humatrope®, Norditropin®, Nutropin®, Nutropin AQ®, Omnitrope®, Saizen®, Tev-Tropin®)

Treatment of short stature associated with Turner syndrome (Genotropin®, Humatrope®, Norditropin®, Nutropin®, Nutropin AQ®, Omnitrope®)

Treatment of Prader-Willi syndrome (Genotropin®, Omnitrope®)

Treatment of growth failure associated with chronic renal insufficiency (CRI) up until the time of renal transplantation (Nutropin®, Nutropin AQ®)

Treatment of growth failure in children born small for gestational age who fail to manifest catch-up growth by 2 years of age (Genotropin®, Omnitrope®) or by 2-4 years of age (Humatrope®, Norditropin®)

Treatment of idiopathic short stature (nongrowth hormone-deficient short stature) defined by height standard deviation score (SDS) ≤-2.25 and growth rate not likely to attain normal adult height (Genotropin®, Humatrope®, Nutropin®, Nutropin AQ®, Omnitrope®)

Treatment of short stature or growth failure associated with short stature homeobox gene (SHOX) deficiency (Humatrope®)

Treatment of short stature associated with Noonan syndrome (Norditropin®)

Adults:

HIV patients with wasting or cachexia with concomitant antiviral therapy (Serostim®)

Replacement of endogenous growth hormone in patients with adult growth hormone deficiency who meet both of the following criteria (Genotropin®, Humatrope®, Norditropin®, Nutropin®, Nutropin AQ®, Omnitrope®, Saizen®):

Biochemical diagnosis of adult growth hormone deficiency by means of a subnormal response to a standard growth hormone stimulation test (peak growth hormone ≤5 mcg/L). Confirmatory testing may not be required in patients with congenital/genetic growth hormone deficiency or multiple pituitary hormone deficiencies due to organic diseases.

and

Adult-onset: Patients who have adult growth hormone deficiency whether alone or with multiple hormone deficiencies (hypopituitarism) as a result of pituitary disease, hypothalamic disease, surgery, radiation therapy, or trauma

or

Childhood-onset: Patients who were growth hormone deficient during childhood, confirmed as an adult before replacement therapy is initiated

Treatment of short-bowel syndrome (Zorbtive®)

General Dosage Range I.M., SubQ: *Children and Adults:* Dosage varies greatly depending on indication

Dosage Forms

Injection, powder for reconstitution:
Genotropin®: 5 mg, 12 mg
Humatrope®: 6 mg, 12 mg, 24 mg
Nutropin®: 5 mg, 10 mg
Omnitrope®: 5.8 mg
Saizen®: 5 mg, 8.8 mg
Serostim®: 4 mg, 5 mg, 6 mg
Tev-Tropin®: 5 mg
Zorbtive®: 8.8 mg

Injection, powder for reconstitution [preservative free]:
Genotropin Miniquick®: 0.2 mg, 0.4 mg, 0.6 mg, 0.8 mg, 1 mg, 1.2 mg, 1.4 mg, 1.6 mg, 1.8 mg, 2 mg

Injection, solution:
Norditropin FlexPro®: 5 mg/1.5 mL (1.5 mL); 10 mg/1.5 mL (1.5 mL); 15 mg/1.5 mL (1.5 mL)
Norditropin® NordiFlex®: 30 mg/3 mL (3 mL)
Nutropin AQ Pen®: 10 mg/2 mL (2 mL); 20 mg/2 mL (2 mL)
Nutropin AQ®: 10 mg/2 mL (2 mL)
Nutropin AQ® NuSpin™: 5 mg/2 mL (2 mL); 10 mg/2 mL (2 mL); 20 mg/2 mL (2 mL)
Omnitrope®: 5 mg/1.5 mL (1.5 mL); 10 mg/1.5 mL (1.5 mL)

Somatuline® Autogel® (Can) *see* lanreotide *on page* *522*
Somatuline® Depot *see* lanreotide *on page* *522*
Somavert® *see* pegvisomant *on page* *700*
Sominex® [OTC] *see* diphenhydramine (systemic) *on page* *292*
Sominex® (Can) *see* diphenhydramine (systemic) *on page* *292*
Sominex® Maximum Strength [OTC] *see* diphenhydramine (systemic) *on page* *292*
Somnote® *see* chloral hydrate *on page* *194*
Som Pam (Can) *see* flurazepam *on page* *398*
Sonata® *see* zaleplon *on page* *958*
Soothe® [OTC] *see* artificial tears *on page* *93*
Soothe® Hydration [OTC] *see* artificial tears *on page* *93*
Soothing Care™ Itch Relief [OTC] *see* pramoxine *on page* *750*

sorafenib (sor AF e nib)

Medication Safety Issues

Sound-alike/look-alike issues:
NexAVAR® may be confused with NexIUM®
SORAfenib may be confused with axitinib, gefitinib, imatinib, SUNItinib, vandetanib, vemurafenib

High alert medication:
This medication is in a class the Institute for Safe Medication Practices (ISMP) includes among its list of drug classes which have a heightened risk of causing significant patient harm when used in error.

Synonyms BAY 43-9006; sorafenib tosylate

Tall-Man SORAfenib

U.S. Brand Names NexAVAR®

Canadian Brand Names Nexavar®

Therapeutic Category Antineoplastic Agent, Tyrosine Kinase Inhibitor; Vascular Endothelial Growth Factor (VEGF) Inhibitor

Use Treatment of advanced renal cell cancer (RCC); treatment of unresectable hepatocellular cancer (HCC)

General Dosage Range Dosage adjustments recommended in patients with hepatic or renal impairment, or who develop toxicities
Oral: *Adults:* 400 mg twice daily

Dosage Forms

Tablet, oral:
NexAVAR®: 200 mg

sorafenib tosylate *see* sorafenib *on page* *850*

sorbitol (SOR bi tole)

Therapeutic Category Genitourinary Irrigant; Laxative

Use Genitourinary irrigant in transurethral prostatic resection or other transurethral resection or other transurethral surgical procedures; diuretic; humectant; sweetening agent; hyperosmotic laxative; facilitate the passage of sodium polystyrene sulfonate through the intestinal tract

General Dosage Range

Oral:

Children 2-11 years: 2 mL/kg (70% solution) as a single dose

Children ≥12 years and Adults: 30-150 mL (70% solution) as a single dose

Rectal:

Children 2-11 years: 30-60 mL (25% to 30% solution) as a single dose

Children ≥12 years and Adults: 120 mL (25% to 30% solution) as a single dose

Topical: *Adults:* 3% to 3.3% as a transurethral irrigation

Dosage Forms

Solution, genitourinary irrigation [preservative free]: 3% (3000 mL, 5000 mL); 3.3% (2000 mL, 4000 mL)

Solution, oral: 70% (30 mL, 473 mL, 480 mL, 3840 mL)

Sore Throat Relief [OTC] *see* benzocaine *on page* 121

Soriatane® *see* acitretin *on page* 33

Sorilux™ *see* calcipotriene *on page* 159

Sorine® *see* sotalol *on page* 851

sotalol (SOE ta lole)

Medication Safety Issues

Sound-alike/look-alike issues:

Sotalol may be confused with Stadol, Sudafed®

Betapace® may be confused with Betapace AF®

High alert medication:

The Institute for Safe Medication Practices (ISMP) includes this medication (I.V. formulation) among its list of drugs which have a heightened risk of causing significant patient harm when used in error.

BEERS Criteria medication:

This drug may be potentially inappropriate for use in geriatric patients (Quality of evidence - high; Strength of recommendation - strong).

Synonyms sotalol hydrochloride

U.S. Brand Names Betapace AF®; Betapace®; Sorine®

Canadian Brand Names Apo-Sotalol®; CO Sotalol; Dom-Sotalol; Med-Sotalol; Mylan-Sotalol; Novo-Sotalol; Nu-Sotalol; PHL-Sotalol; PMS-Sotalol; PRO-Sotalol; ratio-Sotalol; Rhoxal-sotalol; Riva-Sotalol; Rylosol; Sandoz-Sotalol; ZYM-Sotalol

Therapeutic Category Antiarrhythmic Agent, Class II; Antiarrhythmic Agent, Class III; Beta-Adrenergic Blocker, Nonselective

Use Treatment of documented ventricular arrhythmias (ie, sustained ventricular tachycardia), that in the judgment of the physician are life-threatening; maintenance of normal sinus rhythm in patients with symptomatic atrial fibrillation and atrial flutter who are currently in sinus rhythm. Manufacturer states substitutions should not be made for Betapace AF® since Betapace AF® is distributed with a patient package insert specific for atrial fibrillation/flutter.

Injection: Substitution for oral sotalol in those who are unable to take sotalol orally

General Dosage Range Dosage adjustment recommended in patients with renal impairment or who develop toxicities

I.V.: *Adults:* Initial: 75 mg twice daily; Maintenance: 75-150 mg twice daily (maximum: 300 mg/day)

Oral:

Children ≤2 years: Dosage should be adjusted (decreased) by plotting of the child's age on a logarithmic scale; **Note:** Refer to manufacturer's package labeling

Children >2 years: Initial: 90 mg/m^2/day in 3 divided doses; Maintenance: 90-180 mg/m^2/day in 3 divided doses (maximum: 180 mg/m^2/day)

Adults: Initial: 80 mg twice daily; Maintenance: 240-320 mg/day in 2-3 divided doses (maximum: 320 mg/day)

Dosage Forms

Injection, solution: 15 mg/mL (10 mL)

Tablet, oral: 80 mg, 120 mg, 160 mg, 240 mg

Betapace AF®: 80 mg, 120 mg, 160 mg

Betapace®: 80 mg, 120 mg, 160 mg

Sorine®: 80 mg, 120 mg, 160 mg, 240 mg

sotalol hydrochloride *see* sotalol *on page 851*

Sotradecol® *see* sodium tetradecyl *on page 847*

Sotret® *see* isotretinoin *on page 505*

SourceCF® *see* vitamins (multiple/oral) *on page 951*

SourceCF® [OTC] *see* vitamins (multiple/pediatric) *on page 952*

SPA *see* albumin *on page 41*

SPD417 *see* carbamazepine *on page 172*

Spectracef® *see* cefditoren *on page 182*

SPI 0211 *see* lubiprostone *on page 554*

spinosad (SPIN oh sad)

Synonyms NatrOVA

U.S. Brand Names Natroba™

Therapeutic Category Antiparasitic Agent, Topical; Pediculocide

Use Topical treatment of head lice (*Pediculosis capitis*) infestation in adults and children ≥4 years of age

General Dosage Range Topical: *Children ≥4 years old and Adults:* Apply sufficient amount to cover dry scalp and hair; may repeat in 7 days

Dosage Forms

Suspension, topical:

Natroba™: 0.9% (120 mL)

Spiriva® (Can) *see* tiotropium *on page 899*

Spiriva® HandiHaler® *see* tiotropium *on page 899*

spironolactone (speer on oh LAK tone)

Medication Safety Issues

Sound-alike/look-alike issues:

Aldactone® may be confused with Aldactazide®

BEERS Criteria medication:

This drug may be potentially inappropriate for use in geriatric patients (Quality of evidence - moderate; Strength of recommendation - strong).

International issues:

Aldactone: Brand name for spironolactone [U.S., Canada, multiple international markets], but also the brand name for potassium canrenoate [Austria, Czech Republic, Germany, Hungary, Poland]

U.S. Brand Names Aldactone®

Canadian Brand Names Aldactone®; Novo-Spiroton; Teva-Spironolactone

Therapeutic Category Diuretic, Potassium Sparing

Use Management of edema associated with excessive aldosterone excretion; hypertension; primary hyperaldosteronism; hypokalemia; cirrhosis of liver accompanied by edema or ascites; nephrotic syndrome; severe heart failure (NYHA class III-IV) to increase survival and reduce hospitalization when added to standard therapy

General Dosage Range Dosage adjustment recommended in patients with renal impairment

Oral:

Adults: 12.5-400 mg/day in 1-2 divided doses

Elderly: Initial: 25-50 mg/day in 1-2 divided doses

Dosage Forms

Tablet, oral: 25 mg, 50 mg, 100 mg

Aldactone®: 25 mg, 50 mg, 100 mg

spironolactone and hydrochlorothiazide *see* hydrochlorothiazide and spironolactone *on page 453*

SPM 927 *see* lacosamide *on page 517*

Sporanox® *see* itraconazole *on page 507*

Sportscreme® [OTC] *see* trolamine *on page 923*

SPP100 *see* aliskiren *on page 47*
Sprayzoin™ [OTC] *see* benzoin *on page 124*
Sprintec® *see* ethinyl estradiol and norgestimate *on page 361*
Sprix® *see* ketorolac (nasal) *on page 513*
Sprycel® *see* dasatinib *on page 256*
SPS® *see* sodium polystyrene sulfonate *on page 846*
SQV *see* saquinavir *on page 824*
SR-89 *see* strontium-89 *on page 854*
SR33589 *see* dronedarone *on page 317*
Sronyx® *see* ethinyl estradiol and levonorgestrel *on page 357*
SS734 *see* besifloxacin *on page 128*
SSD™ *see* silver sulfadiazine *on page 833*
SSKI® *see* potassium iodide *on page 746*
SSS 10-4 *see* sulfur and sulfacetamide *on page 862*
Stadol *see* butorphanol *on page 156*
Stagesic™ *see* hydrocodone and acetaminophen *on page 454*
Stalevo® *see* levodopa, carbidopa, and entacapone *on page 531*
StanGard® Perio *see* fluoride *on page 393*
stannous fluoride *see* fluoride *on page 393*
Starlix® *see* nateglinide *on page 630*
Statex® (Can) *see* morphine (systemic) *on page 612*
Statobex® (Can) *see* phendimetrazine *on page 711*

stavudine (STAV yoo deen)

Medication Safety Issues

Sound-alike/look-alike issues:

Zerit® may be confused with Zestril®, Ziac®, ZyrTEC®

Synonyms d4T

U.S. Brand Names Zerit®

Canadian Brand Names Zerit®

Therapeutic Category Antiviral Agent

Use Treatment of HIV infection in combination with other antiretroviral agents

General Dosage Range Dosage adjustment recommended in patients with renal impairment.

Oral:

Newborns (Birth to 13 days): 0.5 mg/kg every 12 hours
Children ≥14 days and <30 kg: 1 mg/kg every 12 hours
Children and Adults 30-59 kg: 30 mg every 12 hours
Children and Adults ≥60 kg: 40 mg every 12 hours

Dosage Forms

Capsule, oral: 15 mg, 20 mg, 30 mg, 40 mg
Zerit®: 15 mg, 20 mg, 30 mg, 40 mg

Powder for solution, oral: 1 mg/mL (200 mL)
Zerit®: 1 mg/mL (200 mL)

Stavzor™ *see* valproic acid *on page 934*
Staxyn™ *see* vardenafil *on page 938*
Stelara™ *see* ustekinumab *on page 932*
Stelazine *see* trifluoperazine *on page 919*
Stendra™ *see* avanafil *on page 104*
sterile talc *see* talc (sterile) *on page 867*
Sterile Talc Powder™ *see* talc (sterile) *on page 867*
Sterile Vancomycin Hydrochloride, USP (Can) *see* vancomycin *on page 936*
STI-571 *see* imatinib *on page 474*
Stieprox® (Can) *see* ciclopirox *on page 207*
Stieva-A (Can) *see* tretinoin (topical) *on page 914*
Stimate® *see* desmopressin *on page 264*

Sting-Kill® [OTC] *see* benzocaine *on page 121*
St Joseph® Adult Aspirin [OTC] *see* aspirin *on page 96*
Stop® *see* fluoride *on page 393*
Strattera® *see* atomoxetine *on page 99*

streptomycin (strep toe MYE sin)

Medication Safety Issues

Sound-alike/look-alike issues:

Streptomycin may be confused with streptozocin

Synonyms streptomycin sulfate

Canadian Brand Names Streptomycin for Injection

Therapeutic Category Antibiotic, Aminoglycoside; Antitubercular Agent

Use Part of combination therapy of active tuberculosis; used in combination with other agents for treatment of bacteremia caused by susceptible gram-negative bacilli, brucellosis, chancroid granuloma inguinale, *H. influenzae* (respiratory, endocardial, meningeal infections), *K. pneumoniae*, plague, streptococcal or enterococcal endocarditis, tularemia, urinary tract infections (caused by *A. aerogenes, E. coli, E. faecalis, K. pneumoniae, Proteus* spp)

General Dosage Range Dosage adjustment recommended in patients with renal impairment

I.M.:

Children: Tuberculosis: 20-40 mg/kg given daily (maximum: 1 g daily) **or** 25-30 mg/kg 2-3 times weekly (maximum: 1.5 g daily)

Adults: Tuberculosis: 15 mg/kg/day **or** 25-30 mg/kg 2-3 times weekly; Other indications: 1-2 g daily in 2 divided doses

Dosage Forms

Injection, powder for reconstitution: 1 g

Streptomycin for Injection (Can) *see* streptomycin *on page 854*
streptomycin sulfate *see* streptomycin *on page 854*

streptozocin (strep toe ZOE sin)

Medication Safety Issues

Sound-alike/look-alike issues:

Streptozocin may be confused with streptomycin

High alert medication:

The Institute for Safe Medication Practices (ISMP) includes this medication among its list of drugs which have a heightened risk of causing significant patient harm when used in error.

U.S. Brand Names Zanosar®

Canadian Brand Names Zanosar®

Therapeutic Category Antineoplastic Agent

Use Treatment of metastatic islet cell carcinoma of the pancreas

General Dosage Range Dosage adjustment recommended in patients with renal impairment

I.V.: *Children and Adults:* 1-1.5 g/m^2 weekly for 6 weeks followed by a 4-week rest period **or** 0.5-1 g/m^2 for 5 consecutive days as combination therapy followed by a 4- to 6-week rest period

Dosage Forms

Injection, powder for reconstitution:

Zanosar®: 1 g

Striant® *see* testosterone *on page 881*
Stridex® Essential Care® [OTC] *see* salicylic acid *on page 816*
Stridex® Facewipes To Go® [OTC] *see* salicylic acid *on page 816*
Stridex® Maximum Strength [OTC] *see* salicylic acid *on page 816*
Stridex® Sensitive Skin [OTC] *see* salicylic acid *on page 816*
Strifon Forte® (Can) *see* chlorzoxazone *on page 204*
Stromectol® *see* ivermectin (systemic) *on page 507*
strontium-89 chloride *see* strontium-89 *on page 854*

strontium-89 (STRON shee um atey nine)

Synonyms SR-89; Sr89; strontium chloride SR 89; strontium-89 chloride

U.S. Brand Names Metastron®

Canadian Brand Names Metastron®

Therapeutic Category Radiopharmaceutical

Use Relief of bone pain in patients with skeletal metastases

General Dosage Range I.V.: *Adults:* 148 megabecquerel (4 millicurie) **or** 1.5-2.2 megabecquerel (40-60 microcurie)/kg

Dosage Forms

Injection, solution [preservative free]:
Metastron®: 1 mCi/mL (4 mL)

strontium chloride SR 89 *see* strontium-89 *on page 854*
Strovite® *see* vitamins (multiple/oral) *on page 951*
Strovite® Advance *see* vitamins (multiple/oral) *on page 951*
Strovite® Forte *see* vitamins (multiple/oral) *on page 951*
Strovite® Plus *see* vitamins (multiple/oral) *on page 951*
Stuart Prenatal® [OTC] *see* vitamins (multiple/prenatal) *on page 952*
SU011248 *see* sunitinib *on page 864*
suberoylanilide hydroxamic acid *see* vorinostat *on page 954*
Sublinox™ (Can) *see* zolpidem *on page 966*
Suboxone® *see* buprenorphine and naloxone *on page 150*
Subsys® *see* fentanyl *on page 377*
Subutex® [DSC] *see* buprenorphine *on page 149*
Subutex® (Can) *see* buprenorphine *on page 149*

succimer (SUKS si mer)

Synonyms DMSA

U.S. Brand Names Chemet®

Canadian Brand Names Chemet®

Therapeutic Category Chelating Agent

Use Treatment of lead poisoning in children with serum lead levels >45 mcg/dL

General Dosage Range Oral: *Children and Adults:* 10 mg/kg (or 350 mg/m^2/dose) every 8-12 hours (maximum: 500 mg/dose)

Dosage Forms

Capsule, oral:
Chemet®: 100 mg

succinylcholine (suks in il KOE leen)

Medication Safety Issues

High alert medication:
The Institute for Safe Medication Practices (ISMP) includes this medication among its list of drugs which have a heightened risk of causing significant patient harm when used in error.

Other safety concerns:
United States Pharmacopeia (USP) 2006: The Interdisciplinary Safe Medication Use Expert Committee of the USP has recommended the following:

- Hospitals, clinics, and other practice sites should institute special safeguards in the storage, labeling, and use of these agents and should include these safeguards in staff orientation and competency training.
- Healthcare professionals should be on high alert (especially vigilant) whenever a neuromuscular-blocking agent (NMBA) is stocked, ordered, prepared, or administered.

International issues:
Quelicin [U.S., Brazil, Canada, Indonesia] may be confused with Keflin brand name for cefalotin [Argentina, Brazil, Mexico, Netherlands, Norway]

Synonyms succinylcholine chloride; suxamethonium chloride

U.S. Brand Names Anectine®; Quelicin®

Canadian Brand Names Quelicin®

Therapeutic Category Skeletal Muscle Relaxant

Use To facilitate both rapid sequence and routine endotracheal intubation and to relax skeletal muscles during surgery

Note: Does not relieve pain or produce sedation

General Dosage Range Dosage adjustment recommended in patients with renal or hepatic impairment

I.M.: *Children and Adults:* Up to 3-4 mg/kg (maximum: 150 mg total dose)

I.V.:

Smaller Children: Intermittent: Initial: 2 mg/kg/dose; Maintenance: 0.3-0.6 mg/kg/dose every 5-10 minutes as needed

Older Children and Adolescents: Intermittent: Initial: 1 mg/kg/dose; Maintenance: 0.3-0.6 mg/kg every 5-10 minutes as needed

Adults: Intubation: 0.6 mg/kg (range: 0.3-1.1 mg/kg); Rapid sequence intubation: 1-1.5 mg/kg

Dosage Forms

Injection, solution:

Anectine®: 20 mg/mL (10 mL)

Quelicin®: 20 mg/mL (10 mL)

Injection, solution [preservative free]:

Quelicin®: 100 mg/mL (10 mL)

succinylcholine chloride *see* succinylcholine *on page* 855

Sucraid® *see* sacrosidase *on page* 816

sucralfate (soo KRAL fate)

Medication Safety Issues

Sound-alike/look-alike issues:

Sucralfate may be confused with salsalate

Carafate® may be confused with Cafergot®

Synonyms aluminum sucrose sulfate, basic

U.S. Brand Names Carafate®

Canadian Brand Names Apo-Sucralfate; Dom-Sucralfate; Novo-Sucralate; Nu-Sucralate; PMS-Sucralate; Sucralfate-1; Sulcrate®; Sulcrate® Suspension Plus; Teva-Sucralfate

Therapeutic Category Gastrointestinal Agent, Gastric or Duodenal Ulcer Treatment

Use Short-term (≤8 weeks) management of duodenal ulcers; maintenance therapy for duodenal ulcers

General Dosage Range Oral: *Adults:* 1 g 2-4 times/day

Dosage Forms

Suspension, oral: 1 g/10 mL (10 mL)

Carafate®: 1 g/10 mL (420 mL)

Tablet, oral: 1 g

Carafate®: 1 g

Sucralfate-1 (Can) *see* sucralfate *on page* 856

Sucrets® Children's [OTC] *see* dyclonine *on page* 320

Sucrets® Maximum Strength [OTC] *see* dyclonine *on page* 320

Sucrets® Original [OTC] *see* hexylresorcinol *on page* 448

Sucrets® Regular Strength [OTC] *see* dyclonine *on page* 320

sucrose (SOO krose)

U.S. Brand Names Sweet-Ease® [OTC]; TootSweet™ [OTC]

Therapeutic Category Analgesic, Nonopioid

Use Provide short-term analgesia in infants during immunization administration

Dosage Forms

Solution, oral:

Sweet-Ease® Preserved: 24% (15 mL)

TootSweet™: 24% (0.5 mL, 1 mL, 2 mL, 12 mL)

Solution, oral [preservative free]:

Sweet-Ease Natural®: 24% (15 mL)

Sudafed *see* pseudoephedrine *on page* 771

Sudafed® 12 Hour [OTC] *see* pseudoephedrine *on page* 771

Sudafed® 12 Hour Pressure + Pain [OTC] *see* naproxen and pseudoephedrine *on page* 629

Sudafed® 24 Hour [OTC] *see* pseudoephedrine *on page* 771

Sudafed® Children's [OTC] *see* pseudoephedrine *on page* 771

Sudafed® Children's Cold & Cough [OTC] *see* pseudoephedrine and dextromethorphan *on page* 772

Sudafed® Decongestant (Can) *see* pseudoephedrine *on page 771*
Sudafed® Head Cold and Sinus Extra Strength (Can) *see* acetaminophen and pseudoephedrine *on page 25*
Sudafed® Maximum Strength Nasal Decongestant [OTC] *see* pseudoephedrine *on page 771*
Sudafed PE® Children's [OTC] *see* phenylephrine (systemic) *on page 715*
Sudafed PE® Children's Cold & Cough [OTC] *see* dextromethorphan and phenylephrine *on page 273*
Sudafed PE® Congestion [OTC] *see* phenylephrine (systemic) *on page 715*
Sudafed PE™ Nasal Decongestant [OTC] *see* phenylephrine (systemic) *on page 715*
Sudafed PE® Nighttime Cold [OTC] *see* acetaminophen, diphenhydramine, and phenylephrine *on page 29*
Sudafed PE® Non-Drying Sinus [OTC] *see* guaifenesin and phenylephrine *on page 435*
Sudafed PE® Pressure + Pain [OTC] *see* acetaminophen and phenylephrine *on page 24*
Sudafed PE® Severe Cold [OTC] *see* acetaminophen, diphenhydramine, and phenylephrine *on page 29*
Sudafed PE® Sinus + Allergy [OTC] *see* chlorpheniramine and phenylephrine *on page 200*
Sudafed® Sinus Advance (Can) *see* pseudoephedrine and ibuprofen *on page 773*
SudaTex-G [OTC] *see* guaifenesin and pseudoephedrine *on page 436*
SudoGest [OTC] *see* pseudoephedrine *on page 771*
SudoGest 12 Hour [OTC] *see* pseudoephedrine *on page 771*
SudoGest Children's [OTC] [DSC] *see* pseudoephedrine *on page 771*
Sudogest™ PE [OTC] *see* phenylephrine (systemic) *on page 715*
SudoGest™ Sinus & Allergy [OTC] *see* chlorpheniramine and pseudoephedrine *on page 200*
Sudo-Tab® [OTC] *see* pseudoephedrine *on page 771*
Sufenta® *see* sufentanil *on page 857*

sufentanil (soo FEN ta nil)

Medication Safety Issues

Sound-alike/look-alike issues:

SUFentanil may be confused with alfentanil, fentaNYL

Sufenta® may be confused with Alfenta®, Sudafed®, Survanta®

High alert medication:

The Institute for Safe Medication Practices (ISMP) includes this medication among its list of drugs which have a heightened risk of causing significant patient harm when used in error.

Synonyms sufentanil citrate

Tall-Man SUFentanil

U.S. Brand Names Sufenta®

Canadian Brand Names Sufentanil Citrate Injection, USP; Sufenta®

Therapeutic Category Analgesic, Narcotic; General Anesthetic

Controlled Substance C-II

Use Analgesic supplement in maintenance of general anesthesia; epidural analgesic in conjunction with a local anesthetic

General Dosage Range

I.V.:

Children 2-12 years: 10-25 mcg/kg with 100% O_2; Maintenance: Up to 1-2 mcg/kg total dose

Adults: 1-2 mcg/kg with N_2O/O_2; Maintenance: 5-20 mcg/kg as needed

Epidural: *Adults:* 10-15 mcg (maximum: 3 doses)

Dosage Forms

Injection, solution [preservative free]: 50 mcg/mL (1 mL, 2 mL, 5 mL)

Sufenta®: 50 mcg/mL (1 mL, 2 mL, 5 mL)

sufentanil citrate *see* sufentanil *on page 857*
Sufentanil Citrate Injection, USP (Can) *see* sufentanil *on page 857*
sulamyd *see* sulfacetamide (ophthalmic) *on page 858*
sulamyd *see* sulfacetamide (topical) *on page 858*
Sular® *see* nisoldipine *on page 643*
sulbactam and ampicillin *see* ampicillin and sulbactam *on page 73*

sulconazole (sul KON a zole)

Synonyms sulconazole nitrate

U.S. Brand Names Exelderm®

Canadian Brand Names Exelderm®

Therapeutic Category Antifungal Agent

Use Treatment of superficial fungal infections of the skin, including tinea cruris (jock itch), tinea corporis (ringworm), tinea versicolor, and tinea pedis (athlete's foot, cream only)

General Dosage Range Topical: *Adults:* Apply a small amount to affected area once or twice daily

Dosage Forms

Cream, topical:

Exelderm®: 1% (15 g, 30 g, 60 g)

Solution, topical:

Exelderm®: 1% (30 mL)

sulconazole nitrate *see* sulconazole *on page 858*

Sulcrate® (Can) *see* sucralfate *on page 856*

Sulcrate® Suspension Plus (Can) *see* sucralfate *on page 856*

sulfabenzamide, sulfacetamide, and sulfathiazole

(sul fa BENZ a mide, sul fa SEE ta mide, & sul fa THYE a zole)

Synonyms triple sulfa

U.S. Brand Names V.V.S.®

Therapeutic Category Antibiotic, Vaginal

Use Treatment of *Haemophilus vaginalis* vaginitis

General Dosage Range Intravaginal: *Adults:* Insert 1/4 to 1 applicatorful twice daily

Dosage Forms

Cream, vaginal: Sulfabenzamide 3.7%, sulfacetamide 2.86%, and sulfathiazole 3.42% (78 g with applicator)

V.V.S.®: Sulfabenzamide 3.7%, sulfacetamide 2.86%, and sulfathiazole 3.42% (78 g with applicator)

sulfacetamide (ophthalmic) (sul fa SEE ta mide)

Medication Safety Issues

Sound-alike/look-alike issues:

Bleph®-10 may be confused with Blephamide®

Synonyms sodium sulfacetamide; sulamyd; sulfacetamide sodium

U.S. Brand Names Bleph®-10; Sulfamide

Canadian Brand Names AK Sulf Liq; Bleph 10 DPS; Diosulf™; PMS-Sulfacetamide; Sodium Sulamyd

Therapeutic Category Antibiotic, Ophthalmic

Use Treatment and prophylaxis of conjunctivitis and other superficial ocular infections due to susceptible organisms; adjunctive treatment with systemic sulfonamides for therapy of trachoma

General Dosage Range Ophthalmic: *Children >2 months and Adults:* Solution: Instill 1-2 drops up to every 2-3 hours and at bedtime; Ointment: Instill 1/2" (1.25 cm) ribbon every 3-4 hours and at bedtime

Dosage Forms

Ointment, ophthalmic: 10% (3.5 g)

Solution, ophthalmic: 10% (15 mL)

Bleph®-10: 10% (5 mL)

Sulfamide: 10% (15 mL)

sulfacetamide (topical) (sul fa SEE ta mide)

Medication Safety Issues

Sound-alike/look-alike issues:

Klaron® may be confused with Klor-Con®

Synonyms sodium sulfacetamide; sulamyd; sulfacetamide sodium

U.S. Brand Names Klaron®; Ovace®; Ovace® Plus; Seb-Prev™ [DSC]

Canadian Brand Names Sulfacet-R

Therapeutic Category Acne Products; Antibiotic, Sulfonamide Derivative; Topical Skin Product, Acne

Use

Cleansing gel, wash: Scaling dermatoses (seborrheic dermatitis and seborrhea sicca [dandruff]); bacterial infections of the skin

Lotion: Acne vulgaris

Shampoo: Scaling dermatoses (seborrheic dermatitis and seborrhea sicca [dandruff])

General Dosage Range Topical: *Children ≥12 years and Adults:* Lotion/cleansing gel/wash: Apply to affected areas 1-2 times/day; Shampoo: Wash hair at least twice weekly

Dosage Forms

Cream, topical:

Ovace® Plus: 10% (57 g)

Gel, topical:

Ovace® Plus: 10% (355 mL)

Lotion, topical: 10% (118 mL, 177 mL, 354.8 mL)

Klaron®: 10% (118 mL)

Ovace®: 10% (355 mL)

Pad, topical: 10% (30s)

Shampoo, topical:

Ovace® Plus: 10% (237 mL)

Suspension, topical: 10% (118 mL)

sulfacetamide and prednisolone (sul fa SEE ta mide & pred NIS oh lone)

Medication Safety Issues

Sound-alike/look-alike issues:

Blephamide® may be confused with Bleph®-10

Synonyms prednisolone and sulfacetamide

U.S. Brand Names Blephamide®

Canadian Brand Names AK Cide Oph; Blephamide®; Dioptimyd®

Therapeutic Category Antibiotic/Corticosteroid, Ophthalmic

Use Steroid-responsive inflammatory ocular conditions in which a corticosteroid is indicated and where infection is present or there is a risk of infection

General Dosage Range Ophthalmic: *Children ≥6 years and Adults:*

Ointment: Apply ~1/2" ribbon 3-4 times/day and 1-2 times at night

Solution, suspension: Instill 2 drops every 4 hours

Dosage Forms

Ointment, ophthalmic:

Blephamide®: Sulfacetamide 10% and prednisolone 0.2% (3.5 g)

Solution, ophthalmic: Sulfacetamide 10% and prednisolone 0.25% (5 mL, 10 mL)

Suspension, ophthalmic:

Blephamide®: Sulfacetamide 10% and prednisolone 0.2% (5 mL, 10 mL)

sulfacetamide and sulfur *see* sulfur and sulfacetamide *on page 862*

sulfacetamide sodium *see* sulfacetamide (ophthalmic) *on page 858*

sulfacetamide sodium *see* sulfacetamide (topical) *on page 858*

Sulfacet-R (Can) *see* sulfacetamide (topical) *on page 858*

Sulfacet-R® (Can) *see* sulfur and sulfacetamide *on page 862*

SulfaCleanse™ 8/4 *see* sulfur and sulfacetamide *on page 862*

sulfadiazine (sul fa DYE a zeen)

Medication Safety Issues

Sound-alike/look-alike issues:

SulfADIAZINE may be confused with sulfaSALAzine, sulfiSOXAZOLE

Tall-Man sulf**ADIAZINE**

Therapeutic Category Sulfonamide

Use Treatment of the following conditions (per product labeling): Chancroid, trachoma, inclusion conjunctivitis, nocardiosis, urinary tract infections, toxoplasmosis encephalitis, malaria, meningococcal meningitis, acute otitis media, rheumatic fever (prophylaxis), meningitis (adjunctive)

Refer to current guidelines for appropriate use.

General Dosage Range Oral:
Children >2 months: Initial: 75 mg/kg; Maintenance: 150 mg/kg/day (maximum: 6 g/24 hours)
Children <30 kg and Adults <30 kg: 0.5 g/day (rheumatic fever prophylaxis)
Children ≥30 kg and Adults ≥30 kg: 1 g/day (rheumatic fever prophylaxis)
Adults: 2-4 g/day in divided doses

Dosage Forms
Tablet, oral: 500 mg

sulfadoxine and pyrimethamine (sul fa DOKS een & peer i METH a meen)

Synonyms pyrimethamine and sulfadoxine

U.S. Brand Names Fansidar® [DSC]

Therapeutic Category Antimalarial Agent

Use Treatment of *Plasmodium falciparum* malaria in patients in whom chloroquine resistance is suspected; malaria prophylaxis for travelers to areas where chloroquine-resistant malaria is endemic

General Dosage Range Oral:
Children 2-11 months: 1/4 tablet as a single dose
Children 1-3 years: 1/2 tablet as a single dose
Children 4-8 years: 1 tablet as a single dose
Children 9-14 years: 2 tablets as a single dose
Children >14 years and Adults: 3 tablets as a single dose

sulfamethoxazole and trimethoprim (sul fa meth OKS a zole & trye METH oh prim)

Medication Safety Issues
Sound-alike/look-alike issues:
Bactrim™ may be confused with bacitracin, Bactine®, Bactroban®
Co-trimoxazole may be confused with clotrimazole
Septra® may be confused with Ceptaz, Sectral®
Septra® DS may be confused with Semprex®-D

Synonyms co-trimoxazole; Septra; SMX-TMP; SMZ-TMP; Sulfatrim; TMP-SMX; TMP-SMZ; trimethoprim and sulfamethoxazole

U.S. Brand Names Bactrim™; Bactrim™ DS; Septra® DS

Canadian Brand Names Apo-Sulfatrim®; Apo-Sulfatrim® DS; Apo-Sulfatrim® Pediatric; Novo-Trimel; Novo-Trimel D.S.; Nu-Cotrimox; Septra® Injection

Therapeutic Category Sulfonamide

Use
Oral treatment of urinary tract infections due to *E. coli*, *Klebsiella* and *Enterobacter* sp, *M. morganii*, *P. mirabilis* and *P. vulgaris*; acute otitis media in children; acute exacerbations of chronic bronchitis in adults due to susceptible strains of *H. influenzae* or *S. pneumoniae*; treatment and prophylaxis of *Pneumocystis jirovecii* pneumonia (PCP); traveler's diarrhea due to enterotoxigenic *E. coli*; treatment of enteritis caused by *Shigella flexneri* or *Shigella sonnei*
I.V. treatment of severe or complicated infections when oral therapy is not feasible, for documented PCP, empiric treatment of PCP in immune compromised patients; treatment of documented or suspected shigellosis, typhoid fever, or other infections caused by susceptible bacteria

General Dosage Range Dosage adjustment recommended in patients with renal impairment
I.V.: *Children >2 months and Adults:* 8-20 mg TMP/kg/day divided every 6-12 hours
Oral:
Children >2 months: 6-20 mg TMP/kg/day divided every 6-12 hours **or** 150 mg TMP/m^2/day in divided doses every 12-24 hours for 3-7 days/week (maximum: sulfamethoxazole 1600 mg/day; trimethoprim 320 mg/day)
Adults: 1 or 2 double-strength tablets (sulfamethoxazole 800-1600 mg; trimethoprim 160-320 mg) every 12-24 hours **or** 15-20 mg TMP/kg/day in 3-4 divided doses

Dosage Forms The 5:1 ratio (SMX:TMP) remains constant in all dosage forms.
Injection, solution: Sulfamethoxazole 80 mg and trimethoprim 16 mg per mL (5 mL, 10 mL, 30 mL)
Suspension, oral: Sulfamethoxazole 200 mg and trimethoprim 40 mg per 5 mL
Tablet: Sulfamethoxazole 400 mg and trimethoprim 80 mg
Bactrim™: Sulfamethoxazole 400 mg and trimethoprim 80 mg
Tablet, double-strength: Sulfamethoxazole 800 mg and trimethoprim 160 mg
Bactrim™ DS, Septra® DS: Sulfamethoxazole 800 mg and trimethoprim 160 mg

Sulfamide *see* sulfacetamide (ophthalmic) *on page 858*

Sulfamylon® *see* mafenide *on page* 556

sulfanilamide (sul fa NIL a mide)

Synonyms p-amino-benzenesulfonamide

U.S. Brand Names AVC™

Therapeutic Category Antifungal Agent, Vaginal

Use Treatment of vulvovaginitis caused by *Candida albicans*

General Dosage Range Intravaginal: *Adults:* 1 applicatorful once or twice daily

Dosage Forms

Cream, vaginal:

AVC™: 15% (120 g)

sulfasalazine (sul fa SAL a zeen)

Medication Safety Issues

Sound-alike/look-alike issues:

SulfaSALAzine may be confused with salsalate, sulfADIAZINE, sulfiSOXAZOLE

Azulfidine® may be confused with Augmentin®, azaTHIOprine

Synonyms salicylazosulfapyridine

Tall-Man sulfa**SALA**zine

U.S. Brand Names Azulfidine EN-tabs®; Azulfidine®; Sulfazine; Sulfazine EC

Canadian Brand Names Alti-Sulfasalazine; Salazopyrin En-Tabs®; Salazopyrin®

Therapeutic Category 5-Aminosalicylic Acid Derivative

Use Treatment of mild-to-moderate ulcerative colitis or as adjunctive therapy in severe ulcerative colitis; enteric coated tablets are also used for rheumatoid arthritis (including juvenile idiopathic arthritis [JIA]) in patients who inadequately respond to analgesics and NSAIDs

General Dosage Range Oral:

Delayed release:

Children ≥6 years: Initial: 1/4 to 1/3 of expected maintenance dose; Maintenance: 30-50 mg/kg/day in 2 divided doses (maximum: 2 g/day)

Adults: Initial: 0.5-1 g/day; Maintenance: 2 g/day in 2 divided doses (maximum: 3 g/day)

Immediate release:

Children ≥6 years: Initial: 40-60 mg/kg/day in 3-6 divided doses; Maintenance: 30 mg/kg/day in 4 divided doses

Adults: Initial: 3-4 g/day in evenly divided doses at ≤8-hour intervals; Maintenance: 2 g/day in divided doses at ≤8-hour intervals

Dosage Forms

Tablet, oral: 500 mg

Azulfidine®: 500 mg

Sulfazine: 500 mg

Tablet, delayed release, enteric coated, oral: 500 mg

Azulfidine EN-tabs®: 500 mg

Sulfazine EC: 500 mg

Sulfatrim *see* sulfamethoxazole and trimethoprim *on page* 860

Sulfazine *see* sulfasalazine *on page* 861

Sulfazine EC *see* sulfasalazine *on page* 861

sulfisoxazole and erythromycin *see* erythromycin and sulfisoxazole *on page* 344

sulfur and salicylic acid (SUL fyoor & sal i SIL ik AS id)

Synonyms salicylic acid and sulfur

U.S. Brand Names ala seb [OTC]; Pernox® Lemon [OTC]; Pernox® Regular [OTC]; Sebex [OTC]; Sebulex® [OTC]

Therapeutic Category Antiseborrheic Agent, Topical

Use Therapeutic shampoo for dandruff and seborrheic dermatitis; acne skin cleanser

Dosage Forms

Cleanser, topical [scrub]:

Pernox® Lemon: Sulfur 2% and salicylic acid 1.5% (56 g, 113 g)

Pernox® Regular: Sulfur 2% and salicylic acid 1.5% (113 g)

Shampoo, topical:
ala seb: Sulfur 2% and salicylic acid 2% (118 mL, 355 mL)
Sebex: Sulfur 2% and salicylic acid 2% (118 mL)
Sebulex®: Sulfur 2% and salicylic acid 2% (200 g)

sulfur and sulfacetamide (SUL fur & sul fa SEE ta mide)

Synonyms sodium sulfacetamide and sulfur; sulfacetamide and sulfur; sulfur and sulfacetamide sodium

U.S. Brand Names AVAR™; AVAR™ LS; AVAR™-e; AVAR™-e Green; AVAR™-e LS; BP 10-1; BP Cleansing Wash; Clarifoam™ EF; Claris™; Clenia®; Plexion SCT® [DSC]; Plexion® [DSC]; Prascion®; Prascion® FC; Prascion® RA; Rosanil®; SSS 10-4; SulfaCleanse™ 8/4; Sumadan™; Sumaxin®; Sumaxin® TS; Zencia™

Canadian Brand Names Sulfacet-R®

Therapeutic Category Antiseborrheic Agent, Topical

Use Aid in the treatment of acne vulgaris, acne rosacea, and seborrheic dermatitis

General Dosage Range **Topical:** *Children ≥12 years and Adults:* Apply a thin film 1-3 times/day

Dosage Forms

Aerosol, foam, topical: Sulfur 5% and sulfacetamide 10% (60 g)
Clarifoam™ EF: Sulfur 5% and sulfacetamide 10% (60 g, 100 g)
SSS 10-4: Sulfur 4% and sulfacetamide 10% (100 g)

Cleanser, topical: Sulfur 5% and sulfacetamide 10% (170 g, 340 g)
AVAR™: Sulfur 5% and sulfacetamide 10% (227 g)
AVAR™ LS: Sulfur 2% and sulfacetamide 10% (227 g)
Plexion®, Prascion®: Sulfur 5% and sulfacetamide 10% (170 g, 340 g)
Rosanil®: Sulfur 5% and sulfacetamide 10% (170 g)

Cream, topical:
AVAR™-e, AVAR™-e Green, Prascion® RA: Sulfur 5% and sulfacetamide 10% (45 g)
AVAR™-e LS: Sulfur 2% and sulfacetamide 10% (45 g)
Clenia®: Sulfur 5% and sulfacetamide 10% (28 g)

Gel, topical: Sulfur 5% and sulfacetamide 10% (45 g)

Pad, topical [cleansing cloth]: Sulfur 4% and sulfacetamide 10% (60s)
Plexion®, Prascion® FC: Sulfur 5% and sulfacetamide 10% (30s, 60s)
Sumaxin®: Sulfur 4% and sulfacetamide 10% (60s)

Suspension, topical: Sulfur 4% and sulfacetamide 8% (473 mL)
SulfaCleanse™ 8/4: Sulfur 4% and sulfacetamide 8% (473 mL)
Sumaxin® TS: Sulfur 4% and sulfacetamide 8% (473 mL)

Wash, topical: Sulfur 4% and sulfacetamide 9% (480 mL); Sulfur 4.5% and sulfacetamide 9% (454 g)
BP 10-1: Sulfur 1% and sulfacetamide 10% (170 g)
Sumaxin®: Sulfur 4% and sulfacetamide 9% (473 mL)
Zencia™: Sulfur 4% and sulfacetamide 9% (480 mL)

Wash, topical [emulsion-based]:
BP Cleansing Wash: Sulfur 4% and sulfacetamide 10% (473 mL)
Claris™: Sulfur 4% and sulfacetamide 10% (473 mL)
Sumadan™: Sulfur 4.5% and sulfacetamide 9% (454 g)

sulfur and sulfacetamide sodium *see* sulfur and sulfacetamide *on page 862*

sulindac (SUL in dak)

Medication Safety Issues

Sound-alike/look-alike issues:
Clinoril® may be confused with Cleocin®, Clozaril®

BEERS Criteria medication:
This drug may be potentially inappropriate for use in geriatric patients (Quality of evidence - moderate; Strength of recommendation - strong).

U.S. Brand Names Clinoril®

Canadian Brand Names Apo-Sulin®; Novo-Sundac; Nu-Sulindac; Nu-Sundac; Teva-Sulindac

Therapeutic Category Analgesic, Nonnarcotic; Nonsteroidal Antiinflammatory Drug (NSAID)

Use Management of inflammatory diseases including osteoarthritis, rheumatoid arthritis, acute gouty arthritis, ankylosing spondylitis, acute painful shoulder (bursitis/tendonitis)

General Dosage Range Dosage adjustment recommended in patients with hepatic impairment

Oral: *Adults:* 150-200 mg twice daily (maximum: 400 mg/day)

Dosage Forms

Tablet, oral: 150 mg, 200 mg

Clinoril®: 200 mg

Sumadan™ *see* sulfur and sulfacetamide *on page 862*

sumatriptan (soo ma TRIP tan)

Medication Safety Issues

Sound-alike/look-alike issues:

SUMAtriptan may be confused with saxagliptin, sitaGLIPtin, somatropin, ZOLMitriptan

Synonyms sumatriptan succinate

Tall-Man SUMAtriptan

U.S. Brand Names Alsuma™; Imitrex®; Sumavel® DosePro®

Canadian Brand Names Apo-Sumatriptan®; Ava-Sumatriptan; CO Sumatriptan; Dom-Sumatriptan; Imitrex®; Imitrex® DF; Imitrex® Injection; Imitrex® Nasal Spray; Mylan-Sumatriptan; PHL-Sumatriptan; PMS-Sumatriptan; Riva-Sumatriptan; Sandoz-Sumatriptan; Sumatriptan Injection; Sumatriptan Sun Injection; Sumatryx; Teva-Sumatriptan; Teva-Sumatriptan DF

Therapeutic Category Antimigraine Agent

Use

Intranasal, Oral, SubQ: Acute treatment of migraine with or without aura

SubQ: Acute treatment of cluster headache episodes

General Dosage Range Dosage adjustment recommended for oral route in patients with hepatic impairment

Intranasal: *Adults:* 5-20 mg in one nostril as a single dose (may divide dose into both nostrils); may repeat after 2 hours (maximum: 40 mg/day)

Oral: *Adults:* 25-100 mg as a single dose; may repeat after 2 hours (maximum: 200 mg/day)

SubQ: *Adults:* Initial: Up to 6 mg; may repeat if needed ≥1 hour after initial dose (maximum: Two 6 mg injections per 24-hour period)

Dosage Forms

Injection, solution: 4 mg/0.5 mL (0.5 mL); 6 mg/0.5 mL (0.5 mL)

Alsuma™: 6 mg/0.5 mL (0.5 mL)

Imitrex®: 4 mg/0.5 mL (0.5 mL); 6 mg/0.5 mL (0.5 mL)

Sumavel® DosePro®: 6 mg/0.5 mL (0.5 mL)

Injection, solution [preservative free]: 6 mg/0.5 mL (0.5 mL)

Solution, intranasal: 5 mg/0.1 mL (6s); 20 mg/0.1 mL (6s)

Imitrex®: 5 mg/0.1 mL (6s); 20 mg/0.1 mL (6s)

Tablet, oral: 25 mg, 50 mg, 100 mg

Imitrex®: 25 mg, 50 mg, 100 mg

sumatriptan and naproxen (soo ma TRIP tan & na PROKS en)

Medication Safety Issues

Sound-alike/look-alike issues:

Naproxen may be confused with Natacyn®, Nebcin, neomycin, niacin

SUMAtriptan may be confused with somatropin, ZOLMitriptan

Treximet® may be confused with Trexall™

Synonyms naproxen and sumatriptan; naproxen sodium and sumatriptan; naproxen sodium and sumatriptan succinate; sumatriptan succinate and naproxen; sumatriptan succinate and naproxen sodium

U.S. Brand Names Treximet®

Therapeutic Category Antimigraine Agent; Nonsteroidal Antiinflammatory Drug (NSAID); Serotonin 5-$HT_{1B, 1D}$ Receptor Agonist

Use Acute treatment of migraine with or without aura

General Dosage Range Oral: *Adults:* 1 tablet (sumatriptan 85 mg and naproxen 500 mg); may repeat in 2 hours if needed (maximum: 2 tablets/24 hours)

Dosage Forms

Tablet, oral:

Treximet® 85/500: Sumatriptan 85 mg and naproxen sodium 500 mg

Sumatriptan Injection (Can) *see* sumatriptan *on page 863*

sumatriptan succinate *see* sumatriptan *on page 863*

sumatriptan succinate and naproxen *see* sumatriptan and naproxen *on page 863*
sumatriptan succinate and naproxen sodium *see* sumatriptan and naproxen *on page 863*
Sumatriptan Sun Injection (Can) *see* sumatriptan *on page 863*
Sumatryx (Can) *see* sumatriptan *on page 863*
Sumavel® DosePro® *see* sumatriptan *on page 863*
Sumaxin® *see* sulfur and sulfacetamide *on page 862*
Sumaxin® TS *see* sulfur and sulfacetamide *on page 862*
Summer's Eve® Anti-Itch Maximum Strength [OTC] *see* pramoxine *on page 750*
Summer's Eve® Medicated Douche [OTC] *see* povidone-iodine (topical) *on page 747*

sunitinib (su NIT e nib)

Medication Safety Issues

Sound-alike/look-alike issues:

SUNItinib may be confused with axitinib, dasatinib, erlotinib, gefitinib, imatinib, lapatinib, nilotinib, pazopanib, SORAfenib, vandetanib

High alert medication:

This medication is in a class the Institute for Safe Medication Practices (ISMP) includes among its list of drug classes which have a heightened risk of causing significant patient harm when used in error.

Administration issues:

Dosing schedules vary by indication; some treatment regimens are continuous daily dosing; other treatment schedules are daily dosing for 4 weeks of a 6 week cycle (4 weeks on, 2 weeks off)

Synonyms SU011248; SU11248; sunitinib malate

Tall-Man **SUNI**tinib

U.S. Brand Names Sutent®

Canadian Brand Names Sutent®

Therapeutic Category Antineoplastic Agent, Tyrosine Kinase Inhibitor; Vascular Endothelial Growth Factor (VEGF) Inhibitor

Use Treatment of gastrointestinal stromal tumor (GIST) intolerant to or with disease progression on imatinib; treatment of advanced renal cell cancer (RCC); treatment of advanced, metastatic or unresectable pancreatic neuroendocrine tumors (PNET)

General Dosage Range Dosage adjustment recommended in patients with renal impairment, on concomitant therapy, or who develop toxicities

Oral: *Adults:* 50 mg once daily for 4 weeks of a 6-week treatment cycle **or** 37.5 mg once daily, continuous daily dosing

Dosage Forms

Capsule, oral:

Sutent®: 12.5 mg, 25 mg, 50 mg

sunitinib malate *see* sunitinib *on page 864*
Supartz® *see* hyaluronate and derivatives *on page 450*
Super Calcium 600 [OTC] *see* calcium carbonate *on page 161*
Superdophilus® [OTC] *see* Lactobacillus *on page 518*
Supeudol® (Can) *see* oxycodone *on page 678*
Suplasyn® (Can) *see* hyaluronate and derivatives *on page 450*
Suprane® *see* desflurane *on page 262*
Suprefact® (Can) *see* buserelin *(Canada only) on page 151*
Suprefact® Depot (Can) *see* buserelin *(Canada only) on page 151*
Suprenza™ *see* phentermine *on page 714*
Suprep® Bowel Prep Kit *see* sodium sulfate, potassium sulfate, and magnesium sulfate *on page 847*
Surfaxin® *see* lucinactant *on page 555*
Surgicel® *see* cellulose, oxidized regenerated *on page 188*
Surgicel® Fibrillar *see* cellulose, oxidized regenerated *on page 188*
Surgicel® NuKnit *see* cellulose, oxidized regenerated *on page 188*
Surmontil® *see* trimipramine *on page 921*
Survanta® *see* beractant *on page 128*
Sustiva® *see* efavirenz *on page 324*
Sutent® *see* sunitinib *on page 864*

tacrolimus (systemic) (ta KROE li mus)

Medication Safety Issues

Sound-alike/look-alike issues:

Prograf® may be confused with Gengraf®, PROzac®

Tacrolimus may be confused with everolimus, pimecrolimus, sirolimus, temsirolimus

Synonyms FK506

U.S. Brand Names Hecoria™; Prograf®

Canadian Brand Names Advagraf®; Prograf®

Therapeutic Category Calcineurin Inhibitor; Immunosuppressant Agent

Use

U.S. labeling: Prevention of organ rejection in heart (Prograf® only), and kidney or liver (Hecoria™, Prograf®) transplant recipients

Canadian labeling:

Prograf®: Prevention of organ rejection in heart, kidney, or liver transplant recipients; treatment of refractory rejection in kidney or liver transplant recipients; treatment of active rheumatoid arthritis in adult patients nonresponsive to disease-modifying antirheumatic drug (DMARD) therapy or when DMARD therapy is inappropriate

Advagraf®: Prevention of organ rejection in kidney transplant recipients

General Dosage Range

I.V.:

Children: 0.03-0.05 mg/kg/day as a continuous infusion

Adults: 0.01-0.05 mg/kg/day as a continuous infusion

Oral:

Children: 0.15-0.2 mg/kg/day in divided doses every 12 hours

Adults: 0.075-0.2 mg/kg/day in divided doses every 12 hours

Dosage Forms

Capsule, oral: 0.5 mg, 1 mg, 5 mg

Hecoria™: 0.5 mg, 1 mg, 5 mg

Prograf®: 0.5 mg, 1 mg, 5 mg

Injection, solution:

Prograf®: 5 mg/mL (1 mL)

Dosage Forms - Canada

Capsule, oral:

Advagraf®: 0.5 mg, 1 mg, 3 mg, 5 mg

tacrolimus (topical) (ta KROE li mus)

Medication Safety Issues

Sound-alike/look-alike issues:

Tacrolimus may be confused with everolimus, pimecrolimus, sirolimus, temsirolimus

U.S. Brand Names Protopic®

Canadian Brand Names Protopic®

Therapeutic Category Calcineurin Inhibitor; Topical Skin Product

Use Moderate-to-severe atopic dermatitis in immunocompetent patients not responsive to conventional therapy or when conventional therapy is not appropriate

Canadian labeling: Additional use (not in U.S. labeling): Maintenance therapy to prevent flares and extend flare-free intervals in patients with moderate-to-severe atopic dermatitis who are responsive to initial therapy and experiencing ≥5 flares per year

General Dosage Range Topical:

Children ≥2-15 years: Apply thin layer of 0.03% to affected area twice daily

Children >15 years and Adults: Apply thin layer of 0.03% or 0.1% to affected area twice daily

Dosage Forms

Ointment, topical:

Protopic®: 0.03% (30 g, 60 g, 100 g); 0.1% (30 g, 60 g, 100 g)

Tactuo™ (Can) *see* adapalene and benzoyl peroxide *on page* 36

tadalafil (tah DA la fil)

Medication Safety Issues

Sound-alike/look-alike issues:

Tadalafil may be confused with sildenafil, vardenafil

Adcirca® may be confused with Advair® Diskus®, Advair® HFA, Advicor®

Synonyms GF196960

U.S. Brand Names Adcirca®; Cialis®

Canadian Brand Names Adcirca®; Cialis®

Therapeutic Category Phosphodiesterase (Type 5) Enzyme Inhibitor

Use

Adcirca®: Treatment of pulmonary arterial hypertension (PAH) (WHO Group I) to improve exercise ability

Cialis®: Treatment of erectile dysfunction (ED); treatment of signs and symptoms of benign prostatic hyperplasia (BPH)

General Dosage Range Dosage adjustment recommended in patient with hepatic or renal impairment or on concomitant therapy

Oral: *Adults:* Benign prostatic hyperplasia: 5 mg once daily; Erectile dysfunction: As-needed dosing: 5-20 mg prior to anticipated sexual activity as a single dose (maximum: 1 dose/day); Once-daily dosing: 2.5-5 mg once daily; Pulmonary arterial hypertension: 40 mg once daily

Dosage Forms

Tablet, oral:

Adcirca®: 20 mg

Cialis®: 2.5 mg, 5 mg, 10 mg, 20 mg

tafluprost (TA floo prost)

U.S. Brand Names Zioptan™

Therapeutic Category Ophthalmic Agent, Antiglaucoma; Prostaglandin, Ophthalmic

Use Reduction of intraocular pressure (IOP) in patients with open-angle glaucoma or ocular hypertension

General Dosage Range **Ophthalmic:** *Adults:* One drop in the affected eye(s) once daily

Dosage Forms

Solution, ophthalmic [preservative free]:

Zioptan™: 0.0015% (30s)

Tagamet HB 200® [OTC] *see* cimetidine *on page 209*

Tagitol™ V *see* barium *on page 114*

TAK-375 *see* ramelteon *on page 786*

TAK-390MR *see* dexlansoprazole *on page 268*

TAK-599 *see* ceftaroline fosamil *on page 185*

Talacen *see* pentazocine and acetaminophen *on page 705*

talc *see* talc (sterile) *on page 867*

talc for pleurodesis *see* talc (sterile) *on page 867*

talc (sterile) (talk STARE il)

Synonyms intrapleural talc; sterile talc; talc; talc for pleurodesis

U.S. Brand Names Sclerosol®; Sterile Talc Powder™

Therapeutic Category Sclerosing Agent

Use Prevention of recurrence of malignant pleural effusion in symptomatic patients

General Dosage Range **Intrapleural:** *Adults:* Aerosol: 4-8 g (1-2 cans) as a single dose; Instillation: 5 g

Dosage Forms

Aerosol, powder, intrapleural:

Sclerosol®: 4 g (4 g)

Powder, intrapleural:

Sterile Talc Powder™: USP: 100% (5 g)

taliglucerase alfa (tal i GLOO ser ase AL fa)

U.S. Brand Names Elelyso™

Therapeutic Category Enzyme

Use Long-term enzyme replacement therapy for patients with type 1 Gaucher disease

General Dosage Range **I.V.:** *Adults:* Initial: 60 units/kg every 2 weeks; range: 11-73 units/kg every 2 weeks

Dosage Forms

Injection, powder for reconstitution:

Elelyso™: 200 units

Talwin® *see* pentazocine *on page 705*

Talwin NX *see* pentazocine and naloxone *on page 705*

Tambocor™ *see* flecainide *on page 386*

Tamiflu® *see* oseltamivir *on page 673*

tamoxifen (ta MOKS i fen)

Medication Safety Issues

Sound-alike/look-alike issues:

Tamoxifen may be confused with pentoxifylline, Tambocor™, tamsulosin, temazepam

Synonyms ICI-46474; Nolvadex; tamoxifen citras; tamoxifen citrate

Canadian Brand Names Apo-Tamox®; Mylan-Tamoxifen; Nolvadex®-D; PMS-Tamoxifen; Teva-Tamoxifen

Therapeutic Category Antineoplastic Agent

Use Treatment of metastatic (female and male) breast cancer; adjuvant treatment of breast cancer after primary treatment with surgery and radiation; reduce risk of invasive breast cancer in women with ductal carcinoma *in situ* (DCIS) after surgery and radiation; reduce the incidence of breast cancer in women at high risk

General Dosage Range Oral: *Adults:* 20-40 mg/day

Dosage Forms

Tablet, oral: 10 mg, 20 mg

tamoxifen citras *see* tamoxifen *on page 868*

tamoxifen citrate *see* tamoxifen *on page 868*

tamsulosin (tam SOO loe sin)

Medication Safety Issues

Sound-alike/look-alike issues:

Flomax® may be confused with Flonase®, Flovent®, Foltx®, Fosamax®

Tamsulosin may be confused with tacrolimus, tamoxifen, terazosin

International issues:

Flomax [U.S., Canada, and multiple international markets] may be confused with Flomox brand name for cefcapene [Japan]; Volmax brand name for salbutamol [multiple international markets]

Flomax: Brand name for tamsulosin [U.S., Canada, and multiple international markets], but also the brand name for morniflumate [Italy]

Synonyms tamsulosin hydrochloride

U.S. Brand Names Flomax®

Canadian Brand Names Ava-Tamsulosin CR; Flomax® CR; JAMP-Tamsulosin; Mylan-Tamsulosin; RAN™-Tamsulosin; ratio-Tamsulosin; Sandoz-Tamsulosin; Sandoz-Tamsulosin CR; Teva-Tamsulosin

Therapeutic Category Alpha-Adrenergic Blocking Agent

Use Treatment of signs and symptoms of benign prostatic hyperplasia (BPH)

General Dosage Range Oral: *Adults:* Initial: 0.4 mg once daily; Maintenance: 0.4-0.8 mg once daily

Dosage Forms

Capsule, oral: 0.4 mg

Flomax®: 0.4 mg

tamsulosin and dutasteride *see* dutasteride and tamsulosin *on page 320*

tamsulosin hydrochloride *see* tamsulosin *on page 868*

tamsulosin hydrochloride and dutasteride *see* dutasteride and tamsulosin *on page 320*

Tanac® [OTC] *see* benzocaine *on page 121*

Tandem® DHA *see* vitamins (multiple/prenatal) *on page 952*

Tandem® OB *see* vitamins (multiple/prenatal) *on page 952*

Tanta-Orciprenaline® (Can) *see* metaproterenol *on page 579*

Tantum® (Can) *see* benzydamine *(Canada only) on page 126*

TAP-144 *see* leuprolide *on page 527*

Tapazole® *see* methimazole *on page 583*

tapentadol (ta PEN ta dol)

Medication Safety Issues

Sound-alike/look-alike issues:

Tapentadol may be confused with traMADol

High alert medication:

The Institute for Safe Medication Practices (ISMP) includes this medication among its list of drug classes which have a heightened risk of causing significant patient harm when used in error.

Synonyms CG5503; tapentadol hydrochloride
U.S. Brand Names Nucynta®; Nucynta® ER
Canadian Brand Names Nucynta® IR; Nucynta™ CR
Therapeutic Category Analgesic, Opioid
Controlled Substance C-II
Use
Immediate release formulation: Relief of moderate-to-severe acute pain
Long acting formulation: Relief of moderate-to-severe chronic pain or neuropathic pain associated with diabetic peripheral neuropathy (DPN) when continuous, around-the-clock analgesia is necessary for an extended period of time
General Dosage Range Dosage adjustment recommended in patients with hepatic impairment
Oral:
Immediate release: *Adults:* 50-100 mg every 4-6 hours as needed (maximum: 700 mg/day on day 1; 600 mg/day subsequent days)
Extended release: *Adults:* 50-250 mg twice daily (maximum: 500 mg/day)
Dosage Forms
Tablet, oral:
Nucynta®: 50 mg, 75 mg, 100 mg
Tablet, extended release, oral:
Nucynta® ER: 50 mg, 100 mg, 150 mg, 200 mg, 250 mg
Dosage Forms - Canada
Tablet, controlled release, oral:
Nucynta™ CR: 50 mg, 100 mg, 150 mg, 200 mg, 250 mg

tapentadol hydrochloride *see* tapentadol *on page 868*
Tarceva® *see* erlotinib *on page 341*
Targel® [OTC] (Can) *see* coal tar *on page 228*
Targretin® *see* bexarotene (systemic) *on page 132*
Targretin® *see* bexarotene (topical) *on page 132*
Tarka® *see* trandolapril and verapamil *on page 910*
Taro-Amcinonide (Can) *see* amcinonide *on page 59*
Taro-Carbamazepine Chewable (Can) *see* carbamazepine *on page 172*
Taro-Ciclopirox (Can) *see* ciclopirox *on page 207*
Taro-Ciprofloxacin (Can) *see* ciprofloxacin (systemic) *on page 210*
Taro-Clindamycin (Can) *see* clindamycin (topical) *on page 219*
Taro-Clobetasol (Can) *see* clobetasol *on page 221*
Taro-Enalapril (Can) *see* enalapril *on page 330*
Taro-Fluconazole (Can) *see* fluconazole *on page 388*
Taro-Mometasone (Can) *see* mometasone (topical) *on page 610*
Taro-Phenytoin (Can) *see* phenytoin *on page 719*
Taro-Simvastatin (Can) *see* simvastatin *on page 835*
Taro-Sone (Can) *see* betamethasone *on page 129*
Taro-Warfarin (Can) *see* warfarin *on page 954*
Tarsum® [OTC] *see* coal tar and salicylic acid *on page 229*
Tasigna® *see* nilotinib *on page 642*
Tasmar® *see* tolcapone *on page 903*
Tavist® Allergy [OTC] *see* clemastine *on page 217*
Tavist ND *see* loratadine *on page 549*
Taxol *see* paclitaxel *on page 683*
Taxol® (Can) *see* paclitaxel *on page 683*
Taxotere® *see* docetaxel *on page 303*

tazarotene (taz AR oh teen)

U.S. Brand Names Avage®; Tazorac®
Canadian Brand Names Tazorac®
Therapeutic Category Keratolytic Agent

Use Topical treatment of facial acne vulgaris; topical treatment of stable plaque psoriasis; mitigation (palliation) of facial skin wrinkling, facial mottled hyper-/hypopigmentation, and benign facial lentigines

General Dosage Range **Topical:** *Children ≥12 years and Adults:* Apply a pea-sized amount or thin film **or** 2 mg/cm^2 once daily

Dosage Forms

Cream, topical:
Avage®: 0.1% (30 g)
Tazorac®: 0.05% (30 g, 60 g); 0.1% (30 g, 60 g)

Gel, topical:
Tazorac®: 0.05% (30 g, 100 g); 0.1% (30 g, 100 g)

technetium Tc 99m diethylene triamine penta-acetic acid

(tek NEE shee um tee see nyne tee nyne em dye ETH i leen TRYE a meen PEN ta a SEE tik AS id)

Medication Safety Issues

Other safety concerns:

Radiopharmaceutical: Use appropriate precaution for handling, disposal, and minimizing exposure to patients and healthcare personnel. Use under supervision of experienced personnel. Should be stored in original lead container or adequate radiation shield.

Synonyms 99m-technetium diethylenetriaminepentaacetic acid; ^{99m}Tc; ^{99m}Tc DTPA; ^{99m}Tc-pentetate; Tc-99m-DTPA; Tc-DTPA; technetium Tc 99m pentetate kit

U.S. Brand Names DRAXIMAGE® DTPA

Therapeutic Category Radiopharmaceutical

Use Kidney imaging; brain imaging; renal perfusion assessment; GFR estimation

technetium Tc 99m exametazime

(tek NEE shee um tee see nyne tee nyne em ex a MET a zeem)

Medication Safety Issues

Other safety concerns:

Radiopharmaceutical: Use appropriate precaution for handling, disposal, and minimizing exposure to patients and healthcare personnel. Use under supervision of experienced personnel. Should be stored in original lead container or adequate radiation shield.

Synonyms ^{99m}Tc-exametazime; ^{99m}Tc-HMPAO; Ceretec™; hexamethylpropylene amine oxime; technetium Tc 99m exametazime kit

Therapeutic Category Radiopharmaceutical

Use Evaluation of regional cerebral profusion in stroke patients (with or without methylene blue stabilization); leukocyte-labeled scintigraphy to locate intraabdominal infection and inflammatory bowel disease (without methylene blue stabilization)

technetium Tc 99m gluceptate (tek NEE shee um tee see nyne tee nyne em gloo SEP tate)

Medication Safety Issues

Other safety concerns:

Radiopharmaceutical: Use appropriate precaution for handling, disposal, and minimizing exposure to patients and healthcare personnel. Use under supervision of experienced personnel. Should be stored in original lead container or adequate radiation shield.

Synonyms ^{99m}Tc-GH; ^{99m}Tc-gluceptate; ^{99m}Tc-glucoheptonate; technetium Tc 99m gluceptate kit

U.S. Brand Names DRAXIMAGE® Gluceptate

Therapeutic Category Radiopharmaceutical

Use Evaluation of renal and brain perfusion

technetium Tc 99m-labeled red blood cells

(tek NEE shee um tee see nyne tee nyne em ley buhld red blud sels)

Medication Safety Issues

Other safety concerns:

Radiopharmaceutical: Use appropriate precaution for handling, disposal, and minimizing exposure to patients and healthcare personnel. Use under supervision of experienced personnel. Should be stored in original lead container or adequate radiation shield.

Synonyms ^{99m}Tc-labeled autologous RBCs; ^{99m}Tc-RBCs; technetium Tc 99m-labeled red blood cells kit

U.S. Brand Names UltraTag® RBC

Therapeutic Category Radiopharmaceutical

Use Blood pool imaging agent (including cardiac first pass and gated equilibrium imaging); detection of active lower GI bleeding; evaluation of suspected hemangiomas in liver; specific imaging of spleen to determine presence of functioning tissue

technetium Tc 99m mebrofenin

(tek NEE shee um tee see nyne tee nyne em me broe FEN in)

Medication Safety Issues

Other safety concerns:

Radiopharmaceutical: Use appropriate precaution for handling, disposal, and minimizing exposure to patients and healthcare personnel. Use under supervision of experienced personnel. Should be stored in original lead container or adequate radiation shield.

Synonyms ^{99m}Tc-BRIDA; ^{99m}Tc-bromo-trimethylacetanilido imino diacetic acid; ^{99m}Tc-mebrofenin; technetium Tc 99m mebrofenin kit

U.S. Brand Names Choletec®

Therapeutic Category Radiopharmaceutical

Use Hepatobiliary imaging agent for functional assessment of the hepatobiliary system; acute cholecystitis, chronic biliary tract disorders; common bile duct obstruction; bile extravasation; congenital abnormalities of the biliary tree

technetium Tc 99m medronate (tek NEE shee um tee see nyne tee nyne em ME droe nate)

Medication Safety Issues

Other safety concerns:

Radiopharmaceutical: Use appropriate precaution for handling, disposal, and minimizing exposure to patients and healthcare personnel. Use under supervision of experienced personnel. Should be stored in original lead container or adequate radiation shield.

Synonyms ^{99m}Tc-MDP; ^{99m}Tc-medronate; ^{99m}Tc-methylene diphosphonate; ^{99m}Tc-methylene diphosphonic acid; technetium Tc 99m medronate kit

U.S. Brand Names CIS-MDP™; DRAXIMAGE® MDP-25; MDP Multidose

Therapeutic Category Radiopharmaceutical

Use Skeletal imaging agent to detect areas of altered osteogenesis such as an occult fracture, osteomyelitis, stress fracture, avascular necrosis, bone infarcts, bone graft viability, or unexplained bone pain; identify metastatic bone lesions from breast, prostate, and other cancers

technetium Tc 99m oxidronate (tek NEE shee um tee see nyne tee nyne em ox ID roe nate)

Medication Safety Issues

Other safety concerns:

Radiopharmaceutical: Use appropriate precaution for handling, disposal, and minimizing exposure to patients and healthcare personnel. Use under supervision of experienced personnel. Should be stored in original lead container or adequate radiation shield.

Synonyms ^{99m}Tc-HDP; ^{99m}Tc-hydroxymethylene diphosphonate; ^{99m}Tc-oxidronate; technetium Tc 99m oxidronate kit

U.S. Brand Names Technescan™ HDP

Therapeutic Category Radiopharmaceutical

Use Skeletal imaging agent to detect areas of altered osteogenesis; occult fracture, osteomyelitis, neoplastic disease, stress fracture, avascular necrosis, bone infarcts, bone graft viability, unexplained bone pain

technetium Tc 99m pyrophosphate
(tek NEE shee um tee see nyne tee nyne em pye roe FOS fate)

Medication Safety Issues

Other safety concerns:

Radiopharmaceutical: Use appropriate precaution for handling, disposal, and minimizing exposure to patients and healthcare personnel. Use under supervision of experienced personnel. Should be stored in original lead container or adequate radiation shield.

Synonyms ^{99m}Tc-inorganic pyrophosphate; ^{99m}Tc-PPi; ^{99m}Tc-PYP; ^{99m}Tc-pyrophosphate; technetium Tc 99m pyrophosphate kit

U.S. Brand Names Technescan™ PYP™

Therapeutic Category Radiopharmaceutical

Use Skeletal imaging agent to detect areas of altered osteogenesis; cardiac imaging agent used as an adjunctive agent for the diagnosis of acute myocardial infarction; blood pool imaging agent; detection of GI bleeding sites

technetium Tc 99m succimer (tek NEE shee um tee see nyne tee nyne em SUKS si mer)

Medication Safety Issues

Other safety concerns:

Radiopharmaceutical: Use appropriate precaution for handling, disposal, and minimizing exposure to patients and healthcare personnel. Use under supervision of experienced personnel. Should be stored in original lead container or adequate radiation shield.

Synonyms ^{99m}Tc-DMSA; ^{99m}Tc-succimer; technetium Tc 99m succimer kit

U.S. Brand Names DMSA

Therapeutic Category Radiopharmaceutical

Use Scintigraphic evaluation of renal parenchymal disorders

Tecnal C 1/2 (Can) *see* butalbital, aspirin, caffeine, and codeine *on page 155*

Tecnal C 1/4 (Can) *see* butalbital, aspirin, caffeine, and codeine *on page 155*

Tecta® (Can) *see* pantoprazole *on page 689*

Teflaro™ *see* ceftaroline fosamil *on page 185*

tegaserod (teg a SER od)

Synonyms HTF919; tegaserod maleate

U.S. Brand Names Zelnorm®

Canadian Brand Names Zelnorm® [DSC]

Therapeutic Category Serotonin 5-HT_4 Receptor Agonist

Use Emergency treatment of irritable bowel syndrome with constipation (IBS-C) and chronic idiopathic constipation (CIC) in women (<55 years of age) in which no alternative therapy exists

General Dosage Range Oral: *Adults (females <55 years of age):* 6 mg twice daily

Dosage Forms

Tablet, oral:

Zelnorm®: 2 mg, 6 mg

tegaserod maleate *see* tegaserod *on page 873*

TEGretol® *see* carbamazepine *on page 172*

Tegretol® (Can) *see* carbamazepine *on page 172*

TEGretol®-XR *see* carbamazepine *on page 172*

TEI-6720 *see* febuxostat *on page 374*

Tekamlo™ *see* aliskiren and amlodipine *on page 48*

Tekturna® *see* aliskiren *on page 47*

Tekturna HCT® *see* aliskiren and hydrochlorothiazide *on page 48*

telaprevir (tel A pre vir)

Synonyms LY570310; MP-424; MP424; VRT111950; VX-950; VX950

U.S. Brand Names Incivek™

Canadian Brand Names Incivek™

Therapeutic Category Antiviral Agent; Protease Inhibitor

Use Treatment of genotype 1 chronic hepatitis C (in combination with peginterferon alfa and ribavirin) in adult patients with compensated liver disease (including cirrhosis) who are treatment naive or who have received previous interferon-based treatment, including null or partial responders, and treatment relapsers.

General Dosage Range Oral: Adults: 750 mg 3 times/day

Dosage Forms

Tablet, oral:

Incivek™: 375 mg

telavancin (tel a VAN sin)

Medication Safety Issues

Sound-alike/look-alike issues:

Telavancin may be confused with telithromycin

Vibativ™ may be confused with Viactiv®, Vibramycin®, vigabatrin

Synonyms TD-6424; telavancin hydrochloride

U.S. Brand Names Vibativ™

Therapeutic Category Antibiotic, Miscellaneous

Use Treatment of complicated skin and skin structure infections caused by susceptible gram-positive organisms including methicillin-susceptible or -resistant *Staphylococcus aureus*, vancomycin-susceptible *Enterococcus faecalis*, and *Streptococcus pyogenes*, *Streptococcus agalactiae*, or *Streptococcus anginosus* group

General Dosage Range Dosage adjustment recommended in patients with renal impairment

I.V.: *Adults:* 10 mg/kg every 24 hours

Product Availability Vibativ™: Temporarily not commercially available; anticipated date of availability is unknown.

Dosage Forms

Injection, powder for reconstitution:

Vibativ™: 250 mg, 750 mg

telavancin hydrochloride *see* telavancin *on page 873*

telbivudine (tel BI vyoo deen)

Synonyms L-deoxythymidine; LdT

U.S. Brand Names Tyzeka®

Canadian Brand Names Sebivo®

Therapeutic Category Antiretroviral Agent, Reverse Transcriptase Inhibitor (Nucleoside)

Use Treatment of chronic hepatitis B with evidence of viral replication and either persistent transaminase elevations or histologically-active disease

General Dosage Range Dosage adjustment recommended in patients with renal impairment

Oral: *Children ≥16 years and Adults:* 600 mg once daily

Product Availability Tyzeka® oral solution: FDA approved April 2009; anticipated availability is currently undetermined

Dosage Forms

Tablet, oral:

Tyzeka®: 600 mg

telithromycin (tel ith roe MYE sin)

Medication Safety Issues

Sound-alike/look-alike issues:

Telithromycin may be confused with telavancin

Synonyms HMR 3647

U.S. Brand Names Ketek®

Canadian Brand Names Ketek®

Therapeutic Category Antibiotic, Ketolide

Use Treatment of community-acquired pneumonia (mild-to-moderate) caused by susceptible strains of *Streptococcus pneumoniae* (including multidrug-resistant isolates), *Haemophilus influenzae*, *Chlamydophila pneumoniae*, *Moraxella catarrhalis*, and *Mycoplasma pneumoniae*

General Dosage Range Dosage adjustment recommended in patients with renal impairment

Oral: *Adults:* 800 mg once daily

Dosage Forms

Tablet, oral:

Ketek®: 300 mg, 400 mg

Dosage Forms - Canada

Tablet:

Ketek®: 400 mg

telmisartan (tel mi SAR tan)

U.S. Brand Names Micardis®

Canadian Brand Names Micardis®; Mylan-Telmisartan; Teva-Telmisartan

Therapeutic Category Angiotensin II Receptor Antagonist

Use Treatment of hypertension (may be used alone or in combination with other antihypertensive agents); cardiovascular risk reduction in patients ≥55 years of age unable to take ACE inhibitors and who are at high risk of major cardiovascular events (eg, MI, stroke, death)

General Dosage Range Oral:

Adults: Initial: 40-80 mg once daily; Maintenance: 20-80 mg/day once daily

Elderly: Initial: 20-80 mg once daily

Dosage Forms

Tablet, oral:

Micardis®: 20 mg, 40 mg, 80 mg

telmisartan and amlodipine (tel mi SAR tan & am LOE di peen)

Synonyms amlodipine and telmisartan; amlodipine besylate and telmisartan

U.S. Brand Names Twynsta®

Canadian Brand Names Twynsta®

Therapeutic Category Angiotensin II Receptor Blocker; Calcium Channel Blocker; Calcium Channel Blocker, Dihydropyridine

Use Treatment of hypertension, including initial treatment in patients who will require multiple antihypertensives for adequate control

General Dosage Range Oral: *Adults:* Amlodipine 5-10 mg and telmisartan 40-80 mg once daily (maximum: 10 mg/day [amlodipine]; 80 mg/day [telmisartan])

Dosage Forms

Tablet, oral:

Twynsta® 40/5: Telmisartan 40 mg and amlodipine 5 mg; Twynsta® 40/10: telmisartan 40 mg and amlodipine 10 mg; Twynsta® 80/5: telmisartan 80 mg and amlodipine 5 mg; Twynsta® 80/10: telmisartan 80 mg and amlodipine10 mg

telmisartan and hydrochlorothiazide (tel mi SAR tan & hye droe klor oh THYE a zide)

Synonyms hydrochlorothiazide and telmisartan

U.S. Brand Names Micardis® HCT

Canadian Brand Names Micardis® Plus; Mylan-Telmisartan HCTZ; Teva-Telmisartan HCTZ

Therapeutic Category Antihypertensive Agent, Combination

Use Treatment of hypertension; combination product should not be used for initial therapy

General Dosage Range Oral: *Adults:* Initial: Telmisartan 80 mg and hydrochlorothiazide 12.5-25 mg once daily; Maintenance: Telmisartan 80-160 mg and hydrochlorothiazide 12.5-25 mg once daily

Dosage Forms

Tablet, oral:

Micardis® HCT: 40/12.5: Telmisartan 40 mg and hydrochlorothiazide 12.5 mg; 80/12.5: Telmisartan 80 mg and hydrochlorothiazide 12.5 mg; 80/25: Telmisartan 80 mg and hydrochlorothiazide 25 mg

Dosage Forms - Canada

Tablet, oral:

Micardis® Plus: 80/25: Telmisartan 80 mg and hydrochlorothiazide 25 mg

Telzir® (Can) *see* fosamprenavir *on page 407*

temazepam (te MAZ e pam)

Medication Safety Issues

Sound-alike/look-alike issues:

Temazepam may be confused with flurazepam, LORazepam, tamoxifen

Restoril™ may be confused with Resotran™, RisperDAL®, Vistaril®, Zestril®

BEERS Criteria medication:

This drug may be potentially inappropriate for use in geriatric patients (Quality of evidence - high; Strength of recommendation - strong).

U.S. Brand Names Restoril™

Canadian Brand Names Apo-Temazepam®; CO Temazepam; Dom-Temazepam; Gen-Temazepam; Novo-Temazepam; Nu-Temazepam; PHL-Temazepam; PMS-Temazepam; ratio-Temazepam; Restoril™

Therapeutic Category Benzodiazepine

Controlled Substance C-IV

Use Short-term treatment of insomnia

General Dosage Range Oral:

Adults: 7.5-30 mg at bedtime

Elderly: Initial: 7.5 mg at bedtime

Dosage Forms

Capsule, oral: 7.5 mg, 15 mg, 22.5 mg, 30 mg

Restoril™: 7.5 mg, 15 mg, 22.5 mg, 30 mg

Temodal® (Can) *see* temozolomide *on page 876*

Temodar® *see* temozolomide *on page 876*

Temovate® *see* clobetasol *on page 221*

Temovate E® *see* clobetasol *on page 221*

temozolomide (te moe ZOE loe mide)

Medication Safety Issues

Sound-alike/look-alike issues:

Temodar® may be confused with Tambocor™

Temozolomide may be confused with temsirolimus

High alert medication:

This medication is in a class the Institute for Safe Medication Practices (ISMP) includes among its list of drug classes which have a heightened risk of causing significant patient harm when used in error.

Synonyms SCH 52365; TMZ

U.S. Brand Names Temodar®

Canadian Brand Names Temodal®

Therapeutic Category Antineoplastic Agent, Alkylating Agent

Use Treatment of newly-diagnosed glioblastoma multiforme (initially in combination with radiotherapy, then as maintenance treatment); treatment of refractory anaplastic astrocytoma

Canadian labeling (not an approved indication in the U.S.): Treatment of recurrent or progressive glioblastoma multiforme

General Dosage Range Dosage adjustment recommended in patients who develop toxicities.

I.V., Oral: *Adults:* Dosage varies greatly depending on indication

Dosage Forms

Capsule, oral:

Temodar®: 5 mg, 20 mg, 100 mg, 140 mg, 180 mg, 250 mg

Injection, powder for reconstitution:

Temodar®: 100 mg

Tempra® (Can) *see* acetaminophen *on page* 20

temsirolimus (tem sir OH li mus)

Medication Safety Issues

Sound-alike/look-alike issues:

Temsirolimus may be confused with everolimus, sirolimus, tacrolimus, temozolomide, tesamorelin

High alert medication:

This medication is in a class the Institute for Safe Medication Practices (ISMP) includes among its list of drug classes which have a heightened risk of causing significant patient harm when used in error.

Administration issues:

Temsirolimus requires a two-step dilution process prior to administration. The medication is supplied in a vial containing a total amount of 30 mg in a total volume of 1.2 mL (25 mg/mL). The vial must initially be diluted to 10 mg/mL (with provided 1.8 mL of diluent), then the intended dose should be withdrawn from the 10 mg/mL diluted vial (ie, 2.5 mL for a 25 mg dose) and further diluted for infusion in 250 mL sodium chloride 0.9%. Errors have occurred due to improper preparation.

Temsirolimus, for the treatment of advanced renal cell cancer, is a flat dose (25 mg if no dosage reductions) and is not based on body surface area (BSA).

Synonyms CCI-779

U.S. Brand Names Torisel®

Canadian Brand Names Torisel®

Therapeutic Category Antineoplastic Agent, mTOR Kinase Inhibitor

Use Treatment of advanced renal cell cancer (RCC)

General Dosage Range Dosage adjustment recommended in patients with hepatic impairment, on concomitant therapy, or who develop toxicities

I.V.: *Adults:* 25 mg once weekly

Dosage Forms

Injection, solution:

Torisel®: 25 mg/mL (1.2 mL)

tenecteplase (ten EK te plase)

Medication Safety Issues

Sound-alike/look-alike issues:

TNKase® may be confused with Activase®, t-PA

TNK (occasional abbreviation for TNKase®) is an error-prone abbreviation (mistaken as TPA)

High alert medication:

The Institute for Safe Medication Practices (ISMP) includes this medication (I.V.) among its list of drugs which have a heightened risk of causing significant patient harm when used in error.

U.S. Brand Names TNKase®

Canadian Brand Names TNKase®

Therapeutic Category Thrombolytic Agent

Use Thrombolytic agent used in the management of ST-elevation myocardial infarction (STEMI) for the lysis of thrombi in the coronary vasculature to restore perfusion and reduce mortality.

Recommended criteria for treatment: STEMI: Chest pain ≥20 minutes duration, onset of chest pain within 12 hours of treatment (or within prior 12-24 hours in patients with continuing ischemic symptoms), and S-T segment elevation >0.1 mV in at least two contiguous precordial leads or two adjacent limb leads on ECG or new or presumably new left bundle branch block (LBBB)

General Dosage Range I.V.:

Adults <60 kg: 30 mg as a single dose
Adults ≥60 to <70 kg: 35 mg as a single dose
Adults ≥70 to <80 kg: 40 mg as a single dose
Adults ≥80 to <90 kg: 45 mg as a single dose
Adults ≥90 kg: 50 mg as a single dose

Dosage Forms

Injection, powder for reconstitution [preservative free]:

TNKase®: 50 mg

Tenex® *see* guanfacine *on page* 438

teniposide (ten i POE side)

Medication Safety Issues

Sound-alike/look-alike issues:

Teniposide may be confused with etoposide

High alert medication:

This medication is in a class the Institute for Safe Medication Practices (ISMP) includes among its list of drug classes which have a heightened risk of causing significant patient harm when used in error.

Synonyms EPT; PTG; VM-26

U.S. Brand Names Vumon®

Canadian Brand Names Vumon®

Therapeutic Category Antineoplastic Agent

Use Treatment of refractory childhood acute lymphoblastic leukemia (ALL) in combination with other chemotherapy

General Dosage Range I.V.: *Children:* 165 mg/m^2 twice weekly for 8-9 doses **or** 250 mg/m^2 weekly for 4-8 weeks

Dosage Forms

Injection, solution:

Vumon®: 10 mg/mL (5 mL)

Tenivac™ *see* diphtheria and tetanus toxoids *on page* 295

tenofovir (te NOE fo veer)

Synonyms PMPA; TDF; tenofovir disoproxil fumarate

U.S. Brand Names Viread®

Canadian Brand Names Viread®

Therapeutic Category Antiretroviral Agent, Reverse Transcriptase Inhibitor (Nucleotide)

Use Management of HIV infections in combination with at least two other antiretroviral agents; treatment of chronic hepatitis B virus (HBV) in patients with compensated or decompensated liver disease

General Dosage Range Dosage adjustment recommended in patients with renal impairment

Oral:

Children ≥2 years and Adolescents: 8 mg/kg once daily (maximum: 300 mg once daily)
Adults: 300 mg once daily

Dosage Forms

Powder, oral:

Viread®: 40 mg/g (60 g)

Tablet, oral:

Viread®: 150 mg, 200 mg, 250 mg, 300 mg

tenofovir and emtricitabine *see* emtricitabine and tenofovir *on page* 329

tenofovir disoproxil fumarate *see* tenofovir *on page* 877

tenofovir disoproxil fumarate, efavirenz, and emtricitabine *see* efavirenz, emtricitabine, and tenofovir *on page* 324

tenofovir disoproxil fumarate, rilpivirine, and emtricitabine *see* emtricitabine, rilpivirine, and tenofovir *on page* 329

tenofovir, emtricitabine, and rilpivirine *see* emtricitabine, rilpivirine, and tenofovir *on page* 329

Tenoretic® *see* atenolol and chlorthalidone *on page* 99

Tenormin® *see* atenolol *on page* 99

Tensilon® (Can) *see* edrophonium *on page* 323

Tenuate® (Can) *see* diethylpropion *on page* 283

Tenuate® Dospan® (Can) *see* diethylpropion *on page* 283

Tera-Gel™ [OTC] *see* coal tar *on page* 228

Terazol® (Can) *see* terconazole *on page* 880

Terazol® 3 *see* terconazole *on page* 880

Terazol® 7 *see* terconazole *on page* 880

terazosin (ter AY zoe sin)

Medication Safety Issues

BEERS Criteria medication:

This drug may be potentially inappropriate for use in geriatric patients (Quality of evidence - moderate; Strength of recommendation - strong).

Synonyms Hytrin

Canadian Brand Names Apo-Terazosin®; Dom-Terazosin; Hytrin®; Nu-Terazosin; PHL-Terazosin; PMS-Terazosin; ratio-Terazosin; Teva-Terazosin

Therapeutic Category Alpha-Adrenergic Blocking Agent

Use Management of mild-to-moderate hypertension; alone or in combination with other agents such as diuretics or beta-blockers; benign prostate hyperplasia (BPH)

General Dosage Range Dosage adjustment recommended in patients on concomitant therapy

Oral: *Adults:* Initial: 1 mg at bedtime; Maintenance: 1-20 mg once daily (maximum: 20 mg/day)

Dosage Forms

Capsule, oral: 1 mg, 2 mg, 5 mg, 10 mg

terbinafine (systemic) (TER bin a feen)

Medication Safety Issues

Sound-alike/look-alike issues:

Terbinafine may be confused with terbutaline

LamISIL® may be confused with LaMICtal®, Lomotil®

Synonyms terbinafine hydrochloride

U.S. Brand Names LamISIL®; Terbinex™

Canadian Brand Names Apo-Terbinafine®; Auro-Terbinafine; CO Terbinafine; Dom-Terbinafine; GD-Terbinafine; JAMP-Terbinafine; Lamisil®; Mylan-Terbinafine; Nu-Terbinafine; PHL-Terbinafine; PMS-Terbinafine; Q-Terbinafine; Riva-Terbinafine; Sandoz-Terbinafine; Teva-Terbinafine

Therapeutic Category Antifungal Agent, Oral

Use Treatment of onychomycosis of the toenail or fingernail due to susceptible dermatophytes; treatment of tinea capitis

Canadian labeling: Additional use (not in U.S. labeling): Severe tineal skin infections unresponsive to topical therapy

General Dosage Range

Oral granules: *Children ≥4 years:*

<25 kg: 125 mg once daily for 6 weeks

25-35 kg: 187.5 mg once daily for 6 weeks

>35 kg: 250 mg once daily for 6 weeks

Oral tablet: *Adults:* 250 mg once daily for 6-12 weeks

Dosage Forms

Granules, oral:

LamISIL®: 125 mg/packet (42s); 187.5 mg/packet (14s, 42s)

Tablet, oral: 250 mg

LamISIL®: 250 mg

Terbinex™: 250 mg

Dosage Forms - Canada

Tablet, oral:

LamISIL®: 125 mg

terbinafine (topical) (TER bin a feen)

Medication Safety Issues

Sound-alike/look-alike issues:

Terbinafine may be confused with terbutaline

Synonyms terbinafine hydrochloride

U.S. Brand Names LamISIL AT® [OTC]

Canadian Brand Names Lamisil®

Therapeutic Category Antifungal Agent, Topical

Use Antifungal for the treatment of tinea pedis (athlete's foot), tinea cruris (jock itch), and tinea corporis (ringworm) [OTC/prescription formulations]; tinea versicolor [prescription formulations]

General Dosage Range Topical: *Children ≥12 years and Adults:* Apply to affected area once or twice daily

Dosage Forms

Cream, topical: 1% (12 g, 15 g, 24 g, 30 g)

LamISIL AT® [OTC]: 1% (12 g, 15 g, 24 g, 30 g, 36 g)

Gel, topical:

LamISIL AT® [OTC]: 1% (6 g, 12 g)

Solution, topical:

LamISIL AT® [OTC]: 1% (30 mL)

Dosage Forms - Canada

Cream, topical:

Lamisil®: 1% (15 g, 30 g)

Solution, topical [spray]:

Lamisil®: 1% (30 mL)

terbinafine hydrochloride *see* terbinafine (systemic) *on page 878*

terbinafine hydrochloride *see* terbinafine (topical) *on page 879*

Terbinex™ *see* terbinafine (systemic) *on page 878*

terbutaline (ter BYOO ta leen)

Medication Safety Issues

Sound-alike/look-alike issues:

Brethine may be confused with Methergine®

Terbutaline may be confused with terbinafine, TOLBUTamide

Terbutaline and methylergonovine parenteral dosage forms look similar. Due to their contrasting indications, use care when administering these agents.

Synonyms Brethaire [DSC]; brethine; Bricanyl [DSC]

Canadian Brand Names Bricanyl®

Therapeutic Category Adrenergic Agonist Agent

Use Bronchodilator in reversible airway obstruction and bronchial asthma

General Dosage Range Dosage adjustment recommended in patients with renal impairment

Oral:

Children 12-15 years: 2.5 mg every 6 hours 3 times/day (maximum: 7.5 mg/day)

Children >15 years and Adults: 2.5-5 mg every 6 hours 3 times/day (maximum: 15 mg/day)

SubQ:

Children <12 years: 0.005-0.01 mg/kg/dose to a maximum of 0.4 mg/dose; may repeat in 15-20 minutes

Children ≥12 years and Adults: 0.25 mg/dose; may repeat in 15-30 minutes (maximum: 0.5 mg/4-hour period)

Dosage Forms

Injection, solution: 1 mg/mL (1 mL)

Tablet, oral: 2.5 mg, 5 mg

Dosage Forms - Canada

Powder for oral inhalation:

Bricanyl® Turbuhaler: 500 mcg/actuation [50 or 200 metered actuations]

terconazole (ter KONE a zole)

Medication Safety Issues

Sound-alike/look-alike issues:

Terconazole may be confused with tioconazole

International issues:

Terazol [U.S., Canada] may be confused with Theradol brand name for tramadol [Netherlands]

Synonyms triaconazole

U.S. Brand Names Terazol® 3; Terazol® 7

Canadian Brand Names Terazol®

Therapeutic Category Antifungal Agent

Use Local treatment of vulvovaginal candidiasis

General Dosage Range **Intravaginal:** *Adults:* Insert 1 applicatorful or suppository at bedtime

Dosage Forms

Cream, vaginal: 0.4% (45 g); 0.8% (20 g)

Terazol® 7: 0.4% (45 g)

Terazol® 3: 0.8% (20 g)

Suppository, vaginal: 80 mg (3s)

Terazol® 3: 80 mg (3s)

Terfluzine (Can) *see* trifluoperazine *on page* 919

teriparatide (ter i PAR a tide)

Synonyms parathyroid hormone (1-34); recombinant human parathyroid hormone (1-34); rhPTH(1-34)

U.S. Brand Names Forteo®

Canadian Brand Names Forteo®

Therapeutic Category Diagnostic Agent

Use Treatment of osteoporosis in postmenopausal women at high risk of fracture; treatment of primary or hypogonadal osteoporosis in men at high risk of fracture; treatment of glucocorticoid-induced osteoporosis in men and women at high risk for fracture

General Dosage Range

SubQ: *Adults:* 20 mcg once daily

Dosage Forms

Injection, solution:

Forteo®: 250 mcg/mL (2.4 mL)

Dosage Forms - Canada

Injection, solution:

Forteo®: 250 mcg/mL (3 mL)

Terrell™ *see* isoflurane *on page* 503

Tersa Tar Shp [OTC] (Can) *see* coal tar *on page* 228

Tersi *see* selenium sulfide *on page* 828

tesamorelin (tes a moe REL in)

Medication Safety Issues

Sound-alike/look-alike issues:

Tesamorelin may be confused with temsirolimus

Synonyms tesamorelin acetate; TH9507

U.S. Brand Names Egrifta®

Therapeutic Category Growth Hormone Releasing Factor

Use Reduction of excess abdominal fat in HIV-infected patients with lipodystrophy

General Dosage Range SubQ: *Adults:* 2 mg once daily

Dosage Forms

Injection, powder for reconstitution [preservative free]:

Egrifta®: 1 mg

tesamorelin acetate *see* tesamorelin *on page 881*
TESPA *see* thiotepa *on page 892*
Tessalon® *see* benzonatate *on page 124*
tessalon perles *see* benzonatate *on page 124*
Testim® *see* testosterone *on page 881*
Testopel® *see* testosterone *on page 881*

testosterone (tes TOS ter one)

Medication Safety Issues

Sound-alike/look-alike issues:

Testosterone may be confused with testolactone
Testoderm may be confused with Estraderm®
AndroGel® 1% may be confused with AndroGel® 1.62%
Bio-T-Gel may be confused with T-Gel

BEERS Criteria medication:

This drug may be potentially inappropriate for use in geriatric patients (Quality of evidence - moderate; Strength of recommendation - weak).

Other safety concerns:

Transdermal patch may contain conducting metal (eg, aluminum); remove patch prior to MRI.

Synonyms testosterone cypionate; testosterone enanthate

U.S. Brand Names Androderm®; AndroGel®; Axiron®; Delatestryl®; Depo®-Testosterone; First®-Testosterone; First®-Testosterone MC; Fortesta™; Striant®; Testim®; Testopel®

Canadian Brand Names Andriol®; Androderm®; AndroGel®; Andropository; Delatestryl®; Depotest® 100; Everone® 200; PMS-Testosterone; Testim®

Therapeutic Category Androgen

Controlled Substance C-III

Use

Injection: Androgen replacement therapy in the treatment of delayed male puberty; male hypogonadism (primary or hypogonadotropic); inoperable metastatic female breast cancer (enanthate only)

Pellet: Androgen replacement therapy in the treatment of delayed male puberty; male hypogonadism (primary or hypogonadotropic)

Buccal system, topical gel, topical solution, transdermal system: Male hypogonadism (primary or hypogonadotropic)

Capsule (not available in U.S.): Conditions associated with a deficiency or absence of endogenous testosterone

General Dosage Range

Buccal: *Adults (males):* 30 mg every 12 hours

I.M.: *Adolescents and Adults (males):* 50-400 mg every 2-4 weeks

SubQ: *Adolescents and Adults (males):* 150-450 mg every 3-6 months

Transdermal: *Adults (males):* Androderm®: Apply 2-7.5 mg/day; AndroGel® 1%, Testim®: 5-10 g (50-100 mg testosterone) applied once daily (maximum: 10 g/day); AndroGel® 1.62%: Apply 20.25-81 mg/day; Axiron®: Apply 30-120 mg/day; Fortesta™: Apply 10-70 mg/day

Dosage Forms

Cream, topical:

First®-Testosterone MC: 2% (60 g)

Gel, topical:

AndroGel®: 1% [5 g gel/packet] (30s); 1% [2.5 g gel/packet] (30s); 1% [1.25 g gel/actuation] (75 g); 1.62% [2.5 g gel/packet] (30s); 1.62% [1.25 g gel/actuation] (75 g); 1.62% [1.25 g gel/packet] (30s)

Fortesta™: 10 mg/actuation (60 g)

Testim®: 1% [5 g gel/tube] (30s)

Implant, subcutaneous:

Testopel®: 75 mg (10s, 24s, 100s)

Injection, oil: 200 mg/mL (1 mL, 5 mL, 10 mL)

Delatestryl®: 200 mg/mL (5 mL)

Depo®-Testosterone: 100 mg/mL (10 mL); 200 mg/mL (1 mL, 10 mL)

Mucoadhesive, for buccal application:

Striant®: 30 mg (60s)

Ointment, topical:

First®-Testosterone: 2% (60 g)

Patch, transdermal:

Androderm®: 2 mg/24 hours (60s); 4 mg/24 hours (30s)

Powder, for prescription compounding: USP: 100% (5 g, 25 g)

Solution, topical:

Axiron®: 30 mg/actuation (110 mL)

Dosage Forms - Canada

Capsule, gelatin:

Andriol™: 40 mg (10s)

testosterone cypionate *see* testosterone *on page* *881*

testosterone enanthate *see* testosterone *on page* *881*

Testred® *see* methyltestosterone *on page* *593*

tetanus and diphtheria toxoid *see* diphtheria and tetanus toxoids *on page* *295*

tetanus immune globulin (human) (TET a nus i MYUN GLOB yoo lin HYU man)

Synonyms TIG

U.S. Brand Names HyperTET™ S/D

Canadian Brand Names HyperTET™ S/D

Therapeutic Category Immune Globulin

Use Prophylaxis against tetanus following injury in patients where immunization status is not known or uncertain

The Advisory Committee on Immunization Practices (ACIP) recommends passive immunization with TIG for the following:

- Persons with a wound that is not clean or minor and in whom contraindications to a tetanus-toxoid containing vaccine exist and they have not completed a primary series of tetanus toxoid immunization.
- Persons who are wounded in bombings or similar mass casualty events who have penetrating injuries or nonintact skin exposure and who cannot confirm receipt of a tetanus booster within the previous 5 years. In case of shortage, use should be reserved for persons ≥60 years of age.

General Dosage Range I.M.:

Children <7 years: Prophylaxis: 4 units/kg

Children ≥7 years: Prophylaxis: 250 units

Children: Treatment: 500-6000 units

Adults: Prophylaxis: 250 units; Treatment: 500-6000 units

Dosage Forms

Injection, solution [preservative free]:

HyperTET™ S/D: 250 units/mL (~1 mL)

tetanus toxoid *see* diphtheria and tetanus toxoids, acellular pertussis, poliovirus and *Haemophilus* b conjugate vaccine *on page* *298*

tetanus toxoid (adsorbed) (TET a nus TOKS oyd, ad SORBED)

Medication Safety Issues

Sound-alike/look-alike issues:

Tetanus toxoid products may be confused with influenza virus vaccine and tuberculin products. Medication errors have occurred when tetanus toxoid products have been inadvertently administered instead of tuberculin skin tests (PPD) and influenza virus vaccine. These products are refrigerated and often stored in close proximity to each other.

Synonyms TT

Therapeutic Category Toxoid

Use Active immunization against tetanus when combination antigen preparations are not indicated; tetanus prophylaxis in wound management. **Note:** Tetanus and diphtheria toxoids for adult use (Td) is the preferred immunizing agent for most adults and for children after their seventh birthday. Young children should receive trivalent DTaP (diphtheria/tetanus/acellular pertussis) as part of their childhood immunization program, unless pertussis is contraindicated, then DT is warranted.

General Dosage Range I.M.: *Children ≥7 years and Adults:* Initial: 0.5 mL; repeat at 4-8 weeks after first dose and 6-12 months after second dose

Dosage Forms

Injection, suspension: 5 Lf units/0.5 mL (0.5 mL, 5 mL)

tetanus toxoid, reduced diphtheria toxoid, and acellular pertussis, adsorbed *see* diphtheria and tetanus toxoids, and acellular pertussis vaccine *on page 298*

Tetcaine *see* tetracaine (ophthalmic) *on page 883*

tetrabenazine (tet ra BEN a zeen)

U.S. Brand Names Xenazine®

Canadian Brand Names Nitoman™

Therapeutic Category Monoamine Depleting Agent

Use Treatment of chorea associated with Huntington disease

Canadian labeling: Treatment of hyperkinetic movement disorders, including Huntington chorea, hemiballismus, senile chorea, Tourette syndrome, and tardive dyskinesia

General Dosage Range Dosage adjustment recommended in patients on concomitant therapy or who develop toxicities

Oral: *Adults:* 12.5 mg once daily; Maintenance: 25-100 mg/day in 2-3 divided doses

Dosage Forms

Tablet, oral:

Xenazine®: 12.5 mg, 25 mg

Dosage Forms - Canada

Tablet:

Nitoman™: 25 mg

tetracaine (systemic) (TET ra kane)

Synonyms amethocaine hydrochloride; tetracaine hydrochloride

Canadian Brand Names Pontocaine®

Therapeutic Category Local Anesthetic

Use Spinal anesthesia

General Dosage Range Subarachnoid injection: *Adults:* 2-15 mg (maximum: 20 mg)

Dosage Forms

Injection, solution [preservative free]: 1% [10 mg/mL] (2 mL)

tetracaine (ophthalmic) (TET ra kane)

Synonyms amethocaine hydrochloride; tetracaine hydrochloride

U.S. Brand Names Altacaine; Tetcaine; TetraVisc™; TetraVisc™ FORTE

Canadian Brand Names Pontocaine®

Therapeutic Category Local Anesthetic

Use Local anesthesia for various ophthalmic procedures of short duration (eg, tonometry, gonioscopy); minor ophthalmic surgical procedures (eg, removal of corneal foreign bodies, suture removal); and for various diagnostic purposes (eg, conjunctival scrapings)

General Dosage Range Ophthalmic: *Adults:* Instill 1-2 drops into eye(s); may repeat every 5-10 minutes; do not exceed 5 doses

Dosage Forms

Solution, ophthalmic: 0.5% [5 mg/mL] (2 mL, 15 mL)

Altacaine: 0.5% [5 mg/mL] (15 mL, 30 mL)

Tetcaine: 0.5% [5 mg/mL] (15 mL)

TetraVisc™: 0.5% [5 mg/mL) (0.6 mL, 5 mL)

TetraVisc™ FORTE: 0.5% [5 mg/mL] (0.6 mL, 5 mL)

tetracaine (topical) (TET ra kane)

Synonyms amethocaine hydrochloride; tetracaine hydrochloride

U.S. Brand Names Pontocaine® [DSC]

Canadian Brand Names Ametop™; Pontocaine®

Therapeutic Category Local Anesthetic

Use Applied to nose and throat for diagnostic procedures

General Dosage Range Topical: *Adults:* 0.25% or 0.5% by direct application or nebulization (maximum: 20 mg total)

Dosage Forms

Solution, topical:

Pontocaine®: 2% [20 mg/mL] (30 mL, 118 mL)

tetracaine and lidocaine *see* lidocaine and tetracaine *on page* 539

tetracaine, benzocaine, and butamben *see* benzocaine, butamben, and tetracaine *on page* 123

tetracaine hydrochloride *see* tetracaine (ophthalmic) *on page* 883

tetracaine hydrochloride *see* tetracaine (systemic) *on page* 883

tetracaine hydrochloride *see* tetracaine (topical) *on page* 884

tetracosactide *see* cosyntropin *on page* 239

tetracycline (tet ra SYE kleen)

Medication Safety Issues

Sound-alike/look-alike issues:

Tetracycline may be confused with tetradecyl sulfate

Achromycin may be confused with actinomycin, Adriamycin®

Synonyms achromycin; TCN; tetracycline hydrochloride

Canadian Brand Names Apo-Tetra®; Nu-Tetra

Therapeutic Category Tetracycline Derivative

Use Treatment of susceptible bacterial infections of both gram-positive and gram-negative organisms; also infections due to *Mycoplasma*, *Chlamydia*, and *Rickettsia*; indicated for acne, exacerbations of chronic bronchitis, and treatment of gonorrhea and syphilis in patients who are allergic to penicillin; as part of a multidrug regimen for *H. pylori* eradication to reduce the risk of duodenal ulcer recurrence

General Dosage Range Dosage adjustment recommended in patients with renal impairment

Oral:

Children >8 years: 25-50 mg/kg/day divided every 6 hours

Adults: 250-500 mg 2-4 times/day

Dosage Forms

Capsule, oral: 250 mg, 500 mg

tetracycline hydrochloride *see* tetracycline *on page* 884

tetracycline, metronidazole, and bismuth subcitrate potassium *see* bismuth, metronidazole, and tetracycline *on page* 136

tetracycline, metronidazole, and bismuth subsalicylate *see* bismuth, metronidazole, and tetracycline *on page* 136

tetrahydrocannabinol *see* dronabinol *on page* 316

tetrahydrocannabinol and cannabidiol *(Canada only)*

(TET ra hye droe can NAB e nol & can nab e DYE ol)

Synonyms cannabidiol and tetrahydrocannabinol; delta-9-tetrahydrocannabinol and cannabinol; GW-1000-02; THC and CBD

Canadian Brand Names Sativex®

Therapeutic Category Analgesic, Miscellaneous

Controlled Substance CDSA-II

Use Adjunctive treatment of neuropathic pain or spasticity in multiple sclerosis; adjunctive treatment of moderate-to-severe pain in advanced cancer

General Dosage Range Dosage adjustment recommended in patients who develop toxicities

Buccal: *Adults:* Initial: 1 spray twice daily; Maintenance: Usual maximum: 12 sprays/day

Product Availability Not available in U.S.

Dosage Forms - Canada
Solution, buccal [spray]:
Sativex®: Delta-9 tetrahydrocannabinol 27 mg/mL and cannabidiol 25 mg/mL (5.5 mL, 10 mL)

tetrahydrozoline (nasal) (tet ra hye DROZ a leen)

Synonyms tetrahydrozoline hydrochloride; tetryzoline
U.S. Brand Names Tyzine®; Tyzine® Pediatric
Therapeutic Category Adrenergic Agonist Agent; Imidazoline Derivative
Use Symptomatic relief of nasal congestion
General Dosage Range Intranasal:
Children 2-6 years: Instill 2-3 drops (0.05%) into each nostril every 4-6 hours as needed (maximum: Every 3 hours)
Children >6 years and Adults: Instill 2-4 drops (0.1%) **or** 3-4 sprays (0.1%) into each nostril every 3-4 hours as needed (maximum: Every 3 hours)
Dosage Forms
Solution, intranasal:
Tyzine®: 0.1% (15 mL, 30 mL)
Tyzine® Pediatric: 0.05% (15 mL)

tetrahydrozoline (ophthalmic) (tet ra hye DROZ a leen)

Medication Safety Issues
Sound-alike/look-alike issues:
Visine® may be confused with Visken®
Synonyms tetrahydrozoline hydrochloride; tetryzoline
U.S. Brand Names Murine® Tears Plus [OTC]; Opti-Clear [OTC]; Visine® Advanced Relief [OTC]; Visine® Original [OTC]
Therapeutic Category Adrenergic Agonist Agent; Imidazoline Derivative; Ophthalmic Agent, Vasoconstrictor
Use Symptomatic relief of conjunctival congestion
General Dosage Range Ophthalmic: *Adults:* Instill 1-2 drops in each eye 2-4 times/day
Dosage Forms
Solution, ophthalmic: 0.05% (15 mL); 0.5% (15 mL)
Murine® Tears Plus [OTC]: 0.05% (15 mL)
Opti-Clear [OTC]: 0.05% (15 mL)
Visine® Advanced Relief [OTC]: 0.05% (15 mL, 30 mL)
Visine® Original [OTC]: 0.05% (15 mL, 30 mL)

tetrahydrozoline hydrochloride *see* tetrahydrozoline (nasal) *on page 885*
tetrahydrozoline hydrochloride *see* tetrahydrozoline (ophthalmic) *on page 885*
tetraiodothyronine and triiodothyronine *see* thyroid, desiccated *on page 893*
2,2,2-tetramine *see* trientine *on page 918*

tetrastarch (TET ra starch)

Synonyms etherified starch; HES; HES 130/0.4; hydroxyethyl starch
U.S. Brand Names Voluven®
Canadian Brand Names Volulyte®; Voluven®
Therapeutic Category Plasma Volume Expander, Colloid
Use Blood volume expander used in treatment and prevention of hypovolemia
General Dosage Range I.V. infusion:
Children <2 years: Average dose: 7-25 mL/kg
Children >12 years and Adults: Maximum dose: 50 mL/kg/day (or up to 3500 mL daily in a 70 kg patient)
Dosage Forms
Infusion, premixed in NS:
Voluven®: 6% (500 mL)
Dosage Forms - Canada
Infusion, premixed in isotonic electrolyte solution:
Volulyte®: 6% (250 mL, 500 mL)

TetraVisc™ *see* tetracaine (ophthalmic) *on page 883*

Teva-Venlafaxine XR (Can) *see* venlafaxine *on page 942*
Teva-Zolmitriptan (Can) *see* zolmitriptan *on page 966*
Teva-Zolmitriptan OD (Can) *see* zolmitriptan *on page 966*
Teveten® *see* eprosartan *on page 338*
Teveten® HCT *see* eprosartan and hydrochlorothiazide *on page 338*
Teveten® Plus (Can) *see* eprosartan and hydrochlorothiazide *on page 338*
Tev-Tropin® *see* somatropin *on page 849*
Texacort™ *see* hydrocortisone (topical) *on page 457*
TG *see* thioguanine *on page 890*
T/Gel® Daily Control 2 in 1 Dandruff Shampoo Plus Conditioner [OTC] *see* pyrithione zinc *on page 779*
T/Gel® Daily Control Dandruff Shampoo [OTC] *see* pyrithione zinc *on page 779*
T/Gel Therapeutic Shampoo Extra Strength [OTC] (Can) *see* coal tar *on page 228*
6-TG (error-prone abbreviation) *see* thioguanine *on page 890*
TH9507 *see* tesamorelin *on page 881*

thalidomide (tha LI doe mide)

Medication Safety Issues

Sound-alike/look-alike issues:

Thalidomide may be confused with flutamide, lenalidomide

Thalomid® may be confused with thiamine

High alert medication:

This medication is in a class the Institute for Safe Medication Practices (ISMP) includes among its list of drugs which have a heightened risk of causing significant patient harm when used in error.

International issues:

Thalomid [U.S., Canada] may be confused with Thilomide brand name for lodoxamide [Greece, Turkey]

U.S. Brand Names Thalomid®

Canadian Brand Names Thalomid®

Therapeutic Category Immunosuppressant Agent

Use Treatment of newly-diagnosed multiple myeloma; treatment and maintenance of cutaneous manifestations of erythema nodosum leprosum (ENL)

General Dosage Range Dosage adjustment recommended in patients who develop toxicities

Oral: *Children ≥12 years and Adults:* Initial: 100-300 mg once daily (maximum: 400 mg/day)

Dosage Forms

Capsule, oral:

Thalomid®: 50 mg, 100 mg, 150 mg, 200 mg

Thalitone® *see* chlorthalidone *on page 204*
Thalomid® *see* thalidomide *on page 888*
THAM® *see* tromethamine *on page 924*
THC *see* dronabinol *on page 316*
THC and CBD *see* tetrahydrocannabinol and cannabidiol *(Canada only) on page 884*
The Magic Bullett [OTC] (Can) *see* bisacodyl *on page 134*
Theo-24® *see* theophylline *on page 888*
Theo ER (Can) *see* theophylline *on page 888*
Theolair (Can) *see* theophylline *on page 888*

theophylline (thee OFF i lin)

Synonyms theophylline anhydrous

U.S. Brand Names Elixophyllin® Elixir; Theo-24®

Canadian Brand Names Apo-Theo LA®; Novo-Theophyl SR; PMS-Theophylline; Pulmophylline; ratio-Theo-Bronc; Teva-Theophylline SR; Theo ER; Theolair; Uniphyl

Therapeutic Category Theophylline Derivative

Use Treatment of symptoms and reversible airway obstruction due to chronic asthma, or other chronic lung diseases

Note: The Global Initiative for Asthma Guidelines (2009) and the National Heart, Lung and Blood Institute Guidelines (2007) do not recommend oral theophylline as a long-term control medication for asthma in children ≤5 years of age; use has been shown to be effective as an add-on (but not preferred) agent in older children and adults with severe asthma treated with inhaled or oral glucocorticoids. The guidelines do not recommend theophylline for the treatment of exacerbations of asthma.

The Global Initiative for Chronic Obstructive Lung Disease Guidelines (2009) suggest that while higher doses of slow release formulations of theophylline have been proven to be effective for use in COPD, it is not a preferred agent due to its potential for toxicity.

General Dosage Range

I.V.:

Infants 6-52 weeks: mg/kg/hour = (0.008) (age in weeks) + 0.21

Children 1-9 years: 0.8 mg/kg/hour

Children 9-12 years and Adolescents 12-16 years (cigarette or marijuana smokers): 0.7 mg/kg/hour

Adolescents 12-16 years (nonsmokers): 0.5 mg/kg/hour; maximum 900 mg/day unless serum levels indicate need for larger dose

Adults 16-60 years (otherwise healthy, nonsmokers): 0.4 mg/kg/hour; maximum 900 mg/day unless serum levels indicate need for larger dose

Adults >60 years: 0.3 mg/kg/hour; maximum 400 mg/day unless serum levels indicate need for larger dose

Oral solution:

Full-term Infants and Infants <26 weeks: Total daily dose (mg) = [(0.2 x age in weeks) +5] x (weight in kg); divide dose into 3 equal amounts and administer at 8-hour intervals

Full-term Infants and Infants ≥26 weeks and <52 weeks: Total daily dose (mg) = [(0.2 x age in weeks) +5] x (weight in kg); divide dose into 4 equal amounts and administer at 6-hour intervals

Children ≥1 year and <45 kg: Initial: 10-14 mg/kg/day in divided doses (maximum dose: 300 mg/day); titrate to maintenance dose: 20 mg/kg/day in divided doses every 4-6 hours (maximum dose: 600 mg/day)

Children >45 kg and Adults: Initial: 300 mg/day in divided doses; titrate to maintenance dose: 600 mg/day in divided doses every 6-8 hours

Oral extended release formulations:

Children ≥1 year and <45 kg: Initial: 10-14 mg/kg once daily (maximum dose: 300 mg/day); titrate to maintenance dose: 20 mg/kg once daily (maximum dose: 600 mg/day)

Children >45 kg and Adults: 300-600 mg once daily

Dosage Forms

Capsule, extended release, oral:

Theo-24®: 100 mg, 200 mg, 300 mg, 400 mg

Infusion, premixed in D_5W: 400 mg (500 mL); 800 mg (500 mL)

Solution, oral: 80 mg/15 mL (15 mL, 473 mL)

Elixophyllin® Elixir: 80 mg/15 mL (473 mL)

Tablet, extended release, oral: 100 mg, 200 mg, 300 mg, 400 mg, 450 mg, 600 mg

theophylline anhydrous *see* theophylline *on page* 888

theophylline ethylenediamine *see* aminophylline *on page* 62

TheraCys® *see* BCG *on page* 116

Theraflu® Daytime Severe Cold & Cough [OTC] *see* acetaminophen, dextromethorphan, and phenylephrine *on page* 28

Theraflu® Nighttime Severe Cold & Cough [OTC] *see* acetaminophen, diphenhydramine, and phenylephrine *on page* 29

Theraflu® Sugar-Free Nighttime Severe Cold & Cough [OTC] *see* acetaminophen, diphenhydramine, and phenylephrine *on page* 29

Theraflu® Thin Strips® Multi Symptom [OTC] *see* diphenhydramine (systemic) *on page* 292

Theraflu Warming Relief® Daytime Multi-Symptom Cold [OTC] *see* acetaminophen, dextromethorphan, and phenylephrine *on page* 28

Theraflu Warming Relief® Daytime Severe Cold & Cough [OTC] *see* acetaminophen, dextromethorphan, and phenylephrine *on page* 28

Theraflu® Warming Relief ™ Flu & Sore Throat [OTC] *see* acetaminophen, diphenhydramine, and phenylephrine *on page* 29

Theraflu® Warming Relief™ Nighttime Severe Cold & Cough [OTC] *see* acetaminophen, diphenhydramine, and phenylephrine *on page* 29

Thera-Gel [OTC] *see* coal tar *on page* 228

Thera-Gesic® [OTC] *see* methyl salicylate and menthol *on page* 592
Thera-Gesic® Plus [OTC] *see* methyl salicylate and menthol *on page* 592
Theragran *see* vitamins (multiple/oral) *on page* 951
therapeutic multivitamins *see* vitamins (multiple/oral) *on page* 951
Thera-Sal [OTC] [DSC] *see* salicylic acid *on page* 816
Theratears® [OTC] *see* carboxymethylcellulose *on page* 176
Thermazene® *see* silver sulfadiazine *on page* 833
thiamazole *see* methimazole *on page* 583
thiamin *see* thiamine *on page* 890

thiamine (THYE a min)

Medication Safety Issues

Sound-alike/look-alike issues:

Thiamine may be confused with Tenormin®, Thalomid®, Thorazine

International issues:

Doxal [Brazil] may be confused with Doxil brand name for doxorubicin [U.S.]
Doxal: Brand name for pyridoxine/thiamine [Brazil], but also the brand name for doxepin [Finland]

Synonyms aneurine hydrochloride; thiamin; thiamine hydrochloride; thiaminium chloride hydrochloride; vitamin B_1

Canadian Brand Names Betaxin®

Therapeutic Category Vitamin, Water Soluble

Use Treatment of thiamine deficiency including beriberi, Wernicke encephalopathy, Korsakoff syndrome, neuritis associated with pregnancy, or in alcoholic patients; dietary supplement

General Dosage Range

I.M., I.V.:

Children: 10-25 mg/dose daily (thiamine deficiency)
Adults: 5-30 mg/dose 3 times/day (thiamine deficiency) **or** 50-250 mg/day (Wernicke encephalopathy)

Oral:

Infants: 0.2-0.3 mg/day (adequate intake)
Children: 0.5-1.4 mg/day (recommended daily intake) **or** 5-50 mg/day (thiamine deficiency)
Adults: 1.1-1.4 mg/day (recommended daily intake) **or** 5-30 mg/day in 1-3 divided doses (thiamine deficiency)

Dosage Forms

Injection, solution: 100 mg/mL (2 mL)
Tablet, oral: 50 mg, 100 mg, 250 mg, 500 mg

thiamine hydrochloride *see* thiamine *on page* 890
thiaminium chloride hydrochloride *see* thiamine *on page* 890

thioguanine (thye oh GWAH neen)

Medication Safety Issues

Sound-alike/look-alike issues:

Thioguanine may be confused with thiotepa

High alert medication:

This medication is in a class the Institute for Safe Medication Practices (ISMP) includes among its list of drug classes which have a heightened risk of causing significant patient harm when used in error.

Other safety concerns:

6-thioguanine and 6-TG are error-prone abbreviations (associated with sixfold overdoses of thioguanine)

International issues:

Lanvis [Canada and multiple international markets] may be confused with Lantus brand name for insulin glargine [U.S., Canada, and multiple international markets]

Synonyms 2-amino-6-mercaptopurine; 6-TG (error-prone abbreviation); 6-thioguanine (error-prone abbreviation); TG; tioguanine

U.S. Brand Names Tabloid®

Canadian Brand Names Lanvis®

Therapeutic Category Antineoplastic Agent

Use Treatment of acute myelogenous (nonlymphocytic) leukemia (AML)

Dosage Forms

Tablet, oral:

Tabloid®: 40 mg

6-thioguanine (error-prone abbreviation) *see* thioguanine *on page 890*

Thiola® *see* tiopronin *on page 899*

thiopental (thye oh PEN tal)

Medication Safety Issues

High alert medication:

The Institute for Safe Medication Practices (ISMP) includes this medication among its list of drugs which have a heightened risk of causing significant patient harm when used in error.

Synonyms thiopental sodium

U.S. Brand Names Pentothal® [DSC]

Therapeutic Category Barbiturate

Controlled Substance C-III

Use Induction of anesthesia; control of convulsive states; treatment of elevated intracranial pressure

General Dosage Range Dosage adjustment recommended in patients with renal impairment

I.V.:

Infants <1 year: Anesthesia induction: 5-8 mg/kg

Children 1-12 years: Anesthesia induction: 5-6 mg/kg; Maintenance: 1 mg/kg as needed **or** 1.5-5 mg/kg/dose, repeat as needed

Children >12 years: Maintenance: 1 mg/kg as needed **or** 1.5-5 mg/kg/dose, repeat as needed

Adults: Anesthesia induction: 3-5 mg/kg; Maintenance: 25-100 mg as needed **or** 1.5-5 mg/kg/dose, repeat as needed **or** 75-250 mg/dose, repeat as needed

Product Availability Pentothal® (thiopental injection): Hospira Pharmaceuticals, the sole manufacturer, has discontinued all Pentothal® products. Product is currently unavailable in the U.S. and in Canada.

Dosage Forms

Injection, powder for reconstitution:

Pentothal®: 400 mg, 500 mg, 1 g

thiopental sodium *see* thiopental *on page 891*

thiophosphoramide *see* thiotepa *on page 892*

Thioplex *see* thiotepa *on page 892*

thioridazine (thye oh RID a zeen)

Medication Safety Issues

Sound-alike/look-alike issues:

Thioridazine may be confused with thiothixene, Thorazine

Mellaril may be confused with Elavil, Mebaral®

BEERS Criteria medication:

This drug may be potentially inappropriate for use in geriatric patients (Quality of evidence - moderate; Strength of recommendation - strong).

Synonyms Mellaril; thioridazine hydrochloride

Therapeutic Category Phenothiazine Derivative

Use Management of schizophrenic patients who fail to respond adequately to treatment with other antipsychotic drugs, either because of insufficient effectiveness or the inability to achieve an effective dose due to intolerable adverse effects from those medications

General Dosage Range Oral:

Children >2-12 years: 0.5-3 mg/kg/day in 2-3 divided doses **or** 10-25 mg 2-3 times/day (maximum: 3 mg/kg/day)

Children >12 years and Adults: Initial: 50-100 mg 3 times/day; Maintenance: 150-800 mg/day in 2-4 divided doses (maximum: 800 mg/day) **or** Initial: 25 mg 3 times/day; Maintenance: 20-200 mg/day

Elderly: Initial: 10-25 mg 1-2 times/day; Maintenance: 10-400 mg/day in 1-2 divided doses (maximum: 400 mg/day)

Dosage Forms

Tablet, oral: 10 mg, 25 mg, 50 mg, 100 mg

thioridazine hydrochloride *see* thioridazine *on page 891*

thiosulfuric acid disodium salt *see* sodium thiosulfate *on page 848*

thiotepa (thye oh TEP a)

Medication Safety Issues

Sound-alike/look-alike issues:

Thiotepa may be confused with thioguanine

High alert medication:

This medication is in a class the Institute for Safe Medication Practices (ISMP) includes among its list of drugs which have a heightened risk of causing significant patient harm when used in error.

Administration issues:

Intrathecal medication safety: The American Society of Clinical Oncology (ASCO)/Oncology Nursing Society (ONS) chemotherapy administration safety standards (Jacobson, 2009) encourage the following safety measures for intrathecal chemotherapy:

- Intrathecal medication should not be prepared during the preparation of any other agents
- After preparation, store in an isolated location or container clearly marked with a label identifying as "intrathecal" use only
- Delivery to the patient should only be with other medications intended for administration into the central nervous system

Synonyms TESPA; thiophosphoramide; Thioplex; triethylenethiophosphoramide; TSPA

Therapeutic Category Antineoplastic Agent

Use Treatment of superficial papillary bladder cancer; palliative treatment of adenocarcinoma of breast or ovary; controlling intracavitary effusions caused by metastatic tumors

General Dosage Range Dosage adjustment recommended in patients who develop toxicities

I.V.: *Adults:* 0.3-0.4 mg/kg every 1-4 weeks

Intracavitary: *Adults:* 0.6-0.8 mg/kg

Intravesical: *Adults:* 60 mg retained for 2 hours once weekly for 4 weeks

Dosage Forms

Injection, powder for reconstitution: 15 mg

thiothixene (thye oh THIKS een)

Medication Safety Issues

Sound-alike/look-alike issues:

Thiothixene may be confused with FLUoxetine, thioridazine

Navane® may be confused with Norvasc®, Nubain

BEERS Criteria medication:

This drug may be potentially inappropriate for use in geriatric patients (Quality of evidence - moderate; Strength of recommendation - strong).

Synonyms tiotixene

U.S. Brand Names Navane® [DSC]

Canadian Brand Names Navane®

Therapeutic Category Thioxanthene Derivative

Use Management of schizophrenia

General Dosage Range **Oral:** *Adults:* Initial: 6-10 mg/day in 2-3 divided doses; Maintenance: 20-60 mg/day in 2-3 divided doses (maximum: 60 mg/day)

Dosage Forms

Capsule, oral: 1 mg, 2 mg, 5 mg, 10 mg

thonzonium, neomycin, colistin, and hydrocortisone *see* neomycin, colistin, hydrocortisone, and thonzonium *on page* 633

Thorazine *see* chlorpromazine *on page* 203

Thorets [OTC] *see* benzocaine *on page* 121

Thrive™ [OTC] *see* nicotine *on page* 640

Thrombate III® *see* antithrombin III *on page* 80

Thrombi-Gel® *see* thrombin (topical) *on page* 893

Thrombin-JMI® *see* thrombin (topical) *on page* 893

Thrombin-JMI® Epistaxis Kit *see* thrombin (topical) *on page* 893

Thrombin-JMI® Pump Spray Kit *see* thrombin (topical) *on page* 893

Thrombin-JMI® Syringe Spray Kit *see* thrombin (topical) *on page* 893

thrombin (topical) (THROM bin, TOP i kal)

Medication Safety Issues

Administration issues:

For topical use only. Do not administer intravenously or intra-arterially.

To reduce the risk of intravascular administration, the Institute for Safe Medication Practices (ISMP) has the following recommendations:

- Prepare, label, and dispense topical thrombin from the pharmacy department (including doses used in the operating room).
- Do not leave vial or syringe at bedside.
- Add auxiliary label to all labels and syringes stating "For topical use only - do not inject".
- When appropriate, use solutions which can be applied with an absorbable gelatin sponge or use a dry form on oozing surfaces.
- When appropriate, use spray kits to help differentiate between parenteral products.

U.S. Brand Names Evithrom®; Recothrom®; Thrombi-Gel®; Thrombi-Pad®; Thrombin-JMI®; Thrombin-JMI® Epistaxis Kit; Thrombin-JMI® Pump Spray Kit; Thrombin-JMI® Syringe Spray Kit

Therapeutic Category Hemostatic Agent

Use Hemostasis whenever minor bleeding from capillaries and small venules is accessible

Thrombi-Gel®; Thrombi-Pad®: Temporary control as trauma dressing for moderate-to-severe bleeding wounds; control of surface bleeding from vascular access sites and percutaneous catheter/tubes

General Dosage Range **Topical:** *Children and Adults:* Dose based on severity of bleeding

Dosage Forms

Pad, topical [preservative free]:

Thrombi-Pad® 3x3: ≥200 units

Powder for reconstitution, topical:

Thrombin-JMI®: 5000 units, 20,000 units

Thrombin-JMI® Epistaxis Kit: 5000 units

Thrombin-JMI® Pump Spray Kit: 20,000 units

Thrombin-JMI® Syringe Spray Kit: 5000 units; 20,000 units

Powder for reconstitution, topical [preservative free]:

Recothrom®: 5000 units; 20,000 units

Solution, topical:

Evithrom®: 800-1200 units/mL (2 mL, 5 mL, 20 mL)

Sponge, topical [preservative free]:

Thrombi-Gel® 10: ≥1000 units (10s)

Thrombi-Gel® 40: ≥1000 units (5s)

Thrombi-Gel® 100: ≥2000 units (5s)

Thrombi-Pad® *see* thrombin (topical) *on page 893*

thymocyte stimulating factor *see* aldesleukin *on page 44*

Thymoglobulin® *see* antithymocyte globulin (rabbit) *on page 80*

Thyrogen® *see* thyrotropin alpha *on page 894*

thyroid, desiccated (THYE roid DES i kay tid)

Medication Safety Issues

BEERS Criteria medication:

This drug may be potentially inappropriate for use in geriatric patients (Quality of evidence - low; Strength of recommendation - strong).

Synonyms desiccated thyroid; levothyroxine and liothyronine; tetraiodothyronine and triiodothyronine; thyroid extract; thyroid USP

U.S. Brand Names Armour® Thyroid; Nature-Throid™; Westhroid™

Therapeutic Category Thyroid Product

Use Replacement or supplemental therapy in hypothyroidism; pituitary TSH suppressants (thyroid nodules, thyroiditis, multinodular goiter, thyroid cancer)

General Dosage Range **Oral:**

Children 0-6 months: 15-30 mg/day **or** 4.8-6 mg/kg/day

Children 6-12 months: 30-45 mg/day **or** 3.6-4.8 mg/kg/day

Children 1-5 years: 45-60 mg/day **or** 3-3.6 mg/kg/day

Children 6-12 years: 60-90 mg/day **or** 2.4-3 mg/kg/day

Children >12 years: >90 mg/day **or** 1.2-1.8 mg/kg/day

Adults: Initial: 15-30 mg/day; Maintenance: 60-120 mg/day

Dosage Forms
Tablet, oral:
Armour® Thyroid: 15 mg, 30 mg, 60 mg, 90 mg, 120 mg, 180 mg, 240 mg, 300 mg
Nature-Throid™: 16.25 mg, 32.5 mg, 65 mg, 130 mg, 195 mg
Westhroid™: 32.5 mg, 65 mg, 130 mg

thyroid extract *see* thyroid, desiccated *on page* *893*
thyroid USP *see* thyroid, desiccated *on page* *893*
Thyrolar® *see* liotrix *on page* *542*
ThyroSafe® [OTC] *see* potassium iodide *on page* *746*
Thyroshield® [OTC] *see* potassium iodide *on page* *746*

thyrotropin alpha (thye roe TROH pin AL fa)

Medication Safety Issues
Sound-alike/look-alike issues:
Thyrogen® may be confused with Thyrolar®

Synonyms human thyroid stimulating hormone; recombinant human thyrotropin; Rh-TSH; thyrotropin alpha; TSH

U.S. Brand Names Thyrogen®

Canadian Brand Names Thyrogen®

Therapeutic Category Diagnostic Agent

Use As an adjunctive diagnostic tool for serum thyroglobulin (Tg) testing; adjunctive treatment for radioiodine ablation of thyroid tissue remnants after total or near-total thyroidectomy in patients with well-differentiated thyroid cancer without evidence of metastatic disease

Potential clinical uses include: Patients with an undetectable Tg on thyroid hormone suppressive therapy to exclude the diagnosis of residual or recurrent thyroid cancer, patients requiring serum Tg testing and radioiodine imaging who are unwilling to undergo thyroid hormone withdrawal testing and whose treating physician believes that use of a less sensitive test is justified, patients who are either unable to mount an adequate endogenous TSH response to thyroid hormone withdrawal or in whom withdrawal is medically contraindicated, and patients without evidence of metastatic disease to ablate thyroid remnants (in combination with radioiodine [I^{131}]) following near-total thyroidectomy.

General Dosage Range I.M.: *Children >16 years and Adults:* 0.9 mg, followed 24 hours later by a second 0.9 mg dose

Dosage Forms
Injection, powder for reconstitution:
Thyrogen®: 1.1 mg

thyrotropin alpha *see* thyrotropin alpha *on page* *894*
tiacumicin B *see* fidaxomicin *on page* *383*

tiagabine (tye AG a been)

Medication Safety Issues
Sound-alike/look-alike issues:
TiaGABine may be confused with tiZANidine

Synonyms tiagabine hydrochloride

Tall-Man tia**GAB**ine

U.S. Brand Names Gabitril®

Therapeutic Category Anticonvulsant

Use Adjunctive therapy in adults and children ≥12 years of age in the treatment of partial seizures

General Dosage Range Dosage adjustment recommended in patients on concomitant therapy
Oral:
Children 12-18 years: Initial: 4 mg once daily; Maintenance: 8-32 mg/day in 2-4 divided doses
Adults: Initial: 4 mg once daily; Maintenance: 8-56 mg/day in 2-4 divided doses

Dosage Forms
Tablet, oral:
Gabitril®: 2 mg, 4 mg, 12 mg, 16 mg

tiagabine hydrochloride *see* tiagabine *on page* *894*
Tiamol® (Can) *see* fluocinonide *on page* *392*

tiaprofenic acid *(Canada only)* (tye ah PRO fen ik AS id)

Canadian Brand Names Apo-Tiaprofenic®; Dom-Tiaprofenic; Nu-Tiaprofenic; PMS-Tiaprofenic; Teva-Tiaprofenic Acid

Therapeutic Category Nonsteroidal Antiinflammatory Drug (NSAID)

Use Relief of signs and symptoms of rheumatoid arthritis and osteoarthritis (degenerative joint disease)

General Dosage Range Oral: *Adults:* 300-600 mg/day in 2-3 divided doses (maximum: 600 mg/day)

Product Availability Not available in U.S.

Dosage Forms - Canada

Tablet, oral: 200 mg, 300 mg

Tiazac® *see* diltiazem *on page 288*

Tiazac® XC (Can) *see* diltiazem *on page 288*

ticagrelor (tye KA grel or)

Synonyms AZD6140

U.S. Brand Names Brilinta™

Canadian Brand Names Brilinta™

Therapeutic Category Antiplatelet Agent; Antiplatelet Agent, Cyclopentyltriazolopyrimidine

Use Used in conjunction with aspirin for secondary prevention of thrombotic events in patients with unstable angina (UA), non-ST-elevation myocardial infarction (NSTEMI), or ST-elevation myocardial infarction (STEMI) managed medically or with percutaneous coronary intervention (PCI) and/or coronary artery bypass graft (CABG)

General Dosage Range Oral: *Adults:* Loading dose: 180 mg; Maintenance: 90 mg twice daily

Dosage Forms

Tablet, oral:

Brilinta™: 90 mg

Dosage Forms - Canada

Tablet, oral:

Brilinta®: 90 mg

ticarcillin and clavulanate potassium (tye kar SIL in & klav yoo LAN ate poe TASS ee um)

Synonyms ticarcillin and clavulanic acid

U.S. Brand Names Timentin®

Canadian Brand Names Timentin®

Therapeutic Category Penicillin

Use Treatment of lower respiratory tract, urinary tract, skin and skin structures, bone and joint, gynecologic (endometritis) and intraabdominal (peritonitis) infections, and septicemia caused by susceptible organisms. Clavulanate expands activity of ticarcillin to include beta-lactamase producing strains of *S. aureus*, *H. influenzae*, *Bacteroides* species, and some other gram-negative bacilli

General Dosage Range Dosage adjustment recommended in patients with hepatic or renal impairment

I.V.:

Children and Adults <60 kg: 200-300 mg of ticarcillin component/kg/day in divided doses every 4-6 hours

Children ≥60 kg and Adults: 3.1 g (ticarcillin 3 g plus clavulanic acid 0.1 g) every 4-6 hours (maximum: 24 g of ticarcillin component/day)

Dosage Forms

Infusion [premixed, frozen]:

Timentin®: Ticarcillin 3 g and clavulanic acid 0.1 g (100 mL)

Injection, powder for reconstitution:

Timentin®: Ticarcillin 3 g and clavulanic acid 0.1 g (3.1 g, 31 g)

ticarcillin and clavulanic acid *see* ticarcillin and clavulanate potassium *on page 895*

TICE® BCG *see* BCG *on page 116*

ticlopidine (tye KLOE pi deen)

Medication Safety Issues

BEERS Criteria medication:

This drug may be potentially inappropriate for use in geriatric patients (Quality of evidence - moderate; Strength of recommendation - strong).

Synonyms ticlopidine hydrochloride

Canadian Brand Names Apo-Ticlopidine®; Dom-Ticlopidine; Gen-Ticlopidine; Mylan-Ticlopidine; Novo-Ticlopidine; Nu-Ticlopidine; PMS-Ticlopidine; Sandoz-Ticlopidine; Teva-Ticlopidine

Therapeutic Category Antiplatelet Agent

Use Platelet aggregation inhibitor that reduces the risk of thrombotic stroke in patients who have had a stroke or stroke precursors (**Note:** Due to its association with life-threatening hematologic disorders, ticlopidine should be reserved for patients who are intolerant to aspirin, or who have failed aspirin therapy); adjunctive therapy (with aspirin) following successful coronary stent implantation to reduce the incidence of subacute stent thrombosis.

General Dosage Range Oral: *Adults:* 250 mg twice daily

Dosage Forms

Tablet, oral: 250 mg

ticlopidine hydrochloride *see* ticlopidine *on page* 895

TIG *see* tetanus immune globulin (human) *on page* 882

Tigan® *see* trimethobenzamide *on page* 920

tigecycline (tye ge SYE kleen)

Synonyms GAR-936

U.S. Brand Names Tygacil®

Canadian Brand Names Tygacil®

Therapeutic Category Antibiotic, Glycylcycline

Use Treatment of complicated skin and skin structure infections caused by susceptible organisms, including methicillin-resistant *Staphylococcus aureus* and vancomycin-sensitive *Enterococcus faecalis*; complicated intraabdominal infections (cIAI); community-acquired pneumonia

General Dosage Range Dosage adjustment recommended in patients with hepatic impairment

I.V.: *Adults:* Initial: 100 mg as a single dose; Maintenance: 50 mg every 12 hours

Dosage Forms

Injection, powder for reconstitution:

Tygacil®: 50 mg

Tikosyn® *see* dofetilide *on page* 306

Tilia™ Fe *see* ethinyl estradiol and norethindrone *on page* 359

tiludronate (tye LOO droe nate)

Synonyms tiludronate disodium

U.S. Brand Names Skelid®

Therapeutic Category Bisphosphonate Derivative

Use Treatment of Paget disease of the bone (osteitis deformans) in patients who have a level of serum alkaline phosphatase (SAP) at least twice the upper limit of normal, or who are symptomatic, or who are at risk for future complications of their disease

General Dosage Range Oral: *Adults:* 400 mg once daily

Dosage Forms

Tablet, oral:

Skelid®: 200 mg

tiludronate disodium *see* tiludronate *on page* 896

Tim-AK (Can) *see* timolol (ophthalmic) *on page* 897

Time-C® [OTC] *see* ascorbic acid *on page* 94

Timentin® *see* ticarcillin and clavulanate potassium *on page* 895

timolol (systemic) (TIM oh lol)

Medication Safety Issues

Sound-alike/look-alike issues:

Timolol may be confused with atenolol, Tylenol®

Synonyms timolol maleate

Canadian Brand Names Apo-Timol®; Nu-Timolol; Teva-Timolol

Therapeutic Category Beta-Adrenergic Blocker, Nonselective

Use Treatment of hypertension and angina; to reduce mortality following myocardial infarction; prophylaxis of migraine

General Dosage Range Oral: *Adults:* Initial: 10 mg twice daily; Maintenance: 20-60 mg/day in 2 divided doses (maximum: 60 mg/day)

Dosage Forms

Tablet, oral: 5 mg, 10 mg, 20 mg

timolol (ophthalmic) (TIM oh lol)

Medication Safety Issues

Sound-alike/look-alike issues:

Timolol may be confused with atenolol, Tylenol®

Timoptic® may be confused with Betoptic S®, Talacen, Viroptic®

Other safety concerns:

Bottle cap color change: Timoptic®: Both the 0.25% and 0.5% strengths are now packaged in bottles with yellow caps; previously, the color of the cap on the product corresponded to different strengths.

International issues:

Betimol [U.S.] may be confused with Betanol brand name for metipranolol [Monaco]

Synonyms timolol hemihydrate; timolol maleate

U.S. Brand Names Betimol®; Istalol®; Timolol GFS; Timoptic-XE®; Timoptic®; Timoptic® in OcuDose®

Canadian Brand Names Apo-Timop®; Dom-Timolol; Mylan-Timolol; Novo-Timol; PMS-Timolol; Sandoz-Timolol; Tim-AK; Timolol Maleate-EX; Timoptic-XE®; Timoptic®

Therapeutic Category Beta-Adrenergic Blocker, Nonselective; Ophthalmic Agent, Antiglaucoma

Use Treatment of elevated intraocular pressure such as glaucoma or ocular hypertension

General Dosage Range Ophthalmic:

Gel-forming solution: *Children and Adults:* Instill 1 drop (0.25% or 0.5%) once daily

Solution: *Children and Adults:* Initial: Instill 1 drop (0.25%) twice daily; Maintenance: Instill 1 drop (0.25% or 0.5%) 1-2 times daily (maximum: 2 drops/day [0.5%])

Dosage Forms

Gel forming solution, ophthalmic: 0.25% (5 mL); 0.5% (5 mL)

Timolol GFS: 0.25% (5 mL); 0.5% (5 mL)

Timoptic-XE®: 0.25% (5 mL); 0.5% (5 mL)

Solution, ophthalmic: 0.25% (5 mL, 10 mL, 15 mL); 0.5% (5 mL, 10 mL, 15 mL)

Betimol®: 0.25% (5 mL); 0.5% (5 mL, 10 mL, 15 mL)

Istalol®: 0.5% (2.5 mL, 5 mL)

Timoptic®: 0.25% (5 mL); 0.5% (5 mL, 10 mL)

Solution, ophthalmic [preservative free]:

Timoptic® in OcuDose®: 0.25% (0.2 mL); 0.5% (0.2 mL)

timolol and brimonidine *see* brimonidine and timolol *on page* 141

timolol and dorzolamide *see* dorzolamide and timolol *on page* 310

Timolol GFS *see* timolol (ophthalmic) *on page* 897

timolol hemihydrate *see* timolol (ophthalmic) *on page* 897

timolol maleate *see* timolol (ophthalmic) *on page* 897

timolol maleate *see* timolol (systemic) *on page* 896

timolol maleate and brinzolamide *see* brinzolamide and timolol *(Canada only) on page* 142

timolol maleate and latanoprost *see* latanoprost and timolol *(Canada only) on page* 524

timolol maleate and travoprost *see* travoprost and timolol *(Canada only) on page* 912

Timolol Maleate-EX (Can) *see* timolol (ophthalmic) *on page* 897

Timoptic® *see* timolol (ophthalmic) *on page* 897

Timoptic® in OcuDose® *see* timolol (ophthalmic) *on page* 897

Timoptic-XE® *see* timolol (ophthalmic) *on page* 897

Tinactin® Antifungal [OTC] *see* tolnaftate *on page* 904

Tinactin® Antifungal Deodorant [OTC] *see* tolnaftate *on page* 904

Tinactin® Antifungal Jock Itch [OTC] *see* tolnaftate *on page* 904

Tinaderm [OTC] *see* tolnaftate *on page* 904

Tinamed® Corn and Callus Remover [OTC] *see* salicylic acid *on page* 816

Tinamed® Wart Remover [OTC] *see* salicylic acid *on page* 816

tincture of opium *see* opium tincture *on page* 669

Tindamax® *see* tinidazole *on page 898*
Ting® Cream [OTC] *see* tolnaftate *on page 904*
Ting® Spray Liquid [OTC] *see* tolnaftate *on page 904*
Ting® Spray Powder [OTC] *see* miconazole (topical) *on page 599*

tinidazole (tye NI da zole)

U.S. Brand Names Tindamax®

Therapeutic Category Amebicide; Antibiotic, Miscellaneous; Antiprotozoal, Nitroimidazole

Use Treatment of trichomoniasis caused by *T. vaginalis*; treatment of giardiasis caused by *G. duodenalis* (*G. lamblia*); treatment of intestinal amebiasis and amebic liver abscess caused by *E. histolytica*; treatment of bacterial vaginosis caused by *Bacteroides* spp, *Gardnerella vaginalis*, and *Prevotella* spp in nonpregnant females

General Dosage Range Oral:
Children >3 years: 50 mg/kg/day (maximum: 2 g/day)
Adults: 1-2 g/day

Dosage Forms
Tablet, oral: 250 mg, 500 mg
Tindamax®: 250 mg, 500 mg

tinzaparin (tin ZA pa rin)

Medication Safety Issues
High alert medication:
The Institute for Safe Medication Practices (ISMP) includes this medication among its list of drug classes which have a heightened risk of causing significant patient harm when used in error.

Synonyms tinzaparin sodium

Canadian Brand Names Innohep®

Therapeutic Category Anticoagulant (Other)

Use Treatment of deep vein thrombosis (DVT) and/or pulmonary embolism (PE) (except in patients with severe hemodynamic instability); prevention of venous thromboembolism (VTE) following orthopedic surgery or following general surgery in patients at high risk of VTE; prevention of clotting in indwelling intravenous lines and extracorporeal circuit during hemodialysis (in patients without high bleeding risk)

General Dosage Range Dosage adjustment recommended in renal impairment and extended (>4 hours) hemodialysis sessions.
I.V. or added to hemodialysis circuit: *Adults:* 2250-4500 anti-Xa units
SubQ: *Adults:* 50 anti-Xa units/kg or 3500 anti-Xa units/kg preoperatively; 75-3500 anti-Xa units/kg once daily (maximum: 18,000 anti-Xa units daily)

Dosage Forms - Canada
Injection, solution:
Innohep®: 10,000 anti-Xa units/mL (2 mL)
Innohep®: 20,000 anti-Xa units/mL (0.5 mL, 0.7 mL, 0.9 mL, 2 mL)
Injection, solution [preservative free]:
Innohep®: 10,000 anti-Xa units/mL (0.25 mL, 0.35 mL, 0.45 mL)

tinzaparin sodium *see* tinzaparin *on page 898*

tioconazole (tye oh KONE a zole)

Medication Safety Issues
Sound-alike/look-alike issues:
Tioconazole may be confused with terconazole

U.S. Brand Names 1-Day™ [OTC]; Vagistat®-1 [OTC]

Therapeutic Category Antifungal Agent

Use Local treatment of vulvovaginal candidiasis

General Dosage Range Intravaginal: *Adults:* Insert 1 applicatorful prior to bedtime, as a single dose

Dosage Forms
Ointment, vaginal:
1-Day™ [OTC]: 6.5% (4.6 g)
Vagistat®-1 [OTC]: 6.5% (4.6 g)

tioguanine *see* thioguanine *on page 890*

tiopronin (tye oh PROE nin)

U.S. Brand Names Thiola®

Therapeutic Category Urinary Tract Product

Use Prevention of kidney stone (cystine) formation in patients with severe homozygous cystinuria who have urinary cystine >500 mg/day who are resistant to treatment with high fluid intake, alkali and diet modification, or who have had adverse reactions to penicillamine

General Dosage Range Oral:

Children ≥9 years: Initial: 15 mg/kg/day in 3 divided doses

Adults: Initial: 800 mg/day in 3 divided doses; average dose: 1000 mg/day

Dosage Forms

Tablet, oral:

Thiola®: 100 mg

tiotixene *see* thiothixene *on page* 892

tiotropium (ty oh TRO pee um)

Medication Safety Issues

Sound-alike/look-alike issues:

Spiriva® may be confused with Inspra™, Serevent®

Tiotropium may be confused with ipratropium

Administration issues:

Spiriva® capsules for inhalation are for administration via HandiHaler® device and are **not** for oral use

Synonyms tiotropium bromide monohydrate

U.S. Brand Names Spiriva® HandiHaler®

Canadian Brand Names Spiriva®

Therapeutic Category Anticholinergic Agent

Use Maintenance treatment of bronchospasm associated with COPD (including bronchitis and emphysema); reduction of COPD exacerbations

General Dosage Range Inhalation: *Adults:* Contents of 1 capsule (18 mcg) once daily

Dosage Forms

Powder, for oral inhalation:

Spiriva® HandiHaler®: 18 mcg/capsule (5s, 30s, 90s)

Dosage Forms - Canada

Powder, for oral inhalation:

Spiriva®: 18 mcg/capsule (10s)

tiotropium bromide monohydrate *see* tiotropium *on page* 899

tipranavir (tip RA na veer)

Synonyms PNU-140690E; TPV

U.S. Brand Names Aptivus®

Canadian Brand Names Aptivus®

Therapeutic Category Antiretroviral Agent, Protease Inhibitor

Use Treatment of HIV-1 infections in combination with ritonavir and other antiretroviral agents; limited to highly treatment-experienced or multiprotease inhibitor-resistant patients.

General Dosage Range Dosage adjustment recommended in patients on concomitant therapy

Oral:

Children ≥2 years: 12-14 mg/kg or 290-375 mg/m^2 (maximum: 500 mg/dose) twice daily

Adults: 500 mg twice daily

Dosage Forms

Capsule, soft gelatin, oral:

Aptivus®: 250 mg

Solution, oral:

Aptivus®: 100 mg/mL (95 mL)

tirofiban (tye roe FYE ban)

Medication Safety Issues

Sound-alike/look-alike issues:

Aggrastat® may be confused with Aggrenox®, argatroban

High alert medication:

The Institute for Safe Medication Practices (ISMP) includes this medication among its list of drugs which have a heightened risk of causing significant patient harm when used in error.

Synonyms MK383; tirofiban hydrochloride

U.S. Brand Names Aggrastat®

Canadian Brand Names Aggrastat®

Therapeutic Category Antiplatelet Agent

Use Treatment of acute coronary syndrome (ie, unstable angina/non-ST-elevation myocardial infarction [UA/NSTEMI]) in combination with heparin

General Dosage Range Dosage adjustment recommended in patients with renal impairment

I.V.: *Adults:* Initial: 0.4 mcg/kg/minute for 30 minutes; Maintenance infusion: 0.1 mcg/kg/minute

Dosage Forms

Infusion, premixed in NS [preservative free]:

Aggrastat®: 50 mcg/mL (250 mL)

tirofiban hydrochloride *see* tirofiban *on page* *900*

Tirosint® *see* levothyroxine *on page* *533*

Tisseel *see* fibrin sealant *on page* *383*

Tisseel VH S/D *see* fibrin sealant *on page* *383*

Titralac™ [OTC] *see* calcium carbonate *on page* *161*

Titralac® Plus [OTC] *see* calcium carbonate and simethicone *on page* *163*

Ti-U-Lac® H (Can) *see* urea and hydrocortisone *on page* *931*

TIV *see* influenza virus vaccine (inactivated) *on page* *482*

tizanidine (tye ZAN i deen)

Medication Safety Issues

Sound-alike/look-alike issues:

TiZANidine may be confused with tiaGABine

Zanaflex® may be confused with Xiaflex®

BEERS Criteria medication:

This drug may be potentially inappropriate for use in geriatric patients (Quality of evidence - varies based on comorbidity; Strength of recommendation - varies based on comorbidity)

Other safety concerns:

Zanaflex® capsules and Zanaflex® tablets (or generic tizanidine tablets) are not interchangeable in the fed state

Synonyms Sirdalud®

Tall-Man ti**ZAN**idine

U.S. Brand Names Zanaflex Capsules®; Zanaflex®

Canadian Brand Names Apo-Tizanidine®; Gen-Tizanidine; Mylan-Tizanidine; Zanaflex®

Therapeutic Category Alpha$_2$-Adrenergic Agonist Agent

Use Skeletal muscle relaxant used for treatment of muscle spasticity

General Dosage Range Oral: *Adults:* Initial: 4 mg up to 3 times daily (at 6- to 8-hour intervals); maximum: 36 mg daily

Dosage Forms

Capsule, oral: 2 mg, 4 mg, 6 mg

Zanaflex Capsules®: 2 mg, 4 mg, 6 mg

Tablet, oral: 2 mg, 4 mg

Zanaflex®: 4 mg

TL BPO MX *see* benzoyl peroxide *on page* *124*

TMC-114 *see* darunavir *on page* *255*

TMC125 *see* etravirine *on page* *367*

TMC278 *see* rilpivirine *on page* *801*

TMP *see* trimethoprim *on page* *920*

TMP-SMX *see* sulfamethoxazole and trimethoprim *on page 860*
TMP-SMZ *see* sulfamethoxazole and trimethoprim *on page 860*
TMX-67 *see* febuxostat *on page 374*
TMZ *see* temozolomide *on page 876*
T. N. Dickinson's® Hazelets® [OTC] *see* witch hazel *on page 956*
T. N. Dickinson's® Witch Hazel® Astringent [OTC] *see* witch hazel *on page 956*
T. N. Dickinson's® Witch Hazel® Hemorrhoidal [OTC] *see* witch hazel *on page 956*
TNKase® *see* tenecteplase *on page 876*
TOBI® *see* tobramycin (systemic, oral inhalation) *on page 901*
TOBI® Podhaler® (Can) *see* tobramycin (systemic, oral inhalation) *on page 901*
TobraDex® *see* tobramycin and dexamethasone *on page 902*
Tobradex® (Can) *see* tobramycin and dexamethasone *on page 902*
TobraDex® ST *see* tobramycin and dexamethasone *on page 902*

tobramycin (systemic, oral inhalation) (toe bra MYE sin)

Medication Safety Issues

Sound-alike/look-alike issues:

Tobramycin may be confused with Trobicin®, vancomycin

International issues:

Nebcin [Multiple international markets] may be confused with Naprosyn brand name for naproxen [U.S., Canada, and multiple international markets]; Nubain brand name for nalbuphine [Multiple international markets]

High alert medication:

The Institute for Safe Medication Practices (ISMP) includes this medication (intrathecal administration) among its list of drug classes which have a heightened risk of causing significant patient harm when used in error.

Synonyms tobramycin sulfate

U.S. Brand Names TOBI®

Canadian Brand Names TOBI®; TOBI® Podhaler®; Tobramycin Injection, USP

Therapeutic Category Antibiotic, Aminoglycoside

Use Treatment of documented or suspected infections caused by susceptible gram-negative bacilli, including *Pseudomonas aeruginosa*. Tobramycin solution for inhalation and powder for inhalation (Canadian availability; not available in the U.S.) are indicated for the management of cystic fibrosis patients (>6 years of age) with *Pseudomonas aeruginosa*.

General Dosage Range Dosage adjustment recommended for the I.M. and I.V. routes in patients with renal impairment

I.M.:

Infants and Children <5 years: 2.5 mg/kg every 8 hours
Children ≥5 years: 2-3.3 mg/kg every 6-8 hours
Adults: 1-2.5 mg/kg every 8-12 hours (1 mg/kg used for synergy) **or** 4-7 mg/kg/day as a single daily dose
Elderly: 1.5-5 mg/kg/day in 1-2 divided doses

I.V.:

Infants and Children <5 years: 2.5 mg/kg every 8 hours
Children ≥5 years: 2-3.3 mg/kg every 6-8 hours
Adults: 1-2.5 mg/kg every 8-12 hours (1 mg/kg/dose used for synergy) **or** 4-7 mg/kg/day as a single daily dose
Elderly: 1.5-5 mg/kg/day in 1-2 divided doses **or** 5-7 mg/kg given every 24, 36, or 48 hours based on Cl_{cr}

Inhalation: *Children ≥6 years and Adults:* 300 mg every 12 hours [TOBI®]

Dosage Forms

Infusion, premixed in NS: 80 mg (100 mL)
Injection, powder for reconstitution: 1.2 g
Injection, solution: 10 mg/mL (2 mL, 8 mL); 40 mg/mL (2 mL, 30 mL, 50 mL)
Solution, for nebulization [preservative free]:
TOBI®: 300 mg/5 mL (56s)

Dosage Forms - Canada

Powder, for oral inhalation [capsule]:
TOBI® Podhaler®: 28 mg/capsule (224s)

tobramycin (ophthalmic) (toe bra MYE sin)

Medication Safety Issues

Sound-alike/look-alike issues:

Tobramycin may be confused with Trobicin®, vancomycin

Tobrex® may be confused with TobraDex®

Synonyms tobramycin sulfate

U.S. Brand Names AK-Tob™; Tobrex®

Canadian Brand Names PMS-Tobramycin; Sandoz-Tobramycin; Tobrex®

Therapeutic Category Antibiotic, Aminoglycoside; Antibiotic, Ophthalmic

Use Treatment of superficial ophthalmic infections caused by susceptible bacteria

General Dosage Range **Ophthalmic:** *Children ≥2 months and Adults:* Ointment: Apply 2-3 times/day; for severe infections, apply every 3-4 hours; Solution: Instill 1-2 drops every 2-4 hours

Dosage Forms

Ointment, ophthalmic:

Tobrex®: 0.3% (3.5 g)

Solution, ophthalmic: 0.3% (5 mL)

AK-Tob™: 0.3% (5 mL)

Tobrex®: 0.3% (5 mL)

tobramycin and dexamethasone (toe bra MYE sin & deks a METH a sone)

Medication Safety Issues

Sound-alike/look-alike issues:

TobraDex® may be confused with Tobrex®

Synonyms dexamethasone and tobramycin

U.S. Brand Names TobraDex®; TobraDex® ST

Canadian Brand Names Tobradex®

Therapeutic Category Antibiotic/Corticosteroid, Ophthalmic

Use Treatment of external ocular infection caused by susceptible gram-negative bacteria and steroid responsive inflammatory conditions of the palpebral and bulbar conjunctiva, cornea, and anterior segment of the globe

General Dosage Range **Ophthalmic:** *Children ≥2 years and Adults:* Ointment: Apply ~1/2" ribbon up to 3-4 times/day; Suspension: Instill 1-2 drops every every 4-6 hours, may increase to 1-2 drops every 2 hours for 24-48 hours

Dosage Forms

Ointment, ophthalmic:

TobraDex®: Tobramycin 0.3% and dexamethasone 0.1% (3.5 g)

Suspension, ophthalmic: Tobramycin 0.3% and dexamethasone 0.1% (2.5 mL, 5 mL, 10 mL)

TobraDex®: Tobramycin 0.3% and dexamethasone 0.1% (2.5 mL, 5 mL, 10 mL)

TobraDex® ST: Tobramycin 0.3% and dexamethasone 0.05% (5 mL)

tobramycin and loteprednol etabonate *see* loteprednol and tobramycin *on page* 552

Tobramycin Injection, USP (Can) *see* tobramycin (systemic, oral inhalation) *on page* 901

tobramycin sulfate *see* tobramycin (ophthalmic) *on page* 902

tobramycin sulfate *see* tobramycin (systemic, oral inhalation) *on page* 901

Tobrex® *see* tobramycin (ophthalmic) *on page* 902

tocilizumab (toe si LIZ oo mab)

Synonyms atlizumab; MRA; R-1569; RoActemra®

U.S. Brand Names Actemra®

Canadian Brand Names Actemra®

Therapeutic Category Antirheumatic, Disease Modifying; Interleukin-6 Receptor Antagonist

Use Treatment of moderately- to severely-active rheumatoid arthritis in adult patients who have had an inadequate response to one or more TNF antagonists (as monotherapy or in combination with nonbiological disease-modifying antirheumatic drugs [DMARDs]); treatment of active systemic juvenile idiopathic arthritis (SJIA) (as monotherapy or in combination with methotrexate)

General Dosage Range Dosage adjustment recommended in patients who develop toxicities

I.V.:

Children ≥2 years and <30 kg: 12 mg/kg every 2 weeks

Children ≥2 years and ≥30 kg: 8 mg/kg every 2 weeks

Adults: 4-8 mg/kg every 4 weeks (maximum: 800 mg per infusion)

Dosage Forms

Injection, solution [preservative free]:

Actemra®: 20 mg/mL (4 mL, 10 mL, 20 mL)

Today® [OTC] *see* nonoxynol 9 *on page 647*

Tofranil® *see* imipramine *on page 476*

Tofranil-PM® *see* imipramine *on page 476*

tolazamide (tole AZ a mide)

Medication Safety Issues

Sound-alike/look-alike issues:

TOLAZamide may be confused with TOLBUTamide

Tolinase® may be confused with Orinase

High alert medication:

The Institute for Safe Medication Practices (ISMP) includes this medication among its list of drugs which have a heightened risk of causing significant patient harm when used in error.

Tall-Man **TOLAZ**amide

Therapeutic Category Antidiabetic Agent, Oral

Use Adjunct to diet for the management of mild-to-moderately severe, stable, type 2 diabetes mellitus (noninsulin-dependent, NIDDM)

General Dosage Range Oral: *Adults:* Initial: 100-250 mg/day with first main meal of day; Maintenance: 100-1000 mg/day in 1-2 (doses >500 mg) divided doses (maximum: 1 g/day)

Dosage Forms

Tablet, oral: 250 mg, 500 mg

tolbutamide (tole BYOO ta mide)

Medication Safety Issues

Sound-alike/look-alike issues:

TOLBUTamide may be confused with terbutaline, TOLAZamide

Orinase may be confused with Orabase®, Ornex®, Tolinase®

High alert medication:

The Institute for Safe Medication Practices (ISMP) includes this medication among its list of drugs which have a heightened risk of causing significant patient harm when used in error.

Synonyms Orinase; tolbutamide sodium

Tall-Man **TOLBUT**amide

Canadian Brand Names Apo-Tolbutamide®

Therapeutic Category Antidiabetic Agent, Oral

Use Adjunct to diet for the management of type 2 diabetes mellitus (noninsulin-dependent, NIDDM)

General Dosage Range Oral:

Adults: Initial: 1-2 g/day as a single dose or divided doses; Maintenance: 0.25-3 g/day as a single dose or divided doses

Elderly: Initial: 0.25 g 1-3 times/day; Maintenance: 0.5-2 g/day in 1-3 divided doses (maximum: 3 g/day)

Dosage Forms

Tablet, oral: 500 mg

tolbutamide sodium *see* tolbutamide *on page 903*

tolcapone (TOLE ka pone)

U.S. Brand Names Tasmar®

Therapeutic Category Anti-Parkinson Agent

Use Adjunct to levodopa and carbidopa for the treatment of signs and symptoms of idiopathic Parkinson disease in patients with motor fluctuations not responsive to other therapies

General Dosage Range Oral: *Adults:* Initial: 100 mg 3 times/day; Maintenance: 100-200 mg 3 times/day

Dosage Forms

Tablet, oral:

Tasmar®: 100 mg

Tolectin *see* tolmetin *on page* 904

tolmetin (TOLE met in)

Medication Safety Issues

BEERS Criteria medication:

This drug may be potentially inappropriate for use in geriatric patients (Quality of evidence - moderate; Strength of recommendation - strong).

Synonyms Tolectin; tolmetin sodium

Therapeutic Category Analgesic, Nonnarcotic; Nonsteroidal Antiinflammatory Drug (NSAID)

Use Treatment of rheumatoid arthritis and osteoarthritis, juvenile idiopathic arthritis (JIA)

General Dosage Range Oral:

Children ≥2 years: Initial: 20 mg/kg/day in 3-4 divided doses; Maintenance: 15-30 mg/kg/day in 3-4 divided doses (maximum: 30 mg/kg/day)

Adults: Initial: 400 mg 3 times/day; Maintenance: 600-1800 mg/day in 3 divided doses (maximum: 1.8 g/day)

Dosage Forms

Capsule, oral: 400 mg

Tablet, oral: 200 mg, 600 mg

tolmetin sodium *see* tolmetin *on page* 904

tolnaftate (tole NAF tate)

Medication Safety Issues

Sound-alike/look-alike issues:

Tinactin® may be confused with Talacen

U.S. Brand Names Blis-To-Sol® [OTC]; Mycocide® NS [OTC]; Podactin Powder [OTC]; Tinactin® Antifungal Deodorant [OTC]; Tinactin® Antifungal Jock Itch [OTC]; Tinactin® Antifungal [OTC]; Tinaderm [OTC]; Ting® Cream [OTC]; Ting® Spray Liquid [OTC]

Canadian Brand Names Pitrex

Therapeutic Category Antifungal Agent

Use Treatment of tinea pedis, tinea cruris, tinea corporis

General Dosage Range Topical: *Children ≥2 years and Adults:* Apply to affected areas 2 times/day

Dosage Forms

Aerosol, powder, topical:

Tinactin® Antifungal [OTC]: 1% (133 g)

Tinactin® Antifungal Deodorant [OTC]: 1% (133 g)

Tinactin® Antifungal Jock Itch [OTC]: 1% (133 g)

Aerosol, spray, topical:

Tinactin® Antifungal [OTC]: 1% (150 g)

Ting® Spray Liquid [OTC]: 1% (128 g)

Cream, topical: 1% (15 g, 30 g, 114 g)

Tinactin® Antifungal [OTC]: 1% (15 g, 30 g)

Tinactin® Antifungal Jock Itch [OTC]: 1% (15 g)

Ting® Cream [OTC]: 1% (15 g)

Liquid, topical:

Blis-To-Sol® [OTC]: 1% (30 mL, 55 mL)

Tinactin® Antifungal [OTC]: 1% (59 mL)

Powder, topical: 1% (45 g)

Podactin Powder [OTC]: 1% (60 g)

Tinactin® Antifungal [OTC]: 1% (108 g)

Solution, topical:

Mycocide® NS [OTC]: 1% (30 mL)

Tinaderm [OTC]: 1% (10 mL)

Toloxin® (Can) *see* digoxin *on page* 285

tolterodine (tole TER oh deen)

Medication Safety Issues

Sound-alike/look-alike issues:

Tolterodine may be confused with fesoterodine

Detrol® may be confused with Ditropan

BEERS Criteria medication:

This drug may be potentially inappropriate for use in geriatric patients (Quality of evidence - varies based on comorbidity; Strength of recommendation - varies based on comorbidity)

Synonyms tolterodine tartrate

U.S. Brand Names Detrol®; Detrol® LA

Canadian Brand Names Detrol®; Detrol® LA; Unidet®

Therapeutic Category Anticholinergic Agent

Use Treatment of patients with an overactive bladder with symptoms of urinary frequency, urgency, or urge incontinence

General Dosage Range Dosage adjustment recommended in patients with hepatic or renal impairment and on concomitant therapy

Oral: *Adults:* Extended release capsule: 2-4 mg once daily; Immediate release tablet: 1-2 mg twice daily

Dosage Forms

Capsule, extended release, oral:

Detrol® LA: 2 mg, 4 mg

Tablet, oral: 1 mg, 2 mg

Detrol®: 1 mg, 2 mg

tolterodine tartrate *see* tolterodine *on page* 905

tolvaptan (tol VAP tan)

Synonyms OPC-41061

U.S. Brand Names Samsca™

Canadian Brand Names Samsca™

Therapeutic Category Vasopressin Antagonist

Use Treatment of clinically significant hypervolemic or euvolemic hyponatremia (associated with heart failure, cirrhosis, or SIADH) with either a serum sodium <125 mEq/L or less marked hyponatremia that is symptomatic and resistant to fluid restriction

General Dosage Range Oral: *Adults:* 15-60 mg once daily

Dosage Forms

Tablet, oral:

Samsca™: 15 mg, 30 mg

Dosage Forms - Canada

Tablet, oral:

Samsca™: 15 mg, 30 mg, 60 mg

tomoxetine *see* atomoxetine *on page* 99

Tomudex® (Can) *see* raltitrexed *(Canada only) on page* 786

TootSweet™ [OTC] *see* sucrose *on page* 856

Topactin (Can) *see* fluocinonide *on page* 392

Topamax® *see* topiramate *on page* 906

TopCare® Junior Strength [OTC] *see* ibuprofen *on page* 468

TopCare® Pain Relief PM [OTC] *see* acetaminophen and diphenhydramine *on page* 23

Topicaine® [OTC] *see* lidocaine (topical) *on page* 535

Topicort® *see* desoximetasone *on page* 265

Topicort® Gel (Can) *see* desoximetasone *on page* 265

Topicort® LP *see* desoximetasone *on page* 265

Topicort® Mild (Can) *see* desoximetasone *on page* 265

Topicort® Ointment (Can) *see* desoximetasone *on page* 265

topiramate (toe PYRE a mate)

Medication Safety Issues

Sound-alike/look-alike issues:

Topamax® may be confused with Sporanox®, TEGretol®, TEGretol®-XR, Toprol-XL®

U.S. Brand Names Topamax®

Canadian Brand Names Apo-Topiramate®; CO Topiramate; Dom-Topiramate; Mint-Topiramate; Mylan-Topiramate; Novo-Topiramate; PHL-Topiramate; PMS-Topiramate; PRO-Topiramate; ratio-Topiramate; Sandoz-Topiramate; Topamax®; ZYM-Topiramate

Therapeutic Category Anticonvulsant

Use Monotherapy or adjunctive therapy for partial onset seizures and primary generalized tonic-clonic seizures; adjunctive treatment of seizures associated with Lennox-Gastaut syndrome; prophylaxis of migraine headache

General Dosage Range Dosage adjustment recommended in patients with renal impairment

Oral:

Children 2-9 years: Initial: 25 mg once daily **or** 1-3 mg/kg/day; Maintenance: 150-400 mg/day in 2 divided doses **or** 5-9 mg/kg/day in 2 divided doses

Children 10-16 years: Initial: 25 mg once or twice daily **or** 1-3 mg/kg/day; Maintenance: 5-9 mg/kg/day in 2 divided doses **or** 25-200 mg twice daily

Children ≥17 years: Initial: 25 mg once or twice daily; Maintenance: 100-200 mg twice daily

Adults: Initial: 25-50 mg/day in 1-2 divided doses; Maintenance: 50-200 mg twice daily

Dosage Forms

Capsule, sprinkle, oral: 15 mg, 25 mg

Topamax®: 15 mg, 25 mg

Tablet, oral: 25 mg, 50 mg, 100 mg, 200 mg

Topamax®: 25 mg, 50 mg, 100 mg, 200 mg

topiramate and phentermine *see* phentermine and topiramate *on page* 714

Toposar® *see* etoposide *on page* 366

topotecan (toe poe TEE kan)

Medication Safety Issues

Sound-alike/look-alike issues:

Hycamtin® may be confused with Mycamine®

Topotecan may be confused with irinotecan

High alert medication:

This medication is in a class the Institute for Safe Medication Practices (ISMP) includes among its list of drug classes which have a heightened risk of causing significant patient harm when used in error.

Synonyms hycamptamine; SKF 104864; SKF 104864-A; topotecan hydrochloride

U.S. Brand Names Hycamtin®

Canadian Brand Names Hycamtin®; Topotecan For Injection; Topotecan Hydrochloride For Injection

Therapeutic Category Antineoplastic Agent

Use Treatment of metastatic ovarian cancer, relapsed or refractory small cell lung cancer, recurrent or resistant (stage IVB) cervical cancer (in combination with cisplatin)

General Dosage Range Dosage adjustment recommended in patients with renal impairment or who develop toxicities

Oral: *Adults:* 2.3 mg/m^2/day for 5 days; repeated every 21 days

I.V.: *Adults:* IVPB: 1.5 mg/m^2/day for 5 days; repeated every 21 days **or** 0.75 mg/m^2/day for 3 days; repeated every 21 days

Dosage Forms

Capsule, oral:

Hycamtin®: 0.25 mg, 1 mg

Injection, powder for reconstitution: 4 mg

Hycamtin®: 4 mg

Injection, solution: 1 mg/mL (4 mL)

Topotecan For Injection (Can) *see* topotecan *on page* 906

topotecan hydrochloride *see* topotecan *on page* 906

Topotecan Hydrochloride For Injection (Can) *see* topotecan *on page* 906

Toprol-XL® *see* metoprolol *on page* 595

Topsyn® (Can) *see* fluocinonide *on page* 392

Toradol *see* ketorolac (systemic) *on page 512*

Toradol® (Can) *see* ketorolac (systemic) *on page 512*

Toradol® IM (Can) *see* ketorolac (systemic) *on page 512*

toremifene (tore EM i feen)

Synonyms FC1157a; toremifene citrate

U.S. Brand Names Fareston®

Canadian Brand Names Fareston®

Therapeutic Category Antineoplastic Agent

Use Treatment of metastatic breast cancer in postmenopausal women with estrogen receptor positive or estrogen receptor status unknown

General Dosage Range Oral: *Adults:* 60 mg once daily

Dosage Forms

Tablet, oral:

Fareston®: 60 mg

toremifene citrate *see* toremifene *on page 907*

Torisel® *see* temsirolimus *on page 876*

torsemide (TORE se mide)

Medication Safety Issues

Sound-alike/look-alike issues:

Torsemide may be confused with furosemide

Demadex® may be confused with Denorex®

U.S. Brand Names Demadex®

Therapeutic Category Diuretic, Loop

Use Management of edema associated with heart failure and hepatic or renal disease (including chronic renal failure); treatment of hypertension

General Dosage Range

I.V.: *Adults:* 10-200 mg once daily

Oral: *Adults:* 5-200 mg once daily (maximum: 200 mg/day)

Dosage Forms

Injection, solution: 10 mg/mL (2 mL, 5 mL)

Tablet, oral: 5 mg, 10 mg, 20 mg, 100 mg

Demadex®: 5 mg, 10 mg, 20 mg, 100 mg

tositumomab I-131 *see* tositumomab and iodine I 131 tositumomab *on page 907*

tositumomab and iodine I 131 tositumomab

(toe si TYOO mo mab & EYE oh dyne eye one THUR tee one toe si TYOO mo mab)

Medication Safety Issues

High alert medication:

This medication is in a class the Institute for Safe Medication Practices (ISMP) includes among its list of drug classes which have a heightened risk of causing significant patient harm when used in error.

Synonyms 131 I anti-B1 antibody; 131 I-anti-B1 monoclonal antibody; anti-CD20-murine monoclonal antibody I-131; iodine I 131 tositumomab and tositumomab; tositumomab I-131

U.S. Brand Names Bexxar®

Therapeutic Category Antineoplastic Agent, Monoclonal Antibody; Radiopharmaceutical

Use Treatment of relapsed or refractory CD20 positive, low-grade, follicular, or transformed non-Hodgkin lymphoma (NHL)

General Dosage Range Dosage adjustment recommended in patients who develop toxicities

I.V.:

Tositumomab: *Adults:* Step 1: 450 mg; Step 2: 450 mg

Iodine I-131 tositumomab (given after tositumomab): *Adults:* Step 1: I-131 5 mCi and tositumomab 35 mg; Step 2: I-131 (calculated to deliver 65-75 cGy total body irradiation) and tositumomab 35 mg

Dosage Forms

Kit [dosimetric package]:

Bexxar®: Tositumomab 225 mg/16.1 mL [2 vials], tositumomab 35 mg/2.5 mL [1 vial], and iodine I 131 tositumomab 0.1 mg/mL and 0.61mCi/mL (20 mL) [1 vial]

Kit [therapeutic package]:

Bexxar®: Tositumomab 225 mg/16.1 mL [2 vials], tositumomab 35 mg/2.5 mL [1 vial], and iodine I 131 tositumomab 1.1 mg/mL and 5.6 mCi/mL (20 mL) [1 or 2 vials]

total parenteral nutrition (TOE tal par EN ter al noo TRISH un)

Medication Safety Issues

High alert medication:

The Institute for Safe Medication Practices (ISMP) includes this medication among its list of drugs which have a heightened risk of causing significant patient harm when used in error.

Synonyms Hyperal; hyperalimentation; parenteral nutrition; PN; TPN

Therapeutic Category Caloric Agent; Intravenous Nutritional Therapy

Use Infusion of nutrient solutions into the bloodstream to support nutritional needs during a time when patient is unable to absorb nutrients via the gastrointestinal tract, cannot take adequate nutrition orally or enterally, or have had (or are expected to have) inadequate oral intake for 7-14 days.

General Dosage Range I.V.: Dosage varies greatly depending on indication

Dosage Forms TPN is usually compounded from optimal combinations of macronutrients (water, protein, dextrose, and lipids) and micronutrients (electrolytes, trace elements, and vitamins) to meet the specific nutritional requirements of a patient. Individual hospitals may have designated standard TPN formulas. There are a few commercially-available amino acids with electrolytes solutions; however, these products may not meet an individual's specific nutrition requirements.

Totect® *see* dexrazoxane *on page* 269

Toviaz® *see* fesoterodine *on page* 381

tPA *see* alteplase *on page* 53

TPN *see* total parenteral nutrition *on page* 908

TPV *see* tipranavir *on page* 899

tRA *see* tretinoin (systemic) *on page* 913

trace elements (trase EL e ments)

Synonyms chromium; copper; manganese; neonatal trace metals; selenium; trace metals; trace minerals; zinc

U.S. Brand Names Multitrace®-4; Multitrace®-4 Concentrate; Multitrace®-4 Neonatal; Multitrace®-4 Pediatric; Multitrace®-5; Multitrace®-5 Concentrate; Trace Elements 4 Pediatric

Therapeutic Category Trace Element

Use Prevention and correction of trace metal deficiencies

General Dosage Range I.V.: *Infants, Children, and Adults:* Dosage varies greatly depending on indication

Dosage Forms

Injection, solution [combination products]:

Multitrace®-4: Chromium 4 mcg, copper 0.4 mg, manganese 0.1 mg, and zinc 1 mg per 1 mL (10 mL)

Multitrace®-4 Concentrate: Chromium 10 mcg, copper 1 mg, manganese 0.5 mg, and zinc 5 mg per 1 mL (1 mL, 10 mL)

Multitrace®-4 Neonatal: Chromium 0.85 mcg, copper 0.1 mg, manganese 0.025 mg, and zinc 1.5 mg per 1 mL (2 mL)

Multitrace®-5: Chromium 4 mcg, copper 0.4 mg, manganese 0.1 mg, selenium 20 mcg, and zinc 1 mg per 1 mL (10 mL)

Multitrace®-5 Concentrate: Chromium 10 mcg, copper 1 mg, manganese 0.5 mg, selenium 60 mcg, and zinc 5 mg per 1 mL (1 mL, 10 mL)

Trace Elements 4 Pediatric: Chromium 1 mcg, copper 0.1 mg, manganese 0.03 mg, and zinc 0.5 mg per 1 mL (10 mL)

Injection, solution [combination products, preservative free]:

Multitrace®-4 Pediatric: Chromium 1 mcg, copper 0.1 mg, manganese 0.025 mg, and zinc 1 mg per 1 mL (3 mL)

Trace Elements 4 Pediatric *see* trace elements *on page* 908

trace metals *see* trace elements *on page* 908

trace minerals *see* trace elements *on page* 908

Tracleer® *see* bosentan *on page* 139
Tradjenta™ *see* linagliptin *on page* 539
Trajenta™ (Can) *see* linagliptin *on page* 539
Tramacet (Can) *see* acetaminophen and tramadol *on page* 25

tramadol (TRA ma dole)

Medication Safety Issues

Sound-alike/look-alike issues:

TraMADol may be confused with tapentadol, Toradol®, Trandate®, traZODone, Voltaren®
Ultram® may be confused with Ultane®, Ultracet®, Voltaren®

International issues:

Theradol [Netherlands] may be confused with Foradil brand name for formoterol [U.S., Canada, and multiple international markets], Terazol brand name for terconazole [U.S. and Canada], and Toradol brand name for ketorolac [Canada and multiple international markets]

Trexol [Mexico] may be confused with Trexall brand name for methotrexate [U.S.]; Truxal brand name for chlorprothixene [multiple international markets]

Synonyms tramadol hydrochloride

Tall-Man traMADol

U.S. Brand Names ConZip™; Rybix™ ODT; Ryzolt™; Ultram®; Ultram® ER

Canadian Brand Names Durela™; Ralivia™; Tridural™; Ultram®; Zytram® XL

Therapeutic Category Analgesic, Nonnarcotic

Use Relief of moderate to moderately-severe pain

Extended release formulations are indicated for patients requiring around-the-clock management of moderate to moderately-severe pain for an extended period of time

General Dosage Range Dosage adjustment recommended in patients with hepatic or renal impairment

Oral:

Immediate release:

Children ≥17 years: 50-100 mg every 4-6 hours (maximum: 400 mg/day)
Adults: 50-100 mg every 4-6 hours (maximum: 400 mg/day)
Elderly >75 years: Maximum: 300 mg/day

Extended release: *Adults:* 100-300 once daily (maximum: 300 mg/day)

Dosage Forms

Capsule, variable release, oral: 150 mg [37.5 mg (immediate release) and 112.5 mg (extended release)]

ConZip™: 100 mg [25 mg (immediate release) and 75 mg (extended release)]
ConZip™: 200 mg [50 mg (immediate release) and 150 mg (extended release)]
ConZip™: 300 mg [50 mg (immediate release) and 250 mg (extended release)]

Tablet, oral: 50 mg

Ultram®: 50 mg

Tablet, extended release, oral: 100 mg, 200 mg, 300 mg

Ryzolt™: 100 mg, 200 mg, 300 mg
Ultram® ER: 100 mg, 200 mg, 300 mg

Tablet, orally disintegrating, oral:

Rybix™ ODT: 50 mg

Dosage Forms - Canada

Tablet, extended release:

Ralivia™ ER, Tridural™: 100 mg, 200 mg, 300 mg
Zytram® XL: 75 mg, 100 mg, 150 mg, 200 mg, 300 mg, 400 mg

tramadol hydrochloride *see* tramadol *on page* 909
tramadol hydrochloride and acetaminophen *see* acetaminophen and tramadol *on page* 25
Trandate® *see* labetalol *on page* 516

trandolapril (tran DOE la pril)

U.S. Brand Names Mavik®

Canadian Brand Names Mavik®

Therapeutic Category Angiotensin-Converting Enzyme (ACE) Inhibitor

Use Treatment of hypertension alone or in combination with other antihypertensive agents; treatment of heart failure (HF) or left ventricular (LV) dysfunction after myocardial infarction (MI)

General Dosage Range Dosage adjustment recommended in patients with hepatic or renal impairment

Oral: *Adults:* Initial: 1-2 mg once daily; Maintenance: 1-4 mg once daily

Dosage Forms

Tablet, oral: 1 mg, 2 mg, 4 mg

Mavik®: 1 mg, 2 mg, 4 mg

trandolapril and verapamil (tran DOE la pril & ver AP a mil)

Synonyms verapamil and trandolapril

U.S. Brand Names Tarka®

Canadian Brand Names Tarka®

Therapeutic Category Antihypertensive Agent, Combination

Use Treatment of hypertension; however, not indicated for initial treatment of hypertension

General Dosage Range Dosage adjustment recommended in patients with hepatic or renal impairment

Oral: *Adults:* Trandolapril 1-4 mg and verapamil 180-240 mg once daily

Dosage Forms

Tablet, variable release: Trandolapril 2 mg [immediate release] and verapamil 180 mg [sustained release]; Trandolapril 2 mg [immediate release] and verapamil 240 mg [sustained release]; Trandolapril 4 mg [immediate release] and verapamil 240 mg [sustained release]

Tarka®:

1/240: Trandolapril 1 mg [immediate release] and verapamil 240 mg [sustained release]

2/180: Trandolapril 2 mg [immediate release] and verapamil 180 mg [sustained release]

2/240: Trandolapril 2 mg [immediate release] and verapamil 240 mg [sustained release]

4/240: Trandolapril 4 mg [immediate release] and verapamil 240 mg [sustained release]

tranexamic acid (tran eks AM ik AS id)

Medication Safety Issues

Sound-alike/look-alike issues:

Cyklokapron® may be confused with cycloSPORINE

U.S. Brand Names Cyklokapron®; Lysteda™

Canadian Brand Names Cyklokapron®; Tranexamic Acid Injection BP

Therapeutic Category Antihemophilic Agent

Use

Solution for injection: Short-term use (2-8 days) in hemophilia patients to reduce or prevent hemorrhage and reduce need for replacement therapy during and following tooth extraction

Tablet: Treatment of cyclic heavy menstrual bleeding

General Dosage Range Dosage adjustment recommended in patients with renal impairment

I.V.: *Children and Adults:* Initial: 10 mg/kg as a single dose; Maintenance: 10 mg/kg/dose 3-4 times/day

Oral: *Adults:* 1300 mg 3 times daily (3900 mg/day)

Dosage Forms

Injection, solution: 100 mg/mL (10 mL)

Cyklokapron®: 100 mg/mL (10 mL)

Tablet, oral:

Lysteda™: 650 mg

Tranexamic Acid Injection BP (Can) *see* tranexamic acid *on page 910*

transamine sulphate *see* tranylcypromine *on page 911*

Transderm-V® (Can) *see* scopolamine (systemic) *on page 826*

Transderm-Nitro® (Can) *see* nitroglycerin *on page 645*

Transderm Scōp® *see* scopolamine (systemic) *on page 826*

Trans-Plantar® (Can) *see* salicylic acid *on page 816*

***trans*-retinoic acid** *see* tretinoin (systemic) *on page 913*

***trans*-retinoic acid** *see* tretinoin (topical) *on page 914*

Trans-Ver-Sal® [OTC] *see* salicylic acid *on page 816*

Trans-Ver-Sal® (Can) *see* salicylic acid *on page 816*

***trans* vitamin A acid** *see* tretinoin (systemic) *on page 913*

Tranxene® T-Tab® *see* clorazepate *on page 226*

tranylcypromine (tran il SIP roe meen)

Synonyms transamine sulphate; tranylcypromine sulfate

U.S. Brand Names Parnate®

Canadian Brand Names Parnate®

Therapeutic Category Antidepressant, Monoamine Oxidase Inhibitor

Use Treatment of major depressive episode without melancholia

General Dosage Range Oral: *Adults:* 10-30 mg twice daily (maximum: 60 mg/day)

Dosage Forms

Tablet, oral: 10 mg

Parnate®: 10 mg

tranylcypromine sulfate *see* tranylcypromine *on page 911*

trastuzumab (tras TU zoo mab)

Medication Safety Issues

Sound-alike/look-alike issues:

Trastuzumab may be confused with pertuzumab

High alert medication:

This medication is in a class the Institute for Safe Medication Practices (ISMP) includes among its list of drug classes which have a heightened risk of causing significant patient harm when used in error.

Synonyms anti-c-erB-2; anti-ERB-2; MOAB HER2; rhuMAb HER2

U.S. Brand Names Herceptin®

Canadian Brand Names Herceptin®

Therapeutic Category Antineoplastic Agent

Use Treatment (adjuvant) of HER2 overexpressing breast cancer as part of a combination regimen with doxorubicin, cyclophosphamide, and either paclitaxel or docetaxel; in combination with docetaxel and carboplatin; as a single agent following anthracycline-based combination treatment; treatment of HER2 overexpressing metastatic breast cancer in combination with paclitaxel as first-line treatment or as a single agent in patients who have received prior chemotherapy regimens for treatment of metastatic disease; treatment of HER2 overexpressing metastatic gastric or gastroesophageal junction adenocarcinoma in combination with cisplatin and either capecitabine or fluorouracil in patients who have not received prior treatment for metastatic disease

General Dosage Range Dosage adjustment recommended in patients who develop toxicities

I.V.: *Adults:* Loading dose: 4 mg/kg; Maintenance: 2 mg/kg once weekly **or** Loading dose: 8 mg/kg; Maintenance: 6 mg/kg every 3 weeks

Dosage Forms

Injection, powder for reconstitution:

Herceptin®: 440 mg

Trasylol® (Can) *see* aprotinin *on page 88*

Trav-L-Tabs® [OTC] *see* meclizine *on page 566*

Travasol® *see* amino acid injection *on page 61*

Travatan Z® *see* travoprost *on page 912*

traveler's diarrhea and cholera vaccine *(Canada only)*

(TRAV uh lerz dahy uh REE uh & KOL er uh vak SEEN)

Synonyms *Vibrio cholera* and enterotoxigenic *Escherichia coli* vaccine; cholera and traveler's diarrhea vaccine; cholera vaccine; enterotoxigenic *Escherichia coli* and *Vibrio cholera* vaccine; oral cholera vaccine; traveller's diarrhea vaccine and cholera; WC-rBS

Canadian Brand Names Dukoral®

Therapeutic Category Vaccine

Use Protection against traveler's diarrhea and/or cholera in adults and children ≥2 years of age who will be visiting areas where there is a risk of contracting traveler's diarrhea caused by enterotoxigenic *E. coli* (ETEC) or cholera caused by *V. cholerae* O1 (classical and El Tor biotypes; Inaba and Ogawa serotypes)

General Dosage Range Oral:

Children 2-6 years: Cholera: Primary immunization: 3 doses given at intervals of ≥1 week

Children ≥2 years: ETEC: Primary immunization: 2 doses given at intervals of ≥1 week

Children >6 years: Cholera: Primary immunization: 2 doses given at intervals of ≥1 week

Adults: Cholera: Primary immunization: 2 doses given at intervals of ≥1 week; ETEC: Primary immunization: 2 doses given at intervals of ≥1 week

Product Availability Not available in U.S.

Dosage Forms - Canada

Suspension [vial]:

Dukoral®: 2.5 x 10^{10} of each of the following *Vibrio cholerae* O1 strains: Inaba classic (heat inactivated), Inaba El Tor (formalin inactivated), Ogawa classic (heat inactivated), Ogawa classic (formalin inactivated), and 1 mg recombinant cholera toxin B subunit (rCTB) (3 mL)

traveller's diarrhea vaccine and cholera *see* traveler's diarrhea and cholera vaccine *(Canada only) on page 911*

Travel Tabs [OTC] (Can) *see* dimenhydrinate *on page 289*

travoprost (TRA voe prost)

Medication Safety Issues

Sound-alike/look-alike issues:

Travatan® may be confused with Xalatan®

U.S. Brand Names Travatan Z®

Canadian Brand Names Travatan Z®

Therapeutic Category Prostaglandin, Ophthalmic

Use Reduction of elevated intraocular pressure in patients with open-angle glaucoma or ocular hypertension who are intolerant of the other IOP-lowering medications or insufficiently responsive (failed to achieve target IOP determined after multiple measurements over time) to another IOP-lowering medication

General Dosage Range Ophthalmic: *Adults:* Instill 1 drop into affected eye(s) once daily

Dosage Forms

Solution, ophthalmic:

Travatan Z®: 0.004% (2.5 mL, 5 mL)

travoprost and timolol *(Canada only)* (TRA voe prost & TIM oh lol)

Medication Safety Issues

Sound-alike/look-alike issues:

DuoTrav™ may be confused with DuoNeb®

Synonyms timolol maleate and travoprost

Canadian Brand Names DuoTrav™

Therapeutic Category Beta-Blocker, Nonselective; Ophthalmic Agent, Antiglaucoma; Prostaglandin, Ophthalmic

Use Reduction of intraocular pressure (IOP) in patients with open-angle glaucoma or ocular hypertension who are insufficiently responsive to topical beta-blockers, prostaglandin analogues, or other IOP-reducing agents and in whom combination therapy is appropriate

General Dosage Range Ophthalmic: *Adults:* Instill 1 drop into affected eye(s) once daily

Product Availability Not available in U.S.

Dosage Forms - Canada

Solution, ophthalmic:

DuoTrav™: Travoprost 0.004% and timolol 0.5%: (2.5 mL, 5 mL)

trazodone (TRAZ oh done)

Medication Safety Issues

Sound-alike/look-alike issues:

Desyrel may be confused with deferoxamine, Demerol®, Delsym®, Zestril®

TraZODone may be confused with traMADol, ziprasidone

International issues:

Desyrel [Canada, Turkey] may be confused with Deseril brand name for methysergide [Australia, Belgium, Great Britain, Netherlands]

Synonyms Desyrel; trazodone hydrochloride

Tall-Man tra**ZOD**one

U.S. Brand Names Oleptro™

Canadian Brand Names Apo-Trazodone D®; Apo-Trazodone®; Dom-Trazodone; Mylan-Trazodone; Novo-Trazodone; Nu-Trazodone; Nu-Trazodone D; Oleptro™; PHL-Trazodone; PMS-Trazodone; ratio-Trazodone; Teva-Trazodone; Trazorel®; ZYM-Trazodone

Therapeutic Category Antidepressant, Triazolopyridine

Use Treatment of major depressive disorder

General Dosage Range Oral:

Adults: Immediate release: Initial: 150 mg/day in 3 divided doses; Maintenance: 150-600 mg/day in 3 divided doses; Extended-release: Initial: 150 mg once daily; Maximum dose: 375 mg/day

Elderly: Immediate release: Initial: 25-50 mg at bedtime; Maintenance: 25-150 mg/day at bedtime

Dosage Forms

Tablet, oral: 50 mg, 100 mg, 150 mg, 300 mg

Tablet, extended release, oral:

Oleptro™: 150 mg, 300 mg

trazodone hydrochloride *see* trazodone *on page 912*

Trazorel® (Can) *see* trazodone *on page 912*

Treanda® *see* bendamustine *on page 120*

Trecator® *see* ethionamide *on page 363*

Trelstar® *see* triptorelin *on page 922*

Tremytoine Inj (Can) *see* phenytoin *on page 719*

TRENtal® *see* pentoxifylline *on page 707*

Trental® (Can) *see* pentoxifylline *on page 707*

treprostinil (tre PROST in il)

Synonyms treprostinil sodium

U.S. Brand Names Remodulin®; Tyvaso™

Canadian Brand Names Remodulin®

Therapeutic Category Vasodilator

Use

Injection: Treatment of pulmonary arterial hypertension (PAH) (WHO Group I) in patients with NYHA Class II-IV symptoms to decrease exercise-associated symptoms; to diminish clinical deterioration when transitioning from epoprostenol (I.V.)

Inhalation: Treatment of pulmonary arterial hypertension (PAH) (WHO Group I) in patients with NYHA Class III symptoms to improve exercise ability. **Note:** Nearly all controlled clinical trial experience has been with concomitant bosentan or sildenafil.

General Dosage Range Dosage adjustment recommended for the I.V. infusion and SubQ routes in patients with hepatic impairment

Inhalation: *Adults:* Initial: 18 mcg (or 3 inhalations) every 4 hours 4 times/day; Maintenance: Maximum dose: 54 mcg (or 9 inhalations) 4 times/day

I.V. Infusion, SubQ: *Adults:* Initial: 0.625-1.25 ng/kg/minute; Maintenance: 1.25-40 ng/kg/minute

Dosage Forms

Injection, solution:

Remodulin®: 1 mg/mL (20 mL); 2.5 mg/mL (20 mL); 5 mg/mL (20 mL); 10 mg/mL (20 mL)

Solution, for oral inhalation:

Tyvaso™: 0.6 mg/mL (2.9 mL)

treprostinil sodium *see* treprostinil *on page 913*

Tretin-X® *see* tretinoin (topical) *on page 914*

tretinoin (systemic) (TRET i noyn)

Synonyms *trans* vitamin A acid; *trans*-retinoic acid; all-*trans* retinoic acid; all-*trans* vitamin A acid; ATRA; Ro 5488; tRA; tretinoinum; Vesanoid

Canadian Brand Names Vesanoid®

Therapeutic Category Antineoplastic Agent

Use Induction of remission in patients with acute promyelocytic leukemia (APL), French American British (FAB) classification M3 (including the M3 variant) characterized by t(15;17) translocation and/or PML/RARα gene presence

General Dosage Range Dosage adjustment recommended in patients who develop toxicities

Oral: *Children and Adults:* Induction: 45 mg/m^2/day in 2 divided doses (maximum duration of treatment: 90 days)

Dosage Forms

Capsule, oral: 10 mg

tretinoin (topical) (TRET i noyn)

Medication Safety Issues

Sound-alike/look-alike issues:

Tretinoin may be confused with ISOtretinoin, Tenormin®, triamcinolone, trientine

International issues:

Renova [U.S., Canada] may be confused with Remov brand name for nimesulide [Italy]

Synonyms *trans*-retinoic acid; retinoic acid; vitamin A acid

U.S. Brand Names Atralin™; Avita®; Refissa®; Renova®; Retin-A Micro®; Retin-A®; Tretin-X®

Canadian Brand Names Rejuva-A®; Renova®; Retin-A Micro®; Retin-A®; Retinova®; Stieva-A; Vitamin A Acid

Therapeutic Category Retinoic Acid Derivative

Use Treatment of acne vulgaris; photodamaged skin; palliation of fine wrinkles, mottled hyperpigmentation, and tactile roughness of facial skin as part of a comprehensive skin care and sun avoidance program

General Dosage Range Topical: *Children >12 years and Adults:* Apply once daily **or** every other day

Dosage Forms

Cream, topical: 0.025% (20 g, 45 g); 0.05% (20 g, 40 g, 45 g, 60 g); 0.1% (20 g, 45 g)

Avita®: 0.025% (20 g, 45 g)

Refissa®: 0.05% (40 g)

Renova®: 0.02% (40 g, 44 g, 60 g)

Retin-A®: 0.025% (20 g, 45 g); 0.05% (20 g, 45 g); 0.1% (20 g, 45 g)

Tretin-X®: 0.025% (35 g); 0.0375% (35 g); 0.05% (35 g); 0.1% (35 g)

Gel, topical: 0.01% (15 g, 45 g); 0.025% (15 g, 45 g)

Atralin™: 0.05% (45 g)

Avita®: 0.025% (20 g, 45 g)

Retin-A Micro®: 0.04% (20 g, 45 g, 50 g); 0.1% (20 g, 45 g, 50 g)

Retin-A®: 0.01% (15 g, 45 g); 0.025% (15 g, 45 g)

Tretin-X®: 0.01% (35 g); 0.025% (35 g)

tretinoin and clindamycin *see* clindamycin and tretinoin *on page 219*

tretinoin, fluocinolone acetonide, and hydroquinone *see* fluocinolone, hydroquinone, and tretinoin *on page 392*

tretinoinum *see* tretinoin (systemic) *on page 913*

Trexall™ *see* methotrexate *on page 584*

Treximet® *see* sumatriptan and naproxen *on page 863*

Trezix™ *see* acetaminophen, caffeine, and dihydrocodeine *on page 26*

triaconazole *see* terconazole *on page 880*

Triaderm (Can) *see* triamcinolone (topical) *on page 916*

triamcinolone (systemic) (trye am SIN oh lone)

Medication Safety Issues

Sound-alike/look-alike issues:

Kenalog® may be confused with Ketalar®

Other safety concerns:

TAC (occasional abbreviation for triamcinolone) is an error-prone abbreviation (mistaken as tetracaine-adrenaline-cocaine)

Synonyms triamcinolone acetonide, parenteral; triamcinolone hexacetonide

U.S. Brand Names Aristospan®; Kenalog®-10; Kenalog®-40

Canadian Brand Names Aristospan®

Therapeutic Category Corticosteroid, Inhalant (Oral); Corticosteroid, Systemic

Use

Intraarticular (soft tissue): Acute gouty arthritis, acute/subacute bursitis, acute tenosynovitis, epicondylitis, rheumatoid arthritis, synovitis of osteoarthritis

Intralesional: Alopecia areata, discoid lupus erythematosus, keloids, granuloma annulare lesions (localized hypertrophic, infiltrated, or inflammatory), lichen planus plaques, lichen simplex chronicus plaques, psoriatic plaques, necrobiosis lipoidica diabeticorum, cystic tumors of aponeurosis or tendon (ganglia)

Oral inhalation: Control of bronchial asthma and related bronchospastic conditions

Systemic: Adrenocortical insufficiency, dermatologic diseases, endocrine disorders, gastrointestinal diseases, hematologic and neoplastic disorders, nervous system disorders, nephrotic syndrome, rheumatic disorders, allergic states, respiratory diseases, systemic lupus erythematosus (SLE), and other diseases requiring antiinflammatory or immunosuppressive effects

General Dosage Range

I.M.:

Children 6-12 years: Acetonide: Initial: 40 mg; Range: 2.5-100 mg/day

Children >12 years: Acetonide: Initial: 60 mg; Range: 2.5-100 mg/day

Adults: Acetonide: Initial: 60 mg; Range: 2.5-100 mg/day, may repeat with 20-100 mg when symptoms recur; Multiple sclerosis: 160 mg/day for 1 week, then 64 mg every other day

Intraarticular: *Adults:* Acetonide: 2.5-80 mg; Hexacetonide: 2-20 mg

Intradermal: *Adults:* Acetonide: 1 mg/site

Intralesional: *Adults:* Acetonide: 1-30 mg (usually 1 mg/injection site); Hexacetonide: Up to 0.5 mg/sq inch

Intrasynovial: *Adults:* Acetonide: 5-40 mg

Tendon Sheath: *Adults:* Acetonide: 2.5-10 mg

Dosage Forms

Injection, suspension:

Aristospan®: 5 mg/mL (5 mL); 20 mg/mL (1 mL, 5 mL)

Kenalog®-10: 10 mg/mL (5 mL)

Kenalog®-40: 40 mg/mL (1 mL, 5 mL, 10 mL)

triamcinolone (nasal) (trye am SIN oh lone)

Medication Safety Issues

Sound-alike/look-alike issues:

Nasacort® may be confused with NasalCrom®

Other safety concerns:

TAC (occasional abbreviation for triamcinolone) is an error-prone abbreviation (mistaken as tetracaine-adrenaline-cocaine)

Synonyms triamcinolone acetonide

U.S. Brand Names Nasacort® AQ

Canadian Brand Names Nasacort® AQ; Trinasal®

Therapeutic Category Corticosteroid, Nasal

Use Management of seasonal and perennial allergic rhinitis

General Dosage Range Inhalation:

Nasal inhaler:

Children 6-11 years: 220 mcg/day as 2 sprays in each nostril once daily

Children ≥12 years and Adults: 220-440 mcg/day as 2-4 sprays in each nostril 1-4 times/day

Nasal spray:

Children 2-5 years: 110 mcg/day as 1 spray in each nostril once daily (maximum: 110 mcg/day)

Children 6-11 years: Initial: 110 mcg/day as 1 spray in each nostril once daily; Maintenance: 110-220 mcg/day as 1-2 sprays in each nostril

Children ≥12 years and Adults: 110-220 mcg/day as 1-2 sprays in each nostril once daily

Dosage Forms

Suspension, intranasal: 55 mcg/inhalation (16.5 g)

Nasacort® AQ: 55 mcg/inhalation (16.5 g)

triamcinolone (ophthalmic) (trye am SIN oh lone)

Medication Safety Issues

Other safety concerns:

TAC (occasional abbreviation for triamcinolone) is an error-prone abbreviation (mistaken as tetracaine-adrenaline-cocaine)

Synonyms triamcinolone acetonide

U.S. Brand Names Triesence™

Therapeutic Category Corticosteroid, Ophthalmic

Use

Intavitreal: Treatment of sympathetic ophthalmia, temporal arteritis, uveitis, ocular inflammatory conditions unresponsive to topical corticosteroids

Triesence™: Visualization during vitrectomy

General Dosage Range Intravitreal: *Children and Adults:* Ocular disease: 4 mg as needed; visualization during vitrectomy: 1-4 mg

Dosage Forms

Injection, suspension, ophthalmic:

Triesence™: 40 mg/mL (1 mL)

triamcinolone (topical) (trye am SIN oh lone)

Medication Safety Issues

Sound-alike/look-alike issues:

Kenalog® may be confused with Ketalar®

Other safety concerns:

TAC (occasional abbreviation for triamcinolone) is an error-prone abbreviation (mistaken as tetracaine-adrenaline-cocaine)

U.S. Brand Names Kenalog®; Oralone®; Pediaderm™ TA; Trianex™; Triderm®; Zytopic™

Canadian Brand Names Kenalog®; Oracort; Triaderm

Therapeutic Category Corticosteroid, Topical

Use

Oral topical: Adjunctive treatment and temporary relief of symptoms associated with oral inflammatory lesions and ulcerative lesions resulting from trauma

Topical: Inflammatory dermatoses responsive to steroids

General Dosage Range Topical: *Adults:* Cream, ointment: Apply thin film to affected areas 2-4 times/day; Oral: Press a small dab (about 1/4") to the lesion until a thin film develops; Spray: Apply to affected area 3-4 times/day

Dosage Forms

Aerosol, spray, topical:

Kenalog®: 0.2 mg/2-second spray (63 g, 100 g)

Cream, topical: 0.025% (15 g, 80 g, 454 g); 0.1% (15 g, 30 g, 80 g, 454 g, 2240 g, 2270 g); 0.5% (15 g)

Pediaderm™ TA: 0.1% (30 g)

Triderm®: 0.1% (30 g, 85 g)

Zytopic™: 0.1% (85 g)

Lotion, topical: 0.025% (60 mL); 0.1% (60 mL); 0.1%

Ointment, topical: 0.025% (15 g, 80 g, 454 g); 0.05% (430 g); 0.1% (15 g, 80 g, 454 g); 0.5% (15 g)

Trianex™: 0.05% (17 g, 85 g)

Paste, oral topical: 0.1% (5 g)

Oralone®: 0.1% (5 g)

triamcinolone acetonide *see* triamcinolone (nasal) *on page 915*

triamcinolone acetonide *see* triamcinolone (ophthalmic) *on page 915*

triamcinolone acetonide, parenteral *see* triamcinolone (systemic) *on page 914*

triamcinolone and nystatin *see* nystatin and triamcinolone *on page 658*

triamcinolone hexacetonide *see* triamcinolone (systemic) *on page 914*

Triaminic® Children's Chest & Nasal Congestion [OTC] *see* guaifenesin and phenylephrine *on page 435*

Triaminic® Children's Cold & Allergy [OTC] *see* chlorpheniramine and phenylephrine *on page 200*

Triaminic® Children's Cough Long Acting [OTC] *see* dextromethorphan *on page 272*

Triaminic™ Children's Fever Reducer Pain Reliever [OTC] *see* acetaminophen *on page 20*

Triaminic® Children's Night Time Cold & Cough [OTC] *see* diphenhydramine and phenylephrine *on page 294*

Triaminic® Children's Softchews® Cough & Runny Nose [OTC] *see* dextromethorphan and chlorpheniramine *on page 273*

Triaminic® Children's Thin Strips® Night Time Cold & Cough [OTC] *see* diphenhydramine and phenylephrine *on page 294*

Triaminic® Cold & Allergy (Can) *see* chlorpheniramine and pseudoephedrine *on page 200*

Triaminic® Day Time Cold & Cough [OTC] *see* dextromethorphan and phenylephrine *on page 273*

Triaminic Thin Strips® Children's Cold with Stuffy Nose [OTC] *see* phenylephrine (systemic) *on page* 715

Triaminic Thin Strips® Children's Cough & Runny Nose [OTC] *see* diphenhydramine (systemic) *on page* 292

Triaminic Thin Strips® Children's Long Acting Cough [OTC] *see* dextromethorphan *on page* 272

Triaminic Thin Strips® Children's Day Time Cold & Cough [OTC] *see* dextromethorphan and phenylephrine *on page* 273

triamterene (trye AM ter een)

Medication Safety Issues

Sound-alike/look-alike issues:

Triamterene may be confused with trimipramine

Dyrenium® may be confused with Pyridium®

U.S. Brand Names Dyrenium®

Therapeutic Category Diuretic, Potassium Sparing

Use Alone or in combination with other diuretics in treatment of edema and hypertension; decreases potassium excretion caused by kaliuretic diuretics

General Dosage Range Oral: *Adults:* 50-300 mg/day in 1-2 divided doses (maximum: 300 mg/day)

Dosage Forms

Capsule, oral:

Dyrenium®: 50 mg, 100 mg

triamterene and hydrochlorothiazide *see* hydrochlorothiazide and triamterene *on page* 453

Trianex™ *see* triamcinolone (topical) *on page* 916

Triatec-8 (Can) *see* acetaminophen and codeine *on page* 22

Triatec-8 Strong (Can) *see* acetaminophen and codeine *on page* 22

Triatec-30 (Can) *see* acetaminophen and codeine *on page* 22

triazolam (trye AY zoe lam)

Medication Safety Issues

Sound-alike/look-alike issues:

Triazolam may be confused with alPRAZolam

Halcion® may be confused with halcinonide, Haldol®

BEERS Criteria medication:

This drug may be potentially inappropriate for use in geriatric patients (Quality of evidence - high; Strength of recommendation - strong).

U.S. Brand Names Halcion®

Canadian Brand Names Apo-Triazo®; Gen-Triazolam; Halcion®; Mylan-Triazolam

Therapeutic Category Benzodiazepine

Controlled Substance C-IV

Use Short-term treatment of insomnia

General Dosage Range Dosage adjustment recommended in patients with hepatic impairment

Oral:

Adults: 0.125-0.25 mg at bedtime (maximum: 0.5 mg/day)

Elderly: Initial: 0.125 mg at bedtime (maximum: 0.25 mg/day)

Dosage Forms

Tablet, oral: 0.125 mg, 0.25 mg

Halcion®: 0.25 mg

Tri-B® [OTC] *see* folic acid, cyanocobalamin, and pyridoxine *on page* 404

tribavirin *see* ribavirin *on page* 798

Tribenzor™ *see* olmesartan, amlodipine, and hydrochlorothiazide *on page* 662

Tri Biozene [OTC] *see* bacitracin, neomycin, polymyxin B, and pramoxine *on page* 112

Tri-Buffered Aspirin [OTC] *see* aspirin *on page* 96

tricalcium phosphate *see* calcium phosphate (tribasic) *on page* 166

Tricardio B *see* folic acid, cyanocobalamin, and pyridoxine *on page* 404

TriCare® Prenatal *see* vitamins (multiple/prenatal) *on page* 952

TriCare® Prenatal DHA One® *see* vitamins (multiple/prenatal) *on page 952*

Tri-Chlor® *see* trichloroacetic acid *on page 918*

trichloroacetaldehyde monohydrate *see* chloral hydrate *on page 194*

trichloroacetic acid (trye klor oh a SEE tik AS id)

U.S. Brand Names Tri-Chlor®

Therapeutic Category Keratolytic Agent

Use Chemical used in compounding agents for the treatment of warts, skin resurfacing (chemical peels)

Dosage Forms

Liquid, topical:

Tri-Chlor®: 80% (15 mL)

Trichophyton skin test (trye koe FYE ton skin test)

Therapeutic Category Diagnostic Agent

Use Skin test in diagnosis of Type I hypersensitivity to *Trichophyton* fungus

General Dosage Range Intradermal: *Children and Adults:* 0.1 mL

Dosage Forms

Injection, solution: 1:200 (2 mL)

Tricitrates *see* citric acid, sodium citrate, and potassium citrate *on page 214*

Tricode® AR *see* chlorpheniramine, pseudoephedrine, and codeine *on page 202*

Tricode® GF *see* guaifenesin, pseudoephedrine, and codeine *on page 437*

TriCor® *see* fenofibrate *on page 375*

tricosal *see* choline magnesium trisalicylate *on page 206*

Tri-Cyclen® (Can) *see* ethinyl estradiol and norgestimate *on page 361*

Tri-Cyclen® Lo (Can) *see* ethinyl estradiol and norgestimate *on page 361*

Triderm® *see* triamcinolone (topical) *on page 916*

Tridesilon (Can) *see* desonide *on page 265*

Tridil *see* nitroglycerin *on page 645*

Tridural™ (Can) *see* tramadol *on page 909*

trien *see* trientine *on page 918*

trientine (TRYE en teen)

Medication Safety Issues

Sound-alike/look-alike issues:

Trientine may be confused with TRENtal®, tretinoin

Synonyms 2,2,2-tetramine; trien; trientine hydrochloride; triethylene tetramine dihydrochloride

U.S. Brand Names Syprine®

Canadian Brand Names Syprine®

Therapeutic Category Chelating Agent

Use Treatment of Wilson disease in patients intolerant to penicillamine

General Dosage Range Oral:

Children <12 years: 20 mg/kg **or** 500-750 mg/day in 2-4 divided doses (maximum: 1.5 g/day)

Children ≥12 years and Adults: 750-1500 mg/day in 2-4 divided doses (maximum: 2 g/day)

Dosage Forms

Capsule, oral:

Syprine®: 250 mg

trientine hydrochloride *see* trientine *on page 918*

Triesence™ *see* triamcinolone (ophthalmic) *on page 915*

triethanolamine salicylate *see* trolamine *on page 923*

triethylene tetramine dihydrochloride *see* trientine *on page 918*

triethylenethiophosphoramide *see* thiotepa *on page 892*

trifluoperazine (trye floo oh PER a zeen)

Medication Safety Issues

Sound-alike/look-alike issues:

Trifluoperazine may be confused with trihexyphenidyl

Stelazine may be confused with selegiline

BEERS Criteria medication:

This drug may be potentially inappropriate for use in geriatric patients (Quality of evidence - moderate; Strength of recommendation - strong).

Synonyms Stelazine; trifluoperazine hydrochloride

Canadian Brand Names Apo-Trifluoperazine®; Novo-Trifluzine; PMS-Trifluoperazine; Terfluzine

Therapeutic Category Phenothiazine Derivative

Use Treatment of schizophrenia; short-term treatment of generalized nonpsychotic anxiety

General Dosage Range Oral:

Children 6-12 years: Initial: 1 mg 1-2 times/day; Maintenance: 1-15 mg/day in 1-2 divided doses (maximum: 15 mg/day)

Adults: Inpatient: Initial: 2-5 mg twice daily; Maintenance: 15-40 mg/day in 2 divided doses (maximum: 40 mg/day); Outpatient: Initial: 1-3 mg twice daily (maximum: 40 mg/day)

Dosage Forms

Tablet, oral: 1 mg, 2 mg, 5 mg, 10 mg

trifluoperazine hydrochloride *see* trifluoperazine *on page 919*

trifluorothymidine *see* trifluridine *on page 919*

trifluridine (trye FLURE i deen)

Medication Safety Issues

Sound-alike/look-alike issues:

Viroptic® may be confused with Timoptic®

Synonyms F_3T; trifluorothymidine

U.S. Brand Names Viroptic®

Canadian Brand Names Sandoz-Trifluridine; Viroptic®

Therapeutic Category Antiviral Agent

Use Treatment of primary keratoconjunctivitis and recurrent epithelial keratitis caused by herpes simplex virus types I and II

General Dosage Range Ophthalmic: *Adults:* Initial: Instill 1 drop into affected eye(s) every 2 hours while awake (maximum: 9 drops/day); After re-epithelialization of corneal ulcer: 1 drop every 4 hours (maximum: 21 days of treatment)

Dosage Forms

Solution, ophthalmic: 1% (7.5 mL)

Viroptic®: 1% (7.5 mL)

Triglide® *see* fenofibrate *on page 375*

triglycerides, medium chain *see* medium chain triglycerides *on page 567*

Trihexyphen (Can) *see* trihexyphenidyl *on page 919*

trihexyphenidyl (trye heks ee FEN i dil)

Medication Safety Issues

Sound-alike/look-alike issues:

Trihexyphenidyl may be confused with trifluoperazine

BEERS Criteria medication:

This drug may be potentially inappropriate for use in geriatric patients (Quality of evidence - moderate; Strength of recommendation - strong).

Synonyms Artane; benzhexol hydrochloride; trihexyphenidyl hydrochloride

Canadian Brand Names PMS-Trihexyphenidyl; Trihexyphen; Trihexyphenidyl

Therapeutic Category Anti-Parkinson Agent; Anticholinergic Agent

Use Adjunctive treatment of Parkinson disease; treatment of drug-induced extrapyramidal symptoms

General Dosage Range Oral: *Adults:* Initial: 1 mg/day; Maintenance: 3-15 mg/day in 3-4 divided doses

Dosage Forms

Elixir, oral: 2 mg/5 mL (473 mL)

Tablet, oral: 2 mg, 5 mg

Trihexyphenidyl (Can) *see* trihexyphenidyl *on page 919*
trihexyphenidyl hydrochloride *see* trihexyphenidyl *on page 919*
TriHIBit® [DSC] *see* diphtheria and tetanus toxoids, acellular pertussis and *Haemophilus influenzae* b conjugate vaccine *on page 296*
Trilafon *see* perphenazine *on page 710*
Tri-Legest™ Fe *see* ethinyl estradiol and norethindrone *on page 359*
Trileptal® *see* oxcarbazepine *on page 676*
TriLipix® *see* fenofibric acid *on page 376*
Trilisate *see* choline magnesium trisalicylate *on page 206*
Tri-Luma® *see* fluocinolone, hydroquinone, and tretinoin *on page 392*
TriLyte® *see* polyethylene glycol-electrolyte solution *on page 738*

trimebutine *(Canada only)* (trye me BYOO teen)

Synonyms trimebutine maleate
Canadian Brand Names Modulon®
Therapeutic Category Antispasmodic Agent, Gastrointestinal
Use Treatment and relief of symptoms associated with irritable bowel syndrome (IBS) (spastic colon). In postoperative paralytic ileus in order to accelerate the resumption of the intestinal transit following abdominal surgery.
General Dosage Range Oral: *Children ≥12 years and Adults:* 200 mg 3 times/day
Product Availability Not available in U.S.
Dosage Forms - Canada Tablet, oral: 100 mg, 200 mg

trimebutine maleate *see* trimebutine *(Canada only) on page 920*

trimethobenzamide (trye meth oh BEN za mide)

Medication Safety Issues
Sound-alike/look-alike issues:
Tigan® may be confused with Tiazac®, Ticlid
Trimethobenzamide may be confused with metoclopramide, trimethoprim
BEERS Criteria medication:
This drug may be potentially inappropriate for use in geriatric patients (Quality of evidence - moderate; Strength of recommendation - strong).
Synonyms trimethobenzamide hydrochloride
U.S. Brand Names Tigan®
Canadian Brand Names Tigan®
Therapeutic Category Anticholinergic Agent; Antiemetic
Use Treatment of postoperative nausea and vomiting; treatment of nausea associated with gastroenteritis
General Dosage Range
I.M.: *Adults:* 200 mg 3-4 times/day **or** 200 mg as a single dose, repeat 1 hour later
Oral: *Children >40 kg and Adults:* 300 mg 3-4 times/day
Dosage Forms
Capsule, oral: 300 mg
Tigan®: 300 mg
Injection, solution: 100 mg/mL (20 mL)
Tigan®: 100 mg/mL (20 mL)
Injection, solution [preservative free]: 100 mg/mL (2 mL)
Tigan®: 100 mg/mL (2 mL)

trimethobenzamide hydrochloride *see* trimethobenzamide *on page 920*

trimethoprim (trye METH oh prim)

Synonyms TMP
U.S. Brand Names Primsol®
Canadian Brand Names Apo-Trimethoprim®
Therapeutic Category Antibiotic, Miscellaneous

Use Treatment of urinary tract infections due to susceptible strains of *E. coli*, *P. mirabilis*, *K. pneumoniae*, *Enterobacter* spp and coagulase-negative *Staphylococcus* including *S. saprophyticus*; acute otitis media due to susceptible strains of *S. pneumoniae* and *H. influenzae* in children

General Dosage Range Dosage adjustment recommended in patients with renal impairment

Oral:

Children ≥2 months: 4-12 mg/kg/day in divided doses every 12 hours

Adults: 100 mg once daily **or** 100 mg every 12 hours **or** 200 mg every 24 hours; up to 15mg/kg/day

Dosage Forms

Solution, oral:

Primsol®: 50 mg (base)/5 mL (473 mL)

Tablet, oral: 100 mg

trimethoprim and polymyxin B (trye METH oh prim & pol i MIKS in bee)

Synonyms polymyxin B and trimethoprim

U.S. Brand Names Polytrim®

Canadian Brand Names PMS-Polytrimethoprim; Polytrim™

Therapeutic Category Antibiotic, Ophthalmic

Use Treatment of surface ocular bacterial conjunctivitis and blepharoconjunctivitis

General Dosage Range **Ophthalmic:** *Children ≥2 months and Adults:* Instill 1 drop in affected eye(s) every 3 hours (maximum: 6 doses per day) for 7-10 days

Dosage Forms

Solution, ophthalmic: Trimethoprim 1 mg and polymyxin B 10,000 units per 1 mL (10 mL)

Polytrim®: Trimethoprim 1 mg and polymyxin B 10,000 units per 1 mL (10 mL)

trimethoprim and sulfamethoxazole *see* sulfamethoxazole and trimethoprim *on page 860*

trimipramine (trye MI pra meen)

Medication Safety Issues

Sound-alike/look-alike issues:

Trimipramine may be confused with triamterene

BEERS Criteria medication:

This drug may be potentially inappropriate for use in geriatric patients (Quality of evidence - high [moderate for SIADH]; Strength of recommendation - strong).

Synonyms trimipramine maleate

U.S. Brand Names Surmontil®

Canadian Brand Names Apo-Trimip®; Nu-Trimipramine; Rhotrimine®; Surmontil®

Therapeutic Category Antidepressant, Tricyclic (Tertiary Amine)

Use Treatment of depression

General Dosage Range

Oral:

Adolescents: Initial: 50 mg/day (maximum: 100 mg/day)

Adults: 50-200 mg at bedtime (maximum: 200 mg/day [outpatient] or 300 mg/day [inpatient])

Elderly: 50-100 mg at bedtime (maximum: 100 mg/day)

Dosage Forms

Capsule, oral: 25 mg, 50 mg

Surmontil®: 25 mg, 50 mg, 100 mg

trimipramine maleate *see* trimipramine *on page 921*

Trinasal® (Can) *see* triamcinolone (nasal) *on page 915*

TriNessa® *see* ethinyl estradiol and norgestimate *on page 361*

Trinipatch® (Can) *see* nitroglycerin *on page 645*

Tri-Norinyl® *see* ethinyl estradiol and norethindrone *on page 359*

Triostat® *see* liothyronine *on page 541*

Tripedia *see* diphtheria and tetanus toxoids, and acellular pertussis vaccine *on page 298*

Triphasil® (Can) *see* ethinyl estradiol and levonorgestrel *on page 357*

triple antibiotic *see* bacitracin, neomycin, and polymyxin B *on page 111*

triple sulfa *see* sulfabenzamide, sulfacetamide, and sulfathiazole *on page 858*

Tri-Previfem® *see* ethinyl estradiol and norgestimate *on page 361*

triprolidine and pseudoephedrine (trye PROE li deen & soo doe e FED rin)

Medication Safety Issues

BEERS Criteria medication:

This drug may be potentially inappropriate for use in geriatric patients (Quality of evidence - moderate; Strength of recommendation - strong).

Synonyms pseudoephedrine and triprolidine

U.S. Brand Names Aprodine [OTC]; Pediatex® TD; Silafed [OTC]

Canadian Brand Names Actifed®

Therapeutic Category Antihistamine/Decongestant Combination

Use Temporary relief of nasal congestion, decongest sinus openings, running nose, sneezing, itching of nose or throat and itchy, watery eyes due to common cold, hay fever, or other upper respiratory allergies

General Dosage Range Oral: *Children ≥6 years and Adults:* Dosage varies greatly depending on product

Dosage Forms

Liquid, oral:

Pediatex® TD: Triprolidine 0.938 mg and pseudoephedrine 10 mg per 1 mL

Syrup, oral:

Aprodine [OTC], Silafed [OTC]: Triprolidine 1.25 mg and pseudoephedrine 30 mg per 5 mL

Tablet, oral:

Aprodine [OTC]: Triprolidine 2.5 mg and pseudoephedrine 60 mg

triprolidine, codeine, and pseudoephedrine *see* triprolidine, pseudoephedrine, and codeine *(Canada only) on page 922*

triprolidine, pseudoephedrine, and codeine *(Canada only)*

(trye PROE li deen, soo doe e FED rin, & KOE deen)

Medication Safety Issues

Sound-alike/look-alike issues:

Triacin-C® may be confused with triacetin

High alert medication:

The Institute for Safe Medication Practices (ISMP) includes this medication among its list of drug classes which have a heightened risk of causing significant patient harm when used in error.

BEERS Criteria medication:

This drug may be potentially inappropriate for use in geriatric patients (Quality of evidence - moderate; Strength of recommendation - strong).

Synonyms codeine, pseudoephedrine, and triprolidine; codeine, triprolidine, and pseudoephedrine; Cotridin; pseudoephedrine, codeine, and triprolidine; pseudoephedrine, triprolidine, and codeine; triprolidine, codeine, and pseudoephedrine

Canadian Brand Names CoActifed®; Covan®; ratio-Cotridin

Therapeutic Category Antihistamine/Decongestant/Antitussive

Controlled Substance CDSA-I

Use Symptomatic relief of upper respiratory symptoms and cough

General Dosage Range Oral:

Children 2-6 years: 2.5 mL 4 times/day

Children 7-12 years: 5 mL 4 times/day **or** 1/2 tablet 4 times/day

Children >12 years and Adults: 10 mL 4 times/day **or** 1 tablet 4 times/day

Product Availability Not available in U.S.

Dosage Forms - Canada

Syrup, oral:

CoActifed®, ratio-Cotridin: Triprolidine 2 mg, pseudoephedrine 30 mg, and codeine 10 mg per 5 mL

CoVan®: Triprolidine 2 mg, pseudoephedrine 30 mg, and codeine 10 mg per 5 mL (500 mL)

Tablet, oral:

CoActifed®: Triprolidine 4 mg, pseudoephedrine 60 mg, and codeine 20 mg (50s)

TripTone® [OTC] *see* dimenhydrinate *on page 289*

triptorelin (trip toe REL in)

Synonyms AY-25650; CL-118,532; D-Trp(6)-LHRH; detryptoreline; triptorelin pamoate; tryptoreline

U.S. Brand Names Trelstar®

Canadian Brand Names Trelstar®

Therapeutic Category Luteinizing Hormone-Releasing Hormone Analog

Use Palliative treatment of advanced prostate cancer

General Dosage Range I.M.: *Adults:* 3.75 mg once every 4 weeks **or** 11.25 mg once every 12 weeks **or** 22.5 mg once every 24 weeks

Dosage Forms

Injection, powder for reconstitution:

Trelstar®: 3.75 mg, 11.25 mg, 22.5 mg

triptorelin pamoate *see* triptorelin *on page* *922*

Triquilar® (Can) *see* ethinyl estradiol and levonorgestrel *on page* *357*

tris buffer *see* tromethamine *on page* *924*

Trisenox® *see* arsenic trioxide *on page* *91*

tris(hydroxymethyl)aminomethane *see* tromethamine *on page* *924*

trisodium calcium diethylenetriaminepentaacetate (Ca-DTPA) *see* diethylene triamine pentaacetic acid *on page* *283*

Tri-Sprintec® *see* ethinyl estradiol and norgestimate *on page* *361*

Trivagizole-3® (Can) *see* clotrimazole (topical) *on page* *227*

trivalent inactivated influenza vaccine *see* influenza virus vaccine (inactivated) *on page* *482*

Tri-Vi-Sol® [OTC] *see* vitamins (multiple/pediatric) *on page* *952*

Tri-Vi-Sol® With Iron [OTC] *see* vitamins (multiple/pediatric) *on page* *952*

Trivora® *see* ethinyl estradiol and levonorgestrel *on page* *357*

Trixaicin [OTC] *see* capsaicin *on page* *170*

Trixaicin HP [OTC] *see* capsaicin *on page* *170*

Trizivir® *see* abacavir, lamivudine, and zidovudine *on page* *16*

Trocaine® [OTC] *see* benzocaine *on page* *121*

Trocal® [OTC] [DSC] *see* dextromethorphan *on page* *272*

trolamine (TROLE a meen)

Medication Safety Issues

Sound-alike/look-alike issues:

Myoflex® may be confused with Mycelex

International issues:

Biafine: Brand name for trolamine [multiple international markets], but also the brand name for a topical emulsion [U.S.]

Synonyms TEAS; triethanolamine salicylate; trolamine salicylate

U.S. Brand Names Aspercreme® [OTC]; Flex-Power [OTC]; Mobisyl® [OTC]; Myoflex® [OTC]; Sportscreme® [OTC]

Canadian Brand Names Antiphlogistine Rub A-535 No Odour; Myoflex®

Therapeutic Category Analgesic, Topical

Use Relief of pain of muscular aches, rheumatism, neuralgia, sprains, arthritis on intact skin

General Dosage Range Topical: *Children ≥12 years and Adults:* Apply to affected area as needed up to 3-4 times/day

Dosage Forms

Cream, topical:

Aspercreme® [OTC]: 10% (35 g, 85 g, 142 g)
Flex-Power [OTC]: 10% (57 g, 113 g)
Mobisyl® [OTC]: 10% (100 g, 227 g)
Myoflex® [OTC]: 10% (57 g, 113 g)
Sportscreme® [OTC]: 10% (35 g, 85 g)

Lotion, topical:

Aspercreme® [OTC]: 10% (180 mL)

trolamine salicylate *see* trolamine *on page* *923*

Trombovar® (Can) *see* sodium tetradecyl *on page* *847*

tromethamine (troe METH a meen)

Medication Safety Issues

Sound-alike/look-alike issues:

Tromethamine may be confused with TrophAmine®

Synonyms tris buffer; tris(hydroxymethyl)aminomethane

U.S. Brand Names THAM®

Therapeutic Category Alkalinizing Agent

Use Correction of metabolic acidosis associated with cardiac bypass surgery or cardiac arrest; to correct excess acidity of stored blood that is preserved with acid citrate dextrose (ACD); indicated in infants needing alkalinization after receiving maximum sodium bicarbonate (8-10 mEq/kg/24 hours)

General Dosage Range

I.V.:

Infants: Initial: Approximately 1 mL/kg for each pH unit below 7.4; additional doses determined by changes in PaO_2, pH, and pCO_2

Adults: 3.6-10.8 g (111-333 mL) **or** 9 mL/kg (maximum: 500 mg/kg) **or** 15-77 mL added to each 500 mL of blood

Intraventricular: *Adults:* 3.6-10.8 g (111-333 mL) **or** 9 mL/kg (maximum: 500 mg/kg) **or** 15-77 mL added to each 500 mL of blood

Dosage Forms

Injection, solution:

THAM®: 18 g (500 mL)

Tronolane® Cream [OTC] *see* pramoxine *on page* 750
Tronolane® Suppository [OTC] *see* phenylephrine (topical) *on page* 717
Tropazone™ *see* emollients *on page* 328
TrophAmine® *see* amino acid injection *on page* 61
Tropicacyl® *see* tropicamide *on page* 924

tropicamide (troe PIK a mide)

Synonyms bistropamide

U.S. Brand Names Mydriacyl®; Tropicacyl®

Canadian Brand Names Diotrope®; Mydriacyl®

Therapeutic Category Anticholinergic Agent

Use Short-acting mydriatic used in diagnostic procedures; as well as preoperatively and postoperatively; treatment of some cases of acute iritis, iridocyclitis, and keratitis

General Dosage Range **Ophthalmic:** *Children and Adults:* 0.5%: Instill 1-2 drops 15-20 minutes before exam, may repeat; 1%: Instill 1-2 drops, may repeat in 5 minutes

Dosage Forms

Solution, ophthalmic: 0.5% (15 mL); 1% (2 mL, 3 mL, 15 mL)

Mydriacyl®: 1% (3 mL, 15 mL)

Tropicacyl®: 0.5% (15 mL); 1% (15 mL)

tropicamide and hydroxyamphetamine *see* hydroxyamphetamine and tropicamide *on page* 462
Trosec (Can) *see* trospium *on page* 924

trospium (TROSE pee um)

Medication Safety Issues

BEERS Criteria medication:

This drug may be potentially inappropriate for use in geriatric patients (Quality of evidence - varies based on comorbidity; Strength of recommendation - varies based on comorbidity)

Synonyms trospium chloride

U.S. Brand Names Sanctura®; Sanctura® XR

Canadian Brand Names Sanctura® XR; Trosec

Therapeutic Category Anticholinergic Agent

Use Treatment of overactive bladder with symptoms of urgency, incontinence, and urinary frequency

General Dosage Range Dosage adjustment recommended in patients with renal impairment

Oral:

Adults: Immediate release formulation: 20 mg twice daily; Extended release formulation: 60 mg once daily

Elderly ≥75 years: Immediate release formulation: Initial: 20 mg at bedtime

Dosage Forms

Capsule, extended release, oral:

Sanctura® XR: 60 mg

Tablet, oral: 20 mg

Sanctura®: 20 mg

trospium chloride *see* trospium *on page 924*

Trusopt® *see* dorzolamide *on page 310*

Truvada® *see* emtricitabine and tenofovir *on page 329*

trypsin, balsam Peru, and castor oil (TRIP sin, BAL sam pe RUE, & KAS tor oyl)

Medication Safety Issues

Sound-alike/look-alike issues:

Granulex® may be confused with Regranex®

Synonyms balsam Peru, castor oil, and trypsin; castor oil, trypsin, and balsam Peru

U.S. Brand Names Granulex®; Optase™; TBC; Vasolex™; Xenaderm®

Therapeutic Category Protectant, Topical

Use Treatment of decubitus ulcers, varicose ulcers, debridement of eschar, dehiscent wounds and sunburn; promote wound healing; reduce odor from necrotic wounds

General Dosage Range Topical: *Adults:* Apply a minimum of twice daily or as often as necessary

Dosage Forms

Aerosol, spray, topical:

Granulex®: Trypsin 0.12 mg, balsam Peru 87 mg, and castor oil 788 mg per gram (60 g, 120 g)

TBC: Trypsin 0.1 mg, balsam Peru 72.5 mg, and castor oil 650 mg per 0.82 mL (60 g, 120 g)

Gel, topical:

Optase™: Trypsin 0.12 mg, balsam Peru 87 mg, and castor oil 788 mg per gram (95 g)

Ointment, topical:

Vasolex™: Trypsin 90 USP units, balsam Peru 87 mg, and castor oil 788 mg per gram (5 g, 30 g, 60 g)

Xenaderm®: Trypsin 90 USP units, balsam Peru 87 mg, and castor oil 788 mg per gram (30 g, 60 g)

tryptoreline *see* triptorelin *on page 922*

TSH *see* thyrotropin alpha *on page 894*

TSPA *see* thiotepa *on page 892*

TST *see* tuberculin tests *on page 925*

TT *see* tetanus toxoid (adsorbed) *on page 882*

tuberculin purified protein derivative *see* tuberculin tests *on page 925*

tuberculin skin test *see* tuberculin tests *on page 925*

tuberculin tests (too BER kyoo lin tests)

Medication Safety Issues

Sound-alike/look-alike issues:

Aplisol® may be confused with Anusol®

Administration issues:

Tuberculin products may be confused with tetanus toxoid products, poliovirus vaccine (inactivated), and influenza virus vaccine. Medication errors have occurred when tuberculin skin tests (PPD) have been inadvertently administered instead of tetanus toxoid products and influenza virus vaccine. These products are refrigerated and often stored in close proximity to each other.

Synonyms Mantoux; PPD; TB skin test; TST; tuberculin purified protein derivative; tuberculin skin test

U.S. Brand Names Aplisol®; Tubersol®

Therapeutic Category Diagnostic Agent

Use Skin test in diagnosis of tuberculosis

General Dosage Range Intradermal: *Children and Adults:* 0.1 mL

Dosage Forms

Injection, solution:

Aplisol®: 5 TU/0.1 mL (1 mL, 5 mL)

Tubersol®: 5 TU/0.1 mL (1 mL, 5 mL)

Tubersol® *see* tuberculin tests *on page* 925

Tucks® Anti-Itch [OTC] *see* witch hazel *on page* 956

Tucks® Hemorrhoidal [OTC] *see* pramoxine *on page* 750

Tucks® Take Alongs® [OTC] *see* witch hazel *on page* 956

Tudorza® Pressair® *see* aclidinium *on page* 33

Tums® [OTC] *see* calcium carbonate *on page* 161

Tums® Chews Extra Strength (Can) *see* calcium carbonate *on page* 161

Tums® Dual Action [OTC] *see* famotidine, calcium carbonate, and magnesium hydroxide *on page* 373

Tums® E-X [OTC] *see* calcium carbonate *on page* 161

Tums Extra Strength (Can) *see* calcium carbonate *on page* 161

Tums® Extra Strength Sugar Free [OTC] *see* calcium carbonate *on page* 161

Tums® Quickpak [OTC] *see* calcium carbonate *on page* 161

Tums® Regular Strength (Can) *see* calcium carbonate *on page* 161

Tums® Smoothies™ [OTC] *see* calcium carbonate *on page* 161

Tums Smoothies (Can) *see* calcium carbonate *on page* 161

Tums® Ultra [OTC] *see* calcium carbonate *on page* 161

Tums® Ultra Strength (Can) *see* calcium carbonate *on page* 161

Tusscough DHC™ *see* dihydrocodeine, chlorpheniramine, and phenylephrine *on page* 287

TussiCaps® *see* hydrocodone and chlorpheniramine *on page* 455

Tussigon® *see* hydrocodone and homatropine *on page* 455

Tussionex® *see* hydrocodone and chlorpheniramine *on page* 455

Tusso™-DMR [DSC] *see* guaifenesin, dextromethorphan, and phenylephrine *on page* 437

T-Vites [OTC] *see* vitamins (multiple/oral) *on page* 951

TVP-1012 *see* rasagiline *on page* 789

Twelve Resin-K [OTC] *see* cyanocobalamin *on page* 242

Twilite® [OTC] *see* diphenhydramine (systemic) *on page* 292

Twinject® *see* epinephrine (systemic, oral inhalation) *on page* 334

Twinrix® *see* hepatitis A and hepatitis B recombinant vaccine *on page* 444

Twinrix® Junior (Can) *see* hepatitis A and hepatitis B recombinant vaccine *on page* 444

Twynsta® *see* telmisartan and amlodipine *on page* 874

Ty21a vaccine *see* typhoid vaccine *on page* 928

Tygacil® *see* tigecycline *on page* 896

Tykerb® *see* lapatinib *on page* 523

Tylenol® [OTC] *see* acetaminophen *on page* 20

Tylenol® (Can) *see* acetaminophen *on page* 20

Tylenol #2 *see* acetaminophen and codeine *on page* 22

Tylenol #3 *see* acetaminophen and codeine *on page* 22

Tylenol® 8 Hour [OTC] *see* acetaminophen *on page* 20

Tylenol® Allergy Multi-Symptom Nighttime [OTC] *see* acetaminophen, diphenhydramine, and phenylephrine *on page* 29

Tylenol® Arthritis Pain Extended Relief [OTC] *see* acetaminophen *on page* 20

Tylenol® Children's [OTC] *see* acetaminophen *on page* 20

Tylenol® Children's Meltaways [OTC] *see* acetaminophen *on page* 20

Tylenol® Children's Plus Cold and Allergy [OTC] *see* acetaminophen, diphenhydramine, and phenylephrine *on page* 29

Tylenol Codeine *see* acetaminophen and codeine *on page* 22

Tylenol® Cold & Cough Nighttime [OTC] *see* acetaminophen, dextromethorphan, and doxylamine *on page* 27

typhoid and hepatitis A vaccine *(Canada only)*

(TYE foid & hep a TYE tis aye vak SEEN)

Medication Safety Issues

Sound-alike/look-alike issues:

ViVAXIM® may be confused with Vyvanse™

Synonyms HA; hepatitis A and typhoid vaccine; Typh-1

Canadian Brand Names ViVAXIM®

Therapeutic Category Vaccine, Inactivated (Bacterial); Vaccine, Inactivated (Viral)

Use Active immunization against typhoid fever caused by *Salmonella typhi* and against disease caused by hepatitis A virus (HAV)

National Advisory Committee on Immunizations (NACI) does not recommend use for routine vaccination but does recommend that immunization be considered in the following groups:

- Travelers to areas with a prolonged risk (>4 weeks) of exposure to *S. typhi* or travelers to areas with endemic hepatitis A
- Persons with intimate exposure to a *S. typhi* carrier or who are residing in communities with high endemic rates of hepatitis A virus or at risk of outbreaks
- Laboratory technicians with frequent exposure to *S. typhi* or individuals involved in hepatitis A research or production of hepatitis A vaccine
- Travelers with achlorhydria or hypochlorhydria
- Military personnel, relief workers, or others relocated to areas with high rates of hepatitis A infection
- Persons with lifestyle risks for hepatitis A infection (eg, drug abusers, homosexual men), chronic liver disease, receiving hepatotoxic medication or with disease(s) which may necessitate use of hepatotoxic medications
- Persons with hemophilia A or B treated with plasma-derived clotting factors
- Zookeepers, veterinarians, and researchers who handle nonhuman primates

General Dosage Range I.M.: *Children ≥16 years and Adults:* 1 mL given at least 2 weeks prior to expected exposure; may administer 1 mL booster dose 3 years after previous dose when necessary

Product Availability Not available in the U.S.

Dosage Forms - Canada

Injection, solution:

ViVAXIM®: Purified Vi capsular polysaccharide 25 mcg and hepatitis A virus 160 antigen units per 1 mL [contains polysorbate 80 and neomycin]

typhoid vaccine (TYE foid vak SEEN)

Synonyms Ty21a vaccine; typhoid vaccine live oral Ty21a; Vi vaccine

U.S. Brand Names Typhim Vi®; Vivotif®

Canadian Brand Names Typherix®; Typhim Vi®; Vivotif®

Therapeutic Category Vaccine, Inactivated Bacteria

Use Active immunization against typhoid fever caused by *Salmonella typhi*

Not for routine vaccination. In the United States and Canada, use should be limited to:

- Travelers to areas with a prolonged risk of exposure to *S. typhi*
- Persons with intimate exposure to a *S. typhi* carrier
- Laboratory technicians with exposure to *S. typhi*
- Travelers with achlorhydria or hypochlorhydria (Canadian recommendation)

General Dosage Range

I.M.: *Children ≥2 years and Adults:* 0.5 mL given at least 2 weeks prior to expected exposure; may repeat every 2 years

Oral: *Children ≥6 years and Adults:* 1 capsule on alternate days for a total of 4 doses; may repeat full course every 5 years

Dosage Forms

Capsule, enteric coated:

Vivotif®: Viable *S. typhi* Ty21a 2-6.8 x 10^9 colony-forming units and nonviable *S. typhi* Ty21a 5-50 x 10^9 bacterial cells [contains lactose 100-180 mg/capsule and sucrose 26-130 mg/capsule]

Injection, solution:

Typhim Vi®: Purified Vi capsular polysaccharide 25 mcg/0.5 mL (0.5 mL, 10 mL) [derived from *S. typhi* Ty2 strain]

Dosage Forms - Canada

Injection, solution:

Typherix®: Vi capsular polysaccharide 25 mcg/0.5 mL (0.5 mL) [derived from *S. typhi* Ty2 strain]

typhoid vaccine live oral Ty21a *see* typhoid vaccine *on page 928*
Tysabri® *see* natalizumab *on page 630*
Tyvaso™ *see* treprostinil *on page 913*
Tyzeka® *see* telbivudine *on page 874*
Tyzine® *see* tetrahydrozoline (nasal) *on page 885*
Tyzine® Pediatric *see* tetrahydrozoline (nasal) *on page 885*
506U78 *see* nelarabine *on page 632*
U-90152S *see* delavirdine *on page 259*
UCB-P071 *see* cetirizine *on page 190*
U-Cort® *see* hydrocortisone (topical) *on page 457*
UK-88,525 *see* darifenacin *on page 255*
UK-427,857 *see* maraviroc *on page 562*
UK92480 *see* sildenafil *on page 832*
UK109496 *see* voriconazole *on page 953*
Ulcerease® [OTC] *see* phenol *on page 713*
Ulcidine (Can) *see* famotidine *on page 372*
Ulesfia® *see* benzyl alcohol *on page 127*

ulipristal (ue li PRIS tal)

Medication Safety Issues

Sound-alike/look-alike issues:

Ulipristal may be confused with ursodiol

Synonyms CDB-2914; ulipristal acetate

U.S. Brand Names ella®

Therapeutic Category Contraceptive; Progestin

Use Emergency contraception following unprotected intercourse or possible contraceptive failure

General Dosage Range Oral: *Adults:* 1 tablet (30 mg) as a single dose

Dosage Forms

Tablet, oral:

ella®: 30 mg

ulipristal acetate *see* ulipristal *on page* *928*
Uloric® *see* febuxostat *on page* *374*
Ultane® *see* sevoflurane *on page* *832*
Ultiva® *see* remifentanil *on page* *793*
Ultracaine® DS (Can) *see* articaine and epinephrine *on page* *92*
Ultracaine® DS Forte (Can) *see* articaine and epinephrine *on page* *92*
Ultracet® *see* acetaminophen and tramadol *on page* *25*
Ultra Freeda A-Free [OTC] *see* vitamins (multiple/oral) *on page* *951*
Ultra Freeda Iron-Free [OTC] *see* vitamins (multiple/oral) *on page* *951*
Ultra Freeda With Iron [OTC] *see* vitamins (multiple/oral) *on page* *951*
Ultram® *see* tramadol *on page* *909*
Ultram® ER *see* tramadol *on page* *909*
Ultra Mide 25® [OTC] *see* urea *on page* *930*
UltraMide 25™ (Can) *see* urea *on page* *930*
Ultramop™ (Can) *see* methoxsalen (systemic) *on page* *586*
Ultraprin [OTC] *see* ibuprofen *on page* *468*
Ultraquin™ (Can) *see* hydroquinone *on page* *461*
Ultra-R® *see* barium *on page* *114*
Ultrase® (Can) *see* pancrelipase *on page* *687*
Ultrase® MT (Can) *see* pancrelipase *on page* *687*
UltraTag® RBC *see* technetium Tc 99m-labeled red blood cells *on page* *871*
Ultravate® *see* halobetasol *on page* *440*
Ultravist® *see* iopromide *on page* *496*
Ultresa™ *see* pancrelipase *on page* *687*
Umecta® *see* urea *on page* *930*
Umecta® Nail Film *see* urea *on page* *930*
Umecta PD™ *see* urea *on page* *930*
Unasyn® *see* ampicillin and sulbactam *on page* *73*
Unburn® [OTC] *see* lidocaine (topical) *on page* *535*

undecylenic acid and derivatives (un de sil EN ik AS id & dah RIV ah tivs)

Synonyms zinc undecylenate

U.S. Brand Names Fungi-Nail® [OTC]

Therapeutic Category Antifungal Agent

Use Treatment of athlete's foot (tinea pedis); ringworm (except nails and scalp)

General Dosage Range Topical: *Children ≥2 years and Adults:* Apply twice daily to affected area

Dosage Forms

Solution, topical:

Fungi-Nail® [OTC]: Undecylenic acid 25% (29.57 mL)

Unidet® (Can) *see* tolterodine *on page* *905*
Unipen® (Can) *see* nafcillin *on page* *624*
Uniphyl (Can) *see* theophylline *on page* *888*
Uniretic® *see* moexipril and hydrochlorothiazide *on page* *609*
Unisom®-2 (Can) *see* doxylamine *on page* *315*
Unisom® SleepGels® Maximum Strength [OTC] *see* diphenhydramine (systemic) *on page* *292*
Unisom® SleepMelts™ [OTC] *see* diphenhydramine (systemic) *on page* *292*
Unithroid® *see* levothyroxine *on page* *533*
Univasc® *see* moexipril *on page* *609*

Unna boot *see* zinc gelatin *on page* 963
Unna paste *see* zinc gelatin *on page* 963
Uramaxin® *see* urea *on page* 930
Uramaxin® GT *see* urea *on page* 930
Uramaxin® GT Kit *see* urea *on page* 930
Urasal® (Can) *see* methenamine *on page* 582
urate oxidase *see* rasburicase *on page* 789
urate oxidase, pegylated *see* pegloticase *on page* 699

urea (yoor EE a)

Synonyms carbamide

U.S. Brand Names Aluvea™; Aqua Care® [OTC]; Aquaphilic® with Carbamide [OTC]; BP 50%; Carmol® 10 [OTC]; Carmol® 20 [OTC]; Carmol® 40; Carmol® Deep Cleansing [OTC]; DPM™ [OTC]; Gordon's® Urea [OTC]; Gormel® Ten [OTC]; Gormel® [OTC]; Hydro 35™; Hydro 40™; Kerafoam®; Kerafoam® 42; Keralac™; Keralac™ Nailstik; Kerol™; Kerol™ AD; Kerol™ Redi-Cloths; Kerol™ ZX; Lanaphilic® with Urea [OTC]; Nutraplus® [OTC]; Quinnostik; Rea Lo® 30 [OTC]; Rea Lo® 40; Remeven™; RevitaDERM® 40; Ultra Mide 25® [OTC]; Umecta PD™; Umecta®; Umecta® Nail Film; Uramaxin®; Uramaxin® GT; Uramaxin® GT Kit; Ureacin-10® [OTC]; Ureacin-20® [OTC]; X-Viate™

Canadian Brand Names UltraMide 25™; Uremol®; Urisec®

Therapeutic Category Diuretic, Osmotic; Topical Skin Product

Use Keratolytic agent to soften nails or skin; OTC: Moisturizer for dry, rough skin

General Dosage Range Topical: *Adults:* Apply 1-3 times/day

Dosage Forms

Aerosol, foam, topical:
- Hydro 35™: 35% (150 g)
- Hydro 40™: 40% (150 g)
- Kerafoam® 42: 42% (60 g, 100 g)
- Kerafoam®: 30% (60 g, 100 g)
- Umecta®: 40% (113.4 g)
- Uramaxin®: 20% (100 g)

Cloth, topical:
- Kerol™ Redi-Cloths: 42% (30s)

Cream, topical: 40% (28 g, 30 g, 85 g, 199 g, 210 g); 45% (255 g); 50% (142 g, 255 g)
- Aluvea™: 39% (227 g)
- Aqua Care® [OTC]: 10% (71 g)
- Carmol® 20 [OTC]: 20% (90 g)
- Carmol® 40: 40% (28 g, 85 g, 199 g)
- DPM™ [OTC]: 20% (118 g)
- Gordon's® Urea [OTC]: 40% (30 g)
- Gormel® [OTC]: 20% (75 g, 120 g, 454 g, 2270 g)
- Keralac™: 50% (142 g, 255 g)
- Nutraplus® [OTC]: 10% (85 g)
- Rea Lo® 30 [OTC]: 30% (60 g, 240 g)
- Rea Lo® 40: 40% (60 g, 240 g)
- Remeven™: 50% (142 g, 255 g)
- RevitaDERM® 40: 40% (112 g)
- Uramaxin®: 45% (255 g)
- Ureacin-20® [OTC]: 20% (113 g)
- X-Viate™: 40% (29 g, 85 g, 199 g)

Emulsion, topical: 50% (284 g, 300 g)
- BP 50%: 50% (300 g)
- Kerol™: 50% (284 g)
- Kerol™ AD: 45% (240 mL)
- Umecta PD™: 40% (198.5 g)
- Umecta®: 40% (114 g, 227 g)

Gel, topical: 40% (15 mL); 45% (28 mL); 50% (18 mL)
Carmol® 40: 40% (15 mL)
Keralac™: 50% (18 mL)
Uramaxin®: 45% (28 mL)
Uramaxin® GT: 45% (20 mL)
Uramaxin® GT Kit: 45% (20 mL)
X-Viate™: 40% (15 mL)
Lotion, topical: 35% (207 mL, 325 mL); 45% (454 g)
Aqua Care® [OTC]: 10% (240 mL)
Carmol® 10 [OTC]: 10% (180 mL)
Carmol® 40: 40% (237 mL)
Gormel® Ten [OTC]: 20% (240 mL)
Keralac™: 35% (207 mL, 325 mL)
Nutraplus® [OTC]: 10% (240 mL, 480 mL)
Ultra Mide 25® [OTC]: 25% (236 mL, 240 mL)
Uramaxin®: 45% (480 mL)
Ureacin-10® [OTC]: 10% (237 mL)
X-Viate™: 40% (237 mL)
Ointment, topical: 50% (45 g)
Aquaphilic® with Carbamide [OTC]: 10% (180 g, 454 g); 20% (454 g)
Keralac™: 50% (45 g)
Lanaphilic® with Urea [OTC]: 10% (454 g); 20% (454 g)
Shampoo, topical:
Carmol® Deep Cleansing [OTC]: 10% (240 mL)
Solution, topical: 50% (2.4 mL, 12 mL)
Keralac™ Nailstik: 50% (2.4 mL)
Kerol™ ZX: 50% (12 mL)
Quinnostik: 50% (2.4 mL)
Suspension, topical: 40% (18 mL); 50% (284 g)
Kerol™: 50% (284 g)
Umecta PD™: 40% (255.1 g)
Umecta®: 40% (283 g)
Umecta® Nail Film: 40% (3 mL, 18 mL)

urea and hydrocortisone (yoor EE a & hye droe KOR ti sone)

Synonyms hydrocortisone and urea
U.S. Brand Names Carmol-HC®
Canadian Brand Names Ti-U-Lac® H; Uremol® HC
Therapeutic Category Corticosteroid, Topical
Use Inflammation of corticosteroid-responsive dermatoses
General Dosage Range **Topical:** *Children and Adults:* Apply thin film and rub in well 2-4 times/day
Dosage Forms
Cream:
Carmol-HC®: Urea 10% and hydrocortisone 1% (30 g)

Ureacin-10® [OTC] *see* urea *on page 930*
Ureacin-20® [OTC] *see* urea *on page 930*
urea peroxide *see* carbamide peroxide *on page 173*
Urecholine® *see* bethanechol *on page 131*
Uremol® (Can) *see* urea *on page 930*
Uremol® HC (Can) *see* urea and hydrocortisone *on page 931*
Urex *see* methenamine *on page 582*
Urinary Pain Relief [OTC] *see* phenazopyridine *on page 711*
Urisec® (Can) *see* urea *on page 930*
Urispas *see* flavoxate *on page 386*
Urispas® (Can) *see* flavoxate *on page 386*
Urocit®-K *see* potassium citrate *on page 745*

urofollitropin (yoor oh fol li TROE pin)

Synonyms follicle-stimulating hormone, human; FSH; hFSH

U.S. Brand Names Bravelle®
Canadian Brand Names Bravelle®; Fertinorm® H.P.
Therapeutic Category Gonadotropin; Ovulation Stimulator
Use Ovulation induction in patients who previously received pituitary suppression; development of multiple follicles with Assisted Reproductive Technologies (ART)
General Dosage Range
I.M.: *Adults (females):* Initial: 150 units once daily for 5 days; Maintenance: Up to 450 units/day (maximum: 12 days therapy)
SubQ: *Adults (females):* Initial: 150-225 units once daily for 5 days; Maintenance: Up to 450 units/day (maximum: 12 days therapy)
Dosage Forms
Injection, powder for reconstitution:
Bravelle®: 75 units

Uro-Mag® [OTC] *see* magnesium oxide *on page* 559
Uromax® (Can) *see* oxybutynin *on page* 677
Uromitexan (Can) *see* mesna *on page* 578
Uroxatral® *see* alfuzosin *on page* 47
Urso® (Can) *see* ursodiol *on page* 932
Urso 250® *see* ursodiol *on page* 932
ursodeoxycholic acid *see* ursodiol *on page* 932

ursodiol (ur soe DYE ol)

Medication Safety Issues
Sound-alike/look-alike issues:
Ursodiol may be confused with ulipristal
Synonyms ursodeoxycholic acid
U.S. Brand Names Actigall®; Urso 250®; Urso Forte®
Canadian Brand Names Dom-Ursodiol C; PHL-Ursodiol C; PMS-Ursodiol C; Urso®; Urso® DS
Therapeutic Category Gallstone Dissolution Agent
Use
Actigall®: Gallbladder stone dissolution; prevention of gallstones in obese patients experiencing rapid weight loss
Urso®, Urso Forte®: Primary biliary cirrhosis
General Dosage Range Oral: *Adults:* 8-15 mg/kg/day in 2-4 divided doses **or** 300 mg twice daily
Dosage Forms
Capsule, oral: 300 mg
Actigall®: 300 mg
Tablet, oral: 250 mg, 500 mg
Urso 250®: 250 mg
Urso Forte®: 500 mg

Urso® DS (Can) *see* ursodiol *on page* 932
Urso Forte® *see* ursodiol *on page* 932

ustekinumab (yoo stek in YOO mab)

Medication Safety Issues
Sound-alike/look-alike issues:
Stelara™ may be confused with Aldara®
Ustekinumab may be confused with infliximab, rituximab
Synonyms CNTO 1275
U.S. Brand Names Stelara™
Canadian Brand Names Stelara™
Therapeutic Category Antipsoriatic Agent; Interleukin-12 Inhibitor; Interleukin-23 Inhibitor; Monoclonal Antibody
Use Treatment of moderate-to-severe plaque psoriasis
General Dosage Range Oral: *Adults:* ≤100 kg: 45 mg at 0- and 4 weeks, and then every 12 weeks; >100 kg: 45 mg or 90 mg at 0- and 4 weeks, and then every 12 weeks

Dosage Forms

Injection, solution [preservative free]:

Stelara™: 45 mg/0.5 mL (0.5 mL); 90 mg/mL (1 mL)

Utradol™ (Can) *see* etodolac *on page 365*

Uvadex® *see* methoxsalen (systemic) *on page 586*

vaccinia immune globulin (intravenous)

(vax IN ee a i MYUN GLOB yoo lin IN tra VEE nus)

Synonyms VIGIV

U.S. Brand Names CNJ-016®

Therapeutic Category Immune Globulin

Use Treatment of infectious complications of smallpox (vaccinia virus) vaccination, such as eczema vaccinatum, progressive vaccinia, and severe generalized vaccinia; treatment of vaccinia infections in individuals with concurrent skin conditions or accidental virus exposure to eyes (except vaccinia keratitis), mouth, or other areas where viral infection would pose significant risk

CDC guidelines for use:

Use is recommended for:

- Inadvertent inoculation (considering severity, toxicity of affected person, and pain)
- Eczema vaccinatum
- Generalized vaccinia (severe form or if underlying illness is present)
- Progressive vaccinia

Use may be considered for:

- Severe ocular complications except isolated keratitis

Use is not recommended for:

- Inadvertent inoculation that is not severe
- Mild or limited generalized vaccinia
- Nonspecific rashes, erythema multiforme, or Stevens-Johnson syndrome
- Postvaccinial encephalitis or encephalomyelitis

General Dosage Range I.V.: *Adults:* Initial: 6000 units/kg; may repeat 6000-9000 units/kg if needed (maximum: 24,000 units/kg)

Dosage Forms Injection, solution [preservative free; solvent-detergent treated]:

CNJ-016®: ≥50,000 units/15 mL (15 mL)

vaccinia vaccine *see* smallpox vaccine *on page 839*

Vagifem® *see* estradiol (topical) *on page 348*

Vagifem® 10 (Can) *see* estradiol (topical) *on page 348*

Vagi-Gard® [OTC] *see* povidone-iodine (topical) *on page 747*

Vagistat®-1 [OTC] *see* tioconazole *on page 898*

valacyclovir (val ay SYE kloe veer)

Medication Safety Issues

Sound-alike/look-alike issues:

Valtrex® may be confused with Keflex®, Valcyte®, Zovirax®

ValACYclovir may be confused with acyclovir, valGANciclovir, vancomycin

Synonyms valacyclovir hydrochloride

Tall-Man val**ACY**clovir

U.S. Brand Names Valtrex®

Canadian Brand Names Apo-Valacyclovir®; CO Valacyclovir; DOM-Valacyclovir; Mylan-Valacyclovir; PHL-Valacyclovir; PMS-Valacyclovir; PRO-Valacyclovir; Riva-Valacyclovir; Valtrex®

Therapeutic Category Antiviral Agent

Use Treatment of herpes zoster (shingles) in immunocompetent patients; treatment of first-episode and recurrent genital herpes; suppression of recurrent genital herpes and reduction of transmission of genital herpes in immunocompetent patients; suppression of genital herpes in HIV-infected individuals; treatment of herpes labialis (cold sores); chickenpox in immunocompetent children

General Dosage Range Dosage adjustment recommended in patients with renal impairment

Oral:

Children 2 to <12 years: 20 mg/kg/dose 3 times daily (maximum: 1 g 3 times daily)

Children ≥12 to <18 years: 2 g every 12 hours for 1 day (cold sores) **or** 20 mg/kg/dose 3 times daily (maximum: 1 g 3 times daily) (chickenpox)

Adults: 500 mg to 1 g 1-3 times daily **or** 2 g every 12 hours for 1 day

Dosage Forms

Caplet, oral: 500 mg, 1 g

Valtrex®: 500 mg, 1 g

Tablet, oral: 500 mg, 1 g

valacyclovir hydrochloride *see* valacyclovir *on page* 933

Valcyte® *see* valganciclovir *on page* 934

10-valent pneumococcal nontypeable *Haemophilus influenzae* protein D conjugate vaccine *see* pneumococcal conjugate vaccine (10-valent) *(Canada only) on page* 733

23-valent pneumococcal polysaccharide vaccine *see* pneumococcal polysaccharide vaccine (polyvalent) *on page* 735

valganciclovir (val gan SYE kloh veer)

Medication Safety Issues

Sound-alike/look-alike issues:

Valcyte® may be confused with Valium®, Valtrex®

ValGANciclovir may be confused with valACYclovir

Synonyms valganciclovir hydrochloride

Tall-Man val**GAN**ciclovir

U.S. Brand Names Valcyte®

Canadian Brand Names Valcyte®

Therapeutic Category Antiviral Agent

Use Treatment of cytomegalovirus (CMV) retinitis in patients with acquired immunodeficiency syndrome (AIDS); prevention of CMV disease in high-risk patients (donor CMV positive/recipient CMV negative) undergoing kidney, heart, or kidney/pancreas transplantation

General Dosage Range Dosage adjustment recommended in patients with renal impairment

Oral:

Children 4 months to 16 years: Dose (mg) = 7 x body surface area x creatinine clearance once daily

Children >16 years and Adults: 900 mg 1-2 times/day

Dosage Forms

Powder for solution, oral:

Valcyte®: 50 mg/mL (100 mL)

Tablet, oral:

Valcyte®: 450 mg

valganciclovir hydrochloride *see* valganciclovir *on page* 934

Valisone® Scalp Lotion (Can) *see* betamethasone *on page* 129

Valium® *see* diazepam *on page* 277

Valorin [OTC] *see* acetaminophen *on page* 20

Valorin Extra [OTC] *see* acetaminophen *on page* 20

valproate semisodium *see* divalproex *on page* 302

valproate semisodium *see* valproic acid *on page* 934

valproate sodium *see* valproic acid *on page* 934

valproic acid (val PROE ik AS id)

Medication Safety Issues

Sound-alike/look-alike issues:

Depakene® may be confused with Depakote®

Valproate sodium may be confused with vecuronium

Synonyms 2-propylpentanoic acid; 2-propylvaleric acid; dipropylacetic acid; DPA; valproate semisodium; valproate sodium

U.S. Brand Names Depacon®; Depakene®; Stavzor™

Canadian Brand Names Apo-Valproic®; Depakene®; Epival® I.V.; Mylan-Valproic; PHL-Valproic Acid; PHL-Valproic Acid E.C.; PMS-Valproic Acid; PMS-Valproic Acid E.C.; ratio-Valproic; ratio-Valproic ECC; Rhoxal-valproic; Sandoz-Valproic

Therapeutic Category Anticonvulsant, Miscellaneous; Antimanic Agent; Histone Deacetylase Inhibitor

Use Monotherapy and adjunctive therapy in the treatment of patients with complex partial seizures; monotherapy and adjunctive therapy of simple and complex absence seizures; adjunctive therapy in patients with multiple seizure types that include absence seizures

Stavzor™: Mania associated with bipolar disorder; migraine prophylaxis

General Dosage Range Dosage adjustment recommended in patients with hepatic impairment

I.V.:

Children: Initial: 15 mg/kg/day; Maximum: 60 mg/kg/day

Children ≥10 years and Adults: Initial: 10-15 mg/kg/day; Maximum: 60 mg/kg/day

Oral:

Children: Initial: 15 mg/kg/day; Maximum: 60 mg/kg/day

Children ≥10 years and Adults: Seizures: Initial: 10-15 mg/kg/day; Maximum: 60 mg/kg/day

Children ≥12 years and Adults: Stavzor™: Initial: 250 mg twice daily; Maintenance: Up to 1000 mg/day

Adults: Mania (Stavzor™): Initial: 750 mg/day in divided doses; Maximum recommended dose: 60 mg/kg/day

Dosage Forms

Capsule, softgel, oral: 250 mg

Depakene®: 250 mg

Capsule, softgel, delayed release, oral:

Stavzor™: 125 mg, 250 mg, 500 mg

Injection, solution: 100 mg/mL (5 mL)

Injection, solution [preservative free]: 100 mg/mL (5 mL)

Depacon®: 100 mg/mL (5 mL)

Solution, oral: 250 mg/5 mL (5 mL, 473 mL, 480 mL)

Syrup, oral: 250 mg/5 mL (5 mL, 10 mL, 473 mL, 480 mL)

Depakene®: 250 mg/5 mL (473 mL)

valproic acid derivative *see* divalproex *on page 302*

valrubicin (val ROO bi sin)

Medication Safety Issues

Sound-alike/look-alike issues:

Valrubicin may be confused with DAUNOrubicin, DOXOrubicin, epirubicin, IDArubicin

Valstar® may be confused with valsartan

High alert medication:

The medication is in a class the Institute for Safe Medication Practices (ISMP) includes among its list of drug classes which have a heightened risk of causing significant patient harm when used in error.

Synonyms *N*-trifluoroacetyladriamycin-14-valerate; AD32

U.S. Brand Names Valstar®

Canadian Brand Names Valtaxin®

Therapeutic Category Antineoplastic Agent, Anthracycline

Use Intravesical treatment of BCG-refractory bladder carcinoma *in situ*

General Dosage Range Dosage adjustment recommended in patients who develop toxicities

Intravesical: *Adults:* 800 mg once weekly for 6 weeks

Dosage Forms

Injection, solution [preservative free]:

Valstar®: 40 mg/mL (5 mL)

valsartan (val SAR tan)

Medication Safety Issues

Sound-alike/look-alike issues:

Valsartan may be confused with losartan, Valstar®, Valturna®

Diovan® may be confused with Zyban®

International issues:

Diovan [U.S., Canada, and multiple international markets] may be confused with Dianben, a brand name for metformin [Spain]

U.S. Brand Names Diovan®

Canadian Brand Names CO Valsartan; Diovan®; Ran-Valsartan; Sandoz-Valsartan; Teva-Valsartan
Therapeutic Category Angiotensin II Receptor Antagonist
Use Alone or in combination with other antihypertensive agents in the treatment of essential hypertension; reduction of cardiovascular mortality in patients with left ventricular dysfunction postmyocardial infarction; treatment of heart failure (NYHA Class II-IV)
General Dosage Range Oral:
Children 6-16 years: Initial: 1.3 mg/kg once daily (maximum: 40 mg/day); Maintenance: Up to 2.7 mg/kg; 160 mg
Adults: Initial: 20-40 mg twice daily **or** 80-160 mg once daily; Maintenance: 80-160 mg twice daily (maximum: 320 mg/day)
Dosage Forms
Tablet, oral:
Diovan®: 40 mg, 80 mg, 160 mg, 320 mg

valsartan and aliskiren *see* aliskiren and valsartan *on page 49*
valsartan and amlodipine *see* amlodipine and valsartan *on page 67*

valsartan and hydrochlorothiazide (val SAR tan & hye droe klor oh THYE a zide)

Medication Safety Issues
Sound-alike/look-alike issues:
Diovan® may be confused with Zyban®
Synonyms hydrochlorothiazide and valsartan
U.S. Brand Names Diovan HCT®
Canadian Brand Names Diovan HCT®; Sandoz Valsartan HCT; Teva-Valsartan HCTZ; Valsartan-HCTZ
Therapeutic Category Antihypertensive Agent, Combination
Use Treatment of hypertension
General Dosage Range Oral: *Adults:* Valsartan 80-320 mg and hydrochlorothiazide 12.5-25 mg once daily (maximum: 25 mg/day [hydrochlorothiazide]; 320 mg/day [valsartan])
Dosage Forms
Tablet:
Diovan HCT®: 80 mg/12.5 mg: Valsartan 80 mg and hydrochlorothiazide 12.5 mg; 160 mg/12.5 mg: Valsartan 160 mg and hydrochlorothiazide 12.5 mg; 160 mg/25 mg: Valsartan 160 mg and hydrochlorothiazide 25 mg; 320 mg/12.5 mg: Valsartan 320 mg and hydrochlorothiazide 12.5 mg; 320 mg/25 mg: Valsartan 320 mg and hydrochlorothiazide 25 mg

Valsartan-HCTZ (Can) *see* valsartan and hydrochlorothiazide *on page 936*
valsartan, hydrochlorothiazide, and amlodipine *see* amlodipine, valsartan, and hydrochlorothiazide *on page 68*
Valstar® *see* valrubicin *on page 935*
Valtaxin® (Can) *see* valrubicin *on page 935*
Valtrex® *see* valacyclovir *on page 933*
Valturna® [DSC] *see* aliskiren and valsartan *on page 49*
Val-Vancomycin (Can) *see* vancomycin *on page 936*
Vanceril *see* beclomethasone (oral inhalation) *on page 117*
Vancocin® *see* vancomycin *on page 936*

vancomycin (van koe MYE sin)

Medication Safety Issues
Sound-alike/look-alike issues:
I.V. vancomycin may be confused with INVanz®
Vancomycin may be confused with clindamycin, gentamicin, tobramycin, valACYclovir, vecuronium, Vibramycin®
High alert medication:
The Institute for Safe Medication Practices (ISMP) includes this medication (intrathecal administration) among its list of drug classes which have a heightened risk of causing significant patient harm when used in error.
Synonyms vancomycin hydrochloride
U.S. Brand Names Vancocin®

Canadian Brand Names PMS-Vancomycin; Sterile Vancomycin Hydrochloride, USP; Val-Vancomycin; Vancocin®; Vancomycin Hydrochloride for Injection, USP

Therapeutic Category Antibiotic, Miscellaneous

Use

I.V.: Treatment of patients with infections caused by staphylococcal species and streptococcal species

Oral: Treatment of *C. difficile*-associated diarrhea and treatment of enterocolitis caused by *Staphylococcus aureus* (including methicillin-resistant strains)

General Dosage Range Dosage adjustment recommended in patients with renal impairment

I.V.:

Infants >1 month: 40-60 mg/kg/day in divided doses every 6 hours

Children: 40-60 mg/kg/day in divided doses every 6 hours **or** 20 mg/kg as a single dose

Adults: 30-60 mg/kg/day in divided doses every 6-12 hours **or** 500-750 mg every 6 hours **or** 1000 mg as a single dose

Intracatheter, intraventricular: *Children and Adults:* 2-5 mg/mL instilled into catheter port with a volume sufficient to fill the catheter (2-5 mL)

Intrathecal: *Children and Adults:* 5-20 mg/day

Oral:

Children: 40 mg/kg/day in 3-4 divided doses (maximum: 2000 mg/day)

Adults: 500-2000 mg/day in 3-4 divided doses (maximum: 2000 mg/day)

Dosage Forms

Capsule, oral: 125 mg, 250 mg

Vancocin®: 125 mg, 250 mg

Infusion, premixed iso-osmotic dextrose solution: 500 mg (100 mL); 750 mg (150 mL); 1 g (200 mL)

Injection, powder for reconstitution: 500 mg, 750 mg, 1 g, 5 g, 10 g

vancomycin hydrochloride *see* vancomycin *on page* 936

Vancomycin Hydrochloride for Injection, USP (Can) *see* vancomycin *on page* 936

Vandazole® *see* metronidazole (topical) *on page* 597

vandetanib (van DET a nib)

Medication Safety Issues

Sound-alike/look-alike issues:

Vandetanib may be confused with axitinib, dasatinib, erlotinib, gefitinib, imatinib, lapatinib, nilotinib, pazopanib, SORAfenib, SUNItinib, vemurafenib, vismodegib

High alert medication:

This medication is in a class the Institute for Safe Medication Practices (ISMP) includes among its list of drug classes which have a heightened risk of causing significant patient harm when used in error.

Synonyms AZD6474; Zactima; ZD6474; Zictifa

U.S. Brand Names Caprelsa®

Canadian Brand Names Caprelsa®

Therapeutic Category Antineoplastic Agent, Tyrosine Kinase Inhibitor; Epidermal Growth Factor Receptor (EGFR) Inhibitor; Vascular Endothelial Growth Factor (VEGF) Inhibitor

Use Treatment of metastatic or unresectable locally advanced medullary thyroid cancer (symptomatic or progressive)

General Dosage Range Note: Do not initiate treatment unless QTcF <450 msec. Avoid concomitant use of QT-prolonging agents and strong CYP3A4 inducers. To reduce the risk of QT prolongation, maintain serum calcium and magnesium within normal limits and maintain serum potassium ≥4 mEq/L.

Medullary thyroid cancer, locally advanced or metastatic: Oral: 300 mg once daily, continue treatment until no longer clinically benefiting or until unacceptable toxicity

Dosage Forms

Tablet, oral: 100 mg, 300 mg

Caprelsa®: 100 mg, 300 mg

Vaniqa® *see* eflornithine *on page* 325

Vanos® *see* fluocinonide *on page* 392

Vanoxide-HC® *see* benzoyl peroxide and hydrocortisone *on page* 125

Vanquish® Extra Strength Pain Reliever [OTC] *see* acetaminophen, aspirin, and caffeine *on page* 26

Vantin *see* cefpodoxime *on page* 184

Vaprisol® *see* conivaptan *on page* 235

VAQTA® *see* hepatitis A vaccine *on page 444*

VAR *see* varicella virus vaccine *on page 939*

vardenafil (var DEN a fil)

Medication Safety Issues

Sound-alike/look-alike issues:

Vardenafil may be confused with sildenafil, tadalafil

Levitra® may be confused with Kaletra®, Lexiva®

Synonyms vardenafil hydrochloride

U.S. Brand Names Levitra®; Staxyn™

Canadian Brand Names Levitra®; Staxyn™

Therapeutic Category Phosphodiesterase (Type 5) Enzyme Inhibitor

Use Treatment of erectile dysfunction (ED)

General Dosage Range Dosage adjustment recommended in patients with hepatic impairment or on concomitant therapy

Oral:

Adults: Film-coated tablet (Levitra®): 2.5-20 mg as a single dose (maximum: 1 dose/day); Oral disintegrating tablet (Staxyn™): 10 mg as a single dose (maximum: 10 mg/day)

Elderly ≥65 years: 2.5-5 mg as a single dose (maximum: 1 dose/day)

Dosage Forms

Tablet, oral:

Levitra®: 2.5 mg, 5 mg, 10 mg, 20 mg

Tablet, orally disintegrating, oral:

Staxyn™: 10 mg

vardenafil hydrochloride *see* vardenafil *on page 938*

varenicline (var e NI kleen)

Synonyms varenicline tartrate

U.S. Brand Names Chantix®

Canadian Brand Names Champix®

Therapeutic Category Partial Nicotine Agonist

Use Treatment to aid in smoking cessation

General Dosage Range Dosage adjustment recommended in patients with renal impairment or who develop toxicities

Oral: *Adults:* Days 1-3: 0.5 mg once daily; Days 4-7: 0.5 mg twice daily; Maintenance (≥Day 8): 1 mg twice daily

Dosage Forms

Combination package, oral:

Chantix®: Tablet: 0.5 mg (11s) [white tablets] and Tablet: 1 mg (42s) [light blue tablets]

Tablet, oral:

Chantix®: 0.5 mg, 1 mg

varenicline tartrate *see* varenicline *on page 938*

Varibar® Honey *see* barium *on page 114*

Varibar® Nectar *see* barium *on page 114*

Varibar® Pudding *see* barium *on page 114*

Varibar® Thin Honey *see* barium *on page 114*

Varibar® Thin Liquid *see* barium *on page 114*

varicella, measles, mumps, and rubella vaccine *see* measles, mumps, rubella, and varicella virus vaccine *on page 564*

varicella virus vaccine (var i SEL a VYE rus vak SEEN)

Medication Safety Issues

Sound-alike/look-alike issues:

Varicella virus vaccine has been given in error (instead of the indicated varicella immune globulin) to pregnant women exposed to varicella.

Other safety concerns:

Both varicella vaccine and zoster vaccine are live, attenuated strains of varicella-zoster virus. Their indications, dosing, and composition are distinct. Varicella is indicated in children to prevent chickenpox, while zoster vaccine is indicated in older individuals to prevent reactivation of the virus which causes shingles. Zoster vaccine is **not** a substitute for varicella vaccine and should not be used in children.

Synonyms chickenpox vaccine; VAR; varicella-zoster virus (VZV) vaccine (varicella); VZV vaccine (varicella)

U.S. Brand Names Varivax®

Canadian Brand Names Varilrix®; Varivax® III

Therapeutic Category Vaccine, Live Virus

Use Immunization against varicella in children ≥12 months of age and adults

The ACIP recommends vaccination for all children, adolescents, and adults who do not have evidence of immunity. Vaccination is especially important for:

- Healthcare personnel
- Persons with close contact to those at high risk for severe disease
- Persons living or working in environments where transmission is likely (teachers, child-care workers, residents and staff of institutional settings)
- Persons in environments where transmission has been reported
- Nonpregnant women of childbearing age
- Adolescents and adults in households with children
- International travelers

Postexposure prophylaxis: Vaccination within 3 days (possibly 5 days) after exposure to rash is effective in preventing illness or modifying severity of disease

General Dosage Range SubQ:

Children 12 months to 12 years: 0.5 mL as a single dose; may repeat in ≥3 months

Children ≥13 years and Adults: 2 doses of 0.5 mL separated by 4-8 weeks

Dosage Forms

Injection, powder for reconstitution [preservative free]:

Varivax®: 1350 PFU

Dosage Forms - Canada

Injection, powder for reconstitution [preservative free]:

Varivax® III: 1350 plaque-forming units (PFU)

Injection, powder for reconstitution:

Valrilix®: $10^{3.3}$ plaque-forming units (PFU)

varicella-zoster immune globulin (human)

(var i SEL a- ZOS ter i MYUN GLOB yoo lin HYU man)

Medication Safety Issues

Sound-alike/look-alike issues:

Varicella virus vaccine has been given in error (instead of the indicated varicella immune globulin) to pregnant women exposed to varicella.

Synonyms VZIG

Canadian Brand Names VariZIG™

Therapeutic Category Immune Globulin

Use In pregnant women, for the prevention or reduction in severity of maternal infection within 4 days of exposure to the varicella zoster virus.

General Dosage Range I.M., I.V.: *Adults:* 125 units/10 kg (minimum dose: 125 units; maximum dose: 625 units)

Dosage Forms - Canada

Injection, powder for reconstitution [preservative free]:

VariZIG™: 125 units

varicella-zoster virus (VZV) vaccine (varicella) *see* varicella virus vaccine *on page 939*

varicella-zoster (VZV) vaccine (zoster) *see* zoster vaccine *on page 968*
Varilrix® (Can) *see* varicella virus vaccine *on page 939*
Varivax® *see* varicella virus vaccine *on page 939*
Varivax® III (Can) *see* varicella virus vaccine *on page 939*
VariZIG™ (Can) *see* varicella-zoster immune globulin (human) *on page 939*
Vascepa™ *see* icosapent ethyl *on page 472*
vascular endothelial growth factor trap *see* ziv-aflibercept (systemic) *on page 964*
Vaseretic® *see* enalapril and hydrochlorothiazide *on page 330*
Vasocon® (Can) *see* naphazoline (ophthalmic) *on page 627*
Vasodilan *see* isoxsuprine *on page 506*
Vasolex™ *see* trypsin, balsam Peru, and castor oil *on page 925*

vasopressin (vay soe PRES in)

Medication Safety Issues

High alert medication:

The Institute for Safe Medication Practices (ISMP) includes this medication (I.V. or intraosseous administration) among its list of drugs which have a heightened risk of causing significant patient harm when used in error.

Administration issues:

Use care when prescribing and/or administering vasopressin solutions. Close attention should be given to concentration of solution, route of administration, dose, and rate of administration (units/minute, units/kg/minute, units/kg/hour).

Synonyms 8-arginine vasopressin; ADH; antidiuretic hormone; AVP

U.S. Brand Names Pitressin®

Canadian Brand Names Pressyn®; Pressyn® AR

Therapeutic Category Hormone, Posterior Pituitary

Use Treatment of central diabetes insipidus; differential diagnosis of diabetes insipidus

General Dosage Range I.M., SubQ:

Children: 2.5-10 units 2-4 times/day as needed

Adults: 5-10 units 2-4 times/day as needed

Dosage Forms

Injection, solution: 20 units/mL (0.5 mL, 1 mL, 10 mL)

Pitressin®: 20 units/mL (1 mL)

Vasotec® *see* enalapril *on page 330*
Vasotec® I.V (Can) *see* enalaprilat *on page 330*
Vaxigrip® (Can) *see* influenza virus vaccine (inactivated) *on page 482*
Vazobid-PD™ [OTC] *see* brompheniramine and phenylephrine *on page 144*
VCF® [OTC] *see* nonoxynol 9 *on page 647*
Vectibix® *see* panitumumab *on page 688*
Vectical® *see* calcitriol *on page 160*

vecuronium (vek ue ROE nee um)

Medication Safety Issues

Sound-alike/look-alike issues:

Vecuronium may be confused with valproate sodium, vancomycin

Norcuron® may be confused with Narcan®

High alert medication:

The Institute for Safe Medication Practices (ISMP) includes this medication among its list of drugs which have a heightened risk of causing significant patient harm when used in error.

Other safety concerns:

United States Pharmacopeia (USP) 2006: The Interdisciplinary Safe Medication Use Expert Committee of the USP has recommended the following:

- Hospitals, clinics, and other practice sites should institute special safeguards in the storage, labeling, and use of these agents and should include these safeguards in staff orientation and competency training.
- Healthcare professionals should be on high alert (especially vigilant) whenever a neuromuscular-blocking agent (NMBA) is stocked, ordered, prepared, or administered.

Synonyms Norcuron; ORG NC 45

Canadian Brand Names Norcuron®

Therapeutic Category Skeletal Muscle Relaxant

Use To facilitate endotracheal intubation and to relax skeletal muscles during surgery; to facilitate mechanical ventilation in ICU patients; does not relieve pain or produce sedation

General Dosage Range Dosage adjustment recommended in patients with hepatic impairment

I.V.: *Children ≥1 year and Adults:* Initial: 0.04-0.1 mg/kg; Maintenance: 0.01-0.015 mg/kg every 12-15 minutes **or** 0.8-1.2 mcg/kg/minute as a continuous infusion

Dosage Forms

Injection, powder for reconstitution: 10 mg, 20 mg

VEGF trap *see* aflibercept (ophthalmic) *on page 38*

VEGF trap *see* ziv-aflibercept (systemic) *on page 964*

VEGF trap-eye *see* aflibercept (ophthalmic) *on page 38*

VEGF trap R1R2 *see* ziv-aflibercept (systemic) *on page 964*

velaglucerase alfa (vel a GLOO ser ase AL fa)

Synonyms gene-activated human acid-beta-glucosidase; glcCerase

U.S. Brand Names VPRIV™

Canadian Brand Names VPRIV™

Therapeutic Category Enzyme

Use Long-term enzyme replacement therapy for patients with type 1 Gaucher disease

General Dosage Range I.V.: *Children ≥4 years and Adults:* 15-60 units/kg every other week

Dosage Forms

Injection, powder for reconstitution:

VPRIV™: 400 units

Velban *see* vinblastine *on page 946*

Velcade® *see* bortezomib *on page 139*

Veletri® *see* epoprostenol *on page 338*

Velivet™ *see* ethinyl estradiol and desogestrel *on page 356*

Veltin™ *see* clindamycin and tretinoin *on page 219*

vemurafenib (vem ue RAF e nib)

Medication Safety Issues

Sound-alike/look-alike issues:

Vemurafenib may be confused with axitinib, SORAfenib, vandetanib, vismodegib

High alert medication:

This medication is in a class the Institute for Safe Medication Practices (ISMP) includes among its list of drug classes which have a heightened risk of causing significant patient harm when used in error.

Synonyms BRAF(V600E) kinase inhibitor RO5185426; PLX4032; RG7024; RO5185426

U.S. Brand Names Zelboraf™

Canadian Brand Names Zelboraf™

Therapeutic Category Antineoplastic Agent, BRAF Kinase Inhibitor

Use Treatment of unresectable or metastatic melanoma in patients with a $BRAF^{V600E}$ mutation (as detected by an FDA-approved test)

Note: Not recommended in patients with wild-type BRAF melanoma

General Dosage Range Dosage adjustment recommended in patients who develop toxicities.

Oral: *Adults:* 960 mg twice daily

Dosage Forms

Tablet, oral:

Zelboraf™: 240 mg

venlafaxine (ven la FAX een)

Medication Safety Issues

Sound-alike/look-alike issues:

Effexor® may be confused with Effexor XR®

BEERS Criteria medication:

This drug may be potentially inappropriate for use in geriatric patients (Quality of evidence - moderate; Strength of recommendation - strong).

U.S. Brand Names Effexor XR®; Effexor®

Canadian Brand Names CO Venlafaxine XR; Effexor XR®; GD-Venlafaxine XR; Mylan-Venlafaxine XR; PMS-Venlafaxine XR; Ran-Venlafaxine XR; ratio-Venlafaxine XR; Riva-Venlafaxine XR; Sandoz-Venlafaxine XR; Teva-Venlafaxine XR; Venlafaxine XR

Therapeutic Category Antidepressant, Phenethylamine

Use Treatment of major depressive disorder, generalized anxiety disorder (GAD), social anxiety disorder (social phobia), panic disorder

General Dosage Range Dosage adjustment recommended in patients with hepatic or renal impairment

Oral:

Extended release: *Adults:* Initial: 37.5-75 mg/day once daily; Maintenance: 75-225 mg/day once daily (recommended maximum: 225 mg/day)

Immediate release: *Adults:* Initial: 75 mg/day in 2-3 divided doses; Maintenance: 75-375 mg/day in 2-3 divided doses (recommended maximum: 375 mg/day)

Dosage Forms

Capsule, extended release, oral: 37.5 mg, 75 mg, 150 mg

Effexor XR®: 37.5 mg, 75 mg, 150 mg

Tablet, oral: 25 mg, 37.5 mg, 50 mg, 75 mg, 100 mg

Effexor®: 50 mg

Tablet, extended release, oral: 37.5 mg, 75 mg, 150 mg, 225 mg

Venlafaxine XR (Can) *see* venlafaxine *on page* *942*

Venofer® *see* iron sucrose *on page* *502*

Ventavis® *see* iloprost *on page* *474*

Ventolin® (Can) *see* albuterol *on page* *41*

Ventolin® Diskus (Can) *see* albuterol *on page* *41*

Ventolin® HFA *see* albuterol *on page* *41*

Ventolin® I.V. Infusion (Can) *see* albuterol *on page* *41*

Ventolin® Nebules P.F. (Can) *see* albuterol *on page* *41*

VePesid *see* etoposide *on page* *366*

Vepesid™ (Can) *see* etoposide *on page* *366*

Veracolate® [OTC] *see* bisacodyl *on page* *134*

Veramyst® *see* fluticasone (nasal) *on page* *400*

verapamil (ver AP a mil)

Medication Safety Issues

Sound-alike/look-alike issues:

Calan® may be confused with Colace®, diltiazem

Covera-HS® may be confused with Provera®

Isoptin® may be confused with Isopto® Tears

Verelan® may be confused with Voltaren®

High alert medication:

The Institute for Safe Medication Practices (ISMP) includes this medication (I.V. formulation) among its list of drug classes which have a heightened risk of causing significant patient harm when used in error.

Administration issues:

Significant differences exist between oral and I.V. dosing. Use caution when converting from one route of administration to another.

International issues:

Dilacor [Brazil] may be confused with Dilacor XR brand name for diltiazem [U.S.]

Synonyms iproveratril hydrochloride; verapamil hydrochloride

U.S. Brand Names Calan®; Calan® SR; Covera-HS® [DSC]; Isoptin® SR; Verelan®; Verelan® PM

Canadian Brand Names Apo-Verap®; Apo-Verap® SR; Covera-HS®; Covera®; Dom-Verapamil SR; Isoptin® SR; Mylan-Verapamil; Mylan-Verapamil SR; Novo-Veramil; Novo-Veramil SR; Nu-Verap; Nu-Verap SR; PHL-Verapamil SR; PMS-Verapamil SR; PRO-Verapamil SR; Riva-Verapamil SR; Verapamil Hydrochloride Injection, USP; Verapamil SR; Verelan®

Therapeutic Category Antiarrhythmic Agent, Class IV; Calcium Channel Blocker

Use

Oral: Treatment of hypertension; angina pectoris (vasospastic, chronic stable, unstable) (Calan®, Covera-HS®); supraventricular tachyarrhythmia (PSVT, atrial fibrillation/flutter [rate control])

I.V.: Supraventricular tachyarrhythmia (PSVT, atrial fibrillation/flutter [rate control])

General Dosage Range

I.V.:

Children 1-15 years: 0.1-0.3 mg/kg/dose (maximum: 5 mg/dose); may repeat dose (maximum for second dose: 10 mg)

Adults: Initial dose: 2.5-5 mg; Second dose: 5-10 mg (maximum: 20-30 mg total dose)

Oral:

Extended release:

Adults: 180-480 mg once daily

Elderly: Initial: 100-180 mg once daily

Immediate release: *Adults:* Initial: 80-120 mg 3 times/day; Maintenance: 80-480 mg/day in 2-4 divided doses (maximum: 480 mg/day)

Sustained release:

Adults: 120-480 mg/day in 1-2 divided doses (maximum: 480 mg/day)

Elderly: Initial: 120 mg/day once daily; Maintenance: 120-360 mg/day in 1-2 divided doses

Dosage Forms

Caplet, sustained release, oral:

Calan® SR: 120 mg, 180 mg, 240 mg

Capsule, extended release, oral: 120 mg, 180 mg, 240 mg

Capsule, extended release, controlled onset, oral: 100 mg, 200 mg, 300 mg

Verelan® PM: 100 mg, 200 mg, 300 mg

Capsule, sustained release, oral: 120 mg, 180 mg, 240 mg, 360 mg

Verelan®: 120 mg, 180 mg, 240 mg, 360 mg

Injection, solution: 2.5 mg/mL (2 mL, 4 mL)

Tablet, oral: 40 mg, 80 mg, 120 mg

Calan®: 80 mg, 120 mg

Tablet, extended release, oral: 120 mg, 180 mg, 240 mg

Tablet, sustained release, oral: 120 mg, 180 mg, 240 mg

Isoptin® SR: 120 mg, 180 mg

verapamil and trandolapril *see* trandolapril and verapamil *on page 910*

verapamil hydrochloride *see* verapamil *on page 942*

Verapamil Hydrochloride Injection, USP (Can) *see* verapamil *on page 942*

Verapamil SR (Can) *see* verapamil *on page 942*

Verdeso® *see* desonide *on page 265*

Verdeso™ (Can) *see* desonide *on page 265*

Veregen® *see* sinecatechins *on page 836*

Verelan® *see* verapamil *on page 942*

Verelan® PM *see* verapamil *on page 942*

Veripred™ 20 *see* prednisolone (systemic) *on page 754*

Vermox *see* mebendazole *on page 565*

Vermox® (Can) *see* mebendazole *on page 565*

Versed *see* midazolam *on page 601*

Versel® (Can) *see* selenium sulfide *on page 828*

verteporfin (ver te POR fin)

Synonyms Photodynamic Therapy

U.S. Brand Names Visudyne®

Canadian Brand Names Visudyne®

Therapeutic Category Ophthalmic Agent

Use Treatment of predominantly classic subfoveal choroidal neovascularization due to age-related macular degeneration, presumed ocular histoplasmosis, or pathologic myopia

General Dosage Range I.V.: *Adults:* 6 mg/m^2 body surface area

Dosage Forms

Injection, powder for reconstitution:

Visudyne®: 15 mg

VertiCalm™ [OTC] *see* meclizine *on page* *566*
Vesanoid *see* tretinoin (systemic) *on page 913*
Vesanoid® (Can) *see* tretinoin (systemic) *on page 913*
VESIcare® *see* solifenacin *on page 848*
Vestura™ *see* ethinyl estradiol and drospirenone *on page 356*
Vexol® *see* rimexolone *on page 802*
VFEND® *see* voriconazole *on page 953*
Viactiv® [OTC] *see* vitamins (multiple/oral) *on page 951*
Viactiv® Calcium Flavor Glides™ [OTC] *see* vitamins (multiple/oral) *on page 951*
Viactiv® Flavor Glides [OTC] *see* vitamins (multiple/oral) *on page 951*
Viactiv® for Teens [OTC] *see* vitamins (multiple/oral) *on page 951*
Viactiv® With Calcium [OTC] *see* vitamins (multiple/oral) *on page 951*
Viagra® *see* sildenafil *on page 832*
Vibativ™ *see* telavancin *on page 873*
Vibramycin® *see* doxycycline *on page 314*
Vibra-Tabs® (Can) *see* doxycycline *on page 314*
***Vibrio cholera* and enterotoxigenic *Escherichia coli* vaccine** *see* traveler's diarrhea and cholera vaccine *(Canada only) on page 911*
Vicks® 44® Cough Relief [OTC] *see* dextromethorphan *on page 272*
Vicks® 44E [OTC] *see* guaifenesin and dextromethorphan *on page 434*
Vicks® Casero™ Chest Congestion Relief [OTC] *see* guaifenesin *on page 433*
Vicks® DayQuil® Cold & Flu Multi-Symptom [OTC] *see* acetaminophen, dextromethorphan, and phenylephrine *on page 28*
Vicks® DayQuil® Cough [OTC] *see* dextromethorphan *on page 272*
Vicks® DayQuil® Mucus Control [OTC] *see* guaifenesin *on page 433*
Vicks® DayQuil® Mucus Control DM [OTC] *see* guaifenesin and dextromethorphan *on page 434*
Vicks® DayQuil® Sinex® Daytime Sinus [OTC] *see* acetaminophen and phenylephrine *on page 24*
Vicks® Formula 44® Sore Throat [OTC] *see* phenol *on page 713*
Vicks® Nature Fusion™ Cold & Flu Multi-Symptom Relief [OTC] *see* acetaminophen, dextromethorphan, and phenylephrine *on page 28*
Vicks® Nature Fusion™ Cold & Flu Nighttime Relief [OTC] *see* acetaminophen, dextromethorphan, and doxylamine *on page 27*
Vicks® Nature Fusion™ Cough [OTC] *see* dextromethorphan *on page 272*
Vicks® Nature Fusion™ Cough & Chest Congestion [OTC] *see* guaifenesin and dextromethorphan *on page 434*
Vicks® NyQuil® Cold & Flu Multi-Symptom [OTC] [DSC] *see* acetaminophen, dextromethorphan, and doxylamine *on page 27*
Vicks® NyQuil® Cold & Flu Nighttime Relief [OTC] *see* acetaminophen, dextromethorphan, and doxylamine *on page 27*
Vicks® Pediatric Formula 44E [OTC] *see* guaifenesin and dextromethorphan *on page 434*
Vicks® Sinex® VapoSpray 12-Hour *see* oxymetazoline (nasal) *on page 681*
Vicks® Sinex® VapoSpray 12-Hour UltraFine Mist [OTC] *see* oxymetazoline (nasal) *on page 681*
Vicks® Sinex® VapoSpray Moisturizing 12-Hour UltraFine Mist [OTC] *see* oxymetazoline (nasal) *on page 681*
Vicks® Vitamin C [OTC] *see* ascorbic acid *on page 94*
Vicks® ZzzQuil™ [OTC] *see* diphenhydramine (systemic) *on page 292*
Vicodin® *see* hydrocodone and acetaminophen *on page 454*

Vicodin® ES *see* hydrocodone and acetaminophen *on page 454*

Vicodin® HP *see* hydrocodone and acetaminophen *on page 454*

Vicoprofen® *see* hydrocodone and ibuprofen *on page 456*

Victoza® *see* liraglutide *on page 543*

Victrelis® *see* boceprevir *on page 138*

Vidaza® *see* azacitidine *on page 106*

Videx® *see* didanosine *on page 282*

Videx® EC *see* didanosine *on page 282*

vigabatrin (vye GA ba trin)

Medication Safety Issues

Sound-alike/look-alike issues:

Vigabatrin may be confused with Vibativ™

U.S. Brand Names Sabril®

Canadian Brand Names Sabril®

Therapeutic Category Anticonvulsant

Use Treatment of infantile spasms; refractory complex partial seizures not controlled by usual treatments

Canadian labeling: Additional uses (not in U.S. labeling): Active management of partial or secondary generalized seizures not controlled by usual treatments

General Dosage Range Dosage adjustment recommended in patients with renal impairment

Oral:

Infants: 50-150 mg/kg/day in 2 divided doses

Adults: 1-3 g/day in 2 divided doses

Dosage Forms

Powder for solution, oral:

Sabril®: 500 mg/packet (50s)

Tablet, oral:

Sabril®: 500 mg

Dosage Forms - Canada

Powder for suspension, oral [sachets]:

Sabril®: 0.5 g

Vigamox® *see* moxifloxacin (ophthalmic) *on page 616*

VIGIV *see* vaccinia immune globulin (intravenous) *on page 933*

Viibryd™ *see* vilazodone *on page 945*

vilazodone (vil AZ oh done)

Synonyms EMD 68843; SB659746-A; vilazodone hydrochloride

U.S. Brand Names Viibryd™

Therapeutic Category Antidepressant, Selective Serotonin Reuptake Inhibitor/5-HT_{1A} Receptor Partial Agonist

Use Treatment of major depressive disorder

General Dosage Range Dosage adjustment recommended in patients on concomitant therapy

Oral: *Adults:* 10-40 mg once daily

Dosage Forms

Tablet, oral:

Viibryd™: 10 mg, 20 mg, 40 mg

vilazodone hydrochloride *see* vilazodone *on page 945*

Vimovo™ *see* naproxen and esomeprazole *on page 629*

Vimpat® *see* lacosamide *on page 517*

Vinacal™ *see* vitamins (multiple/prenatal) *on page 952*

Vinate® Care *see* vitamins (multiple/prenatal) *on page 952*

vinblastine (vin BLAS teen)

Medication Safety Issues

Sound-alike/look-alike issues:

VinBLAStine may be confused with vinCRIStine, vinorelbine

High alert medication:

The Institute for Safe Medication Practices (ISMP) includes this medication among its list of drug classes which have a heightened risk of causing significant patient harm when used in error.

Administration issues:

Must be dispensed in overwrap which bears the statement **"Do not remove covering until the moment of injection. Fatal if given intrathecally. For I.V. use only."** Syringes should be labeled: **"Fatal if given intrathecally. For I.V. use only."**

Synonyms Velban; vinblastine sulfate; vincaleukoblastine; VLB

Tall-Man vin**BLAS**tine

Therapeutic Category Antineoplastic Agent

Use Treatment of Hodgkin and non-Hodgkin lymphoma; testicular cancer; breast cancer; mycosis fungoides; Kaposi sarcoma; histiocytosis (Letterer-Siwe disease); choriocarcinoma

General Dosage Range Dosage adjustment recommended in patients with hepatic impairment

I.V.:

Children: Initial dose: 3-6.5 mg/m^2 every 7 days as needed

Adults: Initial: 3.7 mg/m^2; adjust dose every 7 days; Second dose: 5.5 mg/m^2; Third dose: 7.4 mg/m^2; Fourth dose: 9.25 mg/m^2; Fifth dose: 11.1 mg/m^2; Usual range: 5.5-7.4 mg/m^2 every 7 days; Maximum dose: 18.5 mg/m^2

Dosage Forms

Injection, powder for reconstitution: 10 mg

Injection, solution: 1 mg/mL (10 mL)

vinblastine sulfate *see* vinblastine *on page 946*

vincaleukoblastine *see* vinblastine *on page 946*

Vincasar PFS® *see* vincristine *on page 946*

vincristine (vin KRIS teen)

Medication Safety Issues

Sound-alike/look-alike issues:

VinCRIStine may be confused with vinBLAStine, vinorelbine

VinCRIStine conventional may be confused with vinCRIStine liposomal

Oncovin may be confused with Ancobon®

High alert medication:

This medication is in a class the Institute for Safe Medication Practices (ISMP) includes among its list of drug classes which have a heightened risk of causing significant patient harm when used in error.

BEERS Criteria medication:

This drug may be potentially inappropriate for use in geriatric patients (Quality of evidence - moderate; Strength of recommendation - strong).

Administration issues:

For I.V. use only. Fatal if administered by other routes. To prevent fatal inadvertent intrathecal injection, it is recommended that vincristine doses be dispensed in a small minibag. Vincristine should **NOT** be prepared during the preparation of any intrathecal medications. After preparation, keep vincristine in a location **away** from the separate storage location recommended for intrathecal medications. Vincristine should **NOT** be delivered to the patient at the same time with any medications intended for central nervous system administration.

Synonyms leurocristine sulfate; Oncovin; vincristine sulfate

Tall-Man vin**CRIS**tine

U.S. Brand Names Vincasar PFS®

Canadian Brand Names Vincristine Sulfate Injection.

Therapeutic Category Antineoplastic Agent

Use Treatment of acute lymphocytic leukemia (ALL), Hodgkin lymphoma, non-Hodgkin lymphomas, Wilms tumor, neuroblastoma, rhabdomyosarcoma

General Dosage Range Dosage adjustment recommended in patients with hepatic impairment

I.V.:

Children ≤10 kg: 0.05 mg/kg once weekly (maximum: 2 mg/dose)

Children >10 kg: 1.5-2 mg/m^2/dose (maximum: 2 mg/dose)

Adults: 1.4 mg/m^2/dose (maximum: 2 mg/dose)

Dosage Forms

Injection, solution [preservative free]: 1 mg/mL (1 mL, 2 mL)

Vincasar PFS®: 1 mg/mL (1 mL, 2 mL)

vincristine (liposomal) (vin KRIS teen lye po SO mal)

Medication Safety Issues

Sound-alike/look-alike issues:

VinCRIStine liposomal may be confused with vinCRIStine conventional

High alert medication:

This medication is in a class the Institute for Safe Medication Practices (ISMP) includes among its list of drug classes which have a heightened risk of causing significant patient harm when used in error.

BEERS Criteria medication:

Conventional vincristine may be potentially inappropriate for use in geriatric patients (Quality of evidence - moderate; Strength of recommendation - strong).

Administration issues:

Vincristine liposomal and conventional vincristine are **NOT** interchangeable. Dosing differs between formulations; verify intended product and dose prior to preparation and administration.

For I.V. administration only. Intrathecal administration is contraindicated; inadvertent intrathecal administration has resulted in death. Liposomal vincristine should **NOT** be prepared during the preparation of any intrathecal medications. After preparation, keep liposomal vincristine in a location **away** from the separate storage location recommended for intrathecal medications. Liposomal vincristine should **NOT** be delivered to the patient at the same time with any medications intended for central nervous system administration.

Synonyms liposome vincristine; Marqibo®; vincristine sulfate liposome; VSLI

Tall-Man vin**CRIS**tine

Therapeutic Category Antineoplastic Agent, Natural Source (Plant) Derivative; Antineoplastic Agent, Vinca Alkaloid

Use Treatment of relapsed Philadelphia chromosome-negative (Ph-) acute lymphoblastic leukemia (ALL) in adult patients whose disease has progressed after two or more antileukemic therapies

General Dosage Range Dosage adjustment recommended in patients with hepatic impairment or who develop toxicities.

I.V.: *Adults:* 2.25 mg/m^2 once every 7 days

Product Availability Marqibo®: FDA approved August 9, 2012; availability is currently undetermined. Consult prescribing information for additional information.

vincristine sulfate *see* vincristine *on page 946*

Vincristine Sulfate Injection. (Can) *see* vincristine *on page 946*

vincristine sulfate liposome *see* vincristine (liposomal) *on page 947*

vinorelbine (vi NOR el been)

Medication Safety Issues

Sound-alike/look-alike issues:

Vinorelbine may be confused with vinBLAStine, vinCRIStine

High alert medication:

This medication is in a class the Institute for Safe Medication Practices (ISMP) includes among its list of drug classes which have a heightened risk of causing significant patient harm when used in error.

Administration issues:

Vinorelbine is intended **for I.V. use only**: Inadvertent intrathecal administration of other vinca alkaloids has resulted in death. Syringes containing vinorelbine should be labeled **"For I.V. use only. Fatal if given intrathecally."** Vinorelbine should **NOT** be prepared during the preparation of any intrathecal medications. After preparation, store vinorelbine in a location **away** from the separate storage location recommended for intrathecal medications.

Synonyms dihydroxydeoxynorvinkaleukoblastine; vinorelbine tartrate

U.S. Brand Names Navelbine®

Canadian Brand Names Navelbine®; Vinorelbine Injection, USP; Vinorelbine Tartrate for Injection

Therapeutic Category Antineoplastic Agent

Use Treatment of nonsmall cell lung cancer (NSCLC)

General Dosage Range Dosage adjustment recommended in patients with hepatic impairment or who develop toxicities

I.V.: *Adults:* 25-30 mg/m^2/dose every 7 days

Dosage Forms

Injection, solution [preservative free]: 10 mg/mL (1 mL, 5 mL)

Navelbine®: 10 mg/mL (1 mL, 5 mL)

Vinorelbine Injection, USP (Can) *see* vinorelbine *on page 947*
vinorelbine tartrate *see* vinorelbine *on page 947*
Vinorelbine Tartrate for Injection (Can) *see* vinorelbine *on page 947*
Viokace™ *see* pancrelipase *on page 687*
Viokase® (Can) *see* pancrelipase *on page 687*
Viorele *see* ethinyl estradiol and desogestrel *on page 356*
viosterol *see* ergocalciferol *on page 339*
Viracept® *see* nelfinavir *on page 632*
Viramune® *see* nevirapine *on page 637*
Viramune® XR™ *see* nevirapine *on page 637*
Viramune® XR (Can) *see* nevirapine *on page 637*
Virasal® *see* salicylic acid *on page 816*
Virazole® *see* ribavirin *on page 798*
Virdec [OTC] *see* chlorpheniramine and phenylephrine *on page 200*
Virdec DM [OTC] *see* chlorpheniramine, phenylephrine, and dextromethorphan *on page 201*
Viread® *see* tenofovir *on page 877*
Viroptic® *see* trifluridine *on page 919*
Visanne® (Can) *see* dienogest *(Canada only) on page 283*
Viscoat® *see* sodium chondroitin sulfate and sodium hyaluronate *on page 842*
Viscous Lidocaine *see* lidocaine (topical) *on page 535*
Visicol® *see* sodium phosphates *on page 845*
Visine-A® [OTC] *see* naphazoline and pheniramine *on page 627*
Visine® Advanced Allergy (Can) *see* naphazoline and pheniramine *on page 627*
Visine® Advanced Relief [OTC] *see* tetrahydrozoline (ophthalmic) *on page 885*
Visine® L.R.® [OTC] *see* oxymetazoline (ophthalmic) *on page 681*
Visine® Original [OTC] *see* tetrahydrozoline (ophthalmic) *on page 885*
Visipaque™ *see* iodixanol *on page 494*
Viskazide® (Can) *see* pindolol and hydrochlorothiazide *(Canada only) on page 724*
Visken® (Can) *see* pindolol *on page 724*

vismodegib (vis moe DEG ib)

Medication Safety Issues

Sound-alike/look-alike issues:

Vismodegib may be confused with vandetanib, vemurafenib

High alert medication:

This medication is in a class the Institute for Safe Medication Practices (ISMP) includes among its list of drug classes which have a heightened risk of causing significant patient harm when used in error.

Synonyms GDC-0449; hedgehog antagonist GDC-0449

U.S. Brand Names Erivedge™

Therapeutic Category Antineoplastic Agent, Hedgehog Pathway Inhibitor

Use Treatment of metastatic basal cell carcinoma, or locally-advanced basal cell carcinoma that has recurred following surgery or in patients who are not candidates for surgery, and not candidates for radiation therapy

General Dosage Range Oral: *Adults:* 150 mg once daily

Dosage Forms

Capsule, oral:

Erivedge™: 150 mg

Vistaril® *see* hydroxyzine *on page 464*
Vistide® *see* cidofovir *on page 208*
Visudyne® *see* verteporfin *on page 943*
Vita-C® [OTC] *see* ascorbic acid *on page 94*
Vitafol® *see* vitamins (multiple/oral) *on page 951*
Vitafol®-OB [OTC] *see* vitamins (multiple/prenatal) *on page 952*
Vitafol®-OB+DHA [OTC] *see* vitamins (multiple/prenatal) *on page 952*
Vitafol®-PN *see* vitamins (multiple/prenatal) *on page 952*
Vitalets [OTC] *see* vitamins (multiple/pediatric) *on page 952*
vitamin C *see* ascorbic acid *on page 94*
vitamin D_3 and alendronate *see* alendronate and cholecalciferol *on page 45*
vitamin D and calcium carbonate *see* calcium and vitamin D *on page 161*

vitamin A (VYE ta min aye)

Medication Safety Issues

Sound-alike/look-alike issues:

Aquasol® may be confused with Anusol®

Synonyms oleovitamin A

U.S. Brand Names A-25 [OTC]; A-Natural [OTC]; A-Natural-25 [OTC]; Aquasol A®

Therapeutic Category Vitamin, Fat Soluble

Use Treatment and prevention of vitamin A deficiency; parenteral (I.M.) route is indicated when oral administration is not feasible or when absorption is insufficient (malabsorption syndrome); dietary supplement (OTC)

General Dosage Range I.M., Oral: *Children and Adults:* Dosage varies greatly depending on indication

Dosage Forms

Capsule, oral:

A-25 [OTC]: 25,000 units

Capsule, softgel, oral: 10,000 units

A-Natural [OTC]: 10,000 units

A-Natural-25 [OTC]: 25,000 units

Injection, solution:

Aquasol A®: 50,000 units/mL (2 mL)

Tablet, oral: 10,000 units, 15,000 units

vitamin A acid *see* tretinoin (topical) *on page 914*
Vitamin A Acid (Can) *see* tretinoin (topical) *on page 914*

vitamin A and vitamin D (systemic) (VYE ta min aye & VYE ta min dee)

U.S. Brand Names A&D Jr. [OTC]; D-Natural-5 [OTC]

Therapeutic Category Vitamin, Fat Soluble

Use Dietary supplement

General Dosage Range Oral: *Adults:* One tablet or capsule once daily.

Dosage Forms

Capsule, softgel, oral: Vitamin A 1250 units and vitamin D 130 units, Vitamin A 1250 units and vitamin D 135 units, Vitamin A 5,000 units and vitamin D 400 units, Vitamin A 10,000 units and vitamin D 400 units, Vitamin A 25,000 units and vitamin D 1000 units

A&D Jr. [OTC]: Vitamin A 10,000 units and vitamin D 400 units

D-Natural-5 [OTC]: Vitamin A 10,000 units and vitamin D 5000 units

Oil, oral: Vitamin A 5000 units and vitamin D 500 units per 5 mL (120 mL, 473 mL)

Tablet, oral: Vitamin A 10,000 units and vitamin D 400 units

vitamin A and vitamin D (topical) (VYE ta min aye & VYE ta min dee)

Synonyms cod liver oil

U.S. Brand Names A+D® Original [OTC]; Baza® Clear [OTC]; Sween Cream® [OTC]

Therapeutic Category Topical Skin Product

Use Temporary relief of discomfort due to chapped skin or lips, cuts and scrapes, diaper rash, or minor burns

General Dosage Range Topical: *Children and Adults:* Apply to affected areas as needed.

Dosage Forms

Cream, topical:

Sween Cream® [OTC]: (2 g, 14 g, 57 g, 85 g, 142 g, 184 g, 339 g)

Ointment, topical: (0.9 g, 5 g, 60 g, 120 g, 454 g)

A+D® Original [OTC]: (42.5 g); (120 g); (454 g)

Baza® Clear [OTC]: (50 g, 142 g, 227 g)

vitamin B_1 *see* thiamine *on page 890*

vitamin B_2 *see* riboflavin *on page 799*

vitamin B_3 *see* niacin *on page 638*

vitamin B_3 *see* niacinamide *on page 638*

vitamin B_5 *see* pantothenic acid *on page 690*

vitamin B_6 *see* pyridoxine *on page 777*

vitamin B_{12} *see* cyanocobalamin *on page 242*

vitamin B complex combinations (VYE ta min bee KOM pleks kom bi NAY shuns)

Medication Safety Issues

Sound-alike/look-alike issues:

Nephrocaps® may be confused with Nephro-Calci®

Synonyms B complex combinations; B vitamin combinations

Therapeutic Category Vitamin, Water Soluble

Use Dietary supplement

General Dosage Range

Oral: *Adults:* Dosage varies greatly depending on product

Dosage Forms Content varies depending on product used. For more detailed information on ingredients in these and other multivitamins, please refer to package labeling.

vitamin D2 *see* ergocalciferol *on page 339*

Vitamin D3 [OTC] *see* cholecalciferol *on page 205*

vitamin E (VYE ta min ee)

Medication Safety Issues

Sound-alike/look-alike issues:

Aquasol E® may be confused with Anusol®

Synonyms *d*-alpha tocopherol; *dl*-alpha tocopherol

U.S. Brand Names Alph-E [OTC]; Alph-E-Mixed [OTC]; Aqua Gem-E™ [OTC]; Aquasol E® [OTC]; d-Alpha Gems™ [OTC]; E-Gems® Elite [OTC]; E-Gems® Plus [OTC]; E-Gems® [OTC]; E-Gem® Lip Care [OTC]; E-Gem® [OTC]; Ester-E™ [OTC]; Gamma E-Gems® [OTC]; Gamma-E PLUS [OTC]; High Gamma Vitamin E Complete™ [OTC]; Key-E® Kaps [OTC]; Key-E® Powder [OTC]; Key-E® [OTC]

Therapeutic Category Vitamin, Fat Soluble; Vitamin, Topical

Use Dietary supplement

General Dosage Range

Oral:

Infants 1-6 months: Adequate intake: 4 mg

Infants 7-12 months: Adequate intake: 5 mg

Children 1-3 years: RDA: 6 mg; upper limit of intake should not exceed 200 mg/day

Children 4-8 years: RDA: 7 mg; upper limit of intake should not exceed 300 mg/day

Children 9-13 years: RDA: 11 mg; upper limit of intake should not exceed 600 mg/day

Children 14-18 years: RDA: 15 mg; upper limit of intake should not exceed 800 mg/day

Adults: RDA: 15 mg; upper limit of intake should not exceed 1000 mg/day

Pregnant female:

≤18 years: RDA: 15 mg; upper level of intake should not exceed 800 mg/day

19-50 years: RDA: 15 mg; upper level of intake should not exceed 1000 mg/day

Lactating female:

≤18 years: RDA: 19 mg; upper level of intake should not exceed 800 mg/day

19-50 years: RDA: 19 mg; upper level of intake should not exceed 1000 mg/day

Topical: *Adults:* Apply a thin layer over affected area.

Dosage Forms

Capsule, oral: 1000 units

Key-E® Kaps [OTC]: 200 units, 400 units

Capsule, liquid, oral: 400 units
Capsule, softgel, oral: 100 units, 200 units, 400 units, 600 units, 1000 units
Alph-E [OTC]: 200 units, 400 units, 1000 units
Alph-E-Mixed [OTC]: 200 units, 400 units, 1000 units
Aqua Gem-E™ [OTC]: 200 units, 400 units
d-Alpha Gems™ [OTC]: 400 units
E-Gems® [OTC]: 30 units, 100 units, 200 units, 400 units, 600 units, 800 units, 1000 units, 1200 units
E-Gems® Elite [OTC]: 400 units
E-Gems® Plus [OTC]: 200 units, 400 units, 800 units
Ester-E™ [OTC]: 400 units
Gamma E-Gems® [OTC]: 90 units
Gamma-E PLUS [OTC]: 200 units
High Gamma Vitamin E Complete™ [OTC]: 200 units
Cream, topical: 1000 units/120 g (120 g); 100 units/g (57 g, 60 g); 30,000 units/57 g (57 g)
Key-E® [OTC]: 30 units/g (57 g, 120 g, 600 g)
Lip balm, topical:
E-Gem® Lip Care [OTC]: 1000 units/tube
Liquid, oral/topical: 1150 units/1.25 mL (30 mL, 60 mL, 120 mL)
Oil, oral/topical: 100 units/0.25 mL (74 mL)
E-Gem® [OTC]: 10 units/drop (15 mL, 60 mL)
Oil, topical:
Alph-E [OTC]: 28,000 units/30 mL (30 mL)
Ointment, topical:
Key-E® [OTC]: 30 units/g (57 g, 113 g, 500 g)
Powder, oral:
Key-E® Powder [OTC]: (15 g, 75 g, 1000 g)
Solution, oral: 15 units/0.3 mL (30 mL)
Aquasol E® [OTC]: 15 units/0.3 mL (12 mL, 30 mL)
Suppository, rectal/vaginal:
Key-E® [OTC]: 30 units (12s, 24s)
Tablet, oral: 100 units, 200 units, 400 units, 500 units
Key-E® [OTC]: 200 units, 400 units

vitamin G *see* riboflavin *on page 799*
vitamin K_1 *see* phytonadione *on page 722*

vitamins (multiple/injectable) (VYE ta mins, MUL ti pul/in JEK ti bal)

U.S. Brand Names Infuvite® Adult; Infuvite® Pediatric; M.V.I. Adult™; M.V.I.®-12; M.V.I® Pediatric

Therapeutic Category Vitamin

Use Nutritional supplement in patients receiving parenteral nutrition or requiring intravenous administration

General Dosage Range I.V.:
Children ≥3 kg to 11 years: 5 mL/day
Children >11 years and Adults: 10 mL/day

Dosage Forms Content varies depending on product used. For more detailed information on ingredients in these and other multivitamins, please refer to package labeling.

vitamins (multiple/oral) (VYE ta mins, MUL ti pul/OR al)

Medication Safety Issues
Sound-alike/look-alike issues:
Theragran® may be confused with Phenergan®
Viactiv® may be confused with Vibativ™

Synonyms multiple vitamins; Theragran; therapeutic multivitamins; vitamins, multiple (oral); vitamins, multiple (therapeutic); vitamins, multiple with iron

U.S. Brand Names Androvite® [OTC]; CalciFolic-D™; Centamin [OTC]; Centrum Cardio® [OTC]; Centrum Performance® [OTC]; Centrum® Silver® Ultra Men's [OTC]; Centrum® Silver® Ultra Women's [OTC]; Centrum® Silver® [OTC]; Centrum® Ultra Men's [OTC]; Centrum® Ultra Women's [OTC]; Centrum® [OTC]; Diatx®Zn; Drinkables® Fruits and Vegetables [OTC]; Drinkables® MultiVitamins [OTC]; Encora®; Foltrin®; Freedavite [OTC]; Geri-Freeda [OTC]; Geriation [OTC]; Geritol Complete® [OTC]; Geritol Extend® [OTC]; Geritol® Tonic [OTC]; Glutofac®-MX; Gynovite® Plus [OTC]; Hemocyte Plus®; Hi-Kovite [OTC]; Iberet®-500 [OTC] [DSC]; Monocaps [OTC]; Myadec® [OTC]; Nutrimin-Plus [OTC]; Ocuvite® Adult 50+ [OTC]; Ocuvite® Extra® [OTC]; Ocuvite® Lutein [OTC]; Ocuvite® [OTC]; One

A Day® Cholesterol Plus [OTC]; One A Day® Energy [OTC]; One A Day® Essential [OTC]; One A Day® Maximum [OTC]; One A Day® Men's 50+ Advantage [OTC]; One A Day® Men's Health Formula [OTC]; One A Day® Teen Advantage for Her [OTC]; One A Day® Teen Advantage for Him [OTC]; One A Day® Weight Smart® Advanced [OTC]; One A Day® Women's 50+ Advantage [OTC]; One A Day® Women's Active Mind & Body [OTC]; One A Day® Women's [OTC]; Optivite® P.M.T. [OTC]; PreserVision® AREDS [OTC]; PreserVision® Lutein [OTC]; Quintabs [OTC]; Quintabs-M Iron-Free [OTC]; Quintabs-M [OTC]; Renax®; Renax® 5.5; Replace Without Iron [OTC]; Replace [OTC]; Repliva 21/7®; SourceCF®; Strovite®; Strovite® Advance; Strovite® Forte; Strovite® Plus; T-Vites [OTC]; Ultra Freeda A-Free [OTC]; Ultra Freeda Iron-Free [OTC]; Ultra Freeda With Iron [OTC]; Viactiv® Calcium Flavor Glides™ [OTC]; Viactiv® Flavor Glides [OTC]; Viactiv® for Teens [OTC]; Viactiv® With Calcium [OTC]; Viactiv® [OTC]; Vitafol®; Xtramins [OTC]; Yelets [OTC]

Therapeutic Category Vitamin

Use Prevention/treatment of vitamin and mineral deficiencies; labeled for OTC use as a dietary supplement

General Dosage Range Oral: *Adults:* 1 tablet/capsule **or** 5-15 mL once daily

Dosage Forms Content varies depending on product used. For more detailed information on ingredients in these and other multivitamins, please refer to package labeling.

vitamins, multiple (oral) *see* vitamins (multiple/oral) *on page 951*

vitamins (multiple/pediatric) (VYE ta mins, MUL ti pul/pe de AT rik)

Synonyms children's vitamins; multivitamins/fluoride

U.S. Brand Names ADEKs® [OTC]; AquADEKs™ [OTC]; Centrum Kids® [OTC]; Flintstones™ Complete [OTC]; Flintstones™ Gummies [OTC]; Flintstones™ Plus Bone Building Support Gummies [OTC]; Flintstones™ Plus Bone Building Support [OTC]; Flintstones™ Plus Immunity Support Gummies [OTC]; Flintstones™ Plus Immunity Support [OTC]; Flintstones™ Plus Iron [OTC]; Flintstones™ Sour Gummies [OTC]; My First Flintstones™ [OTC]; MyKidz Iron FL™; MyKidz Iron™ [OTC]; One A Day® Kids Jolly Rancher™ Gummies [OTC]; One A Day® Kids Jolly Rancher™ Sour Gummies [OTC]; One A Day® Kids Scooby-Doo!™ Complete [OTC]; One A Day® Kids Scooby-Doo!™ Gummies [OTC]; Poly-Vi-Sol® With Iron [OTC]; Poly-Vi-Sol® [OTC]; SourceCF® [OTC]; Tri-Vi-Sol® With Iron [OTC]; Tri-Vi-Sol® [OTC]; Vitalets [OTC]

Therapeutic Category Vitamin

Use Prevention/treatment of vitamin deficiency; products containing fluoride are used to prevent dental caries; labeled for OTC use as a dietary supplement

General Dosage Range Oral: *Children:* Daily dose varies greatly depending on product

Dosage Forms Content varies depending on product used. For more detailed information on ingredients in these and other multivitamins, please refer to package labeling.

vitamins (multiple/prenatal) (VYE ta mins, MUL ti pul/pree NAY tal)

Medication Safety Issues

Sound-alike/look-alike issues:

PreCare® may be confused with Precose®

Synonyms prenatal vitamins

U.S. Brand Names A-Free Prenatal [OTC]; CitraNatal® Harmony™; CitraNatal™ 90 DHA; CitraNatal™ Assure; CitraNatal™ B-Calm; CitraNatal™ DHA; CitraNatal™ Rx; Concept DHA™; Concept OB™; Duet®; Duet® Balanced DHA[ec]; Femecal OB; Folcaps™ Care One; Foltabs™ Prenatal; Foltabs™ Prenatal Plus DHA; Gesticare® DHA; KPN Prenatal [OTC]; Mini-Prenatal [OTC]; Multi-Nate 30; NataFort® [OTC]; Néevo®; Néevo® DHA; One A Day® Women's Prenatal [OTC]; OptiNate®; Paire OB™ Plus DHA; PreCare®; PreferaOB®; PreferaOB® + DHA; PreferaOB® One™; Prenatabs FA; Prenatal One Daily [OTC]; Prenatal Rx 1; Prenatal With Beta Carotene [OTC]; Prenate DHA™; Prenate Elite®; Prenate Essential™; PreNexa® Premier; PrimaCare® One; Select-OB™; Stuart Prenatal® [OTC]; Tandem® DHA; Tandem® OB; TriCare® Prenatal; TriCare® Prenatal DHA One®; Vinacal™; Vinate® Care; Vitafol®-OB [OTC]; Vitafol®-OB+DHA [OTC]; Vitafol®-PN; VitaPhil + DHA

Therapeutic Category Vitamin

Use Nutritional supplement for use prior to conception, during pregnancy, and postnatal (in lactating and nonlactating women)

General Dosage Range Oral: *Adults:* 1 tablet/capsule once daily **or** 4 teaspoonfuls/day once daily or in divided doses

Dosage Forms Content varies depending on product used. For more detailed information on ingredients in these and other multivitamins, please refer to package labeling.

voriconazole (vor i KOE na zole)

Medication Safety Issues

Sound-alike/look-alike issues:

Voriconazole may be confused with fluconazole

Synonyms UK109496

U.S. Brand Names VFEND®

Canadian Brand Names VFEND®

Therapeutic Category Antifungal Agent

Use Treatment of invasive aspergillosis; treatment of esophageal candidiasis; treatment of candidemia (in nonneutropenic patients); treatment of disseminated *Candida* infections of the skin and viscera; treatment of serious fungal infections caused by *Scedosporium apiospermum* and *Fusarium* spp (including *Fusarium solani*) in patients intolerant of, or refractory to, other therapy

General Dosage Range Dosage adjustment recommended in patients with hepatic impairment

I.V.: *Children ≥12 years and Adults:* Initial: 6 mg/kg every 12 hours for 2 doses; Maintenance: 3-4 mg/kg every 12 hours

Oral: *Children ≥12 years and Adults:* 100-300 mg every 12 hours

Dosage Forms

Injection, powder for reconstitution: 200 mg

VFEND®: 200 mg

Powder for suspension, oral:
VFEND®: 40 mg/mL (70 mL)
Tablet, oral: 50 mg, 200 mg
VFEND®: 50 mg, 200 mg

vorinostat (vor IN oh stat)

Medication Safety Issues

Sound-alike/look-alike issues:
Vorinostat may be confused with Votrient™

High alert medication:
This medication is in a class the Institute for Safe Medication Practices (ISMP) includes among its list of drug classes which have a heightened risk of causing significant patient harm when used in error.

Synonyms SAHA; suberoylanilide hydroxamic acid

U.S. Brand Names Zolinza®

Canadian Brand Names Zolinza®

Therapeutic Category Antineoplastic Agent, Histone Deacetylase Inhibitor

Use Treatment of progressive, persistent, or recurrent cutaneous T-cell lymphoma (CTCL)

General Dosage Range Dosage adjustment recommended in patients who develop toxicities

Oral: *Adults:* 400 mg once daily

Dosage Forms

Capsule, oral:
Zolinza®: 100 mg

VoSoL® *see* acetic acid *on page 31*
VoSol® HC *see* acetic acid, propylene glycol diacetate, and hydrocortisone *on page 31*
VoSpire ER® *see* albuterol *on page 41*
Votrient™ *see* pazopanib *on page 694*
VP-16 *see* etoposide *on page 366*
VP-16-213 *see* etoposide *on page 366*
VPRIV™ *see* velaglucerase alfa *on page 941*
VRT111950 *see* telaprevir *on page 873*
VSL #3® [OTC] *see* Lactobacillus *on page 518*
VSL #3®-DS *see* Lactobacillus *on page 518*
VSLI *see* vincristine (liposomal) *on page 947*
Vumon® *see* teniposide *on page 877*
Vusion® *see* miconazole and zinc oxide *on page 600*
V.V.S.® *see* sulfabenzamide, sulfacetamide, and sulfathiazole *on page 858*
VWF/FVIII concentrate *see* antihemophilic factor/von Willebrand factor complex (human) *on page 78*
VWF:RCo *see* antihemophilic factor/von Willebrand factor complex (human) *on page 78*
vWF:RCof *see* antihemophilic factor/von Willebrand factor complex (human) *on page 78*
VX-770 *see* ivacaftor *on page 507*
VX-950 *see* telaprevir *on page 873*
Vyloma™ (Can) *see* imiquimod *on page 476*
Vytone *see* iodoquinol and hydrocortisone *on page 495*
Vytorin® *see* ezetimibe and simvastatin *on page 370*
Vyvanse® *see* lisdexamfetamine *on page 543*
VZIG *see* varicella-zoster immune globulin (human) *on page 939*
VZV vaccine (varicella) *see* varicella virus vaccine *on page 939*
VZV vaccine (zoster) *see* zoster vaccine *on page 968*

warfarin (WAR far in)

Medication Safety Issues

Sound-alike/look-alike issues:
Coumadin® may be confused with Avandia®, Cardura®, Compazine, Kemadrin

Jantoven® may be confused with Janumet®, Januvia®

High alert medication:

The Institute for Safe Medication Practices (ISMP) includes this medication among its list of drugs which have a heightened risk of causing significant patient harm when used in error.

National Patient Safety Goals:

The Joint Commission on Accreditation of Healthcare Organizations requires healthcare organizations that provide anticoagulant therapy to have a process in place to reduce the risk of anticoagulant-associated patient harm. Patients receiving anticoagulants should receive individualized care through a defined process that includes standardized ordering, dispensing, administration, monitoring and education. This does not apply to routine short-term use of anticoagulants for prevention of venous thromboembolism when the expectation is that the patient's laboratory values will remain within or close to normal values (NPSG.03.05.01).

Synonyms warfarin sodium

U.S. Brand Names Coumadin®; Jantoven®

Canadian Brand Names Apo-Warfarin®; Coumadin®; Mylan-Warfarin; Novo-Warfarin; Taro-Warfarin

Therapeutic Category Anticoagulant (Other)

Use Prophylaxis and treatment of thromboembolic disorders (eg, venous, pulmonary) and embolic complications arising from atrial fibrillation or cardiac valve replacement; adjunct to reduce risk of systemic embolism (eg, recurrent MI, stroke) after myocardial infarction

General Dosage Range

I.V.: *Adults:* 2-5 mg once daily

Oral:

Adults: Initial: 2-5 mg daily for 2 days; Maintenance: 2-10 mg daily

Elderly: Initial: ≤5 mg/day; Maintenance: 2-5 mg/day

Dosage Forms

Injection, powder for reconstitution:

Coumadin®: 5 mg

Tablet, oral: 1 mg, 2 mg, 2.5 mg, 3 mg, 4 mg, 5 mg, 6 mg, 7.5 mg, 10 mg

Coumadin®: 1 mg, 2 mg, 2.5 mg, 3 mg, 4 mg, 5 mg, 6 mg, 7.5 mg, 10 mg

Jantoven®: 1 mg, 2 mg, 2.5 mg, 3 mg, 4 mg, 5 mg, 6 mg, 7.5 mg, 10 mg

warfarin sodium *see* warfarin *on page* 954

Wartec® (Can) *see* podofilox *on page* 735

Wart-Off® Maximum Strength [OTC] *see* salicylic acid *on page* 816

Wax Away [OTC] *see* carbamide peroxide *on page* 173

4-Way® 12 Hour [OTC] *see* oxymetazoline (nasal) *on page* 681

4 Way® Fast Acting [OTC] *see* phenylephrine (nasal) *on page* 716

4 Way® Menthol [OTC] *see* phenylephrine (nasal) *on page* 716

4-Way® Saline Moisturizing Mist [OTC] *see* sodium chloride *on page* 840

WC-rBS *see* traveler's diarrhea and cholera vaccine *(Canada only) on page* 911

Welchol® *see* colesevelam *on page* 232

Wellbutrin® *see* bupropion *on page* 150

Wellbutrin XL® *see* bupropion *on page* 150

Wellbutrin® XL (Can) *see* bupropion *on page* 150

Wellbutrin SR® *see* bupropion *on page* 150

Wellbutrin® SR (Can) *see* bupropion *on page* 150

Westcort® *see* hydrocortisone (topical) *on page* 457

Westhroid™ *see* thyroid, desiccated *on page* 893

wheat dextrin (weet DEKS trin)

Synonyms dextrin; resistant dextrin; resistant maltodextrin

U.S. Brand Names Benefiber® Plus Calcium [OTC]; Benefiber® [OTC]

Therapeutic Category Fiber Supplement; Laxative, Bulk-Producing

Use OTC labeling: Dietary fiber supplement

General Dosage Range Oral: *Children and Adults:* Dosage varies greatly depending on product

Dosage Forms

Caplet, oral:

Benefiber® [OTC]: 1.3 g

Powder, oral:
Benefiber® [OTC]: (80 g, 155 g, 161 g, 245 g, 267 g, 350 g, 477 g, 529 g); 3.5 g/packet (8s, 16s, 28s)
Benefiber® Plus Calcium [OTC]: (424 g)
Tablet, chewable, oral:
Benefiber® [OTC]: 2.7 g
Benefiber® Plus Calcium [OTC]: 2.7 g

Wilate® *see* antihemophilic factor/von Willebrand factor complex (human) *on page 78*
Winpred™ (Can) *see* prednisone *on page 755*
WinRho® SDF *see* Rh_o(D) immune globulin *on page 797*

witch hazel (witch HAY zel)

Synonyms hamamelis water

U.S. Brand Names Dickinson's® Witch Hazel Astringent Cleanser [OTC]; Dickinson's® Witch Hazel Cleansing Astringent [OTC]; Dickinson's® Witch Hazel [OTC]; Medi Pads [OTC]; Preparation H® Medicated Wipes [OTC]; T. N. Dickinson's® Hazelets® [OTC]; T. N. Dickinson's® Witch Hazel® Astringent [OTC]; T. N. Dickinson's® Witch Hazel® Hemorrhoidal [OTC]; Tucks® Anti-Itch [OTC]; Tucks® Take Alongs® [OTC]

Canadian Brand Names Preparation H® Cleansing Pads

Therapeutic Category Astringent

Use After-stool wipe to remove most causes of local irritation; temporary management of vulvitis, pruritus ani and vulva; help relieve the discomfort of simple hemorrhoids, anorectal surgical wounds, and episiotomies

General Dosage Range Topical: *Children ≥12 years and Adults:* Apply to anorectal area as needed up to 6 times daily or after each bowel movement

Dosage Forms

Liquid, topical:
Dickinson's® Witch Hazel Astringent Cleanser [OTC]: 99.5% (3785 mL)
Dickinson's® Witch Hazel Cleansing Astringent [OTC]: 99.5% (59 mL, 237 mL, 473 mL)
T. N. Dickinson's® Witch Hazel® Astringent [OTC]: 100% (59 mL, 237 mL, 473 mL)
Pad, topical:
Dickinson's® Witch Hazel [OTC]: 99% (60s)
Dickinson's® Witch Hazel Cleansing Astringent [OTC]: 99% (20s)
Medi Pads [OTC]: 50% (100s)
Preparation H® Medicated Wipes [OTC]: 50% (8s, 48s, 96s)
T. N. Dickinson's® Hazelets® [OTC]: 100% (50s, 60s)
T. N. Dickinson's® Witch Hazel® Hemorrhoidal [OTC]: 50% (100s)
Tucks® Anti-Itch [OTC]: 50% (40s, 100s)
Towelette, topical:
Tucks® Take Alongs® [OTC]: 50% (12s)

Woman's Laxative [OTC] (Can) *see* bisacodyl *on page 134*
Wound Wash Saline™ [OTC] *see* sodium chloride *on page 840*
WR-2721 *see* amifostine *on page 59*
WR-139007 *see* dacarbazine *on page 250*
WR-139013 *see* chlorambucil *on page 195*
WR-139021 *see* carmustine *on page 178*
Wycillin [DSC] *see* penicillin G procaine *on page 703*
Wycillin® (Can) *see* penicillin G procaine *on page 703*
Wymzya™ Fe *see* ethinyl estradiol and norethindrone *on page 359*
Xalacom™ (Can) *see* latanoprost and timolol *(Canada only) on page 524*
Xalatan® *see* latanoprost *on page 524*
Xalkori® *see* crizotinib *on page 240*
Xalkori™ (Can) *see* crizotinib *on page 240*
Xamiol® (Can) *see* calcipotriene and betamethasone *on page 159*
Xanax® *see* alprazolam *on page 52*
Xanax TS™ (Can) *see* alprazolam *on page 52*
Xanax XR® *see* alprazolam *on page 52*
Xarelto® *see* rivaroxaban *on page 806*

yellow fever vaccine (YEL oh FEE ver vak SEEN)

U.S. Brand Names YF-VAX®

Canadian Brand Names YF-VAX®

Therapeutic Category Vaccine, Live Virus

Use Induction of active immunity against yellow fever virus, primarily among persons traveling or living in areas where yellow fever infection exists and laboratory workers who may be exposed to the virus; vaccination may also be required for some international travelers

The Advisory Committee on Immunization Practices (ACIP) recommends vaccination for:
- Persons traveling to or living in areas at risk for yellow fever transmission
- Persons traveling to countries which require vaccination for international travel
- Laboratory personnel who may be exposed to the yellow fever virus or concentrated preparations of the vaccine

Although the vaccine is approved for use in children ≥9 months of age, the CDC recommends use in children as young as 6 months under unusual circumstances (eg, travel to an area where exposure is unavoidable). Children <6 months of age should **never** receive the vaccine.

General Dosage Range SubQ: *Children ≥9 months and Adults:* Initial: 0.5 mL as a single dose

Dosage Forms

Injection, powder for reconstitution [17D-204 strain]:
YF-VAX®: ≥4.74 Log_{10} plaque-forming units (PFU) per 0.5 mL dose

Yervoy™ *see* ipilimumab *on page 498*
YF-VAX® *see* yellow fever vaccine *on page 957*
YM087 *see* conivaptan *on page 235*
YM905 *see* solifenacin *on page 848*
YM-08310 *see* amifostine *on page 59*
Yodoxin® *see* iodoquinol *on page 494*
Z4942 *see* ifosfamide *on page 473*
Zactima *see* vandetanib *on page 937*
Zaditen® (Can) *see* ketotifen (systemic) *(Canada only) on page 514*
Zaditor® [OTC] *see* ketotifen (ophthalmic) *on page 514*
Zaditor® (Can) *see* ketotifen (ophthalmic) *on page 514*

zafirlukast (za FIR loo kast)

Medication Safety Issues

Sound-alike/look-alike issues:
Accolate® may be confused with Accupril®, Accutane®, Aclovate®

Synonyms ICI-204,219

U.S. Brand Names Accolate®

Canadian Brand Names Accolate®

Therapeutic Category Leukotriene Receptor Antagonist

Use Prophylaxis and chronic treatment of asthma

General Dosage Range Oral:
Children 5-11 years: 10 mg twice daily
Children ≥12 years and Adults: 20 mg twice daily

Dosage Forms

Tablet, oral: 10 mg, 20 mg
Accolate®: 10 mg, 20 mg

zaleplon (ZAL e plon)

Medication Safety Issues

Sound-alike/look-alike issues:
Sonata® may be confused with Soriatane®
Zaleplon may be confused with Zelapar®, Zemplar®, zolpidem, ZyPREXA® Zydis®

BEERS Criteria medication:
This drug may be potentially inappropriate for use in geriatric patients (Quality of evidence - moderate; Strength of recommendation - strong).

U.S. Brand Names Sonata®

Therapeutic Category Hypnotic, Miscellaneous

Controlled Substance C-IV

Use Short-term (7-10 days) treatment of insomnia (has been demonstrated to be effective for up to 5 weeks in controlled trial)

General Dosage Range Dosage adjustment recommended in patients with hepatic impairment

Oral:

Adults: 5-20 mg at bedtime

Elderly: 5 mg at bedtime (maximum: 10 mg/day)

Dosage Forms

Capsule, oral: 5 mg, 10 mg

Sonata®: 5 mg, 10 mg

Zaltrap® *see* ziv-aflibercept (systemic) *on page 964*

Zamicet™ *see* hydrocodone and acetaminophen *on page 454*

Zanaflex® *see* tizanidine *on page 900*

Zanaflex Capsules® *see* tizanidine *on page 900*

zanamivir (za NA mi veer)

Medication Safety Issues

Sound-alike/look-alike issues:

Relenza® may be confused with Albenza®, Aplenzin™

U.S. Brand Names Relenza®

Canadian Brand Names Relenza®

Therapeutic Category Antiviral Agent, Inhalation Therapy

Use Treatment of uncomplicated acute illness due to influenza virus A and B in patients who have been symptomatic for no more than 2 days; prophylaxis against influenza virus A and B

The Advisory Committee on Immunization Practices (ACIP) recommends that **treatment** be considered for the following:

- Persons with severe, complicated or progressive illness
- Hospitalized persons
- Persons at higher risk for influenza complications:
  - Children <2 years of age (highest risk in children <6 months of age)
  - Adults ≥65 years of age
  - Persons with chronic disorders of the pulmonary (including asthma) or cardiovascular systems (except hypertension)
  - Persons with chronic metabolic diseases (including diabetes mellitus), hepatic disease, renal dysfunction, hematologic disorders (including sickle cell disease), or immunosuppression (including immunosuppression caused by medications or HIV)
  - Persons with neurologic/neuromuscular conditions (including conditions such as spinal cord injuries, seizure disorders, cerebral palsy, stroke, mental retardation, moderate to severe developmental delay, or muscular dystrophy) which may compromise respiratory function, the handling of respiratory secretions, or that can increase the risk of aspiration
  - Pregnant or postpartum women (≤2 weeks after delivery)
  - Persons <19 years of age on long-term aspirin therapy
  - American Indians and Alaskan Natives
  - Persons who are morbidly obese (BMI ≥40)
  - Residents of nursing homes or other chronic care facilities
- Use may also be considered for previously healthy, nonhigh-risk outpatients with confirmed or suspected influenza based on clinical judgment when treatment can be started within 48 hours of illness onset.

The ACIP recommends that **prophylaxis** be considered for the following:

- Postexposure prophylaxis may be considered for family or close contacts of suspected or confirmed cases, who are at higher risk of influenza complications, and who have not been vaccinated against the circulating strain at the time of the exposure.
- Postexposure prophylaxis may be considered for unvaccinated healthcare workers who had occupational exposure without protective equipment.
- Preexposure prophylaxis should only be used for persons at very high risk of influenza complications who cannot be otherwise protected at times of high risk for exposure.
- Prophylaxis should also be administered to all eligible residents of institutions that house patients at high risk when needed to control outbreaks.

General Dosage Range Oral inhalation:
Children ≥5 years: Prophylaxis: 10 mg once daily
Children ≥7 years: Treatment: 10 mg twice daily
Adolescents and Adults: Prophylaxis: 10 mg once to twice daily; Treatment: 10 mg twice daily

Dosage Forms
Powder, for oral inhalation:
Relenza®: 5 mg/blister (20s)

Zanosar® *see* streptozocin *on page 854*
Zantac® *see* ranitidine *on page 788*
Zantac 75® [OTC] *see* ranitidine *on page 788*
Zantac 75® (Can) *see* ranitidine *on page 788*
Zantac 150® [OTC] *see* ranitidine *on page 788*
Zantac® EFFERdose® *see* ranitidine *on page 788*
Zantac Maximum Strength Non-Prescription (Can) *see* ranitidine *on page 788*
Zapzyt® [OTC] *see* benzoyl peroxide *on page 124*
Zapzyt® Acne Wash [OTC] *see* salicylic acid *on page 816*
Zapzyt® Pore Treatment [OTC] *see* salicylic acid *on page 816*
Zarah® *see* ethinyl estradiol and drospirenone *on page 356*
Zarontin® *see* ethosuximide *on page 363*
Zaroxolyn® *see* metolazone *on page 594*
Zavesca® *see* miglustat *on page 603*
Z-chlopenthixol *see* zuclopenthixol *(Canada only) on page 969*
ZD1033 *see* anastrozole *on page 75*
ZD1694 *see* raltitrexed *(Canada only) on page 786*
ZD1839 *see* gefitinib *on page 420*
ZD6474 *see* vandetanib *on page 937*
ZD9238 *see* fulvestrant *on page 411*
ZDV *see* zidovudine *on page 961*
ZDV, abacavir, and lamivudine *see* abacavir, lamivudine, and zidovudine *on page 16*
ZDX *see* goserelin *on page 431*
Zeasorb®-AF [OTC] *see* miconazole (topical) *on page 599*
Zebeta® *see* bisoprolol *on page 136*
Zebutal® *see* butalbital, acetaminophen, and caffeine *on page 153*
Zegerid® *see* omeprazole and sodium bicarbonate *on page 666*
Zegerid OTC™ [OTC] *see* omeprazole and sodium bicarbonate *on page 666*
Zelapar® *see* selegiline *on page 828*
Zelboraf™ *see* vemurafenib *on page 941*
Zeldox *see* ziprasidone *on page 964*
Zeldox® (Can) *see* ziprasidone *on page 964*
Zelnorm® *see* tegaserod *on page 873*
Zelnorm® [DSC] (Can) *see* tegaserod *on page 873*
Zemaira® *see* alpha$_1$-proteinase inhibitor *on page 51*
Zemplar® *see* paricalcitol *on page 692*
Zemuron® *see* rocuronium *on page 808*
Zenchent™ *see* ethinyl estradiol and norethindrone *on page 359*
Zenchent Fe™ *see* ethinyl estradiol and norethindrone *on page 359*
Zencia™ *see* sulfur and sulfacetamide *on page 862*
Zenhale™ (Can) *see* mometasone and formoterol *on page 611*
Zenpep® *see* pancrelipase *on page 687*
Zeosa™ *see* ethinyl estradiol and norethindrone *on page 359*
Zerit® *see* stavudine *on page 853*
Zestoretic® *see* lisinopril and hydrochlorothiazide *on page 544*
Zestril® *see* lisinopril *on page 544*
Zetar® [OTC] *see* coal tar *on page 228*

Zetia® *see* ezetimibe *on page* 369
Zetonna™ *see* ciclesonide (nasal) *on page* 207
Zevalin® *see* ibritumomab *on page* 468
Zgesic *see* acetaminophen and phenyltoloxamine *on page* 25
Ziac® *see* bisoprolol and hydrochlorothiazide *on page* 137
Ziagen® *see* abacavir *on page* 16
Ziana® *see* clindamycin and tretinoin *on page* 219

ziconotide (zi KOE no tide)

Medication Safety Issues

High alert medication:

The Institute for Safe Medication Practices (ISMP) includes this medication among its list of drugs which have a heightened risk of causing significant patient harm when used in error.

U.S. Brand Names Prialt®

Therapeutic Category Analgesic, Nonnarcotic; Calcium Channel Blocker, N-Type

Use Management of severe chronic pain in patients requiring intrathecal (I.T.) therapy and who are intolerant or refractory to other therapies

General Dosage Range Dosage adjustment recommended in patients who develop toxicities

I.T.: *Adults:* Initial dose: ≤2.4 mcg/day (0.1 mcg/hour); Maintenance range: 2.4-19.2 mcg/day (0.1-0.8 mcg/hour) (maximum: 19.2 mcg/day [0.8 mcg/hour])

Dosage Forms

Infusion, intrathecal [preservative free]:

Prialt®: 25 mcg/mL (20 mL); 100 mcg/mL (1 mL, 5 mL)

Zictifa *see* vandetanib *on page* 937

zidovudine (zye DOE vyoo deen)

Medication Safety Issues

Sound-alike/look-alike issues:

Azidothymidine may be confused with azaTHIOprine, aztreonam

Retrovir® may be confused with acyclovir, ritonavir

Other safety concerns:

AZT is an error-prone abbreviation (mistaken as azathioprine, aztreonam)

Synonyms azidothymidine; AZT (error-prone abbreviation); compound S; ZDV

U.S. Brand Names Retrovir®

Canadian Brand Names Apo-Zidovudine®; AZT™; Novo-AZT; Retrovir®; Retrovir® (AZT™)

Therapeutic Category Antiviral Agent

Use Treatment of HIV infection in combination with at least two other antiretroviral agents; prevention of maternal/fetal HIV transmission

General Dosage Range Dosage adjustment recommended in patients with renal impairment or who develop toxicities

I.V.:

Infants <30 weeks gestation at birth: 1.5 mg/kg/dose every 12 hours; at 4 weeks of age advance to 2.3 mg/kg/dose every 12 hours

Infants ≥30 weeks and <35 weeks gestation at birth: 1.5 mg/kg/dose every 12 hours; at 15 days of age, advance to 2.3 mg/kg/dose every 12 hours

Infants ≥35 weeks: 3 mg/kg/dose every 12 hour

Children 6 weeks to <12 years: 120 mg/m^2/dose every 6 hours **or** 20 mg/m^2/hour as a continuous infusion

Children ≥12 years and Adults: 1 mg/kg/dose every 4 hours around-the-clock **or** 2 mg/kg bolus followed by 1 mg/kg/hour continuous infusion during labor and delivery

Oral:

Infants <30 weeks gestation at birth: 2 mg/kg/dose every 12 hours; at 4 weeks of age advance to 3 mg/kg/dose every 12 hours

Infants ≥30 weeks and <35 weeks gestation at birth: 2 mg/kg/dose every 12 hours; at 15 days of age, advance to 3 mg/kg/dose every 12 hours

Infants ≥35 weeks: 4 mg/kg/dose twice daily

Children 4 weeks to <18 years: 240 mg/m^2 every 12 hours (maximum 300 mg every 12 hours) **or** 160 mg/m^2/dose every 8 hours (maximum: 200 mg every 8 hours)
4 to <9 kg: 12 mg/kg/dose twice daily **or** 8 mg/kg/dose 3 times/day
≥9 to <30 kg: 9 mg/kg/dose twice daily **or** 6 mg/kg/dose 3 times/day
≥30 kg and Adults: 300 mg twice daily **or** 200 mg 3 times/day

Dosage Forms
Capsule, oral: 100 mg
Retrovir®: 100 mg
Injection, solution [preservative free]:
Retrovir®: 10 mg/mL (20 mL)
Syrup, oral: 10 mg/mL (240 mL)
Retrovir®: 10 mg/mL (240 mL)
Tablet, oral: 300 mg

zidovudine, abacavir, and lamivudine *see* abacavir, lamivudine, and zidovudine *on page 16*
zidovudine and lamivudine *see* lamivudine and zidovudine *on page 520*
Zilactin®-L [OTC] *see* benzyl alcohol *on page 127*
Zilactin®-B [OTC] *see* benzocaine *on page 121*
Zilactin-B® (Can) *see* benzocaine *on page 121*
Zilactin Baby® (Can) *see* benzocaine *on page 121*
Zilactin® Tooth & Gum Pain [OTC] *see* benzocaine *on page 121*

zileuton (zye LOO ton)

U.S. Brand Names Zyflo CR®; Zyflo®
Therapeutic Category 5-Lipoxygenase Inhibitor
Use Prophylaxis and chronic treatment of asthma
General Dosage Range Oral:
Extended release: *Children ≥12 years and Adults:* 1200 mg twice daily
Immediate release: *Children ≥12 years and Adults:* 600 mg 4 times/day
Dosage Forms
Tablet, oral:
Zyflo®: 600 mg [scored]
Tablet, extended release, oral:
Zyflo CR®: 600 mg

Zinacef® *see* cefuroxime *on page 187*
zinc *see* trace elements *on page 908*
Zinc 15 [OTC] *see* zinc sulfate *on page 963*

zinc acetate (zink AS e tate)

U.S. Brand Names Galzin®
Therapeutic Category Trace Element
Use Maintenance treatment of Wilson disease following initial chelation therapy
General Dosage Range Oral:
Children ≥10 years and Adults (pregnant females): 75-150 mg/day in 3 divided doses
Adults (males and nonpregnant females): 150 mg/day in 3 divided doses
Dosage Forms
Capsule, oral:
Galzin®: Elemental zinc 25 mg, Elemental zinc 50 mg

Zincate® [DSC] *see* zinc sulfate *on page 963*

zinc chloride (zink KLOR ide)

Therapeutic Category Trace Element
Use Cofactor for replacement therapy to different enzymes; helps maintain normal growth rates, normal skin hydration, and senses of taste and smell
General Dosage Range I.V.:
Premature infants <1500 g up to 3 kg: 300 mcg/kg/day
Infants (full term) and Children ≤5 years: 100 mcg/kg/day to I.V. fluid
Adults: 2-6 mg/day, up to 12.2 mg/L TPN **or** 17.1 mg/kg of stool or ileostomy output

Dosage Forms

Injection, solution [preservative free]: 1 mg/mL (10 mL)

zinc diethylenetriaminepentaacetate (Zn-DTPA) *see* diethylene triamine penta-acetic acid *on page 283*

zinc diethylene triamine penta-acetic acid (Zn-DTPA) *see* diethylene triamine penta-acetic acid *on page 283*

Zincfrin® (Can) *see* phenylephrine and zinc sulfate *(Canada only) on page 718*

zinc gelatin (zink JEL ah tin)

Synonyms dome paste bandage; Unna boot; Unna paste; zinc gelatin boot

U.S. Brand Names Gelucast®

Therapeutic Category Protectant, Topical

Use As a protectant and to support varicosities and similar lesions of the lower limbs

General Dosage Range Topical: *Adults:* Apply externally as an occlusive boot

Dosage Forms

Bandage: 3" x 10 yards; 4" x 10 yards
Gelucast®: 3" x 10 yards; 4" x 10 yards

zinc gelatin boot *see* zinc gelatin *on page 963*

Zincofax® (Can) *see* zinc oxide *on page 963*

Zincon® [OTC] *see* pyrithione zinc *on page 779*

zinc oxide (zink OKS ide)

Synonyms base ointment; lassar's zinc paste

U.S. Brand Names Ammens® Original Medicated [OTC]; Ammens® Shower Fresh [OTC]; Balmex® [OTC]; Boudreaux's® Butt Paste [OTC]; Critic-Aid Skin Care® [OTC]; Desitin® Creamy [OTC]; Desitin® [OTC]

Canadian Brand Names Zincofax®

Therapeutic Category Topical Skin Product

Use Protective coating for mild skin irritations and abrasions; soothing and protective ointment to promote healing of chapped skin, diaper rash

General Dosage Range Topical: *Children and Adults:* Apply as required to affected areas several times daily

Dosage Forms

Cream, topical:
Balmex® [OTC]: 11.3% (60 g, 120 g, 480 g)

Cream, topical [stick]:
Balmex® [OTC]: 11.3% (56 g)

Ointment, topical: 20% (30 g, 60 g, 454 g); 40% (120 g)
Desitin® [OTC]: 40% (30 g, 60 g, 90 g, 120 g, 270 g, 480 g)
Desitin® Creamy [OTC]: 10% (60 g, 120 g)

Paste, topical:
Boudreaux's® Butt Paste [OTC]: 16% (30 g, 60 g, 120 g, 480 g)
Critic-Aid Skin Care® [OTC]: 20% (71 g, 170 g)

Powder, topical:
Ammens® Original Medicated [OTC], Ammens® Shower Fresh [OTC]: 9.1% (312 g)

zinc oxide and miconazole nitrate *see* miconazole and zinc oxide *on page 600*

zinc sulfate (zink SUL fate)

Medication Safety Issues

Sound-alike/look-alike issues:
$ZnSO_4$ is an error-prone abbreviation (mistaken as morphine sulfate)

Synonyms $ZnSO_4$ (error-prone abbreviation)

U.S. Brand Names Orazinc® 110 [OTC]; Orazinc® 220 [OTC]; Zinc 15 [OTC]; Zincate® [DSC]

Canadian Brand Names Anuzinc; Rivasol

Therapeutic Category Electrolyte Supplement, Oral

Use Zinc supplement (oral and parenteral); may improve wound healing in those who are deficient

General Dosage Range

I.V.:

Premature infants (<1500 g up to 3 kg): 300 mcg/kg/day

Infants (full term) and Children ≤5 years: 100 mcg/kg/day

Adults: 2.5-6 mg/day **or** 12.2 mg/L of TPN **or** 17.1 mg/kg of stool or ileostomy output

Oral: *Children and Adults:* Dosage varies depending on product labeling

Dosage Forms

Capsule, oral: 220 mg

Orazinc® 220 [OTC]: 220 mg

Injection, solution [preservative free]: Elemental zinc 1 mg/mL (10 mL); Elemental zinc 5 mg/mL (5 mL)

Tablet, oral: 220 mg

Orazinc® 110 [OTC]: 110 mg

Zinc 15 [OTC]: 66 mg

zinc sulfate and phenylephrine *see* phenylephrine and zinc sulfate *(Canada only) on page 718*

zinc undecylenate *see* undecylenic acid and derivatives *on page 929*

Zinecard® *see* dexrazoxane *on page 269*

Zioptan™ *see* tafluprost *on page 867*

ziprasidone (zi PRAS i done)

Medication Safety Issues

Sound-alike/look-alike issues:

Ziprasidone may be confused with TraZODone

BEERS Criteria medication:

This drug may be potentially inappropriate for use in geriatric patients (Quality of evidence - moderate; Strength of recommendation - strong).

Synonyms Zeldox; ziprasidone hydrochloride; ziprasidone mesylate

U.S. Brand Names Geodon®

Canadian Brand Names Zeldox®

Therapeutic Category Antipsychotic Agent

Use Treatment of schizophrenia; treatment of acute manic or mixed episodes associated with bipolar disorder with or without psychosis; maintenance treatment of bipolar disorder as an adjunct to lithium or valproate; acute agitation in patients with schizophrenia

General Dosage Range

I.M.: *Adults:* 10 mg every 2 hours **or** 20 mg every 4 hours (maximum: 40 mg/day)

Oral: *Adults:* Initial: 20-40 mg twice daily; Maintenance: 20-80 mg twice daily (maximum: 200 mg/day)

Dosage Forms

Capsule, oral: 20 mg, 40 mg, 60 mg, 80 mg

Geodon®: 20 mg, 40 mg, 60 mg, 80 mg

Injection, powder for reconstitution:

Geodon®: 20 mg

ziprasidone hydrochloride *see* ziprasidone *on page 964*

ziprasidone mesylate *see* ziprasidone *on page 964*

Zipsor® *see* diclofenac (systemic) *on page 279*

Zirgan® *see* ganciclovir (ophthalmic) *on page 419*

Zithranol®-RR *see* anthralin *on page 76*

Zithromax® *see* azithromycin (systemic) *on page 108*

Zithromax® TRI-PAK™ *see* azithromycin (systemic) *on page 108*

Zithromax® Z-PAK® *see* azithromycin (systemic) *on page 108*

ziv-aflibercept (systemic) (ziv a FLIB er sept)

Medication Safety Issues

Sound-alike/look-alike issues:

Ziv-aflibercept may be confused with aflibercept

High alert medication:

This medication is in a class the Institute for Safe Medical Practices (ISMP) includes among its list of drug classes which have a heightened risk of causing significant patient harm when used in error.

Synonyms aflibercept I.V.; vascular endothelial growth factor trap; VEGF trap; VEGF trap R1R2; Zaltrap®

U.S. Brand Names Zaltrap®
Therapeutic Category Antineoplastic Agent; Vascular Endothelial Growth Factor (VEGF) Inhibitor
Use Treatment of metastatic colorectal cancer (in combination with fluorouracil, leucovorin, and irinotecan [FOLFIRI]) in patients who are resistant to or have progressed on an oxaliplatin-based regimen
General Dosage Range Dosage adjustment recommended in patients who develop toxicities.
I.V.: *Adults:* 4 mg/kg every 2 weeks
Dosage Forms
Injection, solution [preservative free]:
Zaltrap®: 25 mg/mL (4 mL, 8 mL)

Zmax® *see* azithromycin (systemic) *on page* *108*
Zmax SR™ (Can) *see* azithromycin (systemic) *on page* *108*
Zn-DTPA *see* diethylene triamine penta-acetic acid *on page* *283*
ZNP® [OTC] *see* pyrithione zinc *on page* *779*
$ZnSO_4$ (error-prone abbreviation) *see* zinc sulfate *on page* *963*
Zocor® *see* simvastatin *on page* *835*
Zofran® *see* ondansetron *on page* *667*
Zofran® ODT *see* ondansetron *on page* *667*
zol 446 *see* zoledronic acid *on page* *965*
Zoladex® *see* goserelin *on page* *431*
Zoladex® LA (Can) *see* goserelin *on page* *431*
zoledronate *see* zoledronic acid *on page* *965*

zoledronic acid (zoe le DRON ik AS id)

Medication Safety Issues
Sound-alike/look-alike issues:
Zometa® may be confused with Zofran®, Zoladex®
Other safety concerns:
Duplicate therapy issues: Reclast® and Aclasta® contain zoledronic acid, which is the same ingredient contained in Zometa®; patients receiving Zometa® should not be treated with Reclast® or Aclasta®
Synonyms CGP-42446; zol 446; zoledronate
U.S. Brand Names Reclast®; Zometa®
Canadian Brand Names Aclasta®; Zometa®
Therapeutic Category Bisphosphonate Derivative
Use
Oncology-related uses: Treatment of hypercalcemia of malignancy (albumin-corrected serum calcium >12 mg/dL); treatment of multiple myeloma; treatment of bone metastases of solid tumors
Nononcology uses: Treatment of Paget disease of bone; treatment of osteoporosis in postmenopausal women (to reduce the incidence of fractures or to reduce the incidence of new clinical fractures in patients with low-trauma hip fracture); prevention of osteoporosis in postmenopausal women, treatment of osteoporosis in men (to increase bone mass); treatment and prevention of glucocorticoid-induced osteoporosis (in patients initiating or continuing prednisone ≥7.5 mg/day [or equivalent] and expected to remain on glucocorticoids for at least 12 months)
General Dosage Range
I.V.: *Adults:*
Zometa®: 4 mg as a single dose or every 3-4 weeks
Reclast®: 5 mg as a single dose, once a year or every 2 years
Dosage Forms
Infusion, premixed:
Reclast®: 5 mg (100 mL)
Zometa®: 4 mg (100 mL)
Injection, solution:
Zometa®: 4 mg/5 mL (5 mL)
Dosage Forms - Canada
Infusion, solution [premixed]:
Aclasta®: 5 mg (100 mL)

Zolinza® *see* vorinostat *on page* *954*

zolmitriptan (zohl mi TRIP tan)

Medication Safety Issues

Sound-alike/look-alike issues:

ZOLMitriptan may be confused with SUMAtriptan

Synonyms 311C90

Tall-Man ZOLMitriptan

U.S. Brand Names Zomig-ZMT®; Zomig®

Canadian Brand Names Mylan-Zolmitriptan; PMS-Zolmitriptan; PMS-Zolmitriptan ODT; Sandoz-Zolmitriptan; Sandoz-Zolmitriptan ODT; Teva-Zolmitriptan; Teva-Zolmitriptan OD; Zolmitriptan ODT; Zomig®; Zomig® Nasal Spray; Zomig® Rapimelt

Therapeutic Category Antimigraine Agent; Serotonin Agonist

Use Acute treatment of migraine with or without aura

General Dosage Range Dosage adjustment recommended in patients with hepatic impairment

Nasal inhalation: *Adults:* 1 spray (5 mg) at the onset of migraine headache; may repeat in 2 hours if no relief (maximum: 10 mg/24 hours)

Oral: *Adults:* 1.25-2.5 mg at the onset of migraine headache; may repeat in 2 hours if no relief (maximum: 10 mg/24 hours)

Dosage Forms

Solution, intranasal:

Zomig®: 5 mg/0.1 mL (0.1 mL)

Tablet, oral:

Zomig®: 2.5 mg, 5 mg

Tablet, orally disintegrating, oral:

Zomig-ZMT®: 2.5 mg, 5 mg

Zolmitriptan ODT (Can) *see* zolmitriptan *on page 966*

Zoloft® *see* sertraline *on page 831*

zolpidem (zole PI dem)

Medication Safety Issues

Sound-alike/look-alike issues:

Ambien® may be confused with Abilify®, Ativan®, Ambi 10®

Sublinox™ may be confused with Suboxone®

Zolpidem may be confused with lorazepam, zaleplon

BEERS Criteria medication:

This drug may be potentially inappropriate for use in geriatric patients (Quality of evidence - moderate; Strength of recommendation - strong).

International issues:

Ambien [U.S., Argentina, Israel] may be confused with Amyben brand name for amiodarone [Great Britain]

Synonyms zolpidem tartrate

U.S. Brand Names Ambien CR®; Ambien®; Edluar™; Intermezzo®; Zolpimist®

Canadian Brand Names Sublinox™

Therapeutic Category Hypnotic, Miscellaneous

Controlled Substance C-IV

Use

Ambien®, Edluar™, Zolpimist®: Short-term treatment of insomnia (with difficulty of sleep onset)

Ambien CR®: Treatment of insomnia (with difficulty of sleep onset and/or sleep maintenance)

Intermezzo®: "As needed" treatment of middle-of-the-night insomnia with ≥4 hours of sleep time remaining.

Sublinox™ (Canadian availability; not available in U.S.): Short-term treatment of insomnia (with difficulty of sleep onset, frequent awakenings, and/or early awakenings)

General Dosage Range Dosage adjustment recommended in patients with hepatic impairment and concomitant medications.

Oral:

Immediate release tablet, spray:

Adults: 10 mg immediately before bedtime

Elderly: 5 mg immediately before bedtime

Sublingual tablet:

Adults: 10 mg immediately before bedtime **or** 1.75 mg (females) or 3.5 mg (males) once per night as needed

Elderly: 5 mg immediately before bedtime **or** 1.75 mg (females and males) once per night as needed

Extended release tablet:

Adults: 12.5 mg immediately before bedtime

Elderly: 6.25 mg immediately before bedtime

Dosage Forms

Solution, oral:

Zolpimist®: 5 mg/actuation (8.2 g)

Tablet, oral: 5 mg, 10 mg

Ambien®: 5 mg, 10 mg

Tablet, sublingual:

Edluar™: 5 mg, 10 mg

Intermezzo®: 1.75 mg, 3.5 mg

Tablet, extended release, oral: 6.25 mg, 12.5 mg

Ambien CR®: 6.25 mg, 12.5 mg

Dosage Forms - Canada

Tablet, sublingual:

Sublinox™: 10 mg

zolpidem tartrate *see* zolpidem *on page 966*
Zolpimist® *see* zolpidem *on page 966*
Zolvit® *see* hydrocodone and acetaminophen *on page 454*
Zometa® *see* zoledronic acid *on page 965*
Zomig® *see* zolmitriptan *on page 966*
Zomig® Nasal Spray (Can) *see* zolmitriptan *on page 966*
Zomig® Rapimelt (Can) *see* zolmitriptan *on page 966*
Zomig-ZMT® *see* zolmitriptan *on page 966*
Zonalon® *see* doxepin (topical) *on page 312*
Zonatuss™ *see* benzonatate *on page 124*
Zonegran® *see* zonisamide *on page 967*

zonisamide (zoe NIS a mide)

Medication Safety Issues

Sound-alike/look-alike issues:

Zonegran® may be confused with SINEquan®

Zonisamide may be confused with lacosamide

U.S. Brand Names Zonegran®

Therapeutic Category Anticonvulsant, Sulfonamide

Use Adjunct treatment of partial seizures in children >16 years of age and adults with epilepsy

General Dosage Range Oral: *Children >16 years and Adults:* Initial: 100 mg/day; Maintenance: 100-600 mg/day (maximum: 600 mg/day)

Dosage Forms

Capsule, oral: 25 mg, 50 mg, 100 mg

Zonegran®: 25 mg, 100 mg

zopiclone *(Canada only)* (ZOE pi clone)

Canadian Brand Names Apo-Zopiclone®; CO Zopiclone; Dom-Zopiclone; Imovane®; Mylan-Zopiclone; Novo-Zopiclone; Nu-Zopiclone; PHL-Zopiclone; PMS-Zopiclone; PRO-Zopiclone; RAN™-Zopiclone; ratio-Zopiclone; Rhovane®; Riva-Zopiclone; Sandoz-Zopiclone

Therapeutic Category Hypnotic, Miscellaneous

Use Short-term and symptomatic relief of insomnia

General Dosage Range Dosage adjustment recommended in patients with hepatic and renal impairment, elderly and debilitated patients, and patients with chronic respiratory insufficiency.

Oral:

Adults: 3.75-7.5 mg once daily at bedtime

Elderly: Initial: 3.75 mg once daily at bedtime

Product Availability Not available in U.S.

Dosage Forms - Canada

Tablet, oral: 5 mg, 7.5 mg

Zorbtive® *see* somatropin *on page 849*
Zorcaine™ *see* articaine and epinephrine *on page 92*
Zortress® *see* everolimus *on page 367*
ZOS *see* zoster vaccine *on page 968*
Zostavax® *see* zoster vaccine *on page 968*

zoster vaccine (ZOS ter vak SEEN)

Medication Safety Issues

Administration issues:

Both varicella vaccine and zoster vaccine are live, attenuated strains of varicella-zoster virus. Their indications, dosing, and composition are distinct. Varicella vaccine is indicated for the prevention of chickenpox, while zoster vaccine is indicated in older individuals to prevent reactivation of the virus which causes shingles. Zoster vaccine is **not** a substitute for varicella vaccine and should not be used in children.

Synonyms shingles vaccine; varicella-zoster (VZV) vaccine (zoster); VZV vaccine (zoster); ZOS

U.S. Brand Names Zostavax®

Canadian Brand Names Zostavax®

Therapeutic Category Vaccine

Use Prevention of herpes zoster (shingles) in patients ≥50 years of age

The Advisory Committee on Immunization Practices (ACIP) recommends routine vaccination of all patients ≥60 years of age, including:

- Patients who report a previous episode of zoster.
- Patients with chronic medical conditions (eg, chronic renal failure, diabetes mellitus, rheumatoid arthritis, chronic pulmonary disease) unless those conditions are contraindications.
- Residents of nursing homes and other long-term care facilities ≥60 years of age, without contraindications.

Although not specifically recommended for their profession, healthcare providers within the recommended age group should also receive the zoster vaccine (CDC, 61[4], 2012)

General Dosage Range SubQ: *Adults ≥50 years:* 0.65 mL as a single dose

Dosage Forms

Injection, powder for reconstitution [preservative free]:

Zostavax®: 19,400 PFU

Zostrix® [OTC] *see* capsaicin *on page 170*
Zostrix® (Can) *see* capsaicin *on page 170*
Zostrix® Diabetic Foot Pain [OTC] *see* capsaicin *on page 170*
Zostrix®-HP [OTC] *see* capsaicin *on page 170*
Zostrix® H.P. (Can) *see* capsaicin *on page 170*
Zosyn® *see* piperacillin and tazobactam *on page 726*
Zovia® *see* ethinyl estradiol and ethynodiol diacetate *on page 357*
Zovirax® *see* acyclovir (systemic) *on page 34*
Zovirax® *see* acyclovir (topical) *on page 35*
Z-Pak *see* azithromycin (systemic) *on page 108*
ZUACTA™ (Can) *see* zucapsaicin *(Canada only) on page 968*

zucapsaicin *(Canada only)* (zu kap SAY sin)

Canadian Brand Names ZUACTA™

Therapeutic Category Analgesic, Topical; Topical Skin Product; Transient Receptor Potential Vanilloid 1 (TRPV1) Agonist

Use In conjunction with an oral NSAID or COX-2 inhibitor for short-term (≤3 months) treatment of severe pain associated with osteoarthritis of the knee that is not controlled by NSAID or COX-2 inhibitor monotherapy

General Dosage Range Topical: *Adults:* Apply a pea-sized amount to each of 3 different locations around affected knee 3 times/day (minimum interval between applications: 4 hours) (maximum: 3 applications/day)

Product Availability Not available in the U.S.

Dosage Forms - Canada

Cream, topical:

Zuacta™: 0.075% (30 g, 60 g)

zuclopenthixol acetate *see* zuclopenthixol *(Canada only) on page 969*

zuclopenthixol *(Canada only)* (zoo kloe pen THIX ol)

Synonyms Z-chlopenthixol; zuclopenthixol acetate; zuclopenthixol decanoate; zuclopenthixol dihydrochloride; zuclopenthixol hydrochloride; zuclopentixol acetate; zuclopentixol decanoate; zuclopentixol hydrochloride

Canadian Brand Names Clopixol-Acuphase®; Clopixol®; Clopixol® Depot

Therapeutic Category Antipsychotic Agent

Use Management of schizophrenia; acetate injection is intended for short-term acute treatment; decanoate injection is for long-term management; hydrochloride tablets may be used in either the initial or maintenance phase

General Dosage Range

I.M.: *Adults:* Acetate: Initial: 50-150 mg, may repeat in 2-3 days (maximum: 4 doses or 400 mg during treatment course; maximum treatment course: 2 weeks); Decanoate: Initial: 100-400 mg every 2 weeks (usual maintenance: 150-300 mg every 2-4 weeks)

Oral: *Adults:* Initial: 10-50 mg/day in 2-3 divided doses; usual dosage range for acute therapy: 20-60 mg/day (maximum: 100 mg/day); usual maintenance dose: 20-40 mg/day

Product Availability Not available in U.S.

Dosage Forms - Canada

Injection:

Clopixol Acuphase®: 50 mg/mL [zuclopenthixol 42.5 mg/mL] (1 mL, 2 mL)

Clopixol® Depot: 200 mg/mL [zuclopenthixol 144.4 mg/mL] (10 mL)

Tablet, oral:

Clopixol®: 10 mg, 25 mg, 40 mg

zuclopenthixol decanoate *see* zuclopenthixol *(Canada only) on page 969*

zuclopenthixol dihydrochloride *see* zuclopenthixol *(Canada only) on page 969*

zuclopenthixol hydrochloride *see* zuclopenthixol *(Canada only) on page 969*

zuclopentixol acetate *see* zuclopenthixol *(Canada only) on page 969*

zuclopentixol decanoate *see* zuclopenthixol *(Canada only) on page 969*

zuclopentixol hydrochloride *see* zuclopenthixol *(Canada only) on page 969*

Zuplenz® *see* ondansetron *on page 667*

Zutripro™ *see* hydrocodone, chlorpheniramine, and pseudoephedrine *on page 457*

Zyban® *see* bupropion *on page 150*

Zyclara® *see* imiquimod *on page 476*

Zydone® *see* hydrocodone and acetaminophen *on page 454*

Zyflo® *see* zileuton *on page 962*

Zyflo CR® *see* zileuton *on page 962*

Zylet® *see* loteprednol and tobramycin *on page 552*

Zyloprim® *see* allopurinol *on page 50*

ZYM-Amlodipine (Can) *see* amlodipine *on page 65*

Zymar™ (Can) *see* gatifloxacin *on page 420*

Zymaxid™ *see* gatifloxacin *on page 420*

ZYM-Carvedilol (Can) *see* carvedilol *on page 179*

ZYM-Cholestyramine-Light (Can) *see* cholestyramine resin *on page 205*

ZYM-Cholestyramine-Regular (Can) *see* cholestyramine resin *on page 205*

ZYM-Clonazepam (Can) *see* clonazepam *on page 223*

ZYM-Cyclobenzaprine (Can) *see* cyclobenzaprine *on page 243*

ZYM-Fluconazole (Can) *see* fluconazole *on page 388*

ZYM-Fluoxetine (Can) *see* fluoxetine *on page 396*

ZYM-Mirtazapine (Can) *see* mirtazapine *on page 606*

ZYM-Ondansetron (Can) *see* ondansetron *on page 667*

ZYM-Pioglitazone (Can) *see* pioglitazone *on page 725*

CHEMOTHERAPY REGIMENS

5 + 2 (Cytarabine-Daunorubicin) (AML Induction)

Use Leukemia, acute myeloid

Regimen

Cytarabine: I.V.: 100 mg/m^2/day continuous infusion days 1 to 5 [total dose/cycle = 500 mg/m^2]

Daunorubicin: I.V.: 45 mg/m^2/day I.V. bolus days 1 and 2 [total dose/cycle = 90 mg/m^2]

May administer a second induction cycle if needed

5 + 2 (Cytarabine-Daunorubicin) (AML Postremission)

Use Leukemia, acute myeloid

Regimen

Cytarabine: I.V.: 100 mg/m^2/day continuous infusion days 1 to 5 [total dose/cycle = 500 mg/m^2]

Daunorubicin: I.V.: 45 mg/m^2/day I.V. bolus days 1 and 2 [total dose/cycle = 90 mg/m^2]

Administer 2 courses

5 + 2 (Cytarabine-Idarubicin) (AML Consolidation)

Use Leukemia, acute myeloid

Regimen

Cytarabine: I.V.: 100 mg/m^2/day continuous infusion days 1 to 5 [total dose/cycle = 500 mg/m^2]

Idarubicin: I.V.: 13 mg/m^2/day I.V. bolus days 1 and 2 [total dose/cycle = 26 mg/m^2]

Administer 2 courses

5 + 2 + 5 (Cytarabine-Daunorubicin-Etoposide) (AML Consolidation)

Use Leukemia, acute myeloid

Regimen

Cytarabine: I.V.: 100 mg/m^2/day continuous infusion days 1 to 5 [total dose/cycle = 500 mg/m^2]

Daunorubicin: I.V.: 50 mg/m^2/day I.V. bolus days 1 and 2 [total dose/cycle = 100 mg/m^2]

Etoposide: I.V.: 75 mg/m^2/day over 1 hour days 1 to 5 [total dose/cycle = 375 mg/m^2]

Administer 2 courses

5 + 2 (Cytarabine-Mitoxantrone) (AML Consolidation)

Use Leukemia, acute myeloid

Regimen

Cytarabine: I.V.: 100 mg/m^2/day continuous infusion days 1 to 5 [total dose/cycle = 500 mg/m^2]

Mitoxantrone: I.V.: 12 mg/m^2/day days 1 and 2 [total dose/cycle = 24 mg/m^2]

Administered every 28 days for a total of 2 cycles

7 + 3 (Cytarabine-Daunorubicin) (AML Induction)

Use Leukemia, acute myeloid

Regimen NOTE: Multiple variations are listed.

Variation 1:

Cytarabine: I.V.: 100 mg/m^2/day continuous infusion days 1 to 7 [total dose/cycle = 700 mg/m^2]

Daunorubicin: I.V.: 45 mg/m^2/day I.V. bolus days 1, 2, and 3 [total dose/cycle = 135 mg/m^2]

May administer a second induction cycle if needed

Variation 2 (≥60 years of age):
  Cytarabine: I.V.: 100 mg/m^2/day continuous infusion days 1 to 7
    [total dose/cycle = 700 mg/m^2]
  Daunorubicin: I.V.: 30 mg/m^2/day days 1, 2, and 3
    [total dose/cycle = 90 mg/m^2]
  May administer a second induction cycle if needed (at a reduced dose of daunorubicin [45 mg/m^2])
Variation 3 (between 17 and 60 years of age):
  Cytarabine: I.V.: 100 mg/m^2/day continuous infusion days 1 to 7
    [total dose/cycle = 700 mg/m^2]
  Daunorubicin: I.V.: 90 mg/m^2/day I.V. bolus days 1, 2, and 3
    [total dose/cycle = 270 mg/m^2]
  May administer a second induction cycle if needed
Variation 4 (<60 years of age):
  Cytarabine: I.V.: 200 mg/m^2/day continuous infusion days 1 to 7
    [total dose/cycle = 1400 mg/m^2]
  Daunorubicin: I.V.: 45 mg/m^2/day I.V. bolus days 1, 2, and 3
    [total dose/cycle = 135 mg/m^2]
  May administer a second induction cycle if needed

7 + 3 (Cytarabine-Idarubicin) (AML Induction)

Use Leukemia, acute myeloid

Regimen NOTE: Multiple variations are listed.

Variation 1:
  Cytarabine: I.V.: 100 mg/m^2/day continuous infusion days 1 to 7
    [total dose/cycle = 700 mg/m^2]
  Idarubicin: I.V.: 12 mg/m^2/day slow I.V. infusion days 1, 2, and 3
    [total dose/cycle = 36 mg/m^2]
  May administer a second induction cycle if needed
Variation 2:
  Cytarabine: I.V.: 100 mg/m^2/day continuous infusion days 1 to 7
    [total dose/cycle = 700 mg/m^2]
  Idarubicin: I.V.: 13 mg/m^2/day slow I.V. infusion days 1, 2, and 3
    [total dose/cycle = 39 mg/m^2]
  May administer a second induction cycle if needed

7 + 3 (Cytarabine-Mitoxantrone) (AML Induction)

Use Leukemia, acute myeloid

Regimen

Induction:
  Cytarabine: I.V.: 100 mg/m^2/day continuous infusion days 1 to 7
    [total dose/cycle = 700 mg/m^2]
  Mitoxantrone: I.V.: 12 mg/m^2/day days 1, 2, and 3
    [total dose/cycle = 36 mg/m^2]
Reinduction if needed:
  Cytarabine: I.V.: 100 mg/m^2/day continuous infusion days 1 to 5
    [total dose/cycle = 500 mg/m^2]
  Mitoxantrone: I.V.: 12 mg/m^2/day days 1 and 2
    [total dose/cycle = 24 mg/m^2]

7 + 3 + 7 (Cytarabine-Daunorubicin-Etoposide) (AML Induction)

Use Leukemia, acute myeloid

Regimen

Cytarabine: I.V.: 100 mg/m^2/day continuous infusion days 1 to 7
  [total dose/cycle = 700 mg/m^2]
Daunorubicin: I.V.: 50 mg/m^2/day days 1, 2, and 3
  [total dose/cycle = 150 mg/m^2]
Etoposide: I.V.: 75 mg/m^2/day over 1 hour days 1 to 7
  [total dose/cycle = 525 mg/m^2]
Up to 3 induction cycles may be given based on individual response

A3 (Neuroblastoma)

Use Neuroblastoma

Regimen

Cycle 1 (New A1):

Cyclophosphamide: I.V.: 1200 mg/m^2 over 6 hours day 1
[total dose/cycle = 1200 mg/m^2]

Doxorubicin: I.V.: 40 mg/m^2 day 3
[total dose/cycle = 40 mg/m^2]

Etoposide: I.V.: 100 mg/m^2/day days 1 to 5
[total dose/cycle = 500 mg/m^2]

Cisplatin: I.V.: 90 mg/m^2 day 5
[total dose/cycle = 90 mg/m^2]

Treatment cycle is 28 days

Cycles 2-5 (A3):

Cyclophosphamide: I.V.: 1200 mg/m^2/day over 6 hours days 1 and 2
[total dose/cycle = 2400 mg/m^2]

Doxorubicin: I.V.: 40 mg/m^2 day 3
[total dose/cycle = 40 mg/m^2]

Etoposide: I.V.: 100 mg/m^2/day days 1 to 5
[total dose/cycle = 500 mg/m^2]

Cisplatin: I.V.: 25 mg/m^2/day continuous infusion days 1 to 5
[total dose/cycle = 125 mg/m^2]

Repeat cycle every 28 days for 5 cycles (total of 6 cycles, cycle 1 administer New A1, cycles 2 to 5 administer A3)

Abiraterone-Prednisone (Prostate Cancer)

Use Prostate cancer

Regimen

Abiraterone acetate: Oral: 1000 mg once a day

Prednisone: Oral: 5 mg twice a day

ABVD Early Stage (Hodgkin)

Use Lymphoma, Hodgkin

Regimen

Doxorubicin: I.V.: 25 mg/m^2/day days 1 and 14
[total dose/cycle = 50 mg/m^2]

Bleomycin: I.V.: 10 units/m^2/day days 1 and 14
[total dose/cycle = 20 units/m^2]

Vinblastine: I.V.: 6 mg/m^2/day days 1 and 14
[total dose/cycle = 12 mg/m^2]

Dacarbazine: I.V.: 375 mg/m^2/day days 1 and 14
[total dose/cycle = 750 mg/m^2]

Repeat cycle every 28 days for a total of 2 cycles

ABVD (Hodgkin)

Use Lymphoma, Hodgkin

Regimen

Doxorubicin: I.V.: 25 mg/m^2/day days 1 and 15
[total dose/cycle = 50 mg/m^2]

Bleomycin: I.V.: 10 units/m^2/day days 1 and 15
[total dose/cycle = 20 units/m^2]

Vinblastine: I.V.: 6 mg/m^2/day days 1 and 15
[total dose/cycle = 12 mg/m^2]

Dacarbazine: I.V.: 375 mg/m^2/day days 1 and 15
[total dose/cycle = 750 mg/m^2]

Repeat cycle every 28 days for 6-8 cycles

AC

Use Breast cancer

Regimen NOTE: Multiple variations are listed.

Variation 1: AC (conventional):

Doxorubicin: I.V.: 60 mg/m^2 day 1
[total dose/cycle = 60 mg/m^2]

Cyclophosphamide: I.V.: 600 mg/m^2 day 1
[total dose/cycle = 600 mg/m^2]

Repeat cycle every 21 days

Variation 2:

Cyclophosphamide: Oral: 200 mg/m^2/day days 3 to 6
[total dose/cycle = 800 mg/m^2]

Doxorubicin: I.V.: 40 mg/m^2 day 1
[total dose/cycle = 40 mg/m^2]

Repeat cycle every 3 weeks for 3 cycles, then every 4 weeks

AC/Paclitaxel (Sequential)

Use Breast cancer

Regimen

Variation 1: AC + Paclitaxel (conventional):

Doxorubicin: I.V.: 60 mg/m^2 day 1
[total dose/cycle = 60 mg/m^2]

Cyclophosphamide: I.V.: 600 mg/m^2 day 1
[total dose/cycle = 600 mg/m^2]

Repeat cycle every 21 days for 4 cycles

followed by

Paclitaxel: I.V.: 175 mg/m^2 day 1
[total dose/cycle = 175 mg/m^2]

Repeat cycle every 21 days for 4 cycles

Variation 2: AC + Paclitaxel (dose dense):

Doxorubicin: I.V.: 60 mg/m^2 day 1
[total dose/cycle = 60 mg/m^2]

Cyclophosphamide: I.V.: 600 mg/m^2 day 1
[total dose/cycle = 600 mg/m^2]

Filgrastim: SubQ: 5 mcg/kg/day days 3 to 10
[total dose/cycle = 40 mcg/kg]

Repeat cycle every 14 days for 4 cycles

followed by

Paclitaxel: I.V.: 175 mg/m^2 day 1
[total dose/cycle = 175 mg/m^2]

Filgrastim: SubQ: 5 mcg/kg/day days 3 to 10
[total dose/cycle = 40 mcg/kg]

Repeat cycle every 14 days for 4 cycles

AC-Paclitaxel-Trastuzumab

Use Breast cancer

Regimen NOTE: Multiple variations are listed.

Variation 1:

Doxorubicin: I.V.: 60 mg/m^2 day 1
[total dose/cycle = 60 mg/m^2]

Cyclophosphamide: I.V.: 600 mg/m^2 day 1
[total dose/cycle = 600 mg/m^2]

Repeat cycle every 21 days for 4 cycles

followed by

Paclitaxel: I.V.: 175 mg/m^2 day 1
[total dose/cycle = 175 mg/m^2]

Trastuzumab: I.V.: 4 mg/kg (loading dose) day 1 (cycle 1 only)
[total dose/cycle = 4 mg/kg]
followed by I.V.: 2 mg/kg/day days 8 and 15 (cycle 1)
[total dose/cycle = 4 mg/kg]
then I.V.: 2 mg/kg/day days 1, 8, and 15 (cycles 2, 3, and 4)
[total dose/cycle = 6 mg/kg]
Repeat cycle every 21 days for 4 cycles
followed by
Trastuzumab: I.V.: 2 mg/kg weekly for 40 weeks
Variation 2:
Doxorubicin: I.V.: 60 mg/m^2 day 1
[total dose/cycle = 60 mg/m^2]
Cyclophosphamide: I.V.: 600 mg/m^2 day 1
[total dose/cycle = 600 mg/m^2]
Repeat cycle every 21 days for 4 cycles
followed by
Paclitaxel: I.V.: 80 mg/m^2day 1 week 13
[total dose/cycle = 80 mg/m^2]
Trastuzumab: I.V.: 4 mg/kg (loading dose) day 1 week 13 only
[total dose/cycle = 4 mg/kg]
followed by
Paclitaxel: I.V.: 80 mg/m^2 weekly
[total dose/cycle = 80 mg/m^2]
Trastuzumab: I.V.: 2 mg/kg /weekly
[total dose/cycle = 2 mg/kg]
Repeat cycle every week for 11 cycles
followed by
Trastuzumab: I.V.: 2 mg/kg/weekly for 40 weeks

AD (Soft Tissue Sarcoma)

Use Soft tissue sarcoma

Regimen

NOTE: Multiple variations are listed.
Variation 1 (metastatic):
Doxorubicin: I.V.: 15 mg/m^2/day continuous infusion days 1 to 4
[total dose/cycle = 60 mg/m^2]
Dacarbazine: I.V.: 187.5 mg/m^2/day continuous infusion days 1 to 4
[total dose/cycle = 750 mg/m^2]
Repeat cycle every 21 days; maximum lifetime doxorubicin dose of 450 mg/m^2
Variation 2 (metastatic):
Doxorubicin: I.V.: 60 mg/m^2 I.V. bolus day 1
[total dose/cycle = 60 mg/m^2]
Dacarbazine: I.V.: 750 mg/m^2/day I.V. bolus day 1
[total dose/cycle = 750 mg/m^2]
Repeat cycle every 21 days; maximum lifetime doxorubicin dose of 450 mg/m^2
Variation 3 (metastatic):
Doxorubicin: I.V.: 15 mg/m^2/day continuous infusion days 1 to 4
[total dose/cycle = 60 mg/m^2]
Dacarbazine: I.V.: 250 mg/m^2/day continuous infusion days 1 to 4
[total dose/cycle = 1000 mg/m^2]
Repeat cycle every 21 days
Variation 4 (metastatic):
Doxorubicin: I.V.: 60 mg/m^2 day 1
[total dose/cycle = 60 mg/m^2]
Dacarbazine: I.V.: 250 mg/m^2/day days 1 to 5
[total dose/cycle = 1250 mg/m^2]
Repeat cycle every 21 days until disease progression; when maximum lifetime doxorubicin dose received, continue with single agent dacarbazine

AI

Use Soft tissue sarcoma

Regimen NOTE: Multiple variations are listed.

Variation 1:

Doxorubicin: I.V.: 25 mg/m^2/day continuous infusion days 1, 2, and 3
[total dose/cycle = 75 mg/m^2]

Ifosfamide: I.V.: 2 g/m^2/day days 1 to 5
[total dose/cycle = 10 g/m^2]

Mesna: I.V.: 400 mg/m^2 day 1
followed by I.V.: 1200 mg/m^2/day continuous infusion days 1 to 5
[total dose/cycle = 6400 mg/m^2]

Repeat cycle every 3 weeks

Variation 2:

Doxorubicin: I.V.: 30 mg/m^2/day continuous infusion days 1, 2, and 3
[total dose/cycle = 90 mg/m^2]

Ifosfamide: I.V.: 2.5 g/m^2/day days 1 to 4
[total dose/cycle = 10 g/m^2]

Mesna: I.V.: 500 mg/m^2 day 1
followed by I.V.: 1500 mg/m^2/day continuous infusion days 1 to 4
[total dose/cycle = 6500 mg/m^2]

Filgrastim: SubQ: 5 mcg/kg/day days 5 through ANC recovery

Repeat cycle every 3 weeks

AP

Use Endometrial cancer

Regimen

Doxorubicin: I.V.: 60 mg/m^2 day 1
[total dose/cycle = 60 mg/m^2]

Cisplatin: I.V.: 60 mg/m^2 day 1
[total dose/cycle = 60 mg/m^2]

Repeat cycle every 21-28 days

Azacitidine (AML Regimen)

Use Leukemia, acute myeloid

Regimen

Azacitidine: SubQ: 75 mg/m^2/day days 1 to 7
[total dose/cycle = 525 mg/m^2]

Repeat cycle every 28 days (for a minimum of 6 cycles [Fenaux, 2010]) as long as tolerated and maintaining response

Azacitidine (MDS Regimen)

Use Myelodysplastic syndrome

Regimen NOTE: Multiple variations are listed.

Variation 1:

Azacitidine: SubQ: 75 mg/m^2/day days 1 to 7
[total dose/cycle = 525 mg/m^2]

Repeat cycle every 28 days

Variation 2:

Azacitidine: I.V.: 75 mg/m^2/day days 1 to 7
[total dose/cycle = 525 mg/m^2]

Repeat cycle every 28 days

Variation 3:

Azacitidine: SubQ: 75 mg/m^2/day days 1 to 5 (Mon-Fri), 2 days of rest (Sat, Sun), then 75 mg/m^2/day days 1 and 2 (Mon, Tues)
[total dose/cycle = 525 mg/m^2]

Repeat cycle every 28 days for a total of 6 cycles

Variation 4:

Azacitidine: SubQ: 50 mg/m²/day days 1 to 5 (Mon-Fri), 2 days of rest (Sat, Sun), then 50 mg/m²/day days 1 to 5 (Mon-Fri)
[total dose/cycle = 500 mg/m²]

Repeat cycle every 28 days for a total of 6 cycles

Variation 5:

Azacitidine: SubQ: 75 mg/m²/day days 1 to 5 (Mon-Fri)
[total dose/cycle = 375 mg/m²]

Repeat cycle every 28 days for a total of 6 cycles

BEACOPP-14 (Hodgkin)

Use Lymphoma, Hodgkin disease

Regimen

Bleomycin: I.V.: 10 units/m² day 8
[total dose/cycle = 10 units/m²]

Etoposide: I.V.: 100 mg/m²/day days 1, 2, and 3
[total dose/cycle = 300 mg/m²]

Doxorubicin: I.V.: 25 mg/m² day 1
[total dose/cycle = 25 mg/m²]

Cyclophosphamide: I.V.: 650 mg/m² day 1
[total dose/cycle = 650 mg/m²]

Vincristine: I.V.: 1.4 mg/m² (maximum dose: 2 mg) day 8
[total dose/cycle = 1.4 mg/m²; maximum: 2 mg]

Procarbazine: Oral: 100 mg/m²/day days 1 to 7
[total dose/cycle = 700 mg/m²]

Prednisone: Oral: 80 mg/m²/day days 1 to 7
[total dose/cycle = 560 mg/m²]

Filgrastim: SubQ: 300 mcg/day (patients <75 kg) or 480 mcg/day (patients ≥75 kg) days 8 to13

Repeat cycle every 14 days for a total of 8 cycles

BEACOPP Escalated (Hodgkin)

Use Lymphoma, Hodgkin disease

Regimen

Bleomycin: I.V.: 10 units/m² day 8
[total dose/cycle = 10 units/m²]

Etoposide: I.V.: 200 mg/m²/day days 1, 2, and 3
[total dose/cycle = 600 mg/m²]

Doxorubicin: I.V.: 35 mg/m² day 1
[total dose/cycle = 35 mg/m²]

Cyclophosphamide: I.V.: 1200 mg/m² day 1
[total dose/cycle = 1200 mg/m²]

Vincristine: I.V.: 1.4 mg/m² (maximum dose: 2 mg) day 8
[total dose/cycle = 1.4 mg/m²: maximum: 2 mg]

Procarbazine: Oral: 100 mg/m²/day days 1 to 7
[total dose/cycle = 700 mg/m²]

Prednisone: Oral: 40 mg/m²/day days 1 to 14
[total dose/cycle = 560 mg/m²]

Filgrastim: SubQ: 300 or 480 mcg/day (depending on weight of 75 kg) day 8 until leukocyte recovery (3 days at >1000/mm³)

Repeat cycle every 21 days for a total of 8 cycles

BEACOPP Escalated Plus Standard (Hodgkin)

Use Lymphoma, Hodgkin

Regimen NOTE: Multiple variations are listed.

Variation 1: BEACOPP Escalated for 4 cycles **followed by** 2 cycles of BEACOPP Standard

BEACOPP Escalated for 4 cycles:

Bleomycin: I.V.: 10 units/m² day 8
[total dose/cycle = 10 units/m²]

Etoposide: I.V.: 200 mg/m²/day days 1, 2, and 3
[total dose/cycle = 600 mg/m²]

Doxorubicin: I.V.: 35 mg/m^2 day 1
[total dose/cycle = 35 mg/m^2]
Cyclophosphamide: I.V.: 1250 mg/m^2 day 1
[total dose/cycle = 1250 mg/m^2]
Vincristine: I.V.: 1.4 mg/m^2 (maximum dose: 2 mg) day 8
[total dose/cycle = 1.4 mg/m^2: maximum: 2 mg]
Procarbazine: Oral: 100 mg/m^2/day days 1 to 7
[total dose/cycle = 700 mg/m^2]
Prednisone: Oral: 40 mg/m^2/day days 1 to 14
[total dose/cycle = 560 mg/m^2]
Filgrastim: SubQ: 300 mcg/day day 8 until neutrophil recovery (>500/mm^3)
Repeat cycle every 21 days for a total of 4 cycles

Followed by BEACOPP Standard for 2 cycles:
Bleomycin: I.V.: 10 units/m^2 day 8
[total dose/cycle = 10 units/m^2]
Etoposide: I.V.: 100 mg/m^2/day days 1, 2, and 3
[total dose/cycle = 300 mg/m^2]
Doxorubicin: I.V.: 25 mg/m^2 day 1
[total dose/cycle = 25 mg/m^2]
Cyclophosphamide: I.V.: 650 mg/m^2 day 1
[total dose/cycle = 650 mg/m^2]
Vincristine: I.V.: 1.4 mg/m^2 (maximum dose: 2 mg) day 8
[total dose/cycle = 1.4 mg/m^2: maximum: 2 mg]
Procarbazine: Oral: 100 mg/m^2/day days 1 to 7
[total dose/cycle = 700 mg/m^2]
Prednisone: Oral: 40 mg/m^2/day days 1 to 14
[total dose/cycle = 560 mg/m^2]
Filgrastim: SubQ: 300 mcg/day day 8 until neutrophil recovery (>500/mm^3)
Repeat cycle every 21 days for a total of 2 cycles

Variation 2: BEACOPP Escalated for 4 cycles **followed by** 4 cycles of BEACOPP Standard

BEACOPP Escalated for 4 cycles:
Bleomycin: I.V.: 10 units/m^2 day 8
[total dose/cycle = 10 units/m^2]
Etoposide: I.V.: 200 mg/m^2/day days 1, 2, and 3
[total dose/cycle = 600 mg/m^2]
Doxorubicin: I.V.: 35 mg/m^2 day 1
[total dose/cycle = 35 mg/m^2]
Cyclophosphamide: I.V.: 1250 mg/m^2 day 1
[total dose/cycle = 1250 mg/m^2]
Vincristine: I.V.: 1.4 mg/m^2 (maximum dose: 2 mg) day 8
[total dose/cycle = 1.4 mg/m^2: maximum: 2 mg]
Procarbazine: Oral: 100 mg/m^2/day days 1 to 7
[total dose/cycle = 700 mg/m^2]
Prednisone: Oral: 40 mg/m^2/day days 1 to 14
[total dose/cycle = 560 mg/m^2]
Filgrastim: SubQ: 300 mcg/day day 8 until neutrophil count >1000/mm^3 for 3 consecutive days)
Repeat cycle every 21 days for a total of 4 cycles

Followed by BEACOPP Standard for 4 cycles:
Bleomycin: I.V.: 10 units/m^2 day 8
[total dose/cycle = 10 units/m^2]
Etoposide: I.V.: 100 mg/m^2/day days 1, 2, and 3
[total dose/cycle = 300 mg/m^2]
Doxorubicin: I.V.: 25 mg/m^2 day 1
[total dose/cycle = 25 mg/m^2]
Cyclophosphamide: I.V.: 650 mg/m^2 day 1
[total dose/cycle = 650 mg/m^2]

Vincristine: I.V.: 1.4 mg/m² (maximum dose: 2 mg) day 8
[total dose/cycle = 1.4 mg/m²: maximum: 2 mg]
Procarbazine: Oral: 100 mg/m²/day days 1 to 7
[total dose/cycle = 700 mg/m²]
Prednisone: Oral: 40 mg/m²/day days 1 to 14
[total dose/cycle = 560 mg/m²]
Filgrastim: SubQ: 300 mcg/day day 8 until neutrophil count >1000/mm³ for 3 consecutive days)
Repeat cycle every 21 days for a total of 4 cycles

BEACOPP Standard (Hodgkin)

Use Lymphoma, Hodgkin disease

Regimen

Bleomycin: I.V.: 10 units/m² day 8
[total dose/cycle = 10 units/m²]
Etoposide: I.V.: 100 mg/m²/day days 1, 2, and 3
[total dose/cycle = 300 mg/m²]
Doxorubicin: I.V.: 25 mg/m² day 1
[total dose/cycle = 25 mg/m²]
Cyclophosphamide: I.V.: 650 mg/m² day 1
[total dose/cycle = 650 mg/m²]
Vincristine: I.V.: 1.4 mg/m² (maximum dose: 2 mg) day 8
[total dose/cycle = 1.4 mg/m²; maximum: 2 mg]
Procarbazine: Oral: 100 mg/m²/day days 1 to 7
[total dose/cycle = 700 mg/m²]
Prednisone: Oral: 40 mg/m²/day days 1 to 14
[total dose/cycle = 560 mg/m²]
Repeat cycle every 21 days for a total of 8 cycles

Bendamustine-Rituximab

Use Lymphoma, non-Hodgkin (mantle cell or low-grade NHL)

Regimen NOTE: Multiple variations are listed.

Variation 1:
Pretreatment:
Rituximab: I.V.: 375 mg/m² 1 week before the start of cycle 1
[total dose/pretreatment = 375 mg/m²]
Cycles:
Rituximab: I.V.: 375 mg/m² day 1
[total dose/cycle = 375 mg/m²]
Bendamustine: I.V.: 90 mg/m² days 2 and 3
[total dose/cycle = 180 mg/m²]
Repeat cycle every 4 weeks for up to 4 cycles
Post-Treatment:
Rituximab: I.V.: 375 mg/m² 4 weeks after the last cycle
[total dose/post-treatment = 375 mg/m²]

Variation 2:
Pretreatment:
Rituximab: I.V.: 375 mg/m² 1 week before the start of cycle 1
[total dose/pretreatment = 375 mg/m²]
Cycles:
Rituximab: I.V.: 375 mg/m² day 1
[total dose/cycle = 375 mg/m²]
Bendamustine: I.V.: 90 mg/m² days 2 and 3
[total dose/cycle = 180 mg/m²]
Repeat cycle every 4 weeks for 4-6 cycles
Post-Treatment:
Rituximab: I.V.: 375 mg/m² 4 weeks after the last cycle
[total dose/post-treatment = 375 mg/m²]

BEP (Ovarian Cancer)

Use Ovarian cancer

Regimen

Bleomycin: I.V.: 20 units/m^2 (maximum dose: 30 units) day 1
[total dose/cycle = 20 units/m^2]

Etoposide: I.V.: 75 mg/m^2/day days 1 to 5
[total dose/cycle = 375 mg/m^2]
or I.V.: 75 mg/m^2/day days 1 to 4 (if received prior radiation therapy)
[total dose/cycle = 300 mg/m^2]

Cisplatin: I.V.: 20 mg/m^2/day days 1 to 5
[total dose/cycle = 100 mg/m^2]

Repeat cycle every 3 weeks for 4 cycles

BEP (Ovarian Cancer, Testicular Cancer)

Use Ovarian cancer; Testicular cancer

Regimen

Bleomycin: I.V.: 30 units/day days 2, 9, and 16
[total dose/cycle = 90 units]

Etoposide: I.V.: 100 mg/m^2/day days 1 to 5
[total dose/cycle = 500 mg/m^2]
or I.V.: 120 mg/m^2/day days 1, 2, and 3
[total dose/cycle = 360 mg/m^2]

Cisplatin: I.V.: 20 mg/m^2/day days 1 to 5
[total dose/cycle = 100 mg/m^2]

Repeat cycle every 21 days

BEP (Testicular Cancer)

Use Testicular cancer

Regimen NOTE: Multiple variations are listed.

Variation 1:

Bleomycin: I.V.: 30 units/day days 1, 8, and 15
[total dose/cycle = 90 units]

Etoposide: I.V.: 100 mg/m^2/day days 1 to 5
[total dose/cycle = 500 mg/m^2]

Cisplatin: I.V.: 20 mg/m^2/day days 1 to 5
[total dose/cycle = 100 mg/m^2]

Repeat cycle every 21 days for 3-4 cycles

Variation 2:

Bleomycin: I.V.: 30 units/day days 2, 9, and 16
[total dose/cycle = 90 units]

Etoposide: I.V.: 100 mg/m^2/day days 1 to 5
[total dose/cycle = 500 mg/m^2]

Cisplatin: I.V.: 20 mg/m^2/day days 1 to 5
[total dose/cycle = 100 mg/m^2]

Repeat cycle every 21 days

Variation 3:

Bleomycin: I.V.: 30 units once weekly
[total dose/cycle = 90 units]

Etoposide: I.V.: 120 mg/m^2/day days 1, 3, and 5
[total dose/cycle = 360 mg/m^2]

Cisplatin: I.V.: 20 mg/m^2/day days 1 to 5
[total dose/cycle = 100 mg/m^2]

Repeat cycle every 21 days

Variation 4:
Bleomycin: I.V.: 30 units/day days 1, 8, and 15
[total dose/cycle = 90 units]
Etoposide: I.V.: 165 mg/m^2/day days 1, 2, and 3
[total dose/cycle = 495 mg/m^2]
Cisplatin: I.V.: 50 mg/m^2/day days 1 and 2
[total dose/cycle = 100 mg/m^2]
Repeat cycle every 21 days

Bevacizumab-Capecitabine (Breast Cancer)

Use Breast cancer

Regimen NOTE: Multiple variations are listed.

Variation 1:
Capecitabine: Oral: 1250 mg/m^2 twice daily days 1 to 14
[total dose/cycle = 35,000 mg/m^2]
Bevacizumab: I.V.: 15 mg/kg day 1
[total dose/cycle = 15 mg/kg]
Repeat cycle every 21 days for up to 35 cycles

Variation 2:
Capecitabine: Oral: 2000 mg/m^2/day days 1 to 14
[total dose/cycle = 28,000 mg/m^2]
Bevacizumab: I.V.: 15 mg/kg day 1
[total dose/cycle = 15 mg/kg]
Repeat cycle every 21 days

Bevacizumab-Cisplatin-Gemcitabine (NSCLC)

Use Lung cancer, nonsmall cell

Regimen

Bevacizumab: I.V.: 7.5 or 15 mg/kg/dose day 1
[total dose/cycle = 7.5 or 15 mg/kg]
Cisplatin: I.V.: 80 mg/m^2/dose day 1
[total dose/cycle = 80 mg/m^2]
Gemcitabine: I.V.: 1250 mg/m^2/dose days 1 and 8
[total dose/cycle = 2500 mg/m^2]
Repeat cycle every 21 days for up to 6 cycles (bevacizumab monotherapy may be continued thereafter until disease progression)

Bevacizumab-Fluorouracil-Leucovorin

Use Colorectal cancer

Regimen

Bevacizumab: I.V.: 5 mg/kg/day days 1, 15, 29, and 43
[total dose/cycle = 20 mg/kg]
Leucovorin: I.V.: 500 mg/m^2/day days 1, 8, 15, 22, 29, and 36
[total dose/cycle = 3000 mg/m^2]
Fluorouracil: I.V.: 500 mg/m^2/day days 1, 8, 15, 22, 29, and 36
[total dose/cycle = 3000 mg/m^2]
Repeat cycle every 56 days

Bevacizumab + FOLFIRI (Colorectal)

Use Colorectal cancer

Regimen

Bevacizumab: I.V.: 5 mg/kg day 1
[total dose/cycle = 5 mg/kg]
Irinotecan: I.V.: 180 mg/m^2 over 90 minutes day 1
[total dose/cycle = 180 mg/m^2]
Leucovorin: I.V.: 400 mg/m^2 over 2 hours day 1
[total dose/cycle = 400 mg/m^2]
Fluorouracil: I.V. bolus: 400 mg/m^2 day 1
followed by I.V.: 2400 mg/m^2 continuous infusion (CI) over 46 hours beginning day 1
[total fluorouracil dose/cycle (bolus and CI) = 2800 mg/m^2]
Repeat cycle every 14 days until disease progression or unacceptable toxicity

Bevacizumab-Interferon Alfa (RCC)

Use Renal cell cancer

Regimen

Interferon Alfa-2b: SubQ: 9 million units on 3 nonconsecutive days per week
[total dose/cycle = 108 million units]
Bevacizumab: I.V.: 10 mg/kg days 1 and 15
[total dose/cycle = 20 mg/kg]
Repeat cycle every 28 days until disease progression or unacceptable toxicity

Bevacizumab-Irinotecan (Glioblastoma)

Use Brain tumors

Regimen **NOTE:** Patients receiving concurrent antiepileptic enzyme-inducing drugs received an increased dose of irinotecan (340 mg/m^2/dose).

Bevacizumab: I.V.: 10 mg/kg day 1
[total dose/cycle = 10 mg/kg]
Irinotecan: I.V.: 125 mg/m^2 day 1
[total dose/cycle = 125 mg/m^2]
Repeat cycle every 14 days

Bevacizumab-Oxaliplatin-Fluorouracil-Leucovorin

Use Colorectal cancer

Regimen

Bevacizumab: I.V.: 10 mg/kg day 1
[total dose/cycle = 10 mg/kg]
Oxaliplatin: I.V.: 85 mg/m^2 day 1
[total dose/cycle = 85 mg/m^2]
Leucovorin: I.V.: 200 mg/m^2/day days 1 and 2
[total dose/cycle = 400 mg/m^2]
Fluorouracil: I.V. bolus: 400 mg/m^2/day days 1 and 2
followed by I.V.: 600 mg/m^2 continuous infusion over 22 hours days 1 and 2
[total dose/cycle = 2000 mg/m^2]
Repeat cycle every 14 days

Bevacizumab (RCC Regimen)

Use Renal cell cancer

Regimen

Bevacizumab: I.V.: 10 mg/kg day 1
[total dose/cycle = 10 mg/kg]
Repeat cycle every 14 days until disease progression or unacceptable toxicity

Bevacizumab + XELOX (Colorectal)

Use Colorectal cancer

Regimen NOTE: Multiple variations are listed.

Variation 1:
Bevacizumab: I.V.: 7.5 mg/kg day 1
[total dose/cycle = 7.5 mg/kg]
Oxaliplatin: I.V.: 130 mg/m^2 day 1
[total dose/cycle = 130 mg/m^2]
Capecitabine: Oral: 850 mg/m^2 twice daily days 1 (beginning with evening dose) to 15 (ending with morning dose)
[total dose/cycle = 23,800 mg/m^2]
Repeat cycle every 21 days

Variation 2:
Bevacizumab: I.V.: 7.5 mg/kg over 30-90 minutes day 1
[total dose/cycle = 7.5 mg/kg]
Oxaliplatin: I.V.: 130 mg/m^2 over 2 hours day 1
[total dose/cycle = 130 mg/m^2]
Capecitabine: Oral: 1000 mg/m^2 twice daily days 1 to 14
[total dose/cycle = 28,000 mg/m^2]
Repeat cycle every 21 days

Bicalutamide-Goserelin

Use Prostate cancer

Regimen

Bicalutamide: Oral: 50 mg/day
[total dose/cycle = 1400 mg]
Goserelin acetate: SubQ: 3.6 mg day 1
[total dose/cycle = 3.6 mg]
Repeat cycle every 28 days

Bicalutamide-Leuprolide

Use Prostate cancer

Regimen

Bicalutamide: Oral: 50 mg/day
[total dose/cycle = 1400 mg]
Leuprolide depot: I.M.: 7.5 mg day 1
[total dose/cycle = 7.5 mg]
Repeat cycle every 28 days

BOLD

Use Melanoma

Regimen

Dacarbazine: I.V.: 200 mg/m^2/day days 1 to 5
[total dose/cycle = 1000 mg/m^2]
Vincristine: I.V.: 1 mg/m^2/day days 1 and 4
[total dose/cycle = 2 mg/m^2]
Bleomycin: I.V.: 15 units/day days 2 and 5
[total dose/cycle = 30 units]
Lomustine: Oral: 80 mg day 1
[total dose/cycle = 80 mg]
Repeat cycle every 4 weeks

BOLD + Interferon

Use Melanoma

Regimen NOTE: Multiple variations are listed.

Variation 1:
Bleomycin: I.V.: 15 units/day days 2 and 5
[total dose/cycle = 30 units]
Vincristine: I.V.: 1 mg/m^2/day days 1 and 4
[total dose/cycle = 2 mg/m^2]
Lomustine: Oral: 80 mg day 1
[total dose/cycle = 80 mg]
Dacarbazine: I.V.: 200 mg/m^2/day days 1 to 5
[total dose/cycle = 1000 mg/m^2]
Interferon Alfa-2b: SubQ: 3 million units/day days 8 to 49 (cycles 1 and 2)
[total dose through day 49 = 126 million units]
followed by SubQ: 6 million units 3 times/week (beginning day 50 and subsequent cycles)
[total dose/cycle = 72 million units]
Repeat cycle every 4 weeks

Variation 2:
Bleomycin: I.V.: 30 units day 1
[total dose/cycle = 30 units]
Vincristine: I.V.: 2 mg day 1
[total dose/cycle = 2 mg]
Lomustine: Oral: 80 mg day 1
[total dose/cycle = 80 mg]
Dacarbazine: I.V.: 700 mg/m^2 day 1
[total dose/cycle = 700 mg/m^2]
Interferon Alfa-2b: SubQ: 3 million units 3 times/week
[total dose/cycle = 36 million units]
Repeat cycle every 4 weeks

Variation 3:
- Bleomycin: I.V.: 15 units/day days 2 and 5
  [total dose/cycle = 30 units]
- Vincristine: I.V.: 1-2 mg/day days 1 and 4
  [total dose/cycle = 2-4 mg]
- Lomustine: Oral: 80 mg day 1
  [total dose/cycle = 80 mg]
- Dacarbazine: I.V.: 200 mg/m^2/day days 1 to 5
  [total dose/cycle = 1000 mg/m^2]
- Interferon Alfa-2b: SubQ: 6 million units 3 times/week, for 6 doses, starting day 8
  [total dose/cycle = 36 million units]
- Repeat cycle every 4 weeks

Variation 4:
- Bleomycin: I.V.: 15 units/day days 2 and 5
  [total dose/cycle = 30 units]
- Vincristine: I.V.: 1 mg/m^2/day (maximum dose: 2 mg) days 1 and 4
  [total dose/cycle = 2 mg/m^2]
- Lomustine: Oral: 80 mg day 1
  [total dose/cycle = 80 mg]
- Dacarbazine: I.V.: 200 mg/m^2/day days 1 to 5
  [total dose/cycle = 1000 mg/m^2]
- Interferon Alfa-2b: SubQ: 3 million units/day days 8, 10, 12, 15, 17, and 19
  [total dose/cycle = 18 million units]
- Repeat cycle every 4 weeks

BOLD (Melanoma)

Use Melanoma

Regimen NOTE: Multiple variations are listed.

Variation 1:
- Bleomycin: SubQ: 7.5 units/day days 1 and 4 (cycle 1 only)
  followed by SubQ: 15 units/day days 1 and 4 (subsequent cycles)
  [total dose/cycle = 45 units; maximum total dose (all cycles): 400 units]
- Vincristine: I.V.: 1 mg/m^2/day days 1 and 5
  [total dose/cycle = 2 mg/m^2]
- Lomustine: Oral: 80 mg/m^2 (maximum dose: 150 mg) day 1
  [total dose/cycle = 80 mg/m^2]
- Dacarbazine: I.V.: 200 mg/m^2/day (maximum dose: 400 mg) days 1 to 5
  [total dose/cycle = 1000 mg/m^2; maximum: 2000 mg]
- Repeat cycle every 4-6 weeks

Variation 2:
- Bleomycin: I.V.: 15 units/day days 1 and 4
  [total dose/cycle = 30 units]
- Vincristine: I.V.: 1 mg/m^2/day days 1 and 5
  [total dose/cycle = 2 mg/m^2]
- Lomustine: Oral: 80 mg/m^2 (maximum dose: 150 mg) day 1
  [total dose/cycle = 80 mg/m^2]
- Dacarbazine: I.V.: 200 mg/m^2/day days 1 to 5
  [total dose/cycle = 1000 mg/m^2]
- Repeat cycle every 4 weeks

Variation 3:
- Bleomycin: I.V.: 15 units/day days 1 and 4
  [total dose/cycle = 30 units]
- Vincristine: I.V.: 1 mg/m^2 day 1
  [total dose/cycle = 1 mg/m^2]
- Lomustine: Oral: 80 mg/m^2 day 3 (odd numbered cycles)
  [total dose/cycle = 80 mg/m^2; every other cycle]
- Dacarbazine: I.V.: 200 mg/m^2/day days 1 to 5
  [total dose/cycle = 1000 mg/m^2]
- Repeat cycle every 4 weeks

Bortezomib-Dexamethasone-Rituximab (Waldenstrom Macroglobulinemia)

Use Waldenstrom Macroglobulinemia

Regimen

Bortezomib: I.V.: 1.3 mg/m^2 days 1, 4, 8, and 11
[total dose/cycle = 5.2 mg/m^2]
Dexamethasone: I.V.: 40 mg days 1, 4, 8, and 11
[total dose/cycle = 160 mg]
Rituximab: I.V.: 375 mg/m^2 day 11
[total dose/cycle = 375 mg/m^2]
Repeat cycle every 21 days for 4 cycles, followed by a 12 week interruption, then repeat cycle every 12 weeks for 4 cycles

Bortezomib-Dexamethasone (Amyloidosis)

Use Systemic light chain amyloidosis

Regimen

Bortezomib: I.V.: 1.3 mg/m^2/dose days 1, 4, 8, and 11
[total dose/cycle = 5.2 mg/m^2]
Dexamethasone: Oral: 40 mg/day days 1 to 4
[total dose/cycle = 160 mg]
Repeat cycle every 21 days

Bortezomib-Dexamethasone (Multiple Myeloma)

Use Multiple myeloma

Regimen NOTE: Multiple variations are listed.

Variation 1:
Cycles 1 and 2:
Bortezomib: I.V.: 1.3 mg/m^2/day days 1, 4, 8, and 11
[total dose/cycle = 5.2 mg/m^2]
Dexamethasone: Oral: 40 mg/day days 1 to 4 and days 9 to 12
[total dose/cycle = 320 mg]
Treatment cycle is 21 days
Cycles 3 and 4:
Bortezomib: I.V.: 1.3 mg/m^2/day days 1, 4, 8, and 11
[total dose/cycle = 5.2 mg/m^2]
Dexamethasone: Oral: 40 mg/day days 1 to 4
[total dose/cycle = 160 mg]
Treatment cycle is 21 days

Variation 2:
Cycles 1 and 2:
Bortezomib: I.V.: 1.3 mg/m^2/day days 1, 4, 8, and 11
[total dose/cycle = 5.2 mg/m^2]
Treatment cycle is 21 days
Cycles 3 through 6 (begin dexamethasone after cycle 2 if partial response not achieved or after cycle 4 if complete response not achieved):
Bortezomib: I.V.: 1.3 mg/m^2/day days 1, 4, 8, and 11
[total dose/cycle = 5.2 mg/m^2]
Dexamethasone: Oral: 40 mg/day days 1 and 2
[total dose/cycle = 80 mg]
Treatment cycle is 21 days (for up to a total of 6 cycles)

Bortezomib-Doxorubicin-Dexamethasone

Use Multiple myeloma

Regimen NOTE: Multiple variations are listed.

Variation 1:
Cycle 1:
Bortezomib: I.V.: 1.3 mg/m^2/day days 1, 4, 8, and 11
[total dose/cycle = 5.2 mg/m^2]
Dexamethasone: Oral: 40 mg/day days 1 to 4, 8 to 11, and 15 to 18
[total dose/cycle = 480 mg]

Doxorubicin: I.V.: 4.5 or 9 mg/m^2/day days 1 to 4
[total dose/cycle = 18 or 36 mg/m^2]
Treatment cycle is 21 days
Cycles 2-4:
Bortezomib: I.V.: 1.3 mg/m^2/day days 1, 4, 8, and 11
[total dose/cycle = 5.2 mg/m^2]
Dexamethasone: Oral: 40 mg/day days 1 to 4
[total dose/cycle = 160 mg]
Doxorubicin: I.V.: 4.5 or 9 mg/m^2/day days 1 to 4
[total dose/cycle = 18 or 36 mg/m^2]
Treatment cycle is 21 days
Variation 2:
Cycle 1:
Bortezomib: I.V.: 1 mg/m^2/day days 1, 4, 8, and 11
[total dose/cycle = 4 mg/m^2]
Dexamethasone: Oral: 40 mg/day days 1 to 4, 8 to 11, and 15 to 18
[total dose/cycle = 480 mg]
Doxorubicin: I.V.: 9 mg/m^2/day days 1 to 4
[total dose/cycle = 36 mg/m^2]
Treatment cycle is 21 days
Cycles 2-4:
Bortezomib: I.V.: 1 mg/m^2/day days 1, 4, 8, and 11
[total dose/cycle = 4 mg/m^2]
Dexamethasone: Oral: 40 mg/day days 1 to 4
[total dose/cycle = 160 mg]
Doxorubicin: I.V.: 9 mg/m^2/day days 1 to 4
[total dose/cycle = 36 mg/m^2]
Treatment cycle is 21 days
Variation 3:
Bortezomib: I.V.: 1.3 mg/m^2/day days 1, 4, 8, and 11
[total dose/cycle = 5.2 mg/m^2]
Dexamethasone: Oral: 40 mg/day days 1 to 4
[total dose/cycle = 160 mg]
Doxorubicin: I.V.: 20 mg/m^2/day days 1 and 4
[total dose/cycle = 40 mg/m^2]
Repeat cycle every 28 days for up to 6 cycles

Bortezomib-Doxorubicin (Liposomal)

Use Multiple myeloma

Regimen

Bortezomib: I.V.: 1.3 mg/m^2/day days 1, 4, 8, and 11
[total dose/cycle = 5.2 mg/m^2]
Doxorubicin (liposomal): I.V.: 30 mg/m^2 day 4
[total dose/cycle = 30 mg/m^2]
Repeat cycle every 21 days for up to 8 cycles

Bortezomib-Doxorubicin (Liposomal)-Dexamethasone

Use Multiple myeloma

Regimen

Bortezomib: I.V.: 1.3 mg/m^2/day days 1, 4, 8, and 11
[total dose/cycle = 5.2 mg/m^2]
Doxorubicin (Liposomal): I.V.: 30 mg/m^2 day 1
[total dose/cycle = 30 mg/m^2]
Dexamethasone: Oral: 40 mg/day days 1 to 4
[total dose/cycle = 160 mg]
Repeat cycle every 28 days for up to 6 cycles

Bortezomib-Melphalan-Prednisone-Thalidomide

Use Multiple myeloma

Regimen

Bortezomib: I.V.: 1-1.3 mg/m^2/day days 1, 4, 15, and 22
[total dose/cycle = 4-5.2 mg/m^2]
Melphalan: Oral: 6 mg/m^2/day days 1 to 5
[total dose/cycle = 30 mg/m^2]
Prednisone: Oral: 60 mg/m^2/day days 1 to 5
[total dose/cycle = 300 mg/m^2]
Thalidomide: Oral: 50 mg/day days 1 to 35
[total dose/cycle = 1750 mg]
Repeat cycle every 35 days for 6 cycles

Bortezomib-Rituximab (Waldenstrom Macroglobulinemia)

Use Waldenstrom Macroglobulinemia

Regimen

Bortezomib: I.V.: 1.6 mg/m^2/day days 1, 8, and 15 (cycles 1 to 6)
[total dose/cycle = 4.8 mg/m^2]
Rituximab: I.V.: 375 mg/m^2/day days 1, 8, 15, and 22 (cycles 1 and 4 only)
[total dose/cycle (cycles 1 and 4 only) = 1500 mg/m^2]
Repeat cycle every 28 days for a total of 6 cycles; bortezomib administered for all 6 cycles and rituximab administered cycles 1 and 4 only

Bortezomib (Waldenstrom Macroglobulinemia)

Use Waldenstrom Macroglobulinemia

Regimen

Bortezomib: I.V.: 1.3 mg/m^2/day days 1, 4, 8, and 11
[total dose/cycle = 5.2 mg/m^2]
Repeat cycle every 21 days until disease progression or until 2 cycles after a complete response

Cabazitaxel-Prednisone (Prostate Cancer)

Use Prostate cancer

Regimen

Cabazitaxel: I.V.: 25 mg/m^2/dose day 1
[total dose/cycle = 25 mg/m^2]
Prednisone: Oral: 10 mg once daily
[total dose/cycle = 210 mg]
Repeat cycle every 21 days

CAF

Use Breast cancer

Regimen NOTE: Multiple variations are listed.

Variation 1:
Cyclophosphamide: Oral: 100 mg/m^2/day days 1 to 14
[total dose/cycle = 1400 mg/m^2]
Doxorubicin: I.V.: 30 mg/m^2/day days 1 and 8
[total dose/cycle = 60 mg/m^2]
Fluorouracil: I.V.: 500 mg/m^2/day days 1 and 8
[total dose/cycle = 1000 mg/m^2]
Repeat cycle every 28 days

Variation 2:
Cyclophosphamide: Oral: 100 mg/m^2/day days 1 to 14
[total dose/cycle = 1400 mg/m^2]
Doxorubicin: I.V.: 25 mg/m^2/day days 1 and 8
[total dose/cycle = 50 mg/m^2]
Fluorouracil: I.V.: 500 mg/m^2/day days 1 and 8
[total dose/cycle = 1000 mg/m^2]
Repeat cycle every 28 days

CAP

Use Bladder cancer

Regimen

Cyclophosphamide: I.V.: 400 mg/m^2 day 1
[total dose = 400 mg/m^2]
Doxorubicin: I.V.: 40 mg/m^2 day 1
[total dose = 40 mg/m^2]
Cisplatin: I.V.: 60 mg/m^2 day 1
[total dose = 60 mg/m^2]
Repeat cycle every 21 days

Capecitabine + Docetaxel (Breast Cancer)

Use Breast cancer

Regimen NOTE: Multiple variations are listed.

Variation 1:
Capecitabine: Oral: 1250 mg/m^2 twice daily days 1 to 14
[total dose/cycle = 35,000 mg/m^2]
Docetaxel: I.V.: 75 mg/m^2 day 1
[total dose/cycle = 75 mg/m^2]
Repeat cycle every 3 weeks

Variation 2:
Capecitabine: Oral: 1000 mg/m^2 twice daily days 2 to 15
[total dose/cycle = 28,000 mg/m^2]
Docetaxel: I.V.: 75 mg/m^2 day 1
[total dose/cycle = 75 mg/m^2]
Repeat cycle every 3 weeks

Variation 3:
Capecitabine: Oral: 937.5 mg/m^2 twice daily days 2 to 15
[total dose/cycle = 26,250 mg/m^2]
Docetaxel: I.V.: 60 mg/m^2 day 1
[total dose/cycle = 60 mg/m^2]
Repeat cycle every 3 weeks

Capecitabine-Docetaxel (Gastric Cancer)

Use Gastric cancer

Regimen NOTE: Multiple variations are listed.

Variation 1:
Capecitabine: Oral: 1000 mg/m^2 twice daily days 1 to 14
[total dose/cycle = 28,000 mg/m^2]
Docetaxel: I.V.: 75 mg/m^2 day 1
[total dose/cycle = 75 mg/m^2]
Repeat cycle every 3 weeks for up to 9 cycles or until disease progression or unacceptable toxicity

Variation 2:
Capecitabine: Oral: 1000 mg/m^2 twice daily days 1 to 14
[total dose/cycle = 28,000 mg/m^2]
Docetaxel: I.V.: 36 mg/m^2 days 1 and 8
[total dose/cycle = 72 mg/m^2]
Repeat cycle every 3 weeks until disease progression or unacceptable toxicity

Variation 3:
Capecitabine: Oral: 825 mg/m^2 twice daily days 1 to 14
[total dose/cycle = 23,100 mg/m^2]
Docetaxel: I.V.: 75 mg/m^2 day 1
[total dose/cycle = 75 mg/m^2]
Repeat cycle every 3 weeks until disease progression

Variation 4:
Capecitabine: Oral: 1250 mg/m^2 twice daily days 1 to 14
[total dose/cycle = 35,000 mg/m^2]
Docetaxel: I.V.: 75 mg/m^2 day 1
[total dose/cycle = 75 mg/m^2]
Repeat cycle every 3 weeks until disease progression for up to a maximum of 6 cycles

Capecitabine-Gemcitabine (Pancreatic)

Use Pancreatic cancer

Regimen NOTE: Multiple variations are listed.

Variation 1:

Gemcitabine: I.V.: 1000 mg/m^2/day over 30 minutes days 1 and 8
[total dose/cycle = 2000 mg/m^2]

Capecitabine: Oral: 650 mg/m^2/dose twice daily days 1 to 14
[total dose/cycle = 18,200 mg/m^2]

Repeat cycle every 21 days until disease progression (maximum duration: 24 weeks)

Variation 2:

Gemcitabine: I.V.: 1000 mg/m^2/day over 30 minutes days 1, 8, and 15
[total dose/cycle = 3000 mg/m^2]

Capecitabine: Oral: 830 mg/m^2/dose twice daily days 1 to 21
[total dose/cycle = 34,860 mg/m^2]

Repeat cycle every 28 days until disease progression or unacceptable toxicity

Capecitabine + Lapatinib (Breast Cancer)

Use Breast cancer

Regimen

Capecitabine: Oral: 1000 mg/m^2 twice daily days 1 to 14
[total dose/cycle = 28,000 mg/m^2]

Lapatinib: Oral: 1250 mg/day days 1 to 21
[total dose/cycle = 26,250 mg]

Repeat cycle every 3 weeks

Capecitabine-Trastuzumab

Use Breast cancer

Regimen NOTE: Multiple variations are listed.

Variation 1:

Cycle 1:

Capecitabine: Oral: 1250 mg/m^2 twice daily days 1 to 14
[total dose/cycle 1 = 35,000 mg/m^2]

Trastuzumab: I.V.: 4 mg/kg (loading dose) day 1 cycle 1
followed by I.V.: 2 mg/kg/day days 8 and 15 cycle 1
[total dose/cycle 1 = 8 mg/kg]

Treatment cycle is 21 days

Subsequent cycles:

Capecitabine: Oral: 1250 mg/m^2 twice daily days 1 to 14
[total dose/cycle = 35,000 mg/m^2]

Trastuzumab: I.V.: 2 mg/kg/day days 1, 8, and 15
[total dose/cycle = 6 mg/kg]

Repeat cycle every 21 days

Variation 2:

Cycle 1:

Capecitabine: Oral: 1250 mg/m^2 twice daily days 1 to 14
[total dose/cycle 1 = 35,000 mg/m^2]

Trastuzumab: I.V.: 8 mg/kg (loading dose) day 1 cycle 1
[total dose/cycle 1 = 8 mg/kg]

Treatment cycle is 21 days

Subsequent cycles:

Capecitabine: Oral: 1250 mg/m^2 twice daily days 1 to 14
[total dose/cycle = 35,000 mg/m^2]

Trastuzumab: I.V.: 6 mg/kg day 1
[total dose/cycle = 6 mg/kg]

Repeat cycle every 21 days

CAPOX (Biliary Cancer)

Use Biliary adenocarcinoma

Regimen

Capecitabine: Oral: 1000 mg/m^2/dose twice daily days 1 to 14
[total dose/cycle = 28,000 mg/m^2]
Oxaliplatin: I.V.: 130 mg/m^2 over 2 hours day 1
[total dose/cycle = 130 mg/m^2]
Repeat cycle every 3 weeks

CAPOX (Pancreatic Cancer)

Use Pancreatic cancer

Regimen NOTE: Multiple variations are listed.

Variation 1 (patients ≤65 years of age or ECOG PS <2):
Capecitabine: Oral: 1000 mg/m^2/dose twice daily days 1 to 14
[total dose/cycle = 28,000 mg/m^2]
Oxaliplatin: I.V.: 130 mg/m^2/dose over 2 hours day 1
[total dose/cycle = 130 mg/m^2]
Repeat cycle every 21 days until disease progression or unacceptable toxicity
Variation 2 (patients >65 years of age or ECOG PS of 2):
Capecitabine: Oral: 750 mg/m^2/dose twice daily days 1 to 14
[total dose/cycle = 21,000 mg/m^2]
Oxaliplatin: I.V.: 110 mg/m^2/dose over 2 hours day 1
[total dose/cycle = 110 mg/m^2]
Repeat cycle every 21 days until disease progression or unacceptable toxicity

Carboplatin-Cetuximab (Head and Neck Cancer)

Use Head and neck cancer

Regimen

Cycle 1:
Cetuximab: I.V.: 400 mg/m^2 (loading dose) day 1 (week 1, cycle 1 only)
[total loading dose = 400 mg/m^2]
followed by I.V.: 250 mg/m^2/day days 8 and 15
[total dose/cycle 1 = 900 mg/m^2]
Carboplatin: I.V.: AUC 5 day 1
[total dose/cycle = AUC = 5]
Treatment cycle is 3 weeks
Subsequent cycles:
Cetuximab: I.V.: 250 mg/m^2/day days 1, 8, and 15
[total dose/cycle = 750 mg/m^2]
Carboplatin: I.V.: AUC 5 day 1
[total dose/cycle = AUC = 5]
Repeat cycle every 3 weeks until disease progression or unacceptable toxicity for up to a maximum of 8 cycles

Carboplatin-Docetaxel (Ovarian)

Use Ovarian cancer

Regimen NOTE: Multiple variations are listed.

Variation 1:
Docetaxel: I.V.: 60 mg/m^2 over 60 minutes day 1
[total dose/cycle = 60 mg/m^2]
Carboplatin: I.V.: AUC 6 over 30 minutes day 1
[total dose/cycle = AUC = 6]
Repeat cycle every 21 days for 6 cycles
Variation 2:
Docetaxel: I.V.: 75 mg/m^2 over 60 minutes day 1
[total dose/cycle = 75 mg/m^2]
Carboplatin: I.V.: AUC 5 over 30-60 minutes day 1
[total dose/cycle = AUC = 5]
Repeat cycle every 21 days for 6 cycles

Variation 3:

Docetaxel: I.V.: 35 mg/m^2 over 60 minutes days 1, 8, and 15
[total dose/cycle = 105 mg/m^2]

Carboplatin: I.V.: AUC 2 over 30 minutes days 1, 8, and 15
[total dose/cycle = AUC = 6]

Repeat cycle every 28 days until disease progression or unacceptable toxicity or 2 cycles post complete response

Carboplatin-Docetaxel (Unknown Primary)

Use Unknown primary (adenocarcinoma)

Regimen

Docetaxel: I.V.: 65 mg/m^2 over 1 hour day 1
[total dose/cycle = 65 mg/m^2]

Carboplatin: I.V.: AUC 6 over 20 minutes day 1
[total dose/cycle = AUC = 6]

Repeat cycle every 21 days for up to a total of 8 cycles

Carboplatin-Doxorubicin (Liposomal) (Ovarian)

Use Ovarian cancer

Regimen NOTE: Multiple variations are listed.

Variation 1:

Doxorubicin (liposomal): I.V.: 30 mg/m^2 day 1
[total dose/cycle = 30 mg/m^2]

Carboplatin: I.V.: AUC 5 day 1
[total dose/cycle = AUC = 5]

Repeat cycle every 28 days until disease progression or unacceptable toxicity

Variation 2:

Doxorubicin (liposomal): I.V.: 30 mg/m^2 over 60 minutes day 1
[total dose/cycle = 30 mg/m^2]

Carboplatin: I.V.: AUC 5 over 30 minutes day 1
[total dose/cycle = AUC = 5]

Repeat cycle every 21 days for 6 cycles

Carboplatin-Etoposide-Paclitaxel (Unknown Primary)

Use Unknown primary, adenocarcinoma

Regimen

Paclitaxel: I.V.: 200 mg/m^2 over 1 hour day 1
[total dose/cycle = 200 mg/m^2]

Carboplatin: I.V.: AUC 6 over 20-30 minutes day 1
[total dose/cycle = AUC = 6]

Etoposide: Oral: 50 mg/day days 1, 3, 5, 7, and 9
and Oral: 100 mg/day days 2, 4, 6, 8, and 10
[total dose/cycle = 750 mg]

Repeat cycle every 21 days for a total of 4-8 cycles

Carboplatin-Etoposide (Retinoblastoma)

Use Retinoblastoma

Regimen

Etoposide: I.V.: 100 mg/m^2/day over 1 hour days 1 to 5
[total dose/cycle = 500 mg/m^2]

Carboplatin: I.V.: 160 mg/m^2/day over 1 hour days 1 to 5
[total dose/cycle = 800 mg/m^2]

Repeat cycle in 21 to 28 days for a total of 2 cycles

Carboplatin-Etoposide (Small Cell Lung Cancer)

Use Lung cancer, small cell

Regimen NOTE: Multiple variations are listed.

Variation 1 (limited stage with thoracic radiotherapy):

Carboplatin: I.V.: AUC 6 over 1 hour day 1
[total dose/cycle = AUC = 6]

Etoposide: I.V.: 100 mg/m²/day over 2 hours days 1, 2, and 3
[total dose/cycle = 300 mg/m²]
Repeat cycle every 21 days for 6 cycles
Variation 2 (extensive):
Carboplatin: I.V.: AUC 5 day 1
[total dose/cycle = AUC = 5]
Etoposide: I.V.: 100 mg/m²/day days 1, 2, and 3
[total dose/cycle = 300 mg/m²]
Repeat cycle every 21 days for 6 cycles
Variation 3 (elderly, limited, and extensive):
Carboplatin: I.V.: AUC 5 over 1 hour day 1
[total dose/cycle = AUC = 5]
Etoposide: I.V.: 100 mg/m²/day over 1 hour days 1, 2, and 3
[total dose/cycle = 300 mg/m²]
Repeat cycle every 28 days for 4 cycles

Carboplatin-Etoposide-Vincristine (Retinoblastoma)

Use Retinoblastoma

Regimen NOTE: Multiple variations are listed.
Variation 1 (<1 year of age):
Carboplatin: I.V.: 20 mg/kg day 1
[total dose/cycle = 20 mg/kg]
Etoposide Phosphate: I.V.: 5 mg/kg day 1
[total dose/cycle = 5 mg/kg]
Vincristine: I.V.: 0.05 mg/kg day 1
[total dose/cycle = 0.05 mg/kg]
Variation 2 (age >1 year):
Carboplatin: I.V.: 550-600 mg/m² day 1
[total dose/cycle = 550-600 mg/m²]
Etoposide Phosphate: I.V.: 150 mg/m² day 1
[total dose/cycle = 150 mg/m²]
Vincristine: I.V.: 1.5-2 mg/m² day 1
[total dose/cycle = 1.5-2 mg/m²]
Variation 3 (≤36 months of age):
Carboplatin: I.V.: 18.6 mg/kg day 1
[total dose/cycle = 18.6 mg/kg]
Etoposide: I.V.: 5 mg/kg days 1 and 2
[total dose/cycle = 10 mg/kg]
Vincristine: I.V.: 0.05 mg/kg day 1 (maximum dose: 2 mg)
[total dose/cycle = 0.05 mg/kg; maximum dose: 2 mg]
Repeat cycle every 28 days for a total of 6 cycles
Variation 4 (>36 months of age):
Carboplatin: I.V.: 560 mg/m² day 1
[total dose/cycle = 560 mg/m²]
Etoposide: I.V.: 150 mg/m² days 1 and 2
[total dose/cycle = 300 mg/m²]
Vincristine: I.V.: 1.5 mg/m² day 1 (maximum dose: 2 mg)
[total dose/cycle = 1.5 mg/m²; maximum dose: 2 mg]
Repeat cycle every 28 days for a total of 6 cycles

Carboplatin-Gemcitabine (Ovarian)

Use Ovarian cancer

Regimen
Gemcitabine: I.V.: 1000 mg/m²/day days 1 and 8
[total dose/cycle = 2000 mg/m²]
Carboplatin: I.V.: AUC 4 day 1
[total dose/cycle = AUC = 4]
Repeat cycle every 21 days for 6-10 cycles

Carboplatin-Gemcitabine-Paclitaxel (Unknown Primary)

Use Unknown primary (adenocarcinoma)

Regimen

Paclitaxel: I.V.: 200 mg/m^2 over 1 hour day 1
[total dose/cycle = 200 mg/m^2]
Carboplatin: I.V.: AUC 5 over 20-30 minutes day 1
[total dose/cycle = AUC = 5]
Gemcitabine: I.V.: 1000 mg/m^2/day days 1 and 8
[total dose/cycle = 2000 mg/m^2]
Repeat cycle every 21 days for a total of 4 cycles
Followed by:
Paclitaxel: I.V.: 70 mg/m^2 days 1, 8, 15, 22, 29, 36
[total dose/cycle = 420 mg/m^2]
Repeat cycle every 56 days for a total of 3 cycles

Carboplatin-Irinotecan (Small Cell Lung Cancer)

Use Lung cancer, small cell

Regimen NOTE: Multiple variations are listed.

Variation 1:
Carboplatin: I.V.: AUC 5 (Calvert formula) day 1
[total dose/cycle = AUC = 5]
Irinotecan: I.V.: 175 mg/m^2 day 1
[total dose/cycle = 175 mg/m^2]
Repeat cycle every 21 days for a total of 4 cycles
Variation 2:
Carboplatin: I.V.: AUC 5 (Calvert formula) over 1 hour day 1
[total dose/cycle = AUC = 5]
Irinotecan: I.V.: 50 mg/m^2/day over 30 minutes days 1, 8, and 15
[total dose/cycle = 150 mg/m^2]
Repeat cycle every 28 days

Carboplatin-Paclitaxel (Cervical Cancer)

Use Cervical cancer

Regimen NOTE: Multiple variations are listed.

Variation 1:
Paclitaxel: I.V.: 175 mg/m^2 over 3 hours day 1 (reduce to 155 mg/m^2 over 3 hours day 1 if prior pelvic irradiation)
[total dose/cycle = 175 (or 155) mg/m^2]
Carboplatin: I.V.: AUC 5 or 6 day 1
[total dose/cycle = AUC = 5 or 6]
Repeat cycle every 28 days for up to a total of 6-9 cycles
Variation 2:
Paclitaxel: I.V.: 175 mg/m^2 over 3 hours day 1
[total dose/cycle = 175 mg/m^2]
Carboplatin: I.V.: AUC 5 day 1
[total dose/cycle = AUC = 5]
Repeat cycle every 21 days for 6-9 cycles

Carboplatin-Paclitaxel (Ovarian)

Use Ovarian cancer

Regimen NOTE: Multiple variations are listed.

Variation 1:
Paclitaxel: I.V.: 175 mg/m^2 over 3 hours day 1
[total dose/cycle = 175 mg/m^2]
Carboplatin: I.V.: AUC 7.5 day 1
[total dose/cycle = AUC = 7.5]
Repeat cycle every 21 days for a total of 6 cycles

Variation 2:
Paclitaxel: I.V.: 175-185 mg/m^2 over 3 hours day 1
[total dose/cycle = 175-185 mg/m^2]
Carboplatin: I.V.: AUC 5-6 day 1
[total dose/cycle = AUC = 5-6]
Repeat cycle every 21 days

Variation 3:
Paclitaxel: I.V.: 175 mg/m^2 over 3 hours day 1
[total dose/cycle = 175 mg/m^2]
Carboplatin: I.V.: AUC 5 day 1
[total dose/cycle = AUC = 5]
Repeat cycle every 21 days

Variation 4:
Paclitaxel: I.V.: 175 mg/m^2 over 3 hours day 1
[total dose/cycle = 175 mg/m^2]
Carboplatin: I.V.: AUC 7.5 over 30 minutes day 1
[total dose/cycle = AUC = 7.5]
Repeat cycle every 21 days for 3-6 cycles

Variation 5:
Paclitaxel: I.V.: 80 mg/m^2 over 1 hour days 1, 8, and 15
[total dose/cycle = 240 mg/m^2]
Carboplatin: I.V.: AUC 6 over 1 hour day 1
[total dose/cycle = AUC = 6]
Repeat cycle every 21 days for a total of 6 cycles

Carboplatin-Paclitaxel (Unknown Primary)

Use Unknown primary (adenocarcinoma)

Regimen

Carboplatin: I.V.: Target AUC 6 day 1
[total dose/cycle = AUC = 6]
followed by
Paclitaxel: I.V.: 200 mg/m^2 infused over 3 hours day 1
[total dose/cycle = 200 mg/m^2]
Filgrastim: SubQ: 300 mcg/day days 5 to 12
[total dose/cycle = 2400 mcg]
Repeat cycle every 21 days for a total of 6 or 8 cycles

Carboplatin-Pemetrexed (Mesothelioma)

Use Malignant pleural mesothelioma

Regimen

Pemetrexed: I.V.: 500 mg/m^2 over 10 minutes day 1
[total dose/cycle = 500 mg/m^2]
Carboplatin: I.V.: AUC 5 over 30 minutes day 1 (start 30 minutes after pemetrexed)
[total dose/cycle = AUC = 5]
Repeat cycle every 21 days

Carboplatin-Pemetrexed (NSCLC)

Use Lung cancer, nonsmall cell

Regimen

Pemetrexed: I.V.: 500 mg/m^2 day 1
[total dose/cycle = 500 mg/m^2]
Carboplatin: I.V.: AUC 5 day 1
[total dose/cycle = AUC = 5]
Repeat cycle every 21 days for a maximum of 4 cycles

Carboplatin-Vincristine (Retinoblastoma)

Use Retinoblastoma

Regimen NOTE: Multiple variations are listed.

Variation 1 (GFR >50 mL/minute/m^2):
Carboplatin: I.V.: 560 mg/m^2 day 1
[total dose/cycle = 560 mg/m^2]

Vincristine: I.V.: 0.05 mg/kg day 1
[total dose/cycle = 0.05 mg/kg]
Repeat for up to a total of 8 cycles
Variation 2 (GFR <50 mL/minute/m^2):
Carboplatin: I.V.: AUC 6.5 day 1
[total dose/cycle = AUC 6.5]
Vincristine: I.V.: 0.05 mg/kg day 1
[total dose/cycle = 0.05 mg/kg]
Repeat for up to a total of 8 cycles

Carbo-Tax (NSCLC)

Use Lung cancer, nonsmall cell

Regimen

Paclitaxel: I.V.: 135-215 mg/m^2 infused over 24 hours day 1
[total dose/cycle = 135-215 mg/m^2]
or I.V.: 175 mg/m^2 infused over 3 hours day 1
[total dose/cycle = 175 mg/m^2]
followed by
Carboplatin: I.V.: Target AUC 7.5
[total dose/cycle = AUC = 7.5]
Repeat cycle every 21 days

CaT (NSCLC)

Use Lung cancer, nonsmall cell

Regimen NOTE: Multiple variations are listed.

Variation 1:
Paclitaxel: I.V.: 175 mg/m^2 day 1
[total dose/cycle = 175 mg/m^2]
or I.V.: 135 mg/m^2 continuous infusion day 1
[total dose/cycle = 135 mg/m^2]
Carboplatin: I.V.: AUC 7.5 day 1 or 2
[total dose/cycle = AUC = 7.5]
Repeat cycle every 21 days
Variation 2:
Paclitaxel: I.V.: 225 mg/m^2 day 1
[total dose/cycle = 225 mg/m^2]
Carboplatin: I.V.: AUC 6 day 1
[total dose/cycle = AUC = 6]
Repeat cycle every 21 days

CAV-P/VP (Neuroblastoma)

Use Neuroblastoma

Regimen

Note: The interval between courses is not fixed; the next course to begin upon hematologic recovery (ANC ≥500/mm^3 and platelets ≥100,000/mm^3)
Course 1, 2, 4, and 6 (CAV):
Cyclophosphamide: I.V.: 70 mg/kg/day over 6 hours days 1 and 2
[total dose/cycle = 140 mg/kg]
Doxorubicin: I.V.: 25 mg/m^2/day continuous infusion days 1, 2, and 3
[total dose/cycle = 75 mg/m^2]
Vincristine: I.V.: 0.033 mg/kg/day continuous infusion days 1, 2, and 3
[total dose/cycle = 0.099 mg/kg]
Vincristine: I.V.: 1.5 mg/m^2 bolus day 9
[total dose/cycle = 1.5 mg/m^2]
Course 3, 5, and 7 (P/VP):
Etoposide: I.V.: 200 mg/m^2/day over 2 hours days 1, 2, and 3
[total dose/cycle = 600 mg/m^2]
Cisplatin: I.V.: 50 mg/m^2/day over 1 hour days 1 to 4
[total dose/cycle = 200 mg/m^2]

CCDT (Melanoma)

Use Melanoma

Regimen

Dacarbazine: I.V.: 220 mg/m^2/day days 1, 2, and 3, every 21 to 28 days
[total dose/cycle = 660 mg/m^2]
Carmustine: I.V.: 150 mg/m^2 day 1, every 42 to 56 days
[total dose/cycle = 150 mg/m^2]
Cisplatin: I.V.: 25 mg/m^2/day days 1, 2, and 3, every 21 to 28 days
[total dose/cycle = 75 mg/m^2]
Tamoxifen: Oral: 20 mg/day (use of tamoxifen is optional)

CDDP/VP-16

Use Brain tumors

Regimen

Cisplatin: I.V.: 90 mg/m^2 day 1
[total dose/cycle = 90 mg/m^2]
Etoposide: I.V.: 150 mg/m^2/day days 3 and 4
[total dose/cycle = 300 mg/m^2]
Repeat cycle every 21 days

CE-CAdO (Neuroblastoma)

Use Neuroblastoma

Regimen

Variation 1:
Cycles 1 and 2 (CE):
Carboplatin: I.V.: 200 mg/m^2/day days 1, 2, and 3
[total dose/cycle = 600 mg/m^2]
Etoposide: I.V.: 150 mg/m^2/day days 1, 2, and 3
[total dose/cycle = 450 mg/m^2]
Repeat CE cycle once at 21 days, then follow with
Cycles 3 and 4 (CAdO):
Cyclophosphamide: I.V.: 300 mg/m^2/day days 1 to 5
[total dose/cycle = 1500 mg/m^2]
Doxorubicin: I.V.: 60 mg/m^2 day 5
[total dose/cycle = 60 mg/m^2]
Vincristine: I.V.: 1.5 mg/m^2 (maximum dose: 2 mg) days 1 and 5
[total dose/cycle = 3 mg/m^2 (maximum: 2 mg/dose)]
Repeat CAdO cycle once at 21 days
Variation 2:
Cycles 1 and 2 (CE):
Carboplatin: I.V.: 6.6 mg/kg/day days 1, 2, and 3
[total dose/cycle = 19.8 mg/kg]
Etoposide: I.V.: 5 mg/kg/day days 1, 2, and 3
[total dose/cycle = 15 mg/kg]
Repeat CE cycle once, then follow with
Cycles 3 and 4 (CAdO):
Cyclophosphamide: I.V.: 10 mg/kg/day days 1 to 5
[total dose/cycle = 50 mg/kg]
Doxorubicin: I.V.: 2 mg/kg day 5
[total dose/cycle = 2 mg/kg]
Vincristine: I.V.: 0.05 mg/kg days 1 and 5
[total dose/cycle = 0.1 mg/kg]
Repeat CAdO cycle once

CEF

Use Breast cancer

Regimen

Cyclophosphamide: Oral: 75 mg/m^2/day days 1 to 14
[total dose/cycle = 1050 mg/m^2]
Epirubicin: I.V.: 60 mg/m^2/day days 1 and 8
[total dose/cycle = 120 mg/m^2]
Fluorouracil: I.V.: 500 mg/m^2/day days 1 and 8
[total dose/cycle = 1000 mg/m^2]
Repeat cycle every 28 days

CEPP(B)

Use Lymphoma, non-Hodgkin

Regimen

Cyclophosphamide: I.V.: 600-650 mg/m^2/day days 1 and 8
[total dose/cycle = 1200-1300 mg/m^2]
Etoposide: I.V.: 70-85 mg/m^2/day days 1, 2, and 3
[total dose/cycle = 210-255 mg/m^2]
Procarbazine: Oral: 60 mg/m^2/day days 1 to 10
[total dose/cycle = 600 mg/m^2]
Prednisone: Oral: 60 mg/m^2/day days 1 to 10
[total dose/cycle = 600 mg/m^2]
Bleomycin: I.V.: 15 units/m^2/day days 1 and 15 (Bleomycin is sometimes omitted)
[total dose/cycle = 30 units/m^2]
Repeat cycle every 28 days

Cetuximab (Biweekly)-Irinotecan

Use Colorectal cancer

Regimen

Cycle 1:
Cetuximab: I.V.: 500 mg/m^2 over 120 minutes day 1 (cycle 1 only)
[total dose/cycle = 500 mg/m^2]
Irinotecan: I.V.: 180 mg/m^2 day 1
[total dose/cycle = 180 mg/m^2]
Subsequent cycles:
Cetuximab: I.V.: 500 mg/m^{2}over 60 minutes day 1
[total dose/cycle = 500 mg/m^2]
Irinotecan: I.V.: 180 mg/m^2 day 1
[total dose/cycle = 180 mg/m^2]
Repeat cycle every 14 days

Cetuximab-Carboplatin-Fluorouracil (Head and Neck Cancer)

Use Head and neck cancer

Regimen

Cycle 1:
Cetuximab: I.V.: 400 mg/m^2 (loading dose) day 1 (week 1, cycle 1 only)
[total loading dose = 400 mg/m^2]
followed by I.V.: 250 mg/m^2/day days 8 and 15
[total dose/cycle 1 = 900 mg/m^2]
Carboplatin: I.V.: AUC 5 day 1
[total dose/cycle = AUC = 5]
Fluorouracil: I.V.: 1000 mg/m^2/day continuous infusion days 1 to 4
[total dose/cycle = 4000 mg/m^2]
Treatment cycle is 3 weeks

Subsequent cycles:

Cetuximab: I.V.: 250 mg/m^2/day days 1, 8, and 15
[total dose/cycle = 750 mg/m^2]

Carboplatin: I.V.: AUC 5 day 1
[total dose/cycle = AUC = 5]

Fluorouracil: I.V.: 1000 mg/m^2/day continuous infusion days 1 to 4
[total dose/cycle = 4000 mg/m^2]

Repeat cycle every 3 weeks for a total of up to 6 cycles (cetuximab monotherapy may be continued thereafter until disease progression or unacceptable toxicity)

Cetuximab-Cisplatin-Fluorouracil (Head and Neck Cancer)

Use Head and neck cancer

Regimen

Cycle 1:

Cetuximab: I.V.: 400 mg/m^2 (loading dose) day 1 (week 1, cycle 1 only)
[total loading dose = 400 mg/m^2]
followed by I.V.: 250 mg/m^2/day days 8 and 15
[total dose/cycle 1 = 900 mg/m^2]

Cisplatin: I.V.: 100 mg/m^2 day 1
[total dose/cycle = 100 mg/m^2]

Fluorouracil: I.V.: 1000 mg/m^2/day continuous infusion days 1 to 4
[total dose/cycle = 4000 mg/m^2]

Treatment cycle is 3 weeks

Subsequent cycles:

Cetuximab: I.V.: 250 mg/m^2/day days 1, 8, and 15
[total dose/cycle = 750 mg/m^2]

Cisplatin: I.V.: 100 mg/m^2 day 1
[total dose/cycle = 100 mg/m^2]

Fluorouracil: I.V.: 1000 mg/m^2/day continuous infusion days 1 to 4
[total dose/cycle = 4000 mg/m^2]

Repeat cycle every 3 weeks for a total of up to 6 cycles (cetuximab monotherapy may be continued thereafter until disease progression or unacceptable toxicity)

Cetuximab-Cisplatin-Vinorelbine

Use Lung cancer, nonsmall cell

Regimen

Cycle 1:

Cetuximab: I.V.: 400 mg/m^2 (loading dose) day 1 (week 1, cycle 1 only)
[total loading dose = 400 mg/m^2]
followed by I.V.: 250 mg/m^2/dose days 8 and 15
[total dose/cycle 1 = 900 mg/m^2]

Cisplatin: I.V.: 80 mg/m^2/dose day 1
[total dose/cycle = 80 mg/m^2]

Vinorelbine: I.V.: 25 mg/m^2/dose days 1 and 8
[total dose/cycle = 50 mg/m^2]

Treatment cycle is 3 weeks

Subsequent cycles:

Cetuximab: I.V.: 250 mg/m^2/day days 1, 8, and 15
[total dose/cycle = 750 mg/m^2]

Cisplatin: I.V.: 80 mg/m^2 day 1
[total dose/cycle = 80 mg/m^2]

Vinorelbine: I.V.: 25 mg/m^2/dose days 1 and 8
[total dose/cycle = 50 mg/m^2]

Repeat cycle every 3 weeks

Cetuximab (Colorectal Regimen)

Use Colorectal cancer

Regimen

Cycle 1:

Cetuximab: I.V.: 400 mg/m^2 (loading dose) over 120 minutes day 1 (week 1, cycle 1 only)

followed by I.V.: 250 mg/m^2/day over 60 minutes days 8, 15, and 22 (cycle 1)

[total dose/cycle 1 = 1150 mg/m^2]

Treatment cycle is 28 days

Subsequent cycles:

Cetuximab: I.V.: 250 mg/m^2/day over 60 minutes days 1, 8, 15, and 22

[total dose/cycle = 1000 mg/m^2]

Repeat cycle every 28 days until disease progression or unacceptable toxicity

Cetuximab + FOLFIRI (Colorectal)

Use Colorectal cancer

Regimen

Cycle 1:

Cetuximab: I.V.: 400 mg/m^2 (loading dose) over 120 minutes day 1 (week 1, cycle 1 only)

followed by I.V.: 250 mg/m^2/day over 60 minutes day 8

[total dose/cycle 1 = 650 mg/m^2]

Irinotecan: I.V.: 180 mg/m^2 over 30-90 minutes day 1

[total dose/cycle = 180 mg/m^2]

Leucovorin (racemic): I.V.: 400 mg/m^2 over 120 minutes day 1

[total dose/cycle = 400 mg/m^2]

Fluorouracil: I.V. bolus: 400 mg/m^2 day 1

followed by I.V.: 2400 mg/m^2 continuous infusion (CI) over 46 hours beginning day 1

[total fluorouracil dose/cycle (bolus and CI) = 2800 mg/m^2]

Treatment cycle is 14 days

Subsequent cycles:

Cetuximab: I.V.: 250 mg/m^2/day over 60 minutes days 1 and 8

[total dose/cycle = 500 mg/m^2]

Irinotecan: I.V.: 180 mg/m^2 over 30-90 minutes day 1

[total dose/cycle = 180 mg/m^2]

Leucovorin (racemic): I.V.: 400 mg/m^2 over 120 minutes day 1

[total dose/cycle = 400 mg/m^2]

Fluorouracil: I.V. bolus: 400 mg/m^2 day 1

followed by I.V.: 2400 mg/m^2 CI over 46 hours beginning day 1

[total fluorouracil dose/cycle (bolus and CI) = 2800 mg/m^2]

Repeat cycle every 14 days until disease progression or unacceptable toxicity

Cetuximab-FOLFOX4

Use Colorectal cancer

Regimen

Cycle 1:

Cetuximab: I.V.: 400 mg/m^2 (loading dose) day 1 (week 1, cycle 1 only)

followed by I.V.: 250 mg/m^2/day day 8

[total dose/cycle 1 = 650 mg/m^2]

Oxaliplatin: I.V.: 85 mg/m^2 (over 2 hours) day 1

[total dose/cycle = 85 mg/m^2]

Leucovorin: I.V.: 200 mg/m^2/day (over 2 hours) days 1 and 2

[total dose/cycle = 400 mg/m^2]

Fluorouracil: I.V. bolus: 400 mg/m^2/day days 1 and 2

followed by I.V.: 600 mg/m^2 continuous infusion (over 22 hours) days 1 and 2

[total dose/cycle = 2000 mg/m^2]

Note: Bolus fluorouracil and continuous infusion are both given on each day.

Treatment cycle is 14 days

Subsequent cycles:
Cetuximab: I.V.: 250 mg/m^2/day days 1 and 8
[total dose/cycle = 500 mg/m^2]
Oxaliplatin: I.V.: 85 mg/m^2 day 1
[total dose/cycle = 85 mg/m^2]
Leucovorin: I.V.: 200 mg/m^2/day (over 2 hours) days 1 and 2
[total dose/cycle = 400 mg/m^2]
Fluorouracil: I.V. bolus: 400 mg/m^2/day days 1 and 2
followed by I.V.: 600 mg/m^2 continuous infusion (over 22 hours) days 1 and 2
[total dose/cycle = 2000 mg/m^2]
Note: Bolus fluorouracil and continuous infusion are both given on each day.
Repeat cycle every 14 days

Cetuximab-Irinotecan (Colorectal)

Use Colorectal cancer

Regimen NOTE: Multiple variations are listed.

Variation 1:
Cycle 1:
Cetuximab: I.V.: 400 mg/m^2 (loading dose) day 1 (week 1, cycle 1 only)
followed by I.V.: 250 mg/m^2/day days 8, 15, 22, 29, and 36
[total dose/cycle 1 = 1650 mg/m^2]
Irinotecan: I.V.: 125 mg/m^2/day days 1, 8, 15, and 22
[total dose/cycle = 500 mg/m^2]
Treatment cycle is 42 days (6 weeks)
Subsequent cycles:
Cetuximab: I.V.: 250 mg/m^2/day days 1, 8, 15, 22, 29, and 36
[total dose/cycle = 1500 mg/m^2]
Irinotecan: I.V.: 125 mg/m^2/day days 1, 8, 15, and 22
[total dose/cycle = 500 mg/m^2]
Repeat cycle every 42 days (6 weeks) until disease progression or unacceptable toxicity

Variation 2:
Cycle 1:
Cetuximab: I.V.: 400 mg/m^2 (loading dose) day 1 (week 1, cycle 1 only)
followed by I.V.: 250 mg/m^2/day days 8 and 15
[total dose/cycle 1 = 900 mg/m^2]
Irinotecan: I.V.: 350 mg/m^2 day 1
[total dose/cycle = 350 mg/m^2]
Treatment cycle is 21 days
Subsequent cycles:
Cetuximab: I.V.: 250 mg/m^2/day days 1, 8, and 15
[total dose/cycle = 750 mg/m^2]
Irinotecan: I.V.: 350 mg/m^2 day 1
[total dose/cycle = 350 mg/m^2]
Repeat cycle every 21 days until disease progression or unacceptable toxicity

CEV

Use Rhabdomyosarcoma

Regimen

Carboplatin: I.V.: 500 mg/m^2 day 1
[total dose/cycle = 500 mg/m^2]
Epirubicin: I.V.: 150 mg/m^2 day 1
[total dose/cycle = 150 mg/m^2]
Vincristine: I.V.: 1.5 mg/m^2/day days 1 and 7
[total dose/cycle = 3 mg/m^2]
Repeat cycle every 21 days

CHAMOCA (Modified Bagshawe Regimen)

Use Gestational trophoblastic tumor

Regimen NOTE: Multiple variations are listed.

Variation 1:
Hydroxyurea: Oral: 500 mg every 6 hours, for 4 doses, day 1 (start at 6 AM)
[total dose/cycle = 2000 mg]

Dactinomycin: I.V.: 0.2 mg/day days 1, 2, and 3 (give at 7 PM)
followed by I.V.: 0.5 mg/day days 4 and 5 (give at 7 PM)
[total dose/cycle = 1.6 mg]
Cyclophosphamide: I.V.: 500 mg/m^2/day days 3 and 8 (give at 7 PM)
[total dose/cycle = 1000 mg/m^2]
Vincristine: I.V.: 1 mg/m^2 (maximum dose: 2 mg) day 2 (give at 7 AM)
[total dose/cycle = 1 mg/m^2; maximum: 2 mg]
Methotrexate: I.V. bolus: 100 mg/m^2 day 2 (give at 7 PM)
followed by I.V.: 200 mg/m^2 continuous infusion over 12 hours day 2
[total dose/cycle = 300 mg/m^2]
Leucovorin: I.M.: 14 mg every 6 hours, for 6 doses, days 3, 4, and 5 (begin at 7 PM on day 3; start 24 hours after the start of methotrexate)
[total dose/cycle = 84 mg]
Doxorubicin: I.V.: 30 mg/m^2 day 8 (give at 7 PM)
[total dose/cycle = 30 mg/m^2]
Repeat cycle every 18 days or as toxicity permits (cycle may be repeated 10 days after last treatment)

Variation 2:
Hydroxyurea: Oral: 500 mg every 12 hours, for 4 doses, days 1 and 2 (usually started in early morning)
[total dose/cycle = 2000 mg]
Dactinomycin: I.V.: 10 mcg/kg/day days 5, 6, and 7
[total dose/cycle = 30 mcg/kg]
Vincristine: I.V.: 1 mg/m^2 day 3
[total dose/cycle = 1 mg/m^2]
Methotrexate: I.V. bolus: 100 mg/m^2 day 3
followed by I.V.: 200 mg/m^2 continuous infusion over 12 hours day 3
[total dose/cycle = 300 mg/m^2]
Leucovorin: I.M.: 10 mg/m^2 every 12 hours, for 4 doses, days 4 and 5 (start 24 hours after the start of methotrexate)
[total dose/cycle = 40 mg/m^2]
Cyclophosphamide: I.V.: 600 mg/m^2 day 5
[total dose/cycle = 600 mg/m^2]
Doxorubicin: I.V.: 30 mg/m^2 day 10
[total dose/cycle = 30 mg/m^2]
Repeat cycle every 3 weeks

Variation 3:
Hydroxyurea: Oral: 500 mg every 12 hours, for 4 doses, days 1 and 2 (usually started in early morning)
[total dose/cycle = 2000 mg/m^2]
Vincristine: I.V.: 1 mg/m^2 day 3
[total dose/cycle = 1 mg/m^2]
Methotrexate: I.V. bolus: 100 mg/m^2 day 3
followed by I.V.: 200 mg/m^2continuous infusion over 12 hours day 3
[total dose/cycle = 300 mg/m^2]
Leucovorin: I.M.: 14 mg every 6 hours, for 6 doses, days 4, 5, and 6 (start 24 hours after start of methotrexate)
[total dose/cycle = 84 mg]
Dactinomycin: I.V.: 0.2 mg/day days 2, 3, and 4
followed by I.V.: 0.5 mg/day days 5 and 6
[total dose/cycle = 1.6 mg]
Cyclophosphamide: I.V.: 500 mg/m^2 day 4
[total dose/cycle = 500 mg/m^2]
Doxorubicin: I.V.: 30 mg/m^2 day 9
[total dose/cycle = 30 mg/m^2]
Melphalan: I.V.: 6 mg/m^2 day 9
[total dose/cycle = 6 mg/m^2]
Repeat cycle approximately every 3 weeks

Variation 4:
Hydroxyurea: Oral: 500 mg 4 times/day, for 4 doses, day 1
[total dose/cycle = 2000 mg/m^2]
Vincristine: I.V.: 1 mg/m^2 day 2
[total dose/cycle = 1 mg/m^2]

Methotrexate: I.V. bolus: 100 mg/m^2 day 2
followed by I.V.: 200 mg/m^2 continuous infusion over 12 hours day 2
[total dose/cycle = 300 mg/m^2]
Leucovorin: I.M.: 14 mg every 6 hours, for 6 doses, days 3, 4, and 5 (start 24 hours after the start of methotrexate)
[total dose/cycle = 84 mg]
Dactinomycin: I.V.: 0.2 mg days 1, 2, and 3
followed by I.V.: 0.5 mg days 4 and 5
[total dose/cycle = 1.6 mg]
Cyclophosphamide: I.V.: 500 mg/m^2 day 3
[total dose/cycle = 500 mg/m^2]
Cyclophosphamide: I.V.: 300 mg/m^2 on day 8
[total dose/cycle = 300 mg/m^2]
Doxorubicin: I.V.: 30 mg/m^2 day 8
[total dose/cycle = 30 mg/m^2]
Repeat cycle approximately every 3 weeks

CHAMOMA (Bagshawe Regimen)

Use Gestational trophoblastic tumor

Regimen

Hydroxyurea: Oral: 500 mg every 12 hours, for 4 doses, days 1 and 2
[total dose/cycle = 2000 mg]
Vincristine: I.V.: 1 mg/m^2 day 3
[total dose/cycle = 1 mg/m^2]
Methotrexate: I.V. bolus: 100 mg/m^2 day 3
followed by I.V.: 200 mg/m^2 continuous infusion over 12 hours day 3
[total dose/cycle = 300 mg/m^2]
Leucovorin: I.M.: 12 mg/m^2 every 12 hours, for 4 doses, days 4 and 5 (start 12 hours after the end of methotrexate infusion)
[total dose/cycle = 48 mg/m^2]
Dactinomycin: I.V.: 10 mcg/kg/day days 5, 6, and 7
[total dose/cycle = 30 mcg/kg]
Cyclophosphamide: I.V.: 600 mg/m^2 day 5
[total dose/cycle = 600 mg/m^2]
Doxorubicin: I.V.: 30 mg/m^2 day 10
[total dose/cycle = 30 mg/m^2]
Melphalan: I.V.: 6 mg/m^2 day 10
[total dose/cycle = 6 mg/m^2]
Repeat cycle approximately every 3 weeks

ChIVPP (Hodgkin)

Use Lymphoma, Hodgkin disease

Regimen NOTE: Multiple variations are listed.

Variation 1:
Chlorambucil: Oral: 6 mg/m^2/day (maximum dose: 10 mg/day) days 1 to 14
[total dose/cycle = 84 mg/m^2; maximum: 140 mg/cycle]
Vinblastine: I.V.: 6 mg/m^2/day (maximum dose: 10 mg/dose) days 1 and 8
[total dose/cycle = 12 mg/m^2; maximum: 20 mg/cycle]
Procarbazine: Oral: 100 mg/m^2/day (maximum dose: 150 mg/day) days 1 to 14
[total dose/cycle = 1400 mg/m^2; maximum: 2100 mg/cycle]
Prednisone or Prednisolone: Oral: 40 mg/day days 1 to 14
[total dose/cycle = 560 mg]
Repeat cycle every 28 days to complete remission plus 2 cycles; minimum of 6 cycles, maximum of 8 cycles

Variation 2:

Chlorambucil: Oral: 6 mg/m^2/day days 1 to 14
[total dose/cycle = 84 mg/m^2]

Vinblastine: I.V.: 6 mg/m^2/day days 1 and 8
[total dose/cycle = 12 mg/m^2]

Procarbazine: Oral: 100 mg/m^2/day days 1 to 14
[total dose/cycle = 1400 mg/m^2]

Prednisone: Oral: 40 mg/day days 1 to 14
[total dose/cycle = 560 mg]

Repeat cycle every 28 days for 6 cycles

CP (Leukemia)

Use Leukemia, chronic lymphocytic

Regimen

Chlorambucil: Oral: 30 mg/m^2 day 1
[total dose/cycle = 30 mg/m^2]

Prednisone: Oral: 80 mg/day days 1 to 5
[total dose/cycle = 400 mg]

Repeat cycle every 14 days until disease progression for a maximum duration of 9 months (if no response at 9 months), 15 months (if complete response at 9 months), or 18 months (if partial response at 9 months)

CHOP (NHL)

Use Lymphoma, non-Hodgkin

Regimen NOTE: Multiple variations are listed.

Variation 1:

Cyclophosphamide: I.V.: 750 mg/m^2 day 1
[total dose/cycle = 750 mg/m^2]

Doxorubicin: I.V.: 50 mg/m^2 day 1
[total dose/cycle = 50 mg/m^2]

Vincristine: I.V.: 1.4 mg/m^2 (maximum dose: 2 mg) day 1
[total dose/cycle = 1.4 mg/m^2; maximum: 2 mg]

Prednisone: Oral: 100 mg/day days 1 to 5
[total dose/cycle = 500 mg]

Repeat cycle every 21 days for 6 to 8 cycles

Variation 2 (dose intensity/dose-dense):

Cyclophosphamide: I.V.: 1600 mg/m^2 day 1
[total dose/cycle = 1600 mg/m^2]

Doxorubicin: I.V.: 65 mg/m^2 day 1
[total dose/cycle = 65 mg/m^2]

Vincristine: I.V.: 1.4 mg/m^2 day 1
[total dose/cycle = 1.4 mg/m^2]

Prednisone: Oral: 100 mg/day days 1 to 5
[total dose/cycle = 500 mg]

Filgrastim: SubQ: 5 mcg/kg days 2 to 11 or until ANC >10,000/mm^3

Repeat cycle every 14 days for 6 cycles

Variation 3 (dose-dense):

Cyclophosphamide: I.V.: 750 mg/m^2 day 1
[total dose/cycle = 750 mg/m^2]

Doxorubicin: I.V.: 50 mg/m^2 day 1
[total dose/cycle = 50 mg/m^2]

Vincristine: I.V.: 2 mg day 1
[total dose/cycle = 2 mg]

Prednisone: Oral: 100 mg/day days 1 to 5
[total dose/cycle = 500 mg]

Filgrastim: SubQ: 300 mcg/day (<75 kg patient) or 480 mcg/day (≥75 kg patient) days 4 to 13

Repeat cycle every 14 days for 6 cycles

Variation 4 (localized disease; chemotherapy plus radiotherapy):
Cyclophosphamide: I.V.: 750 mg/m^2 day 1
[total dose/cycle = 750 mg/m^2]
Doxorubicin: I.V.: 50 mg/m^2 day 1
[total dose/cycle = 50 mg/m^2]
Vincristine: I.V.: 1.4 mg/m^2 (maximum dose: 2 mg) day 1
[total dose/cycle = 1.4 mg/m^2; maximum: 2 mg]
Prednisone: Oral: 100 mg/day days 1 to 5
[total dose/cycle = 500 mg]
Repeat cycle every 21 days for 3 cycles followed by radiation therapy
Variation 5 (HIV-associated NHL):
Cyclophosphamide: I.V.: 750 mg/m^2 day 1
[total dose/cycle = 750 mg/m^2]
Doxorubicin: I.V.: 50 mg/m^2 day 1
[total dose/cycle = 50 mg/m^2]
Vincristine: I.V.: 1.4 mg/m^2 (maximum dose: 2 mg) day 1
[total dose/cycle = 1.4 mg/m^2; maximum: 2 mg]
Prednisone: Oral: 100 mg/day days 1 to 5
[total dose/cycle = 500 mg]
Filgrastim: SubQ: 300 mcg/day (<70 kg patient) or 480 mcg/day (>70 kg patient) days 4 to 13
Repeat cycle every 21 days; minimum of 4 cycles or 2 cycles beyond complete remission

CISCA

Use Bladder cancer

Regimen
Cyclophosphamide: I.V.: 650 mg/m^2 day 1
[total dose = 650 mg/m^2]
Doxorubicin: I.V.: 50 mg/m^2 day 1
[total dose = 50 mg/m^2]
Cisplatin: I.V.: 100 mg/m^2 day 2
[total dose = 100 mg/m^2]
Repeat cycle every 21-28 days

Cisplatin-Capecitabine (Esophageal Cancer)

Use Esophageal cancer

Regimen
Cisplatin: I.V.: 80 mg/m^2 over 2 hours day 1
[total dose/cycle = 80 mg/m^2]
Capecitabine: Oral: 1000 mg/m^2/dose twice daily, days 1 to 14
[total dose/cycle = 28,000 mg/m^2]
Repeat cycle every 3 weeks until disease progression or unacceptable toxicity

Cisplatin-Capecitabine (Gastric Cancer)

Use Gastric cancer

Regimen
Cisplatin: I.V.: 80 mg/m^2 over 2 hours day 1
[total dose/cycle = 80 mg/m^2]
Capecitabine: Oral: 1000 mg/m^2/dose twice daily, days 1 to 14
[total dose/cycle = 28,000 mg/m^2]
Repeat cycle every 3 weeks until disease progression or unacceptable toxicity

Cisplatin-Cetuximab (Head and Neck Cancer)

Use Head and neck cancer

Regimen NOTE: Multiple variations are listed.
Variation 1:
Cycle 1:
Cetuximab: I.V.: 400 mg/m^2 (loading dose) day 1 (week 1, cycle 1 only)
[total loading dose = 400 mg/m^2]
followed by I.V.: 250 mg/m^2/day days 8, 15, and 22
[total dose/cycle 1 = 1150 mg/m^2]

Cisplatin: I.V.: 100 mg/m^2 day 1
[total dose/cycle = 100 mg/m^2]
Treatment cycle is 4 weeks
Subsequent cycles:
Cetuximab: I.V.: 250 mg/m^2/day days 1, 8, 15, and 22
[total dose/cycle = 1000 mg/m^2]
Cisplatin: I.V.: 100 mg/m^2 day 1
[total dose/cycle = 100 mg/m^2]
Repeat cycle every 4 weeks
Variation 2:
Cycle 1:
Cetuximab: I.V.: 400 mg/m^2 (loading dose) day 1 (week 1, cycle 1 only)
[total loading dose = 400 mg/m^2]
followed by I.V.: 250 mg/m^2/day days 8 and 15
[total dose/cycle 1 = 900 mg/m^2]
Cisplatin: I.V.: 75-100 mg/m^2 day 1
[total dose/cycle = 75-100 mg/m^2]
Treatment cycle is 3 weeks
Subsequent cycles:
Cetuximab: I.V.: 250 mg/m^2/day days 1, 8, and 15
[total dose/cycle = 750 mg/m^2]
Cisplatin: I.V.: 75-100 mg/m^2 day 1
[total dose/cycle = 75-100 mg/m^2]
Repeat cycle every 3 weeks

Cisplatin-Cytarabine-Dexamethasone (NHL Regimen)

Use Lymphoma, non-Hodgkin

Regimen NOTE: Multiple variations are listed.
Variation 1:
Dexamethasone: I.V. or Oral: 40 mg/day days 1 to 4
[total dose/cycle = 160 mg]
Cisplatin: I.V.: 100 mg/m^2 over 24 hours day 1
[total dose/cycle = 100 mg/m^2]
Cytarabine: I.V.: 2000 mg/m^2 every 12 hours for 2 doses day 2 (begins at the end of the cisplatin infusion)
[total dose/cycle = 4000 mg/m^2]
Repeat cycle every 3-4 weeks for 6-10 cycles
Variation 2 (patients >70 years of age):
Dexamethasone: I.V. or Oral: 40 mg/day days 1 to 4
[total dose/cycle = 160 mg]
Cisplatin: I.V.: 100 mg/m^2 over 24 hours day 1
[total dose/cycle = 100 mg/m^2]
Cytarabine: I.V.: 1000 mg/m^2 every 12 hours for 2 doses day 2 (begins at the end of the cisplatin infusion)
[total dose/cycle = 2000 mg/m^2]
Repeat cycle every 3-4 weeks for 6-10 cycles

Cisplatin-Dacarbazine-Interferon Alfa-2b-Aldesleukin

Use Melanoma

Regimen
Cisplatin: I.V.: 25 mg/m^2/day days 1, 2, and 3
[total dose/cycle = 75 mg/m^2]
Dacarbazine: 250 mg/m^2/day days 1, 2, and 3
[total dose/cycle = 750 mg/m^2]
Interferon Alfa-2b: SubQ: 5 million units/m^2/day days 6, 8, 10, 13, and 15
[total dose/cycle = 25 million units/m^2]
Aldesleukin: I.V.: 18 million units/m^2/day days 6 to 10, 13, 14, and 15
[total dose/cycle = 144 million units/m^2]
Repeat cycle every 28 days

Cisplatin-Docetaxel (Unknown Primary)

Use Unknown primary (adenocarcinoma)

Regimen

Docetaxel: I.V.: 75 mg/m^2 over 1 hour day 1
[total dose/cycle = 75 mg/m^2]
Cisplatin: I.V.: 75 mg/m^2 over 1 hour day 1
[total dose/cycle = 75 mg/m^2]
Repeat cycle every 21 days for up to a total of 8 cycles

Cisplatin-Doxorubicin-Etoposide-Cyclophosphamide (Neuroblastoma)

Use Neuroblastoma

Regimen

Cisplatin: I.V.: 60 mg/m^2 over 6 hours day 0
[total dose/cycle = 60 mg/m^2]
Doxorubicin: I.V.: 30 mg/m^2 day 2
[total dose/cycle = 30 mg/m^2]
Etoposide: I.V.: 100 mg/m^2/day days 2 and 5
[total dose/cycle = 200 mg/m^2]
Cyclophosphamide: I.V.: 1000 mg/m^2/day days 3 and 4
[total dose/cycle = 2000 mg/m^2]
Repeat cycle every 28 days for a total of 5 cycles

Cisplatin-Etoposide (NSCLC)

Use Lung cancer, nonsmall cell

Regimen NOTE: Multiple variations are listed.

Variation 1:
Cisplatin: I.V.: 80 mg/m^2 day 1
[total dose/cycle = 80 mg/m^2]
Etoposide: I.V.: 100 mg/m^2/day days 1, 2, and 3
[total dose/cycle = 300 mg/m^2]
Repeat cycle every 21 days for a total of 4 cycles

Variation 2:
Cisplatin: I.V.: 100 mg/m^2 day 1
[total dose/cycle = 100 mg/m^2]
Etoposide: I.V.: 100 mg/m^2/day days 1, 2, and 3
[total dose/cycle = 300 mg/m^2]
Repeat cycle every 28 days for a total of 3 cycles

Variation 3:
Cisplatin: I.V.: 100 mg/m^2 day 1
[total dose/cycle = 100 mg/m^2]
Etoposide: I.V.: 100 mg/m^2/day days 1, 2, and 3
[total dose/cycle = 300 mg/m^2]
Repeat cycle every 28 days for a total of 4 cycles

Variation 4:
Cisplatin: I.V.: 120 mg/m^2/day days 1, 29, and 71
[total dose/treatment = 360 mg/m^2]
Etoposide: I.V.: 100 mg/m^2/day days 1, 2, 3, 29, 30, 31, 71, 72, and 73
[total dose/treatment = 900 mg/m^2]

Variation 5:
Cisplatin: I.V.: 75 mg/m^2 day 1
[total dose/cycle = 75 mg/m^2]
Etoposide: I.V.: 100 mg/m^2/day days 1, 2, and 3
[total dose/cycle = 300 mg/m^2]
Repeat cycle every 21 days for up to 10 cycles

Cisplatin-Fluorouracil (Bladder Cancer)

Use Bladder cancer

Regimen In combination with radiation therapy

Note: Begin infusion(s) 2 hours before radiation therapy on days 1, 3, 15, and 17:

Cisplatin: I.V.: 15 mg/m²/day over 2 hours days 1, 2, 3, 15, 16, and 17
[total dose/cycle = 90 mg/m²]

Fluorouracil: I.V.: 400 mg/m²/day over 2 hours days 1, 2, 3, 15, 16, and 17
[total dose/cycle = 2400 mg/m²]

Cisplatin-Fluorouracil (Cervical Cancer)

Use Cervical cancer

Regimen NOTE: Multiple variations are listed.

Variation 1 (with concurrent radiation therapy):

Cisplatin: I.V.: 75 mg/m² day 1
[total dose/cycle = 75 mg/m²]

Fluorouracil: I.V.: 1000 mg/m²/day continuous infusion days 1 to 4 (96 hours)
[total dose/cycle = 4000 mg/m²]

Repeat cycle every 21 days for a total 3 cycles

Variation 2 (with concurrent radiation therapy):

Cisplatin: I.V.: 50 mg/m² day 1 starting 4 hours before radiotherapy
[total dose/cycle = 50 mg/m²]

Fluorouracil: I.V.: 1000 mg/m²/day continuous infusion days 2 to 5 (96 hours)
[total dose/cycle = 4000 mg/m²]

Repeat cycle every 28 days for a total of 2 cycles

Variation 3 (cycles 1 and 2 are with concurrent radiation therapy):

Cisplatin: I.V.: 70 mg/m² day 1
[total dose/cycle = 70 mg/m²]

Fluorouracil: I.V.: 1000 mg/m²/day continuous infusion days 1 to 4 (96 hours)
[total dose/cycle = 4000 mg/m²]

Repeat cycle every 21 days for a total of 4 cycles

Cisplatin-Fluorouracil (Esophageal Cancer)

Use Esophageal cancer

Regimen NOTE: Multiple variations are listed.

Variation 1:

Cisplatin: I.V.: 100 mg/m²/dose day 1
[total dose/cycle = 100 mg/m²]

Fluorouracil: I.V.: 1000 mg/m²/day continuous infusion days 1 to 5
[total dose/cycle = 5000 mg/m²]

Repeat cycle every 28 days until disease progression or unacceptable toxicity.

Variation 2:

Cycles 1 to 3 (prior to surgery):

Cisplatin: I.V.: 100 mg/m²/dose day 1
[total dose/cycle = 100 mg/m²]

Fluorouracil: I.V.: 1000 mg/m²/day continuous infusion days 1 to 5
[total dose/cycle = 5000 mg/m²]

Treatment cycles 1-3 are 28 days each

Cycles 4 and 5 (postoperative):

Cisplatin: I.V.: 75 mg/m²/dose day 1
[total dose/cycle = 75 mg/m²]

Fluorouracil: I.V.: 1000 mg/m²/day continuous infusion days 1 to 5
[total dose/cycle = 5000 mg/m²]

Treatment cycles 4 and 5 are 28 days each

Variation 3 (in combination with radiation therapy):
Cycle 1:
Cisplatin: I.V.: 75 mg/m^2/dose day 1
[total dose/cycle = 75 mg/m^2]
Fluorouracil: I.V.: 1000 mg/m^2/day continuous infusion days 1 to 4
[total dose/cycle = 4000 mg/m^2]
Treatment cycle is 28 days
Cycles 2 to 4:
Cisplatin: I.V.: 75 mg/m^2/dose day 1
[total dose/cycle = 75 mg/m^2]
Fluorouracil: I.V.: 1000 mg/m^2/day continuous infusion days 1 to 4
[total dose/cycle = 4000 mg/m^2]
Repeat cycle every 21 days for 3 more cycles (total of 4 cycles)
Variation 4 (in combination with radiation therapy):
Cisplatin: I.V.: 100 mg/m^2/dose day 1
[total dose/cycle = 100 mg/m^2]
Fluorouracil: I.V.: 1000 mg/m^2/day continuous infusion days 1 to 4
[total dose/cycle = 4000 mg/m^2]
Repeat cycle every 28 days for total of 2 cycles
Variation 5 (in combination with radiation therapy):
Cisplatin: I.V.: 75 mg/m^2/dose day 1
[total dose/cycle = 75 mg/m^2]
Fluorouracil: I.V.: 1000 mg/m^2/day continuous infusion days 1 to 4
[total dose/cycle = 4000 mg/m^2]
Repeat cycle every 28 days for 4 cycles
Variation 6 (in combination with radiation therapy):
Cycles 1 and 2:
Cisplatin: I.V.: 75 mg/m^2/dose day 1
[total dose/cycle = 75 mg/m^2]
Fluorouracil: I.V.: 1000 mg/m^2/day continuous infusion days 1 to 4
[total dose/cycle = 4000 mg/m^2]
Treatment cycles 1 and 2 are 28 days each; cycle 2 is followed by a 2-week rest
Cycles 3 and 4 (begin cycle 3 at week 11):
Cisplatin: I.V.: 75 mg/m^2/dose day 1
[total dose/cycle = 75 mg/m^2]
Fluorouracil: I.V.: 1000 mg/m^2/day continuous infusion days 1 to 4
[total dose/cycle = 4000 mg/m^2]
Treatment cycles 3 and 4 are 28 days each
Variation 7 (in combination with radiation therapy):
Cycles 1 to 4:
Cisplatin: I.V.: 15 mg/m^2/day days 1 to 5
[total dose/cycle = 75 mg/m^2]
Fluorouracil: I.V.: 800 mg/m^2/day continuous infusion days 1 to 5
[total dose/cycle = 4000 mg/m^2]
Repeat cycles 1-4 every 21 days; cycle 4 is followed by a 1-week rest
Cycles 5 (begin cycle 5 at week 14):
Cisplatin: I.V.: 15 mg/m^2/day days 1 to 5
[total dose/cycle = 75 mg/m^2]
Fluorouracil: I.V.: 800 mg/m^2/day continuous infusion days 1 to 5
[total dose/cycle = 4000 mg/m^2]
Variation 8:
Cisplatin: I.V.: 80 mg/m^2/dose day 1
[total dose/cycle = 80 mg/m^2]
Fluorouracil: I.V.: 800 mg/m^2/day continuous infusion days 1 to 5
[total dose/cycle = 4000 mg/m^2]
Repeat cycle every 21 days until disease progression or unacceptable toxicity.

Cisplatin-Fluorouracil (Gastric Cancer)

Use Gastric cancer

Regimen NOTE: Multiple variations are listed.
Variation 1:
Cisplatin: I.V.: 100 mg/m^2 day 1
[total dose/cycle = 100 mg/m^2]

Fluorouracil: I.V.: 1000 mg/m^2/day continuous infusion days 1 to 5
[total dose/cycle = 5000 mg/m^2]
Repeat cycle every 4 weeks until disease progression or unacceptable toxicity
Variation 2:
Cisplatin: I.V.: 80 mg/m^2 over 2 hours day 1
[total dose/cycle = 80 mg/m^2]
Fluorouracil: I.V.: 800 mg/m^2/day continuous infusion days 1 to 5
[total dose/cycle = 4000 mg/m^2]
Repeat cycle every 21 days until disease progression or unacceptable toxicity
Variation 3:
Fluorouracil: I.V.: 1000 mg/m^2/day continuous infusion days 1 to 5
[total dose/cycle = 5000 mg/m^2]
Cisplatin: I.V.: 100 mg/m^2 day 2
[total dose/cycle = 100 mg/m^2]
Repeat cycle every 4 weeks

Cisplatin-Fluorouracil (Head and Neck Cancer)

Use Head and neck cancer
Regimen NOTE: Multiple variations are listed.
Variation 1:
Cisplatin: I.V.: 100 mg/m^2 day 1
[total dose/cycle = 100 mg/m^2]
Fluorouracil: I.V.: 1000 mg/m^2/day continuous infusion days 1 to 4
[total dose/cycle = 4000 mg/m^2]
Repeat cycle every 3 weeks
Variation 2:
Cisplatin: I.V.: 100 mg/m^2 day 1
[total dose/cycle = 100 mg/m^2]
Fluorouracil: I.V.: 1000 mg/m^2/day continuous infusion days 1 to 4
[total dose/cycle = 4000 mg/m^2]
Repeat cycle every 3 or 4 weeks
Variation 3:
Cisplatin: I.V.: 100 mg/m^2 day 1
[total dose/cycle = 100 mg/m^2]
Fluorouracil: I.V.: 1000 mg/m^2/day continuous infusion days 1 to 5
[total dose/cycle = 5000 mg/m^2]
Repeat cycle every 3 or 4 weeks
Variation 4:
Cisplatin: I.V.: 60 mg/m^2 day 1
[total dose/cycle = 60 mg/m^2]
Fluorouracil: I.V.: 800 mg/m^2/day continuous infusion days 1 to 5
[total dose/cycle = 4000 mg/m^2]
Repeat cycle every 14 days
Variation 5:
Cisplatin: I.V.: 20 mg/m^2/day days 1 to 5
[total dose/cycle = 100 mg/m^2]
Fluorouracil: I.V.: 200 mg/m^2/day days 1 to 5
[total dose/cycle = 1000 mg/m^2]
Repeat cycle every 3 weeks
Variation 6:
Cisplatin: I.V.: 80 mg/m^2 continuous infusion day 1
[total dose/cycle = 80 mg/m^2]
Fluorouracil: I.V.: 800 mg/m^2/day continuous infusion days 2 to 6
[total dose/cycle = 4000 mg/m^2]
Repeat cycle every 3 weeks
Variation 7:
Cisplatin: I.V.: 75 mg/m^2 day 1
[total dose/cycle = 75 mg/m^2]
Fluorouracil: I.V.: 1000 mg/m^2/day continuous infusion days 1 to 4
[total dose/cycle = 4000 mg/m^2]
Repeat cycle every 4 weeks

Variation 8:
Cisplatin: I.V.: 120 mg/m^2 day 1
[total dose/cycle = 120 mg/m^2]
Fluorouracil: I.V.: 1000 mg/m^2/day continuous infusion days 1 to 5
[total dose/cycle = 5000 mg/m^2]
Repeat cycle every 3 weeks
Variation 9:
Cisplatin: I.V.: 25 mg/m^2/day continuous infusion days 1 to 4
[total dose/cycle = 100 mg/m^2]
Fluorouracil: I.V.: 1000 mg/m^2/day days 1 to 4
[total dose/cycle = 4000 mg/m^2]
Repeat cycle every 3 weeks
Variation 10:
Fluorouracil: I.V.: 350 mg/m^2/day continuous infusion days 1 to 5
[total dose/cycle = 1750 mg/m^2]
Cisplatin: I.V.: 50 mg/m^2 day 6
[total dose/cycle = 50 mg/m^2]
Repeat cycle every 3 weeks
Variation 11:
Cisplatin: I.V.: 5 mg/m^2/day continuous infusion days 1 to 14
[total dose/cycle = 70 mg/m^2]
Fluorouracil: I.V.: 200 mg/m^2/day continuous infusion days 1 to 14
[total dose/cycle = 2800 mg/m^2]
With concurrent radiation therapy, cycle does not repeat
Variation 12 (administer during the final 2 weeks of radiation therapy; weeks 6 and 7):
Cisplatin: I.V.: 10 mg/m^2/day days 1 to 5 beginning week 6
[total dose/week = 50 mg/m^2]
Fluorouracil: I.V.: 400 mg/m^2/day continuous infusion days 1 to 5 beginning week 6
[total dose/week = 2000 mg/m^2]
Repeat cycle one time in week 7
Variation 13:
Cisplatin: I.V.: 100 mg/m^2/day day 1 (concurrent with radiation therapy)
[total dose/cycle = 100 mg/m^2]
Repeat cycle every 3 weeks for a total of 3 cycles
Followed by (postradiation chemotherapy; begin 4 weeks after radiotherapy or the last cisplatin dose):
Cisplatin: I.V.: 80 mg/m^2 day 1
[total dose/cycle = 80 mg/m^2]
Fluorouracil: I.V.: 1000 mg/m^2/day continuous infusion days 1 to 4
[total dose/cycle = 4000 mg/m^2]
Repeat cycle every 4 weeks for a total of 3 cycles

Cisplatin-Gemcitabine (Cervical Cancer)

Use Cervical cancer

Regimen NOTE: Multiple variations are listed.
Variation 1:
Gemcitabine: I.V.: 1250 mg/m^2/day days 1 and 8
[total dose/cycle = 2500 mg/m^2]
Cisplatin: I.V.: 50 mg/m^2 day 1
[total dose/cycle = 50 mg/m^2]
Repeat cycle every 21 days for up to a total of 6 cycles
Variation 2:
Gemcitabine: I.V.: 1000 mg/m^2/day days 1 and 8
[total dose/cycle = 2000 mg/m^2]
Cisplatin: I.V.: 50 mg/m^2 day 1
[total dose/cycle = 50 mg/m^2]
Repeat cycle every 21 days for up to a total of 6 cycles; responders may continue beyond 6 cycles

Cisplatin-Gemcitabine (Mesothelioma)

Use Malignant pleural mesothelioma

Regimen NOTE: Multiple variations are listed.
Variation 1:
Cisplatin: I.V.: 100 mg/m^2 over 1 hour day 1
[total dose/cycle = 100 mg/m^2]

Gemcitabine: I.V.: 1000 mg/m²/day over 30 minutes days 1, 8, and 15
[total dose/cycle = 3000 mg/m²]
Repeat cycle every 28 days for up to a total of 6 cycles
Variation 2:
Gemcitabine: I.V.: 1250 mg/m²/day over 30 minutes days 1 and 8
[total dose/cycle = 2500 mg/m²]
Cisplatin: I.V.: 80 mg/m² over 3 hours day 1
[total dose/cycle = 80 mg/m²]
Repeat cycle every 21 days for up to a total of 6 cycles
Variation 3:
Gemcitabine: I.V.: 1000 mg/m²/day over 30 minutes days 1, 8, and 15
[total dose/cycle = 3000 mg/m²]
Cisplatin: I.V.: 30 mg/m²/day over 30 minutes days 1, 8, and 15
[total dose/cycle = 90 mg/m²]
Repeat cycle every 28 days

Cisplatin-Gemcitabine (Pancreatic)

Use Pancreatic cancer

Regimen NOTE: Multiple variations are listed.
Variation 1:
Cisplatin: I.V.: 50 mg/m²/day over 1 hour days 1 and 15
[total dose/cycle = 100 mg/m²]
Gemcitabine: I.V.: 1000 mg/m²/day over 30 minutes days 1 and 15
[total dose/cycle = 2000 mg/m²]
Repeat cycle every 28 days
Variation 2:
Cycle 1:
Cisplatin: I.V.: 25 mg/m²/day days 1, 8, 15, 29, 36, and 43 (cycle 1 only)
[total dose/cycle 1 = 150 mg/m²]
Gemcitabine: I.V.: 1000 mg/m²/day over 30 minutes days 1, 8, 15, 22, 29, 36, and 43 (cycle 1 only), 1 hour after cisplatin
[total dose/cycle 1 = 7000 mg/m²]
Treatment cycle is 56 days
Subsequent cycles:
Cisplatin: I.V.: 25 mg/m²/day days 1, 8, and 15
[total dose/cycle = 75 mg/m²]
Gemcitabine: I.V.: 1000 mg/m²/day over 30 minutes days 1, 8, and 15, 1 hour after cisplatin
[total dose/cycle = 3000 mg/m²]
Repeat cycle every 28 days until disease progression or unacceptable toxicity

Cisplatin-Gemcitabine (Unknown Primary)

Use Unknown primary (adenocarcinoma)

Regimen
Gemcitabine: I.V.: 1250 mg/m²/day days 1 and 8
[total dose/cycle = 2500 mg/m²]
Cisplatin: I.V.: 100 mg/m² day 1
[total dose/cycle = 100 mg/m²]
Repeat cycle every 21 days

Cisplatin-Irinotecan (NSCLC)

Use Lung cancer, nonsmall cell

Regimen
Cisplatin: I.V.: 80 mg/m² day 1
[total dose/cycle = 80 mg/m²]
Irinotecan: I.V.: 60 mg/m²/dose days 1, 8, and 15
[total dose/cycle = 180 mg/m²]
Repeat cycle every 28 days for at least 3 more cycles or until disease progression or unacceptable toxicity

Cisplatin-Irinotecan (Small Cell Lung Cancer)

Use Lung cancer, small cell

Regimen NOTE: Multiple variations are listed.

Variation 1:

Cisplatin: I.V.: 60 mg/m^2 day 1
[total dose/cycle = 60 mg/m^2]

Irinotecan: I.V.: 60 mg/m^2/day days 1, 8, and 15
[total dose/cycle = 180 mg/m^2]

Repeat cycle every 28 days for 4 cycles

Variation 2:

Cisplatin: I.V.: 30 mg/m^2/day days 1 and 8
[total dose/cycle = 60 mg/m^2]

Irinotecan: I.V.: 65 mg/m^2/day days 1 and 8
[total dose/cycle = 130 mg/m^2]

Repeat cycle every 21 days for at least 4 cycles

Cisplatin-Paclitaxel (Cervical Cancer)

Use Cervical cancer

Regimen

Paclitaxel: I.V.: 135 mg/m^2 continuous infusion over 24 hours day 1
[total dose/cycle = 135 mg/m^2]

Cisplatin: I.V.: 50 mg/m^2 day 2
[total dose/cycle = 50 mg/m^2]

Repeat cycle every 21 days for up to a total of 6 cycles; responders may continue beyond 6 cycles

Cisplatin-Paclitaxel (Head and Neck Cancer)

Use Head and neck cancer

Regimen NOTE: Multiple variations are listed.

Variation 1 (with concurrent radiation therapy):

Paclitaxel: I.V.: 30 mg/m^2 day 1
[total dose/week = 30 mg/m^2]

Cisplatin: I.V.: 20 mg/m^2 day 2
[total dose/week = 20 mg/m^2]

Repeat every week for a total of 7 weeks

Variation 2:

Paclitaxel: I.V.: 175 mg/m^2 dose over 3 hours day 1
[total dose/cycle = 175 mg/m^2]

Cisplatin: I.V.: 75 mg/m^2/dose day 1
[total dose/cycle = 75 mg/m^2]

Repeat cycle every 3 weeks

Cisplatin-Paclitaxel (Intraperitoneal Regimen)

Use Ovarian cancer

Regimen Note: I.P. therapies administered in 2 liters warmed saline

Paclitaxel: I.V.: 135 mg/m^2 continuous infusion (over 24 hours) day 1
[total dose/cycle = 135 mg/m^2]

Cisplatin: I.P.: 100 mg/m^2 day 2
[total dose/cycle = 100 mg/m^2]

Paclitaxel: I.P.: 60 mg/m^2 day 8
[total dose/cycle = 60 mg/m^2]

Repeat cycle every 21 days for 6 cycles

Cisplatin-Paclitaxel (Ovarian Cancer)

Use Ovarian cancer

Regimen

Paclitaxel: I.V.: 135 mg/m^2 continuous infusion over 24 hours day 1
[total dose/cycle = 135 mg/m^2]

Cisplatin: I.V.: 75 mg/m^2 day 2
[total dose/cycle = 75 mg/m^2]

Repeat cycle every 21 days for a total of 6 cycles

Cisplatin-Pemetrexed (Mesothelioma)

Use Malignant pleural mesothelioma

Regimen

Pemetrexed: I.V.: 500 mg/m^2 over 10 minutes day 1
[total dose/cycle = 500 mg/m^2]

Cisplatin: I.V.: 75 mg/m^2 over 2 hours day 1 (start 30 minutes after pemetrexed)
[total dose/cycle = 75 mg/m^2]

Repeat cycle every 21 days

Cisplatin-Pemetrexed (NSCLC)

Use Lung cancer, nonsmall cell

Regimen

Pemetrexed: I.V.: 500 mg/m^2 day 1
[total dose/cycle = 500 mg/m^2]

Cisplatin: I.V.: 75 mg/m^2 day 1
[total dose/cycle = 75 mg/m^2]

Repeat cycle every 21 days for up to 6 cycles

Cisplatin-Raltitrexed (Mesothelioma)

Use Malignant pleural mesothelioma

Regimen

Raltitrexed: I.V.: 3 mg/m^2 over 15 minutes day 1
[total dose/cycle = 3 mg/m^2]

Cisplatin: I.V.: 80 mg/m^2 over 1-2 hours day 1
[total dose/cycle = 80 mg/m^2]

Repeat cycle every 21 days until disease progression or unacceptable toxicity.

Cisplatin-Topotecan (Cervical Cancer)

Use Cervical cancer

Regimen NOTE: Multiple variations are listed.

Variation 1 (Body surface area capped at 2 m^2 maximum):

Topotecan: I.V.: 0.75 mg/m^2/day days 1, 2, and 3
[total dose/cycle = 2.25 mg/m^2]

Cisplatin: I.V.: 50 mg/m^2 day 1 only
[total dose/cycle = 50 mg/m^2]

Repeat cycle every 21 days for up to a total of 6 cycles; responders may continue beyond 6 cycles

Variation 2:

Topotecan: I.V.: 0.75 mg/m^2/day days 1, 2, and 3
[total dose/cycle = 2.25 mg/m^2]

Cisplatin: I.V.: 50 mg/m^2 day 1 only
[total dose/cycle = 50 mg/m^2]

Repeat cycle every 21 days for up to a total of 6 cycles; responders may continue beyond 6 cycles

Cisplatin-Vinblastine-Dacarbazine (Melanoma)

Use Melanoma

Regimen NOTE: Multiple variations are listed.

Variation 1:

Cisplatin: I.V.: 20 mg/m^2/day days 2 to 5
[total dose/cycle = 80 mg/m^2]

Vinblastine: I.V.: 1.6 mg/m^2/day days 1 to 5
[total dose/cycle = 8 mg/m^2]

Dacarbazine: I.V.: 800 mg/m^2 day 1
[total dose/cycle = 800 mg/m^2]

Repeat cycle every 21 days

Variation 2:
Cisplatin: I.V.: 20 mg/m^2/day days 1 to 4
[total dose/cycle = 80 mg/m^2]
Vinblastine: I.V.: 2 mg/m^2/day days 1 to 4
[total dose/cycle = 8 mg/m^2]
Dacarbazine: I.V.: 800 mg/m^2 day 1
[total dose/cycle = 800 mg/m^2]
Repeat cycle every 21 days

Cisplatin-Vinblastine (NSCLC)

Use Lung cancer, nonsmall cell

Regimen NOTE: Multiple variations are listed.

Variation 1:
Cisplatin: I.V.: 80 mg/m^2/day days 1, 22, 43, and 64
[total dose/treatment = 320 mg/m^2]
Vinblastine: I.V.: 4 mg/m^2/day days 1, 8, 15, 22, 29, 43, and 57
[total dose/treatment = 28 mg/m^2]
Variation 2:
Cisplatin: I.V.: 100 mg/m^2/day days 1, 29, and 57
[total dose/treatment = 300 mg/m^2]
Vinblastine: I.V.: 4 mg/m^2/day days 1, 8, 15, 22, 29, 43, and 57
[total dose/treatment = 28 mg/m^2]
Variation 3:
Cisplatin: I.V.: 100 mg/m^2/day days 1, 29, 57, and 85
[total dose/treatment = 400 mg/m^2]
Vinblastine: I.V.: 4 mg/m^2/day days 1, 8, 15, 22, 29, 43, 57, 71, and 85
[total dose/treatment = 36 mg/m^2]
Variation 4:
Cisplatin: I.V.: 120 mg/m^2/day days 1, 29, and 71
[total dose/treatment = 360 mg/m^2]
Vinblastine: I.V.: 4 mg/m^2/day days 1, 8, 15, 22, 29, 43, 57, and 71
[total dose/treatment = 32 mg/m^2]

Cisplatin-Vinorelbine (Cervical Cancer)

Use Cervical cancer

Regimen NOTE: Multiple variations are listed.

Variation 1:
Cisplatin: I.V.: 50 mg/m^2 day 1
[total dose/cycle = 50 mg/m^2]
Vinorelbine: I.V.: 30 mg/m^2/day days 1 and 8
[total dose/cycle = 60 mg/m^2]
Repeat cycle every 21 days for up to a total of 6 cycles; responders may continue beyond 6 cycles
Variation 2:
Cisplatin: I.V.: 80 mg/m^2 day 1
[total dose/cycle = 80 mg/m^2]
Vinorelbine: I.V.: 25 mg/m^2/day days 1 and 8
[total dose/cycle = 50 mg/m^2]
Repeat cycle every 21 days for a total of 3-6 cycles

CLAG (AML Induction)

Use Leukemia, acute myeloid

Regimen

Cladribine: I.V.: 5 mg/m^2/day over 2 hours days 1 to 5
[total dose/cycle = 25 mg/m^2]
Cytarabine: I.V.: 2 g/m^2/day over 4 hours days 1 to 5 (begin 2 hours after cladribine)
[total dose/cycle = 10 g/m^2]
Filgrastim: SubQ: 300 mcg daily days 0 to 5 (start 24 hours prior to chemotherapy; for a total of 6 days)
[total dose/cycle = 1800 mcg]
May administer a second induction cycle if needed

CLAG-M (AML Induction)

Use Leukemia, acute myeloid

Regimen

Cladribine: I.V.: 5 mg/m^2/day over 2 hour days 1 to 5
[total dose/cycle = 25 mg/m^2]
Cytarabine: I.V.: 2 g/m^2/day over 4 hours days 1 to 5 (begin 2 hours after cladribine)
[total dose/cycle = 10 g/m^2]
Mitoxantrone: I.V.: 10 mg/m^2/day days 1 to 3
[total dose/cycle = 30 mg/m^2]
Filgrastim: SubQ: 300 mcg daily days 0 to 5 (start 24 hours prior to chemotherapy; for a total of 6 days)
[total dose/cycle = 1800 mcg]
May administer a second induction cycle if needed

Clofarabine (AML Consolidation)

Use Leukemia, acute myeloid

Regimen

Clofarabine: I.V.: 20 mg/m^2/day over 1 hour days 1 to 5
[total dose/cycle = 100 mg/m^2]
Up to a maximum total of 6 cycles (including induction/reinduction) may be administered

Clofarabine (AML Induction)

Use Leukemia, acute myeloid

Regimen

Induction:
Clofarabine: I.V.: 30 mg/m^2/day over 1 hour days 1 to 5
[total dose/cycle = 150 mg/m^2]
Reinduction (if needed) after day 28 of induction:
Clofarabine: I.V.: 20 mg/m^2/day over 1 hour days 1 to 5
[total dose/cycle = 100 mg/m^2]

Clofarabine-Cytarabine (AML Consolidation)

Use Leukemia, acute myeloid

Regimen

Clofarabine: I.V.: 30 mg/m^2/day infusion over 1 hour on days 1, 2, and 3
[total dose/cycle = 90 mg/m^2]
Cytarabine: SubQ: 20 mg/m^2/day days 1 to 7 (4 hours after clofarabine on days 1, 2, and 3)
[total dose/cycle = 140 mg/m^2]
Repeat cycle every 4 to 7 weeks; up to a total of 12 consolidation cycles may be administered

Clofarabine-Cytarabine (AML Induction)

Use Leukemia, acute myeloid

Regimen

Clofarabine: I.V.: 30 mg/m^2/day infusion over 1 hour on days 1 to 5
[total dose/cycle = 150 mg/m^2]
Cytarabine: SubQ: 20 mg/m^2/day days 1 to 14 (4 hours after clofarabine on days 1 to 5)
[total dose/cycle = 280 mg/m^2]
A second induction cycle may be administered if needed

CMF

Use Breast cancer

Regimen NOTE: Multiple variations are listed.

Variation 1:
Methotrexate: I.V.: 40 mg/m^2/day days 1 and 8
[total dose/cycle = 80 mg/m^2]
Fluorouracil: I.V.: 600 mg/m^2/day days 1 and 8
[total dose/cycle = 1200 mg/m^2]
Cyclophosphamide: Oral: 100 mg/m^2/day days 1 to 14
[total dose/cycle = 1400 mg/m^2]
Repeat cycle every 28 days

Variation 2 (>60 years of age):
Methotrexate: I.V.: 30 mg/m^2/day days 1 and 8
[total dose/cycle = 60 mg/m^2]
Fluorouracil: I.V.: 400 mg/m^2/day days 1 and 8
[total dose/cycle = 800 mg/m^2]
Cyclophosphamide: Oral: 100 mg/m^2/day days 1 to 14
[total dose/cycle = 1400 mg/m^2]
Repeat cycle every 28 days

CMF-IV

Use Breast cancer

Regimen

Cyclophosphamide: I.V.: 600 mg/m^2 day 1
[total dose/cycle = 600 mg/m^2]
Methotrexate: I.V.: 40 mg/m^2 day 1
[total dose/cycle = 40 mg/m^2]
Fluorouracil: I.V.: 600 mg/m^2 day 1
[total dose/cycle = 600 mg/m^2]
Repeat cycle every 21 or 28 days

C-MOPP/ABV Hybrid (Hodgkin)

Use Lymphoma, Hodgkin

Regimen

Cyclophosphamide: I.V.: 650 mg/m^2/day day 1
[total dose/cycle = 650 mg/m^2]
Vincristine: I.V.: 1.4 mg/m^2/day (maximum dose: 3 mg) day 1
[total dose/cycle = 1.4 mg/m^2; maximum dose/cycle: 3 mg]
Procarbazine: Oral: 100 mg/m^2/day days 1 to 7
[total dose/cycle = 700 mg/m^2]
Prednisone: Oral: 40 mg/m^2/day days 1 to 14
[total dose/cycle = 560 mg/m^2]
Doxorubicin: I.V.: 35 mg/m^2/day day 8
[total dose/cycle = 35 mg/m^2]
Bleomycin: I.V.: 10 units/m^2/day day 8
[total dose/cycle = 10 units/m^2]
Vinblastine: I.V.: 6 mg/m^2/day day 8
[total dose/cycle = 6 mg/m^2]
Repeat cycles every 28 days for a total of 8 cycles

CMV

Use Bladder cancer

Regimen

Cisplatin: I.V.: 100 mg/m^2 infused over 4 hours (start at least 12 hours after methotrexate) day 2
[total dose = 100 mg/m^2]
Methotrexate: I.V.: 30 mg/m^2/day days 1 and 8
[total dose = 60 mg/m^2]
Vinblastine: I.V.: 4 mg/m^2/day days 1 and 8
[total dose = 8 mg/m^2]
Repeat cycle every 21 days

CNOP

Use Lymphoma, non-Hodgkin

Regimen

Cyclophosphamide: I.V.: 750 mg/m^2 day 1
[total dose/cycle = 750 mg/m^2]
Mitoxantrone: I.V.: 10 mg/m^2 day 1
[total dose/cycle = 10 mg/m^2]
Vincristine: I.V.: 1.4 mg/m^2 day 1
[total dose/cycle = 1.4 mg/m^2]
Prednisone: Oral: 50 mg/m^2/day days 1 to 5
[total dose/cycle = 250 mg/m^2]
Repeat cycle every 21 days

CODOX-M

Use Lymphoma, non-Hodgkin

Regimen NOTE: Multiple variations are listed.

Variation 1:

Cyclophosphamide: I.V.: 800 mg/m^2 day 1
followed by I.V.: 200 mg/m^2/day days 2 to 5
[total dose/cycle = 1600 mg/m^2]
Vincristine: I.V.: 1.5 mg/m^2/dose (no maximum dose) days 1 and 8
[total dose/cycle = 3 mg/m^2]
Doxorubicin: I.V.: 40 mg/m^2/dose day 1
[total dose/cycle = 40 mg/m^2]
Methotrexate: I.V.: 1200 mg/m^2 (loading dose) over 1 hour
followed by I.V.: 240 mg/m^2/hour for 23 hours day 10
[total dose/cycle = 6720 mg/m^2]
Leucovorin: I.V.: 192 mg/m^2/dose day 11 (begin 36 hours after the start of methotrexate infusion)
followed by I.V.: 12 mg/m^2/dose every 6 hours until methotrexate level <5 x 10^{-8}M
Cytarabine: I.T.: 70 mg/dose (adjust to age-appropriate dose if <3 years of age) day 1
[total dose/cycle = 70 mg]
Methotrexate: I.T.: 12 mg/dose (adjust to age-appropriate dose if <3 years of age) day 3
[total dose/cycle = 12 mg]
Repeat cycle when ANC >1000/m^3 for a total of three cycles

Variation 2:

Cyclophosphamide: I.V.: 800 mg/m^2/dose day 1
followed by I.V.: 200 mg/m^2/dose days 2 to 5
[total dose/cycle = 1600 mg/m^2]
Vincristine: I.V.: 1.5 mg/m^2/dose (maximum dose: 2 mg) days 1 and 8
[total dose/cycle = 3 mg/m^2; maximum: 4 mg/cycle]
Doxorubicin: I.V.: 40 mg/m^2/dose day 1
[total dose/cycle = 40 mg/m^2]
Methotrexate: I.V.: 1200 mg/m^2 (loading dose) over 1 hour
followed by I.V.: 240 mg/m^2/hour for 23 hours day 10
[total dose/cycle = 6720 mg/m^2]
Leucovorin: I.V.: 192 mg/m^2/dose day 11 (begin 36 hours after the start of methotrexate infusion)
followed by I.V.: 12 mg/m^2/dose every 6 hours until methotrexate level <5 x 10^{-8}M
Cytarabine: I.T.: 70 mg/dose days 1 and 3
[total dose/cycle = 140 mg]
Methotrexate: I.T.: 12 mg/dose day 15
[total dose/cycle = 12 mg]
Leucovorin: Oral: 15 mg/dose day 16 (24 hours after I.T. methotrexate)
Filgrastim: 5 mcg/kg/day beginning day 13, continue until ANC >1000/mm^3
Repeat cycle when ANC >1000/mm^3 for a total of three cycles

Variation 3:

Cyclophosphamide: I.V.: 800 mg/m^2/dose days 1 and 2
[total dose/cycle = 1600 mg/m^2]
Vincristine: I.V.: 1.4 mg/m^2/dose (maximum dose: 2 mg) days 1 and 10
[total dose/cycle = 2.8 mg/m^2; maximum: 4 mg/cycle]
Doxorubicin: I.V.: 50 mg/m^2/dose day 1
[total dose/cycle = 50 mg/m^2]
Methotrexate: I.V.: 3 g/m^2 day 10
[total dose/cycle = 3 g/m^2]
Leucovorin: I.V.: 200 mg/m^2/dose day 11
followed by Oral, I.V.: 15 mg/m^2/dose every 6 hours until methotrexate level <0.1 Mmol/L
Cytarabine: I.T.: 50 mg/dose day 1
[total dose/cycle = 50 mg]
Hydrocortisone: I.T.: 50 mg/dose day 1
[total dose/cycle = 50 mg]
Methotrexate: I.T.: 12 mg/dose day 1
[total dose/cycle = 12 mg]
Filgrastim: SubQ: Dose not specified; days 3 to 8 and day 12 until ANC >1000/mm^3
Repeat cycle when ANC >1000/mm^3 for a total of three cycles

CODOX-M/IVAC

Use Lymphoma, non-Hodgkin (Burkitt)

Regimen NOTE: Multiple variations are listed.

Variation 1:

CODOX-M (Cycles 1 and 3; cycles begin when ANC >1000/mm^3)

Cyclophosphamide: I.V.: 800 mg/m^2/dose day 1
followed by I.V.: 200 mg/m^2/dose days 2 to 5
[total dose/cycle = 1600 mg/m^2]

Vincristine: I.V.: 1.5 mg/m^2/dose (no maximum dose) days 1 and 8 (cycle 1) and days 1, 8, and 15 (cycle 3)
[total dose/cycle = 3-4.5 mg/m^2]

Doxorubicin: I.V.: 40 mg/m^2/dose day 1
[total dose/cycle = 40 mg/m^2]

Methotrexate: I.V.: 1200 mg/m^2 (loading dose) over 1 hour
followed by I.V.: 240 mg/m^2/hour for 23 hours day 10
[total dose/cycle = 6720 mg/m^2]

Leucovorin: I.V.: 192 mg/m^2/dose day 11 (begin 36 hours after the start of methotrexate infusion)
followed by I.V.: 12 mg/m^2/dose every 6 hours until methotrexate level <5 x 10^{-8}M

Cytarabine: I.T.: 70 mg/dose (adjust to age-appropriate dose if <3 years of age) days 1 and 3
[total dose/cycle = 140 mg]

Methotrexate: I.T.: 12 mg/dose (adjust to age-appropriate dose if <3 years of age) day 15
[total dose/cycle = 12 mg]

Sargramostim: SubQ: 7.5 mcg/kg/day beginning day 13, continue until ANC >1000/mm^3

Note: If CNS disease present, administer additional I.T. treatment in cycle 1: Cytarabine 70 mg/dose (adjust to age-appropriate dose if <3 years of age) on day 5 and methotrexate 12 mg/dose (adjust to age-appropriate dose if <3 years of age) on day 17

IVAC (Cycles 2 and 4; cycles begin when ANC >1000/mm^3)

Ifosfamide: I.V.: 1500 mg/m^2/dose days 1 to 5
[total dose/cycle = 7500 mg/m^2]

Mesna: I.V.: 360 mg/m^2/dose every 3 hours days 1 to 5

Etoposide: I.V.: 60 mg/m^2/dose days 1 to 5
[total dose/cycle = 300 mg/m^2]

Cytarabine: I.V.: 2 g/m^2/dose every 12 hours, for 4 doses, days 1 and 2
[total dose/cycle = 8 g/m^2]

Methotrexate: I.T.: 12 mg/dose day 5
[total dose/cycle = 12 mg]

Sargramostim: SubQ: 7.5 mcg/kg/day beginning day 7, continue until ANC >1000/mm^3

Note: If CNS disease present, administer additional I.T. treatment in cycle 2: Cytarabine 70 mg/dose (adjust to age-appropriate dose if <3 years of age) on days 7 and 9

Variation 2:

CODOX-M (Cycles 1 and 3; cycles begin when ANC >1000/mm^3)

Cyclophosphamide: I.V.: 800 mg/m^2/dose day 1
followed by I.V.: 200 mg/m^2/dose days 2 to 5
[total dose/cycle = 1600 mg/m^2]

Vincristine: I.V.: 1.5 mg/m^2/dose (maximum dose: 2 mg) days 1 and 8
[total dose/cycle = 3 mg/m^2; maximum: 4 mg/cycle]

Doxorubicin: I.V.: 40 mg/m^2/dose day 1
[total dose/cycle = 40 mg/m^2]

Methotrexate: I.V.: 300 mg/m^2 (100 mg/m^2 if >65 years of age) (loading dose) over 1 hour
followed by I.V.: 2700 mg/m^2 (900 mg/m^2 if >65 years of age) over 23 hours day 10
[total dose/cycle = 3000 mg/m^2 (1000 mg/m^2 if >65 years of age)]

Leucovorin: I.V.: 15 mg/m^2/dose every 3 hours beginning day 11 (begin 36 hours after the start of methotrexate infusion) for 5 doses
followed by I.V.: 15 mg/m^2/dose every 6 hours until methotrexate level <5 x 10^{-8}M

Cytarabine: I.T.: 70 mg/dose days 1 and 3
[total dose/cycle = 140 mg]

Methotrexate: I.T.: 12 mg/dose day 15
[total dose/cycle = 12 mg]

Leucovorin: Oral: 15 mg/dose day 16 (24 hours after I.T. methotrexate)

Filgrastim: SubQ: 5 mcg/kg/day beginning day 13, continue until ANC >1000/mm^3

Note: If CNS disease present, administer additional I.T. treatment: Cytarabine 70 mg/dose on day 5 and methotrexate 12 mg/dose (with leucovorin rescue) on day 17

IVAC (Cycles 2 and 4; cycles begin when ANC >1000/mm^3)

Ifosfamide: I.V.: 1500 mg/m^2/dose (1000 mg/m^2/dose if >65 years of age) days 1 to 5
[total dose/cycle = 7500 mg/m^2 (5000 mg/m^2 if >65 years of age)]

Mesna: I.V.: 300 mg/m^2/dose (200 mg/m^2/dose if >65 years of age) mixed with each ifosfamide dose **followed by** I.V.: 300 mg/m^2/dose (200 mg/m^2/dose if >65 years of age) every 4 hours for 2 doses/day days 1 to 5
[total dose/cycle = 4500 mg/m^2 (3000 mg/m^2/dose if >65 years of age)]

Etoposide: I.V.: 60 mg/m^2/dose days 1 to 5
[total dose/cycle = 300 mg/m^2]

Cytarabine: I.V.: 2 g/m^2/dose (1 g/m^2/dose if >65 years of age) every 12 hours, for 4 doses, days 1 and 2
[total dose/cycle = 8 g/m^2 (4 g/m^2 if >65 years of age)]

Methotrexate: I.T.: 12 mg day 5
[total dose/cycle = 12 mg]

Leucovorin: Oral: 15 mg/dose day 6 (24 hours after I.T. methotrexate)

Filgrastim: SubQ: 5 mcg/kg/day beginning day 7, continue until ANC >1000/mm^3

Note: If CNS disease present, administer additional I.T. treatment: Cytarabine 70 mg/dose on days 7 and 9

Variation 3:

CODOX-M (Cycles 1 and 3; cycles begin when ANC >1000/mm^3)

Cyclophosphamide: I.V.: 800 mg/m^2/dose day 1
followed by I.V.: 200 mg/m^2/dose days 2 to 5
[total dose/cycle = 1600 mg/m^2]

Vincristine: I.V.: 1.5 mg/m^2/dose (maximum dose: 2 mg) days 1 and 8
[total dose/cycle = 3 mg/m^2; maximum: 4 mg/cycle]

Doxorubicin: I.V.: 40 mg/m^2/dose day 1
[total dose/cycle = 40 mg/m^2]

Methotrexate: I.V.: 1200 mg/m^2 (loading dose) over 1 hour
followed by I.V.: 240 mg/m^2/hour for 23 hours day 10
[total dose/cycle = 6720 mg/m^2]

Leucovorin: I.V.: 192 mg/m^2/dose day 11 (begin 36 hours after the start of methotrexate infusion)
followed by I.V.: 12 mg/m^2/dose every 6 hours until methotrexate level <5 x 10^{-8}M

Cytarabine: I.T.: 70 mg/dose days 1 and 3
[total dose/cycle = 140 mg]

Methotrexate: I.T.: 12 mg/dose day 15
[total dose/cycle = 12 mg]

Leucovorin: Oral: 15 mg/dose day 16 (24 hours after I.T. methotrexate)

Filgrastim: SubQ: 5 mcg/kg/day beginning day 13, continue until ANC >1000/mm^3

Note: If CNS disease present, administer additional I.T. treatment in cycle 1: Cytarabine 70 mg/dose (15 mg if via Ommaya reservoir) on day 5 and methotrexate 12.5 mg/dose (2 mg if via Ommaya reservoir) on day 17

IVAC (Cycles 2 and 4; cycles begin when ANC >1000/mm^3)

Ifosfamide: I.V.: 1500 mg/m^2/dose days 1 to 5
[total dose/cycle = 7500 mg/m^2]

Mesna: I.V.: 360 mg/m^2/dose mixed with each ifosfamide dose
followed by I.V.: 360 mg/m^2/dose every 3 hours for 7 doses/day days 1 to 5
[total dose/cycle = 14,400 mg/m^2]

Etoposide: I.V.: 60 mg/m^2/dose days 1 to 5
[total dose/cycle = 300 mg/m^2]

Cytarabine: I.V.: 2 g/m^2/dose every 12 hours, for 4 doses, days 1 and 2
[total dose/cycle = 8 g/m^2]

Methotrexate: I.T.: 12 mg/dose day 5
[total dose/cycle = 12 mg]

Leucovorin: Oral: 15 mg/dose day 6 (24 hours after I.T. methotrexate)

Filgrastim: SubQ: 5 mcg/kg/day beginning day 7, continue until ANC >1000/mm^3

Note: If CNS disease present, administer additional I.T. treatment in cycle 2: Cytarabine 70 mg/dose (15 mg if via Ommaya reservoir) on days 7 and 9

Variation 4:

CODOX-M (Cycles 1 and 3; cycles begin when ANC >1000/mm^3)

Cyclophosphamide: I.V.: 800 mg/m^2/dose days 1 and 2
[total dose/cycle = 1600 mg/m^2]

Vincristine: I.V.: 1.4 mg/m^2/dose (maximum dose: 2 mg) days 1 and 10
[total dose/cycle = 2.8 mg/m^2; maximum: 4 mg/cycle]

Doxorubicin: I.V.: 50 mg/m^2/dose day 1
[total dose/cycle = 50 mg/m^2]

Methotrexate: I.V.: 3 g/m^2 day 10
[total dose/cycle = 3 g/m^2]

Leucovorin: I.V.: 200 mg/m^2/dose day 11
followed by Oral, I.V.: 15 mg/m^2/dose every 6 hours until methotrexate level <0.1 Mmol/L

Cytarabine: I.T.: 50 mg/dose days 1 and 3
[total dose/cycle = 100 mg]

Hydrocortisone: I.T.: 50 mg/dose days 1 and 3
[total dose/cycle = 100 mg]

Methotrexate: I.T.: 12 mg/dose day 1
[total dose/cycle = 12 mg]

Filgrastim: SubQ: Dose not specified, days 3 to 8 and day 12 until ANC >1000 mm^3

Note: If CNS disease present, administer additional I.T. treatment in cycle 1: Cytarabine 50 mg/dose on day 5 and methotrexate 12 mg/dose on day 10

IVAC (Cycles 2 and 4; cycles begin when ANC >1000/mm^3)

Ifosfamide: I.V.: 1500 mg/m^2/dose days 1 to 5
[total dose/cycle = 7500 mg/m^2]

Mesna: I.V.: 1500 mg/m^2/day (in divided doses) days 1 to 5
[total dose/cycle = 7500 mg/m^2]

Etoposide: I.V.: 60 mg/m^2/dose days 1 to 5
[total dose/cycle = 300 mg/m^2]

Cytarabine: I.V.: 2 g/m^2/dose every 12 hours, for 4 doses, days 1 and 2
[total dose/cycle = 8 g/m^2]

Methotrexate: I.T.: 12 mg/dose day 5
[total dose/cycle = 12 mg]

Hydrocortisone: I.T.: 50 mg/dose day 5
[total dose/cycle = 50 mg]

Filgrastim: SubQ: Dose not specified, daily beginning day 6 until ANC >1000 mm^3

Note: If CNS disease present, administer additional I.T. treatment in cycle 2: Cytarabine 50 mg/dose on days 3 and 5

COMLA

Use Lymphoma, non-Hodgkin

Regimen

Cyclophosphamide: I.V.: 1500 mg/m^2 day 1
[total dose/cycle = 1500 mg/m^2]

Vincristine: I.V.: 1.4 mg/m^2/day (maximum dose: 2 mg) days 1, 8, and 15
[total dose/cycle = 4.2 mg/m^2]

Methotrexate: I.V.: 120 mg/m^2/day days 22, 29, 36, 43, 50, 57, 64, and 71
[total dose/cycle = 960 mg/m^2]

Leucovorin: Oral: 25 mg/m^2 every 6 hours for 4 doses (beginning 24 hours after each methotrexate dose)
[total dose/cycle = 800 mg/m^2]

Cytarabine: I.V.: 300 mg/m^2/day days 22, 29, 36, 43, 50, 57, 64, and 71
[total dose/cycle = 2400 mg/m^2]

Repeat cycle every 85 days

COP-BLAM

Use Lymphoma, non-Hodgkin

Regimen

Cyclophosphamide: I.V.: 400 mg/m^2 day 1
[total dose/cycle = 400 mg/m^2]

Vincristine: I.V.: 1 mg/m^2 day 1
[total dose/cycle = 1 mg/m^2]

Prednisone: Oral: 40 mg/m^2/day days 1 to 10
[total dose/cycle = 400 mg/m^2]

Bleomycin: I.V.: 15 mg day 14
[total dose/cycle = 15 mg]
Doxorubicin: I.V.: 40 mg/m^2 day 1
[total dose/cycle = 40 mg/m^2]
Procarbazine: Oral: 100 mg/m^2/day days 1 to 10
[total dose/cycle = 1000 mg/m^2]

COPE

Use Brain tumors

Regimen

Cycle A:
Vincristine: I.V.: 0.065 mg/kg/day (maximum dose: 1.5 mg) days 1 and 8
[total dose/cycle = 0.13 mg/kg]
Cyclophosphamide: I.V.: 65 mg/kg day 1
[total dose/cycle = 65 mg/kg]
Cycle B:
Cisplatin: I.V.: 4 mg/kg day 1
[total dose/cycle = 4 mg/kg]
Etoposide: I.V.: 6.5 mg/kg/day days 3 and 4
[total dose/cycle = 13 mg/kg]
Repeat cycle every 28 days in the following sequence: AABAAB

COPP

Use Lymphoma, non-Hodgkin

Regimen

Cyclophosphamide: I.V.: 450-650 mg/m^2/day days 1 and 8
[total dose/cycle = 900-1300 mg/m^2]
Vincristine: I.V.: 1.4-2 mg/m^2/day (maximum dose: 2 mg) days 1 and 8
[total dose/cycle = 2.8-4 mg/m^2]
Procarbazine: Oral: 100 mg/m^2/day days 1 to 14
[total dose/cycle = 1400 mg/m^2]
Prednisone: Oral: 40 mg/m^2/day days 1 to 14
[total dose/cycle = 560 mg/m^2]
Repeat cycle every 3-4 weeks

Crizotinib (NSCLC Regimen)

Use Lung cancer, nonsmall cell

Regimen

Crizotinib: Oral: 250 mg twice daily days 1 to 28
[total dose/cycle = 14,000 mg]
Repeat cycle every 28 days until disease progression or unacceptable toxicity

CVD-Interleukin-Interferon (Melanoma)

Use Melanoma

Regimen NOTE: Multiple variations are listed.

Variation 1:
Cisplatin: I.V.: 20 mg/m^2/day days 1 to 4 and 22 to 25
[total dose/cycle = 160 mg/m^2]
Vinblastine: I.V.: 1.5 mg/m^2/day days 1 to 4 and 22 to 25
[total dose/cycle = 12 mg/m^2]
Dacarbazine: I.V.: 800 mg/m^2/day days 1 and 22
[total dose/cycle = 1600 mg/m^2]
Aldesleukin: I.V.: 9 million units/m^2/day continuous infusion days 5 to 8, 17 to 20, and 26 to 29
[total dose/cycle = 108 million units/m^2]
Interferon alfa-2b: SubQ: 5 million units/m^2/day days 5 to 9, 17 to 21, and 26 to 30
[total dose/cycle = 75 million units/m^2]
Repeat every 42 days (maximum of five 21-day cycles for cytokine [interleukin and interferon] component)

Variation 2:

Cisplatin: I.V.: 20 mg/m^2/day days 1 to 4
[total dose/cycle = 80 mg/m^2]

Vinblastine: I.V.: 1.6 mg/m^2/day days 1 to 4
[total dose/cycle = 6.4 mg/m^2]

Dacarbazine: I.V.: 800 mg/m^2 day 1
[total dose/cycle = 800 mg/m^2]

Aldesleukin: I.V.: 9 million units/m^2/day continuous infusion days 1 to 4
[total dose/cycle = 36 million units/m^2]

Interferon alfa-2a: SubQ: 5 million units/m^2/day days 1 to 5, 7, 9, 11, and 13
[total dose/cycle = 45 million units/m^2]

Repeat cycle every 21 days for a total of 6 cycles

Variation 3:

Cisplatin: I.V.: 20 mg/m^2/day days 1 to 4
[total dose/cycle = 80 mg/m^2]

Vinblastine: I.V.: 1.2 mg/m^2/day days 1 to 4
[total dose/cycle = 4.8 mg/m^2]

Dacarbazine: I.V.: 800 mg/m^2 day 1
[total dose/cycle = 800 mg/m^2]

Aldesleukin: I.V.: 9 million units/m^2/day continuous infusion days 1 to 4
[total dose/cycle = 36 million units/m^2]

Interferon alfa-2b: SubQ: 5 million units/m^2/day days 1 to 5, 8, 10, and 12
[total dose/cycle = 40 million units/m^2]

Repeat cycle every 21 days (maximum: 4 cycles)

CVP (Leukemia)

Use Leukemia, chronic lymphocytic

Regimen NOTE: Multiple variations are listed.

Variation 1:

Cyclophosphamide: Oral: 300 or 400 mg/m^2/day days 1 to 5
[total dose/cycle = 1500 or 2000 mg/m^2]

Vincristine: I.V.: 1.4 mg/m^2 (maximum dose: 2 mg) day 1
[total dose/cycle = 1.4 mg/m^2]

Prednisone: Oral: 100 mg/m^2/day days 1 to 5
[total dose/cycle = 500 mg/m^2]

Repeat cycle every 21 days

Variation 2:

Cyclophosphamide: I.V.: 800 mg/m^2 day 1
[total dose/cycle = 800 mg/m^2]

Vincristine: I.V.: 1.4 mg/m^2 (maximum dose: 2 mg) day 1
[total dose/cycle = 1.4 mg/m^2]

Prednisone: Oral: 100 mg/m^2/day days 1 to 5
[total dose/cycle = 500 mg/m^2]

Repeat cycle every 21 days

CVP (Lymphoma, non-Hodgkin)

Use Lymphoma, non-Hodgkin

Regimen NOTE: Multiple variations are listed.

Variation 1:

Cyclophosphamide: I.V.: 750 mg/m^2 day 1
[total dose/cycle = 750 mg/m^2]

Vincristine: I.V.: 1.2 mg/m^2 day 1
[total dose/cycle = 1.2 mg/m^2]

Prednisone: Oral: 40 mg/m^2/day days 1 to 5
[total dose/cycle = 200 mg/m^2]

Repeat cycle every 21 days for up to 10 cycles

Variation 2:

Cyclophosphamide: I.V.: 750 mg/m^2 day 1
[total dose/cycle = 750 mg/m^2]

Vincristine: I.V.: 1.2 mg/m^2 day 1 (maximum dose: 2 mg)
[total dose/cycle = 1.2 mg/m^2 (maximum: 2 mg)]

Prednisone: Oral: 40 mg/m^2/day days 1 to 5
[total dose/cycle = 200 mg/m^2]
Repeat cycle every 28 days for up to 8 cycles
Variation 3:
Cyclophosphamide: I.V.: 750 mg/m^2 day 1
[total dose/cycle = 750 mg/m^2]
Vincristine: I.V.: 1.4 mg/m^2 day 1 (maximum dose: 2 mg)
[total dose/cycle = 1.4 mg/m^2 (maximum: 2 mg)]
Prednisone: Oral: 40 mg/m^2/day days 1 to 5
[total dose/cycle = 200 mg/m^2]
Repeat cycle every 21 days for up to 8 cycles
Variation 4:
Cyclophosphamide: Oral: 400 mg/m^2/day days 1 to 5
[total dose/cycle = 2000 mg/m^2]
Vincristine: I.V.: 1.4 mg/m^2 day 1 (maximum dose: 2 mg)
[total dose/cycle = 1.4 mg/m^2 (maximum: 2 mg)]
Prednisone: Oral: 100 mg/m^2/day days 1 to 5
[total dose/cycle = 500 mg/m^2]
Repeat cycle every 21 days

Cyclophosphamide-Fludarabine-Alemtuzumab-Rituximab (CLL)

Use Leukemia, chronic lymphocytic

Regimen

Variation 1:
Cyclophosphamide: I.V.: 200 mg/m^2/day days 3, 4, and 5
[total dose/cycle = 600 mg/m^2]
Fludarabine: I.V.: 20 mg/m^2/day days 3, 4, and 5
[total dose/cycle = 60 mg/m^2]
Rituximab: I.V.: 375-500 mg/m^2/dose day 2
[total dose/cycle = 375-500 mg/m^2]
Alemtuzumab: I.V.: 30 mg/dose days 1, 3, and 5
[total dose/cycle = 90 mg]
Repeat cycle every 28 days for up to a total of 6 cycles
Variation 2:
Cyclophosphamide: I.V.: 200 mg/m^2/day days 3, 4, and 5
[total dose/cycle = 600 mg/m^2]
Fludarabine: I.V.: 20 mg/m^2/day days 3, 4, and 5
[total dose/cycle = 60 mg/m^2]
Rituximab: I.V.: 375-500 mg/m^2/dose day 2
[total dose/cycle = 375-500 mg/m^2]
Alemtuzumab: I.V.: 30 mg/dose days 1, 3, and 5
[total dose/cycle = 90 mg]
Pegfilgrastim: SubQ: 6 mg with each cycle
Repeat cycle every 28 days for a total of 6 cycles
Variation 3:
Cyclophosphamide: I.V.: 250 mg/m^2/day days 3, 4, and 5
[total dose/cycle = 750 mg/m^2]
Fludarabine: I.V.: 25 mg/m^2/day days 3, 4, and 5
[total dose/cycle = 75 mg/m^2]
Rituximab: I.V.: 375-500 mg/m^2/dose day 2
[total dose/cycle = 375-500 mg/m^2]
Alemtuzumab: I.V.: 30 mg/dose days 1, 3, and 5
[total dose/cycle = 90 mg]
Repeat cycle every 28 days for a total of 6 cycles

Cytarabine (High Dose)-Daunorubicin (AML Induction)

Use Leukemia, acute myeloid

Regimen

Cytarabine: I.V.: 2 g/m^2/day over 1 hour every 12 hours days 1 to 6 (12 total doses)
[total dose/cycle = 24 g/m^2]
Daunorubicin: I.V.: 45 mg/m^2/day I.V. bolus days 7 to 9
[total dose/cycle = 135 mg/m^2]

Cytarabine (High Dose)-Daunorubicin-Etoposide (AML Induction)

Use Leukemia, acute myeloid

Regimen

Daunorubicin: I.V.: 50 mg/m²/day days 1, 2, and 3
[total dose/cycle = 150 mg/m²]

Cytarabine: I.V.: 3 g/m²/dose over 3 hours every 12 hours days 1, 3, 5, and 7 (8 total doses)
[total dose/cycle = 24 g/m²]

Etoposide: I.V.: 75 mg/m²/day days 1 to 7
[total dose/cycle = 525 mg/m²]

Up to 3 induction cycles may be given based on individual response

Cytarabine (High-Dose Single-Agent AML Induction Regimen)

Use Leukemia, acute myeloid

Regimen NOTE: Multiple variations are listed.

Variation 1 (ages 14 to 50 years):
Cytarabine: I.V.: 3 g/m² over 2 hours every 12 hours days 1 to 6 (total of 12 doses)
[total dose/cycle = 36 g/m²]
May administer a second induction cycle if needed

Variation 2 (ages >50 years):
Cytarabine: I.V.: 2 g/m² over 2 hours every 12 hours days 1 to 6 (total of 12 doses)
[total dose/cycle = 24 g/m²]
May administer a second induction cycle if needed

Cytarabine (Single-Agent AML Consolidation Regimen)

Use Leukemia, acute myeloid

Regimen NOTE: Multiple variations are listed.

Variation 1:
Cytarabine: I.V.: 3 g/m² over 3 hours every 12 hours on days 1, 3, and 5 (total of 6 doses)
[total dose/cycle = 18 g/m²]
Repeat cycle every 4 to 5 weeks (depending on marrow recovery) for a total of 4 postremission cycles

Variation 2:
Cytarabine: I.V.: 400 mg/m²/day continuous infusion on days 1 to 5
[total dose/cycle = 2000 mg/m²]
Repeat cycle every 4 to 5 weeks (depending on marrow recovery) for a total of 4 postremission cycles

Variation 3:
Cytarabine: I.V.: 100 mg/m²/day continuous infusion on days 1 to 5
[total dose/cycle = 500 mg/m²]
Repeat cycle every 4 to 5 weeks (depending on marrow recovery) for a total of 4 postremission cycles

Variation 4 (≥60 years of age):
Cytarabine: I.V.: 100 mg/m²/day continuous infusion on days 1 to 5
[total dose/cycle = 500 mg/m²]
Repeat cycle every 28 days for a total of 4 consolidation cycles

Variation 5 (≤50 years of age):
Cytarabine: I.V.: 3 g/m² every 12 hours on days 1 to 3 (total of 6 doses)
[total dose/cycle = 18 g/m²]
Administer a total of 3 consolidation cycles

Variation 6 (>50 years of age)
Cytarabine: I.V.: 2 g/m² every 12 hours on days 1 to 3 (total of 6 doses)
[total dose/cycle = 12 g/m²]
Administer a total of 3 consolidation cycles

Variation 7(>65 years of age):
Cytarabine: SubQ: 10 mg/m²/dose every 12 hours days 1 to 14
[total dose/cycle = 280 mg/m²]
Repeat cycle every 6 weeks for 18 months

Cytarabine (SubQ Single-Agent AML Induction Regimen)

Use Leukemia, acute myeloid

Regimen NOTE: Multiple variations are listed.

Variation 1 (>50 years of age):

Cytarabine: SubQ: 20 mg/m^2/day days 1 to 14
[total dose/cycle = 280 mg/m^2]

Repeat cycle every 28 days for at least 4 cycles

Variation 2 (>65 years of age):

Cytarabine: SubQ: 10 mg/m^2/day every 12 hours days 1 to 21
[total dose/cycle = 420 mg/m^2]

After 15 days, a second induction course may be administered if needed

CYVADIC

Use Sarcoma

Regimen

Cyclophosphamide: I.V.: 500 mg/m^2 day 1
[total dose/cycle = 500 mg/m^2]

Vincristine: I.V.: 1.4 mg/m^2/day days 1 and 5
[total dose/cycle = 2.8 mg/m^2]

Doxorubicin: I.V.: 50 mg/m^2 day 1
[total dose/cycle = 50 mg/m^2]

Dacarbazine: I.V.: 250 mg/m^2/day days 1 to 5
[total dose/cycle = 1250 mg/m^2]

Repeat cycle every 21 days

Dacarbazine-Carboplatin-Aldesleukin-Interferon

Use Melanoma

Regimen

Dacarbazine: I.V.: 750 mg/m^2/day days 1 and 22
[total dose/cycle = 1500 mg/m^2]

Carboplatin: I.V.: 400 mg/m^2/day days 1 and 22
[total dose/cycle = 800 mg/m^2]

Aldesleukin: SubQ: 4,800,000 units every 8 hours days 36 and 57
[total dose/cycle = 28,800,000 units]

then 4,800,000 units every 12 hours days 37 and 58
[total dose/cycle = 19,200,000 units]

then 4,800,000 units/day days 38 to 40, 43 to 47, 50 to 54, 59 to 61, 65 to 68, 71 to 75
[total dose/cycle = 120,000,000 units]

Interferon alpha-2a: SubQ: 6,000,000 units days 38, 40, 43, 45, 47, 50, 52, 54, 59, 61, 64, 66, 68, 71, 73, and 75
[total dose/cycle = 96,000,000 units]

Repeat cycle every 78 days for 3 cycles

Dartmouth Regimen

Use Melanoma

Regimen NOTE: Multiple variations are listed.

Variation 1:

Cisplatin: I.V.: 25 mg/m^2/day days 1, 2, and 3
[total dose/cycle = 75 mg/m^2]

Dacarbazine: I.V.: 220 mg/m^2/day days 1, 2, and 3
[total dose/cycle = 660 mg/m^2]

Carmustine: I.V.: 150 mg/m^2 day 1 (every other cycle)
[total dose/cycle = 150 mg/m^2; every other cycle]

Tamoxifen: Oral: 10 mg twice daily (begin 1 week before chemotherapy)
[total dose/cycle = 420 mg]

Repeat cycle every 21 days

Variation 2:
Carmustine: I.V.: 150 mg/m^2 day 1
[total dose/cycle = 150 mg/m^2]
Cisplatin: I.V.: 25 mg/m^2/day days 1, 2, 3, 22, 23, and 24
[total dose/cycle = 150 mg/m^2]
Dacarbazine: I.V.: 220 mg/m^2/day days 1, 2, 3, 22, 23, and 24
[total dose/cycle = 1320 mg/m^2]
Tamoxifen: Oral: 10 mg twice daily days 1 to 42
[total dose/cycle = 840 mg]
Repeat cycle every 42 days
Variation 3:
Carmustine: I.V.: 150 mg/m^2 day 1
[total dose/cycle = 150 mg/m^2]
Cisplatin: I.V.: 25 mg/m^2/day days 1, 2, 3, 22, 23, and 24
[total dose/cycle = 150 mg/m^2]
Dacarbazine: I.V.: 220 mg/m^2/day days 1, 2, 3, 22, 23, and 24
[total dose/cycle = 1320 mg/m^2]
Tamoxifen: Oral: 160 mg/day days -6 to 0 (cycle 1 only)
[total dose/cycle = 1120 mg]
followed by Oral: 40 mg/day days 1 to 42
[total dose/cycle = 1680 mg]
Repeat cycle every 42 days
Variation 4:
Carmustine: I.V.: 150 mg/m^2 day 1
[total dose/cycle = 150 mg/m^2]
Cisplatin: I.V.: 25 mg/m^2/day days 1, 2, 3, 29, 30, and 31
[total dose/cycle = 150 mg/m^2]
Dacarbazine: I.V.: 220 mg/m^2/day days 1, 2, 3, 29, 30, and 31
[total dose/cycle = 1320 mg/m^2]
Tamoxifen: Oral: 10-20 mg twice daily days 1 to 56
[total dose/cycle = 1120-2240 mg]
Repeat cycle every 56 days
Variation 5:
Cisplatin: I.V.: 25 mg/m^2/day days 1, 2, and 3
[total dose/cycle = 75 mg/m^2]
Dacarbazine: I.V.: 220 mg/m^2/day days 1, 2, and 3
[total dose/cycle = 660 mg/m^2]
Carmustine: I.V.: 100 mg/m^2 day 1 (give in cycles 1, 3, and 6 **only**)
[total dose/cycles 1, 3, and 6 = 100 mg/m^2]
Tamoxifen: Oral: 160 mg loading dose immediately before cycle 1
[total dose/loading dose + cycle 1 = 580 mg]
followed by Oral: 20 mg daily days 1 to 21
[total dose/subsequent cycles = 420 mg]
Repeat cycle every 21 days
Note: Tamoxifen is continued until 3 weeks after last cycle.

Dasatinib (CML Regimen)

Use Leukemia, chronic myelogenous

Regimen NOTE: Multiple variations are listed.
Variation 1 (chronic phase):
Dasatinib: Oral: 100 mg once daily
[total dose/cycle = 2800 mg]
Repeat cycle every 28 days until disease progression or unacceptable toxicity
Variation 2 (accelerated and blast phase resistant or intolerant to imatinib):
Dasatinib: Oral: 140 mg once daily
[total dose/cycle = 3920 mg]
Repeat cycle every 28 days until disease progression or unacceptable toxicity

DD-4A (Wilms Tumor)

Use Wilms tumor

Regimen

Dactinomycin: I.V.: 45 mcg/kg day 1 of weeks 0, 6, 12, 18, 24, 30, 36, 42, 48, and 54
[total dose = 450 mcg/kg]
Doxorubicin: I.V.: 45 mg/m^2 days 1 of weeks 3 and 9
Followed by
Doxorubicin: I.V.: 30 mg/m^2 days 1 of weeks 15, 21, 27, 33, 39, 45, and 51
[total dose = 300 mg/m^2]
Vincristine: I.V.: 1.5 mg/m^2 day 1 of weeks 1 to 10
Followed by
Vincristine: I.V.: 2 mg/m^2 day 1 of weeks 12, 15, 18, 21, 24, 27, 30, 33, 36, 39, 42, 45, 48, 51, and 54
[total dose = 45 mg/m^2]
Treatment course duration is week 0 through week 54

Decitabine (AML Regimen)

Use Leukemia, acute myeloid

Regimen

Decitabine: I.V.: 20 mg/m^2/day over 1 hour days 1 to 5
[total dose/cycle = 100 mg/m^2]
Repeat cycle every 28 days

Decitabine (MDS Regimen)

Use Myelodysplastic syndrome

Regimen NOTE: Multiple variations are listed.

Variation 1:
Decitabine: I.V.: 20 mg/m^2/day over 1 hour days 1 to 5
[total dose/cycle = 100 mg/m^2]
Repeat cycle every 28 days
Variation 2:
Decitabine: I.V.: 15 mg/m^2/dose over 3 hours every 8 hours days 1 to 3 (total of 45 mg/m^2/day)
[total dose/cycle = 135 mg/m^2]
Repeat cycle every 6 weeks

Dexa-BEAM (Hodgkin)

Use Lymphoma, Hodgkin

Regimen

Dexamethasone: Oral: 8 mg every 8 hours days 1 to 10
[total dose/cycle = 240 mg]
Carmustine: I.V.: 60 mg/m^2 day 2
[total dose/cycle = 60 mg/m^2]
Etoposide: I.V.: 75 mg/m^2/day days 4 to 7
[total dose/cycle = 300 mg/m^2]
Cytarabine: I.V.: 100 mg/m^2/dose every 12 hours days 4 to 7 (total of 8 doses)
[total dose/cycle = 800 mg/m^2]
Melphalan: I.V.: 20 mg/m^2 day 3
[total dose/cycle = 20 mg/m^2]
Repeat cycle every 28 days; consider stem cell transplantation after 2 cycles in responding patients and a maximum of 4 cycles (total) in nontransplant candidates

DHAP (Hodgkin)

Use Lymphoma, Hodgkin

Regimen

Salvage treatment:
Dexamethasone: I.V.: 40 mg/day days 1 to 4
[total dose/cycle = 160 mg]
Cisplatin: I.V.: 100 mg/m^2 continuous infusion for 24 hours day 1
[total dose/cycle = 100 mg/m^2]

Cytarabine: I.V.: 2000 mg/m^2 over 3 hours every 12 hours day 2 (total of 2 doses) [total dose/cycle = 4000 mg/m^2]
Filgrastim: SubQ: 5 mcg/kg/day beginning 24 hours after last dose of cytarabine, continue until leukocytes ≥2500/mm^3 for 3 days
Administer 2 cycles

Docetaxel-Bevacizumab

Use Breast cancer

Regimen NOTE: Multiple variations are listed.
Variation 1:
Docetaxel: I.V.: 100 mg/m^2 day 1
[total dose/cycle = 100 mg/m^2]
Bevacizumab: I.V.: 7.5 mg/kg day 1
[total dose/cycle = 7.5 mg/kg]
Repeat cycle every 21 days (administer docetaxel for up to 9 cycles, bevacizumab until disease progression or unacceptable toxicity)
Variation 2:
Docetaxel: I.V.: 100 mg/m^2 day 1
[total dose/cycle = 100 mg/m^2]
Bevacizumab: I.V.: 15 mg/kg day 1
[total dose/cycle = 15 mg/kg]
Repeat cycle every 21 days (administer docetaxel for up to 9 cycles, bevacizumab until disease progression or unacceptable toxicity)

Docetaxel-Cisplatin

Use Lung cancer, nonsmall cell

Regimen
Docetaxel: I.V.: 75 mg/m^2 day 1
[total dose/cycle = 75 mg/m^2]
Cisplatin: I.V.: 75 mg/m^2 day 1
[total dose/cycle = 75 mg/m^2]
Repeat cycle every 21 days

Docetaxel-Cisplatin-Fluorouracil (Gastric/Esophageal Cancer)

Use Esophageal cancer; Gastric cancer

Regimen NOTE: Multiple variations are listed.
Variation 1:
Docetaxel: I.V.: 75 mg/m^2 day 1
[total dose/cycle = 75 mg/m^2]
Cisplatin: I.V.: 75 mg/m^2 day 1
[total dose/cycle = 75 mg/m^2]
Fluorouracil: I.V.: 750 mg/m^2/day continuous infusion days 1 to 5
[total dose/cycle = 3750 mg/m^2]
Repeat cycle every 21 days until disease progression or unacceptable toxicity
Variation 2:
Docetaxel: I.V.: 75 mg/m^2 day 1
[total dose/cycle = 75 mg/m^2]
Cisplatin: I.V.: 75 mg/m^2 over 4 hours day 1
[total dose/cycle = 75 mg/m^2]
Fluorouracil: I.V.: 300 mg/m^2/day continuous infusion days 1 to 14
[total dose/cycle = 4200 mg/m^2]
Repeat cycle every 21 days until disease progression or unacceptable toxicity for up to a maximum of 8 cycles

Docetaxel-Cisplatin-Fluorouracil (Head and Neck Cancer)

Use Head and neck cancer

Regimen NOTE: Multiple variations are listed.
Variation 1:
Docetaxel: I.V.: 75 mg/m^2 day 1
[total dose/cycle = 75 mg/m^2]

Cisplatin: I.V.: 75 mg/m^2 day 1
[total dose/cycle = 75 mg/m^2]
Fluorouracil: I.V.: 750 mg/m^2/day continuous infusion days 1 to 5
[total dose/cycle = 3750 mg/m^2]
Repeat cycle every 21 days for 4 cycles

Variation 2:
Docetaxel: I.V.: 75 mg/m^2 day 1
[total dose/cycle = 75 mg/m^2]
Cisplatin: I.V.: 75-100 mg/m^2 day 1
[total dose/cycle = 75-100 mg/m^2]
Fluorouracil: I.V.: 1000 mg/m^2/day continuous infusion days 1 to 4
[total dose/cycle = 4000 mg/m^2]
Repeat cycle every 21 days for total of 3 cycles

Docetaxel-Cisplatin-Fluorouracil (Unknown Primary)

Use Unknown primary (squamous cell)

Regimen
Docetaxel: I.V.: 75 mg/m^2 day 1
[total dose/cycle = 75 mg/m^2]
Cisplatin: I.V.: 75 mg/m^2 day 1
[total dose/cycle = 75 mg/m^2]
Fluorouracil: I.V.: 750 mg/m^2/day continuous infusion days 1 to 5
[total dose/cycle = 3750 mg/m^2]
Repeat cycle every 21 days for a total of 3 cycles

Docetaxel-Cyclophosphamide (TC)

Use Breast cancer

Regimen
Docetaxel: I.V.: 75 mg/m^2 day 1
[total dose/cycle = 75 mg/m^2]
Cyclophosphamide: I.V.: 600 mg/m^2 day 1
[total dose/cycle = 600 mg/m^2]
Repeat cycle every 21 days for 4 cycles

Docetaxel-Doxorubicin (Breast Cancer)

Use Breast cancer

Regimen
Doxorubicin: I.V.: 50 mg/m^2 day 1
[total dose/cycle = 50 mg/m^2]
Docetaxel: I.V.: 75 mg/m^2 day 1
[total dose/cycle = 75 mg/m^2]
Repeat cycle every 3 weeks for up to 8 cycles

Docetaxel-FEC

Use Breast cancer

Regimen
Cycles 1, 2, and 3:
Docetaxel: I.V.: 80-100 mg/m^2 day 1
[total dose/cycle = 80-100 mg/m^2]
Repeat cycle every 21 days for 3 cycles

Cycles 4, 5, and 6 (FEC):
Fluorouracil: I.V.: 600 mg/m^2 day 1
[total dose/cycle = 600 mg/m^2]
Epirubicin: I.V.: 60 mg/m^2 day 1
[total dose/cycle = 60 mg/m^2]
Cyclophosphamide: I.V.: 600 mg/m^2 day 1
[total dose/cycle = 600 mg/m^2]
Repeat FEC cycle every 21 days for total of 3 cycles

Docetaxel-Gemcitabine (Unknown Primary)

Use Unknown primary (adenocarcinoma)

Regimen

Gemcitabine: I.V.: 1000 mg/m^2/day over 30 minutes days 1 and 8
[total dose/cycle = 2000 mg/m^2]
Docetaxel: I.V.: 75 mg/m^2 over 1 hour day 8
[total dose/cycle = 75 mg/m^2]
Repeat cycle every 21 days for up to a total of 6 cycles

Docetaxel (NSCLC Regimen)

Use Lung cancer, nonsmall cell

Regimen NOTE: Multiple variations are listed.

Variation 1:
Docetaxel: I.V.: 75 mg/m^2 over 1 hour day 1
[total dose/cycle = 75 mg/m^2]
Repeat cycle every 21 days
Variation 2:
Docetaxel: I.V.: 35 mg/m^2 days 1, 8, and 15
[total dose/cycle = 105 mg/m^2]
Repeat cycle every 28 days for a maximum of 8 cycles
Variation 3:
Docetaxel: I.V.: 36 mg/m^2/day over 1 hour days 1, 8, 15, 22, 29, and 36
[total dose/cycle = 216 mg/m^2]
Repeat cycle every 56 days for up to 4 cycles
Variation 4 (maintenance therapy):
Docetaxel: I.V.: 75 mg/m^2 over 1 hour day 1
[total dose/cycle = 75 mg/m^2]
Repeat cycle every 21 days for a maximum of 6 cycles

Docetaxel (Ovarian Regimen)

Use Ovarian cancer

Regimen

Docetaxel: I.V.: 100 mg/m^2 over 1 hour day 1
[total dose/cycle = 100 mg/m^2]
Repeat cycle every 21 days

Docetaxel-Oxaliplatin-Fluorouracil (Esophageal Cancer)

Use Esophageal cancer

Regimen

Docetaxel: I.V.: 50 mg/m^2 day 1
[total dose/cycle = 50 mg/m^2]
Oxaliplatin: I.V.: 85 mg/m^2 day 1
[total dose/cycle = 85 mg/m^2]
Fluorouracil: I.V.: 2400 mg/m^2 continuous infusion over 46 hours starting day 1
[total dose/cycle = 2400 mg/m^2]
Repeat cycle every 14 days.

Docetaxel-Oxaliplatin-Leucovorin-Fluorouracil (Esophageal Cancer)

Use Esophageal cancer

Regimen

Docetaxel: I.V.: 50 mg/m^2 day 1
[total dose/cycle = 50 mg/m^2]
Oxaliplatin: I.V.: 85 mg/m^2 day 1
[total dose/cycle = 85 mg/m^2]
Leucovorin: I.V.: 200 mg/m^2 day 1
[total dose/cycle = 200 mg/m^2]
Fluorouracil: I.V.: 2600 mg/m^2/day continuous infusion over 24 hours day 1
[total dose/cycle = 2600 mg/m^2]
Repeat cycle every 14 days until disease progression or unacceptable toxicity for up to a total of 8 cycles.

Docetaxel-Oxaliplatin (Ovarian Cancer)

Use Ovarian cancer

Regimen

Docetaxel: I.V.: 75 mg/m^2/dose over 60 minutes day 1
[total dose/cycle = 75 mg/m^2]
Oxaliplatin: I.V.: 100 mg/m^2/dose over 2 hours day 1
[total dose/cycle = 100 mg/m^2]
Repeat cycle every 21 days

Docetaxel-Prednisone

Use Prostate cancer

Regimen

Docetaxel: I.V.: 75 mg/m^2 day 1
[total dose/cycle = 75 mg/m^2]
Prednisone: Oral: 5 mg twice daily
[total dose/cycle = 210 mg]
Repeat cycle every 21 days for up to 10 cycles

Docetaxel (Small Cell Lung Cancer Regimen)

Use Lung cancer, small cell

Regimen

Docetaxel: I.V.: 100 mg/m^2 over 1 hour day 1
[total dose/cycle = 100 mg/m^2]
Repeat cycle every 21 days

Docetaxel-Trastuzumab

Use Breast cancer

Regimen

Cycle 1:
Docetaxel: I.V.: 100 mg/m^2 day 1
[total dose/cycle 1 = 100 mg/m^2]
Trastuzumab: I.V.: 4 mg/kg (loading dose) day 1 cycle 1
followed by I.V.: 2 mg/kg/day days 8 and 15 cycle 1
[total dose/cycle 1 = 8 mg/kg]
Treatment cycle is 21 days
Subsequent cycles:
Docetaxel: I.V.: 100 mg/m^2 day 1
[total dose/cycle = 100 mg/m^2]
Trastuzumab: I.V.: 2 mg/kg/day days 1, 8, and 15
[total dose/cycle = 6 mg/kg]
Repeat cycle every 21 days for a total of at least 6 cycles (continue weekly trastuzumab until disease progression)

Docetaxel-Trastuzumab-Carboplatin

Use Breast cancer

Regimen

Cycle 1:
Trastuzumab: I.V.: 4 mg/kg (loading dose) day 1 cycle 1
followed by I.V.: 2 mg/kg/day days 8 and 15 cycle 1
[total dose/cycle 1 = 8 mg/kg]
Docetaxel: I.V.: 75 mg/m^2 day 2
[total dose/cycle 1 = 75 mg/m^2]
Carboplatin: I.V.: AUC 6 day 2
[total dose/cycle 1 = AUC = 6]
Treatment cycle is 21 days

Subsequent cycles:
Trastuzumab: I.V.: 2 mg/kg/day days 1, 8, and 15
[total dose/cycle = 6 mg/kg]
Docetaxel: I.V.: 75 mg/m^2 day 1
[total dose/cycle = 75 mg/m^2]
Carboplatin: I.V.: AUC 6 day 1
[total dose/cycle = AUC = 6]
Repeat cycle every 21 days for a total of ~6 cycles (continue weekly trastuzumab for 1 year after chemotherapy, or until disease progression or unacceptable toxicity)

Docetaxel-Trastuzumab-Cisplatin

Use Breast cancer

Regimen

Cycle 1:
Trastuzumab: I.V.: 4 mg/kg (loading dose) day 1 cycle 1
followed by I.V.: 2 mg/kg/day days 8 and 15 cycle 1
[total dose/cycle 1 = 8 mg/kg]
Docetaxel: I.V.: 75 mg/m^2 day 2
[total dose/cycle 1 = 75 mg/m^2]
Cisplatin: I.V.: 75 mg/m^2 day 2
[total dose/cycle 1 = 75 mg/m^2]
Treatment cycle is 21 days
Subsequent cycles:
Trastuzumab: I.V.: 2 mg/kg/day days 1, 8, and 15
[total dose/cycle = 6 mg/kg]
Docetaxel: I.V.: 75 mg/m^2 day 1
[total dose/cycle = 75 mg/m^2]
Cisplatin: I.V.: 75 mg/m^2 day 1
[total dose/cycle = 75 mg/m^2]
Repeat cycle every 21 days for a total of ~6 cycles (continue weekly trastuzumab for 1 year after chemotherapy, or until disease progression or unacceptable toxicity)

Docetaxel-Trastuzumab-FEC

Use Breast cancer

Regimen

Cycle 1:
Trastuzumab: I.V.: 4 mg/kg (loading dose) day 1 cycle 1
followed by I.V.: 2 mg/kg/day days 8 and 15 cycle 1
[total dose/cycle 1 = 8 mg/kg]
Docetaxel: I.V.: 80-100 mg/m^2 day 1
[total dose/cycle 1 = 80-100 mg/m^2]
Treatment cycle is 21 days
Cycles 2 and 3:
Trastuzumab: I.V.: 2 mg/kg/day days 1, 8, and 15
[total dose/cycle = 6 mg/kg]
Docetaxel: I.V.: 80-100 mg/m^2 day 1
[total dose/cycle = 80-100 mg/m^2]
Treatment cycle is 21 days
Cycles 4, 5, and 6 (FEC):
Fluorouracil: I.V.: 600 mg/m^2 day 1
[total dose/cycle = 600 mg/m^2]
Epirubicin: I.V.: 60 mg/m^2 day 1
[total dose/cycle = 60 mg/m^2]
Cyclophosphamide: I.V.: 600 mg/m^2 day 1
[total dose/cycle = 600 mg/m^2]
Repeat FEC cycle every 21 days for total of 3 cycles

Docetaxel (Weekly Regimen)

Use Prostate cancer

Regimen

Docetaxel: I.V.: 40 mg/m^2 days 1, 8, and 15
[total dose/cycle = 120 mg/m^2]
Repeat cycle every 4 weeks

Docetaxel (Weekly)-Trastuzumab

Use Breast cancer

Regimen

Cycle 1:
Docetaxel: I.V.: 35 mg/m^2/day days 1, 8, and 15
[total dose/cycle 1 = 105 mg/m^2]
Trastuzumab: I.V.: 4 mg/kg (loading dose) day 0 cycle 1
followed by I.V.: 2 mg/kg/day days 8 and 15 cycle 1
[total dose/cycle 1 = 8 mg/kg]
Treatment cycle is 28 days
Subsequent cycles:
Docetaxel: I.V.: 35 mg/m^2/day days 1, 8, and 15
[total dose/cycle = 105 mg/m^2]
Trastuzumab: I.V.: 2 mg/kg/day days 1, 8, and 15
[total dose/cycle = 6 mg/kg]
Repeat cycle every 28 days

Dox-CMF (Sequential)

Use Breast cancer

Regimen

Doxorubicin: I.V.: 75 mg/m^2 day 1
[total dose/cycle = 75 mg/m^2]
Repeat cycle every 21 days for 4 cycles
followed by (after completing Cycle 4)
Cyclophosphamide: I.V.: 600 mg/m^2 day 1
[total dose/cycle = 600 mg/m^2]
Methotrexate: I.V.: 40 mg/m^2 day 1
[total dose/cycle = 40 mg/m^2]
Fluorouracil: I.V.: 600 mg/m^2 day 1
[total dose/cycle = 600 mg/m^2]
Repeat cycle every 21 days for 8 cycles

Doxorubicin + Ketoconazole

Use Prostate cancer

Regimen

Doxorubicin: I.V.: 20 mg/m^2 continuous infusion day 1
[total dose/cycle = 20 mg/m^2]
Ketoconazole: Oral: 400 mg 3 times/day days 1 to 7
[total dose/cycle = 8400 mg]
Repeat cycle every 7 days

Doxorubicin + Ketoconazole/Estramustine + Vinblastine

Use Prostate cancer

Regimen

Doxorubicin: I.V.: 20 mg/m^2/day days 1, 15, and 29
[total dose/cycle = 60 mg/m^2]
Ketoconazole: Oral: 400 mg 3 times/day days 1 to 7, 15 to 21, and 29 to 35
[total dose/cycle = 25,200 mg]
Estramustine: Oral: 140 mg 3 times/day days 8 to 14, 22 to 28, and 36 to 42
[total dose/cycle = 8820 mg]
Vinblastine: I.V.: 5 mg/m^2/day days 8, 22, and 36
[total dose/cycle = 15 mg/m^2]
Repeat cycle every 8 weeks

Doxorubicin (Liposomal) (Ovarian Regimen)

Use Ovarian cancer

Regimen NOTE: Multiple variations are listed.

Variation 1:

Doxorubicin (liposomal): I.V.: 50 mg/m^2 over 60 minutes day 1
[total dose/cycle = 50 mg/m^2]

Repeat cycle every 28 days until disease progression or unacceptable toxicity

Variation 2:

Doxorubicin (liposomal): I.V.: 40 mg/m^2 over 60 minutes day 1
[total dose/cycle = 40 mg/m^2]

Repeat cycle every 28 days until disease progression or unacceptable toxicity

Doxorubicin (Liposomal)-Docetaxel (Breast Cancer)

Use Breast cancer

Regimen

Doxorubicin (liposomal): I.V.: 30 mg/m^2 over 1 hour day 1
[total dose/cycle = 30 mg/m^2]

Docetaxel: I.V.: 60 mg/m^2 over 1 hour day 1
[total dose/cycle = 60 mg/m^2]

Repeat cycle every 3 weeks until disease progression or unacceptable toxicity

Doxorubicin (Liposomal)-Vincristine-Dexamethasone

Use Multiple myeloma

Regimen NOTE: Multiple variations are listed.

Variation 1:

Doxorubicin, liposomal: I.V.: 40 mg/m^2 day 1
[total dose/cycle = 40 mg/m^2]

Vincristine: I.V.: 2 mg day 1
[total dose/cycle = 2 mg]

Dexamethasone: Oral or I.V.: 40 mg/day days 1 to 4
[total dose/cycle = 160 mg]

Repeat cycle every 4 weeks

Variation 2:

Doxorubicin, liposomal: I.V.: 40 mg/m^2 day 1
[total dose/cycle = 40 mg/m^2]

Vincristine: I.V.: 1.4 mg/m^2 (maximum dose: 2 mg) day 1
[total dose/cycle = 1.4 mg/m^2; maximum: 2 mg]

Dexamethasone: Oral: 40 mg/day days 1 to 4
[total dose/cycle = 160 mg]

Repeat cycle every 4 weeks

DTPACE

Use Multiple myeloma

Regimen

Dexamethasone: Oral: 40 mg/day days 1 to 4
[total dose/cycle = 160 mg]

Thalidomide: Oral: 400 mg/day
[total dose/cycle = 11,200 - 16,800 mg]

Cisplatin: I.V.: 10 mg/m^2/day continuous infusion days 1 to 4
[total dose/cycle = 40 mg/m^2]

Doxorubicin: I.V.: 10 mg/m^2/day continuous infusion days 1 to 4
[total dose/cycle = 40 mg/m^2]

Cyclophosphamide: I.V.: 400 mg/m^2 continuous infusion days 1 to 4
[total dose/cycle = 1600 mg/m^2]

Etoposide: I.V.: 40 mg/m^2 continuous infusion days 1 to 4
[total dose/cycle = 160 mg/m^2]

Repeat cycle every 4-6 weeks

DVP

Use Leukemia, acute lymphocytic

Regimen Induction:

Daunorubicin: I.V.: 25 mg/m^2/day days 1, 8, and 15
[total dose/cycle = 75 mg/m^2]
Vincristine: I.V.: 1.5 mg/m^2/day (maximum dose: 2 mg) days 1, 8, 15, and 22
[total dose/cycle = 6 mg/m^2]
Prednisone: Oral: 60 mg/m^2/day days 1 to 28 then taper over next 14 days
[total dose/cycle = 1680 mg/m^2 + taper over next 14 days]
Administer single cycle; used in conjunction with intrathecal chemotherapy

EC (NSCLC)

Use Lung cancer, nonsmall cell

Regimen

Etoposide: I.V.: 120 mg/m^2/day days 1, 2, and 3
[total dose/cycle = 360 mg/m^2]
Carboplatin: I.V.: AUC 6 day 1
[total dose/cycle = AUC = 6]
Repeat cycle every 21-28 days

EE-4A (Wilms Tumor)

Use Wilms tumor

Regimen

Dactinomycin: I.V.: 45 mcg/kg day 1 of weeks 0, 3, 6, 9, 12, 15, and 18
[total dose = 315 mcg/kg]
Vincristine: I.V.: 1.5 mg/m^2 day 1 of weeks 1 to 10
Followed by
Vincristine: I.V.: 2 mg/m^2 day 1 of weeks 12, 15, and 18
[total dose = 21 mg/m^2]
Treatment course duration is week 0 through week 18

EMA/CO

Use Gestational trophoblastic tumor

Regimen NOTE: Multiple variations are listed.

Variation 1:
Etoposide: I.V.: 100 mg/m^2/day days 1 and 2
[total dose/cycle = 200 mg/m^2]
Methotrexate: I.V.: 300 mg/m^2 continuous infusion over 12 hours day 1
[total dose/cycle = 300 mg/m^2]
Dactinomycin: I.V. push: 0.5 mg/day days 1 and 2
[total dose/cycle = 1 mg]
Leucovorin: Oral, I.M.: 15 mg twice daily for 2 days (start 24 hours after the start of methotrexate) days 2 and 3
[total dose/cycle = 60 mg]
Alternate weekly with:
Cyclophosphamide: I.V.: 600 mg/m^2 day 1
[total dose/cycle = 600 mg/m^2]
Vincristine: I.V. push: 0.8 mg/m^2 (maximum dose: 2 mg) day 1
[total dose/cycle = 0.8 mg/m^2]
Repeat cycle every 2 weeks

Variation 2:
Dactinomycin: I.V.: 0.5 mg/day days 1 and 2
[total dose/cycle = 1 mg]
Etoposide: I.V.: 100 mg/m^2/day days 1 and 2
[total dose/cycle = 200 mg/m^2]
Methotrexate: I.V. bolus: 100 mg/m^2 then 200 mg/m^2 continuous infusion over 12 hours day 1
[total dose/cycle = 300 mg/m^2]
Leucovorin: Oral, I.M.: 15 mg every 12 hours for 4 doses (start 24 hours after methotrexate) days 2 and 3
[total dose/cycle = 60 mg]

Vincristine: I.V.: 1 mg/m^2 day 8
[total dose/cycle = 1 mg/m^2]
Cyclophosphamide: I.V.: 600 mg/m^2 day 8
[total dose/cycle = 600 mg/m^2]
Repeat cycle every 2 weeks
Variation 3:
Dactinomycin: I.V.: 0.5 mg/day days 1 and 2
[total dose/cycle = 1 mg]
Etoposide: I.V.: 100 mg/m^2/day days 1 and 2
[total dose/cycle = 200 mg/m^2]
Methotrexate: I.V.: 300 mg/m^2 continuous infusion over 12 hours day 1
[total dose/cycle = 300 mg/m^2]
Leucovorin: Oral, I.M.: 15 mg every 12 hours for 4 doses (start 24 hours after start of methotrexate) days 2 and 3
[total dose/cycle = 60 mg]
Vincristine: I.V.: 1 mg/m^2 day 8
[total dose/cycle = 1 mg/m^2]
Cyclophosphamide: I.V.: 600 mg/m^2 day 8
[total dose/cycle = 600 mg/m^2]
Repeat cycle every 2 weeks
Variation 4:
Dactinomycin: I.V.: 0.35 mg/m^2/day days 1 and 2
[total dose/cycle = 0.7 mg/m^2]
Etoposide: I.V.: 100 mg/m^2/day days 1 and 2
[total dose/cycle = 200 mg/m^2]
Methotrexate: I.V. bolus: 100 mg/m^2 then 200 mg/m^2 continuous infusion over 12 hours day 1
[total dose/cycle = 300 mg/m^2]
Leucovorin: Oral, I.M.: 15 mg every 12 hours for 4 doses (start 24 hours after start of methotrexate) days 2 and 3
[total dose/cycle = 60 mg]
Vincristine: I.V.: 1 mg/m^2 day 8
[total dose/cycle = 1 mg/m^2]
Cyclophosphamide: I.V.: 600 mg/m^2 day 8
[total dose/cycle = 600 mg/m^2]
Repeat cycle every 2 weeks
Variation 5 (patients with brain metastases):
Dactinomycin: I.V.: 0.5 mg/day days 1 and 2
[total dose/cycle = 1 mg]
Etoposide:I.V.: 100 mg/m^2/day days 1 and 2
[total dose/cycle = 200 mg/m^2]
Methotrexate: I.V.: 1 g/m^2 continuous infusion over 12 hours day 1
[total dose/cycle = 1 g/m^2]
Leucovorin: I.M.: 20 mg/m^2 every 6 hours for 12 doses (start 24 hours after start of methotrexate) days 2, 3, and 4
[total dose/cycle = 240 mg/m^2]
Vincristine: I.V.: 1 mg/m^2 day 8
[total dose/cycle = 1 mg/m^2]
Cyclophosphamide: I.V.: 600 mg/m^2 day 8
[total dose/cycle = 600 mg/m^2]
Repeat cycle every 2 weeks
Variation 6 (patients with brain metastases):
Dactinomycin: I.V.: 0.5 mg/day days 1 and 2
[total dose/cycle = 1 mg]
Etoposide: I.V.: 100 mg/m^2/day days 1 and 2
[total dose/cycle = 200 mg/m^2]
Methotrexate: I.V.: 1 g/m^2 continuous infusion over 12 hours day 1
[total dose/cycle = 1 g/m^2]
Leucovorin: Oral, I.M.: 30 mg/m^2 every 12 hours for 6 doses (start 32 hours after start of methotrexate) days 2, 3, and 4
[total dose/cycle = 180 mg/m^2]
Vincristine: I.V.: 1 mg/m^2 day 8
[total dose/cycle = 1 mg/m^2]

Cyclophosphamide: I.V.: 600 mg/m^2 day 8
[total dose/cycle = 600 mg/m^2]
Repeat cycle every 2 weeks
Variation 7:
Dactinomycin: I.V.: 0.5 mg/day days 1 and 2
[total dose/cycle = 1 mg]
Etoposide: I.V.: 100 mg/m^2/day days 1 and 2
[total dose/cycle = 200 mg/m^2]
Methotrexate: I.V.: 1 g/m^2 continuous infusion over 24 hours day 1
[total dose/cycle = 1 g/m^2]
Leucovorin: Oral, I.M.: 15 mg every 8 hours for 9 doses (start 32 hours after start of methotrexate) days 2, 3, and 4
[total dose/cycle = 135 mg/m^2]
Vincristine: I.V.: 1 mg/m^2 day 8
[total dose/cycle = 1 mg/m^2]
Cyclophosphamide: I.V.: 600 mg/m^2 day 8
[total dose/cycle = 600 mg/m^2]
Repeat cycle every 2 weeks
Variation 8 (patients with lung metastases):
Dactinomycin: I.V.: 0.5 mg/day days 1 and 2
[total dose/cycle = 1 mg]
Etoposide: I.V.: 100 mg/m^2/day days 1 and 2
[total dose/cycle = 200 mg/m^2]
Methotrexate: I.V. bolus: 100 mg/m^2 then 200 mg/m^2 continuous infusion over 12 hours day 1
[total dose/cycle = 300 mg/m^2]
Leucovorin: Oral, I.M.: 15 mg every 12 hours for 4 doses (start 24 hours after start of methotrexate) days 2 and 3
[total dose/cycle = 60 mg]
Vincristine: I.V.: 1 mg/m^2 day 8
[total dose/cycle = 1 mg/m^2]
Cyclophosphamide: I.V.: 600 mg/m^2 day 8
[total dose/cycle = 600 mg/m^2]
Methotrexate: I.T.: 10 mg day 1 (every other cycle)
[total dose/cycle = 10 mg, every other cycle]
Repeat cycle every 2 weeks
Variation 9 (patients with lung metastases):
Dactinomycin: I.V.: 0.5 mg/day days 1 and 2
[total dose/cycle = 1 mg]
Etoposide: I.V.: 100 mg/m^2/day days 1 and 2
[total dose/cycle = 200 mg/m^2]
Methotrexate: I.V. bolus: 100 mg/m^2 then 200 mg/m^2 continuous infusion over 12 hours day 1
[total dose/cycle = 300 mg/m^2]
Leucovorin: Oral, I.M.: 15 mg every 12 hours for 4 doses (start 24 hours after start of methotrexate) days 2 and 3
[total dose/cycle = 60 mg]
Vincristine: I.V.: 1 mg/m^2 day 8
[total dose/cycle = 1 mg/m^2]
Cyclophosphamide: I.V.: 600 mg/m^2 day 8
[total dose/cycle = 600 mg/m^2]
Methotrexate: I.T.: 12.5 mg day 8
[total dose/cycle = 12.5 mg]
Repeat cycle every 2 weeks

EP/EMA

Use Gestational trophoblastic tumor
Regimen NOTE: Multiple variations are listed.
Variation 1:
Etoposide: I.V.: 150 mg/m^2 day 1
[total dose/cycle = 150 mg/m^2]
Cisplatin: I.V.: 25 mg/m^2 infused over 4 hours for 3 consecutive doses, day 1
[total dose/cycle = 75 mg/m^2]

Alternate weekly with:

Etoposide: I.V.: 100 mg/m^2 day 1
[total dose/cycle = 100 mg/m^2]

Methotrexate: I.V.: 300 mg/m^2 infused over 12 hours day 1
[total dose/cycle = 300 mg/m^2]

Dactinomycin: I.V. push: 0.5 mg day 1
[total dose/cycle = 0.5 mg]

Leucovorin: Oral, I.M.: 15 mg twice daily for 2 days (start 24 hours after the start of methotrexate) days 2 and 3
[total dose/cycle = 60 mg]

Variation 2:

Dactinomycin: I.V.: 0.5 mg/day days 1 and 2
[total dose/cycle = 1 mg]

Etoposide: I.V.: 100 mg/m^2/day days 1 and 2
[total dose/cycle = 200 mg/m^2]

Methotrexate: I.V.: 300 mg/m^2 continuous infusion over 12 hours day 1
[total dose/cycle = 300 mg/m^2]

Leucovorin: Oral, I.M.: 15 mg every 12 hours for 4 doses (start 24 hours after start of methotrexate) days 2 and 3
[total dose/cycle = 60 mg]

Etoposide: I.V.: 150 mg/m^2 day 8
[total dose/cycle = 150 mg/m^2]

Cisplatin: I.V.: 75 mg/m^2 day 8
[total dose/cycle = 75 mg/m^2]

Repeat cycle every 2 weeks

Epirubicin-Cisplatin-Capecitabine (Esophageal Cancer)

Use Esophageal cancer

Regimen

Epirubicin: I.V.: 50 mg/m^2 day 1
[total dose/cycle = 50 mg/m^2]

Cisplatin: I.V.: 60 mg/m^2 day 1
[total dose/cycle = 60 mg/m^2]

Capecitabine: Oral: 625 mg/m^2 twice daily days 1 to 21
[total dose/cycle = 26,250 mg/m^2]

Repeat cycle every 21 days for up to 8 cycles

Epirubicin-Cisplatin-Fluorouracil (Gastric/Esophageal Cancer)

Use Esophageal cancer; Gastric cancer

Regimen NOTE: Multiple variations are listed.

Variation 1:

Epirubicin: I.V.: 50 mg/m^2 day 1
[total dose/cycle = 50 mg/m^2]

Cisplatin: I.V.: 60 mg/m^2 day 1
[total dose/cycle = 60 mg/m^2]

Fluorouracil: I.V.: 200 mg/m^2/day continuous infusion days 1 to 21
[total dose/cycle = 4200 mg/m^2]

Repeat cycle every 3 weeks for up to a maximum of 8 cycles

Variation 2:

Epirubicin: I.V.: 50 mg/m^2 day 1
[total dose/cycle = 50 mg/m^2]

Cisplatin: I.V.: 60 mg/m^2 day 1
[total dose/cycle = 60 mg/m^2]

Fluorouracil: I.V.: 200 mg/m^2/day continuous infusion days 1 to 21
[total dose/cycle = 4200 mg/m^2]

Repeat cycle every 3 weeks for up to 6 cycles (3 cycles before surgery and 3 cycles postoperatively)

Epirubicin-Oxaliplatin-Capecitabine

Use Esophageal cancer; Gastric cancer

Regimen

Epirubicin: I.V.: 50 mg/m^2 day 1
[total dose/cycle = 50 mg/m^2]
Oxaliplatin: I.V.: 130 mg/m^2 day 1
[total dose/cycle = 130 mg/m^2]
Capecitabine: Oral: 625 mg/m^2 twice daily days 1 to 21
[total dose/cycle = 26,250 mg/m^2]
Repeat cycle every 21 days for up to 8 cycles

Epirubicin-Oxaliplatin-Fluorouracil (Esophageal Cancer)

Use Esophageal cancer

Regimen

Epirubicin: I.V.: 50 mg/m^2 day 1
[total dose/cycle = 50 mg/m^2]
Oxaliplatin: I.V.: 130 mg/m^2 day 1
[total dose/cycle = 130 mg/m^2]
Fluorouracil: I.V.: 200 mg/m^2/day continuous infusion days 1 to 21
[total dose/cycle = 4200 mg/m^2]
Repeat cycle every 21 days for up to 8 cycles

EP (NSCLC)

Use Lung cancer, nonsmall cell

Regimen

Etoposide: I.V.: 80-120 mg/m^2/day days 1, 2, and 3
[total dose/cycle = 240-360 mg/m^2]
Cisplatin: I.V.: 80-100 mg/m^2 day 1
[total dose/cycle = 80-100 mg/m^2]
Repeat cycle every 21-28 days

EPOCH Dose-Adjusted (AIDS-Related Lymphoma)

Use Lymphoma, AIDS-related

Regimen

Etoposide: I.V.: 50 mg/m^2/day continuous infusion days 1 to 4
[total dose/cycle = 200 mg/m^2]
Vincristine: I.V.: 0.4 mg/m^2/day continuous infusion days 1 to 4
[total dose/cycle = 1.6 mg/m^2]
Doxorubicin: I.V.: 10 mg/m^2/day continuous infusion days 1 to 4
[total dose/cycle = 40 mg/m^2]
Cyclophosphamide: I.V.: 375 mg/m^2 day 5 for CD4+ cells ≥100/mm^3 **or** 187 mg/m^2 day 5 for CD4+ cells <100/mm^3
[total dose/cycle = 187-375 mg/m^2]
Prednisone: Oral: 60 mg/m^2/day days 1 to 5
[total dose/cycle = 300 mg/m^2]
Filgrastim: SubQ: 5 mcg/kg/day beginning day 6; continue until ANC >5000/mm^3 (past nadir)
Repeat cycle every 21 days for 6 cycles with cyclophosphamide dose adjusted based on previous cycle nadir according to the following schedule:
Nadir ANC >500/mm^3: Increase cyclophosphamide dose by 187 mg/m^2 above previous cycle dose (maximum dose: 750 mg/m^2)
Nadir ANC <500/mm^3 or platelet <25,000/mm^3: Decrease cyclophosphamide dose by 187 mg/m^2 below previous cycle dose

EPOCH Dose-Adjusted (NHL)

Use Lymphoma, non-Hodgkin

Regimen

Etoposide: I.V.: 50 mg/m^2/day continuous infusion days 1 to 4
[total dose/cycle = 200 mg/m^2]

Vincristine: I.V.: 0.4 mg/m^2/day continuous infusion days 1 to 4
[total dose/cycle = 1.6 mg/m^2]

Doxorubicin: I.V.: 10 mg/m^2/day continuous infusion days 1 to 4
[total dose/cycle = 40 mg/m^2]

Cyclophosphamide: I.V.: 750 mg/m^2 day 5
[total dose/cycle = 750 mg/m^2]

Prednisone: Oral: 60 mg/m^2 twice daily days 1 to 5
total dose/cycle = 600 mg/m^2]

Filgrastim: SubQ: 5 mcg/kg/day beginning day 6; continue until ANC >5000/mm^3

Repeat cycle every 21 days with etoposide, doxorubicin, and cyclophosphamide dose adjustments (based on CBC 2 times/week) according to the following schedule:

Nadir ANC ≥500/mm^3: 20% increase (above previous cycle) for etoposide, doxorubicin, and cyclophosphamide

Nadir ANC <500/mm^3 (on 1 or 2 measurements): Same doses as previous cycle

Nadir ANC <500/mm^3 (on ≥3 measurements) or nadir platelet <25,000/mm^3 (on 1 measurement): 20% decrease below previous cycle for etoposide, doxorubicin, and cyclophosphamide (dosing adjustments below starting dose levels only apply to cyclophosphamide)

EPOCH (Dose-Adjusted)-Rituximab (NHL)

Use Lymphoma, non-Hodgkin

Regimen NOTE: Multiple variations are listed.

Variation 1:

Rituximab: I.V.: 375 mg/m^2 day 1
[total dose/cycle = 375 mg/m^2]

Etoposide: I.V.: 50 mg/m^2/day continuous infusion days 1 to 4
[total dose/cycle = 200 mg/m^2]

Vincristine: I.V.: 0.4 mg/m^2/day continuous infusion days 1 to 4
[total dose/cycle = 1.6 mg/m^2]

Doxorubicin: I.V.: 10 mg/m^2/day continuous infusion days 1 to 4
[total dose/cycle = 40 mg/m^2]

Cyclophosphamide: I.V.: 750 mg/m^2 day 5
[total dose/cycle = 750 mg/m^2]

Prednisone: Oral: 60 mg/m^2 twice daily days 1 to 5
[total dose/cycle = 600 mg/m^2]

Filgrastim: SubQ: 5 mcg/kg/day beginning day 6; continue until ANC >5000/mm^3

Repeat cycle every 21 days (for at least 2 cycles beyond best response; minimum of 6 cycles) with etoposide, doxorubicin, and cyclophosphamide dose adjustments (based on CBC 2 times/week) according to the following schedule:

Nadir ANC ≥500/mm^3: 20% increase (above previous cycle) for etoposide, doxorubicin, and cyclophosphamide

Nadir ANC <500/mm^3 (on 1 or 2 measurements): Same doses as previous cycle

Nadir ANC <500/mm^3 (on ≥3 measurements): 20% decrease below previous cycle for etoposide, doxorubicin, and cyclophosphamide (dosing adjustments below starting dose levels only apply to cyclophosphamide)

Variation 2:

Rituximab: I.V.: 375 mg/m^2 day 1
[total dose/cycle = 375 mg/m^2]

Etoposide: I.V.: 50 mg/m^2/day continuous infusion days 1 to 4
[total dose/cycle = 200 mg/m^2]

Vincristine: I.V.: 0.4 mg/m^2/day continuous infusion days 1 to 4
[total dose/cycle = 1.6 mg/m^2]

Doxorubicin: I.V.: 10 mg/m^2/day continuous infusion days 1 to 4
[total dose/cycle = 40 mg/m^2]

Cyclophosphamide: I.V.: 750 mg/m^2 day 5
[total dose/cycle = 750 mg/m^2]

Prednisone: Oral: 60 mg/m^2/day days 1 to 5
[total dose/cycle = 300 mg/m^2]
Filgrastim: SubQ: 5 mcg/kg/day beginning day 6; continue until ANC >500/mm^3
Repeat cycle every 21 days (for 6-8 cycles); refer to variation 1 for dose adjustments

EPOCH (NHL)

Use Lymphoma, non-Hodgkin

Regimen NOTE: Multiple variations are listed.

Variation 1:

Etoposide: I.V.: 50 mg/m^2/day continuous infusion days 1 to 4
[total dose/cycle = 200 mg/m^2]
Vincristine: I.V.: 0.4 mg/m^2/day continuous infusion days 1 to 4
[total dose/cycle = 1.6 mg/m^2]
Doxorubicin: I.V.: 10 mg/m^2/day continuous infusion days 1 to 4
[total dose/cycle = 40 mg/m^2]
Cyclophosphamide: I.V.: 750 mg/m^2 day 5
[total dose/cycle = 750 mg/m^2]
Prednisone: Oral: 60 mg/m^2/day days 1 to 5
[total dose/cycle = 300 mg/m^2]
Repeat cycle (with cyclophosphamide dose adjustments if needed based on ANC) every 21 days (best response seen in a median of 4 cycles)

Variation 2:

Etoposide: I.V.: 50 mg/m^2/day continuous infusion days 1 to 4
[total dose/cycle = 200 mg/m^2]
Vincristine: I.V.: 0.4 mg/m^2/day continuous infusion days 1 to 4
[total dose/cycle = 1.6 mg/m^2]
Doxorubicin: I.V.: 10 mg/m^2/day continuous infusion days 1 to 4
[total dose/cycle = 40 mg/m^2]
Cyclophosphamide: I.V.: 750 mg/m^2 day 6
[total dose/cycle = 750 mg/m^2]
Prednisone: Oral: 60 mg/m^2/day days 1 to 6
[total dose/cycle = 360 mg/m^2]
Repeat cycle (with cyclophosphamide dose adjustments if needed based on ANC) every 21 days (best response seen in a median of 4 cycles)

EPOCH-Rituximab (NHL)

Use Lymphoma, non-Hodgkin

Regimen

Rituximab: I.V.: 375 mg/m^2 day 1
[total dose/cycle = 375 mg/m^2]
Etoposide: I.V.: 65 mg/m^2/day continuous infusion days 2, 3, and 4
[total dose/cycle = 195 mg/m^2]
Vincristine: I.V.: 0.5 mg/m^2/day continuous infusion days 2, 3, and 4
[total dose/cycle = 1.5 mg/m^2]
Doxorubicin: I.V.: 15 mg/m^2/day continuous infusion days 2, 3, and 4
[total dose/cycle = 45 mg/m^2]
Cyclophosphamide: I.V.: 750 mg/m^2 day 5
[total dose/cycle = 750 mg/m^2]
Prednisone: Oral: 60 mg/m^2/day days 1 to 14
[total dose/cycle = 840 mg/m^2]
Repeat cycle every 21 days for 4-6 cycles

EP/PE

Use Lung cancer, nonsmall cell

Regimen

Etoposide: I.V.: 120 mg/m^2/day days 1, 2, and 3
[total dose/cycle = 360 mg/m^2]
Cisplatin: I.V.: 60-120 mg/m^2 day 1
[total dose/cycle = 60-120 mg/m^2]
Repeat cycle every 21-28 days

EP (Small Cell Lung Cancer)

Use Lung cancer, small cell

Regimen NOTE: Multiple variations are listed.

Variation 1: (limited stage with concurrent thoracic radiotherapy)
Etoposide: I.V.: 120 mg/m^2/day days 1, 2, and 3
[total dose/cycle = 360 mg/m^2]
Cisplatin: I.V.: 60 mg/m^2 day 1
[total dose/cycle = 60 mg/m^2]
Repeat cycle every 21 days for 4 cycles

Variation 2: (limited stage with concurrent thoracic radiotherapy)
Etoposide: I.V.: 100 mg/m^2/day days 1, 2, and 3
[total dose/cycle = 300 mg/m^2]
Cisplatin: I.V.: 80 mg/m^2 day 1
[total dose/cycle = 80 mg/m^2]
Repeat cycle every 28 days for 4 cycles

Variation 3: (extensive)
Etoposide: I.V.: 100 mg/m^2 day 1
[total I.V. dose/cycle = 100 mg/m^2]
followed by: Etoposide: Oral: 200 mg/m^2/day days 2, 3, and 4
[total oral dose/cycle = 600 mg/m^2]
Cisplatin: I.V.: 75 mg/m^2 day 1
[total dose/cycle = 75 mg/m^2]
Repeat cycle every 21 days for a maximum of 5 cycles

Variation 4: (extensive)
Etoposide: I.V.: 80 mg/m^2/day days 1, 2, and 3
[total dose/cycle = 240 mg/m^2]
Cisplatin: I.V.: 80 mg/m^2 day 1
[total dose/cycle = 80 mg/m^2]
Repeat cycle every 21 days for maximum of 8 cycles

Variation 5: (extensive)
Etoposide: I.V.: 100 mg/m^2/day days 1, 2, and 3
[total dose/cycle = 300 mg/m^2]
Cisplatin: I.V.: 25 mg/m^2/day days 1, 2, and 3
[total dose/cycle = 75 mg/m^2]
Repeat cycle every 21 to 28 days for 6 cycles

Variation 6: (extensive)
Etoposide: I.V.: 80 mg/m^2/day days 1 to 5
[total dose/cycle = 400 mg/m^2]
Cisplatin: I.V.: 20 mg/m^2/day days 1 to 5
[total dose/cycle = 100 mg/m^2]
Repeat cycle every 21 days for 4 cycles

EP (Testicular Cancer)

Use Testicular cancer

Regimen NOTE: Multiple variations are listed.

Variation 1:
Etoposide: I.V.: 100 mg/m^2/day days 1 to 5
[total dose/cycle = 500 mg/m^2]
Cisplatin: I.V.: 20 mg/m^2/day days 1 to 5
[total dose/cycle = 100 mg/m^2]
Repeat cycle every 21 days

Variation 2:
Etoposide: I.V.: 120 mg/m^2/day days 1, 2, and 3
[total dose/cycle = 360 mg/m^2]
Cisplatin: I.V.: 20 mg/m^2/day days 1 to 5
[total dose/cycle = 100 mg/m^2]
Repeat cycle every 3 or 4 weeks

Variation 3:
Etoposide: I.V.: 120 mg/m^2/day days 1, 3, and 5
[total dose/cycle = 360 mg/m^2]
Cisplatin: I.V.: 20 mg/m^2/day days 1 to 5
[total dose/cycle = 100 mg/m^2]
Repeat cycle every 3 weeks

Erlotinib-Gemcitabine (Pancreatic)

Use Pancreatic cancer

Regimen

Cycle 1:
Gemcitabine: I.V.: 1000 mg/m^2/day over 30 minutes days 1, 8, 15, 22, 29, 36, and 43 (cycle 1 only)
[total dose/cycle 1 = 7000 mg/m^2]
Erlotinib: Oral: 100 mg once daily days 1 to 56
[total dose/cycle 1 = 5600 mg]
Treatment cycle is 56 days
Subsequent cycles:
Gemcitabine: I.V.: 1000 mg/m^2/day over 30 minutes days 1, 8, and 15
[total dose/cycle = 3000 mg/m^2]
Erlotinib: Oral: 100 mg once daily days 1 to 28
[total dose/cycle = 2800 mg]
Repeat cycle every 28 days

ESHAP

Use Lymphoma, non-Hodgkin

Regimen NOTE: Multiple variations are listed.

Variation 1:
Etoposide: I.V.: 40 mg/m^2/day days 1 to 4
[total dose/cycle = 160 mg/m^2]
Methylprednisolone: I.V.: 250-500 mg/day days 1 to 5
[total dose/cycle = 1250-2500 mg]
Cytarabine: I.V.: 2000 mg/m^2 day 5
[total dose/cycle = 2000 mg/m^2]
Cisplatin: I.V.: 25 mg/m^2/day continuous infusion days 1 to 4
[total dose/cycle = 100 mg/m^2]
Repeat cycle every 21-28 days
Variation 2:
Etoposide: I.V.: 40 mg/m^2/day days 1 to 4
[total dose/cycle = 160 mg/m^2]
Methylprednisolone: I.V.: 500 mg/day days 1 to 5
[total dose/cycle = 2500 mg]
Cytarabine: I.V.: 2000 mg/m^2 day 5
[total dose/cycle = 2000 mg/m^2]
Cisplatin: I.V.: 25 mg/m^2/day continuous infusion days 1 to 4
[total dose/cycle = 100 mg/m^2]
Repeat cycle every 21-28 days
Variation 3:
Etoposide: I.V.: 60 mg/m^2/day days 1 to 4
[total dose/cycle = 240 mg/m^2]
Methylprednisolone: I.V.: 500 mg/day days 1 to 4
[total dose/cycle = 2000 mg]
Cytarabine: I.V.: 2000 mg/m^2 day 5
[total dose/cycle = 2000 mg/m^2]
Cisplatin: I.V.: 25 mg/m^2/day continuous infusion days 1 to 4
[total dose/cycle = 100 mg/m^2]
Repeat cycle every 21 days

ESHAP (Hodgkin)

Use Lymphoma, Hodgkin

Regimen

Etoposide: I.V.: 40 mg/m^2/day days 1 to 4
[total dose/cycle = 160 mg/m^2]

Methylprednisolone: I.V.: 500 mg/day days 1 to 4
[total dose/cycle = 2000 mg]
Cisplatin: I.V.: 25 mg/m^2/day days 1 to 4
[total dose/cycle = 100 mg/m^2]
Cytarabine: I.V.: 2000 mg/m^2 day 5
[total dose/cycle = 2000 mg/m^2]
Filgrastim: SubQ: 5 mcg/kg/day days 6 to 18
Repeat cycle every 21 to 28 days for 3 cycles (if transplant candidate) or 6 cycles (nontransplant candidate)

Estramustine + Docetaxel

Use Prostate cancer

Regimen NOTE: Multiple variations are listed.

Variation 1:
Docetaxel: I.V.: 20-80 mg/m^2 day 2
[total dose/cycle = 20-80 mg/m^2]
Estramustine: Oral: 280 mg 3 times/day days 1 to 5
[total dose/cycle = 4200 mg]
Repeat cycle every 21 days

Variation 2:
Docetaxel: I.V.: 20-80 mg/m^2 day 2
[total dose/cycle = 20-80 mg/m^2]
Estramustine: Oral: 14 mg/kg/day days 1 to 21
[total dose/cycle = 294 mg/kg]
Repeat cycle every 21 days

Variation 3:
Docetaxel: I.V.: 35 mg/m^2/day days 2 and 9
[total dose/cycle = 70 mg/m^2]
Estramustine: Oral: 420 mg 3 times/day for 4 doses, then 280 mg 3 times/day for 5 doses days 1, 2, 3, 8, 9, and 10
[total dose/cycle = 6160 mg]
Repeat cycle every 21 days

Variation 4:
Docetaxel: I.V.: 60 mg/m^2 day 2 cycle 1
[total dose/cycle = 60 mg/m^2]
followed by I.V.: 60-70 mg/m^2 day 2 (subsequent cycles)
[total dose/cycle = 60-70 mg/m^2]
Estramustine: Oral: 280 mg 3 times/day days 1 to 5
[total dose/cycle = 4200 mg]
Repeat cycle every 21 days for up to 12 cycles

Estramustine + Docetaxel + Calcitriol

Use Prostate cancer

Regimen

Cycle 1:
Calcitriol: Oral: 60 mcg (in divided doses) day 1
[total dose/cycle = 60 mcg]
Estramustine: Oral: 280 mg 3 times/day days 1 to 5
[total dose/cycle = 4200 mg]
Docetaxel: I.V.: 60 mg/m^2 day 2
[total dose/cycle = 60 mg/m^2]
Treatment cycle is 21 days

Subsequent cycles:
Calcitriol: Oral: 60 mcg (in divided doses) day 1
[total dose/cycle = 60 mcg]
Estramustine: Oral: 280 mg 3 times/day days 1 to 5
[total dose/cycle = 4200 mg]
Docetaxel: I.V.: 70 mg/m^2 day 2
[total dose/cycle = 70 mg/m^2]
Repeat cycle every 21 days for up to 12 cycles

Estramustine + Docetaxel + Carboplatin

Use Prostate cancer

Regimen

Docetaxel: I.V.: 70 mg/m^2 day 2
[total dose/cycle = 70 mg/m^2]
Estramustine: Oral: 280 mg 3 times/day days 1 to 5
[total dose/cycle = 4200 mg]
Carboplatin: I.V.: Target AUC 5 day 2
[total dose/cycle = AUC = 5]
Repeat cycle every 3 weeks

Estramustine + Docetaxel + Hydrocortisone

Use Prostate cancer

Regimen

Docetaxel: I.V.: 70 mg/m^2 day 2
[total dose/cycle = 70 mg/m^2]
Estramustine: Oral: 10 mg/kg/day days 1 to 5
[total dose/cycle = 50 mg/kg]
Hydrocortisone: Oral: 40 mg daily
[total dose/cycle = 840 mg]
Repeat cycle every 3 weeks

Estramustine + Docetaxel + Prednisone

Use Prostate cancer

Regimen

Estramustine: Oral: 280 mg 3 times/day days 1 to 5 and days 7 to 11
[total dose/cycle = 8400 mg]
Docetaxel: I.V.: 70 mg/m^2 day 2
[total dose/cycle = 70 mg/m^2]
Prednisone: Oral: 10 mg daily
[total dose/cycle = 210 mg]
Repeat cycle every 21 days for up to 6 cycles

Estramustine + Etoposide

Use Prostate cancer

Regimen NOTE: Multiple variations are listed.

Variation 1:
Estramustine: Oral: 15 mg/kg/day days 1 to 21
[total dose/cycle = 315 mg/kg]
Etoposide: Oral: 50 mg/m^2/day days 1 to 21
[total dose/cycle = 1050 mg/m^2]
Repeat cycle every 4 weeks

Variation 2:
Estramustine: Oral: 10 mg/kg/day days 1 to 21
[total dose/cycle = 210 mg/kg]
Etoposide: Oral: 50 mg/m^2/day days 1 to 21
[total dose/cycle = 1050 mg/m^2]
Repeat cycle every 4 weeks

Variation 3:
Estramustine: Oral: 140 mg 3 times/day days 1 to 21
[total dose/cycle = 8820 mg]
Etoposide: Oral: 50 mg/m^2/day days 1 to 21
[total dose/cycle = 1050 mg/m^2]
Repeat cycle every 4 weeks

Estramustine-Paclitaxel

Use Prostate cancer

Regimen NOTE: Multiple variations are listed.

Variation 1:

Paclitaxel: I.V.: 30-35 mg/m^2/day continuous infusion (given in 2-3 divided doses daily) either days 1 to 4 or days 2 to 5

[total dose/cycle = 120-140 mg/m^2]

Estramustine: Oral: 600 mg/m^2/day days 1 to 21

[total dose/cycle = 12,600 mg/m^2]

Repeat cycle every 21 days

Variation 2:

Paclitaxel: I.V. 60-107 mg/m^2 infused over 3 hours weekly for 6 weeks

[total dose/cycle = 360-642 mg/m^2]

Estramustine: Oral: 280 mg twice daily 3 days/week for 6 weeks

[total dose/cycle = 3360 mg]

Repeat cycle every 8 weeks

Variation 3:

Paclitaxel: I.V. 150 mg/m^2/day days 2, 9, and 16

[total dose/cycle = 450 mg/m^2]

Estramustine: Oral: 280 mg 3 times/day days 1, 2, 3, 8, 9, 10, 15, 16, and 17

[total dose/week = 7560 mg/m^2]

Repeat cycle every 4 weeks

Variation 4:

Paclitaxel: I.V.: 100 mg/m^2/day days 2, 9, and 16

[total dose/cycle = 300 mg/m^2]

Estramustine: Oral: 280 mg 3 times/day days 1, 2, 3, 8, 9, 10, 15, 16, and 17

[total dose/cycle = 7560 mg]

Repeat cycle every 4 weeks

Estramustine-Vinblastine

Use Prostate cancer

Regimen NOTE: Multiple variations are listed.

Variation 1:

Estramustine: Oral: 10 mg/kg/day days 1 to 42

[total dose/cycle = 420 mg/kg]

Vinblastine: I.V.: 4 mg/m^2/day days 1, 8, 15, 22, 29, and 36

[total dose/cycle = 24 mg/m^2]

Repeat cycle every 8 weeks

Variation 2:

Estramustine: Oral: 600 mg/m^2/day days 1 to 42

[total dose/cycle = 25,200 mg/m^2]

Vinblastine: I.V.: 4 mg/m^2/day days 1, 8, 15, 22, 29, and 36

[total dose/cycle = 24 mg/m^2]

Repeat cycle every 8 weeks

Estramustine + Vinorelbine

Use Prostate cancer

Regimen NOTE: Multiple variations are listed.

Variation 1:

Estramustine: Oral: 140 mg 3 times/day days 1 to 14

[total dose/cycle = 5880 mg]

Vinorelbine: I.V.: 25 mg/m^2/day days 1 and 8

[total dose/cycle = 50 mg/m^2]

Repeat cycle every 21 days

Variation 2:

Estramustine: Oral: 280 mg 3 times/day days 1, 2, and 3

[total dose/cycle = 2520 mg/m^2]

Vinorelbine: I.V.: 15 or 20 mg/m^2 day 2

[total dose/cycle = 15 or 20 mg/m^2]

Repeat cycle weekly for 8 weeks, then every other week

Etoposide-Carboplatin (Ovarian Cancer)

Use Ovarian cancer

Regimen

Etoposide: I.V.: 120 mg/m^2/day days 1, 2, and 3
[total dose/cycle = 360 mg/m^2]
Carboplatin: I.V.: 400 mg/m^2 day 1
[total dose/cycle = 400 mg/m^2]
Repeat cycle every 28 days for a total of 3 cycles

Etoposide (Ovarian Regimen)

Use Ovarian cancer

Regimen NOTE: Multiple variations are listed.

Variaition 1: (no prior radiation therapy)
Etoposide: Oral: 50 mg/m^2/day days 1 to 21
[total dose/cycle = 1050 mg/m^2]
Repeat cycle every 28 days
Variation 2: (prior radiation therapy)
Etoposide: Oral: 30 mg/m^2/day days 1 to 21
[total dose/cycle = 630 mg/m^2]
Repeat cycle every 28 days

Everolimus-Exemestane (Breast)

Use Breast cancer

Regimen

Everolimus: Oral: 10 mg once daily
Exemestane: Oral: 25 mg once daily
Continue until disease progression or unacceptable toxicity

Everolimus (RCC Regimen)

Use Renal cell cancer

Regimen

Everolimus: Oral: 10 mg once daily
[total dose/cycle = 280 mg]
Repeat cycle every 28 days until disease progression or unacceptable toxicity

FAC

Use Breast cancer

Regimen NOTE: Multiple variations are listed.

Variation 1:
Fluorouracil: I.V.: 500 mg/m^2/day days 1 and 8
[total dose/cycle = 1000 mg/m^2]
or 500 mg/m^2 day 1
[total dose/cycle = 500 mg/m^2]
Doxorubicin: I.V.: 50 mg/m^2 day 1
[total dose/cycle = 50 mg/m^2]
Cyclophosphamide: I.V.: 500 mg/m^2 day 1
[total dose/cycle = 500 mg/m^2]
Repeat cycle every 21-28 days
Variation 2:
Fluorouracil: I.V.: 200 mg/m^2/day days 1, 2, and 3
[total dose/cycle = 600 mg/m^2]
Doxorubicin: I.V.: 40 mg/m^2 day 1
[total dose/cycle = 40 mg/m^2]
Cyclophosphamide: I.V.: 400 mg/m^2 day 1
[total dose/cycle = 400 mg/m^2]
Repeat cycle every 28 days

Variation 3:

Fluorouracil: I.V.: 400 mg/m^2/day days 1 and 8
[total dose/cycle = 800 mg/m^2]
Doxorubicin: I.V.: 40 mg/m^2 day 1
[total dose/cycle = 40 mg/m^2]
Cyclophosphamide: I.V.: 400 mg/m^2 day 1
[total dose/cycle = 400 mg/m^2]
Repeat cycle every 28 days

Variation 4:

Fluorouracil: I.V.: 600 mg/m^2/day days 1 and 8
[total dose/cycle = 1200 mg/m^2]
Doxorubicin: I.V.: 60 mg/m^2 day 1
[total dose/cycle = 60 mg/m^2]
Cyclophosphamide: I.V.: 600 mg/m^2 day 1
[total dose/cycle = 600 mg/m^2]
Repeat cycle every 28 days

Variation 5:

Fluorouracil: I.V.: 300 mg/m^2/day days 1 and 8
[total dose/cycle = 600 mg/m^2]
Doxorubicin: I.V.: 30 mg/m^2 day 1
[total dose/cycle = 30 mg/m^2]
Cyclophosphamide: I.V.: 300 mg/m^2 day 1
[total dose/cycle = 300 mg/m^2]
Repeat cycle every 28 days

FEC

Use Breast cancer

Regimen

Fluorouracil: I.V.: 500 mg/m^2 day 1
[total dose/cycle = 500 mg/m^2]
Cyclophosphamide: I.V.: 500 mg/m^2 day 1
[total dose/cycle = 500 mg/m^2]
Epirubicin: I.V.: 100 mg/m^2 day 1
[total dose/cycle = 100 mg/m^2]
Repeat cycle every 21 days

FL

Use Prostate cancer

Regimen NOTE: Multiple variations are listed.

Variation 1:

Flutamide: Oral: 250 mg every 8 hours
[total dose/cycle = 21,000 mg]
Leuprolide acetate: SubQ: 1 mg/day
[total dose/cycle = 28 mg]
Repeat cycle every 28 days

Variation 2:

Flutamide: Oral: 250 mg every 8 hours
[total dose/cycle = 67,500 mg]
Leuprolide acetate depot: I.M.: 22.5 mg day 1
[total dose/cycle = 22.5 mg]
Repeat cycle every 3 months

FLAG (AML Induction)

Use Leukemia, acute myeloid

Regimen NOTE: Multiple variations are listed.

Variation 1:

Fludarabine: I.V.: 30 mg/m^2/day over 30 minutes days 1 to 5
[total dose/cycle = 150 mg/m^2]
Cytarabine: I.V.: 2 g/m^2/day over 4 hours days 1 to 5 (begin 4 hours after fludarabine infusion)
[total dose/cycle = 10 g/m^2]

Filgrastim: SubQ: 300 mcg 12 hours prior to start of fludarabine then 300 mcg/day days 2 through 5 [total dose/cycle = 1500 mcg]

followed by Filgrastim: SubQ: 300 mcg/day beginning one week after the end of treatment and continuing until complete neutrophil recovery

Variation 2:

Fludarabine: I.V.: 30 mg/m^2/day over 30 minutes days 1 to 5 [total dose/cycle = 150 mg/m^2]

Cytarabine: I.V.: 2 g/m^2/day over 4 hours days 1 to 5 (begin 3.5 hours after end of fludarabine infusion) [total dose/cycle = 10 g/m^2]

Filgrastim: SubQ: 5 mcg/kg/day beginning 24 hours prior to start of fludarabine and continuing until ANC >500 mm^3

May repeat cycle one time for partial remission

Variation 3:

Fludarabine: I.V.: 30 mg/m^2/day over 30 minutes days 1 to 5 [total dose/cycle = 150 mg/m^2]

Cytarabine: I.V.: 2 g/m^2/day over 2 hours days 1 to 5 (begin 4 hours after the start of fludarabine infusion) [total dose/cycle = 10 g/m^2]

Filgrastim: SubQ or I.V.: 300 mcg/day beginning the day prior to start of chemotherapy and continuing during chemotherapy and until ANC >1000 mm^3

May receive a second cycle

Variation 4:

Fludarabine: I.V.: 25 mg/m^2/day over 30 minutes days 1 to 5 [total dose/cycle = 125 mg/m^2]

Cytarabine: I.V.: 2 g/m^2/day over 4 hours days 1 to 5 (begin 4 hours after start of fludarabine infusion) [total dose/cycle = 10 g/m^2]

Filgrastim: SubQ: 5 mcg/kg/day beginning 24 hours prior to start of cytarabine and continuing until ANC >500 mm^3

May repeat cycle in patients with complete remission and partial remission

FLAG-IDA (AML Induction)

Use Leukemia, acute myeloid

Regimen NOTE: Multiple variations are listed.

Variation 1:

Fludarabine: I.V.: 30 mg/m^2/day over 30 minutes days 1 to 5 [total dose/cycle = 150 mg/m^2]

Cytarabine: I.V.: 2 g/m^2/day over 4 hours days 1 to 5 (begin 4 hours after the start of fludarabine) [total dose/cycle = 10 g/m^2]

Idarubicin: I.V.: 10 mg/m^2/day days 1, 2, and 3 [total dose/cycle = 30 mg/m^2]

Filgrastim: SubQ: 5 mcg/kg from day 6 until ANC >500/mm^3

Variation 2:

Fludarabine: I.V.: 30 mg/m^2/day over 30 minutes days 1 to 5 [total dose/cycle = 150 mg/m^2]

Cytarabine: I.V.: 2 g/m^2/day over 2 hours days 1 to 5 (begin 4 hours after the start of fludarabine infusion) [total dose/cycle = 10 g/m^2]

Idarubicin: I.V.: 8 mg/m^2/day over 30 minutes days 1, 2, and 3 [total dose/cycle = 24 mg/m^2]

Filgrastim: SubQ or I.V.: 300 mcg/day beginning the day prior to start of chemotherapy and continuing during chemotherapy and until ANC >1000/mm^3

May receive up to 2 cycles

Variation 3:

Fludarabine: I.V.: 30 mg/m^2/day over 30 minutes days 1 to 4 [total dose/cycle = 120 mg/m^2]

Cytarabine: I.V.: 2 g/m^2/day over 4 hours days 1 to 4 (begin 4 hours after fludarabine treatment) [total dose/cycle = 8 g/m^2]

Idarubicin: I.V.: 10 mg/m^2/day days 1, 2, and 3 [total dose/cycle = 30 mg/m^2]

Filgrastim: SubQ: see article for dose and frequency

FLOX (Colorectal)

Use Colorectal cancer

Regimen

Oxaliplatin: I.V.: 85 mg/m^2 over 2 hours days 1, 15, and 29
[total dose/cycle = 255 mg/m^2]

Leucovorin: I.V.: 500 mg/m^2/day over 2 hours weekly for 6 weeks on days 1, 8, 15, 22, 29, and 36
[total dose/cycle = 3000 mg/m^2]

Fluorouracil: I.V.: 500 mg/m^2/day bolus (1 hour after beginning the leucovorin infusion) weekly for 6 weeks on days 1, 8, 15, 22, 29, and 36
[total dose/cycle = 3000 mg/m^2]

Repeat cycle every 8 weeks for a total of 3 cycles

Fludarabine-Alemtuzumab (CLL)

Use Leukemia, chronic lymphocytic

Regimen

Prior to Cycle 1 (days -14 to -1):

Alemtuzumab dose escalation (on consecutive days): I.V.: 3 mg/dose/day (repeat until tolerated); when tolerated, increase to 10 mg/dose/day (repeat until tolerated); when tolerated, increase to 30 mg/dose

Cycle 1 (begin when alemtuzumab successfully escalated to 30 mg, but no more than 14 days from dose escalation protocol):

Alemtuzumab: I.V.: 30 mg/dose over 2 hours days 1, 2, and 3
[total dose/cycle = 90 mg]

Fludarabine: I.V.: 30 mg/m^2/day over 15-30 minutes days 1, 2, and 3 (begin with alemtuzumab at full dose)
[total dose/cycle = 90 mg/m^2]

Repeat cycle in 28 days

Cycles 2-4:

Alemtuzumab: I.V.: 30 mg/dose (over 4 hours day 1; over 2 hours days 2 and 3) days 1, 2, and 3
[total dose/cycle = 90 mg]

Fludarabine: I.V.: 30 mg/m^2/day over 15-30 minutes days 1, 2, and 3
[total dose/cycle = 90 mg/m^2]

Repeat cycle every 28 days; may administer an additional 2 cycles (cycles 5 and 6) if respond (and tolerate)

Fludarabine-Cyclophosphamide (CLL)

Use Leukemia, chronic lymphocytic

Regimen NOTE: Multiple variations are listed.

Variation 1:

Fludarabine: I.V.: 25 mg/m^2/day days 1, 2, and 3
[total dose/cycle = 75 mg/m^2]

Cyclophosphamide: I.V.: 250 mg/m^2/day days 1, 2, and 3
[total dose/cycle = 750 mg/m^2]

Repeat cycle every 4 weeks for up to 6 cycles

Variation 2:

Fludarabine: I.V.: 30 mg/m^2/day days 1, 2, and 3
[total dose/cycle = 90 mg/m^2]

Cyclophosphamide: I.V.: 250 mg/m^2/day days 1, 2, and 3
[total dose/cycle = 750 mg/m^2]

Repeat cycle every 4 weeks for up to 6 cycles

Variation 3:

Cyclophosphamide: I.V.: 600 mg/m^2 day 1
[total dose/cycle = 600 mg/m^2]

Fludarabine: I.V.: 20 mg/m^2/day days 1 to 5
[total dose/cycle = 100 mg/m^2]

Repeat cycle every 4 weeks for up to 6 cycles

Variation 4:

Fludarabine: I.V.: 30 mg/m^2/day days 1, 2, and 3
[total dose/cycle = 90 mg/m^2]

Cyclophosphamide: I.V.: 300 mg/m^2/day days 1, 2, and 3
[total dose/cycle = 900 mg/m^2]

Repeat cycle every 4 weeks for up to 6 cycles

Variation 5:
Fludarabine: I.V.: 30 mg/m^2/day days 1, 2, and 3
[total dose/cycle = 90 mg/m^2]
Cyclophosphamide: I.V.: 300 mg/m^2/day days 1, 2, and 3
[total dose/cycle = 900 mg/m^2]
Repeat cycle every 4-6 weeks for up to 6 cycles

Fludarabine-Cyclophosphamide-Mitoxantrone-Rituximab

Use Lymphoma, non-Hodgkin

Regimen NOTE: Multiple variations are listed.

Consider pretherapy cytoreduction with cyclophosphamide 200 mg/m^2/day for 3-5 days for patients with high tumor burden and/or lymphocytes >20,000/mm^3

Variation 1:
Rituximab: I.V.: 375 mg/m^2/dose day 1
[total dose/cycle = 375 mg/m^2]
Fludarabine: I.V.: 25 mg/m^2/day days 2, 3, and 4
[total dose/cycle = 75 mg/m^2]
Cyclophosphamide: I.V.: 200 mg/m^2/day days 2, 3, and 4
[total dose/cycle = 600 mg/m^2]
Mitoxantrone: I.V.: 8 mg/m^2/dose day 2
[total dose/cycle = 8 mg/m^2]
Repeat cycle every 28 days for total of 4 cycles

Variation 2 (with maintenance rituximab):
Rituximab: I.V.: 375 mg/m^2/dose day 1
[total dose/cycle = 375 mg/m^2]
Fludarabine: I.V.: 25 mg/m^2/day days 2, 3, and 4
[total dose/cycle = 75 mg/m^2]
Cyclophosphamide: I.V.: 200 mg/m^2/day days 2, 3, and 4
[total dose/cycle = 600 mg/m^2]
Mitoxantrone: I.V.: 8 mg/m^2/dose day 2
[total dose/cycle = 8 mg/m^2]
Repeat cycle every 28 days for total of 4 cycles
followed by:
Maintenance rituximab (begin 3 months after completion of cycle 4):
Rituximab: I.V.: 375 mg/m^2/dose day 1, 8, 15, and 22
[total dose/cycle = 1500 mg/m^2]
Repeat maintenance cycle (once) in 6 months

Fludarabine-Cyclophosphamide (NHL-Mantle Cell)

Use Lymphoma, non-Hodgkin (mantle cell)

Regimen NOTE: Multiple variations are listed.

Variation 1:
Fludarabine: I.V.: 20 mg/m^2/day days 1 to 5
[total dose/cycle = 100 mg/m^2]
Cyclophosphamide: I.V.: 800 mg/m^2/dose day 1
[total dose/cycle = 800 mg/m^2]
Repeat cycle every 3-4 weeks for up to a total of 5 cycles

Variation 2:
Fludarabine: I.V.: 20 mg/m^2/day days 1 to 5
[total dose/cycle = 100 mg/m^2]
Cyclophosphamide: I.V.: 1000 mg/m^2/dose day 1
[total dose/cycle = 1000 mg/m^2]
Repeat cycle every 3-4 weeks for up to a total of 5 cycles

Variation 3:
Fludarabine: I.V.: 25 mg/m^2/day days 1 to 4
[total dose/cycle = 100 mg/m^2]
Cyclophosphamide: I.V.: 1000 mg/m^2/dose day 1
[total dose/cycle = 1000 mg/m^2]
Repeat cycle every 3-4 weeks for up to a total of 5 cycles

Fludarabine-Cyclophosphamide-Rituximab (CLL)

Use Leukemia, chronic lymphocytic

Regimen

Cycle 1:
- Rituximab: I.V.: 375 mg/m^2 day 1
  [total dose/cycle = 375 mg/m^2]
- Fludarabine: I.V.: 25 mg/m^2/day days 2, 3, and 4
  [total dose/cycle = 75 mg/m^2]
- Cyclophosphamide: I.V.: 250 mg/m^2/day days 2, 3, and 4
  [total dose/cycle = 750 mg/m^2]
- Treatment cycle is 4 weeks

Cycles 2-6:
- Rituximab: I.V.: 500 mg/m^2 day 1
  [total dose/cycle = 500 mg/m^2]
- Fludarabine: I.V.: 25 mg/m^2/day days 1, 2, and 3
  [total dose/cycle = 75 mg/m^2]
- Cyclophosphamide: I.V.: 250 mg/m^2/day days 1, 2, and 3
  [total dose/cycle = 750 mg/m^2]
- Repeat cycle every 4 weeks

Fludarabine-Cyclophosphamide-Rituximab (NHL-Follicular)

Use Lymphoma, non-Hodgkin (Follicular lymphoma)

Regimen

Cycle 1:
- Rituximab: I.V.: 375 mg/m^2 day 15
  [total dose/cycle = 375 mg/m^2]
- Fludarabine: I.V.: 25 mg/m^2/day days 1, 2, and 3
  [total dose/cycle = 75 mg/m^2]
- Cyclophosphamide: I.V.: 300 mg/m^2/day days 1, 2, and 3
  [total dose/cycle = 900 mg/m^2]
- Treatment cycle is 3 weeks

Cycles 2-4:
- Rituximab: I.V.: 375 mg/m^2 day 1
  [total dose/cycle = 375 mg/m^2]
- Fludarabine: I.V.: 25 mg/m^2/day days 1, 2, and 3
  [total dose/cycle = 75 mg/m^2]
- Cyclophosphamide: I.V.: 300 mg/m^2/day days 1, 2, and 3
  [total dose/cycle = 900 mg/m^2]
- Each treatment cycle is 3 weeks

Fludarabine-Mitoxantrone

Use Lymphoma, non-Hodgkin

Regimen

- Fludarabine: I.V.: 25 mg/m^2/day days 1, 2, and 3
  [total dose/cycle = 75 mg/m^2]
- Mitoxantrone: I.V.: 10 mg/m^2/dose day 1
  [total dose/cycle = 10 mg/m^2]
- Repeat cycle every 21 days for total of 6 cycles

Fludarabine-Mitoxantrone-Dexamethasone (NHL)

Use Lymphoma, non-Hodgkin

Regimen

- Fludarabine: I.V.: 25 mg/m^2/day days 1, 2, and 3
  [total dose/cycle = 75 mg/m^2]
- Mitoxantrone: I.V.: 10 mg/m^2/dose day 1
  [total dose/cycle = 10 mg/m^2]
- Dexamethasone: I.V. or Oral: 20 mg/day days 1 to 5
  [total dose/cycle = 100 mg]
- Repeat cycle every 28 days for up to a total of 8 cycles

Fludarabine-Mitoxantrone-Dexamethasone-Rituximab

Use Lymphoma, non-Hodgkin

Regimen

Cycle 1:

Rituximab: I.V.: 375 mg/m^2/day days 1 and 8
[total dose/cycle = 750 mg/m^2]

Fludarabine: I.V.: 25 mg/m^2/day days 1, 2, and 3
[total dose/cycle = 75 mg/m^2]

Mitoxantrone: I.V.: 10 mg/m^2/dose day 1
[total dose/cycle = 10 mg/m^2]

Dexamethasone: I.V. or Oral: 20 mg/m^2/day days 1 to 5
[total dose/cycle = 100 mg/m^2]

Treatment cycle is 28 days

Cycles 2-5:

Rituximab: I.V.: 375 mg/m^2 day 1
[total dose/cycle = 375 mg/m^2]

Fludarabine: I.V.: 25 mg/m^2/day days 2, 3, and 4
[total dose/cycle = 75 mg/m^2]

Mitoxantrone: I.V.: 10 mg/m^2/dose day 2
[total dose/cycle = 10 mg/m^2]

Dexamethasone: I.V. or Oral: 20 mg/m^2/day days 1 to 5
[total dose/cycle = 100 mg/m^2]

Repeat cycle every 28 days

Cycles 6-8:

Fludarabine: I.V.: 25 mg/m^2/day days 1, 2, and 3
[total dose/cycle = 75 mg/m^2]

Mitoxantrone: I.V.: 10 mg/m^2/dose day 1
[total dose/cycle = 10 mg/m^2]

Dexamethasone: I.V. or Oral: 20 mg/m^2/day days 1 to 5
[total dose/cycle = 100 mg/m^2]

Repeat cycle every 28 days

followed by:

Interferon maintenance:

Interferon alfa-2b: SubQ: 3 million units/m^2 days 1 to 14
[total dose/cycle = 42 million units/m^2]

Dexamethasone: Oral: 8 mg/day days 1, 2, and 3
[total dose/cycle = 24 mg]

Repeat cycle every month for 1 year

Fludarabine-Mitoxantrone-Rituximab

Use Lymphoma, non-Hodgkin

Regimen

Fludarabine: I.V.: 25 mg/m^2/day days 1, 2, and 3
[total dose/cycle = 75 mg/m^2]

Mitoxantrone: I.V.: 10 mg/m^2/dose day 1
[total dose/cycle = 10 mg/m^2]

Repeat cycle every 21 days for total of 6 cycles

followed by:

Sequential rituximab (after completion of cycle 6):

Rituximab: I.V.: 375 mg/m^2/dose weekly for 4 doses
[total dose/4 weeks = 1500 mg/m^2]

Fludarabine-Rituximab (CLL)

Use Leukemia, chronic lymphocytic

Regimen

Rituximab: I.V.: 375 mg/m^2/day days 1 and 4 (cycle 1); day 1 (cycles 2 to 6)

Fludarabine: I.V.: 25 mg/m^2/day days 1 to 5

Repeat cycle every 4 weeks

Fludarabine-Rituximab (NHL-Follicular)

Use Lymphoma, non-Hodgkin (follicular lymphoma)

Regimen

Week 1:
Rituximab: I.V.: 375 mg/m^2/dose for 2 doses 4 days apart
[total dose/week = 750 mg/m^2]
Week 2:
Fludarabine: I.V.: 25 mg/m^2/day days 1 to 5
[total dose/week = 125 mg/m^2]
Week 5:
Rituximab: I.V.: 375 mg/m^2/dose day 5
[total dose/week = 375 mg/m^2]
Week 6:
Fludarabine: I.V.: 25 mg/m^2/day days 1 to 5
[total dose/week = 125 mg/m^2]
Week 10:
Fludarabine: I.V.: 25 mg/m^2/day days 1 to 5
[total dose/week = 125 mg/m^2]
Week 13:
Rituximab: I.V.: 375 mg/m^2/dose day 5
[total dose/week = 375 mg/m^2]
Week 14:
Fludarabine: I.V.: 25 mg/m^2/day days 1 to 5
[total dose/week = 125 mg/m^2]
Week 18:
Fludarabine: I.V.: 25 mg/m^2/day days 1 to 5
[total dose/week = 125 mg/m^2]
Week 21:
Rituximab: I.V.: 375 mg/m^2/dose day 5
[total dose/week = 375 mg/m^2]
Week 22:
Fludarabine: I.V.: 25 mg/m^2/day days 1 to 5
[total dose/week = 125 mg/m^2]
Week 26:
Rituximab: I.V.: 375 mg/m^2/dose for 2 doses 4 days apart
[total dose/week = 750 mg/m^2]

Fluorouracil-Carboplatin (Head and Neck Cancer)

Use Head and neck cancer

Regimen NOTE: Multiple variations are listed.

Variation 1:
Fluorouracil: I.V.: 600 mg/m^2/day continuous infusion days 1 to 4
[total dose/cycle = 2400 mg/m^2]
Carboplatin: I.V.: 70 mg/m^2/day days 1 to 4
[total dose/cycle = 280 mg/m^2]
Repeat cycle every 3 weeks for 3 cycles
Variation 2:
Fluorouracil: I.V.: 1000 mg/m^2/day continuous infusion days 1 to 4
[total dose/cycle = 4000 mg/m^2]
Carboplatin: I.V.: 300 mg/m^2/dose day 1 (may escalate to 360 mg/m^2/dose in future cycles for grade 0 or 1 hematologic toxicity)
[total dose/cycle = 300-360 mg/m^2]
Repeat cycle every 28 weeks
Variation 3:
Carboplatin: I.V.: 400 mg/m^2 day 1
[total dose/cycle = 400 mg/m^2]
Fluorouracil: I.V.: 1000 mg/m^2/day continuous infusion days 1 to 4
[total dose/cycle = 4000 mg/m^2]
Repeat cycle every 28 days for a total of 2 or 3 cycles

Fluorouracil-Hydroxyurea (Head and Neck Cancer)

Use Head and neck cancer

Regimen NOTE: Administered with concurrent radiation therapy

Fluorouracil: I.V.: 800 mg/m^2/day continuous infusion days 1 to 5
[total dose/cycle = 4000 mg/m^2]

Hydroxyurea: Oral: 1000 mg/dose every 12 hours for 11 doses beginning day 1
[total dose/cycle = 11,000 mg]

Repeat cycle every other week for a total therapy duration of 13 weeks

Fluorouracil-Leucovorin

Use Colorectal cancer

Regimen NOTE: Multiple variations are listed.

Variation 1 (Mayo Regimen):
Fluorouracil: I.V.: 370-425 mg/m^2/day days 1 to 5
[total dose/cycle = 1850-2125 mg/m^2]
Leucovorin: I.V.: 20 mg/m^2/day days 1 to 5
[total dose/cycle = 100 mg/m^2]
Repeat cycle at 4 weeks, 8 weeks, and every 5 weeks thereafter

Variation 2:
Fluorouracil: I.V.: 400 mg/m^2/day days 1 to 5
[total dose/cycle = 2000 mg/m^2]
Leucovorin: I.V.: 20 mg/m^2/day days 1 to 5
[total dose/cycle = 100 mg/m^2]
Repeat cycle every 28 days

Variation 3:
Fluorouracil: I.V.: 500 mg/m^2 day 1
[total dose/cycle = 500 mg/m^2]
Leucovorin: I.V.: 20 mg/m^2 (2-hour infusion) day 1
[total dose/cycle = 20 mg/m^2]
Repeat cycle weekly

Variation 4:
Fluorouracil: I.V.: 600 mg/m^2 weekly for 6 weeks
[total dose/cycle = 3600 mg/m^2]
Leucovorin: I.V.: 500 mg/m^2 (3-hour infusion) weekly for 6 weeks
[total dose/cycle = 3000 mg/m^2]
Repeat cycle every 8 weeks

Variation 5:
Fluorouracil: I.V.: 600 mg/m^2 weekly for 6 weeks
[total dose/cycle = 3600 mg/m^2]
Leucovorin: I.V.: 500 mg/m^2 (2-hour infusion) weekly for 6 weeks
[total dose/cycle = 3000 mg/m^2]
Repeat cycle every 8 weeks

Variation 6:
Fluorouracil: I.V.: 600 mg/m^2 weekly
[total dose/cycle = 600 mg/m^2]
Leucovorin: I.V.: 500 mg/m^2 (2-hour infusion) weekly
[total dose/cycle = 500 mg/m^2]
Repeat cycle weekly

Variation 7:
Fluorouracil: I.V.: 2600 mg/m^2 continuous infusion over 24 hours day 1
[total dose/cycle = 2600 mg/m^2]
Leucovorin: I.V.: 500 mg/m^2 continuous infusion over 24 hours day 1
[total dose/cycle = 500 mg/m^2]
Repeat cycle weekly

Variation 8:
Fluorouracil: I.V.: 2600 mg/m^2 continuous infusion over 24 hours day 1
[total dose/cycle = 2600 mg/m^2]
Leucovorin: I.V.: 300 mg/m^2 (maximum dose: 500 mg) continuous infusion over 24 hours day 1
[total dose/cycle = 300 mg/m^2; maximum: 500 mg]
Repeat cycle weekly

Variation 9:
Fluorouracil: I.V.: 2600 mg/m^2 continuous infusion over 24 hours once weekly for 6 weeks
[total dose/cycle = 15,600 mg/m^2]
Leucovorin: I.V.: 500 mg/m^2 over 2 hours once weekly for 6 weeks
[total dose/cycle = 3000 mg/m^2]
Repeat cycle every 8 weeks

Variation 10:
Fluorouracil: I.V.: 2300 mg/m^2 continuous infusion over 24 hours day 1
[total dose/cycle = 2300 mg/m^2]
Leucovorin: I.V.: 50 mg/m^2 continuous infusion over 24 hours day 1
[total dose/cycle = 50 mg/m^2]
Repeat cycle weekly

Variation 11:
Fluorouracil: I.V.: 200 mg/m^2/day continuous infusion days 1 to 14
[total dose/cycle = 2800 mg/m^2]
Leucovorin: I.V.: 5 mg/m^2/day continuous infusion days 1 to 14
[total dose/cycle = 70 mg/m^2]
Repeat cycle every 28 days

Variation 12:
Cycle 1:
Fluorouracil: I.V.: 200 mg/m^2/day continuous infusion for 4 weeks
[total dose/cycle = 5600 mg/m^2]
Leucovorin: I.V.: 20 mg/m^2/day days 1, 8, 15, 22
[total dose/cycle = 80 mg/m^2]
Treatment cycle is 6 weeks
Subsequent cycles (starting week 7):
Fluorouracil: 200 mg/m^2 continuous infusion days 1 to 21
[total dose/cycle = 4200 mg/m^2]
Leucovorin: I.V.: 20 mg/m^2/day days 1, 8, and 15
[total dose/cycle = 60 mg/m^2]
Repeat cycle every 4 weeks

Fluorouracil-Leucovorin-Irinotecan (Saltz Regimen)

Use Colorectal cancer

Regimen

Fluorouracil: I.V.: 500 mg/m^2/day days 1, 8, 15, and 22
[total dose/cycle = 2000 mg/m^2]
Leucovorin: I.V.: 20 mg/m^2/day days 1, 8, 15, and 22
[total dose/cycle = 80 mg/m^2]
Irinotecan: I.V.: 125 mg/m^2/day days 1, 8, 15, and 22
[total dose/cycle = 500 mg/m^2]
Repeat cycle every 42 days

Fluorouracil-Leucovorin-Oxaliplatin (Esophageal Cancer)

Use Esophageal Cancer

Regimen NOTE: Multiple variations are listed.

Variation 1:
Oxaliplatin: I.V.: 85 mg/m^2/dose over 2 hours day 1
[total dose/cycle = 85 mg/m^2]
Leucovorin: I.V.: 200 mg/m^2/dose over 2 hours day 1
[total dose/cycle = 200 mg/m^2]
Fluorouracil: I.V.: 2600 mg/m^2/dose continuous infusion over 24 hours day 1
[total dose/cycle = 2600 mg/m^2]
Repeat cycle every 2 weeks until disease progression or unacceptable toxicity.

Variation 2:
Oxaliplatin: I.V.: 85 mg/m^2/dose over 2 hours day 1
[total dose/cycle = 85 mg/m^2]
Leucovorin: I.V.: 500 mg/m^2/day over 2 hours days 1 and 2
[total dose/cycle = 1000 mg/m^2]

Fluorouracil: I.V. bolus: 400 mg/m²/day days 1 and 2
followed by I.V.: 600 mg/m²/day continuous infusion over 22 hours days 1 and 2
[total dose/cycle = 2000 mg/m²]
Repeat cycle every 2 weeks for 4 cycles (if achieve stable disease or response, continue until disease progression or unacceptable toxicity).

Variation 3:
Oxaliplatin: I.V.: 85 mg/m²/dose day 1
[total dose/cycle = 85 mg/m²]
Leucovorin: I.V.: 200 mg/m²/day over 2 hours days 1 and 2
[total dose/cycle = 400 mg/m²]
Fluorouracil: I.V. bolus: 400 mg/m²/day days 1 and 2
followed by I.V.: 600 mg/m²/day continuous infusion over 22 hours days 1 and 2
[total dose/cycle = 2000 mg/m²]
Repeat cycle every 2 weeks for 6 cycles (3 cycles with radiation therapy and 3 cycles after completion of radiation therapy).

Fluorouracil-Leucovorin-Oxaliplatin (Gastric Cancer)

Use Gastric cancer

Regimen NOTE: Multiple variations are listed.

Variation 1:
Oxaliplatin: I.V.: 85 mg/m²/dose over 2 hours day 1
[total dose/cycle = 85 mg/m²]
Leucovorin: I.V.: 200 mg/m²/dose over 2 hours day 1
[total dose/cycle = 200 mg/m²]
Fluorouracil: I.V.: 2600 mg/m²/dose continuous infusion over 24 hours day 1
[total dose/cycle = 2600 mg/m²]
Repeat cycle every 2 weeks until disease progression or unacceptable toxicity

Variation 2:
Oxaliplatin: I.V.: 100 mg/m²/dose over 2 hours day 1
[total dose/cycle = 100 mg/m²]
Leucovorin: I.V.: 400 mg/m²/dose over 2 hours day 1
[total dose/cycle = 400 mg/m²]
Fluorouracil: I.V. bolus: 400 mg/m²/dose over 10 minutes day 1
followed by I.V.: 3000 mg/m² continuous infusion over 46 hours beginning day 1
[total dose/cycle = 3400 mg/m²]
Repeat cycle every 2 weeks until disease progression or unacceptable toxicity for at least 6 cycles

Variation 3:
Oxaliplatin: I.V.: 85 mg/m²/dose over 2 hours day 1
[total dose/cycle = 85 mg/m²]
Leucovorin: I.V.: 500 mg/m²/dose over 2 hours day 1
[total dose/cycle = 500 mg/m²]
Fluorouracil: I.V.: 2600 mg/m²/dose continuous infusion over 24 hours day 1
[total dose/cycle = 2600 mg/m²]
Repeat cycle every 2 weeks until disease progression or unacceptable toxicity

Fluorouracil-Mitomycin (Anal Cancer)

Use Anal cancer

Regimen NOTE: Multiple variations are listed.

Variation 1 (in combination with radiotherapy):
Fluorouracil: I.V.: 1000 mg/m²/day continuous infusion days 1 to 4 and days 29 to 32
[total dose/cycle = 8000 mg/m²]
Mitomycin: I.V.: 10 mg/m²/day (maximum dose: 20 mg) days 1 and 29
[total dose/cycle = 20 mg/m²; maximum: 40 mg]

Variation 2 (in combination with radiotherapy):
Fluorouracil: I.V.: 1000 mg/m²/day continuous infusion days 1 to 4
[total dose/cycle = 4000 mg/m²]
Mitomycin: I.V.: 10 mg/m²/dose (maximum dose: 20 mg) day 1
[total dose/cycle = 10 mg/m²; maximum: 20 mg]
Repeat cycle in 28 days (total of 2 cycles)

FOLFIRI (Colorectal Cancer)

Use Colorectal cancer

Regimen NOTE: Multiple variations are listed.

Variation 1:

Cycles 1 and 2:

Irinotecan: I.V.: 180 mg/m^2 over 90 minutes day 1
[total dose/cycle = 180 mg/m^2]

Leucovorin: I.V.: 400 mg/m^2 over 2 hours day 1
[total dose/cycle = 400 mg/m^2]

Fluorouracil: I.V. bolus: 400 mg/m^2 day 1
followed by I.V.: 2400 mg/m^2 continuous infusion (over 46 hours) beginning day 1
[total fluorouracil dose/cycle = 2800 mg/m^2]

Repeat cycle in 14 days

Subsequent cycles:

Irinotecan: I.V.: 180 mg/m^2 over 90 minutes day 1
[total dose/cycle = 180 mg/m^2]

Leucovorin: I.V.: 400 mg/m^2 over 2 hours day 1
[total dose/cycle = 400 mg/m^2]

Fluorouracil: I.V. bolus: 400 mg/m^2 day 1
followed by I.V.: 3000 mg/m^2 continuous infusion (over 46 hours) beginning day 1
[total fluorouracil dose/cycle = 3400 mg/m^2]

Repeat cycle every 14 days until disease progression or unacceptable toxicity

Variation 2:

Irinotecan: I.V.: 180 mg/m^2 over 90 minutes day 1
[total dose/cycle = 180 mg/m^2]

Leucovorin: I.V.: 200 mg/m^2/day over 2 hours days 1 and 2
[total dose/cycle = 400 mg/m^2]

Fluorouracil: I.V. bolus: 400 mg/m^2/day days 1 and 2
followed by I.V.: 600 mg/m^2/day continuous infusion (over 22 hours each day) on days 1 and 2
[total fluorouracil dose/cycle = 2000 mg/m^2]

Repeat cycle every 14 days until disease progression or unacceptable toxicity

Variation 3:

Irinotecan: I.V.: 180 mg/m^2 over 1 hour day 1
[total dose/cycle = 180 mg/m^2]

Leucovorin: I.V.: 100 mg/m^2/day over 2 hours days 1 and 2
[total dose/cycle = 200 mg/m^2]

Fluorouracil: I.V. bolus: 400 mg/m^2/day days 1 and 2
followed by I.V.: 600 mg/m^2/day continuous infusion (over 22 hours each day) on days 1 and 2
[total fluorouracil dose/cycle = 2000 mg/m^2]

Repeat cycle every 14 days for up to 12 cycles or until disease progression or unacceptable toxicity

Variation 4:

Irinotecan: I.V.: 180 mg/m^2 over 90 minutes day 1
[total dose/cycle = 180 mg/m^2]

Leucovorin: I.V.: 400 mg/m^2 over 2 hours day 1
[total dose/cycle = 400 mg/m^2]

Fluorouracil: I.V. bolus: 400 mg/m^2 day 1
followed by I.V.: 2400 mg/m^2 continuous infusion (over 46 hours) beginning day 1
[total fluorouracil dose/cycle = 2800 mg/m^2]

Repeat cycle every 14 days until disease progression or unacceptable toxicity

FOLFIRINOX (Pancreatic)

Use Pancreatic cancer

Regimen

Oxaliplatin: I.V.: 85 mg/m^2 over 2 hours day 1
[total dose/cycle = 85 mg/m^2]

Leucovorin: I.V.: 400 mg/m^2 over 2 hours day 1
[total dose/cycle = 400 mg/m^2]

Irinotecan: I.V.: 180 mg/m^2 over 90 minutes day 1
[total dose/cycle = 180 mg/m^2]

Fluorouracil: I.V. bolus: 400 mg/m^2 day 1
followed by I.V.: 2400 mg/m^2 continuous infusion (CI) over 46 hours beginning day 1
[total fluorouracil dose/cycle (bolus and CI) = 2800 mg/m^2]
Note: Bolus and CI fluorouracil are both given on day 1
Repeat cycle every 14 days until disease progression or unacceptable toxicity, 12 cycles recommended

FOLFOX 1 (Colorectal)

Use Colorectal cancer

Regimen

Oxaliplatin: I.V.: 130 mg/m^2 over 2 hours day 1 (every other cycle)
[total dose/cycle = 130 mg/m^2]
Leucovorin: I.V.: 500 mg/m^2/day over 2 hours days 1 and 2
[total dose/cycle = 1000 mg/m^2]
Fluorouracil: I.V.: 1500-2000 mg/m^2/day continuous infusion over 22 hours days 1 and 2
[total dose/cycle = 3000-4000 mg/m^2]
Repeat cycle every 14 days until disease progression or unacceptable toxicity

FOLFOX 2 (Colorectal)

Use Colorectal cancer

Regimen

Oxaliplatin: I.V.: 100 mg/m^2 over 2 hours day 1
[total dose/cycle = 100 mg/m^2]
Leucovorin: I.V.: 500 mg/m^2/day over 2 hours days 1 and 2
[total dose/cycle = 1000 mg/m^2]
Fluorouracil: I.V.: 1500-2000 mg/m^2/day continuous infusion over 22 hours days 1 and 2
[total dose/cycle = 3000-4000 mg/m^2]
Repeat cycle every 14 days until disease progression or unacceptable toxicity

FOLFOX 3 (Colorectal)

Use Colorectal cancer

Regimen

Oxaliplatin: I.V.: 85 mg/m^2 over 2 hours day 1
[total dose/cycle = 85 mg/m^2]
Leucovorin: I.V.: 500 mg/m^2/day over 2 hours days 1 and 2
[total dose/cycle = 1000 mg/m^2]
Fluorouracil: I.V.: 1500-2000 mg/m^2/day continuous infusion over 22 hours days 1 and 2
[total dose/cycle = 3000-4000 mg/m^2]
Repeat cycle every 14 days until disease progression or unacceptable toxicity

FOLFOX 4

Use Colorectal cancer

Regimen

Oxaliplatin: I.V.: 85 mg/m^2 day 1
[total dose/cycle = 85 mg/m^2]
Leucovorin: I.V.: 200 mg/m^2/day days 1 and 2
[total dose/cycle = 400 mg/m^2]
Fluorouracil: I.V. bolus: 400 mg/m^2/day days 1 and 2
[total dose/cycle = 800 mg/m^2]
followed by I.V.: 600 mg/m^2 continuous infusion (over 22 hours) days 1 and 2
[total dose/cycle = 1200 mg/m^2]
Note: Bolus fluorouracil and continuous infusion are both given on each day.
Repeat cycle every 14 days

FOLFOX 6

Use Colorectal cancer

Regimen

Oxaliplatin: I.V.: 100 mg/m^2 day 1
[total dose/cycle = 100 mg/m^2]
Leucovorin: I.V.: 400 mg/m^2 day 1
[total dose/cycle = 400 mg/m^2]

Fluorouracil: I.V. bolus: 400 mg/m^2 day 1
[total dose/cycle = 400 mg/m^2]
followed by I.V.: 2.4-3 g/m^2 continuous infusion (46 hours) extending over days 1 and 2
[total dose/cycle = 2.4-3 g/m^2]
Repeat cycle every 14 days

FOLFOX 7

Use Colorectal cancer

Regimen

Oxaliplatin: I.V.: 130 mg/m^2 day 1
[total dose/cycle = 130 mg/m^2]
Leucovorin: I.V.: 400 mg/m^2 day 1
[total dose/cycle = 400 mg/m^2]
Fluorouracil: I.V. bolus: 400 mg/m^2 day 1
[total dose/cycle = 400 mg/m^2]
followed by I.V.: 2.4 g/m^2 continuous infusion (46 hours) extending over days 1 and 2
[total dose/cycle = 2.4 g/m^2]
Repeat cycle every 14 days

FOLFOXIRI (Colorectal)

Use Colorectal cancer

Regimen

Irinotecan: I.V.: 165 mg/m^2 over 1 hour day 1
[total dose/cycle = 165 mg/m^2]
Oxaliplatin: I.V.: 85 mg/m^2 over 2 hours day 1
[total dose/cycle = 85 mg/m^2]
Leucovorin: I.V.: 200 mg/m^2 over 2 hours day 1
[total dose/cycle = 200 mg/m^2]
Fluorouracil: I.V.: 3200 mg/m^2 continuous infusion over 48 hours beginning day 1
[total dose/cycle = 3200 mg/m^2]
Repeat cycle every 14 days for a maximum of 12 cycles

FOLFOX (Pancreatic)

Use Pancreatic cancer

Regimen

Oxaliplatin: I.V.: 100 mg/m^2 day 1
[total dose/cycle = 100 mg/m^2]
Leucovorin: I.V.: 400 mg/m^2 day 1
[total dose/cycle = 400 mg/m^2]
Fluorouracil: I.V. bolus: 400 mg/m^2 day 1
followed by I.V.: 3000 mg/m^2 continuous infusion (CI) over 46 hours beginning day 1
[total fluorouracil dose/cycle (bolus and CI) = 3400 mg/m^2]
Repeat cycle every 14 days until disease progression or unacceptable toxicity

FU-LV-CPT-11

Use Colorectal cancer

Regimen NOTE: Multiple variations are listed.

Variation 1:
Irinotecan: I.V.: 350 mg/m^2 day 1
[total dose/cycle = 350 mg/m^2]
Leucovorin: I.V.: 20 mg/m^2/day days 22 to 26
[total dose/cycle = 100 mg/m^2]
Fluorouracil: I.V.: 425 mg/m^2/day days 22 to 26
[total dose/cycle = 2125 mg/m^2]
Repeat cycle every 6 weeks

Variation 2:
Irinotecan: I.V.: 80 mg/m^2 day 1
[total dose/cycle = 80 mg/m^2]
Fluorouracil: I.V.: 2300 mg/m^2 continuous infusion day 1
[total dose/cycle = 2300 mg/m^2]
Leucovorin: I.V.: 500 mg/m^2 day 1
[total dose/cycle = 500 mg/m^2]
Repeat cycle weekly
or
Irinotecan: I.V.: 180 mg/m^2 day 1
[total dose/cycle = 180 mg/m^2]
Leucovorin: I.V.: 200 mg/m^2/day days 1 and 2
[total dose/cycle = 400 mg/m^2]
Fluorouracil: I.V.: 400 mg/m^2/day days 1 and 2
[total dose/cycle = 800 mg/m^2]
followed by I.V.: 600 mg/m^2/day continuous infusion days 1 and 2
[total dose/cycle = 1200 mg/m^2]
Repeat cycle every 2 weeks
Variation 3:
Irinotecan: I.V.: 175 mg/m^2 day 1
[total dose/cycle = 175 mg/m^2]
Leucovorin: I.V.: 250 mg/m^2 day 2
[total dose/cycle = 250 mg/m^2]
Fluorouracil: I.V.: 950 mg/m^2 day 2
[total dose/cycle = 950 mg/m^2]
or
Irinotecan: I.V.: 200 mg/m^2 day 1
[total dose/cycle = 200 mg/m^2]
Leucovorin: I.V.: 250 mg/m^2 day 2
[total dose/cycle = 250 mg/m^2]
Fluorouracil: I.V.: 850 mg/m^2 day 2
[total dose/cycle = 850 mg/m^2]
Repeat cycle every other week

FZ

Use Prostate cancer

Regimen NOTE: Multiple variations are listed.
Variation 1:
Flutamide: Oral: 250 mg every 8 hours
[total dose/cycle = 21,000 mg]
Goserelin acetate: SubQ: 3.6 mg day 1
[total dose/cycle = 3.6 mg]
Repeat cycle every 28 days
Variation 2:
Flutamide: Oral: 250 mg every 8 hours
[total dose/cycle = 67,500 mg]
Goserelin acetate: SubQ: 10.8 mg day 1
[total dose/cycle = 10.8 mg]
Repeat cycle every 3 months

GDP (Hodgkin)

Use Lymphoma, Hodgkin

Regimen
Gemcitabine: I.V.: 1000 mg/m^2 over 30 minutes days 1 and 8
[total dose/cycle = 2000 mg/m^2]
Dexamethasone: Oral: 40 mg/day (divided doses) days 1 to 4
[total dose/cycle = 160 mg]
Cisplatin: I.V.: 75 mg/m^2 over 1 hour day 1, administer after gemcitabine
[total dose/cycle = 75 mg/m^2]
Repeat cycle every 21 days; consider stem cell transplantation after 2 cycles in responding patients; and a maximum of 6 cycles in nontransplant candidates

Gemcitabine-Capecitabine (Biliary Cancer)

Use Biliary adenocarcinoma

Regimen

Gemcitabine: I.V.: 1000 mg/m^2/day over 30 minutes days 1 and 8
[total dose/cycle = 2000 mg/m^2]
Capecitabine: Oral: 650 mg/m^2 twice daily days 1 to 14
[total dose/cycle = 18,200 mg/m^2]
Repeat cycle every 21 days until disease progression or unacceptable toxicity

Gemcitabine-Capecitabine (RCC)

Use Renal cell cancer

Regimen NOTE: Multiple variations are listed.

Variation 1:
Gemcitabine: I.V.: 1000 mg/m^2/day days 1, 8, and 15
[total dose/cycle = 3000 mg/m^2]
Capecitabine: Oral: 830 mg/m^2/dose twice daily on days 1 to 21
[total dose/cycle = 34,860 mg/m^2]
Repeat cycle every 28 days

Variation 2 (for patients with Cl_{cr} 30-50 mL/minute):
Gemcitabine: I.V.: 1000 mg/m^2/day days 1, 8, and 15
[total dose/cycle = 3000 mg/m^2]
Capecitabine: Oral: 622 mg/m^2/dose twice daily on days 1 to 21
[total dose/cycle = 26,124 mg/m^2]
Repeat cycle every 28 days

Variation 3:
Gemcitabine: I.V.: 1200 mg/m^2/day days 1 and 8
[total dose/cycle = 2400 mg/m^2]
Capecitabine: Oral: 1300 mg/m^2/dose twice daily on days 1 to 14
[total dose/cycle = 36,400 mg/m^2]
Repeat cycle every 21 days for up to 6 cycles

Gemcitabine-Carboplatin (Bladder Cancer)

Use Bladder cancer

Regimen

Gemcitabine: I.V.: 1000 mg/m^2/day days 1 and 8
[total dose/cycle = 2000 mg/m^2]
Carboplatin: I.V.: AUC 5 day 1
[total dose/cycle = AUC = 5]
Repeat cycle every 21 days for up to 6 cycles

Gemcitabine-Carboplatin (NSCLC)

Use Lung cancer, nonsmall cell

Regimen NOTE: Multiple variations are listed.

Variation 1:
Gemcitabine: I.V.: 1000 mg/m^2/dose days 1, 8, and 15
[total dose/cycle = 3000 mg/m^2]
Carboplatin: I.V.: AUC 5 day 1
[total dose/cycle = AUC = 5]
Repeat cycle every 28 days for up to 4 cycles

Variation 2:
Gemcitabine: I.V.: 1000 or 1100 mg/m^2/day days 1 and 8
[total dose/cycle = 2000 or 2200 mg/m^2]
Carboplatin: I.V.: AUC 5 day 8
[total dose/cycle = AUC = 5]
Repeat cycle every 28 days

Gemcitabine-Cisplatin (Biliary Cancer)

Use Biliary adenocarcinoma

Regimen NOTE: Multiple variations are listed.

Variation 1:

Gemcitabine: I.V.: 1250 mg/m^2/dose days 1 and 8
[total dose/cycle = 2500 mg/m^2]

Cisplatin: I.V.: 75 mg/m^2/dose day 1
[total dose/cycle = 75 mg/m^2]

Repeat cycle every 3 weeks

Variation 2:

Gemcitabine: I.V.: 1000 mg/m^2/dose days 1 and 8
[total dose/cycle = 2000 mg/m^2]

Cisplatin: I.V.: 70 mg/m^2/dose day 1
[total dose/cycle = 70 mg/m^2]

Repeat cycle every 3 weeks (maximum: 6 cycles)

Gemcitabine-Cisplatin (Bladder Cancer)

Use Bladder cancer

Regimen

Gemcitabine: I.V.: 1000 mg/m^2/day days 1, 8, and 15
[total dose/cycle = 3000 mg/m^2]

Cisplatin: I.V.: 70 mg/m^2 day 2
[total dose/cycle = 70 mg/m^2]

Repeat cycle every 28 days for 6 cycles

Gemcitabine-Cisplatin (NSCLC)

Use Lung cancer, nonsmall cell

Regimen NOTE: Multiple variations are listed.

Variation 1:

Gemcitabine: I.V.: 1000 mg/m^2/day days 1, 8, and 15
[total dose/cycle = 3000 mg/m^2]

Cisplatin: I.V.: 100 mg/m^2 day 1
[total dose/cycle = 100 mg/m^2]

Repeat cycle every 28 days

Variation 2:

Gemcitabine: I.V.: 1250 mg/m^2/day days 1 and 8
[total dose/cycle = 2500 mg/m^2]

Cisplatin: I.V.: 100 mg/m^2 day 1
[total dose/cycle = 100 mg/m^2]

Repeat cycle every 21 days

Variation 3:

Gemcitabine: I.V.: 1000 mg/m^2/day days 1 and 8
[total dose/cycle = 2000 mg/m^2]

Cisplatin: I.V.: 80 mg/m^2 day 1
[total dose/cycle = 80 mg/m^2]

Repeat cycle every 21 days

Variation 4:

Gemcitabine: I.V.: 1250 mg/m^2/day days 1 and 8
[total dose/cycle = 2500 mg/m^2]

Cisplatin: I.V.: 75 mg/m^2 day 1
[total dose/cycle = 75 mg/m^2]

Repeat cycle every 21 days for up to 6 cycles

Variation 5:

Gemcitabine: I.V.: 1000 mg/m^2/day days 1, 8, and 15
[total dose/cycle = 3000 mg/m^2]

Cisplatin: I.V.: 100 mg/m^2 day 15
[total dose/cycle = 100 mg/m^2]

Repeat cycle every 28 days

Variation 6:
Gemcitabine: I.V.: 1000 mg/m^2/day days 1, 8, and 15
[total dose/cycle = 3000 mg/m^2]
Cisplatin: I.V.: 100 mg/m^2 day 2
[total dose/cycle = 100 mg/m^2]
Repeat cycle every 28 days for 5 cycles
Variation 7:
Gemcitabine: I.V.: 1200 mg/m^2/day days 1, 8, and 15
[total dose/cycle = 3600 mg/m^2]
Cisplatin: I.V.: 100 mg/m^2 day 15
[total dose/cycle = 100 mg/m^2]
Repeat cycle every 28 days for up to 6 cycles
Variation 8 (patients ≥70 years of age):
Gemcitabine: I.V.: 1000 mg/m^2/day days 1 and 8
[total dose/cycle = 2000 mg/m^2]
Cisplatin: I.V.: 60 mg/m^2 day 1
[total dose/cycle = 60 mg/m^2]
Repeat cycle every 21 days for up to 6 cycles

Gemcitabine-Docetaxel (Sarcoma)

Use Osteosarcoma; Soft tissue sarcoma

Regimen
Gemcitabine: I.V.: 675 mg/m^2/day days 1 and 8
[total dose/cycle = 1350 mg/m^2]
Docetaxel: I.V.: 100 mg/m^2 day 8
[total dose/cycle = 100 mg/m^2]
Repeat cycle every 21 days

Gemcitabine Fixed Dose Rate (Pancreatic Regimen)

Use Pancreatic cancer

Regimen
Gemcitabine: I.V.: 1500 mg/m^2/day over 150 minutes (10 mg/m^2/minute) days 1, 8, and 15
[total dose/cycle = 4500 mg/m^2]
Repeat cycle every 28 days until disease progression or unacceptable toxicity

Gemcitabine-Fluorouracil (RCC)

Use Renal cell cancer

Regimen
Gemcitabine: I.V.: 600 mg/m^2/day days 1, 8, and 15
[total dose/cycle = 1800 mg/m^2]
Fluorouracil: I.V.: 150 mg/m^2/day continuous infusion days 1 to 21
[total dose/cycle = 3150 mg/m^2]
Repeat cycle every 28 days for at least 2 cycles

Gemcitabine (Hodgkin Regimen)

Use Lymphoma, Hodgkin

Regimen NOTE: Multiple variations are listed.
Variation 1:
Gemcitabine: I.V.: 1250 mg/m^2/day over 30 minutes days 1, 8, and 15
[total dose/cycle = 3750 mg/m^2]
Repeat cycles every 28 days
Variation 2:
Gemcitabine: I.V.: 1200 mg/m^2/day over 30 minutes days 1, 8, and 15
[total dose/cycle = 3600 mg/m^2]
Repeat cycles every 28 days for a total of 6 cycles
Variation 3:
Cycle 1:
Gemcitabine: I.V.: 1000 mg/m^2/day over 30 minutes weekly for 7 weeks, followed by one week rest
[total dose/cycle = 7000 mg/m^2]
Treatment cycle is 8 weeks

Subsequent Cycles:

Gemcitabine: I.V.: 1000 mg/m^2/day over 30 minutes days 1, 8, and 15 [total dose/cycle = 3000 mg/m^2]

Repeat cycle every 28 days until disease progression or drug intolerance

Gemcitabine (Mesothelioma Regimen)

Use Malignant pleural mesothelioma

Regimen

Gemcitabine: I.V.: 1250 mg/m^2/day over 30 minutes days 1, 8, and 15 [total dose/cycle = 3750 mg/m^2]

Repeat cycle every 28 days for up to a total of 10 cycles

Gemcitabine (Ovarian Regimen)

Use Ovarian cancer

Regimen NOTE: Multiple variations are listed.

Variation 1:

Gemcitabine: I.V.: 1000 mg/m^2/dose over 30-60 minutes days 1 and 8 [total dose/cycle = 2000 mg/m^2]

Repeat cycle every 21 days until disease progression or unacceptable toxicity

Variation 2:

Gemcitabine: I.V.: 1000 mg/m^2/dose over 30 minutes days 1, 8, and 15 [total dose/cycle = 3000 mg/m^2]

Repeat cycle every 28 days until disease progression or unacceptable toxicity

Gemcitabine-Oxaliplatin (Pancreatic)

Use Pancreatic cancer

Regimen

Gemcitabine: I.V.: 1000 mg/m^2 over 100 minutes (10 mg/m^2/minute) day 1 [total dose/cycle = 1000 mg/m^2]

Oxaliplatin: I.V.: 100 mg/m^2 over 2 hours day 2 [total dose/cycle = 100 mg/m^2]

Repeat cycle every 14 days until disease progression or unacceptable toxicity

Gemcitabine-Oxaliplatin-Rituximab (NHL)

Use Lymphoma, non-Hodgkin

Regimen

Oxaliplatin: I.V.: 100 mg/m^2/dose day 1 [total dose/cycle = 100 mg/m^2]

Gemcitabine: I.V.: 1000 mg/m^2/dose day 1 [total dose/cycle = 1000 mg/m^2]

Rituximab: I.V.: 375 mg/m^2/dose day 1 [total dose/cycle = 375 mg/m^2]

Repeat cycle every 3 weeks (for a total of 6-8 cycles)

Gemcitabine-Paclitaxel (Breast Cancer)

Use Breast cancer

Regimen

Paclitaxel: I.V.: 175 mg/m^2 (infused over 3 hours) day 1 [total dose/cycle = 175 mg/m^2]

Gemcitabine: I.V.: 1250 mg/m^2/day days 1 and 8 [total dose/cycle = 2500 mg/m^2]

Repeat cycle every 21 days until disease progression or unacceptable toxicity

Gemcitabine-Paclitaxel (Ovarian Cancer)

Use Ovarian cancer

Regimen

Paclitaxel: I.V.: 110 mg/m^2/dose over 1 hour days 1, 8, and 15 [total dose/cycle = 330 mg/m^2]

Gemcitabine: I.V.: 1000 mg/m^2/dose days 1, 8, and 15 [total dose/cycle = 3000 mg/m^2]

Repeat cycle every 4 weeks for a maximum of 6 cycles

Gemcitabine-Paclitaxel (Protein Bound) (Pancreatic)

Use Pancreatic cancer

Regimen

Gemcitabine: I.V.: 1000 mg/m^2/day days 1, 8, and 15
[total dose/cycle = 3000 mg/m^2]
Paclitaxel (Protein Bound): I.V.: 125 mg/m^2/day days 1, 8, and 15
[total dose/cycle = 375 mg/m^2]
Repeat cycle every 28 days until disease progression or unacceptable toxicity

Gemcitabine (Small Cell Lung Cancer Regimen)

Use Lung cancer, small cell

Regimen NOTE: Multiple variations are listed.

Variation 1:
Gemcitabine: I.V.: 1000 mg/m^2/day over 30 minutes days 1, 8, and 15
[total dose/cycle = 3000 mg/m^2]
Repeat cycle every 28 days

Variation 2:
Gemcitabine: I.V.: 1250 mg/m^2/day over 30 minutes days 1 and 8
[total dose/cycle = 2500 mg/m^2]
Repeat cycle every 21 days

Gemcitabine Standard Infusion (Pancreatic Regimen)

Use Pancreatic cancer

Regimen

Cycle 1:
Gemcitabine: I.V.: 1000 mg/m^2/day over 30 minutes days 1, 8, 15, 22, 29, 36, and 43 (cycle 1 only)
[total dose/cycle 1 = 7000 mg/m^2]
Treatment cycle is 56 days

Subsequent cycles:
Gemcitabine: I.V.: 1000 mg/m^2/day over 30 minutes days 1, 8, and 15
[total dose/cycle = 3000 mg/m^2]
Repeat cycle every 28 days until disease progression or unacceptable toxicity

Gemcitabine-Vinorelbine (NSCLC)

Use Lung cancer, nonsmall cell

Regimen NOTE: Multiple variations are listed.

Variation 1:
Gemcitabine: I.V.: 1200 mg/m^2/day days 1 and 8
[total dose/cycle = 2400 mg/m^2]
Vinorelbine: I.V.: 30 mg/m^2/day days 1 and 8
[total dose/cycle = 60 mg/m^2]
Repeat cycle every 21 days for 6 cycles

Variation 2:
Gemcitabine: I.V.: 1000 mg/m^2/day days 1, 8, and 15
[total dose/cycle = 3000 mg/m^2]
Vinorelbine: I.V.: 20 mg/m^2/day days 1, 8, and 15
[total dose/cycle = 60 mg/m^2]
Repeat cycle every 28 days for a maximum of 6 cycles

Variation 3:
Gemcitabine: I.V.: 800 mg/m^2/day days 1, 8, and 15
[total dose/cycle = 2400 mg/m^2]
Vinorelbine: I.V.: 20 mg/m^2/day days 1, 8, and 15
[total dose/cycle = 60 mg/m^2]
Repeat cycle every 28 days for up to 6 cycles

Gemcitabine-Vinorelbine (Sarcoma)

Use Soft tissue sarcoma

Regimen NOTE: Multiple variations are listed.

Variation 1:

Vinorelbine: I.V.: 25 mg/m^2/dose over 10 minutes days 1 and 8
[total dose/cycle = 50 mg/m^2]

Gemcitabine: I.V.: 800 mg/m^2/dose over 90 minutes days 1 and 8
[total dose/cycle = 1600 mg/m^2]

Repeat cycle every 21 days until disease progression or unacceptable toxicity

Variation 2 (modification for toxicity):

Vinorelbine: I.V.: 25 mg/m^2/dose over 10 minutes days 1 and 15
[total dose/cycle = 50 mg/m^2]

Gemcitabine: I.V.: 800 mg/m^2/dose over 90 minutes days 1 and 15
[total dose/cycle = 1600 mg/m^2]

Repeat cycle every 28 days until disease progression or unacceptable toxicity

GEMOX (Biliary Cancer)

Use Biliary adenocarcinoma

Regimen

Gemcitabine: I.V.: 1000 mg/m^2 day 1
[total dose/cycle = 1000 mg/m^2]

Oxaliplatin: I.V.: 100 mg/m^2 day 2
[total dose/cycle = 100 mg/m^2]

Repeat cycle every 2 weeks

GEMOX (Testicular Cancer)

Use Testicular cancer

Regimen NOTE: Multiple variations are listed.

Variation 1:

Gemcitabine: I.V.: 1000 mg/m^2/day over 30 minutes days 1 and 8
[total dose/cycle = 2000 mg/m^2]

Oxaliplatin: I.V.: 130 mg/m^2 over 2 hours day 1
[total dose/cycle = 130 mg/m^2]

Repeat cycle every 21 days for a total of at least 2 cycles (maximum: 6 cycles)

Variation 2:

Gemcitabine: I.V.: 1250 mg/m^2/day over 30 minutes days 1 and 8
[total dose/cycle = 2500 mg/m^2]

Oxaliplatin: I.V.: 130 mg/m^2 over 2 hours day 1
[total dose/cycle = 130 mg/m^2]

Repeat cycle every 21 days for a maximum of 6 cycles

GVD (Hodgkin)

Use Lymphoma, Hodgkin disease

Regimen NOTE: Multiple variations are listed.

Variation 1 (for transplant-naive patients):

Vinorelbine: I.V.: 20 mg/m^2/day over 6-10 minutes days 1 and 8
[total dose/cycle = 40 mg/m^2]

Gemcitabine: I.V.: 1000 mg/m^2/day over 30 minutes days 1 and 8
[total dose/cycle = 2000 mg/m^2]

Doxorubicin liposomal: I.V.: 15 mg/m^2/day over 30-60 minutes days 1 and 8
[total dose/cycle = 30 mg/m^2]

Repeat cycle every 21 days for a total of 2 to 6 cycles

Variation 2 (for patients with prior transplant):

Vinorelbine: I.V.: 15 mg/m^2/day over 6-10 minutes days 1 and 8
[total dose/cycle = 30 mg/m^2]

Gemcitabine: I.V.: 800 mg/m^2/day over 30 minutes days 1 and 8
[total dose/cycle = 1600 mg/m^2]

Doxorubicin liposomal: I.V.: 10 mg/m^2/day over 30-60 minutes days 1 and 8
[total dose/cycle = 20 mg/m^2]

Repeat cycle every 21 days for a total of 2 to 6 cycles

HDMTX

Use Osteosarcoma

Regimen

Methotrexate: I.V.: 12 g/m^2/week for 2-12 weeks
[total dose/cycle = 24-144 g/m^2]
Leucovorin calcium rescue: Oral, I.V.: 15 mg/m^2 every 6 hours (beginning 30 hours after the beginning of the 4-hour methotrexate infusion) for 10 doses; **serum methotrexate levels must be monitored**
[total dose/cycle = 150 mg/m^2]

Hydroxyurea (AML Regimen)

Use Leukemia, acute myeloid

Regimen

Hydroxyurea: Oral: 25 mg/kg/dose 4 times/day for a maximum of 30 days
[total maximum dose/cycle = 3000 mg/kg]
Administer treatment until achievement of bone marrow aplasia, for a maximum of 30 days

Hyper-CVAD + Imatinib

Use Leukemia, acute lymphocytic

Regimen

Cycle A: (Cycles 1, 3, 5, and 7)
Imatinib: Oral: 400 mg/day days 1 to 14
[total dose/cycle = 5600 mg]
Cyclophosphamide: I.V.: 300 mg/m^2 every 12 hours, for 6 doses, days 1, 2, and 3
[total dose/cycle = 1800 mg/m^2]
Mesna: I.V. 600 mg/m^2/day continuous infusion days 1, 2, and 3
[total dose/cycle = 1800 mg/m^2]
Vincristine: I.V.: 2 mg/day days 4 and 11
[total dose/cycle = 4 mg]
Doxorubicin: I.V.: 50 mg/m^2/day continuous infusion day 4
[total dose/cycle = 50 mg/m^2]
Dexamethasone: Oral, I.V.: 40 mg/day days 1 to 4 and 11 to 14
[total dose/cycle = 320 mg]
Cycle B: (Cycles 2, 4, 6, and 8)
Imatinib: Oral: 400 mg/day days 1 to 14
[total dose/cycle = 5600 mg]
Methotrexate: I.V.: 1 g/m^2/day continuous infusion day 1
[total dose/cycle = 1 g/m^2]
Leucovorin: I.V.: 50 mg then 15 mg every 6 hours, for 8 doses (start 12 hours after the end of the methotrexate infusion)
[total dose/cycle = 170 mg]
Cytarabine: I.V.: 3 g/m^2 every 12 hours for 4 doses, days 2 and 3
[total dose/cycle = 12 g/m^2]
Repeat every 6 weeks in the following sequence: ABABABAB

CNS Prophylaxis

Methotrexate: I.T.: 12 mg/day day 2
[total dose/cycle = 12 mg/day]
or 6 mg into Ommaya day 2
[total dose/cycle = 6 mg/day]
Cytarabine: I.T.: 100 mg/day day 7 or 8
[total dose/cycle = 100 mg/day]
Repeat cycle every 3 weeks for 3 or 4 cycles

Maintenance (POMP)

Imatinib: Oral: 600 mg/day
[total dose/cycle = 18,000 mg]
Vincristine: I.V.: 2 mg/day day 1
[total dose/cycle = 2 mg]
Prednisone: Oral: 200 mg/day days 1 to 5
[total dose/cycle = 1000 mg/m^2]
Repeat cycle every month (except months 6 and 13) for 13 months

Intensification

Imatinib: Oral: 400 mg/day days 1 to 14
[total dose/cycle = 5600 mg]
Cyclophosphamide: I.V.: 300 mg/m^2 every 12 hours, for 6 doses, days 1, 2, and 3
[total dose/cycle = 1800 mg/m^2]
Mesna: I.V.: 600 mg/m^2/day continuous infusion days 1, 2, and 3
[total dose/cycle = 1800 mg/m^2]
Vincristine: I.V.: 2 mg/day days 4 and 11
[total dose/cycle = 4 mg]
Doxorubicin: 50 mg/m^2/day continuous infusion day 4
[total dose/cycle = 50 mg/m^2]
Dexamethasone: I.V. or Oral: 40 mg/day days 1 to 4 and 11 to 14
[total dose/cycle = 320 mg]
Cycle is given in months 6 and 13 during maintenance

Hyper-CVAD (Leukemia, Acute Lymphocytic)

Use Leukemia, acute lymphocytic

Regimen NOTE: Multiple variations are listed.

Variation 1:

Cycle A: (Cycles 1, 3, 5, and 7)
Cyclophosphamide: I.V.: 300 mg/m^2 every 12 hours, for 6 doses, days 1, 2, and 3
[total dose/cycle = 1800 mg/m^2]
Mesna: I.V.: 1200 mg/m^2/day continuous infusion days 1, 2, and 3
[total dose/cycle = 3600 mg/m^2]
Vincristine: I.V.: 2 mg/day days 4 and 11
[total dose/cycle = 4 mg]
Doxorubicin: I.V.: 50 mg/m^2 day 4
[total dose/cycle = 50 mg/m^2]
Dexamethasone: (route not specified): 40 mg/day days 1 to 4 and 11 to 14
[total dose/cycle = 320 mg]

Cycle B: (Cycles 2, 4, 6, and 8)
Methotrexate: I.V.: 1 g/m^2 continuous infusion day 1
[total dose/cycle = 1g/m^2]
Leucovorin: (route not specified): 15 mg every 6 hours, for 8 doses (start 12 hours after end of methotrexate infusion)
[total dose/cycle = 120 mg]
Cytarabine: I.V.: 3 g/m^2 every 12 hours, for 4 doses, days 2 and 3
[total dose/cycle = 12 g/m^2]
Methylprednisolone: I.V.: 50 mg twice daily, for 6 doses, days 1, 2, and 3
[total dose/cycle = 300 mg/m^2]
Repeat every 6 weeks in the following sequence: ABABABAB

CNS Prophylaxis

Methotrexate: I.T.: 12 mg/day day 2
[total dose/cycle = 12 mg]
or 6 mg/day into Ommaya day 2
[total dose/cycle = 6 mg]
Cytarabine: I.T: 100 mg day 8
[total dose/cycle = 100 mg]
Repeat cycle every 3 weeks

Maintenance (POMP)

Mercaptopurine: Oral: 50 mg 3 times/day
[total dose/cycle = 4200-4650 mg]
Vincristine: I.V.: 2 mg day 1
[total dose/cycle = 2 mg]
Methotrexate: Oral: 20 mg/m^2/day days 1, 8, 15, and 22
[total dose/cycle = 80 mg/m^2]
Prednisone: Oral: 200 mg/day days 1 to 5
[total dose/cycle = 1000 mg/m^2]
or
Mercaptopurine: I.V.: 1 g/m^2/day days 1 to 5
[total dose/cycle = 5 g/m^2]
Vincristine: I.V.: 2 mg day 1
[total dose/cycle = 2 mg]

Methotrexate: I.V.: 10 mg/m^2/day days 1 to 5
[total dose/cycle = 50 mg/m^2]
Prednisone: Oral: 200 mg/day days 1 to 5
[total dose/cycle = 1000 mg/m^2]
Repeat cycles every month for 2 years

Variation 2:

Cycle A: (Cycles 1, 3, 5, and 7)
Cyclophosphamide: I.V.: 300 mg/m^2 every 12 hours, for 6 doses, days 1, 2, and 3
[total dose/cycle = 1800 mg/m^2]
Mesna: I.V.: 600 mg/m^2/day continuous infusion days 1, 2, and 3
[total dose/cycle = 1800 mg/m^2]
Vincristine: I.V.: 2 mg/day days 4 and 11
[total dose/cycle = 4 mg]
Doxorubicin: I.V.: 50 mg/m^2 day 4
[total dose/cycle = 50 mg/m^2]
Dexamethasone: Oral, I.V.: 40 mg/day days 1 to 4 and 11 to 14
[total dose/cycle = 320 mg]

Cycle B: (Cycles 2, 4, 6, and 8)
Methotrexate: I.V.: 1 g/m^2 continuous infusion day 1
[total dose/cycle = 1 g/m^2]
Leucovorin: I.V.: 50 mg (start 12 hours after end of methotrexate infusion)
followed by I.V.: 15 mg every 6 hours, for 8 doses
[total dose/cycle = 170 mg]
Cytarabine: I.V.: 3 g/m^2 every 12 hours, for 4 doses, days 2 and 3
[total dose/cycle = 12 g/m^2]
Repeat every 6 weeks in the following sequence: ABABABAB

CNS Prophylaxis
Methotrexate: I.T.: 12 mg day 2
[total dose/cycle = 12 mg]
or 6 mg into Ommaya day 2
[total dose/cycle = 6 mg]
Cytarabine: I.T.: 100 mg day 7
[total dose/cycle = 100 mg]
Repeat cycle every 3 weeks

Variation 3:

Cycle A: (Cycles 1, 3, 5, and 7)
Cyclophosphamide: I.V.: 300 mg/m^2 every 12 hours, for 6 doses, days 1, 2, and 3
[total dose/cycle = 1800 mg/m^2]
Mesna: I.V.: 600 mg/m^2/day continuous infusion days 1, 2, and 3
[total dose/cycle = 1800 mg/m^2]
Vincristine: I.V.: 2 mg/day days 4 and 11
[total dose/cycle = 4 mg]
Doxorubicin: I.V.: 50 mg/m^2 continuous infusion day 4
[total dose/cycle = 50 mg/m^2]
Dexamethasone: Oral, I.V.: 40 mg/day days 1 to 4 and 11 to 14
[total dose/cycle = 320 mg]

Cycle B: (Cycles 2, 4, 6, and 8)
Methotrexate: I.V.: 200 mg/m^2 day 1
followed by I.V.: 800 mg/m^2 continuous infusion day 1
[total dose/cycle = 1 g/m^2]
Leucovorin: I.V.: 50 mg (start 12 hours after end of methotrexate infusion)
followed by I.V.: 15 mg every 6 hours, for 8 doses
[total dose/cycle = 170 mg/m^2]
Cytarabine: I.V.: 3 g/m^2 every 12 hours, for 4 doses, days 2 and 3
[total dose/cycle = 12 g/m^2]
Repeat every 6 weeks in the following sequence: ABABABAB

CNS Prophylaxis
Methotrexate: I.T.: 12 mg day 2
[total dose/cycle = 12 mg]
or 6 mg into Ommaya day 2
[total dose/cycle = 6 mg]

Cytarabine: I.T.: 100 mg day 7 **or** 8
[total dose/cycle = 100 mg]
Repeat cycles every 3 weeks for 6 or 8 cycles

Maintenance (POMP)

Mercaptopurine: Oral: 50 mg 3 times/day
[total dose/cycle = 4200-4650 mg]
Vincristine: I.V.: 2 mg day 1
[total dose/cycle = 2 mg]
Methotrexate: Oral, I V: 20 mg/m^2/ day days 1, 8, 15, and 22
[total dose/cycle = 80 mg/m^2]
Prednisone: Oral: 200 mg/day days 1 to 5
[total dose/cycle = 1000 mg/m^2]

or

Mercaptopurine: I.V.: 1 g/m^2/day days 1 to 5
[total dose/cycle = 5 g/m^2]
Vincristine: I.V.: 2 mg day 1
[total dose/cycle = 2 mg]
Methotrexate: I.V.: 10 mg/m^2/day days 1 to 5
[total dose/cycle = 50 mg/m^2]
Prednisone: Oral: 200 mg/day days 1 to 5
[total dose/cycle = 1000 mg]
Repeat cycles every month (except months 7 and 11 or 9 and 12) for 2 years

Intensification

Etoposide: I.V.: 100 mg/m^2/day days 1 to 5
[total dose/cycle = 500 mg/m^2]
Pegaspargase: I.V.: 2500 units/m^2 day 1
[total dose/cycle = 2500 units/m^2]
Given during months 9 and 12 of maintenance

or

Methotrexate: I.V.: 100 mg/m^2/day days 1, 8, 15, and 22
[total dose/cycle = 400 mg/m^2]
Asparaginase: I.V.: 20,000 units/day days 2, 9, 16, and 23
[total dose/cycle = 80,000 units]
Given during months 7 and 11 of maintenance

Variation 4:

Cycle A: (Cycles 1, 3, 5, and 7)
Cyclophosphamide: I.V.: 300 mg/m^2 every 12 hours, for 6 doses, days 1, 2, and 3
[total dose/cycle = 1800 mg/m^2]
Mesna: I.V.: 600 mg/m^2/day continuous infusion days 1, 2, and 3
[total dose/cycle = 1800 mg/m^2]
Vincristine: I.V.: 2 mg/day days 4 and 11
[total dose/cycle = 4 mg]
Doxorubicin: I.V.: 50 mg/m^{2}day 4
[total dose/cycle = 50 mg/m^2]
Dexamethasone: (route not specified): 40 mg/day days 1 to 4 and 11 to 14
[total dose/cycle = 320 mg]

Cycle B: (Cycles 2, 4, 6, and 8)
Methotrexate: I.V.: 200 mg/m^2 day 1
followed by I.V.: 800 mg/m^2 continuous infusion day 1
[total dose/cycle = 1 g/m^2]
Leucovorin: (route not specified): 15 mg every 6 hours, for 8 doses (start 24 hours after end of methotrexate infusion)
[total dose/cycle = 120 mg]
Cytarabine: I.V.: 3 g/m^2 every 12 hours, for 4 doses, days 2 and 3
[total dose/cycle = 12 g/m^2]
Repeat every 6 weeks in the following sequence: ABABABAB

CNS Prophylaxis

Methotrexate: I.T.: 12 mg day 2
[total dose/cycle = 12 mg]
Cytarabine: I.T.: 100 mg day 8
[total dose/cycle = 100 mg]
Repeat cycle every 3 weeks for 4 or 8 cycles

Maintenance (POMP)

Mercaptopurine: Oral: 50 mg 3 times/day
[total dose/cycle = 4200-4650 mg]
Vincristine: I.V.: 2 mg day 1
[total dose/cycle = 2 mg]
Methotrexate: Oral: 20 mg/m^2/day days 1, 8, 15, and 22
[total dose/cycle = 80 mg/m^2]
Prednisone: Oral: 200 mg/day days 1 to 5
[total dose/cycle = 1000 mg/m^2]

or

Mercaptopurine: I.V.: 1 g/m^2/day days 1 to 5
[total dose/cycle = 5 g/m^2]
Vincristine: I.V.: 2 mg day 1
[total dose/cycle = 2 mg]
Methotrexate: I.V.: 10 mg/m^2/day days 1 to 5
[total dose/cycle = 50 mg/m^2]
Prednisone: Oral: 200 mg/day days 1 to 5
[total dose/cycle = 1000 mg/m^2]

or

Interferon alfa: SubQ: 5 million units/m^2 daily
[total dose/cycle = 140-155 million units/m^2]
Cytarabine: SubQ: 10 mg daily
[total dose/cycle = 280-310 mg]
Repeat cycles every month for 2 years

Variation 5:

Cycle A: (Cycles 1, 4, 6, and 8)
Cyclophosphamide: I.V.: 300 mg/m^2 every 12 hours, for 6 doses, days 1, 2, and 3
[total dose/cycle = 1800 mg/m^2]
Mesna: I.V.: 600 mg/m^2/day continuous infusion days 1, 2, and 3
[total dose/cycle = 1800 mg/m^2]
Vincristine: I.V.: 2 mg/day days 4 and 11
[total dose/cycle = 4 mg]
Doxorubicin: I.V.: 50 mg/m^2 continuous infusion day 4
[total dose/cycle = 50 mg/m^2]
Dexamethasone: Oral, I.V.: 40 mg/day days 1 to 4 and 11 to 14
[total dose/cycle = 320 mg]

Cycle B: (Cycles 3, 5, 7, and 9)
Methotrexate: I.V.: 200 mg/m^2 day 1
followed by I.V.: 800 mg/m^2 continuous infusion day 1
[total dose/cycle = 1 g/m^2]
Leucovorin: I.V.: 50 mg (start 12 hours after end of methotrexate infusion)
followed by I.V.: 15 mg every 6 hours, for 8 doses
[total dose/cycle = 170 mg]
Cytarabine: I.V.: 3 g/m^2 every 12 hours, for 4 doses, days 2 and 3
[total dose/cycle = 12 g/m^2]

Cycle C: Liposomal Daunorubicin/Cytarabine (Cycle 2):
Daunorubicin, liposomal: I.V.: 150 mg/m^2/day days 1 and 2
[total dose/cycle = 300 mg/m^2]
Cytarabine: I.V.: 1.5 g/m^2/day continuous infusion days 1 and 2
[total dose/cycle = 3 g/m^2]
Prednisone: Oral: 200 mg/day days 1 to 5
[total dose/cycle = 1000 mg]
Administer in the following sequence: ACBABABA (Cycle C does not repeat)

CNS Prophylaxis

Methotrexate: I.T.: 12 mg day 2
[total dose/cycle = 12 mg]
or 6 mg into Ommaya day 2
[total dose/cycle = 6 mg]
Cytarabine: I.T.: 100 mg day 7 **or** 8
[total dose/cycle = 100 mg]
Repeat cycle every 3 weeks for 6 or 8 cycles

Maintenance (POMP)

Mercaptopurine: I.V.: 1 g/m^2/day days 1 to 5
[total dose/cycle = 5 g/m^2]
Vincristine: I.V.: 2 mg day 1
[total dose/cycle = 2 mg]
Methotrexate: I.V.: 10 mg/m^2/day days 1 to 5
[total dose/cycle = 50 mg/m^2]
Prednisone: Oral: 200 mg/day days 1 to 5
[total dose/cycle = 1000 mg]
Repeat cycles monthly, except months 6, 7, 18, and 19 for 3 years

Intensification

Methotrexate: I.V.: 100 mg/m^2/day days 1, 8, 15, and 22
[total dose/cycle = 400 mg/m^2]
Asparaginase: I.V.: 20,000 units/day days 2, 9, 16, and 23
[total dose/cycle = 80,000 units]
Given during months 6 and 18 of maintenance
Cyclophosphamide: I.V.: 300 mg/m^2 every 12 hours, for 6 doses, days 1, 2, and 3
[total dose/cycle = 1800 mg/m^2]
Mesna: I.V.: 600 mg/m^2/day continuous infusion days 1, 2, and 3
[total dose/cycle = 1800 mg/m^2]
Vincristine: I.V.: 2 mg/day days 4 and 11
[total dose/cycle = 4 mg]
Doxorubicin: I.V.: 50 mg/m^2/day continuous infusion day 4
[total dose/cycle = 50 mg/m^2]
Dexamethasone: Oral, I.V.: 40 mg/day days 1 to 4 and 11 to 14
[total dose/cycle = 320 mg]
Given during months 7 and 19 of maintenance

Hyper-CVAD (Lymphoma, non-Hodgkin)

Use Lymphoma, non-Hodgkin

Regimen

Cycle A: (Cycles 1, 3, 5, and 7)
Cyclophosphamide: I.V.: 300 mg/m^2 every 12 hours, for 6 doses, days 1, 2, and 3
[total dose/cycle = 1800 mg/m^2]
Vincristine: I.V.: 2 mg/day days 4 and 11
[total dose/cycle = 4 mg]
Doxorubicin: I.V.: 25 mg/m^2/day continuous infusion days 4 and 5
[total dose/cycle = 50 mg/m^2]
Dexamethasone: Oral, I.V.: 40 mg/day days 1 to 4 and 11 to 14
[total dose/cycle = 320 mg]
Cycle B: (Cycles 2, 4, 6, and 8)
Methotrexate: I.V.: 200 mg/m^2 day 1
followed by I.V.: 800 mg/m^2 continuous infusion day 1
[total dose/cycle = 1 g/m^2]
Leucovorin: Oral: 50 mg
followed by Oral: 15 mg every 6 hours, for 8 doses (start 24 hours after end of methotrexate infusion)
[total dose/cycle = 170 mg]
Cytarabine: I.V.: 3 g/m^2 every 12 hours, for 4 doses, days 2 and 3
[total dose/cycle = 12 g/m^2]
Repeat every 6 weeks in the following sequence: ABABABAB

Hyper-CVAD (Multiple Myeloma)

Use Multiple myeloma

Regimen

Cyclophosphamide: I.V.: 300 mg/m^2 every 12 hours, for 6 doses, days 1, 2, and 3
[total dose/cycle = 1800 mg/m^2]
Mesna: I.V.: 600 mg/m^2/day continuous infusion days 1, 2, and 3
[total dose/cycle = 1800 mg/m^2]
Doxorubicin: I.V.: 25 mg/m^2/day continuous infusion days 4 and 5
[total dose/cycle = 50 mg/m^2]
Vincristine: I.V.: 1 mg/day continuous infusion days 4 and 5
followed by I.V.: 2 mg day 11
[total dose/cycle = 4 mg]

Dexamethasone: Oral, I.V.: 20 mg/m^2/day days 1 to 5 and 11 to 14
[total dose/cycle = 180 mg/m^2]
Repeat cycle once if ≥50% reduction in myeloma protein
Maintenance
Cyclophosphamide: Oral: 125 mg/m^2 every 12 hours, for 10 doses, days 1 to 5
[total dose/cycle = 1250 mg/m^2]
Dexamethasone: Oral: 20 mg/m^2/day days 1 to 5
[total dose/cycle = 100 mg/m^2]
Repeat maintenance cycle every 5 weeks

Hyper-CVAD + Rituximab

Use Lymphona, non-Hodgkin (mantle cell)

Regimen

Cycle A: (Cycles 1, 3, 5 [and 7, if needed])
Rituximab: I.V.: 375 mg/m^2 day 1
[total dose/cycle = 375 mg/m^2]
Cyclophosphamide: I.V.: 300 mg/m^2 every 12 hours, for 6 doses, days 2, 3, and 4
[total dose/cycle = 1800 mg/m^2]
Mesna: I.V.: 600 mg/m^2 continuous infusion days 2, 3, and 4
[total dose/cycle = 1800 mg/m^2]
Vincristine: I.V.: 1.4 mg/m^2 (maximum dose: 2 mg) days 5 and 12
[total dose/cycle = 2.8 mg/m^2; maximum: 4 mg]
Doxorubicin: I.V.: 16.7 mg/m^2 continuous infusion days 5, 6, and 7
[total dose/cycle = 50.1 mg/m^2]
Dexamethasone: Oral, I.V.: 40 mg/day days 2 to 5 and 12 to 15
[total dose/cycle = 320 mg]
Cycle B: (Cycles 2, 4, 6 [and 8, if needed])
Rituximab: I.V.: 375 mg/m^2 day 1
[total dose/cycle = 375 mg/m^2]
Methotrexate: I.V.: 200 mg/m^2 day 2
followed by I.V.: 800 mg/m^2 continuous infusion day 2
[total dose/cycle = 1000 mg/m^2]
Leucovorin: Oral: 50 mg (start 12 hours after the end of the methotrexate infusion)
followed by Oral: 15 mg every 6 hours, for 8 doses
[total dose/cycle = 170 mg]
Cytarabine: I.V.: 3 g/m^2 every 12 hours, for 4 doses, day 3 and 4
[total dose/cycle = 12 g/m^2]
Repeat every 6 weeks in the following sequence: ABABABAB

ICE (Hodgkin)

Use Lymphoma, Hodgkin

Regimen

Etoposide: I.V.: 100 mg/m^2/day days 1 to 3
[total dose/cycle = 300 mg/m^2]
Carboplatin: I.V.: AUC 5 day 2 (maximum dose: 800 mg)
[total dose/cycle = AUC 5, maximum dose/cycle: 800 mg]
Ifosfamide: I.V.: 5 g/m^2/day continuous infusion for 24 hours day 2
[total dose/cycle = 5 g/m^2]
Mesna: I.V.: 5 g/m^2/day continuous infusion for 24 hours day 2
[total dose/cycle = 5 g/m^2]
Filgrastim: 5 mcg/kg/day days 5 to 12 (except during PBPC mobilization)
Repeat cycle every 14 days for 2 cycles

ICE (Lymphoma, non-Hodgkin)

Use Lymphoma, non-Hodgkin

Regimen

Etoposide: I.V.: 100 mg/m^2/day days 1, 2, and 3
[total dose/cycle = 300 mg/m^2]
Carboplatin: I.V.: AUC 5 (maximum dose: 800 mg) day 2
[total dose/cycle = AUC = 5]

Ifosfamide: I.V.: 5000 mg/m^2 continuous infusion day 2
[total dose/cycle = 5000 mg/m^2]
Mesna: I.V.: 5000 mg/m^2 continuous infusion day 2
[total dose/cycle = 5000 mg/m^2]
Filgrastim: SubQ: 5 mcg/kg/day days 5-12 (cycles 1 and 2 only)
[total dose/cycle = 40 mcg/kg]
followed by SubQ: 10 mcg/kg/day day 5 through completion of leukaphoresis (cycle 3 only)
Repeat cycle every 2 weeks for 3 cycles

ICE (Sarcoma)

Use Osteosarcoma; Soft tissue sarcoma

Regimen

Ifosfamide: I.V.: 1500 mg/m^2/day days 1, 2, and 3
[total dose/cycle = 4500 mg/m^2]
Carboplatin: I.V.: 300-635 mg/m^2 day 3
[total dose/cycle = 300-635 mg/m^2]
Etoposide: I.V.: 100 mg/m^2/day days 1, 2, and 3
[total dose/cycle = 300 mg/m^2]
Mesna: I.V.: 500 mg/m^2 prior to each ifosfamide, and every 3 hours for 2 more doses/day days 1, 2, and 3
[total dose/cycle = 4500 mg/m^2]
Repeat cycle every 21-28 days

IE

Use Soft tissue sarcoma

Regimen

Etoposide: I.V.: 100 mg/m^2/day days 1, 2, and 3
[total dose/cycle = 300 mg/m^2]
Ifosfamide: I.V.: 2500 mg/m^2/day days 1, 2, and 3
[total dose/cycle = 7500 mg/m^2]
Mesna: I.V.: 500 mg/m^2 prior to ifosfamide, after ifosfamide, and every 4 hours for 3 more doses (total of 5 doses/day) days 1, 2, and 3
[total dose/cycle = 7500 mg/m^2]
Repeat cycle every 28 days

IGEV (Hodgkin)

Use Lymphoma, Hodgkin

Regimen

Ifosfamide: I.V.: 2000 mg/m^2/day over 2 hours days 1 to 4
[total dose/cycle = 8000 mg/m^2]
Mesna: I.V.: 2600 mg/m^2/day days 1 to 4
[total dose/cycle = 10,400 mg/m^2]
Gemcitabine: I.V.: 800 mg/m^2 days 1 and 4
[total dose/cycle = 1600 mg/m^2]
Vinorelbine: I.V.: 20 mg/m^2 day 1
[total dose/cycle = 20 mg/m^2]
Prednisolone: I.V.: 100 mg days 1 to 4
[total dose/cycle = 400 mg/m^2]
Filgrastim: Days 7 to 12 of each course or up to apheresis in the course of mobilization
Repeat cycle every 21 days for a total of 4 cycles

Imatinib (CML Regimen)

Use Leukemia, chronic myelogenous

Regimen NOTE: Multiple variations are listed.

Variation 1 (chronic phase):
Imatinib: Oral: 400 mg once daily
[total dose/cycle = 11,200 mg]
Repeat cycle every 28 days until disease progression or unacceptable toxicity
Variation 2 (accelerated phase and blast crisis):
Imatinib: Oral: 600 mg once daily
[total dose/cycle = 16,800 mg]
Repeat cycle every 28 days until disease progression or unacceptable toxicity

Variation 3 (chronic phase high dose):
Imatinib: Oral: 400 mg twice daily
[total dose/cycle = 22,400 mg]
Repeat cycle every 28 days until disease progression or unacceptable toxicity

IMVP-16

Use Lymphoma, non-Hodgkin

Regimen

Ifosfamide: I.V.: 4 g/m^2 continuous infusion over 24 hours day 1
[total dose/cycle = 4 g/m^2]
Mesna: I.V.: 800 mg/m^2 bolus prior to ifosfamide, then 4 g/m^2 continuous infusion over 12 hours concurrent with ifosfamide, then 2.4 g/m^2 continuous infusion over 12 hours after ifosfamide infusion day 1
[total dose/cycle = 7.2 g/m^2]
Methotrexate: I.V.: 30 mg/m^2/day days 3 and 10
[total dose/cycle = 60 mg/m^2]
Etoposide: I.V.: 100 mg/m^2/day days 1, 2, and 3
[total dose/cycle = 300 mg/m^2]
Repeat cycle every 21-28 days

Interleukin 2-Interferon Alfa-2 (RCC)

Use Renal cell cancer

Regimen

Induction (2 cycles):
Aldesleukin: I.V.: 18 million units/m^2/day continuous infusion days 1 to 5 and days 12 to 16
[total dose/cycle = 180 million units/m^2]
Repeat aldesleukin induction cycle one time (total of 2 cycles) after a 3-week rest between cycles
Interferon Alfa-2: SubQ: 6 million units/dose 3 times weekly continuously (no rest break) during induction cycles
[total dose/week = 18 million units/week]
Maintenance (begin after a 3-week aldesleukin rest):
Aldesleukin: I.V.: 18 million units/m^2/day continuous infusion days 1 to 5
[total dose/cycle = 90 million units/m^2]
Repeat aldesleukin maintenance cycle 3 times (total of 4 maintenance cycles) after 3-week rest between cycles
Interferon Alfa-2: SubQ: 6 million units/dose 3 times weekly continuously (no rest break) during maintenance cycles
[total dose/week = 18 million units/week]

IPA

Use Hepatoblastoma

Regimen

Ifosfamide: I.V.: 500 mg/m^2 day 1
[total dose/cycle = 500 mg/m^2]
followed by I.V.: 1000 mg/m^2/day continuous infusion days 1 to 3
[total dose/cycle = 3000 mg/m^2]
Cisplatin: I.V.: 20 mg/m^2/day days 4 to 8
[total dose/cycle = 100 mg/m^2]
Doxorubicin: I.V.: 30 mg/m^2/day continuous infusion days 9 and 10
[total dose/cycle = 60 mg/m^2]
Repeat cycle every 21 days

Irinotecan-Capecitabine (Esophageal Cancer)

Use Esophageal cancer

Regimen NOTE: Multiple variations are listed.

Variation 1:
Irinotecan: I.V.: 250 mg/m^2/dose day 1
[total dose/cycle = 250 mg/m^2]
Capecitabine: Oral: 1000 mg/m^2/dose twice daily days 1 to 14
[total dose/cycle = 28000 mg/m^2]
Repeat cycle every 21 days until disease progression or unacceptable toxicity

Variation 2:
Irinotecan: I.V.: 250 mg/m^2/dose day 1
[total dose/cycle = 250 mg/m^2]
Capecitabine: Oral: 1000 mg/m^2/dose twice daily days 1 to 14
[total dose/cycle = 28000 mg/m^2]
Repeat cycle every 21 days for up to 24 weeks

Irinotecan-Capecitabine (Gastric Cancer)

Use Gastric cancer

Regimen NOTE: Multiple variations are listed.

Variation 1:
Irinotecan: I.V.: 250 mg/m^2/dose day 1
[total dose/cycle = 250 mg/m^2]
Capecitabine: Oral: 1000 mg/m^2/dose twice daily days 1 to 14
[total dose/cycle = 28000 mg/m^2]
Repeat cycle every 21 days until disease progression or unacceptable toxicity

Variation 2:
Irinotecan: I.V.: 250 mg/m^2/dose day 1
[total dose/cycle = 250 mg/m^2]
Capecitabine: Oral: 1000 mg/m^2/dose twice daily days 1 to 14
[total dose/cycle = 28000 mg/m^2]
Repeat cycle every 21 days for up to 24 weeks

Irinotecan-Cisplatin (Esophageal Cancer)

Use Esophageal cancer

Regimen NOTE: Multiple variations are listed.

Variation 1:
Cisplatin: I.V.: 30 mg/m^2/dose days 1, 8, 15, and 22
[total dose/cycle = 120 mg/m^2]
Irinotecan: I.V.: 65 mg/m^2/dose days 1, 8, 15, and 22
[total dose/cycle = 260 mg/m^2]
Repeat cycle every 6 weeks until disease progression.

Variation 2 (with concurrent radiation therapy):
Cisplatin: I.V.: 30 mg/m^2/dose on day 1 and 8
[total dose/cycle = 60 mg/m^2]
Irinotecan: I.V.: 65 mg/m^2/dose day 1 and 8
[total dose/cycle = 130 mg/m^2]
Treatment cycle is 21 days; cycle is not repeated.

Variation 3:
Cisplatin: I.V.: 30 mg/m^2/dose on days 1, 8, 22, and 29
[total dose/cycle = 120 mg/m^2]
Irinotecan: I.V.: 50 mg/m^2/dose on days 1, 8, 22, and 29
[total dose/cycle = 200 mg/m^2]
Administered (with concurrent radiation therapy) over one 5-week treatment cycle.
Followed by: Postoperative therapy:
Cisplatin: I.V.: 30 mg/m^2/dose on days 1 and 8
[total dose/cycle = 60 mg/m^2]
Irinotecan: I.V.: 65 mg/m^2/dose on days 1 and 8
[total dose/cycle = 130 mg/m^2]
Repeat postop cycle every 21 days for a total of 3 cycles.

Variation 4:
Cisplatin: I.V.: 30 mg/m^2/dose on day 1 and 8
[total dose/cycle = 60 mg/m^2]
Irinotecan: I.V.: 65 mg/m^2/dose day 1 and 8
[total dose/cycle = 130 mg/m^2]
Repeat cycle every 21 days.

Irinotecan-Cisplatin (Gastric Cancer)

Use Gastric cancer

Regimen

Irinotecan: I.V.: 65 mg/m^2/dose over 90 minutes days 1, 8, 15, and 22
[total dose/cycle = 260 mg/m^2]

Cisplatin: I.V.: 30 mg/m^2/dose over 1 hour days 1, 8, 15, and 22
[total dose/cycle = 120 mg/m^2]

Repeat cycle every 6 weeks until disease progression or unacceptable toxicity

Irinotecan-Fluorouracil-Leucovorin (Esophageal Cancer)

Use Esophageal cancer

Regimen NOTE: Multiple variations are listed.

Variation 1:

Irinotecan: I.V.: 80 mg/m^2/dose days 1, 8, 15, 22, 29, and 36
[total dose/week = 480 mg/m^2]

Fluorouracil: I.V.: 2000 mg/m^2/dose continuous infusion over 24 hours days 1, 8, 15, 22, 29, and 36
[total dose/cycle = 12,000 mg/m^2]

Leucovorin: I.V.: 500 mg/m^2/dose continuous infusion over 24 hours days 1, 8, 15, 22, 29, and 36
[total dose/week = 3000 mg/m^2]

Repeat cycle every 8 weeks until disease progression or unacceptable toxicity.

Variation 2:

Irinotecan: I.V.: 80 mg/m^2/dose day 1
[total dose/cycle = 80 mg/m^2]

Leucovorin: I.V.: 500 mg/m^2/dose over 2 hours day 1
[total dose/cycle = 500 mg/m^2]

Fluorouracil: I.V.: 2000 mg/m^2/dose continuous infusion over 22 hours day 1 (begin immediately after leucovorin)
[total dose/cycle = 2000 mg/m^2]

Repeat every week for 6 weeks followed by a 1-week rest, continue until disease progression or unacceptable toxicity.

Irinotecan-Leucovorin-Fluorouracil (Gastric Cancer)

Use Gastric cancer

Regimen NOTE: Multiple variations are listed.

Variation 1:

Irinotecan: I.V.: 80 mg/m^2/dose day 1
[total dose/week = 80 mg/m^2]

Leucovorin: I.V.: 500 mg/m^2/dose over 2 hours day 1
[total dose/week = 500 mg/m^2]

Fluorouracil: I.V.: 2000 mg/m^2/dose continuous infusion over 22 hours day 1
[total dose/week = 2000 mg/m^2]

Repeat cycle weekly for 6 weeks followed by a 1-week rest; repeat until disease progression or unacceptable toxicity

Variation 2:

Irinotecan: I.V.: 180 mg/m^2/dose day 1
[total dose/cycle = 180 mg/m^2]

Leucovorin: I.V.: 200 mg/m^2/dose over 2 hours days 1 and 2
[total dose/cycle = 400 mg/m^2]

Fluorouracil: I.V. bolus: 400 mg/m^2 days 1 and 2
followed by I.V.: 600 mg/m^2/dose continuous infusion over 22 hours days 1 and 2
[total dose/cycle = 2000 mg/m^2]

Repeat cycle every 14 days for at least 4 cycles or until disease progression or unacceptable toxicity

Irinotecan (Small Cell Lung Cancer Regimen)

Use Lung cancer, small cell

Regimen

Irinotecan: I.V.: 100 mg/m^2/day over 90 minutes days 1, 8, 15, and 22
[total dose/cycle = 400 mg/m^2]

Repeat cycle every 28 days

Irinotecan-Temozolomide (Ewing Sarcoma)

Use Ewing sarcoma

Regimen

Irinotecan: I.V.: 20 mg/m^2/dose days 1 to 5 and days 8 to 12
[total dose/cycle = 200 mg/m^2]
Temozolomide: Oral: 100 mg/m^2/dose days 1 to 5
[total dose/cycle = 500 mg/m^2]
Repeat cycle every 21 days

Ixabepilone-Capecitabine

Use Breast cancer

Regimen

Capecitabine: Oral: 1000 mg/m^2 twice daily days 1 to 14
[total dose/cycle = 28,000 mg/m^2]
Ixabepilone: I.V.: 40 mg/m^2 day 1
[total dose/cycle = 40 mg/m^2]
Repeat cycle every 3 weeks

Lapatinib-Letrozole (Breast Cancer)

Use Breast cancer

Regimen

Lapatinib: Oral: 1500 mg/day days 1 to 28
[total dose/cycle = 42,000 mg]
Letrozole: Oral: 2.5 mg/day days 1 to 28
[total dose/cycle = 70 mg]
Repeat cycle every 28 days until disease progression

Lapatinib-Trastuzumab (Breast Cancer)

Use Breast cancer

Regimen

Week 1:
Trastuzumab: I.V.: 4 mg/kg (loading dose) day 1
[total dose/week 1 = 4 mg/kg]
Lapatinib: Oral: 1000 mg/day days 1 to 7
[total dose/week = 7000 mg]
Subsequent weeks:
Trastuzumab: I.V.: 2 mg/kg day 1
[total dose/week = 2 mg/kg]
Lapatinib: Oral: 1000 mg/day days 1 to 7
[total dose/week = 7000 mg]
Repeat weekly

Larson Regimen (ALL)

Use Leukemia, acute lymphocytic

Regimen NOTE: Multiple variations are listed.

Variation 1 (CALGB 8811):
Induction, patients <60 years of age (4-week cycle):
Cyclophosphamide: I.V.: 1200 mg/m^2 day 1
[total dose/cycle = 1200 mg/m^2]
Daunorubicin: I.V.: 45 mg/m^2/dose days 1, 2, and 3
[total dose/cycle = 135 mg/m^2]
Vincristine: I.V.: 2 mg/dose days 1, 8, 15, and 22
[total dose/cycle = 8 mg]
Prednisone: Oral: 60 mg/m^2/dose days 1 to 21
[total dose/cycle = 1260 mg/m^2]
Asparaginase: SubQ: 6000 units/m^2/dose days 5, 8, 11, 15, 18, and 22
[total dose/cycle = 36,000 units/m^2]

Induction, patients ≥60 years of age (4-week cycle):
Cyclophosphamide: I.V.: 800 mg/m^2 day 1
[total dose/cycle = 800 mg/m^2]
Daunorubicin: I.V.: 30 mg/m^2/dose days 1, 2, and 3
[total dose/cycle = 90 mg/m^2]
Vincristine: I.V.: 2 mg/dose days 1, 8, 15, and 22
[total dose/cycle = 8 mg]
Prednisone: Oral: 60 mg/m^2/dose days 1 to 7
[total dose/cycle = 420 mg/m^2]
Asparaginase: SubQ: 6000 units/m^2/dose days 5, 8, 11, 15, 18, and 22
[total dose/cycle = 36,000 units/m^2]
Early intensification (4-week cycle; repeat cycle once):
Methotrexate: I.T.: 15 mg/dose day 1
[total dose/cycle = 15 mg]
Cyclophosphamide: I.V.: 1000 mg/m^2 day 1
[total dose/cycle = 1000 mg/m^2]
Mercaptopurine: Oral: 60 mg/m^2/dose days 1 to 14
[total dose/cycle = 840 mg/m^2]
Cytarabine: SubQ: 75 mg/m^2/dose days 1 to 4 and 8 to 11
[total dose/cycle = 600 mg/m^2]
Vincristine: I.V.: 2 mg/dose days 15 and 22
[total dose/cycle = 4 mg]
Asparaginase: SubQ: 6000 units/m^2/dose days 15, 18, 22, and 25
[total dose/cycle = 24,000 units/m^2]
CNS prophylaxis/interim maintenance (12 week duration; with cranial irradiation days 1 to 12):
Methotrexate: I.T.: 15 mg/dose days 1, 8, 15, 22, and 29
[total dose/cycle = 75 mg]
Mercaptopurine: Oral: 60 mg/m^2/dose days 1 to 70
[total dose/cycle = 4200 mg/m^2]
Methotrexate: Oral: 20 mg/m^2/dose days 36, 43, 50, 57, and 64
[total dose/cycle = 100 mg/m^2]
Late intensification (8-week cycle):
Doxorubicin: I.V.: 30 mg/m^2/dose days 1, 8, and 15
[total dose/cycle = 90 mg/m^2]
Vincristine: I.V.: 2 mg/dose days 1, 8, and 15
[total dose/cycle = 6 mg]
Dexamethasone: Oral: 10 mg/m^2/dose days 1 to 14
[total dose/cycle = 140 mg/m^2]
Cyclophosphamide: I.V.: 1000 mg/m^2 day 29
[total dose/cycle = 1000 mg/m^2]
Thioguanine: Oral: 60 mg/m^2/dose days 29 to 42
[total dose/cycle = 840 mg/m^2]
Cytarabine: SubQ: 75 mg/m^2/dose days 29 to 32 and 36 to 39
[total dose/cycle = 600 mg/m^2]
Maintenance (continue until 24 months from diagnosis):
Vincristine: I.V. 2 mg/dose day 1 every 4 weeks
[total dose/4 weeks = 2 mg]
Prednisone: Oral: 60 mg/m^2/dose days 1 to 5 every 4 weeks
[total dose/4 weeks = 300 mg/m^2]
Methotrexate: Oral: 20 mg/m^2/dose days 1, 8, 15, and 22
[total dose/phase = 80 mg/m^2]
Mercaptopurine: Oral: 60 mg/m^2/dose days 1 to 28
[total dose/phase = 1680 mg/m^2]
Variation 2 (with G-CSF; CALGB 9111):
Induction, patients <60 years of age (4-week cycle):
Cyclophosphamide: I.V.: 1200 mg/m^2 day 1
[total dose/cycle = 1200 mg/m^2]
Daunorubicin: I.V.: 45 mg/m^2/dose days 1, 2, and 3
[total dose/cycle = 135 mg/m^2]
Vincristine: I.V.: 2 mg/dose days 1, 8, 15, and 22
[total dose/cycle = 8 mg]
Prednisone: Oral: 60 mg/m^2/dose days 1 to 21
[total dose/cycle = 1260 mg/m^2]

Asparaginase: SubQ, I.M.: 6000 units/m^2/dose days 5, 8, 11, 15, 18, and 22
[total dose/cycle = 36,000 units/m^2]
Filgrastim: SubQ: 5 mcg/kg/day starting day 4; continue for at least 7 days and until ANC ≥1000/mm^3 on two draws, 24 hours apart

Induction, patients ≥60 years of age (4-week cycle):
Cyclophosphamide: I.V.: 800 mg/m^2 day 1
[total dose/cycle = 800 mg/m^2]
Daunorubicin: I.V.: 30 mg/m^2/dose days 1, 2, and 3
[total dose/cycle = 90 mg/m^2]
Vincristine: I.V.: 2 mg/dose days 1, 8, 15, and 22
[total dose/cycle = 8 mg]
Prednisone: Oral: 60 mg/m^2/dose days 1 to 7
[total dose/cycle = 420 mg/m^2]
Asparaginase: SubQ, I.M.: 6000 units/m^2/dose days 5, 8, 11, 15, 18, and 22
[total dose/cycle = 36,000 units/m^2]
Filgrastim: SubQ: 5 mcg/kg/day starting day 4; continue for at least 7 days and until ANC ≥1000/mm^3 on two draws, 24 hours apart

Early intensification (4-week cycle; repeat cycle once):
Methotrexate: I.T.: 15 mg/dose day 1
[total dose/cycle = 15 mg]
Cyclophosphamide: I.V.: 1000 mg/m^2 day 1
[total dose/cycle = 1000 mg/m^2]
Mercaptopurine: Oral: 60 mg/m^2/dose days 1 to 14
[total dose/cycle = 840 mg/m^2]
Cytarabine: SubQ: 75 mg/m^2/dose days 1 to 4 and 8 to 11
[total dose/cycle = 600 mg/m^2]
Vincristine: I.V.: 2 mg/dose days 15 and 22
[total dose/cycle = 4 mg]
Asparaginase: SubQ, I.M.: 6000 units/m^2/dose days 15, 18, 22, and 25
[total dose/cycle = 24,000 units/m^2]
Filgrastim: SubQ: 5 mcg/kg/day starting day 2; continue at least 14 days and until ANC ≥5000/mm^3 on two draws, 24 hours apart

CNS prophylaxis/interim maintenance (12-week duration; with cranial irradiation days 1 to 12):
Methotrexate: I.T.: 15 mg/dose days 1, 8, 15, 22, and 29
[total dose/cycle = 75 mg]
Mercaptopurine: Oral: 60 mg/m^2/dose days 1 to 70
[total dose/cycle = 4200 mg/m^2]
Methotrexate: Oral: 20 mg/m^2/dose days 36, 43, 50, 57, and 64
[total dose/cycle = 100 mg/m^2]

Late intensification (8-week cycle):
Doxorubicin: I.V.: 30 mg/m^2/dose days 1, 8, and 15
[total dose/cycle = 90 mg/m^2]
Vincristine: I.V.: 2 mg/dose days 1, 8, and 15
[total dose/cycle = 6 mg]
Dexamethasone: Oral: 10 mg/m^2/dose days 1 to 14
[total dose/cycle = 140 mg/m^2]
Cyclophosphamide: I.V.: 1000 mg/m^2 day 29
[total dose/cycle = 1000 mg/m^2]
Thioguanine: Oral: 60 mg/m^2/dose days 29 to 42
[total dose/cycle = 840 mg/m^2]
Cytarabine: SubQ: 75 mg/m^2/dose days 29 to 32 and 36 to 39
[total dose/cycle = 600 mg/m^2]

Maintenance (continue until 24 months from diagnosis):
Vincristine: I.V.: 2 mg/dose day 1 every 4 weeks
[total dose/4 weeks = 2 mg]
Prednisone: Oral: 60 mg/m^2/dose days 1 to 5 every 4 weeks
[total dose/4 weeks = 300 mg/m^2]
Methotrexate: Oral: 20 mg/m^2/dose days 1, 8, 15, and 22
[total dose/phase = 80 mg/m^2]
Mercaptopurine: Oral: 60 mg/m^2/dose days 1 to 28
[total dose/phase = 1680 mg/m^2]

Lenalidomide-Dexamethasone

Use Multiple myeloma

Regimen

Lenalidomide: Oral: 25 mg/day days 1 to 21
[total dose/cycle = 525 mg]
Dexamethasone: Oral: 40 mg/day days 1 to 4, 9 to 12, and 17 to 20 (cycles 1 to 4)
[total dose/cycle = 480 mg]
Dexamethasone: Oral 40 mg/day days 1 to 4 (cycle 5 and beyond)
[total dose/cycle = 160 mg]
Repeat cycle every 28 days

Lenalidomide-Dexamethasone (Low Dose)

Use Multiple myeloma

Regimen

Lenalidomide: Oral: 25 mg/day days 1 to 21
[total dose/cycle = 525 mg]
Dexamethasone: Oral: 40 mg/day days 1, 8, 15, and 22
[total dose/cycle = 160 mg]
Repeat cycle every 28 days

Linker Protocol (ALL)

Use Leukemia, acute lymphocytic

Regimen

Remission induction:

Daunorubicin: I.V.: 50 mg/m^2/day days 1, 2, and 3
[total dose/cycle = 150 mg/m^2]
Vincristine: I.V.: 2 mg/day days 1, 8, 15, and 22
[total dose/cycle = 8 mg]
Prednisone: Oral: 60 mg/m^2/day days 1 to 28
[total dose/cycle = 1680 mg/m^2]
Asparaginase: I.M.: 6000 units/m^2/day days 17 to 28
[total dose/cycle = 72,000 units/m^2]

If residual leukemia in bone marrow on day 14:

Daunorubicin: I.V.: 50 mg/m^2 day 15
[total dose/cycle = 50 mg/m^2]

If residual leukemia in bone marrow on day 28:

Daunorubicin: I.V.: 50 mg/m^2/day days 29 and 30
[total dose/cycle = 100 mg/m^2]
Vincristine: I.V.: 2 mg/day days 29 and 36
[total dose/cycle = 4 mg]
Prednisone: Oral: 60 mg/m^2/day days 29 to 42
[total dose/cycle = 840 mg/m^2]
Asparaginase: I.M.: 6000 units/m^2/day days 29 to 35
[total dose/cycle = 42,000 units/m^2]

Consolidation therapy:

Treatment A (cycles 1, 3, 5, and 7)

Daunorubicin: I.V.: 50 mg/m^2/day days 1 and 2
[total dose/cycle = 100 mg/m^2]
Vincristine: I.V.: 2 mg/day days 1 and 8
[total dose/cycle = 4 mg]
Prednisone: Oral: 60 mg/m^2/day days 1 to 14
[total dose/cycle = 840 mg/m^2]
Asparaginase: I.M.: 12,000 units/m^2/day days 2, 4, 7, 9, 11, and 14
[total dose/cycle = 72,000 units/m^2]

Treatment B (cycles 2, 4, 6, and 8)

Teniposide: I.V.: 165 mg/m^2/day days 1, 4, 8, and 11
[total dose/cycle = 660 mg/m^2]
Cytarabine: I.V.: 300 mg/m^2/day days 1, 4, 8, and 11
[total dose/cycle = 1200 mg/m^2]

Treatment C (cycle 9)
Methotrexate: I.V.: 690 mg/m^2 continuous infusion over 42 hours day 1
[total dose/cycle = 690 mg/m^2]
Leucovorin: I.V.: 15 mg/m^2 every 6 hours for 12 doses (start at end of methotrexate infusion)
[total dose/cycle = 180 mg/m^2]
Administer remission induction regimen for one cycle only. Repeat consolidation cycle every 28 days.

MACOP-B

Use Lymphoma, non-Hodgkin

Regimen

Methotrexate: I.V. bolus: 100 mg/m^2 weeks 2, 6, 10
followed by I.V.: 300 mg/m^2 over 4 hours weeks 2, 6, and 10
[total dose/cycle = 1200 mg/m^2]
Doxorubicin: I.V.: 50 mg/m^2 weeks 1, 3, 5, 7, 9, and 11
[total dose/cycle = 300 mg/m^2]
Cyclophosphamide: I.V.: 350 mg/m^2 weeks 1, 3, 5, 7, 9, and 11
[total dose/cycle = 2100 mg/m^2]
Vincristine: I.V.: 1.4 mg/m^2 (maximum dose: 2 mg) weeks 2, 4, 6, 8, 10, and 12
[total dose/cycle = 8.4 mg/m^2; maximum: 12 mg]
Bleomycin: I.V.: 10 units/m^2 weeks 4, 8, and 12
[total dose/cycle = 30 units/m^2]
Prednisone: Oral: 75 mg/day for 12 weeks, then taper over 2 weeks
Leucovorin calcium: Oral: 15 mg/m^2 every 6 hours, for 6 doses (beginning 24 hours after methotrexate) weeks 2, 6, and 10
[total dose/cycle = 270 mg/m^2]
Administer one cycle

MAID (Sarcoma)

Use Sarcoma

Regimen NOTE: Multiple variations are listed.

Variation 1:
Mesna: I.V.: 2000 mg/m^2/day continuous infusion days 1 to 4
[total dose/cycle = 8000 mg/m^2]
Doxorubicin: I.V.: 15 mg/m^2/day continuous infusion days 1 to 4
[total dose/cycle = 60 mg/m^2]
Ifosfamide: I.V.: 2000 mg/m^2/day continuous infusion days 1, 2, and 3
[total dose/cycle = 6000 mg/m^2]
Dacarbazine: I.V.: 250 mg/m^2/day continuous infusion days 1 to 4
[total dose/cycle = 1000 mg/m^2]
Repeat cycle every 21 days until disease progression or until maximum lifetime cumulative doxorubicin dose of 450 mg/m^2

Variation 2:
Mesna: I.V.: 2500 mg/m^2/day continuous infusion days 1 to 4
[total dose/cycle = 10,000 mg/m^2]
Doxorubicin: I.V.: 20 mg/m^2/day continuous infusion days 1, 2, and 3
[total dose/cycle = 60 mg/m^2]
Ifosfamide: I.V.: 2500 mg/m^2/day continuous infusion days 1, 2, and 3
[total dose/cycle = 7500 mg/m^2]
Dacarbazine: I.V.: 300 mg/m^2/day continuous infusion days 1, 2, and 3
[total dose/cycle = 900 mg/m^2]
Repeat cycle every 21 days (delay 1 week for leukopenia or thrombocytopenia)

Variation 3 (if prior pelvic irradiation):
Mesna: I.V.: 2500 mg/m^2/day continuous infusion days 1 to 4
[total dose/cycle = 10,000 mg/m^2]
Doxorubicin: I.V.: 20 mg/m^2/day continuous infusion days 1, 2, and 3
[total dose/cycle = 60 mg/m^2]
Ifosfamide: I.V.: 1500 mg/m^2/day continuous infusion days 1, 2, and 3
[total dose/cycle = 4500 mg/m^2]
Dacarbazine: I.V.: 300 mg/m^2/day continuous infusion days 1, 2, and 3
[total dose/cycle = 900 mg/m^2]
Repeat cycle every 21 days (delay 1 week for leukopenia or thrombocytopenia)

Variation 4:
Mesna: I.V.: 2500 mg/m^2/day continuous infusion days 1 to 4
[total dose/cycle = 10,000 mg/m^2]
Doxorubicin: I.V.: 15 mg/m^2/day continuous infusion days 1 to 4
[total dose/cycle = 60 mg/m^2]
Ifosfamide: I.V.: 2000 mg/m^2/day continuous infusion days 1, 2, and 3
[total dose/cycle = 6000 mg/m^2]
Dacarbazine: I.V.: 250 mg/m^2/day continuous infusion days 1 to 4
[total dose/cycle = 1000 mg/m^2]
Repeat cycle every 21 days (or when adequate hematologic recovery)

m-BACOD

Use Lymphoma, non-Hodgkin

Regimen

Methotrexate: I.V.: 200 mg/m^2/day days 8 and 15
[total dose/cycle = 400 mg/m^2]
Leucovorin calcium: Oral: 10 mg/m^2 every 6 hours for 8 doses (beginning 24 hours after each methotrexate dose) days 9 and 16
[total dose/cycle = 160 mg/m^2]
Bleomycin: I.V.: 4 units/m^2 day 1
[total dose/cycle = 4 units/m^2]
Doxorubicin: I.V.: 45 mg/m^2 day 1
[total dose/cycle = 45 mg/m^2]
Cyclophosphamide: I.V.: 600 mg/m^2 day 1
[total dose/cycle = 600 mg/m^2]
Vincristine: I.V.: 1 mg/m^2 day 1
[total dose/cycle = 1 mg/m^2]
Dexamethasone: Oral: 6 mg/m^2/day days 1 to 5
[total dose/cycle = 30 mg/m^2]
Repeat cycle every 21 days

MEC (AML Induction)

Use Leukemia, acute myeloid

Regimen

Variation 1:
Mitoxantrone: I.V.: 12 mg/m^2/day over 30 minutes days 1, 2, and 3
[total dose/cycle = 36 mg/m^2]
Cytarabine: I.V.: 500 mg/m^2/day continuous infusion days 1, 2, and 3 and days 8, 9, and 10
[total dose/cycle = 3000 mg/m^2]
Etoposide: I.V.: 200 mg/m^2/day continuous infusion days 8, 9, and 10
[total dose/cycle = 600 mg/m^2]
May administer a second induction cycle if needed
Variation 2:
Etoposide: I.V.: 80 mg/m^2/day over 1 hour days 1 to 6
[total dose/cycle = 480 mg/m^2]
Cytarabine: I.V.: 1 g/m^2/day over 6 hours days 1 to 6
[total dose/cycle = 6 g/m^2]
Mitoxantrone: I.V.: 6 mg/m^2/day I.V. bolus days 1 to 6 (3 hours after the end of the cytarabine infusion)
[total dose/cycle = 36 mg/m^2]

MEC-G (AML Induction)

Use Leukemia, acute myeloid

Regimen

Variation 1:
Mitoxantrone: I.V.: 12 mg/m^2/day days 1, 2, and 3
[total dose/cycle = 36 mg/m^2]
Cytarabine: I.V.: 500 mg/m^2/day continuous infusion days 1, 2, and 3 and days 8, 9, and 10
[total dose/cycle = 3000 mg/m^2]
Etoposide: I.V.: 200 mg/m^2/day continuous infusion days 8, 9, and 10
[total dose/cycle = 600 mg/m^2]
Sargramostim: I.V.: 5 mcg/kg/day over 6 hours days 4 to 8

Variation 2:
Mitoxantrone: I.V.: 12 mg/m^2/day I.V. bolus days 1, 2, and 3
[total dose/cycle = 36 mg/m^2]
Cytarabine: I.V.: 500 mg/m^2/day continuous infusion days 1, 2, and 3 and days 8, 9, and 10
[total dose/cycle = 3000 mg/m^2]
Etoposide: I.V.: 200 mg/m^2/day continuous infusion days 8, 9, and 10
[total dose/cycle = 600 mg/m^2]
Filgrastim: SubQ: 5 mcg/kg/day starting on day 4 til ANC >500/mm^3 for 2 consecutive days
Administer one cycle only

Melphalan-Prednisone-Bortezomib (Multiple Myeloma)

Use Multiple myeloma

Regimen NOTE: Multiple variations are listed.

Variation 1:
Bortezomib: I.V.: 1.3 mg/m^2/day days 1, 4, 8, 11, 22, 25, 29, and 32
[total dose/cycle = 10.4 mg/m^2]
Melphalan: Oral: 9 mg/m^2/day days 1 to 4
[total dose/cycle = 36 mg/m^2]
Prednisone: Oral: 60 mg/m^2/day days 1 to 4
[total dose/cycle = 240 mg/m^2]
Repeat cycle every 42 days for 4 cycles
followed by
Bortezomib: I.V.: 1.3 mg/m^2/day days 1, 8, 22, and 29
[total dose/cycle = 5.2 mg/m^2]
Melphalan: Oral: 9 mg/m^2/day days 1 to 4
[total dose/cycle = 36 mg/m^2]
Prednisone: Oral: 60 mg/m^2/day days 1 to 4
[total dose/cycle = 240 mg/m^2]
Repeat cycle every 42 days for 5 cycles

Variation 2:
Bortezomib: I.V.: 1-1.3 mg/m^2/day days 1, 4, 8, 11, 22, 25, 29, and 32
[total dose/cycle = 8-10.4 mg/m^2]
Melphalan: Oral: 9 mg/m^2/day days 1 to 4
[total dose/cycle = 36 mg/m^2]
Prednisone: Oral: 60 mg/m^2/day days 1 to 4
[total dose/cycle = 240 mg/m^2]
Repeat cycle every 42 days for 4 cycles
followed by
Bortezomib: I.V.: 1-1.3 mg/m^2/day days 1, 8, 15, and 22
[total dose/cycle = 4-5.2 mg/m^2]
Melphalan: Oral: 9 mg/m^2/day days 1 to 4
[total dose/cycle = 36 mg/m^2]
Prednisone: Oral: 60 mg/m^2/day days 1 to 4
[total dose/cycle = 240 mg/m^2]
Repeat cycle every 35 days for 5 cycles

Melphalan-Prednisone (Multiple Myeloma)

Use Multiple myeloma

Regimen NOTE: Multiple variations are listed.

Variation 1:
Melphalan: Oral: 0.25 mg/kg/dose days 1 to 4
[total dose/cycle = 1 mg/kg]
Prednisone: Oral: 2 mg/kg/dose days 1 to 4
[total dose/cycle = 8 mg/kg]
Repeat cycle every 6 weeks for a total of 12 cycles

Variation 2:
Melphalan: Oral: 4 mg/m^2/dose days 1 to 7
[total dose/cycle = 28 mg/m^2]
Prednisone: Oral: 40 mg/m^2/dose days 1 to 7
[total dose/cycle = 280 mg/m^2]
Repeat cycle every 4 weeks for a total of 6 cycles

Variation 3:
Melphalan: Oral: 9 mg/m^2/dose days 1 to 4
[total dose/cycle = 36 mg/m^2]
Prednisone: Oral: 60 mg/m^2/dose days 1 to 4
[total dose/cycle = 240 mg/m^2]
Repeat cycle every 6 weeks for a total of 9 cycles
Variation 4:
Melphalan: Oral: 6 mg/m^2/dose days 1 to 7
[total dose/cycle = 42 mg/m^2]
Prednisone: Oral: 60 mg/m^2/dose days 1 to 7
[total dose/cycle = 420 mg/m^2]
Repeat cycle every 4 weeks for a total of 6 cycles
Followed by (in responders):
Interferon alfa: SubQ: 3 million units/dose 3 times/week until relapse
Dexamethasone: Oral: 40 mg/dose days 1 to 4 every 2 months until relapse

Melphalan-Prednisone-Thalidomide (Multiple Myeloma)

Use Multiple myeloma

Regimen NOTE: Multiple variations are listed.
Variation 1:
Melphalan: Oral: 4 mg/m^2/day days 1 to 7
[total dose/cycle = 28 mg/m^2]
Prednisone: Oral: 40 mg/m^2/day days 1 to 7
[total dose/cycle = 280 mg/m^2]
Thalidomide: Oral: 100 mg/day days 1 to 28
[total dose/cycle = 2800 mg]
Repeat cycle every 28 days for 6 cycles
followed by
Thalidomide: Oral: 100 mg daily (as maintenance)
Variation 2:
Melphalan: Oral: 0.25 mg/kg/dose days 1 to 4
[total dose/cycle = 1 mg/kg]
Prednisone: Oral: 2 mg/kg/dose days 1 to 4
[total dose/cycle = 8 mg/kg]
Thalidomide: Oral: 100-400 mg/day days 1 to 42
[total dose/cycle = 4200-16,800 mg]
Repeat cycle every 6 weeks for a total of 12 cycles (discontinue thalidomide on day 4 of the last cycle)

Methotrexate-Vinblastine (Desmoid Tumor)

Use Soft tissue sarcoma (desmoid tumor)

Regimen
Methotrexate: I.V.: 30 mg/m^2 every 7-10 days
[total dose/treatment = 30 mg/m^2]
Vinblastine: I.V.: 6 mg/m^2 every 7-10 days
[total dose/treatment = 6 mg/m^2]
Continue treatment for 1 year (52 treatments)

MINE

Use Lymphoma, non-Hodgkin

Regimen
Mesna: I.V.: 1.33 g/m^2/day concurrent with ifosfamide dose, then 500 mg orally (4 hours after each ifosfamide infusion) days 1, 2, and 3
[total dose/cycle = 3.99 g/m^2/1500 mg]
Ifosfamide: I.V.: 1.33 g/m^2/day days 1, 2, and 3
[total dose/cycle = 3.99 g/m^2]
Mitoxantrone: I.V.: 8 mg/m^2 day 1
[total dose/cycle = 8 mg/m^2]
Etoposide: I.V.: 65 mg/m^2/day days 1, 2, and 3
[total dose/cycle = 195 mg/m^2]
Repeat cycle every 28 days

MINE-ESHAP (Hodgkin)

Use Lymphoma, Hodgkin

Regimen

Refractory disease (alternate MINE regimen with ESHAP regimen for a total of 2 MINE cycles and 2 ESHAP cycles):

MINE Regimen:

Mesna: I.V.: 2250 mg/m^2/day days 1, 2, and 3
[total dose/cycle = 6750 mg/m^2]

Ifosfamide: I.V.: 1500 mg/m^2/day days 1, 2, and 3
[total dose/cycle = 4500 mg/m^2]

Mitoxantrone: I.V.: 10 mg/m^2 day 1
[total dose/cycle = 10 mg/m^2]

Etoposide: I.V.: 80 mg/m^2/day days 1, 2, and 3
[total dose/cycle = 240 mg/m^2]

Treatment cycle is 28 days

ESHAP Regimen:

Etoposide: I.V.: 40 mg/m^2/day days 1 to 4
[total dose/cycle = 160 mg/m^2]

Methylprednisolone: I.V.: 250 mg/day days 1 to 4
[total dose/cycle = 1000 mg]

Cisplatin: I.V.: 25 mg/m^2/day continuous infusion over 21 hours days 1 to 4
[total dose/cycle = 100 mg/m^2]

Cytarabine: I.V.: 2000 mg/m^2 day 5
[total dose/cycle = 2000 mg/m^2]

Treatment cycle is 28 days

MINE-ESHAP (NHL)

Use Lymphoma, non-Hodgkin

Regimen

Relapsed NHL (In patients achieving a complete remission, administer 6 cycles of MINE regimen, followed by 3 cycles of ESHAP regimen):

MINE regimen:

Mesna: I.V.: 1330 mg/m^2/day over 1 hour days 1, 2, and 3
[total I.V. dose/cycle = 4000 mg/m^2]

Followed by Mesna: Oral: 500 mg (4 hours after ifosfamide) days 1, 2, and 3
[total oral dose/cycle = 1500 mg]

Ifosfamide: I.V.: 1330 mg/m^2/day over 1 hour days 1, 2, and 3
[total dose/cycle = 4000 mg/m^2]

Mitoxantrone: I.V.: 8 mg/m^2 day 1
[total dose/cycle = 8 mg/m^2]

Etoposide: I.V.: 65 mg/m^2/day over 1 hour days 1, 2, and 3
[total dose/cycle = 195 mg/m^2]

Repeat MINE cycle every 21 days for 6 cycles, followed by 3 cycles of ESHAP

ESHAP Regimen:

Etoposide: I.V.: 60 mg/m^2/day over 1 hour days 1 to 4
[total dose/cycle = 240 mg/m^2]

Methylprednisolone: I.V.: 500 mg/day days 1 to 4
[total dose/cycle = 2000 mg]

Cisplatin: I.V.: 25 mg/m^2/day continuous infusion days 1 to 4
[total dose/cycle = 100 mg/m^2]

Cytarabine: I.V.: 2000 mg/m^2 over 2 hours day 5
[total dose/cycle = 2000 mg/m^2]

Repeat ESHAP cycle every 21 days for 3 cycles

mini-BEAM (Hodgkin)

Use Lymphoma, Hodgkin disease

Regimen

Carmustine: I.V.: 60 mg/m^2 over 30 minutes day 1
[total dose/cycle = 60 mg/m^2]

Etoposide: I.V.: 75 mg/m^2/day over 30 minutes days 2 to 5
[total dose/cycle = 300 mg/m^2]

Cytarabine: I.V.: 100 mg/m^2 every 12 hours days 2 to 5 (total of 8 doses)
[total dose/cycle = 800 mg/m^2]
Melphalan: I.V.: 30 mg/m^2 over 15 minutes day 6
[total dose/cycle = 30 mg/m^2]
Repeat cycle every 4 to 6 weeks

Mitoxantrone-Etoposide (AML Induction)

Use Leukemia, acute myeloid

Regimen

Mitoxantrone: I.V.: 10 mg/m^2/day over ≤15 minutes days 1 to 5
[total dose/cycle = 50 mg/m^2]
Etoposide: I.V.: 100 mg/m^2/day over 30 minutes days 1 to 5
[total dose/cycle = 500 mg/m^2]
May administer a second induction cycle if needed

Mitoxantrone + Hydrocortisone

Use Prostate cancer

Regimen

Mitoxantrone: I.V.: 14 mg/m^2 day 1
[total dose/cycle = 14 mg/m^2]
Hydrocortisone: Oral: 40 mg daily
[total dose/cycle = 840 mg]
Repeat cycle every 3 weeks

Mitoxantrone-Prednisone (Prostate Cancer)

Use Prostate cancer

Regimen NOTE: Multiple variations are listed.

Variation 1:
Mitoxantrone: I.V.: 12 mg/m^2 day 1
[total dose/cycle = 12 mg/m^2]
Prednisone: Oral: 5 mg twice daily
[total dose/cycle = 210 mg]
Repeat cycle every 21 days for up to a total of 10 cycles

Variation 2:
Cycle 1:
Mitoxantrone: I.V.: 12 mg/m^2 day 1
[total dose/cycle = 12 mg/m^2]
Prednisone: Oral: 5 mg twice daily
[total dose/cycle = 210 mg]
Treatment cycle is 21 days
Cycle 2 and beyond:
Mitoxantrone: I.V.: 12-14 mg/m^2 day 1 (increase to 14 mg/m^2 if no grade 3/4 adverse events)
[total dose/cycle = 12-14 mg/m^2]
Prednisone: Oral: 5 mg twice daily
[total dose/cycle = 210 mg]
Repeat cycle every 21 days for up to a maximum cumulative mitoxantrone dose of 144 mg/m^2

Variation 3:
Cycle 1:
Mitoxantrone: I.V.: 12 mg/m^2 day 1
[total dose/cycle = 12 mg/m^2]
Prednisone: Oral: 5 mg twice daily
[total dose/cycle = 210 mg]
Treatment cycle is 21 days
Cycles 2-8:
Mitoxantrone: I.V.: 12-14 mg/m^2 day 1 (increase to 14 mg/m^2 if granulocyte nadir is >1000/mm^3 and platelet nadir >50,000/ mm^3)
[total dose/cycle = 12-14 mg/m^2]
Prednisone: Oral: 5 mg twice daily
[total dose/cycle = 210 mg]
Treatment cycle is 21 days for up to a total of 8 cycles

MOPP/ABVD (Hodgkin)

Use Lymphoma, Hodgkin disease

Regimen NOTE: Multiple variations are listed.

Variation 1:

Mechlorethamine: I.V.: 6 mg/m^2/day days 1 and 8
[total dose/cycle = 12 mg/m^2]
Vincristine: I.V.: 1.4 mg/m^2/day days 1 and 8
[total dose/cycle = 2.8 mg/m^2]
Procarbazine: Oral: 100 mg/m^2/day days 1 to 14
[total dose/cycle = 1400 mg/m^2]
Prednisone: Oral: 40 mg/m^2/day days 1 to 14 (during cycles 1, 4, 7, and 10 **only**)
[total dose/cycle = 560 mg/m^2]
Doxorubicin: I.V.: 25 mg/m^2/day days 29 and 43
[total dose/cycle = 50 mg/m^2]
Bleomycin: I.V.: 10 units/m^2/day days 29 and 43
[total dose/cycle = 20 units/m^2]
Vinblastine: I.V.: 6 mg/m^2/day days 29 and 43
[total dose/cycle = 12 mg/m^2]
Dacarbazine: I.V.: 375 mg/m^2/day days 29 and 43
[total dose/cycle = 750 mg/m^2]
Repeat cycle every 56 days for a total of 6 cycles.

Variation 2:

Mechlorethamine: I.V.: 6 mg/m^2/day days 1 and 8
[total dose/cycle = 12 mg/m^2]
Vincristine: I.V.: 1.4 mg/m^2/day (maximum dose: 2 mg) days 1 and 8
[total dose/cycle = 2.8 mg/m^2; maximum dose/cycle: 4 mg]
Procarbazine: Oral: 100 mg/m^2/day days 1 to 14
[total dose/cycle = 1400 mg/m^2]
Prednisone: Oral: 40 mg/m^2/day days 1 to 14 (during cycles 1 and 7 **only**)
[total dose/cycle = 560 mg/m^2]
Doxorubicin: I.V.: 25 mg/m^2/day days 29 and 43
[total dose/cycle = 50 mg/m^2]
Bleomycin: I.V.: 10 units/m^2/day days 29 and 43
[total dose/cycle = 20 units/m^2]
Vinblastine: I.V.: 6 mg/m^2/day days 29 and 43
[total dose/cycle = 12 mg/m^2]
Dacarbazine: I.V.: 375 mg/m^2/day days 29 and 43
[total dose/cycle = 750 mg/m^2]
Repeat cycle every 56 days for a total of 6 cycles.

MOPP/ABV Hybrid (Hodgkin)

Use Lymphoma, Hodgkin disease

Regimen

Mechlorethamine: I.V.: 6 mg/m^2 day 1
[total dose/cycle = 6 mg/m^2]
Vincristine: I.V.: 1.4 mg/m^2 (maximum dose: 2 mg) day 1
[total dose/cycle = 1.4 mg/m^2; maximum: 2 mg/cycle]
Procarbazine: Oral: 100 mg/m^2/day days 1 to 7
[total dose/cycle = 700 mg/m^2]
Prednisone: Oral: 40 mg/m^2/day days 1 to 14
[total dose/cycle = 560 mg/m^2]
Doxorubicin: I.V.: 35 mg/m^2 day 8
[total dose/cycle = 35 mg/m^2]
Bleomycin: I.V.: 10 units/m^2 day 8
[total dose/cycle = 10 units/m^2]
Vinblastine: I.V.: 6 mg/m^2 day 8
[total dose/cycle = 6 mg/m^2]
Repeat cycle every 28 days for a maximum of 8 cycles

MOPP (Hodgkin)

Use Lymphoma, Hodgkin

Regimen NOTE: Multiple variations are listed.

Variation 1:

Mechlorethamine: I.V.: 6 mg/m^2/day days 1 and 8
[total dose/cycle = 12 mg/m^2]

Vincristine: I.V.: 1.4 mg/m^2/day days 1 and 8
[total dose/cycle = 2.8 mg/m^2]

Procarbazine: Oral: 100 mg/m^2/day days 1 to 14
[total dose/cycle = 1400 mg/m^2]

Prednisone: Oral: 40 mg/m^2/day days 1 to 14 (cycles 1 and 4)
[total dose/cycle = 560 mg/m^2]

Repeat cycle every 28 days for 6 cycles

Variation 2:

Mechlorethamine: I.V.: 6 mg/m^2/day days 1 and 8
[total dose/cycle = 12 mg/m^2]

Vincristine: I.V.: 1.4 mg/m^2/day (maximum dose: 2 mg) days 1 and 8
[total dose/cycle = 2.8 mg/m^2; maximum dose/cycle: 4 mg]

Procarbazine: Oral: 100 mg/m^2/day days 1 to 14
[total dose/cycle = 1400 mg/m^2]

Prednisone: Oral: 40 mg/m^2/day days 1 to 14 (cycles 1 and 4)
[total dose/cycle = 560 mg/m^2]

Repeat cycle every 28 days for 6-8 cycles

MOPP (Medulloblastoma)

Use Brain tumors

Regimen

Mechlorethamine: I.V.: 3 mg/m^2/day days 1 and 8
[total dose/cycle = 6 mg/m^2]

Vincristine: I.V.: 1.4 mg/m^2/day (maximum dose: 2 mg) days 1 and 8
[total dose/cycle = 2.8 mg/m^2]

Prednisone: Oral: 40 mg/m^2/day days 1 to 10
[total dose/cycle = 400 mg/m^2]

Procarbazine: Oral: 50 mg day 1
[total dose/cycle = 50 mg]

followed by Oral: 100 mg day 2
[total dose/cycle = 100 mg]

followed by Oral: 100 mg/m^2/day days 3 to 10
[total dose/cycle = 800 mg/m^2]

Repeat cycle every 28 days

MTX/6-MP/VP (Maintenance)

Use Leukemia, acute lymphocytic

Regimen

Methotrexate: Oral: 20 mg/m^2 weekly
[total dose/cycle = 80 mg/m^2]

Mercaptopurine: Oral: 75 mg/m^2/day
[total dose/cycle = 2250 mg/m^2]

Vincristine: I.V.: 1.5 mg/m^2 day 1
[total dose/cycle = 1.5 mg/m^2]

Prednisone: Oral: 40 mg/m^2/day days 1 to 5
[total dose/cycle = 200 mg/m^2]

Repeat monthly for 2-3 years

MTX-CDDPAdr

Use Osteosarcoma

Regimen

Cisplatin: I.V.: 75 mg/m^2 day 1 of cycles 1-7, then 120 mg/m^2 for cycles 8, 9, and 10

Doxorubicin: I.V.: 25 mg/m^2/day days 1, 2, and 3 of cycles 1 to 7

Methotrexate: I.V.: 12 g/m^2/day days 21 and 28

Leucovorin calcium rescue: I.V.: 20 mg/m^2 every 3 hours (beginning 16 hours after completion of methotrexate) for 8 doses, then orally every 6 hours for 8 doses

M-VAC (Bladder Cancer)

Use Bladder cancer

Regimen NOTE: Multiple variations are listed.

Variation 1:

Methotrexate: I.V.: 30 mg/m^2/day days 1, 15, and 22
[total dose/cycle = 90 mg/m^2]

Vinblastine: I.V.: 3 mg/m^2/day days 2, 15, and 22
[total dose/cycle = 9 mg/m^2]

Doxorubicin: I.V.: 30 mg/m^2 day 2
[total dose/cycle = 30 mg/m^2]

Cisplatin: I.V.: 70 mg/m^2 day 2
[total dose/cycle = 70 mg/m^2]

Repeat cycle every 4 weeks

Variation 2:

Methotrexate: I.V.: 40 or 50 mg/m^2/day days 1, 15, and 22
[total dose/cycle = 120 or 150 mg/m^2]

Vinblastine: I.V.: 4 or 5 mg/m^2/day days 2, 15, and 22
[total dose/cycle = 12 or 15 mg/m^2]

Doxorubicin: I.V.: 40 or 50 mg/m^2 day 2
[total dose/cycle = 40 or 50 mg/m^2]

Cisplatin: I.V.: 100 mg/m^2 day 2
[total dose/cycle = 100 mg/m^2]

Repeat cycle every 4 weeks

Variation 3:

Methotrexate: I.V.: 30 mg/m^2/day days 1, 15, and 22
[total dose/cycle = 90 mg/m^2]

Vinblastine: I.V.: 3 mg/m^2 day 2
[total dose/cycle = 3 mg/m^2]

Doxorubicin: I.V.: 30 mg/m^2 day 2
[total dose/cycle = 30 mg/m^2]

Cisplatin: I.V.: 70 mg/m^2 day 2
[total dose/cycle = 70 mg/m^2]

Repeat cycle every 4 weeks

Variation 4:

Methotrexate: I.V.: 60 mg/m^2 day 1
[total dose/cycle = 60 mg/m^2]
followed by I.V.: 30 mg/m^2 day 16
[total dose/cycle = 30 mg/m^2]

Vinblastine: I.V.: 4 mg/m^2/day days 2 and 16
[total dose/cycle = 8 mg/m^2]

Doxorubicin: I.V.: 60 mg/m^2 day 2
[total dose/cycle = 60 mg/m^2]

Cisplatin: I.V.: 100 mg/m^2 day 2
[total dose/cycle = 100 mg/m^2]

Repeat cycle every 23 days

Variation 5:

Methotrexate: I.V.: 30 mg/m^2/day days 1, 16, and 23
[total dose/cycle = 90 mg/m^2]

Vinblastine: I.V.: 4 mg/m^2/day days 1, 16, and 23
[total dose/cycle = 12 mg/m^2]

Doxorubicin: I.V.: 60 mg/m^2 day 2
[total dose/cycle = 60 mg/m^2]

Cisplatin: I.V.: 100 mg/m^2 day 2
[total dose/cycle = 100 mg/m^2]

Repeat cycle every 23 days

Variation 6:
Methotrexate: I.V.: 30 or 35 mg/m^2 day 1
[total dose/cycle = 30 or 35 mg/m^2]
Vinblastine: I.V.: 3 or 3.5 mg/m^2 day 2
[total dose/cycle = 3 or 3.5 mg/m^2]
Doxorubicin: I.V.: 30 or 35 mg/m^2 day 2
[total dose/cycle = 30 or 35 mg/m^2]
Cisplatin: I.V.: 70 or 80 mg/m^2 day 2
[total dose/cycle = 70 or 80 mg/m^2]
Repeat cycle every 2 weeks
Variation 7:
Methotrexate: I.V.: 30 mg/m^2 day 1
[total dose/cycle = 30 mg/m^2]
Vinblastine: I.V.: 3 mg/m^2 day 2
[total dose/cycle = 3 mg/m^2]
Doxorubicin: I.V.: 30 mg/m^2 day 2
[total dose/cycle = 30 mg/m^2]
Cisplatin: I.V.: 70 mg/m^2 day 2
[total dose/cycle = 70 mg/m^2]
Repeat cycle every 14 days
Variation 8:
Methotrexate: I.V.: 30 mg/m^2/day days 1, 15, and 22
[total dose/cycle = 90 mg/m^2]
Vinblastine: I.V.: 3 mg/m^2/day days 1, 15, and 22
[total dose/cycle = 9 mg/m^2]
Doxorubicin: I.V.: 45 mg/m^2 day 2
[total dose/cycle = 45 mg/m^2]
Cisplatin: I.V.: 70 mg/m^2 day 2
[total dose/cycle = 70 mg/m^2]
Repeat cycle every 4 weeks
Variation 9:
Methotrexate: I.V.: 40 mg/m^2/day days 1 and 15
[total dose/cycle = 80 mg/m^2]
Vinblastine: I.V.: 4 mg/m^2/day days 1, 16, and 23
[total dose/cycle = 12 mg/m^2]
Doxorubicin: I.V.: 60 mg/m^2 day 2
[total dose/cycle = 60 mg/m^2]
Cisplatin: I.V.: 100 mg/m^2 day 2
[total dose/cycle = 100 mg/m^2]
Repeat cycle every 23 days
Variation 10:
Methotrexate: I.V.: 30 mg/m^2/day days 1, 15, and 22
[total dose/cycle = 90 mg/m^2]
Vinblastine: I.V.: 3 mg/m^2/day days 1, 16, and 22
[total dose/cycle = 9 mg/m^2]
Doxorubicin: I.V.: 30 mg/m^2 day 1
[total dose/cycle = 30 mg/m^2]
Cisplatin: I.V.: 70 mg/m^2 day 1
[total dose/cycle = 70 mg/m^2]
Repeat cycle every 4 weeks
Variation 11:
Methotrexate: I.V.: 30 mg/m^2/day days 1, 15, and 22
[total dose/cycle = 90 mg/m^2]
Vinblastine: I.V.: 3 mg/m^2/day days 2, 15, and 22
[total dose/cycle = 9 mg/m^2]
Doxorubicin: I.V.: 30 mg/m^2 day 2
[total dose/cycle = 30 mg/m^2]
Cisplatin: I.V.: 70 mg/m^2 day 2
[total dose/cycle = 70 mg/m^2]
Leucovorin: Oral: 15 mg every 6 hours for 4 doses days 2, 16, and 23
[total dose/cycle = 180 mg]
Repeat cycle every 4 weeks

Variation 12:
Methotrexate: I.V.: 30 mg/m^2/day days 1 and 15
[total dose/cycle = 60 mg/m^2]
Vinblastine: I.V.: 3 mg/m^2/day days 2 and 15
[total dose/cycle = 6 mg/m^2]
Doxorubicin: I.V.: 30 or 40 mg/m^2 day 3
[total dose/cycle = 30 or 40 mg/m^2]
Cisplatin: I.V.: 70 mg/m^2 day 2
[total dose/cycle = 70 mg/m^2]
Repeat cycle every 4 weeks

Variation 13:
Methotrexate: I.V.: 30 mg/m^2/day days 1 and 15
[total dose/cycle = 60 mg/m^2]
Vinblastine: I.V.: 3 mg/m^2/day days 2 and 15
[total dose/cycle = 6 mg/m^2]
Doxorubicin: I.V.: 30 or 40 mg/m^2 day 2
[total dose/cycle = 30 or 40 mg/m^2]
Cisplatin: I.V.: 70 mg/m^2 day 2
[total dose/cycle = 70 mg/m^2]
Repeat cycle every 4 weeks

New A1 (Neuroblastoma)

Use Neuroblastoma

Regimen

Cyclophosphamide: I.V.: 1200 mg/m^2 over 6 hours day 1
[total dose/cycle = 1200 mg/m^2]
Doxorubicin: I.V.: 40 mg/m^2 day 3
[total dose/cycle = 40 mg/m^2]
Etoposide: I.V.: 100 mg/m^2/day days 1 to 5
[total dose/cycle = 500 mg/m^2]
Cisplatin: I.V.: 90 mg/m^2 day 5
[total dose/cycle = 90 mg/m^2]
Repeat cycle every 28 days for up to a total of 6 cycles

Nilotinib (CML Regimen)

Use Leukemia, chronic myelogenous

Regimen NOTE: Multiple variations are listed.

Variation 1 (newly diagnosed chronic phase):
Nilotinib: Oral: 300 mg twice daily
[total dose/cycle = 16,800 mg]
Repeat cycle every 28 days until disease progression or unacceptable toxicity

Variation 2 (chronic or accelerated phase resistant or intolerant to imatinib):
Nilotinib: Oral: 400 mg twice daily
[total dose/cycle = 22,400 mg]
Repeat cycle every 28 days until disease progression or unacceptable toxicity

OFAR (CLL)

Use Leukemia, chronic lymphocytic

Regimen

Cycle 1:
Oxaliplatin: I.V.: 25 mg/m^2/dose day 1 to 4
[total dose/cycle = 100 mg/m^2]
Fludarabine: I.V.: 30 mg/m^2/dose days 2 and 3
[total dose/cycle = 60 mg/m^2]
Cytarabine: I.V.: 1000 mg/m^2/dose over 2 hours days 2 and 3
[total dose/cycle = 2000 mg/m^2]
Rituximab: I.V.: 375 mg/m^2 day 3
[total dose/cycle = 375 mg/m^2]
Treatment cycle is 4 weeks

Cycles 2-6:
Oxaliplatin: I.V.: 25 mg/m^2/dose day 1 to 4
[total dose/cycle = 100 mg/m^2]
Fludarabine: I.V.: 30 mg/m^2/dose days 2 and 3
[total dose/cycle = 60 mg/m^2]
Cytarabine: I.V.: 1000 mg/m^2/dose over 2 hours days 2 and 3
[total dose/cycle = 2000 mg/m^2]
Rituximab: I.V.: 375 mg/m^2 day 1
[total dose/cycle = 375 mg/m^2]
Repeat cycle every 4 weeks (maximum: 6 cycles)

Oxaliplatin-Cytarabine-Dexamethasone (NHL Regimen)

Use Lymphoma, non-Hodgkin

Regimen
Dexamethasone: I.V. or Oral: 40 mg/day days 1 to 4
[total dose/cycle = 160 mg]
Oxaliplatin: I.V.: 130 mg/m^2 over 2 hours day 1
[total dose/cycle = 130 mg/m^2]
Cytarabine: I.V.: 2000 mg/m^2 over 3 hours every 12 hours for 2 doses day 2
[total dose/cycle = 4000 mg/m^2]
Repeat cycle every 3 weeks

Oxaliplatin-Fluorouracil (Esophageal Cancer)

Use Esophageal cancer

Regimen In combination with radiation therapy:
Oxaliplatin: I.V.: 85 mg/m^2/day over 2 hours days 1, 15, and 29
[total dose/cycle = 255 mg/m^2]
Fluorouracil: I.V.: 180 mg/m^2/day continuous infusion days 8 to 42
[total dose/cycle = 6300 mg/m^2]

PAC (CAP)

Use Ovarian cancer

Regimen
Cisplatin: I.V.: 50 mg/m^2 day 1
[total dose/cycle = 50 mg/m^2]
Doxorubicin: I.V.: 50 mg/m^2 day 1
[total dose/cycle = 50 mg/m^2]
Cyclophosphamide: I.V.: 1000 mg/m^2 day 1
[total dose/cycle = 1000 mg/m^2]
Repeat cycle every 21 days for 8 cycles

PA-CI

Use Hepatoblastoma

Regimen NOTE: Multiple variations are listed.
Variation 1:
Cisplatin: I.V.: 90 mg/m^2 day 1
[total dose/cycle = 90 mg/m^2]
Doxorubicin: I.V.: 20 mg/m^2/day continuous infusion days 2 to 5
[total dose/cycle = 80 mg/m^2]
Repeat cycle every 21 days
Variation 2:
Cisplatin: I.V.: 20 mg/m^2/day days 1 to 4
[total dose/cycle = 80 mg/m^2]
Doxorubicin: I.V.: 100 mg/m^2 continuous infusion day 1
[total dose/cycle = 100 mg/m^2]
Repeat cycle every 21-28 days

Paclitaxel-Bevacizumab

Use Breast cancer

Regimen

Paclitaxel: I.V.: 90 mg/m^2/day days 1, 8, and 15
[total dose/cycle = 270 mg/m^2]
Bevacizumab: I.V.: 10 mg/kg/day days 1 and 15
[total dose/cycle = 20 mg/kg]
Repeat cycle every 28 days

Paclitaxel-Carboplatin-Bevacizumab

Use Lung cancer, nonsquamous, nonsmall cell

Regimen

Paclitaxel: I.V.: 200 mg/m^2 infused over 3 hours day 1
[total dose/cycle = 200 mg/m^2]
followed by
Carboplatin: I.V.: Target AUC 6 day 1
[total dose/cycle = AUC = 6]
followed by
Bevacizumab: I.V.: 15 mg/kg day 1
[total dose/cycle = 15 mg/kg]
Repeat cycle every 21 days for 6 cycles

Paclitaxel-Carboplatin (Bladder Cancer)

Use Bladder cancer

Regimen

Paclitaxel: I.V.: 200 mg/m^2 or 225 mg/m^2 day 1
[total dose/cycle = 200 or 225 mg/m^2]
Carboplatin: I.V.: AUC 5-6 day 1
[total dose/cycle = AUC = 5-6]
Repeat cycle every 21 days

Paclitaxel-Carboplatin (Esophageal Cancer)

Use Esophageal cancer

Regimen

Paclitaxel: I.V.: 50 mg/m^2/dose over 1 hour days 1, 8, 15, 22, and 29
[total dose/cycle = 250 mg/m^2]
Carboplatin: I.V.: AUC = 2 days 1, 8, 15, 22, and 29
[total dose/cycle = AUC = 10]
Administer with concurrent radiation therapy; cycle does not repeat.

Paclitaxel-Carboplatin-Gemcitabine

Use Bladder cancer

Regimen

Paclitaxel: I.V.: 200 mg/m^2 day 1
[total dose/cycle = 200 mg/m^2]
Gemcitabine: I.V.: 1000 mg/m^2/day days 1 and 8
[total dose/cycle = 2000 mg/m^2]
Carboplatin: I.V.: AUC 5 day 1
[total dose/cycle = AUC = 5]
Repeat cycle every 21 days

Paclitaxel-Cetuximab

Use Head and neck cancer

Regimen

Week 1:
Paclitaxel: I.V.: 80 mg/m^2 day 1
[total dose/week 1 = 80 mg/m^2]
Cetuximab: I.V.: 400 mg/m^2 (loading dose) day 1 (week 1 only)
[total loading dose (week 1) = 400 mg/m^2]

Subsequent weeks:
Paclitaxel: I.V.: 80 mg/m^2 day 1
[total dose/week = 80 mg/m^2]
Cetuximab: I.V.: 250 mg/m^2 day 1
[total dose/week = 250 mg/m^2]

Paclitaxel-Cisplatin (Esophageal Cancer)

Use Esophageal cancer

Regimen NOTE: Multiple variations are listed.

Variation 1:
Paclitaxel: I.V.: 50 mg/m^2/dose over 1 hour days 1, 8, 15, 22, and 29
[total dose/cycle = 250 mg/m^2]
Cisplatin: I.V.: 30 mg/m^2/dose days 1, 8, 15, 22, and 29
[total dose/cycle = 150 mg/m^2]
Administered (with concurrent radiation therapy) over one 5-week treatment cycle.
Followed by: Postoperative therapy:
Paclitaxel: I.V.: 175 mg/m^2/dose day 1
[total dose/cycle = 175 mg/m^2]
Cisplatin: I.V.: 75 mg/m^2/dose day 1
[total dose/cycle = 75 mg/m^2]
Repeat postop cycle every 21 days for a total of 3 cycles.

Variation 2:
Paclitaxel: I.V.: 60 mg/m^2/dose over 3 hours days 1, 8, 15, and 22
[total dose/cycle = 240 mg/m^2]
Cisplatin: I.V.: 75 mg/m^2/dose over 2 hours day 1
[total dose/cycle = 75 mg/m^2]
Filgrastim: SubQ: 5 mcg/kg/day starting day 23; continue until ANC >10,000/mm^3
Administer with concurrent radiation therapy; cycle does not repeat.

Variation 3:
Paclitaxel: I.V.: 90 mg/m^2/dose over 3 hours day 1
[total dose/cycle = 90 mg/m^2]
Cisplatin: I.V.: 50 mg/m^2/dose over 1 hour day 1
[total dose/cycle = 50 mg/m^2]
Repeat cycle every 14 days until disease progression or unacceptable toxicity.

Paclitaxel-Cisplatin-Fluorouracil (Esophageal Cancer)

Use Esophageal cancer

Regimen

Paclitaxel: I.V.: 175 mg/m^2 over 3 hours day 1
[total dose/cycle = 175 mg/m^2]
Cisplatin: I.V.: 20 mg/m^2/day days 1 to 5 for cycles 1, 2, and 3
[total dose/cycle = 100 mg/m^2]
then 15 mg/m^2/day days 1 to 5
[total dose/cycle = 75 mg/m^2]
Fluorouracil: I.V.: 750 mg/m^2/day continuous infusion days 1 to 5
[total dose/cycle = 3750 mg/m^2]
Repeat cycle every 28 days

Paclitaxel-Cisplatin-Fluorouracil (Unknown Primary)

Use Unknown primary (squamous cell)

Regimen

Paclitaxel: I.V.: 175 mg/m^2 over 3 hours day 1
[total dose/cycle = 175 mg/m^2]
Cisplatin: I.V.: 100 mg/m^2 day 2
[total dose/cycle = 100 mg/m^2]
Fluorouracil: I.V.: 500 mg/m^2/day continuous infusion days 2 to 6
[total dose/cycle = 2500 mg/m^2]
Repeat cycle every 21 days for a total of 3 cycles

Paclitaxel + Estramustine + Carboplatin

Use Prostate cancer

Regimen

Paclitaxel: I.V.: 100 mg/m^2 day 3 each week
[total dose/cycle = 400 mg/m^2]
Estramustine: Oral: 10 mg/kg/day days 1 to 5 each week
[total dose/cycle = 200 mg/kg]
Carboplatin: I.V.: Target AUC 6 day 3
[total dose/cycle = AUC = 6]
Repeat cycle every 28 days

Paclitaxel + Estramustine + Etoposide

Use Prostate cancer

Regimen

Paclitaxel: I.V.: 135 mg/m^2 day 2
[total dose/cycle = 135 mg/m^2]
Estramustine: Oral: 280 mg 3 times/day days 1 to 14
[total dose/cycle = 11,760 mg]
Etoposide: Oral: 100 mg/day days 1 to 14
[total dose/cycle = 1400 mg]
Repeat cycle every 21 days

Paclitaxel-Fluorouracil (Esophageal Cancer)

Use Esophageal cancer

Regimen

Paclitaxel: I.V.: 45 mg/m^2/dose over 3 hours day 1
[total dose/cycle = 45 mg/m^2]
Fluorouracil: I.V.: 300 mg/m^2/day continuous infusion days 1 to 5
[total dose/cycle = 1500 mg/m^2]
Repeat cycle weekly for 5 weeks; administer concurrent with radiation therapy; cycle does not repeat.

Paclitaxel-Gemcitabine

Use Bladder cancer

Regimen

Paclitaxel: I.V.: 200 mg/m^2 day 1
[total dose/cycle = 200 mg/m^2]
Gemcitabine: I.V.: 1000 mg/m^2/day days 1, 8, and 15
[total dose/cycle = 3000 mg/m^2]
Repeat cycle every 21 days for a maximum of 6 cycles

Paclitaxel-Ifosfamide-Cisplatin

Use Testicular cancer

Regimen

Paclitaxel: I.V.: 250 mg/m^2 continuous infusion day 1
[total dose/cycle = 250 mg/m^2]
Ifosfamide: I.V.: 1500 mg/m^2/day days 2 to 5
[total dose/cycle = 6000 mg/m^2]
Cisplatin: I.V.: 25 mg/m^2/day days 2 to 5
[total dose/cycle = 100 mg/m^2]
Mesna: I.V.: 500 mg/m^2 prior to ifosfamide and every 4 hours for 2 doses, days 2 to 5
[total dose/cycle = 6000 mg/m^2]
Repeat cycle every 21 days for 4 cycles

Paclitaxel Maintenance (Ovarian Cancer)

Use Ovarian cancer

Regimen

Paclitaxel: I.V.: 175 mg/m^2 over 3 hours day 1
[total dose/cycle = 175 mg/m^2]
Repeat cycle every 28 days for 12 cycles

Paclitaxel (Ovarian Regimen)

Use Ovarian cancer

Regimen NOTE: Multiple variations are listed.

Variation 1:

Paclitaxel: I.V.: 80 mg/m^2/day days 1, 8, and 15
[total dose/cycle = 240 mg/m^2]

Repeat cycle every 28 days for 6-9 cycles or until disease progression or unacceptable toxicity

Variation 2:

Paclitaxel: I.V.: 80 mg/m^2/day over 1 hour days 1, 8, 15, and 21
[total dose/cycle = 320 mg/m^2]

Repeat cycle every 28 days for 3 cycles

followed by

Paclitaxel: I.V.: 80 mg/m^2/day days 1, 8, and 15
[total dose/cycle = 240 mg/m^2]

Repeat cycle every 28 days until disease progression or unacceptable toxicity

Variation 3:

Paclitaxel: I.V.: 175 mg/m^2 over 3 hours day 1
[total dose/cycle = 175 mg/m^2]

Repeat cycle every 21 days for 6-10 cycles

Variation 4 (heavily pretreated or poor performance status patients):

Paclitaxel: I.V.: 135 mg/m^2 over 3 hours day 1
[total dose/cycle = 135 mg/m^2]

Repeat cycle every 21 days for 6-10 cycles

Paclitaxel (Protein Bound) (NSCLC Regimen)

Use Lung cancer, nonsmall cell

Regimen NOTE: Multiple variations are listed:

Variation 1:

Paclitaxel (Protein Bound): I.V.: 260 mg/m^2 over 30 minutes day 1
[total dose/cycle = 260 mg/m^2]

Repeat cycle every 21 days until disease progression or unacceptable toxicity

Variation 2:

Paclitaxel (Protein Bound): I.V.: 125 mg/m^2/day over 30 minutes days 1, 8, and 15
[total dose/cycle = 375 mg/m^2]

Repeat cycle every 28 days until disease progression or unacceptable toxicity

Paclitaxel (Small Cell Lung Cancer Regimen)

Use Lung cancer, small cell

Regimen NOTE: Multiple variations are listed.

Variation 1:

Paclitaxel: I.V.: 175 mg/m^2 over 3 hours day 1
[total dose/cycle = 175 mg/m^2]

Repeat cycle every 21 days

Variation 2:

Paclitaxel: I.V.: 80 mg/m^2/day over 1 hour days 1, 8, 15, 22, 29, and 36
[total dose/cycle = 480 mg/m^2]

Repeat cycle every 56 days

Paclitaxel-Vinorelbine

Use Breast cancer

Regimen NOTE: Multiple variations are listed.

Variation 1:

Paclitaxel: I.V.: 135 mg/m^2 day 1
[total dose/cycle = 135 mg/m^2]

Vinorelbine: I.V.: 30 mg/m^2 day 1
[total dose/cycle = 30 mg/m^2]

Repeat cycle every 21 days

Variation 2:
Paclitaxel: I.V.: 150 mg/m^2 day 1
[total dose/cycle = 150 mg/m^2]
Vinorelbine: I.V.: 25 mg/m^2 day 1
[total dose/cycle = 25 mg/m^2]
Repeat cycle every 21 days
Variation 3:
Paclitaxel: I.V.: 135 mg/m^2 day 1
[total dose/cycle = 135 mg/m^2]
Vinorelbine: I.V.: 30 mg/m^2/day days 1 and 8
[total dose/cycle = 60 mg/m^2]
Repeat cycle every 28 days

Panitumumab (Colorectal Regimen)

Use Colorectal cancer

Regimen
Panitumumab: I.V.: 6 mg/kg over 60 minutes day 1
[total dose/cycle = 6 mg/kg]
Repeat cycle every 14 days until disease progression or unacceptable toxicity

Panitumumab + FOLFIRI (Colorectal)

Use Colorectal cancer

Regimen
Panitumumab: I.V.: 6 mg/kg over 30-60 minutes day 1
[total dose/cycle = 6 mg/kg]
Irinotecan: I.V.: 180 mg/m^2 day 1
[total dose/cycle = 180 mg/m^2]
Leucovorin (racemic): I.V.: 400 mg/m^2 day 1
[total dose/cycle = 400 mg/m^2]
Fluorouracil: I.V. bolus: 400 mg/m^2 day 1
followed by I.V.: 2400 mg/m^2 continuous infusion (CI) over 46 hours beginning day 1
[total fluorouracil dose/cycle (bolus and CI) = 2800 mg/m^2]
Repeat cycle every 14 days until disease progression or unacceptable toxicity

Panitumumab + FOLFOX4 (Colorectal)

Use Colorectal cancer

Regimen
Panitumumab: I.V.: 6 mg/kg over 30-60 minutes day 1
[total dose/cycle = 6 mg/kg]
Oxaliplatin: I.V.: 85 mg/m^2 day 1
[total dose/cycle = 85 mg/m^2]
Leucovorin: I.V.: 200 mg/m^2/day days 1 and 2
[total dose/cycle = 400 mg/m^2]
Fluorouracil: I.V. bolus: 400 mg/m^2/day days 1 and 2
followed by I.V.: 600 mg/m^2 continuous infusion (CI) over 22 hours days 1 and 2
[total fluorouracil dose/cycle (bolus and CI) = 2000 mg/m^2]
Note: Bolus fluorouracil and continuous infusion fluorouracil are both given on each day
Repeat cycle every 14 days until disease progression or unacceptable toxicity

Pazopanib (RCC Regimen)

Use Renal cell cancer

Regimen
Pazopanib: Oral: 800 mg once daily
[total dose/cycle = 22,400 mg]
Repeat cycle every 28 days until disease progression or unacceptable toxicity

Pazopanib (Soft Tissue Sarcoma Regimen)

Use Soft tissue sarcoma

Regimen
Pazopanib: Oral: 800 mg once daily
[total dose/cycle = 22,400 mg]
Repeat cycle every 28 days until disease progression or unacceptable toxicity

Pazopanib (Thyroid Cancer Regimen)

Use Thyroid cancer

Regimen

Pazopanib: Oral: 800 mg once daily
[total dose/cycle = 22,400 mg]
Repeat cycle every 28 days until disease progression or unacceptable toxicity

PC (NSCLC)

Use Lung cancer, nonsmall cell

Regimen NOTE: Multiple variations are listed.

Variation 1:
Paclitaxel: I.V.: 175-225 mg/m^2 day 1
[total dose/cycle = 175-225 mg/m^2]
Carboplatin: I.V.: Target AUC 5-7 day 1
[total dose/cycle = AUC = 5-7]
Repeat cycle every 21 days for 2-8 cycles

Variation 2:
Paclitaxel: I.V.: 175 mg/m^2 day 1
[total dose/cycle = 175 mg/m^2]
Cisplatin: I.V.: 80 mg/m^2 day 1
[total dose/cycle = 80 mg/m^2]
Repeat cycle every 21 days

Variation 3:
Paclitaxel: I.V.: 135 mg/m^2 continuous infusion day 1
[total dose/cycle = 135 mg/m^2]
Carboplatin: I.V.: AUC 7.5 day 2
[total dose/cycle = AUC = 7.5]
Repeat cycle every 21 days

Variation 4:
Paclitaxel: I.V.: 135 mg/m^2 continuous infusion day 1
[total dose/cycle = 135 mg/m^2]
Cisplatin: I.V.: 75 mg/m^2 day 2
[total dose/cycle = 75 mg/m^2]
Repeat cycle every 21 days

PCR

Use Leukemia, chronic lymphocytic

Regimen NOTE: Multiple variations are listed.

Variation 1:
Cycle 1:
Cyclophosphamide: I.V.: 600 mg/m^2 day 1
[total dose/cycle = 600 mg/m^2]
Pentostatin: I.V.: 4 mg/m^2 day 1
[total dose/cycle = 4 mg/m^2]
Treatment cycle is 3 weeks
Cycles 2-6:
Cyclophosphamide: I.V.: 600 mg/m^2 day 1
[total dose/cycle = 600 mg/m^2]
Pentostatin: I.V.: 4 mg/m^2 day 1
[total dose/cycle = 4 mg/m^2]
Rituximab: I.V.: 375 mg/m^2 day 1
[total dose/cycle = 375 mg/m^2]
Repeat cycle every 3 weeks

Variation 2:
Cycle 1:
Pentostatin: I.V.: 2 mg/m^2 day 1
[total dose/cycle = 2 mg/m^2]
Cyclophosphamide: I.V.: 600 mg/m^2 day 1
[total dose/cycle = 600 mg/m^2]

Rituximab: I.V.: 100 mg/m^2 day 1 only
followed by I.V.: 375 mg/m^2/day days 3 and 5 only
[total dose/cycle 1 = 850 mg/m^2]
Treatment cycle is 3 weeks
Cycles 2-6:
Pentostatin: I.V.: 2 mg/m^2 day 1
[total dose/cycle = 2 mg/m^2]
Cyclophosphamide: I.V.: 600 mg/m^2 day 1
[total dose/cycle = 600 mg/m^2]
Rituximab: I.V.: 375 mg/m^2 day 1
[total dose/cycle = 375 mg/m^2]
Repeat cycle every 3 weeks

PCV (Brain Tumor Regimen)

Use Brain tumors

Regimen NOTE: Multiple variations are listed.

Variation 1:
Lomustine: Oral: 110 mg/m^2 day 1
[total dose/cycle = 110 mg/m^2]
Procarbazine: Oral: 60 mg/m^2/day days 8 to 21
[total dose/cycle = 840 mg/m^2]
Vincristine: I.V.: 1.4 mg/m^2/day (maximum dose: 2 mg) days 8 and 29
[total dose/cycle = 2.8 mg/m^2; maximum: 4 mg]
Repeat cycle every 6 weeks for a total of 6 cycles

Variation 2:
Lomustine: Oral: 110 mg/m^2 day 1
[total dose/cycle = 110 mg/m^2]
Procarbazine: Oral: 60 mg/m^2/day days 8 to 21
[total dose/cycle = 840 mg/m^2]
Vincristine: I.V.: 1.4 mg/m^2/day (maximum dose: 2 mg) days 8 and 29
[total dose/cycle = 2.8 mg/m^2; maximum: 4 mg]
Repeat cycle every 6 weeks for a total of 7 cycles

Variation 3:
Procarbazine: Oral: 75 mg/m^2/day days 8 to 21
[total dose/cycle = 1050 mg/m^2]
Lomustine: Oral: 130 mg/m^2 day 1
[total dose/cycle = 130 mg/m^2]
Vincristine: I.V.: 1.4 mg/m^2/day (no maximum) days 8 and 29
[total dose/cycle = 2.8 mg/m^2; no maximum]
Repeat cycle every 6 weeks for a total of 6 cycles

Variation 4:
Procarbazine: Oral: 75 mg/m^2/day days 8 to 21
[total dose/cycle = 1050 mg/m^2]
Lomustine: Oral: 130 mg/m^2 day 1
[total dose/cycle = 130 mg/m^2]
Vincristine: I.V.: 1.4 mg/m^2/day (no maximum) days 8 and 29
[total dose/cycle = 2.8 mg/m^2; no maximum]
Repeat cycle every 6 weeks for up to a total of 4 cycles

Variation 5:
Lomustine: Oral: 110 mg/m^2 day 1
[total dose/cycle = 110 mg/m^2]
Procarbazine: Oral: 60 mg/m^2/day days 8 to 21
[total dose/cycle = 840 mg/m^2]
Vincristine: I.V.: 1.4 mg/m^2/day days 8 and 29
[total dose/cycle = 2.8 mg/m^2]
Repeat cycle every 6-8 weeks for 1 year

Pemetrexed (Bladder Cancer Regimen)

Use Bladder cancer

Regimen
Pemetrexed: I.V.: 500 mg/m^2 infused over 10 minutes day 1
[total dose/cycle = 500 mg/m^2]
Repeat cycle every 21 days

Pemetrexed (Mesothelioma Regimen)

Use Malignant pleural mesothelioma

Regimen

Pemetrexed: I.V.: 500 mg/m^2 over 10 minutes day 1
[total dose/cycle = 500 mg/m^2]
Repeat cycle every 21 days

Pemetrexed (NSCLC Regimen)

Use Lung cancer, nonsmall cell

Regimen NOTE: Multiple variations are listed.

Variation 1 (second-line):
Pemetrexed: I.V.: 500 mg/m^2 over 10 minutes day 1
[total dose/cycle = 500 mg/m^2]
Repeat cycle every 21 days until disease progression or unacceptable toxicity
Variation 2 (maintenance therapy):
Pemetrexed: I.V.: 500 mg/m^2 day 1
[total dose/cycle = 500 mg/m^2]
Repeat cycle every 21 days until disease progression or unacceptable toxicity

Pemetrexed (Ovarian Regimen)

Use Ovarian cancer

Regimen NOTE: Multiple variations are listed.

Variation 1:
Pemetrexed: I.V.: 500 mg/m^2 day 1
[total dose/cycle = 500 mg/m^2]
Repeat cycle every 21 days
Variation 2 (no prior radiation):
Pemetrexed: I.V.: 900 mg/m^2 over 10 minutes day 1
[total dose/cycle = 900 mg/m^2]
Repeat cycle every 21 days until disease progression or unacceptable toxicity
Variation 3 (prior radiation):
Pemetrexed: I.V.: 700 mg/m^2 over 10 minutes day 1
[total dose/cycle = 700 mg/m^2]
Repeat cycle every 21 days until disease progression or unacceptable toxicity

Pentostatin-Cyclophosphamide

Use Leukemia, chronic lymphocytic

Regimen

Cyclophosphamide: I.V.: 600 mg/m^2 day 1
[total dose/cycle = 600 mg/m^2]
Pentostatin: I.V.: 4 mg/m^2 day 1
[total dose/cycle = 4 mg/m^2]
Repeat cycle every 3 weeks for up to 6 cycles

POC

Use Brain tumors

Regimen

Prednisone: Oral: 40 mg/m^2/day days 1 to 14
[total dose/cycle = 560 mg/m^2]
Vincristine: I.V.: 1.5 mg/m^2/day (maximum dose: 2 mg) days 1, 8, and 15
[total dose/cycle = 4.5 mg/m^2]
Lomustine: Oral: 100 mg/m^2 day 1
[total dose/cycle = 100 mg/m^2]
Repeat cycle every 6 weeks

POG-8651

Use Osteosarcoma

Regimen

(Surgery at week 10)

Methotrexate: I.V.: 12 g/m^2 weeks 0, 1, 5, 6, 13, 14, 18, 19, 23, 24, 37, and 38
[total dose/cycle = 144 g/m^2]

Leucovorin: (route not specified): 15 mg every 6 hours for 10 doses, weeks 0, 1, 5, 6, 13, 14, 18, 19, 23, 24, 37, and 38
[total dose/cycle = 1800 mg]

Doxorubicin: I.V.: 37.5 mg/m^2/dose days 1 and 2 of weeks 2, 7, 25, and 28
followed by I.V.: 30 mg/m^2/dose days 1, 2, and 3 of week 20
[total dose/cycle = 390 mg/m^2]

Cisplatin: I.V.: 60 mg/m^2/day days 1 and 2, weeks 2, 7, 25, and 28
[total dose/cycle = 480 mg/m^2]

Cyclophosphamide: I.V.: 600 mg/m^2/day days 1, 2, and 3, weeks 15, 31, 34, 39, and 42
[total dose/cycle = 9000 mg/m^2]

Bleomycin: I.V.: 15 units/m^2/day days 1, 2, and 3, weeks 15, 31, 34, 39, and 42
[total dose/cycle = 225 units/m^2]

Dactinomycin: I.V.: 0.6 mg/m^2/day days 1, 2, and 3, weeks 15, 31, 34, 39, and 42
[total dose/cycle = 9 mg/m^2]

or

(Surgery at week 0)

Methotrexate: 12 g/m^2 weeks 3, 4, 8, 9, 13, 14, 18, 19, 23, 24, 37, and 38
[total dose/cycle = 144 g/m^2]

Leucovorin: (route not specified): 15 mg every 6 hours for 10 doses, weeks 3, 4, 8, 9, 13, 14, 18, 19, 23, 24, 37, and 38
[total dose/cycle = 1800 mg]

Doxorubicin: I.V.: 37.5 mg/m^2/day days 1 and 2, weeks 5, 10, 25, and 28 and 30 mg/m^2 days 1, 2, and 3, week 20
[total dose/cycle = 390 mg/m^2]

Cisplatin: I.V.: 60 mg/m^2/day days 1 and 2, weeks 5, 10, 25, and 28
[total dose/cycle = 480 mg/m^2]

Cyclophosphamide: I.V.: 600 mg/m^2/day days 1, 2, and 3, weeks 15, 31, 34, 39, and 42
[total dose/cycle = 9000 mg/m^2]

Bleomycin: I.V.: 15 units/m^2/day days 1, 2, and 3, weeks 15, 31, 34, 39, and 42
[total dose/cycle = 225 units/m^2]

Dactinomycin: I.V.: 0.6 mg/m^2/day days 1, 2, and 3, weeks 15, 31, 34, 39, and 42
[total dose/cycle = 9 mg/m^2]

POMP

Use Leukemia, acute lymphocytic

Regimen Maintenance:

Mercaptopurine: Oral: 50 mg 3 times/day
[total dose/cycle = 4200-4650 mg]

Methotrexate: Oral: 20 mg/m^2 once weekly
[total dose/cycle = 80 mg/m^2]

Vincristine: I.V.: 2 mg day 1
[total dose/cycle = 2 mg]

Prednisone: Oral: 200 mg/day days 1 to 5
[total dose/cycle = 1000 mg]

Repeat cycle monthly for 2 years

Pro-MACE-CytaBOM

Use Lymphoma, non-Hodgkin

Regimen

Prednisone: Oral: 60 mg/m^2/day days 1 to 14
[total dose/cycle = 840 mg/m^2]

Doxorubicin: I.V.: 25 mg/m^2 day 1
[total dose/cycle = 25 mg/m^2]

Cyclophosphamide: I.V.: 650 mg/m^2 day 1
[total dose/cycle = 650 mg/m^2]
Etoposide: I.V.: 120 mg/m^2 day 1
[total dose/cycle = 120 mg/m^2]
Cytarabine: I.V.: 300 mg/m^2 day 8
[total dose/cycle = 300 mg/m^2]
Bleomycin: I.V.: 5 units/m^2 day 8
[total dose/cycle = 5 units/m^2]
Vincristine: I.V.: 1.4 mg/m^2 (maximum dose: 2 mg) day 8
[total dose/cycle = 1.4 mg/m^2]
Methotrexate: I.V.: 120 mg/m^2 day 8
[total dose/cycle = 120 mg/m^2]
Leucovorin: Oral: 25 mg/m^2 every 6 hours for 4 doses (start 24 hours after methotrexate dose) day 9
[total dose/cycle = 100 mg/m^2]
Repeat cycle every 21 days

PVA (POG 8602)

Use Leukemia, acute lymphocytic

Regimen

Induction:

Prednisone: Oral: 40 mg/m^2/day (maximum dose: 60 mg) given in 3 divided doses days 0 to 28
[total dose/cycle = 1160 mg/m^2]
Vincristine: I.V.: 1.5 mg/m^2/day (maximum dose: 2 mg) days 0, 7, 14, and 21
[total dose/cycle = 6 mg/m^2; maximum: 8 mg]
Asparaginase: I.M.: 6000 units/m^2 3 times per week for 2 weeks
[total dose/cycle = 36,000 units/m^2]
Intrathecal therapy (triple): Days 0 and 22
Leucovorin: Route and dose not specified: Single dose 24 hours after every intrathecal treatment days 1 and 23
Administer one cycle only

CNS consolidation:

Mercaptopurine: Oral: 75 mg/m^2/day days 29 to 43
[total dose/cycle = 1125 mg/m^2]
Intrathecal therapy (triple): Days 29 and 36
Leucovorin: Route and dose not specified: Single dose 24 hours after every intrathecal treatment days 30 and 37
Administer one cycle only

Intensification:

Regimen A:

Methotrexate: I.V.: 1000 mg/m^2 continuous infusion over 24 hours day 1
[total dose/cycle = 1000 mg/m^2]
Cytarabine: I.V.: 1000 mg/m^2 continuous infusion over 24 hours day 1 (start 12 hours after start of methotrexate)
[total dose/cycle = 1000 mg/m^2]
Leucovorin: I.M., I.V., or Oral: 30 mg/m^2 at 24 and 36 hours after the start of methotrexate
[total dose/cycle = 60 mg/m^2]
followed by I.M., I.V., or Oral: 3 mg/m^2 at 48, 60, and 72 hours after the start of methotrexate
[total dose/cycle = 9 mg/m^2]
Repeat cycle every 3 weeks for 6 cycles (administered weeks 7, 10, 13, 16, 19, and 22)
Intrathecal therapy (triple): Weeks 9, 12, 15, and 18
Leucovorin: Route and dose not specified: Single dose 24 hours after every intrathecal treatment weeks 9, 12, 15, and 18

or

Regimen B:

Methotrexate: I.V.: 1000 mg/m^2 continuous infusion over 24 hours day 1
[total dose/cycle = 1000 mg/m^2]
Cytarabine: I.V.: 1000 mg/m^2 continuous infusion over 24 hours day 1 (start 12 hours after methotrexate)
[total dose/cycle = 1000 mg/m^2]

Leucovorin: I.M., I.V., or Oral: 30 mg/m^2 at 24 and 36 hours after the start of methotrexate
[total dose/cycle = 60 mg/m^2]
followed by I.M., I.V., or Oral: 3 mg/m^2 at 48, 60, and 72 hours after the start of methotrexate
[total dose/cycle = 9 mg/m^2]
Repeat cycle every 12 weeks for 6 cycles (administer weeks 7, 19, 31, 43, 55, and 67)
Intrathecal therapy (triple): Weeks 9, 12, 15, and 18
Leucovorin: Route and dose not specified: Single dose 24 hours after every intrathecal treatment weeks 9, 12, 15, and 18

Maintenance:

Regimen A:

Methotrexate: I.M.: 20 mg/m^2 weekly, weeks 25 to 156
[total dose/cycle = 2640 mg/m^2]
Mercaptopurine: Oral: 75 mg/m^2 daily, weeks 25 to 156
[total dose/cycle = 69,300 mg/m^2]
Intrathecal therapy (triple): Every 8 weeks, weeks 26 through 105
Leucovorin: Route and dose not specified: Single dose 24 hours after every intrathecal treatment weeks 26 through 105
Prednisone: Oral: 40 mg/m^2/day (maximum dose: 60 mg) days 1 to 7 (given in 3 divided doses), weeks 8, 17, 25, 41, 57, 73, 89, and 105
[total dose/cycle = 2240 mg/m^2; maximum: 3360 mg]
Vincristine: I.V.: 1.5 mg/m^2/day (maximum dose: 2 mg) day 1, weeks 8, 9, 17, 18, 25, 26, 41, 42, 57, 58, 73, 74, 89, 90, 105, and 106
[total dose/cycle = 24 mg/m^2; maximum: 32 mg]

or

Regimen B:

Methotrexate: I.M.: 20 mg/m^2 weekly, weeks 22-28, 34-40, 46-52, and 58-64
[total dose/cycle = 560 mg/m^2]
Mercaptopurine: Oral: 75 mg/m^2 daily for 7 weeks, weeks 22-28, 34-40, 46-52, and 58-64
[total dose/cycle = 14700 mg/m^2]

followed by

Methotrexate: I.M.: 20 mg/m^2 weekly, weeks 70 to 156
[total dose/cycle = 1720 mg/m^2]
Mercaptopurine: Oral: 75 mg/m^2 daily, weeks 70 to 156
[total dose/cycle = 45,150 mg/m^2]
Intrathecal therapy (triple): Every 8 weeks, weeks 26 through 105
Leucovorin: Route and dose not specified: Single dose 24 hours after every intrathecal treatment weeks 26 through 105
Prednisone: Oral: 40 mg/m^2/day (maximum dose: 60 mg) days 1 to 7 (given in 3 divided doses), weeks 8, 17, 25, 41, 57, 73, 89, and 105
[total dose/cycle = 2240 mg/m^2]
Vincristine: I.V.: 1.5 mg/m^2/day (maximum dose: 2 mg) day 1, weeks 8, 9, 17, 18, 25, 26, 41, 42, 57, 58, 73, 74, 89, 90, 105, and 106
[total dose/cycle = 24 mg/m^2; maximum dose: 32 mg]

PVB

Use Testicular cancer

Regimen NOTE: Multiple variations are listed.

Variation 1:
Cisplatin: I.V.: 20 mg/m^2/day days 1 to 5
[total dose/cycle = 100 mg/m^2]
Vinblastine: I.V.: 0.2 mg/kg/day days 1 and 2
[total dose/cycle = 0.4 mg/kg]
Bleomycin: I.V.: 30 units/day days 2, 9, and 16
[total dose/cycle = 90 units]
Repeat cycle every 3 weeks

Variation 2:
Cisplatin: I.V.: 20 mg/m^2/day days 1 to 5
[total dose/cycle = 100 mg/m^2]
Vinblastine: I.V.: 0.15 mg/kg/day days 1 and 2
[total dose/cycle = 0.3 mg/kg]
Bleomycin: I.V.: 30 units/day days 2, 9, and 16
[total dose/cycle = 90 units]
Repeat cycle every 3 weeks

Variation 3:
Cisplatin: I.V.: 20 mg/m^2/day days 1 to 5
[total dose/cycle = 100 mg/m^2]
Vinblastine: I.V.: 6 mg/m^2/day days 1 and 2
[total dose/cycle = 12 mg/m^2]
Bleomycin: I.M.: 30 units/day days 2, 9, and 16
[total dose/cycle = 90 units]
Repeat cycle every 3 weeks

PVDA

Use Leukemia, acute lymphocytic

Regimen Induction:
Prednisone: Oral: 60 mg/m^2/day days 1 to 28
[total dose/cycle = 1680 mg/m^2]
Vincristine: I.V.: 1.5 mg/m^2/day days 1, 8, 15, and 22
[total dose/cycle = 6 mg/m^2]
Daunorubicin: I.V.: 25 mg/m^2/day days 1, 8, 15, and 22
[total dose/cycle = 100 mg/m^2]
Asparaginase: I.M., SubQ, or I.V.: 5000 units/m^2/day days 1 to 14
[total dose/cycle = 70,000 units/m^2]
Administer one cycle only; used in conjunction with intrathecal chemotherapy

R-CVP

Use Lymphoma, non-Hodgkin

Regimen
Rituximab: I.V.: 375 mg/m^2 day 1
[total dose/cycle = 375 mg/m^2]
Cyclophosphamide: I.V.: 750 mg/m^2 day 1
[total dose/cycle = 750 mg/m^2]
Vincristine: I.V.: 1.4 mg/m^2 day 1
[total dose/cycle = 1.4 mg/m^2]
Prednisone: Oral: 40 mg/m^2/day days 1 to 5
[total dose/cycle = 200 mg/m^2]
Repeat cycle every 21 days

Regimen I (Wilms Tumor)

Use Wilms' tumor

Regimen NOTE: Multiple variations are listed.
Variation 1 (patients ≤30 kg):
Vincristine: I.V.: 0.05 mg/kg (maximum dose: 2 mg) I.V. push day 1 of weeks 1, 2, 4 to 8, 10 and 11
followed by
Vincristine 0.067 mg/kg (maximum dose: 2 mg) I.V. push day 1 of weeks 12, 13, 18, and 24
[total dose = 0.718 mg/kg; maximum: 26 mg]
Doxorubicin: I.V.: 1.5 mg/kg I.V. push day 1 of weeks 0, 6, 12, 18, and 24
[total dose = 7.5 mg/kg]
Cyclophosphamide: I.V.: 14.7 mg/kg/day days 1 to 5 of weeks 3, 9, 15, and 21
[total dose = 294 mg/kg]
Mesna: I.V.: 3 mg/kg/dose 4 doses/day (after cyclophosphamide) days 1 to 5 of weeks 3, 9, 15, and 21
[total dose = 240 mg/kg]
Cyclophosphamide: I.V.: 14.7 mg/kg/day days 1 to 3 of weeks 6, 12, 18, and 24
[total dose = 176.4 mg/kg]
Mesna: I.V.: 3 mg/kg/dose 4 doses/day (after cyclophosphamide) days 1 to 3 of weeks 6, 12, 18, and 24
[total dose = 144 mg/kg]
Etoposide: I.V.: 3.3 mg/kg/day days 1 to 5 of weeks 3, 9, 15, and 21
[total dose = 66 mg/kg]
Filgrastim: SubQ: 5 mcg/kg/day beginning 24 hours after last dose of chemotherapy and continued until ANC ≥10,000/mm^3 or for a minimum of 1 week
Treatment course duration is week 0 through week 24

Variation 2 (patients >30 kg):
Vincristine: I.V.: 1.5 mg/m^2 (maximum dose: 2 mg) I.V. push day 1 of weeks 1, 2, 4 to 8, 10 and 11
followed by
Vincristine 2 mg/m^2 (maximum dose: 2 mg) I.V. push days 1 of weeks 12, 13, 18, and 24
[total dose = 21.5 mg/m^2; maximum: 26 mg]
Doxorubicin: I.V.: 45 mg/m^2 I.V. push day 1 of weeks 0, 6, 12, 18, and 24
[total dose = 225 mg/m^2]
Cyclophosphamide: I.V.: 440 mg/m^2/day days 1 to 5 of weeks 3, 9, 15, and 21
[total dose = 8800 mg/m^2]
Mesna: I.V.: 90 mg/m^2/dose 4 doses/day (after cyclophosphamide) days 1 to 5 of weeks 3, 9, 15, and 21
[total dose = 7200 mg/m^2]
Cyclophosphamide: I.V.: 440 mg/m^2/day days 1 to 3 of weeks 6, 12, 18, and 24
[total dose = 5280 mg/m^2]
Mesna: I.V.: 90 mg/m^2/dose 4 doses/day (after cyclophosphamide) days 1 to 3 of weeks 6, 12, 18, and 24
[total dose = 4320 mg/m^2]
Etoposide: I.V.: 100 mg/m^2/day days 1 to 5 of weeks 3, 9, 15, and 21
[total dose = 2000 mg/m^2]
Filgrastim: SubQ: 5 mcg/kg/day beginning 24 hours after last dose of chemotherapy and continued until ANC ≥10,000/mm^3 or for a minimum of 1 week
Treatment course duration is week 0 through week 24

RICE

Use Lymphoma, non-Hodgkin

Regimen
Rituximab: I.V.: 375 mg/m^2/day days 2 and 1 (cycle 1)
[total dose/cycle = 750 mg/m^2]
Rituximab: I.V.: 375 mg/m^2 day 1 (cycles 2 and 3)
[total dose/cycle = 375 mg/m^2]
Etoposide: I.V.: 100 mg/m^2/day days 3, 4, and 5
[total dose/cycle = 300 mg/m^2]
Carboplatin: I.V.: AUC = 5 (maximum dose: 800 mg) day 4
[total dose/cycle = AUC = 5]
Ifosfamide: I.V.: 5000 mg/m^2 continuous infusion day 4
[total dose/cycle = 5000 mg/m^2]
Mesna: I.V.: 5000 mg/m^2 continuous infusion day 4
[total dose/cycle = 5000 mg/m^2]
Filgrastim: SubQ: 5 mcg/kg/day days 7 to 14 (cycles 1 and 2)
[total dose/cycle = 40 mcg/kg]
Filgrastim: SubQ: 10 mcg/kg/day days 7 to 14 (cycle 3)
[total dose/cycle = 80 mcg/kg]
Repeat cycle every 2 weeks

Rituximab-CHOP (NHL)

Use Lymphoma, non-Hodgkin

Regimen NOTE: Multiple variations are listed.
Variation 1 (diffuse large B-cell lymphoma):
Rituximab: I.V.: 375 mg/m^2 day 1
[total dose/cycle = 375 mg/m^2]
Cyclophosphamide: I.V.: 750 mg/m^2 day 1
[total dose/cycle = 750 mg/m^2]
Doxorubicin: I.V.: 50 mg/m^2 day 1
[total dose/cycle = 50 mg/m^2]
Vincristine: I.V.: 1.4 mg/m^2 (maximum dose: 2 mg) day 1
[total dose/cycle = 1.4 mg/m^2; maximum: 2 mg]
Prednisone: Oral: 40 mg/m^2/day days 1 to 5
[total dose/cycle = 200 mg/m^2]
Repeat cycle every 21 days for a total of 8 cycles

Variation 2 (low-grade or follicular lymphoma):
Rituximab: I.V.: 375 mg/m^2 administer 7 and 2 days prior to the start of cycle 1 of CHOP, 2 days prior to the start of cycles 3 and 5 of CHOP, and after the 6th cycle of CHOP on days 134 and 141 (total of 6 doses of rituximab)
CHOP:
Cyclophosphamide: I.V.: 750 mg/m^2 day 1
[total dose/cycle = 750 mg/m^2]
Doxorubicin: I.V.: 50 mg/m^2 day 1
[total dose/cycle = 50 mg/m^2]
Vincristine: I.V.: 1.4 mg/m^2 (maximum dose: 2 mg) day 1
[total dose/cycle = 1.4 mg/m^2; maximum: 2 mg]
Prednisone: Oral: 100 mg/m^2/day days 1 to 5
[total dose/cycle = 500 mg/m^2]
Repeat each CHOP cycle every 21 days for a total of 6 CHOP cycles
Variation 3 (dose-dense R-CHOP in aggressive CD20-expressing B-cell lymphomas):
Pre-treatment (to improve performance status and diminish adverse effects to cycle 1):
Vincristine: I.V.: 1 mg 1 week before cycle 1
Prednisone: Oral: 100 mg/day for 7 days 1 week before cycle 1
Rituximab: I.V.: 375 mg/m^2 day 1
[total dose/cycle = 375 mg/m^2]
Cyclophosphamide: I.V.: 750 mg/m^2 day 1
[total dose/cycle = 750 mg/m^2]
Doxorubicin: I.V.: 50 mg/m^2 day 1
[total dose/cycle = 50 mg/m^2]
Vincristine: I.V.: 2 mg day 1
[total dose/cycle = 2 mg]
Prednisone: Oral: 100 mg/day days 1 to 5
[total dose/cycle = 500 mg]
Filgrastim (dose and route not specified): Daily beginning day 4 until leukocyte recovery
Repeat cycle every 14 days for a total of 6 cycles
Variation 4 (diffuse large B-cell lymphoma):
Rituximab: I.V.: 375 mg/m^2 days -7, 1, 22, and 43
[total dose/cycle = 1400 mg/m^2]
Cyclophosphamide: I.V.: 750 mg/m^2 days 3, 24, and 45
[total dose/cycle = 2250 mg/m^2]
Doxorubicin: I.V.: 50 mg/m^2 days 3, 24, and 45
[total dose/cycle = 150 mg/m^2]
Vincristine: I.V.: 1.4 mg/m^2 (maximum dose: 2 mg) days 3, 24, and 45
[total dose/cycle = 4.2 mg/m^2; maximum: 6 mg/cycle]
Prednisone: Oral: 100 mg/day for 5 days starting on days 3, 24, and 45
[total dose/cycle = 1500 mg]
Cycle does not repeat; followed by radiation therapy beginning on day 66
Variation 5 (diffuse large B-cell lymphoma):
Rituximab: I.V.: 375 mg/m^2 administer 7 and 3 days prior to the start of cycle 1 of CHOP, 2 days prior to the start of cycles 3 and 5 of CHOP, and 2 days before cycle 7 (if administered)
CHOP:
Cyclophosphamide: I.V.: 750 mg/m^2 day 1
[total dose/cycle = 750 mg/m^2]
Doxorubicin: I.V.: 50 mg/m^2 day 1
[total dose/cycle = 50 mg/m^2]
Vincristine: I.V.: 1.4 mg/m^2 (maximum dose: 2 mg) day 1
[total dose/cycle = 1.4 mg/m^2; maximum: 2 mg]
Prednisone: Oral: 100 mg/m^2/day days 1 to 5
[total dose/cycle = 500 mg/m^2]
Repeat each CHOP cycle every 21 days for a total of 6 CHOP cycles
Variation 6 (mantle cell lymphoma):
Rituximab: I.V.: 375 mg/m^2 day 0 (administer the day before CHOP)
[total dose/cycle = 375 mg/m^2]
Cyclophosphamide: I.V.: 750 mg/m^2 day 1
[total dose/cycle = 750 mg/m^2]
Doxorubicin: I.V.: 50 mg/m^2 day 1
[total dose/cycle = 50 mg/m^2]

Vincristine: I.V.: 1.4 mg/m^2 (maximum dose: 2 mg) day 1
[total dose/cycle = 1.4 mg/m^2; maximum: 2 mg]
Prednisone: Oral: 100 mg/m^2/day days 1 to 5
[total dose/cycle = 500 mg/m^2]
Repeat cycle every 21 days for a total of 6 cycles

Variation 7 (follicular lymphoma):
Rituximab: I.V.: 375 mg/m^2 day 0 (administer the day before CHOP)
[total dose/cycle = 375 mg/m^2]
Cyclophosphamide: I.V.: 750 mg/m^2 day 1
[total dose/cycle = 750 mg/m^2]
Doxorubicin: I.V.: 50 mg/m^2 day 1
[total dose/cycle = 50 mg/m^2]
Vincristine: I.V.: 1.4 mg/m^2 (maximum dose: 2 mg) day 1
[total dose/cycle = 1.4 mg/m^2; maximum: 2 mg]
Prednisone: Oral: 100 mg/m^2/day days 1 to 5
[total dose/cycle = 500 mg/m^2]
Repeat cycle every 21 days for a total of 6-8 cycles

Variation 8 (follicular lymphoma):
Rituximab: I.V.: 375 mg/m^2 day 1
[total dose/cycle = 375 mg/m^2]
Cyclophosphamide: I.V.: 750 mg/m^2 day 1
[total dose/cycle = 750 mg/m^2]
Doxorubicin: I.V.: 50 mg/m^2 day 1
[total dose/cycle = 50 mg/m^2]
Vincristine: I.V.: 1.4 mg/m^2 (maximum dose: 2 mg) day 1
[total dose/cycle = 1.4 mg/m^2; maximum: 2 mg]
Prednisone: Oral: 100 mg/day days 1 to 5
[total dose/cycle = 500 mg]
Repeat cycle every 21 days for a total of 6 cycles
followed by (maintenance rituximab):
Rituximab: I.V.: 375 mg/m^2 day 1
[total dose/cycle = 375 mg/m^2]
Repeat every 3 months until relapse or for a maximum of 2 years

Sorafenib (RCC Regimen)

Use Renal cell cancer

Regimen NOTE: Multiple variations are listed.

Variation 1 (refractory):
Sorafenib: Oral: 400 mg twice daily
Continue until disease progression or unacceptable toxicity.

Variation 2 (first-line):
Sorafenib: Oral: 400 mg twice daily; if disease progression, may escalate to 600 mg twice daily
Continue until disease progression or unacceptable toxicity.

Stanford V (Hodgkin)

Use Lymphoma, Hodgkin disease

Regimen NOTE: Multiple variations are listed.

Variation 1:
Mechlorethamine: I.V.: 6 mg/m^2/dose weeks 1, 5, and 9
[total dose/cycle = 18 mg/m^2]
Doxorubicin: I.V.: 25 mg/m^2/dose weeks 1, 3, 5, 7, 9, and 11
[total dose/cycle = 150 mg/m^2]
Vinblastine: I.V.: 6 mg/m^2/dose weeks 1, 3, 5, 7, 9, and 11
[total dose/cycle = 36 mg/m^2]
Vincristine: I.V.: 1.4 mg/m^2/dose (maximum dose: 2 mg) weeks 2, 4, 6, 8, 10, and 12
[total dose/cycle = 8.4 mg/m^2; maximum: 12 mg]
Bleomycin: I.V.: 5 units/m^2/dose weeks 2, 4, 6, 8, 10, and 12
[total dose/cycle = 30 units/m^2]

Etoposide: I.V.: 60 mg/m^2/day for 2 consecutive days, weeks 3, 7, and 11
[total dose/cycle = 360 mg/m^2]
Prednisone: Oral: 40 mg/m^2 every other day for 10 weeks
[total dose prior to taper = 1400 mg/m^2]
followed by tapering of prednisone dose during weeks 11 and 12
Treatment cycle is 12 weeks
Variation 2:
Mechlorethamine: I.V.: 6 mg/m^2/dose weeks 1 and 5
[total dose/cycle = 12 mg/m^2]
Doxorubicin: I.V.: 25 mg/m^2/dose weeks 1, 3, 5, and 7
[total dose/cycle = 100 mg/m^2]
Vinblastine: I.V.: 6 mg/m^2/dose weeks 1, 3, 5, and 7
[total dose/cycle = 24 mg/m^2]
Vincristine: I.V.: 1.4 mg/m^2/dose (maximum dose: 2 mg) weeks 2, 4, 6, and 8
[total dose/cycle = 5.6 mg/m^2; maximum: 8 mg]
Bleomycin: I.V.: 5 units/m^2/dose weeks 2, 4, 6, and 8
[total dose/cycle = 20 units/m^2]
Etoposide: I.V.: 60 mg/m^2/day days 15 and 16 and 43 and 44
[total dose/cycle = 240 mg/m^2]
Prednisone: Oral: 40 mg/m^2 days 1 to 36
[total dose prior to taper = 1440 mg/m^2]
followed by tapering of prednisone dose during weeks 7 and 8
Treatment cycle is 8 weeks

Sunitinib (RCC Regimen)

Use Renal cell cancer

Regimen

Sunitinib: Oral: 50 mg once daily for 4 weeks, followed by 2 weeks of rest
[total dose/cycle = 1400 mg]
Repeat cycle every 6 weeks until disease progression or unacceptable toxicity

TAC

Use Breast cancer

Regimen NOTE: Multiple variations are listed.

Variation 1:
Docetaxel: I.V.: 75 mg/m^2 day 1
[total dose/cycle = 75 mg/m^2]
Doxorubicin: I.V.: 50 mg/m^2 day 1
[total dose/cycle = 50 mg/m^2]
Cyclophosphamide: I.V.: 500 mg/m^2 day 1
[total dose/cycle = 500 mg/m^2]
Repeat cycle every 3 weeks
Variation 2:
Docetaxel: I.V.: 60 mg/m^2 day 1
[total dose/cycle = 60 mg/m^2]
Doxorubicin: I.V.: 60 mg/m^2 day 1
[total dose/cycle = 60 mg/m^2]
Cyclophosphamide: I.V.: 600 mg/m^2 day 1
[total dose/cycle = 600 mg/m^2]
Repeat cycle every 3 weeks

Temozolomide-Rituximab (CNS Lymphoma)

Use Primary CNS lymphoma

Regimen NOTE: Multiple variations are listed.

Variation 1:
Combination therapy (cycles 1-4):
Rituximab: I.V.: 375 mg/m^2/dose day 1
[total dose/cycle = 375 mg/m^2]
Temozolomide: Oral: 150 mg/m^2/day days 1 to 5
[total dose/cycle = 750 mg/m^2]
Repeat cycle every 28 days for a total of 4 cycles

followed by
Maintenance therapy:
Temozolomide: Oral: 150 mg/m^2/day days 1 to 5
[total dose/cycle = 750 mg/m^2]
Repeat cycle every 28 days for a total of 8 cycles
Variation 2:
Combination therapy (cycles 1 and 2):
Rituximab: I.V.: 750 mg/m^2/dose days 1, 8, 15, and 22
[total dose/cycle = 3000 mg/m^2]
Temozolomide: Oral: 150 mg/m^2/day days 1 to 7
[total dose/cycle = 1050 mg/m^2]
Repeat cycle every 28 days for a total of 2 cycles
followed by
Maintenance therapy:
Temozolomide: Oral: 150 mg/m^2/day days 1 to 5
[total dose/cycle = 750 mg/m^2]
Repeat cycle every 28 days

Temsirolimus (RCC Regimen)

Use Renal cell cancer

Regimen
Temsirolimus: I.V.: 25 mg over 30 minutes day 1
[total dose/cycle = 25 mg]
Repeat cycle every week until disease progression or unacceptable toxicity

Thalidomide-Dexamethasone (MM)

Use Multiple myeloma

Regimen NOTE: Multiple variations are listed.
Variation 1 (refractory):
Thalidomide: Oral: 100 mg/day days 1 to 28
[total dose/cycle = 2800 mg]
Dexamethasone: Oral: 40 mg/day days 1 to 4
[total dose/cycle = 160 mg]
Repeat cycle every 28 days
Variation 2 (refractory):
Thalidomide: Oral: 200 mg/day days 1 to 14 (cycle 1)
followed by Oral: 400 mg/day days 15 to 28 (cycle 1)
[total dose/cycle = 8400 mg]
Thalidomide: Oral: 400 mg/day days 1 to 28 (subsequent cycles)
[total dose/cycle = 11,200 mg]
Dexamethasone: Oral: 20 mg/m^2/day days 1 to 4, 9 to 12, and 17 to 20 (cycle 1)
[total dose/cycle = 240 mg/m^2]
followed by Oral: 20 mg/m^2/day days 1 to 4 (subsequent cycles)
[total dose/cycle = 80 mg/m^2]
Repeat cycle every 28 days
Variation 3 (newly diagnosed):
Thalidomide: Oral: 200 mg/day days 1 to 28
[total dose/cycle = 5600 mg]
Dexamethasone: Oral: 40 mg/day days 1 to 4, 9 to 12, and 17 to 20
[total dose/cycle = 480 mg]
Repeat cycle every 28 days
Variation 4 (newly diagnosed):
Thalidomide: Oral: 50 mg/day days 1 to 14
followed by Oral: 100 mg/day days 15 to 28 (cycle 1)
[total dose/cycle 1 = 2100 mg]
followed by Oral: 200 mg/day days 1 to 28 (starting with cycle 2 and subsequent cycles)
[total dose/cycle = 5600 mg]
Dexamethasone: Oral: 40 mg/day days 1 to 4, 9 to 12, and 17 to 20 (cycles 1 to 4)
[total dose/cycle 1 to 4 = 480 mg]
followed by Oral: 40 mg/day days 1 to 4 (starting with cycle 5 and subsequent cycles)
[total dose/cycle = 160 mg]
Repeat cycle every 28 days until disease progression or unacceptable toxicity

Variation 5 (newly diagnosed):
Thalidomide: Oral: 100 mg/day days 1 to 14
followed by Oral: 200 mg/day days 15 to 28 (cycle 1)
[total dose/cycle = 4200 mg]
followed by Oral: 200 mg/day days 1 to 28 (starting with cycle 2 and subsequent cycles)
[total dose/cycle = 5600 mg]
Dexamethasone: Oral: 40 mg/day days 1 to 4, 9 to 12, and 17 to 20 (odd cycles)
[total dose/cycle = 480 mg]
Dexamethasone: Oral: 40 mg/day days 1 to 4 (even cycles)
[total dose/cycle = 160 mg]
Repeat cycle every 28 days for a total of 4 cycles
Variation 6 (newly diagnosed induction):
Thalidomide: Oral: 50 mg/day; may escalate by 50 mg per week to a maximum dose of 400 mg/day
[total dose/cycle = up to 14,000 mg]
Dexamethasone: Oral: 40 mg/day days 1 to 4, 9 to 12, and 17 to 20
[total dose/cycle = 480 mg]
Repeat cycle every 35 days for a total of 3 cycles

Topotecan-Cyclophosphamide (Ewing Sarcoma)

Use Ewing sarcoma

Regimen

Cyclophosphamide: I.V.: 250 mg/m^2/dose days 1 to 5
[total dose/cycle = 1250 mg/m^2]
Topotecan: I.V.: 0.75 mg/m^2/dose days 1 to 5
[total dose/cycle = 3.75 mg/m^2]
Repeat cycle every 21 days

Topotecan Intravenous (Small Cell Lung Cancer Regimen)

Use Lung cancer, small cell

Regimen

Topotecan: I.V.: 1.5 mg/m^2/day over 30 minutes days 1 to 5
[total dose/cycle = 7.5 mg/m^2]
Repeat cycle every 21 days

Topotecan (Oral)-Cisplatin

Use Lung cancer, small cell

Regimen

Topotecan: Oral: 1.7 mg/m^2/day days 1 to 5
[total dose/cycle = 8.5 mg/m^2]
Cisplatin: I.V.: 60 mg/m^2 day 5 only
[total dose/cycle = 60 mg/m^2]
Repeat cycle every 21 days for 4 cycles (or for 2 cycles beyond best response)

Topotecan Oral Regimen (Ovarian Cancer)

Use Ovarian cancer

Regimen

Topotecan: Oral: 2.3 mg/m^2/day days 1 to 5
[total dose/cycle = 11.5 mg/m^2]
Repeat cycle every 21 days until disease progression or for at least 4 cycles after achieve stable disease

Topotecan Oral (Small Cell Lung Cancer Regimen)

Use Lung cancer, small cell

Regimen

Topotecan: Oral: 2.3 mg/m^2/day days 1 to 5
[total dose/cycle = 11.5 mg/m^2]
Repeat cycle every 21 days

Trabectedin-Doxorubicin (Liposomal) (Ovarian Cancer)

Use Ovarian cancer

Regimen

Doxorubicin (liposomal): I.V.: 30 mg/m^2 over 90 minutes day 1
[total dose/cycle = 30 mg/m^2]
Trabectedin: I.V.: 1.1 mg/m^2 over 3 hours (via central line) day 1
[total dose/cycle = 1.1 mg/m^2]
Repeat cycle every 3 weeks until disease progression or for 2 cycles beyond confirmed complete response.

Trastuzumab-Cisplatin-Capecitabine (Gastric Cancer)

Use Gastric cancer

Regimen

Cycle 1:
Capecitabine: Oral: 1000 mg/m^2/dose twice daily days 1 to 14
[total dose/cycle = 28,000 mg/m^2]
Cisplatin: I.V.: 80 mg/m^2/dose day 1
[total dose/cycle = 80 mg/m^2]
Trastuzumab: I.V.: 8 mg/kg/dose (loading dose) day 1
[total dose/cycle 1 = 8 mg/kg]
Treatment cycle is 21 days
Cycles 2-6:
Capecitabine: Oral: 1000 mg/m^2/dose twice daily days 1 to 14
[total dose/cycle = 28,000 mg/m^2]
Cisplatin: I.V.: 80 mg/m^2/dose day 1
[total dose/cycle = 80 mg/m^2]
Trastuzumab: I.V.: 6 mg/kg/dose day 1
[total dose/cycle = 6 mg/kg]
Treatment cycle is 21 days
Subsequent cycles:
Trastuzumab: I.V.: 6 mg/kg/dose day 1
[total dose/cycle = 6 mg/kg]
Repeat cycle every 3 weeks until disease progression or unacceptable toxicity

Trastuzumab-Cisplatin-Fluorouracil (Gastric Cancer)

Use Gastric cancer

Regimen

Cycle 1:
Fluorouracil: I.V.: 800 mg/m^2/day continuous infusion days 1 to 5
[total dose/cycle = 4000 mg/m^2]
Cisplatin: I.V.: 80 mg/m^2/dose day 1
[total dose/cycle = 80 mg/m^2]
Trastuzumab: I.V.: 8 mg/kg/dose (loading dose) day 1
[total dose/cycle 1 = 8 mg/kg]
Treatment cycle is 21 days
Cycles 2-6:
Fluorouracil: I.V.: 800 mg/m^2/day continuous infusion days 1 to 5
[total dose/cycle = 4000 mg/m^2]
Cisplatin: I.V.: 80 mg/m^2/dose day 1
[total dose/cycle = 80 mg/m^2]
Trastuzumab: I.V.: 6 mg/kg/dose day 1
[total dose/cycle = 6 mg/kg]
Treatment cycle is 21 days
Subsequent cycles:
Trastuzumab: I.V.: 6 mg/kg/dose day 1
[total dose/cycle = 6 mg/kg]
Repeat cycle every 3 weeks until disease progression or unacceptable toxicity

Trastuzumab-Paclitaxel

Use Breast cancer

Regimen NOTE: Multiple variations are listed.

Variation 1:

Cycle 1:

Paclitaxel: I.V.: 175 mg/m^2 day 1
[total dose/cycle = 175 mg/m^2]

Trastuzumab: I.V.: 4 mg/kg (loading dose) day 1
followed by I.V.: 2 mg/kg/day days 8 and 15
[total dose/cycle 1 = 8 mg/kg]

Treatment cycle is 21 days

Subsequent cycles:

Paclitaxel: I.V.: 175 mg/m^2 day 1
[total dose/cycle = 175 mg/m^2]

Trastuzumab: I.V.: 2 mg/kg/day days 1, 8, and 15
[total dose/cycle = 6 mg/kg]

Repeat cycle every 21 days for a total of at least 6 cycles

Variation 2:

Cycle 1:

Trastuzumab: I.V.: 4 mg/kg (loading dose) day 1
followed by I.V.: 2 mg/kg/day days 8 and 15
[total dose/cycle 1 = 8 mg/kg]

Paclitaxel: I.V.: 175 mg/m^2 day 2
[total dose/cycle = 175 mg/m^2]

Treatment cycle is 21 days

Subsequent cycles:

Trastuzumab: I.V.: 2 mg/kg/day days 1, 8, and 15
[total dose/cycle = 6 mg/kg]

Paclitaxel: I.V.: 175 mg/m^2 day 2
[total dose/cycle = 175 mg/m^2]

Repeat cycle every 21 days for a total of at least 6 cycles (continue weekly trastuzumab after chemotherapy until disease progression or unacceptable toxicity)

Trastuzumab-Paclitaxel-Carboplatin

Use Breast cancer

Regimen

Cycle 1:

Trastuzumab: I.V.: 4 mg/kg (loading dose) day 1
followed by I.V.: 2 mg/kg/day days 8 and 15
[total dose/cycle 1 = 8 mg/kg]

Paclitaxel: I.V.: 175 mg/m^2 day 2
[total dose/cycle = 175 mg/m^2]

Carboplatin: I.V.: AUC 6 day 2
[total dose/cycle = AUC = 6]

Treatment cycle is 21 days

Subsequent cycles:

Trastuzumab: I.V.: 2 mg/kg/day days 1, 8, and 15
[total dose/cycle = 6 mg/kg]

Paclitaxel: I.V.: 175 mg/m^2 day 2
[total dose/cycle = 175 mg/m^2]

Carboplatin: I.V.: AUC 6 day 2
[total dose/cycle = AUC = 6]

Repeat cycle every 21 days for a total of at least 6 cycles (continue weekly trastuzumab after chemotherapy until disease progression or unacceptable toxicity)

Trastuzumab-Paclitaxel (Weekly)

Use Breast cancer

Regimen NOTE: Multiple variations are listed.

Variation 1:

Week 1:

Trastuzumab: I.V.: 4 mg/kg (loading dose) day 1

[total dose/week 1 = 4 mg/kg]

Paclitaxel: I.V.: 90 mg/m^2 day 2

[total dose/week 1 = 90 mg/m^2]

Subsequent weeks:

Paclitaxel: I.V.: 90 mg/m^2 day 1

[total dose/week = 90 mg/m^2]

Trastuzumab: I.V.: 2 mg/kg day 1

[total dose/week = 2 mg/kg]

Repeat weekly

Variation 2:

Week 1:

Trastuzumab: I.V.: 4 mg/kg (loading dose) day 1

[total dose/week 1 = 4 mg/kg]

Paclitaxel: I.V.: 80 mg/m^2 day 1

[total dose/week 1 = 80 mg/m^2]

Subsequent weeks:

Trastuzumab: I.V.: 2 mg/kg day 1

[total dose/week = 2 mg/kg]

Paclitaxel: I.V.: 80 mg/m^2 day 1

[total dose/week = 80 mg/m^2]

Repeat weekly

Tretinoin-Arsenic Trioxide (APL)

Use Leukemia, acute promyelocytic

Regimen

Induction (continue until <5% blasts in marrow and no abnormal promyelocytes):

Tretinoin: Oral: 45 mg/m^2/day (in 2 divided doses) day 1 up to day 85

[total induction dose = up to 3825 mg/m^2]

Arsenic Trioxide: I.V.: 0.15 mg/kg/day over 1 hour beginning day 10 up to day 85

[total induction dose = up to 11.25 mg/kg]

Postremission therapy (beginning with complete remission):

Tretinoin: Oral: 45 mg/m^2/day weeks 1, 2, 5, 6, 9, 10, 13, 14, 17, 18, 21, 22, 25, 26

[total postremission dose = 4410 mg/m^2]

Arsenic Trioxide: I.V.: 0.15 mg/kg/day Monday through Friday weeks 1 to 4, 9 to 12, 17 to 20, and 25 to 28

[total postremission dose = 12 mg/kg]

Tretinoin-Daunorubicin (APL)

Use Leukemia, acute promyelocytic

Regimen

Induction:

Tretinoin: Oral: 45 mg/m^2/day (in 2 divided doses) day 1 until hematologic complete remission

Daunorubicin: I.V.: 60 mg/m^2/day days 1, 2, and 3

[total dose/cycle = 180 mg/m^2]

Consolidation:

Course 1:

Daunorubicin: I.V.: 60 mg/m^2/day days 1, 2, and 3

[total dose/cycle = 180 mg/m^2]

Course 2:

Daunorubicin: I.V.: 45 mg/m^2/day days 1, 2, and 3

[total dose/cycle = 135 mg/m^2]

Maintenance:

Mercaptopurine: Oral: 90 mg/m^2 daily
[total dose/cycle = 8100 mg/m^2 (90 days)]
Methotrexate: Oral: 15 mg/m^2 weekly
[total dose/cycle = 180 mg/m^2]
Tretinoin: Oral: 45 mg/m^2/day (in 2 divided doses) days 1 to 15
[total dose/cycle = 675 mg/m^2]
Repeat cycle every 3 months for 2 years

Tretinoin-Daunorubicin-Cytarabine (APL)

Use Leukemia, acute promyelocytic

Regimen NOTE: Multiple variations are listed.

Variation 1 (patients ≤60 years of age and WBC <10,000/mm^3):

Induction:

Tretinoin: Oral: 45 mg/m^2/day (in 2 divided doses) day 1 until hematologic complete remission
Daunorubicin: I.V.: 60 mg/m^2/day days 1, 2, and 3
[total dose/cycle = 180 mg/m^2]
Cytarabine: I.V.: 200 mg/m^2/day days 3 to 10
[total dose/cycle = 1400 mg/m^2]

Consolidation:

Course 1:
Daunorubicin: I.V.: 60 mg/m^2/day days 1, 2, and 3
[total dose/cycle = 180 mg/m^2]
Cytarabine: I.V.: 200 mg/m^2/day days 1 to 7
[total dose/cycle = 1400 mg/m^2]

Course 2:
Daunorubicin: I.V.: 45 mg/m^2/day days 1, 2, and 3
[total dose/cycle = 135 mg/m^2]
Cytarabine: I.V.: 1000 mg/m^2/dose every 12 hours for 8 doses
[total dose/cycle = 8000 mg/m^2]

Maintenance:

Mercaptopurine: Oral: 90 mg/m^2 daily
[total dose/cycle = 8100 mg/m^2 (90 days)]
Methotrexate: Oral: 15 mg/m^2 weekly
[total dose/cycle = 180 mg/m^2]
Tretinoin: Oral: 45 mg/m^2/day (in 2 divided doses) days 1 to 15
[total dose/cycle = 675 mg/m^2]
Repeat cycle every 3 months for 2 years

Variation 2 (patients ≤60 years of age and WBC ≥10,000/mm^3):

Induction:

Tretinoin: Oral: 45 mg/m^2/day (in 2 divided doses) day 1 until hematologic complete remission
Daunorubicin: I.V.: 60 mg/m^2/day days 1, 2, and 3
[total dose/cycle = 180 mg/m^2]
Cytarabine: I.V.: 200 mg/m^2/day days 3 to 10
[total dose/cycle = 1400 mg/m^2]

Consolidation:

Course 1:
Daunorubicin: I.V.: 60 mg/m^2/day days 1, 2, and 3
[total dose/cycle = 180 mg/m^2]
Cytarabine: I.V.: 200 mg/m^2/day days 1 to 7
[total dose/cycle = 1400 mg/m^2]

Course 2:
Daunorubicin: I.V.: 45 mg/m^2/day days 1, 2, and 3
[total dose/cycle = 135 mg/m^2]
Cytarabine: I.V.: 2000 mg/m^2/dose every 12 hours for 10 doses
[total dose/cycle = 20,000 mg/m^2]

Intrathecal prophylaxis: Five intrathecal injections: First dose in between induction and consolidation and 2 doses during each consolidation phase:
Methotrexate (preservative free): I.T.: 15 mg
Cytarabine (preservative free): I.T.: 50 mg
Corticosteroids (preservative free): I.T.: Dose unspecified

Maintenance:

Mercaptopurine: Oral: 90 mg/m^2 daily

[total dose/cycle = 8100 mg/m^2 (90 days)]

Methotrexate: Oral: 15 mg/m^2 weekly

[total dose/cycle = 180 mg/m^2]

Tretinoin: Oral: 45 mg/m^2/day (in 2 divided doses) days 1 to 15

[total dose/cycle = 675 mg/m^2]

Repeat cycle every 3 months for 2 years

Variation 3 (patients >60 years of age and WBC >10,000/mm^3):

Induction:

Tretinoin: Oral: 45 mg/m^2/day (in 2 divided doses) day 1 until hematologic complete remission

Daunorubicin: I.V.: 60 mg/m^2/day days 1, 2, and 3

[total dose/cycle = 180 mg/m^2]

Cytarabine: I.V.: 200 mg/m^2/day days 3 to 10

[total dose/cycle = 1400 mg/m^2]

Consolidation:

Course 1:

Daunorubicin: I.V.: 60 mg/m^2/day days 1, 2, and 3

[total dose/cycle = 180 mg/m^2]

Cytarabine: I.V.: 200 mg/m^2/day days 1 to 7

[total dose/cycle = 1400 mg/m^2]

Course 2:

Daunorubicin: I.V.: 45 mg/m^2/day days 1, 2, and 3

[total dose/cycle = 135 mg/m^2]

Cytarabine: I.V.: 1000 mg/m^2/dose every 12 hours for 8 doses

[total dose/cycle = 8,000 mg/m^2]

Intrathecal prophylaxis: Five intrathecal injections: First dose in between induction and consolidation and 2 doses during each consolidation phase:

Methotrexate (preservative free): I.T.: 15 mg

Cytarabine (preservative free): I.T.: 50 mg

Corticosteroids (preservative free): I.T.: Dose unspecified

Maintenance:

Mercaptopurine: Oral: 90 mg/m^2 daily

[total dose/cycle = 8100 mg/m^2 (90 days)]

Methotrexate: Oral: 15 mg/m^2 weekly

[total dose/cycle = 180 mg/m^2]

Tretinoin: Oral: 45 mg/m^2/day (in 2 divided doses) days 1 to 15

[total dose/cycle = 675 mg/m^2]

Repeat cycle every 3 months for 2 years

Tretinoin-Idarubicin (APL)

Use Leukemia, acute promyelocytic

Regimen NOTE: Multiple variations are listed.

Variation 1:

Induction:

Tretinoin: Oral: 45 mg/m^2/day (in 2 divided doses) day 1 up to 90 days

[total dose/cycle = up to 4050 mg/m^2]

≤20 years: Oral: 25 mg/m^2/day (in 2 divided doses) day 1 up to 90 days

[total dose/cycle = up to 2250 mg/m^2]

Idarubicin: I.V.: 12 mg/m^2/day days 2, 4, 6, and 8 (omit day 8 for patients >70 years of age)

[total dose/cycle = 36-48 mg/m^2]

Consolidation (administer courses sequentially at 1-month intervals for 3 months):

Course 1:

Idarubicin: I.V.: 5 mg/m^2/day days 1 to 4

[total dose/cycle = 20 mg/m^2]

or

Idarubicin: I.V.: 7 mg/m^2/day days 1 to 4

[total dose/cycle = 28 mg/m^2]

Tretinoin: Oral: 45 mg/m^2/day (in 2 divided doses) days 1 to 15

[total dose/cycle = 675 mg/m^2]

Course 2:
  Mitoxantrone: I.V.: 10 mg/m^2/day days 1 to 5
    [total dose/cycle = 50 mg/m^2]
  or
  Mitoxantrone: I.V.: 10 mg/m^2/day days 1 to 5
    [total dose/cycle = 50 mg/m^2]
  Tretinoin: Oral: 45 mg/m^2/day (in 2 divided doses) days 1 to 15
    [total dose/cycle = 675 mg/m^2]
Course 3:
  Idarubicin: I.V.: 12 mg/m^2 day 1
    [total dose/cycle = 12 mg/m^2]
  or
  Idarubicin: I.V.: 12 mg/m^2/day days 1 and 2
    [total dose/cycle = 24 mg/m^2]
  Tretinoin: Oral: 45 mg/m^2/day (in 2 divided doses) days 1 to 15
    [total dose/cycle = 675 mg/m^2]

Maintenance:
  Mercaptopurine: Oral: 50 mg/m^2 daily
    [total dose/cycle = 4500 mg/m^2 (90 days)]
  Methotrexate: I.M.: 15 mg/m^2 weekly
    [total dose/cycle = 180 mg/m^2]
  Tretinoin: Oral: 45 mg/m^2/day (in 2 divided doses) days 1 to 15
    [total dose/cycle = 675 mg/m^2]
  Repeat cycle every 3 months for 2 years

Variation 2:

Induction:
  Tretinoin: Oral: 45 mg/m^2/day (in 2 divided doses) day 1 up to 90 days
    [total dose/cycle = up to 4050 mg/m^2]
      <15 years: Oral: 25 mg/m^2/day (in 2 divided doses) day 1 up to 90 days
        [total dose/cycle = up to 2250 mg/m^2]
  Idarubicin: I.V.: 12 mg/m^2/day days 2, 4, 6, and 8
    [total dose/cycle = 48 mg/m^2]

Consolidation (administer courses sequentially at 1-month intervals for 3 months):
Course 1:
  Idarubicin: I.V.: 5 mg/m^2/day days 1 to 4
    [total dose/cycle = 20 mg/m^2]
Course 2:
  Mitoxantrone: I.V.: 10 mg/m^2/day days 1 to 5
    [total dose/cycle = 50 mg/m^2]
Course 3:
  Idarubicin: I.V.: 12 mg/m^2 day 1
    [total dose/cycle = 12 mg/m^2]

Maintenance:
  Mercaptopurine: Oral: 90 mg/m^2 daily
    [total dose/cycle = 8100 mg/m^2(90 days)]
  Methotrexate: I.M.: 15 mg/m^2 weekly
    [total dose/cycle = 180 mg/m^2]
  Tretinoin: Oral: 45 mg/m^2/day (in 2 divided doses) days 1 to 15
    [total dose/cycle = 675 mg/m^2]
  Repeat cycle every 3 months for 2 years

Variation 3 (patients ≥60 years of age):

Induction:
  Tretinoin: Oral: 45 mg/m^2/day (in 2 divided doses) day 1 up to 90 days
    [total dose/cycle = up to 4050 mg/m^2]
  Idarubicin: I.V.: 12 mg/m^2/day days 2, 4, 6, and 8 (omit day 8 for patients ≥70 years of age)
    [total dose/cycle = 36-48 mg/m^2]

Consolidation (administer courses sequentially at 1-month intervals for 3 months):
Course 1:
  Idarubicin: I.V.: 5 mg/m^2/day days 1 to 4
    [total dose/cycle = 20 mg/m^2]
  Tretinoin: Oral: 45 mg/m^2/day (in 2 divided doses) days 1 to 15 (if intermediate or high risk)
    [total dose/cycle = 675 mg/m^2]

Course 2:
Mitoxantrone: I.V.: 10 mg/m^2/day days 1 to 5
[total dose/cycle = 50 mg/m^2]
Tretinoin: Oral: 45 mg/m^2/day (in 2 divided doses) days 1 to 15 (if intermediate or high risk)
[total dose/cycle = 675 mg/m^2]
Course 3:
Idarubicin: I.V.: 12 mg/m^2 day 1
[total dose/cycle = 12 mg/m^2]
Tretinoin: Oral: 45 mg/m^2/day (in 2 divided doses) days 1 to 15 (if intermediate or high risk)
[total dose/cycle = 675 mg/m^2]

Maintenance:
Mercaptopurine: Oral: 50 mg/m^2 daily
[total dose/cycle = 4500 mg/m^2 (90 days)]
Methotrexate: I.M.: 15 mg/m^2 weekly
[total dose/cycle = 180 mg/m^2]
Tretinoin: Oral: 45 mg/m^2/day (in 2 divided doses) days 1 to 15
[total dose/cycle = 675 mg/m^2]
Repeat cycle every 3 months for 2 years

VAC Alternating With IE (Ewing Sarcoma)

Use Ewing sarcoma

Regimen

Cycle A (odd numbered cycles):
Cyclophosphamide: I.V.: 1200 mg/m^2 day 1 (followed by mesna; dose not specified)
[total dose/cycle = 1200 mg/m^2]
Vincristine: I.V.: 2 mg/m^2 (maximum dose: 2 mg) day 1
[total dose/cycle = 2 mg/m^2; maximum: 2 mg]
Doxorubicin: I.V.: 75 mg/m^2 day 1, for 5 cycles (maximum cumulative dose: 375 mg/m^2)
[total dose/cycle = 75 mg/m^2; maximum cumulative dose: 375 mg/m^2]
Dactinomycin: I.V.: 1.25 mg/m^2 day 1, begin cycle 11 (after reaching maximum cumulative doxorubicin dose)
[total dose/cycle = 1.25 mg/m^2]
Cycle B (even numbered cycles):
Ifosfamide: I.V.: 1800 mg/m^2/day days 1 to 5 (given with mesna)
[total dose/cycle = 9000 mg/m^2]
Etoposide: I.V.: 100 mg/m^2/day days 1 to 5
[total dose/cycle = 500 mg/m^2]
Alternate Cycles A and B, administering a cycle every 3 weeks (alternating in the following sequence: ABABAB) for 17 cycles

VAC Pulse

Use Rhabdomyosarcoma

Regimen

Vincristine: I.V.: 2 mg/m^2/dose (maximum dose: 2 mg/dose) every 7 days, for 12 weeks
Dactinomycin: I.V.: 0.015 mg/kg/day (maximum dose: 0.5 mg/day) days 1 to 5, every 3 months for 5 courses
Cyclophosphamide: Oral, I.V.: 10 mg/kg/day for 7 days, repeat every 6 weeks

VAC (Rhabdomyosarcoma)

Use Rhabdomyosarcoma

Regimen

Induction (weeks 1 to 17):
Vincristine: I.V. push: 1.5 mg/m^2 (maximum dose: 2 mg) day 1 of weeks 1 to 13, then one dose at week 17
Dactinomycin: I.V. push: 0.015 mg/kg/day (maximum dose: 0.5 mg) days 1 to 5 of weeks 1, 4, 7, and 17
Cyclophosphamide: I.V.: 2.2 g/m^2 day 1 of weeks 1, 4, 7, 10, 13, and 17
Continuation (weeks 21 to 44):
Vincristine: I.V. push: 1.5 mg/m^2 (maximum dose: 2 mg) day 1 of weeks 21 to 26, 30 to 35, and 39 to 44
Dactinomycin: I.V. push: 0.015 mg/kg/day (maximum dose: 0.5 mg) days 1 to 5 of weeks 21, 24, 30, 33, 39, and 42
Cyclophosphamide: I.V.: 2.2 g/m^2 day 1 of weeks 21, 24, 30, 33, 39, and 42

VAD

Use Multiple myeloma

Regimen

Vincristine: I.V.: 0.4 mg/day continuous infusion days 1 to 4
[total dose/cycle = 1.6 mg]
Doxorubicin: I.V.: 9 mg/m^2/day continuous infusion days 1 to 4
[total dose/cycle = 36 mg/m^2]
Dexamethasone: Oral: 40 mg/day days 1 to 4, 9 to 12, and 17 to 20
[total dose/cycle = 480 mg]
Repeat cycle every 28-35 days

VAD/CVAD

Use Leukemia, acute lymphocytic

Regimen Induction cycle:

Vincristine: I.V.: 0.4 mg/day continuous infusion days 1 to 4 and 24 to 27
[total dose/cycle = 3.2 mg]
Doxorubicin: I.V.: 12 mg/m^2/day continuous infusion days 1 to 4 and 24 to 27
[total dose/cycle = 96 mg/m^2]
Dexamethasone: Oral: 40 mg/day days 1 to 4, 9 to 12, 17 to 20, 24 to 27, 32 to 35, and 40 to 43
[total dose/cycle = 960 mg]
Cyclophosphamide: I.V.: 1 g/m^2 day 24
[total dose/cycle = 1 g/m^2]
Administer one cycle only

VAD (Wilms Tumor)

Use Wilms' tumor

Regimen NOTE: Multiple variations are listed.

Variation 1 (Stage III favorable disease; children ≥1 year):
Vincristine: I.V.: 1.5 mg/m^2 weekly for 10 to 11 weeks
followed by
Vincristine: I.V.: 1.5 mg/m^2 every 3 weeks
Dactinomycin: I.V.: 1.5 mg/m^2 every 6 weeks
Doxorubicin: I.V.: 40 mg/m^2 every 6 weeks
NOTE: Alternate dactinomycin and doxorubicin; administer dactinomycin at 3 weeks and doxorubicin in 3 weeks
Treatment continued for 1 year

Variation 2 (Stage III favorable disease; children <1 year):
Vincristine: I.V.: 0.75 mg/m^2 weekly for 10 to 11 weeks
followed by
Vincristine: I.V.: 0.75 mg/m^2 every 3 weeks
Dactinomycin: I.V.: 0.75 mg/m^2 every 6 weeks
Doxorubicin: I.V.: 20 mg/m^2 every 6 weeks
NOTE: Alternate dactinomycin and doxorubicin; administer dactinomycin at 3 weeks and doxorubicin in 3 weeks
Treatment continued for 1 year

VAMP (Hodgkin)

Use Lymphoma, Hodgkin

Regimen NOTE: Patients < 21 years old

Vinblastine: I.V.: 6 mg/m^2/day days 1 and 15
[total dose/cycle = 12 mg/m^2]
Doxorubicin: I.V.: 25 mg/m^2/day days 1 and 15
[total dose/cycle = 50 mg/m$^{2]}$
Methotrexate: I.V.: 20 mg/m^2/day days 1 and 15
[total dose/cycle = 40 mg/m^2]
Prednisone: Oral: 40 mg/m^2/day days 1 to 14 (omit after mediastinal radiation)
[total dose/cycle = 560 mg/m^2]
Repeat cycle every 28 days for a total of 4 cycles

VBMCP (Multiple Myeloma)

Use Multiple myeloma

Regimen NOTE: Multiple variations are listed.

Variation 1:

Vincristine: I.V.: 1.2 mg/m^2 day 1
[total dose/cycle = 1.2 mg/m^2]

Carmustine: I.V.: 20 mg/m^2 day 1
[total dose/cycle = 20 mg/m^2]

Melphalan: Oral: 8 mg/m^2/day days 1 to 4
[total dose/cycle = 32 mg/m^2]

Cyclophosphamide: I.V.: 400 mg/m^2 day 1
[total dose/cycle = 400 mg/m^2]

Prednisone: Oral: 40 mg/m^2/day days 1 to 7
[total dose/cycle = 280 mg/m^2]

Repeat cycle every 35 days for up to 2 years or until disease progression

Variation 2:

Vincristine: I.V.: 1.2 mg/m^2 (maximum dose: 2 mg) day 1
[total dose/cycle = 1.2 mg/m^2; maximum: 2 mg]

Carmustine: I.V.: 20 mg/m^2 day 1
[total dose/cycle = 20 mg/m^2]

Melphalan: Oral: 8 mg/m^2/day days 1 to 4
[total dose/cycle = 32 mg/m^2]

Cyclophosphamide: I.V.: 400 mg/m^2 day 1
[total dose/cycle = 400 mg/m^2]

Prednisone: Oral: 40 mg/m^2/day days 1 to 7 (all cycles)
[total dose/cycle = 280 mg/m^2]

followed by Oral: 20 mg/m^2/day days 8 to 14 (first 3 cycles only)
[total dose/cycle = 140 mg/m^2]

Repeat cycle every 35 days

VBP

Use Testicular cancer

Regimen

Vinblastine: I.V.: 0.15 mg/kg/day days 1 and 2
[total dose/cycle = 0.3 mg/kg]

Bleomycin: I.V.: 30 units/day days 2, 9, and 16
[total dose/cycle = 90 units]

Cisplatin: I.V.: 20 mg/m^2/day days 1 to 5
[total dose/cycle = 100 mg/m^2]

Repeat cycle every 21 days for 4 cycles

VCAP

Use Multiple myeloma

Regimen

Vincristine: I.V.: 1 mg/m^2 (maximum dose: 1.5 mg) day 1
[total dose/cycle = 1 mg/m^2]

Cyclophosphamide: Oral: 125 mg/m^2/day days 1 to 4
[total dose/cycle = 500 mg/m^2]

Doxorubicin: I.V.: 30 mg/m^2 day 1
[total dose/cycle = 30 mg/m^2]

Prednisone: Oral: 60 mg/m^2/day days 1 to 4
[total dose/cycle = 240 mg/m^2]

Repeat cycle every 21 days for 6-12 months

VIM-D (Hodgkin)

Use Lymphoma, Hodgkin disease

Regimen

Etoposide: I.V.: 100 mg/m^2 over 30 minutes day 1
[total dose/cycle = 100 mg/m^2]

Ifosfamide: I.V.: 4 g/m^2 continuous infusion over 24 hours day 1
[total dose/cycle = 4 g/m^2]

Mesna: I.V.: 1 g/m^2 I.V. bolus day 1
followed by: Mesna: I.V.: 6 g/m^2 continuous infusion over 36 hours
[total dose/cycle = 7 g/m^2]
Mitoxantrone: I.V.: 10 mg/m^2 I.V. bolus day 1
[total dose/cycle = 10 mg/m^2]
Dexamethasone: Oral: 40 mg/day days 1 to 5
[total dose/cycle = 200 mg]
Repeat cycle every 28 days; treat 3 cycles post remission

Vinblastine (Hodgkin Regimen)

Use Lymphoma, Hodgkin

Regimen

Vinblastine: I.V.: 4-6 mg/m^2/day I.V. bolus day 1
[total dose/cycle = 4-6 mg/m^2]
Repeat cycle every 1 to 2 weeks until disease progression

Vincristine-Dactinomycin-Cyclophosphamide (Ovarian Cancer)

Use Ovarian cancer (germ cell tumor)

Regimen NOTE: Multiple variations are listed.

Variation 1:
Vincristine: I.V.: 1.5 mg/m^2 (maximum dose: 2 mg) days 1, 8, 15, and 22 for 2-3 cycles
[total dose/cycle = 6 mg/m^2 (maximum: 8 mg)] for 2-3 cycles
Dactinomycin: I.V.: 300 mcg/m^2/day days 1 to 5
[total dose/cycle = 1500 mcg/m^2]
Cyclophosphamide: I.V.: 150 mg/m^2/day days 1 to 5
[total dose/cycle = 750 mg/m^2]
Repeat cycle every 4 weeks for at least 10 cycles; vincristine is only administered for 8-12 weeks

Variation 2:
Vincristine: I.V.: 1-1.5 mg/m^2 day 1
[total dose/cycle = 1-1.5 mg/m^2]
Dactinomycin: I.V.: 500 mcg/day days 1 to 5
[total dose/cycle = 2500 mcg]
Cyclophosphamide: I.V.: 5-7 mg/kg/day days 1 to 5
[total dose/cycle = 25-35 mg/kg]
Repeat cycle every 4 weeks for up to 12 cycles

Vinorelbine-Cisplatin

Use Lung cancer, nonsmall cell

Regimen NOTE: Multiple variations are listed.

Variation 1:
Cisplatin: I.V.: 50 mg/m^2/day days 1 and 8
[total dose/cycle = 100 mg/m^2]
Vinorelbine: I.V.: 25 mg/m^2/day days 1, 8, 15, and 22
[total dose/cycle = 100 mg/m^2]
Repeat cycle every 28 days for total of 4 cycles

Variation 2:
Vinorelbine: I.V.: 25 mg/m^2/day days 1, 8, 15, and 22
[total dose/cycle = 100 mg/m^2]
Cisplatin: I.V.: 100 mg/m^2 day 1
[total dose/cycle = 100 mg/m^2]
Repeat cycle every 28 days

Variation 3:
Vinorelbine: I.V.: 30 mg/m^2 weekly
Cisplatin: I.V.: 120 mg/m^2/day days 1 and 29, then once every 6 weeks

Variation 4:
Vinorelbine: I.V.: 30 mg/m^2/day days 1, 8, and 15
[total dose/cycle = 90 mg/m^2]
Cisplatin: I.V.: 80 mg/m^2 day 1
[total dose/cycle = 80 mg/m^2]
Repeat cycle every 21 days for total of 4 cycles
Note: Vinorelbine treatment is discontinued after day 1 of cycle 4

Variation 5:

Vinorelbine: I.V.: 30 mg/m^2/day days 1, 8, 15, and 22

[total dose/cycle = 120 mg/m^2]

Cisplatin: I.V.: 100 mg/m^2 day 1

[total dose/cycle = 100 mg/m^2]

Repeat cycle every 28 days for total of 3 or 4 cycles

Note: Vinorelbine treatment is discontinued after day 1 of last treatment cycle

Vinorelbine-FEC

Use Breast cancer

Regimen

Cycles 1 and 2:

Vinorelbine: I.V.: 25 mg/m^2/day days 1, 8, and 15

[total dose/cycle = 75 mg/m^2]

Treatment cycle is 21 days

Cycle 3:

Vinorelbine: I.V.: 25 mg/m^2/day days 1 and 8

[total dose/cycle 3 = 50 mg/m^2]

Treatment cycle is 21 days

Cycles 4, 5, and 6 (FEC):

Fluorouracil: I.V.: 600 mg/m^2 day 1

[total dose/cycle = 600 mg/m^2]

Epirubicin: I.V.: 60 mg/m^2 day 1

[total dose/cycle = 60 mg/m^2]

Cyclophosphamide: I.V.: 600 mg/m^2 day 1

[total dose/cycle = 600 mg/m^2]

Repeat FEC cycle every 21 days for total of 3 cycles

Vinorelbine (Hodgkin Regimen)

Use Lymphoma, Hodgkin

Regimen

Vinorelbine: I.V.: 30 mg/m^2/day day 1

[total dose/cycle = 30 mg/m^2]

Repeat cycle every 7 days, maximum of 24 doses

Vinorelbine (Mesothelioma Regimen)

Use Malignant pleural mesothelioma

Regimen

Vinorelbine: I.V.: 30 mg/m^2 (maximum dose: 60 mg) over 5 minutes weekly on days 1, 8, 15, 22, 29, and 36

[total dose/cycle = 180 mg/m^2]

Repeat cycle every 42 days

Vinorelbine (Ovarian Regimen)

Use Ovarian cancer

Regimen

Vinorelbine: I.V.: 30 mg/m^2/day days 1 and 8

[total dose/cycle = 60 mg/m^2]

Repeat cycle every 21 days

Vinorelbine (Small Cell Lung Cancer Regimen)

Use Lung cancer, small cell

Regimen NOTE: Multiple variations are listed:

Variation 1:

Vinorelbine: I.V.: 30 mg/m^2 day 1

[total dose/cycle = 30 mg/m^2]

Repeat cycle every 7 days until disease progression or unacceptable toxicity

Variation 2:

Vinorelbine: I.V.: 25 mg/m^2 day 1

[total dose/cycle = 25 mg/m^2]

Repeat cycle every 7 days until disease progression, no response after 4 cycles, or unacceptable toxicity

Vinorelbine-Trastuzumab

Use Breast cancer

Regimen

Week 1:

Trastuzumab: I.V.: 4 mg/kg (loading dose) day 1 week 1
[total dose/week 1 = 4 mg/kg]

Vinorelbine: I.V.: 25 mg/m^2 day 1
[total dose/week 1 = 25 mg/m^2]

Subsequent weeks:

Trastuzumab: I.V.: 2 mg/kg (loading dose) day 1
[total dose/week = 2 mg/kg]

Vinorelbine: I.V.: 25 mg/m^2 day 1
[total dose/week = 25 mg/m^2]

Repeat weekly

Vinorelbine-Trastuzumab-FEC

Use Breast cancer

Regimen

Cycle 1:

Trastuzumab: I.V.: 4 mg/kg (loading dose) day 1 cycle 1
followed by I.V.: 2 mg/kg/day days 8 and 15 cycle 1
[total dose/cycle 1 = 8 mg/kg]

Vinorelbine: I.V.: 25 mg/m^2/day days 1, 8, and 15
[total dose/cycle 1 = 75 mg/m^2]

Treatment cycle is 21 days

Cycle 2:

Trastuzumab: I.V.: 2 mg/kg/day days 1, 8, and 15
[total dose/cycle = 6 mg/kg]

Vinorelbine: I.V.: 25 mg/m^2/day days 1, 8, and 15
[total dose/cycle 2 = 75 mg/m^2]

Treatment cycle is 21 days

Cycle 3:

Trastuzumab: I.V.: 2 mg/kg/day days 1, 8, and 15
[total dose/cycle = 6 mg/kg]

Vinorelbine: I.V.: 25 mg/m^2/day days 1 and 8
[total dose/cycle 3 = 50 mg/m^2]

Treatment cycle is 21 days

Cycles 4, 5, and 6 (FEC):

Fluorouracil: I.V.: 600 mg/m^2 day 1
[total dose/cycle = 600 mg/m^2]

Epirubicin: I.V.: 60 mg/m^2 day 1
[total dose/cycle = 60 mg/m^2]

Cyclophosphamide: I.V.: 600 mg/m^2 day 1
[total dose/cycle = 600 mg/m^2]

Repeat FEC cycle every 21 days for total of 3 cycles

VIP (Etoposide) (Testicular Cancer)

Use Testicular cancer

Regimen NOTE: Multiple variations are listed.

Variation 1:

Etoposide: I.V.: 75 mg/m^2/day days 1 to 5
[total dose/cycle = 375 mg/m^2]

Ifosfamide: I.V.: 1200 mg/m^2/day days 1 to 5
[total dose/cycle = 6000 mg/m^2]

Cisplatin: I.V.: 20 mg/m^2/day days 1 to 5
[total dose/cycle = 100 mg/m^2]

Mesna: I.V.: 400 mg/m^2 day 1 only
followed by I.V.: 1200 mg/m^2/day continuous infusion days 1 to 5
[total dose/cycle = 6400 mg/m^2]
Repeat cycle every 21 days for 4 cycles

Variation 2:
Etoposide: I.V.: 100 mg/m^2/day days 1 to 5
[total dose/cycle = 500 mg/m^2]
Ifosfamide: I.V.: 1200 mg/m^2/day days 1 to 5
[total dose/cycle = 6000 mg/m^2]
Cisplatin: I.V.: 20 mg/m^2/day days 1 to 5
[total dose/cycle = 100 mg/m^2]
Mesna: I.V.: 200 mg/m^2 every 4 hours, for 3 doses each day, days 1, 2, and 3
[total dose/cycle = 1800 mg/m^2]
Repeat cycle every 21 days

Variation 3:
Ifosfamide: I.V.: 2500 mg/m^2/day days 1 and 2
[total dose/cycle = 5000 mg/m^2]
Mesna: I.V.: 2400 mg/m^2/day days 1 and 2
[total dose/cycle = 4800 mg/m^2]
Etoposide: I.V.: 100 mg/m^2/day days 3, 4, and 5
[total dose/cycle = 300 mg/m^2]
Cisplatin: I.V.: 40 mg/m^2/day days 3, 4, and 5
[total dose/cycle = 120 mg/m^2]
Repeat cycle every 21 days

Variation 4:
Etoposide: I.V.: 75 mg/m^2/day days 1 to 5
[total dose/cycle = 375 mg/m^2]
Ifosfamide: I.V.: 1200 mg/m^2/day days 1 to 5
[total dose/cycle = 6000 mg/m^2]
Cisplatin: I.V.: 20 mg/m^2/day days 1 to 5
[total dose/cycle = 100 mg/m^2]
Mesna: I.V.: 120 mg/m^2 day 1 only
followed by I.V.: 1200 mg/m^2/day continuous infusion days 1 to 5
[total dose/cycle = 6120 mg/m^2]
Repeat cycle every 21 days for 4 cycles

VIP (Vinblastine) (Testicular Cancer)

Use Testicular cancer

Regimen NOTE: Multiple variations are listed.

Variation 1:
Vinblastine: I.V.: 0.11 mg/kg/day days 1 and 2
[total dose/cycle = 0.22 mg/kg]
Ifosfamide: I.V.: 1200 mg/m^2/day days 1 to 5
[total dose/cycle = 6000 mg/m^2]
Cisplatin: I.V.: 20 mg/m^2/day days 1 to 5
[total dose/cycle = 100 mg/m^2]
Mesna: I.V.: 400 mg/m^2 day 1
followed by I.V.: 1200 mg/m^2/day continuous infusion days 1 to 5
[total dose/cycle = 6400 mg/m^2]
Repeat cycle every 21 days for 4 cycles

Variation 2:
Vinblastine: I.V.: 6 mg/m^2/day days 1 and 2
[total dose/cycle = 12 mg/m^2]
Ifosfamide: I.V.: 1500 mg/m^2/day days 1 to 5
[total dose/cycle = 7500 mg/m^2]
Cisplatin: I.V.: 20 mg/m^2/day days 1 to 5
[total dose/cycle = 100 mg/m^2]
Mesna: I.V.: 300 mg/m^2 3 times/day days 1 to 5
[total dose/cycle = 4500 mg/m^2]
Repeat cycle every 21 days for 4 cycles

XELOX (Colorectal)

Use Colorectal cancer

Regimen NOTE: Multiple variations are listed.

Variation 1 (adjuvant):

Oxaliplatin: I.V.: 130 mg/m^2 over 2 hours day 1
[total dose/cycle = 130 mg/m^2]

Capecitabine: Oral: 1000 mg/m^2 twice daily days 1 to 14
[total dose/cycle = 28,000 mg/m^2]

Repeat cycle every 21 days for 8 cycles

Variation 2 (metastatic):

Oxaliplatin: I.V.: 130 mg/m^2 over 2 hours day 1
[total dose/cycle = 130 mg/m^2]

Capecitabine: Oral: 1000 mg/m^2 twice daily days 1 (beginning with evening dose) to 15 (ending with morning dose)
[total dose/cycle = 28,000 mg/m^2]

Repeat cycle every 21 days

Variation 3 (metastatic):

Oxaliplatin: I.V.: 130 mg/m^2 day 1
[total dose/cycle = 130 mg/m^2]

Capecitabine: Oral: 850 mg/m^2 twice daily days 1 (beginning with evening dose) to 15 (ending with morning dose)
[total dose/cycle = 23,800 mg/m^2]

Repeat cycle every 21 days

CHEMOTHERAPY REGIMEN INDEX

AMYLOIDOSIS

BRAIN TUMORS

Neuroblastoma

Primary CNS Lymphoma

BREAST CANCER

GASTROINTESTINAL

Anal Cancer

Biliary Adenocarcinoma

Colorectal Cancer

Esophageal Cancer

Gastric Cancer

HEAD AND NECK CANCER

HEMATOLOGIC/LEUKEMIA

Leukemia, Acute Lymphocytic

Leukemia, Acute Myeloid

Leukemia, Acute Promyelocytic

Leukemia, Chronic Lymphocytic

MALIGNANT PLEURAL MESOTHELIOMA

MELANOMA

MULTIPLE MYELOMA

MYELODYSPLASTIC SYNDROME

RETINOBLASTOMA

SARCOMA

Osteosarcoma

Rhabdomyosarcoma

APPENDIX TABLE OF CONTENTS

Visit thePoint http://thepoint.lww.com/QL2013 for exclusive access to:

- Apothecary/Metric Conversions
- Pounds/Kilograms Conversion
- Temperature Conversion
- Pharmaceutical Manufacturers and Distributors
- Multivitamin Products

Refer to the inside front cover of this book for your online access code.

ABBREVIATIONS & SYMBOLS COMMONLY USED IN MEDICAL ORDERS

Abbreviations Which May Be Used in This Reference

Abbreviation	Meaning
5-HT	5-hydroxytryptamine
AAP	American Academy of Pediatrics
ABG	arterial blood gases
ABW	adjusted body weight
AACT	American Academy of Clinical Toxicology
ACC	American College of Cardiology
ACE	angiotensin converting enzyme
ACLS	advanced cardiac life support
ACOG	American College of Obstetricians and Gynecologists
ACTH	adrenocorticotrophic hormone
ADH	alcohol dehydrogenase
ADHD	attention-deficit/hyperactivity disorder
ADLs	activities of daily living
AED	antiepileptic drug
AHA	American Heart Association
AIDS	acquired immune deficiency syndrome
AIMS	Abnormal Involuntary Movement Scale
ALS	amyotrophic lateral sclerosis
ALT	alanine aminotransferase
AMA	American Medical Association
ANC	absolute neutrophil count
aPTT	activated partial thromboplastin
ARB	angiotensin receptor blocker
ARDS	acute respiratory distress syndrome
AST	aspartate aminotransferase
AUC	area under the curve
BDI	Beck Depression Inventory
BEC	blood ethanol concentration
BLS	basic life support
BMI	body mass index
BMT	bone marrow transplant
BP	blood pressure
BPH	benign prostatic hyperplasia
BPRS	Brief Psychiatric Rating Scale
BSA	body surface area
BUN	blood urea nitrogen
CABG	coronary artery bypass graft
CAD	coronary artery disease
CAN	Canadian
CAPD	continuous ambulatory peritoneal dialysis
CAS	chemical abstract service
CBC	complete blood count
CBT	cognitive behavioral therapy
Cl_{cr}	creatinine clearance

Abbreviations Which May Be Used in This Reference *(continued)*

Abbreviation	Meaning
CDC	Centers for Disease Control and Prevention
CF	cystic fibrosis
CGI	Clinical Global Impression
CHD	coronary heart disease
CHF	congestive heart failure; chronic heart failure
CIE	chemotherapy-induced emesis
C-II	schedule two controlled substance
C-III	schedule three controlled substance
C-IV	schedule four controlled substance
C-V	schedule five controlled substance
CIV	continuous I.V. infusion
C_{max}	maximum plasma concentration
C_{min}	minimum plasma concentration
CMV	cytomegalovirus
CNS	central nervous system or coagulase negative staphylococcus
COLD	chronic obstructive lung disease
COPD	chronic obstructive pulmonary disease
COX	cyclooxygenase
CPK	creatine phosphokinase
CRF	chronic renal failure
CRP	C-reactive protein
CRRT	continuous renal replacement therapy
CSF	cerebrospinal fluid
CSII	continuous subcutaneous insulin infusion
CT	computed tomography
CVA	cerebrovascular accident
CVVH	continuous venovenous hemofiltration
CVVHD	continuous venovenous hemodialysis
CVVHDF	continuous venovenous hemodiafiltration
CYP	cytochrome
D_5W	dextrose 5% in water
DBP	diastolic blood pressure
DEHP	di(3-ethylhexyl)phthalate
DIC	disseminated intravascular coagulation
DM	diabetes mellitus
DMARD	disease modifying antirheumatic drug
DSC	discontinued
DSM-IV	Diagnostic and Statistical Manual
DVT	deep vein thrombosis
EBV	Epstein-Barr virus
ECG	electrocardiogram
ECMO	extracorporeal membrane oxygenation
ECT	electroconvulsive therapy
ED	emergency department
EEG	electroencephalogram
EF	ejection fraction
EG	ethylene glycol
EGA	estimated gestational age
EIA	enzyme immunoassay

Abbreviations Which May Be Used in This Reference *(continued)*

Abbreviation	Meaning
ELISA	enzyme-linked immunosorbent assay
EPS	extrapyramidal side effects
ESR	erythrocyte sedimentation rate
ESRD	end stage renal disease
EtOH	alcohol
FDA	Food and Drug Administration
FTT	failure to thrive
GABA	gamma-aminobutyric acid
GAD	generalized anxiety disorder
GERD	gastroesophageal reflux disease
GFR	glomerular filtration rate
GGT	gamma-glutamyltransferase
GI	gastrointestinal
GU	genitourinary
GVHD	graft versus host disease
HAM-A	Hamilton Anxiety Scale
HAM-D	Hamilton Depression Scale
HDL	high density lipoprotein
HF	heart failure
HFSA	Heart Failure Society of America
HIV	human immunodeficiency virus
HMG-CoA	3-hydroxy-3-methylglutaryl-coenzyme A
HOCM	hypertrophic obstructive cardiomyopathy
HPA	hypothalamic-pituitary-adrenal
HSV	herpes simplex virus
HTN	hypertension
HUS	hemolytic uremic syndrome
IBD	inflammatory bowel disease
IBS	irritable bowel syndrome
IBW	ideal body weight
ICD	implantable cardioverter defibrillator
ICH	intracranial hemorrhage
ICP	intracranial pressure
IDDM	insulin dependent diabetes mellitus
IDSA	Infectious Diseases Society of America
IHSS	idiopathic hypertrophic subaortic stenosis
I.M.	intramuscular
INR	international normalized ration
Int. unit	international unit
IOP	intraocular pressure
IUGR	intrauterine growth retardation
I.V.	intravenous
JIA	juvenile idiopathic arthritis
JNC	Joint National Committee
KIU	kallikrein inhibitor unit
LAMM	L-α-acetyl methadol
LDH	lactate dehydrogenase
LDL	low density lipoprotein
LFT	liver function test

Abbreviations Which May Be Used in This Reference *(continued)*

Abbreviation	Meaning
LGA	large for gestational age
LR	lactated ringers
LVEF	left ventricular ejection fraction
LVH	left ventricular hypertrophy
MADRS	Montgomery Asbery Depression Rating Scale
MAOIs	monamine oxidase inhibitors
MDD	major depressive disorder
MDRD	modification of diet in renal disease
MDRSP	multidrug resistant *streptococcus pneumoniae*
mEq	milliequivalent
mg	milligram
MI	myocardial infarction
mL	milliliter
mm	millimeter
mM	millimolar
mm Hg	millimeters of mercury
MMSE	mini mental status examination
M/P	milk to plasma ratio
MPS I	mucopolysaccharidosis I
MRHD	maximum recommended human dose
MRI	magnetic resonance imaging
MUGA	multiple gated acquisition scan
NAS	neonatal abstinence syndrome
NF	National Formulary
NFD	Nephrogenic fibrosing dermopathy
ng	nanogram
NIDDM	Noninsulin dependent diabetes mellitus
NKA	no known allergies
NKDA	No known drug allergies
NMDA	n-methyl-d-aspartic acid
NMS	neuroleptic malignant syndrome
NNRTI	nonnucleoside reverse transcriptase inhibitor
NRTI	nucleoside reverse transcriptase inhibitor
NS	normal saline
NSAID	nonsteroidal antiinflammatory drug
NSF	nephrogenic systemic fibrosis
NSTEMI	Non-ST-elevation myocardial infarction
OA	osteoarthritis
OCD	obsessive-compulsive disorder
OHSS	ovarian hyperstimulation syndrome
OTC	over-the-counter
PAT	paroxysmal atrial tachycardia
PD	Parkinson disease; peritoneal dialysis
PDA	patent ductus arteriosus
PDE-5	phosphodiesterase-5
PE	pulmonary embolus
PEG tube	percutaneous endoscopic gastrostomy tube
PHN	post-herpetic neuralgia
PID	pelvic inflammatory disease

Abbreviations Which May Be Used in This Reference *(continued)*

Abbreviation	Meaning
PMDD	premenstrual dysphoric disorder
PONV	postoperative nausea and vomiting
PPN	peripheral parenteral nutrition
PROM	premature rupture of membranes
PSVT	paroxysmal supraventricular tachycardia
PT	prothrombin time
PTSD	post-traumatic stress disorder
PTT	partial thromboplastin time
PUD	peptic ulcer disease
PVD	peripheral vascular disease
QT_c	corrected QT interval
QT_c-F	corrected QT interval by Fredricia formula
RA	rheumatoid arthritis
REM	rapid eye movement
RPLS	reversible posterior leukoencephalopathy syndrome
SA	sinoatrial
SAD	seasonal affective disorder
SAH	subarachnoid hemorrhage
SBE	subacute bacterial endocarditis
SBP	systolic blood pressure
S_{Cr}	serum creatinine
SERM	selective estrogen receptor modulator
SGA	small for gestational age
SGOT	serum glutamic oxaloacetic aminotransferase
SGPT	serum glutamic pyruvate transaminase
SI	International System of Units or Systeme international d'Unites
SIADH	syndrome of inappropriate antidiuretic hormone secretion
SLE	systemic lupus erythematosus
SNRI	serotonin norepinephrine reuptake inhibitor
SSKI	saturated solution of potassium iodide
SSRIs	selective serotonin reuptake inhibitors
STD	sexually transmitted disease
STEM I	ST-elevation myocardial infarction
SubQ	subcutaneous
supp	suppository
SVT	supraventricular tachycardia
SWFI	sterile water for injection
syr	syrup
$T_{1/2}$	half-life
tab	tablet
TB	tuberculosis
TC	total cholesterol
TCA	tricyclic antidepressant
TD	tardive dyskinesia
TG	triglyceride
TIA	transient ischemic attack
TMA	thrombotic microangiopathy
T_{max}	time to maximum observed concentration, plasma
TNF	Tumor necrosis factor

Abbreviations Which May Be Used in This Reference *(continued)*

Abbreviation	Meaning
TPN	total parenteral nutrition
tr, tinct	tincture
tsp	teaspoonful
UC	ulcerative colitis
ULN	upper limits of normal
URI	upper respiratory infection
USAN	United States Adopted Names
USP	United States Pharmacopeia
UTI	urinary tract infection
UV	ultraviolet
V_d	volume of distribution
VEGF	vascular endothelial growth factor
VF	ventricular fibrillation
VT	ventricular tachycardia
VTE	venous thromboembolism
vWD	von Willebrand disease
VZV	varicella zoster virus
YBOC	Yale Brown Obsessive-Compulsive Scale
YMRS	Young Mania Rating Scale

Common Weights, Measures, or Apothecary Abbreviations

Abbreviation	Meaning
<[1]	less than
>[1]	greater than
≤	less than or equal to
≥	greater than or equal to
ac	before meals or food
ad	to, up to
ad lib	at pleasure
AM	morning
AMA	against medical advice
amp	ampul
amt	amount
aq	water
aq. dest.	distilled water
ASAP	as soon as possible
a.u.[1]	each ear
bid	twice daily
bm	bowel movement
C	Celsius, centigrade
cal	calorie
cap	capsule
cc[1]	cubic centimeter
cm	centimeter
comp	compound
cont	continue
d	day

Common Weights, Measures, or Apothecary Abbreviations *(continued)*

Abbreviation	Meaning
d/c[1]	discharge
dil	dilute
disp	dispense
div	divide
dtd	give of such a dose
Dx	diagnosis
elix, el	elixir
emp	as directed
et	and
ex aq	in water
F	Fahrenheit
f, ft	make, let be made
g	gram
gr	grain
gtt	a drop
h	hour
hs[1]	at bedtime
kcal	kilocalorie
kg	kilogram
L	liter
liq	a liquor, solution
M	molar
mcg	microgram
m. dict	as directed
mEq	milliequivalent
mg	milligram
microL	microliter
mL	milliliter
mm	millimeter
mM	millimolar
mm Hg	millimeters of mercury
ng	nanogram
no.	number
noc	in the night
non rep	do not repeat, no refills
NPO	nothing by mouth
NV	nausea and vomiting
O, Oct	a pint
o.d.[1]	right eye
o.l.	left eye
o.s.[1]	left eye
o.u.[1]	each eye, both eyes together
pc, post cib	after meals
PM	afternoon or evening
P.O.	by mouth
P.R.	rectally
prn	as needed
pulv	a powder
q	every

Common Weights, Measures, or Apothecary Abbreviations *(continued)*

Abbreviation	Meaning
qad	every other day
qd[1,2]	every day, daily
qh	every hour
qid	four times a day
qod[1,2]	every other day
qs	a sufficient quantity
qs ad	a sufficient quantity to make
Rx	take, a recipe
SL	sublingual
stat	at once, immediately
SubQ	subcutaneous
supp	suppository
syr	syrup
tab	tablet
tal	such
tid	three times a day
tr, tinct	tincture
trit	triturate
tsp	teaspoon
u.d.	as directed
ung	ointment
v.o.	verbal order
w.a.	while awake
x3	3 times
x4	4 times

[1]ISMP error-prone abbreviation.

[2]JCAHO Do Not Use list.

Additional abbreviations used and defined within a specific monograph or text piece may only apply to that text.

REFERENCES

The Institute for Safe Medication Practices (ISMP) list of Error-Prone Abbreviations, Symbols, and Dose Designations. Available at http://www.ismp.org/Tools/errorproneabbreviations.pdf

The Joint Commission Official "Do Not Use" list. Available at http://www.jointcommission.org/PatientSafety/DoNotUseList

NORMAL LABORATORY VALUES FOR ADULTS

CHEMISTRY

Test	Values	Remarks
Serum / Plasma		
Acetone	Negative	
Albumin	3.2-5 g/dL	
Alcohol, ethyl	Negative	
Aldolase	1.2-7.6 IU/L	
Ammonia	20-70 mcg/dL	Specimen to be placed on ice as soon as collected.
Amylase	30-110 units/L	
Bilirubin, direct	0-0.3 mg/dL	
Bilirubin, total	0.1-1.2 mg/dL	
Calcium	8.6-10.3 mg/dL	
Calcium, ionized	2.24-2.46 mEq/L	
Chloride	95-108 mEq/L	
Cholesterol, total	≤200 mg/dL	Fasted blood required – normal value affected by dietary habits. This reference range is for a general adult population.
HDL cholesterol	40-60 mg/dL	Fasted blood required – normal value affected by dietary habits.
LDL cholesterol	<160 mg/dL	If triglyceride is >400 mg/dL, LDL cannot be calculated accurately (Friedewald equation). Target LDL-C depends on patient's risk factors.
CO_2	23-30 mEq/L	
Creatine kinase (CK) isoenzymes		
CK-BB	0%	
CK-MB (cardiac)	0%-3.9%	
CK-MM (muscle)	96%-100%	
CK-MB levels must be both ≥4% and 10 IU/L to meet diagnostic criteria for CK-MB positive result consistent with myocardial injury.		
Creatine phosphokinase (CPK)	8-150 IU/L	
Creatinine	0.5-1.4 mg/dL	
Ferritin	13-300 ng/mL	
Folate	3.6-20 ng/dL	
GGT (gamma-glutamyltranspeptidase)		
male	11-63 IU/L	
female	8-35 IU/L	
GLDH	To be determined	
Glucose (preprandial)	<115 mg/dL	Goals different for diabetics.
Glucose, fasting	60-110 mg/dL	Goals different for diabetics.
Glucose, nonfasting (2-h postprandial)	<120 mg/dL	Goals different for diabetics.
Hemoglobin A_{1c}	<8	
Hemoglobin, plasma free	<2.5 mg/100 mL	
Hemoglobin, total glycosolated (Hb A_1)	4%-8%	
Iron	65-150 mcg/dL	
Iron binding capacity, total (TIBC)	250-420 mcg/dL	
Lactic acid	0.7-2.1 mEq/L	Specimen to be kept on ice and sent to lab as soon as possible.
Lactate dehydrogenase (LDH)	56-194 IU/L	

CHEMISTRY *(continued)*

Test	Values	Remarks
Lactate dehydrogenase (LDH) isoenzymes		
LD_1	20%-34%	
LD_2	29%-41%	
LD_3	15%-25%	
LD_4	1%-12%	
LD_5	1%-15%	
Flipped LD_1/LD_2 ratios (>1 may be consistent with myocardial injury) particularly when considered in combination with a recent CK-MB positive result.		
Lipase	23-208 units/L	
Magnesium	1.6-2.5 mg/dL	Increased by slight hemolysis.
Osmolality	289-308 mOsm/kg	
Phosphatase, alkaline		
adults 25-60 y	33-131 IU/L	
adults ≥61 y	51-153 IU/L	
infancy-adolescence	Values range up to 3-5 times higher than adults	
Phosphate, inorganic	2.8-4.2 mg/dL	
Potassium	3.5-5.2 mEq/L	Increased by slight hemolysis.
Prealbumin	>15 mg/dL	
Protein, total	6.5-7.9 g/dL	
AST	<35 IU/L (20-48)	
ALT (10-35)	<35 IU/L	
Sodium	134-149 mEq/L	
Thyroid stimulating hormone (TSH)		
adults ≤20 y	0.7-6.4 mIU/L	
21-54 y	0.4-4.2 mIU/L	
55-87 y	0.5-8.9 mIU/L	
Transferrin	>200 mg/dL	
Triglycerides	45-155 mg/dL	Fasted blood required.
Troponin I	<1.5 ng/mL	
Urea nitrogen (BUN)	7-20 mg/dL	
Uric acid		
male	2-8 mg/dL	
female	2-7.5 mg/dL	
Cerebrospinal Fluid		
Glucose	50-70 mg/dL	
Protein	15-45 mg/dL	CSF obtained by lumbar puncture.
Note: Bloody specimen gives erroneously high value due to contamination with blood proteins		
Urine (24-hour specimen is required for all these tests unless specified)		
Amylase	32-641 units/L	The value is in units/L and **not** calculated for total volume.
Amylase, fluid (random samples)		Interpretation of value left for physician, depends on the nature of fluid.
Calcium	Depends upon dietary intake	
Creatine		
male	150 mg/24 h	Higher value on children and during pregnancy.
female	250 mg/24 h	
Creatinine	1000-2000 mg/24 h	
Creatinine clearance (endogenous)		
male	85-125 mL/min	
female	75-115 mL/min	A blood sample must accompany urine specimen.

CHEMISTRY *(continued)*

Test	Values	Remarks
Glucose	1 g/24 h	
5-hydroxyindoleacetic acid	2-8 mg/24 h	
Iron	0.15 mg/24 h	Acid washed container required.
Magnesium	146-209 mg/24 h	
Osmolality	500-800 mOsm/kg	With normal fluid intake.
Oxalate	10-40 mg/24 h	
Phosphate	400-1300 mg/24 h	
Potassium	25-120 mEq/24 h	Varies with diet; the interpretation of urine electrolytes and osmolality should be left for the physician.
Sodium	40-220 mEq/24 h	
Porphobilinogen, qualitative	Negative	
Porphyrins, qualitative	Negative	
Proteins	0.05-0.1 g/24 h	
Salicylate	Negative	
Urea clearance	60-95 mL/min	A blood sample must accompany specimen.
Urea N	10-40 g/24 h	Dependent on protein intake.
Uric acid	250-750 mg/24 h	Dependent on diet and therapy.
Urobilinogen	0.5-3.5 mg/24 h	For qualitative determination on random urine, send sample to urinalysis section in Hematology Lab.
Xylose absorption test		
children	16%-33% of ingested xylose	
Feces		
Fat, 3-day collection	<5 g/d	Value depends on fat intake of 100 g/d for 3 days preceding and during collection.
Gastric Acidity		
Acidity, total, 12 h	10-60 mEq/L	Titrated at pH 7.

Blood Gases

	Arterial	Capillary	Venous
pH	7.35-7.45	7.35-7.45	7.32-7.42
pCO_2 (mm Hg)	35-45	35-45	38-52
pO_2 (mm Hg)	70-100	60-80	24-48
HCO_3 (mEq/L)	19-25	19-25	19-25
TCO_2 (mEq/L)	19-29	19-29	23-33
O_2 saturation (%)	90-95	90-95	40-70
Base excess (mEq/L)	-5 to +5	-5 to +5	-5 to +5

HEMATOLOGY

Complete Blood Count

Age	Hgb (g/dL)	Hct (%)	RBC (mill/mm^3)	RDW
0-3 d	15.0-20.0	45-61	4.0-5.9	<18
1-2 wk	12.5-18.5	39-57	3.6-5.5	<17
1-6 mo	10.0-13.0	29-42	3.1-4.3	<16.5
7 mo to 2 y	10.5-13.0	33-38	3.7-4.9	<16
2-5 y	11.5-13.0	34-39	3.9-5.0	<15
5-8 y	11.5-14.5	35-42	4.0-4.9	<15
13-18 y	12.0-15.2	36-47	4.5-5.1	<14.5
Adult male	13.5-16.5	41-50	4.5-5.5	<14.5
Adult female	12.0-15.0	36-44	4.0-4.9	<14.5

Age	MCV (fL)	MCH (pg)	MCHC (%)	Plts (x 10^3/mm^3)
0-3 d	95-115	31-37	29-37	250-450
1-2 wk	86-110	28-36	28-38	250-450
1-6 mo	74-96	25-35	30-36	300-700
7 mo to 2 y	70-84	23-30	31-37	250-600
2-5 y	75-87	24-30	31-37	250-550
5-8 y	77-95	25-33	31-37	250-550
13-18 y	78-96	25-35	31-37	150-450
Adult male	80-100	26-34	31-37	150-450
Adult female	80-100	26-34	31-37	150-450

WBC and Differential

Age	WBC (x 10^3/mm^3)	Segs	Bands	Lymphs	Monos
0-3 d	9.0-35.0	32-62	10-18	19-29	5-7
1-2 wk	5.0-20.0	14-34	6-14	36-45	6-10
1-6 mo	6.0-17.5	13-33	4-12	41-71	4-7
7 mo to 2 y	6.0-17.0	15-35	5-11	45-76	3-6
2-5 y	5.5-15.5	23-45	5-11	35-65	3-6
5-8 y	5.0-14.5	32-54	5-11	28-48	3-6
13-18 y	4.5-13.0	34-64	5-11	25-45	3-6
Adults	4.5-11.0	35-66	5-11	24-44	3-6

Age	Eosinophils	Basophils	Atypical Lymphs	No. of NRBCs
0-3 d	0-2	0-1	0-8	0-2
1-2 wk	0-2	0-1	0-8	0
1-6 mo	0-3	0-1	0-8	0
7 mo to 2 y	0-3	0-1	0-8	0
2-5 y	0-3	0-1	0-8	0
5-8 y	0-3	0-1	0-8	0
13-18 y	0-3	0-1	0-8	0
Adults	0-3	0-1	0-8	0

Segs = segmented neutrophils.
Bands = band neutrophils.
Lymphs = lymphocytes.
Monos = monocytes.

Erythrocyte Sedimentation Rates and Reticulocyte Counts

Sedimentation rate, Westergren	Children	0-20 mm/h
	Adult male	0-15 mm/h
	Adult female	0-20 mm/h
Sedimentation rate, Wintrobe	Children	0-13 mm/h
	Adult male	0-10 mm/h
	Adult female	0-15 mm/h
Reticulocyte count	Newborns	2%-6%
	1-6 mo	0%-2.8%
	Adults	0.5%-1.5%

ACQUIRED IMMUNODEFICIENCY SYNDROME (AIDS) - LAB TESTS AND APPROVED DRUGS FOR HIV INFECTION AND AIDS-RELATED CONDITIONS

This list of tests is not intended in any way to suggest patterns of physician's orders, nor is it complete. These tests may support possible clinical diagnoses or rule out other diagnostic possibilities.

Acid-Fast Stain
Acid-Fast Stain, Modified, *Nocardia* Species
Antimicrobial Susceptibility Testing, Fungi
Antimicrobial Susceptibility Testing, Mycobacteria
Babesiosis Serological Test
Bacteremia Detection, Buffy Coat Micromethod
Bacterial Culture, Blood
Bacterial Culture, Bronchoscopy Specimen
Bacterial Culture, Sputum
Bacterial Culture, Stool
Bacterial Culture, Throat
Bacterial Culture, Urine, Clean Catch
Beta$_2$-Microglobulin
Blood and Fluid Precautions, Specimen Collection
Bronchial Washings Cytology
Bronchoalveolar Lavage Cytology
Brushings Cytology
Candida Antigen
Candidiasis Serologic Test
Cat Scratch Disease Serology
CD4/CD8 Enumeration
Cerebrospinal Fluid Cytology
Cryptococcal Antigen Titer
Cryptosporidium Diagnostic Procedures
Cytomegalic Inclusion Disease Cytology
Cytomegalovirus Antibody
Cytomegalovirus Antigen Detection
Cytomegalovirus Culture
Cytomegalovirus DNA Detection
Darkfield Examination, Syphilis
Electron Microscopy
Folic Acid, Serum
Fungal Culture, Biopsy or Body Fluid
Fungal Culture, Blood
Fungal Culture, Cerebrospinal Fluid
Fungal Culture, Sputum
Fungal Culture, Stool
Fungal Culture, Urine
Hemoglobin A$_2$
Hepatitis B Surface Antigen
Herpes Cytology
Herpes Simplex Virus Antigen Detection
Herpes Simplex Virus Culture
Histopathology
Histoplasmosis Antibody
Histoplasmosis Antigen
HIV-1/HIV-2 Serology
HTLV-I/II Antibody
Human Immunodeficiency Virus Culture
Human Immunodeficiency Virus DNA Amplification
Human Immunodeficiency Virus, Rapid Test, Qualitative
Human Immunodeficiency Virus, Resistance/Susceptibility Testing
Human Immunodeficiency Virus, Viral Load Assay
India Ink Preparation
Inhibitor, Lupus, Phospholipid Type

KOH Preparation
Leishmaniasis Serological Test
Leukocyte Immunophenotyping
Lymphocyte Enumeration Test
Lymphocyte Transformation Test
Microsporidia Diagnostic Procedures
Mycobacteria by DNA Probe
Mycobacterial Culture, Biopsy or Body Fluid
Mycobacterial Culture, Cerebrospinal Fluid
Mycobacterial Culture, Cutaneous and Subcutaneous Tissue
Mycobacterial Culture, Sputum
Mycobacterial Culture, Stool
Neisseria gonorrhoeae Culture and Smear
Nocardia Culture
Ova and Parasites, Stool
p24 Antigen
Platelet Count
Pneumocystis carinii Preparation
Pneumocystis Immunofluorescence
Polymerase Chain Reaction
Red Blood Cell Indices
Risks of Transfusion
Skin Biopsy
Sputum Cytology
Toxoplasmosis Serology
VDRL, Serum
Viral Culture
Viral Culture, Blood
Viral Culture, Body Fluid
Viral Culture, Central Nervous System Symptoms
Viral Culture, Dermatological Symptoms
Viral Culture, Tissue
Virus, Direct Detection by Fluorescent Antibody
White Blood Count

FDA-APPROVED AND INVESTIGATIONAL ANTIRETROVIRAL DRUGS

Antiretroviral Drugs

Generic Name	Also Known As	Brand Name	FDA Status
NUCLEOSIDE/NUCLEOTIDE ANALOG REVERSE TRANSCRIPTASE INHIBITORS (NRTIs)			
abacavir	ABC	Ziagen®	Approved
apricitabine	AVX754	—	Investigational
didanosine	ddI	Videx®; Videx® EC	Approved
elvucitabine	ACH-126,443; Beta-L-Fd4C	—	Investigational
emtricitabine	FTC	Emtriva®	Approved
entecavir	ETV	Baraclude®	Approved
lamiVUDine	3TC	Epivir®	Approved
stavudine	d4T	Zerit®	Approved
tenofovir	TDF	Viread®	Approved
zidovudine	ZDV	Retrovir®	Approved
—	RCV	Racivir	Investigational
NONNUCLEOSIDE REVERSE TRANSCRIPTASE INHIBITORS (NNRTIs)			
delavirdine	DLV	Rescriptor®	Approved
efavirenz	EFV	Sustiva®	Approved
etravirine	TMC 125	Intelence™	Approved
nevirapine	NVP	Viramune®	Approved
rilpivirine	TMC 278	Edurant™	Approved
PROTEASE INHIBITORS (PIs)			
atazanavir	ATV	Reyataz®	Approved
darunavir	DRV	Prezista™	Approved
fosamprenavir	FPV	Lexiva®	Approved
indinavir	IDV	Crixivan®	Approved
lopinavir and ritonavir	LPV/RTV	Kaletra®	Approved
nelfinavir	NFV	Viracept®	Approved
ritonavir	RTV	Norvir®	Approved
saquinavir	SQV	Invirase®	Approved
tipranavir	TPV	Aptivus®	Approved
FIXED-DOSE COMBINATION PRODUCTS			
abacavir and lamivudine	ABC/3TC	Epzicom®, Kivexa™	Approved
abacavir, lamivudine, and zidovudine	ABC/3TC/ZDV	Trizivir®	Approved
efavirenz, emtricitabine and tenofovir	EFV/FTC/TDF	Atripla™	Approved
emtricitabine and tenofovir	FTC/TDF	Truvada®	Approved
zidovudine and lamivudine	ZDV/3TC	Combivir®	Approved
FUSION INHIBITORS			
enfuvirtide	ENF	Fuzeon®	Approved
—	TNX-355	—	Investigational
CHEMOKINE CORECEPTOR ANTAGONIST			
maraviroc	MVC	Selzentry™	Approved
vicriviroc	SCH-417690; SCH-D	—	Investigational
—	PRO 140	—	Investigational
—	INCB9741	—	Investigational

Antiretroviral Drugs *(continued)*

Generic Name	Also Known As	Brand Name	FDA Status
INTEGRASE INHIBITORS			
elvitegravir	GS-9137	—	Investigational
raltegravir	RAL	Isentress™	Approved
—	GSK364735	—	Investigational
MATURATION INHIBITORS			
bevirimat	PA-457	—	Investigational

DRUGS USED TO TREAT COMPLICATIONS OF HIV / AIDS

Brand Name	Generic Name (Synonym)	Use
Abelcet®, AmBisome®	amphotericin B, ABLC	Antifungal for aspergillosis
Bactrim™, Septra®	sulfamethoxazole and trimethoprim, SMZ/TMP	Antiprotozoal antibiotic used to treat and prevent *Pneumocystis carinii* pneumonia
Biaxin®	clarithromycin	Antibiotic used to treat and prevent *Mycobacterium avium*
Cytovene®	ganciclovir, DHPG	Antiviral used to treat CMV retinitis
DaunoXome®	daunorubicin citrate (liposomal)	Chemotherapy for Kaposi sarcoma
Diflucan®	fluconazole	Antifungal for candidiasis, cryptococcal meningitis
Doxil®	DOXOrubicin (liposomal)	Chemotherapy for Kaposi sarcoma
Eraxis™	anidulafungin	Antifungal (intravenous), used to treat *Candida* infections in the esophagus (candidiasis), blood stream (candidemia), and other forms of *Candida* infections, including abdominal abscesses and peritonitis (inflammation of the lining of the abdominal cavity)
Famvir®	famciclovir	Antiviral used to treat herpes
Foscavir®	foscarnet	Antiviral used to treat herpes and CMV retinitis
Gamimune® N	immune globulin, gamma globulin, IGIV	Immune booster used to prevent bacterial infections in children
Intron® A	interferon alfa-2b	Treat Kaposi sarcoma and hepatitis C
Marinol®	dronabinol	Treat loss of appetite
Megace®	megestrol acetate	Treat loss of appetite and weight
Mepron®	atovaquone	Antiprotozoal antibiotic used to treat and prevent *Pneumocystis carinii* pneumonia
Mycobutin®	rifabutin	Antimycobacterial used to prevent *Mycobacterium avium*
NebuPent®	pentamidine	Antiprotozoal antibiotic used to prevent *Pneumocystis carinii* pneumonia
Neutrexin®	trimetrexate glucuronate and leucovorin	Antiprotozoal antibiotic used to treat *Pneumocystis carinii* pneumonia
Panretin® Gel	alitretinoin gel 0.1%	AIDS-related Kaposi sarcoma
Procrit®, Epogen®	erythropoietin, EPO	Treat anemia related to AZT therapy
Roferon-A®	interferon alfa-2a	Treat Kaposi sarcoma and hepatitis C
Serostim®	somatropin rDNA	Treat weight loss
Sporanox®	itraconazole	Antifungal used to treat blastomycosis, histoplasmosis, aspergillosis, and candidiasis
Taxol®	PACLitaxel	Kaposi sarcoma
Valcyte™	valGANciclovir	Antiviral used to treat CMV retinitis
VFEND®	voriconazole	Antifungal for invasive aspergillosis and serious fungal infections due to *Fusarium sporotrichoides* and *Scedosporium apiospermum*, and Esophageal Candidiasis
Vistide®	cidofovir, HPMPC	Antiviral used to treat cytomegalovirus (CMV)
Vitrasert® Implant	ganciclovir insert	Antiviral used to treat CMV retinitis
Vitravene™ intravitreal injection	fomivirsen sodium injection	Antiviral used to treat CMV retinitis
Zithromax®	azithromycin	Antibiotic used to treat *Mycobacterium avium*

NEW DRUGS ADDED SINCE LAST EDITION

Brand Name	Generic Name	Use
ala seb [OTC]	sulfur and salicylic acid	Dandruff; seborrheic dermatitis; acne
Amyvid™	florbetapir F18	Imaging agent (brain)
—	artesunate	Malaria
AstrinGyn®	ferric subsulfate	Hemostatic agent
Belviq®	lorcaserin	Chronic weight management
Choletec®	technetium Tc 99m mebrofenin	Imaging agent (hepatobiliary)
CIS-MDP™	technetium Tc 99m medronate	Imaging agent (skeletal)
DaTscan™	ioflupane I 123	Imaging agent (brain)
DMSA	technetium Tc 99m succimer	Imaging agent (renal)
DRAXIMAGE® DTPA	technetium Tc 99m diethylene triamine penta-acetic acid	Imaging agent
DRAXIMAGE® Gluceptate	technetium Tc 99m gluceptate	Imaging agent (renal and brain perfusion)
DRAXIMAGE® MDP-25	technetium Tc 99m medronate	Imaging agent (skeletal)
Dymista™	azelastine and fluticasone	Rhinitis (seasonal)
edarbyclor™	azilsartan and chlorthalidone	Hypertension
Elelyso™	taliglucerase alfa	Type 1 Gaucher disease
Erivedge™	vismodegib	Metastatic basal cell carcinoma
Erwinaze™	asparaginase (*Erwinia*)	Acute lymphoblastic leukemia (ALL)
Exparel™	bupivacaine (liposomal)	Postoperative analgesia
Eylea™	aflibercept (ophthalmic)	Neovascular (wet) age-related macular degeneration (AMD)
Ferriprox®	deferiprone	Iron overload
Firazyr®	icatibant	Hereditary angioedema (HAE)
—	fludeoxyglucose F 18	Imaging agent (brain)
—	gallium citrate Ga-67	Imaging agent (carcinomas)
Indium DTPA In 111	pentetate indium disodium in 111	Imaging agent (cisterography)
—	indium in-111 pentetreotide	Imaging agent (metastatic tumors)
Inlyta®	axitinib	Advanced renal cell cancer (RCC)
Jakafi™	ruxolitinib	Myelofibrosis
Jentadueto™	linagliptin and metformin	Type 2 diabetes mellitus (noninsulin dependent, NIDDM)
Juvisync™	sitagliptin and simvastatin	Type 2 diabetes mellitus (noninsulin dependent, NIDDM); hypercholesterolemia; hyperlipidemia
Kalydeco™	ivacaftor	Cystic fibrosis (CF)
Kyprolis™	carfilzomib	Multiple myeloma
MDP Multidose	technetium Tc 99m medronate	Imaging agent (skeletal)
Megatope	iodinated I 131 albumin	Imaging agent (cardiac output)
MenHibrix®	meningococcal polysaccharide (groups C and Y) and *Haemophilus* b tetanus toxoid conjugate vaccine	Active immunization

(continued)

Brand Name	Generic Name	Use
Mitosol®	mitomycin (ophthalmic)	Glaucoma
Neupro®	rotigotine	Idiopathic Parkinson disease (early-stage to advanced-stage disease); moderate-to-severe primary restless legs syndrome (RLS)
Omeclamox-Pak®	omeprazole, clarithromycin, and amoxicillin	*H. pylori* infection
Omontys®	peginesatide	Anemia
Perjeta™	pertuzumab	HER2-positive metastatic breast cancer
Pernox® Lemon [OTC]	sulfur and salicylic acid	Dandruff; seborrheic dermatitis; acne
Pernox® Regular [OTC]	sulfur and salicylic acid	Dandruff; seborrheic dermatitis; acne
Picato®	ingenol mebutate	Actinic keratosis
Prepopik™	sodium picosulfate, magnesium oxide, and citric acid	Bowel cleansing
Qsymia™	phentermine and topiramate	Chronic weight management
Quadramet®	samarium Sm 153 lexidronam	Pain (metastatic bone lesions)
Sebex [OTC]	sulfur and salicylic acid	Dandruff; seborrheic dermatitis; acne
Sebulex® [OTC]	sulfur and salicylic acid	Dandruff; seborrheic dermatitis; acne
Sklice™	ivermectin (topical)	Head lice
—	sodium iodide I^{123}	Imaging agent (thyroid function)
—	sodium nitrite	Cyanide poisoning
Stendra™	avanafil	Erectile dysfunction (ED)
Surfaxin®	lucinactant	Respiratory distress syndrome (RDS)
Sweet-Ease® [OTC]; TootSweet™ [OTC]	sucrose	Analgesia
Technescan™ HDP	technetium Tc 99m oxidronate	Imaging agent (skeletal)
Technescan™ PYP™	technetium Tc 99m pyrophosphate	Imaging agent (skeletal)
—	technetium Tc 99m exametazime	Imaging agent
Tudorza® Pressair®	aclidinium	COPD
UltraTag® RBC	technetium Tc 99m-labeled red blood cells	Imaging agent (blood pool)
Vascepa™	icosapent ethyl	Hypertriglyceridemia
Volumex HSA I-131	iodinated I 131 albumin	Imaging agent (cardiac output)
Xalkori®	crizotinib	Metastatic nonsmall cell lung cancer (NSCLC)
Zaltrap®	ziv-aflibercept	Metastatic colorectal cancer
Zioptan™	tafluprost	Glaucoma

PENDING DRUGS OR DRUGS IN CLINICAL TRIALS

Proposed Brand Name or Synonym	Generic Name	Use
Adasuve™	staccato loxapine	Schizophrenia
AEZS-130	—	Adult growth hormone deficiency
AGO 178	agomelatine	Depression
BCI-540	sabcomeline	Depression
CMC-544	inotuzumab ozogamicin	B-cell non-Hodgkin lymphoma (NHL)
Cobicistat™	elvitegravir, cobicistat, emtricitabine, and tenofovir disoproxil fumarate	HIV
E2007	perampanel	Partial-onset seizures
F2695	levomilnacipran	Depression
GW823296	orvepitant	Depression
—	laquinimod	Multiple sclerosis (MS)
Lu-31-130	zicronapine	Psychosis
MK-4305	suvorexant	Insomnia
Nesina™	alogliptin	Type 2 diabetes
—	ocriplasmin (microplasmin)	Symptomatic vitreomacular adhesion
PSI-938	—	Chronic hepatitis C virus (HCV)
RGH-188	caripazine	Schizophrenia
RX-10100	serdaxin	Parkinson disease
Sollpura™	liprotamase	Exocrine pancreatic replacement
TSC	trans sodium crocetinate	Brain carcinoma

INDICATION / THERAPEUTIC CATEGORY INDEX

Local Anesthetic, Ophthalmic

ANESTHESIA (OPHTHALMIC)

Diagnostic Agent

Local Anesthetic

ANGINA PECTORIS

Beta-Adrenergic Blocker

Calcium Channel Blocker

BRADYCARDIA

Anticholinergic Agent

Antidote

BREAST ENGORGEMENT (POSTPARTUM)

Androgen

Estrogen Derivative

BRONCHIECTASIS

Adrenergic Agonist Agent

Alpha/Beta Agonist

Mucolytic Agent

BRONCHIOLITIS

Antiviral Agent

BRONCHITIS

Adrenergic Agonist Agent

CACHEXIA

Growth Hormone

CALCIUM CHANNEL BLOCKER TOXICITY

Electrolyte Supplement, Oral

CANDIDIASIS

Antifungal Agent

Protectant, Topical

CARCINOMA

Androgen

Antiandrogen

Antineoplastic Agent

CONSTIPATION

Antihistamine/Decongestant Combination

Antitussive

Antitussive/Decongestant

Antitussive/Decongestant/Expectorant

Antitussive/Expectorant

Cold Preparation

Cough Preparation

Decongestant

Sympathomimetic

CROHN DISEASE

5-Aminosalicylic Acid Derivative

Antirheumatic, Disease Modifying

Corticosteroid, Systemic

Gastrointestinal Agent, Miscellaneous

Monoclonal Antibody

Monoclonal Antibody, Selective Adhesion-Molecule Inhibitor

Tumor Necrosis Factor (TNF) Blocking Agent

CROUP

Alpha/Beta Agonist

Immune Response Modifier

Immunosuppressant Agent

Topical Skin Product

DIVERTICULITIS

Amebicide

Antibiotic, Aminoglycoside

Antibiotic, Cephalosporin (Second Generation)

Antibiotic, Lincosamide

Antibiotic, Miscellaneous

Antiprotozoal, Nitroimidazole

Carbapenem (Antibiotic)

Cephalosporin (Second Generation)

Penicillin

EDEMA

Antihypertensive Agent, Combination

Diuretic, Combination

Diuretic, Loop

GASTRITIS

Antacid

Histamine H_2 Antagonist

GASTROESOPHAGEAL REFLUX DISEASE (GERD)

Gastrointestinal Agent, Prokinetic

Histamine H_2 Antagonist

Proton Pump Inhibitor

HYPERCHOLESTEROLEMIA

Antidiabetic Agent, Dipeptidyl Peptidase IV (DPP-IV) Inhibitor

Antihyperlipidemic Agent, Miscellaneous

Antilipemic Agent, 2-Azetidinone

Antilipemic Agent, Fibric Acid

Antilipemic Agent, HMG-CoA Reductase Inhibitor

Antilipemic Agent, Miscellaneous

Bile Acid Sequestrant

HMG-CoA Reductase Inhibitor

Angiotensin II Receptor Antagonist

Angiotensin II Receptor Blocker

Angiotensin II Receptor Blocker Combination

Angiotensin-Converting Enzyme (ACE) Inhibitor

Beta-Adrenergic Blocker, Nonselective

Beta-Blocker, Beta-1 Selective

Beta-Blocker With Intrinsic Sympathomimetic Activity

Calcium Channel Blocker

IRON-DEFICIENCY ANEMIA

Electrolyte Supplement, Oral

Iron Salt

IRON OVERLOAD

Antidote

Chelating Agent

IRON POISONING

Antidote

IRRITABLE BOWEL SYNDROME (IBS)

Anticholinergic Agent

Antispasmodic Agent, Gastrointestinal

Calcium Antagonist

Gastrointestinal Agent, Miscellaneous

5-HT_3 Receptor Antagonist

Laxative

Serotonin 5-HT_4 Receptor Agonist

OBSESSIVE-COMPULSIVE DISORDER (OCD)

Antidepressant, Selective Serotonin Reuptake Inhibitor

Antidepressant, Tricyclic (Tertiary Amine)

OCULAR INFLAMMATION

Analgesic, Nonnarcotic

Antibiotic/Corticosteroid, Ophthalmic

Corticosteroid, Ophthalmic

Nonsteroidal Antiinflammatory Drug (NSAID), Ophthalmic

OCULAR REDNESS

Adrenergic Agonist Agent

Alpha$_1$ Agonist

Alpha/Beta Agonist

Antihistamine/Decongestant Combination

Imidazoline Derivative

Ophthalmic Agent, Antiglaucoma

Ophthalmic Agent, Mydriatic

Ophthalmic Agent, Vasoconstrictor

OVERACTIVE BLADDER

Anticholinergic Agent

OVULATION INDUCTION

Ovulation Stimulator

PAGET DISEASE OF BONE

Bisphosphonate Derivative

Polypeptide Hormone

PAIN

Analgesic Combination (Opioid)

Analgesic, Miscellaneous

Analgesic, Narcotic

Analgesic, Nonnarcotic

Analgesic, Nonopioid

Analgesic, Opioid

PAIN (ANOGENITAL)

Anesthetic/Corticosteroid

PAIN (BONE)

Radiopharmaceutical

PAIN (DIABETIC NEUROPATHY NEURALGIA)

Analgesic, Topical

PAIN (LUMBAR PUNCTURE)

Analgesic, Topical

PAIN (METASTATIC BONE LESIONS)

Radiopharmaceutical

PAIN (NEUROPATHIC)

Analgesic, Miscellaneous

PAIN (OCULAR)

Nonsteroidal Antiinflammatory Drug (NSAID), Ophthalmic

PAIN (POSTOPERATIVE)

Analgesic, Nonopioid

PAIN (SKIN GRAFT HARVESTING)

Analgesic, Topical

PAIN (VENIPUNCTURE)

Analgesic, Topical

PANCREATIC EXOCRINE INSUFFICIENCY

Enzyme

PANCREATIC EXOCRINE INSUFFICIENCY (DIAGNOSTIC)

Diagnostic Agent

PANIC DISORDER

Antidepressant, Phenethylamine

Antidepressant, Selective Serotonin Reuptake Inhibitor

Benzodiazepine

Contraceptive, Progestin Only

Progestin

Immunosuppressant Agent

Interleukin-12 Inhibitor

Interleukin-23 Inhibitor

Keratolytic Agent

SEDATION

Alpha-Adrenergic Agonist - Central-Acting (Alpha$_2$-Agonists)

Anesthetic, Gas

Barbiturate

Benzodiazepine

General Anesthetic

Neuroleptic Agent

Sedative

SEIZURES

Anticonvulsant

Anticonvulsant, Miscellaneous

Anticonvulsant, Neuronal Potassium Channel Opener

Anticonvulsant, Sulfonamide

Anticonvulsant, Triazole Derivative

Electrolyte Supplement, Oral

Hydantoin

Antifungal Agent, Oral

Antifungal Agent, Topical

Antifungal/Corticosteroid

Disinfectant

TOPICAL ANESTHESIA

Analgesic, Topical

Local Anesthetic

ZOLLINGER-ELLISON SYNDROME

ZOLLINGER-ELLISON SYNDROME (DIAGNOSTIC)